Directions for accessing your
Oxford University Press Digital Course Materials

From Neuron to Brain
SIXTH EDITION

A. Robert Martin
David A. Brown
Mathew E. Diamond
Antonino Cattaneo
Francisco F. De-Miguel

Carefully scratch off the silver coating to see your personal redemption code.

Your OUP digital course materials can be delivered several different ways, depending on how your instructor has elected to incorporate them into his or her course.

BEFORE REGISTERING FOR ACCESS, be sure to check with your instructor to ensure that you register using the proper method.

VIA YOUR SCHOOL'S LEARNING MANAGEMENT SYSTEM

Use this method if your instructor has integrated these resources into your school's Learning Management System (LMS)—Blackboard, Canvas, Brightspace, Moodle, or other.

> Log in to your instructor's course within your school's LMS.

> When you click a link to a resource that is access-protected, you will be prompted to register for access.

> Follow the on-screen instructions.

> Enter your personal redemption code (or purchase access) when prompted.

VIA OXFORD learning cloud

Use this method only if your instructor has specifically instructed you to enroll in an Oxford Learning Cloud course. **NOTE:** *If your instructor is using these resources within your school's LMS, use the Learning Management System instructions.*

> Visit the course invitation URL provided by your instructor.

> If you already have an oup.instructure.com account you will be added to the course automatically; if not, create an account by providing your name and email.

> When you click a link to a resource in the course that is access-protected, you will be prompted to register.

> Follow the on-screen instructions, entering your personal redemption code where prompted.

For assistance with code redemption, Oxford Learning Cloud registration, or if you redeemed your code using the wrong method for your course, please contact our customer support team at **learninglinkdirect.support@oup.com** or 855-281-8749.

OXFORD
UNIVERSITY PRESS

From Neuron to Brain

SIXTH EDITION

To NESSA
With much love,
Bob

From Neuron to Brain

SIXTH EDITION

A. Robert Martin
Emeritus, University of Colorado School of Medicine

David A. Brown
University College of London

Mathew E. Diamond
International School for Advanced Studies, Trieste, Italy

Antonino Cattaneo
*Scuola Normale Superiore, Pisa, Italy and
Rita Levi-Montalcini European Brain Research Institute,
Rome, Italy*

Francisco F. De-Miguel
*Institute for Cellular Physiology at the Universidad
Nacional Autónoma de México*

With a Foreword by

John G. Nicholls
International School for Advanced Studies, Trieste, Italy

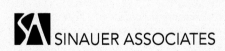

SINAUER ASSOCIATES

NEW YORK   OXFORD
OXFORD UNIVERSITY PRESS

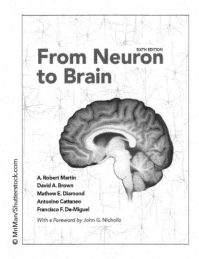

ABOUT THE COVER

The cover image is derived from a magnetic resonance image of a living human brain (sagittal section) © MriMan/Shutterstock.com. Neurons (background) are from the Third Edition cover, designed by Laszlo Meszoly.

Oxford University Press is a department of the University of Oxford. It furthers the University's objective of excellence in research, scholarship, and education by publishing worldwide. Oxford is a registered trade mark of Oxford University Press in the UK and certain other countries.

Published in the United States of America by Oxford University Press
198 Madison Avenue, New York, NY 10016, United States of America

Address editorial correspondence to:
Sinauer Associates
23 Plumtree Road
Sunderland, MA 01375 USA

Address orders, sales, license, permissions, and translation inquiries to:
Oxford University Press USA
2001 Evans Road
Cary, NC 27513 USA
Orders: 1-800-445-9714

ACCESSIBLE COLOR CONTENT   Every opportunity has been taken to ensure that the content herein is fully accessible to those who have difficulty perceiving color. Exceptions are cases where the colors provided are expressly required because of the purpose of the illustration.

Library of Congress Cataloging-in-Publication Data

Names: Martin, A. Robert, 1928– author.
Title: From Neuron to Brain / A. Robert Martin, Emeritus, University of Colorado School of Medicine, David A. Brown, University College London, Mathew E. Diamond, International School for Advanced Studies, Trieste, Italy, Antonino Cattaneo, Scuola Normale Superiore, Florence, Italy, Francisco Fernández De-Miguel, Universidad Nacional Autónoma de México, Mexico City, Mexico ; with a foreword by John G. Nicholls International School for Advanced Studies, Trieste, Italy.
Description: Sixth edition. | Sunderland, Massachusetts : Oxford University Press/Sinauer, [2021] | Previous edition cataloged under: Nicholls, John G. | Includes bibliographical references and index. | Summary: "For the instructor of Introduction to Neuroscience or Neurobiology courses with students who are intimidated by the study of the brain, our textbook *From Neuron to Brain* is designed to present difficult material on the nervous system through the process of experimentation. Lines of research are followed from the inception of an idea to new findings being made in laboratories and clinics today, allowing students to follow the path of experimentation toward an understanding of how the nervous system works. Nicholls et al. have built a readable and informative text that explains how nerve cells go about their business of transmitting signals, how the signals are put together, and how higher function emerges from this integration, all in an accessible and exciting way that will appeal to students. *From Neuron to Brain*, Sixth Edition and its exploration of the intricate workings of the nervous system will be of interest to instructors teaching undergraduate, graduate, and medical school courses in neuroscience"-- Provided by publisher.
Identifiers: LCCN 2020028672 (print) | LCCN 2020028673 (ebook) | ISBN 9781605354392 (hardback) | ISBN 9780197542774 (paperback) | ISBN 9781605359335 (epub)
Subjects: LCSH: Neurophysiology. | Brain. | Neurons.
Classification: LCC QP355.2 .K83 2021 (print) | LCC QP355.2 (ebook) | DDC 612.8--dc23
LC record available at https://lccn.loc.gov/2020028672
LC ebook record available at https://lccn.loc.gov/2020028673

9 8 7 6 5 4 3 2 1
Printed in the United States of America

Foreword to the Sixth Edition

There were several reasons for Stephen Kuffler to think of writing *From Neuron to Brain*. Steve, as he was known to all his colleagues and friends, had created the first department of neurobiology at Harvard Medical School. Research and teaching went from cellular and chemical mechanisms to higher functions. The lectures by Furshpan, Potter, Kravitz, Hubel, Wiesel, and their colleagues were coherent and inspiring. Steve realised that there was no book of that sort and decided to write one with me. Steve and I had worked together in the lab and written a review with great pleasure and success: The book would be a way for us to continue to collaborate.

Our aim was to write a book that could be read by people with little background knowledge, people who wanted to find out how the nervous system works, physicists, chemists, molecular biologists, professionals as well as undergraduates, graduates and medical students. Our dream reader would read the book from cover to cover. To make the text readable, each chapter would try to tell an interesting story. Inevitably, we would have to be selective and leave out all sorts of important material. The basis for what to include was personal…our own taste. We'd describe how actual experiments were done and who did them. Readers could make up their own minds about the evidence. We aimed to make the text clear enough to be read without consulting figures and the figures clear enough to be understood without the text.

The first edition took several years, six or so. We were both doing research and devoted only summers to writing full time at the Marine Biological Lab at Woods Hole and the Salk Institute at La Jolla.

The way Steve wrote was similar to his approach to experiments—a great deal of time devoted to thinking and formulating ideas and then—Zap!—write! Here is an example: We spent a full three weeks just on the title before we wrote anything. After all, we thought, the title should encompass the spirit and contents of the book. For each chapter, one of us wrote the first draft and the other went over it, back and forth again and again, hoping that our readers would not find out who had written what. I remember one occasion when I was in despair about a biophysical problem that had been dealt with beautifully and clearly in Bernard Katz's marvellous book *Nerve, Muscle and Synapse*. Steve consoled me. "Look, we're never going to write as well as Bernard, so let's just do our best."

Writing everything by hand was a laborious task. Even harder was changing things in the typed version (done by what is now an extinct species, our secretaries). Alterations had to be short enough to keep the page intact, additions compensated for by deletions, or the whole chapter had to be repaginated. During the preparation of the first edition, Xeroxing became available for the first time and that made figures far easier to reproduce and modify.

When the text and rough figures were ready, there came the search for a publisher. The major publishers wanted *From Neuron to Brain* because there was at that time no other book like it (Katz's book did not deal with the central nervous system). We knew that we wanted the book to look attractive with fine, uncluttered illustrations, and abundant references to back up all our statements, albeit placed discretely. We also wanted color, unusual at that time, because it would help to make the illustrations clear. In the end we chose Andy Sinauer who was just starting with a handful of books, a choice that we never regretted. He became our friend and understood our desire to produce a pleasing book. He worked with us on the production of the first edition from start to finish, not only correcting and modifying but adding new ideas. And the same on every subsequent edition.

It was after the preparation of the first edition that the explosion of molecular biology transformed the study of the nervous system. When Steve died, close friends, first Bob Martin, then Bruce Wallace, and I prepared new editions. Later other colleagues with special skills joined in, all of whom prepared chapters and read the entire text as if each was the sole author. With time, new advances, such as word processing, PubMed, and full color, became available, yet Andy Sinauer himself, and later Sydney Carroll, kept the spirit of the book alive.

It is a privilege and honor for me to have contributed to *From Neuron to Brain* in past editions and a source of regret that I am no longer able to do so. My congratulations to Francisco, Bob, David, Mathew, and Antonino. Heartfelt thanks to them and to Andy, our dear friend and guide.

John Nicholls

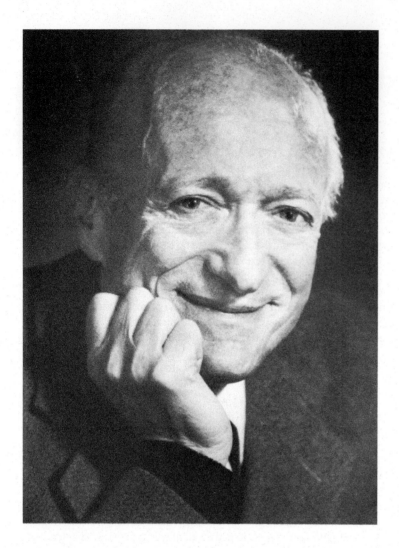

This book is dedicated to the memory of our friend and colleague, Steve Kuffler.

In a career that spanned 40 years, Stephen Kuffler made experiments on fundamental problems and laid paths for future research to follow. A feature of his work is the way in which the right problem was tackled using the right preparation. Examples are his studies on denervation, stretch receptors, efferent control, inhibition, GABA and peptides as transmitters, integration in the retina, glial cells, and the analysis of synaptic transmission. What gave papers by Stephen Kuffler a special quality were the clarity, the beautiful figures, and the underlying excitement. Moreover, he himself had done *every* experiment he described. Stephen Kuffler's work exemplified and introduced a multidisciplinary approach to the study of the nervous system. At Harvard he created the first department of neurobiology, in which he brought together people from different disciplines who developed new ways of thinking. Those who knew him remember a unique combination of tolerance, firmness, kindness, and good sense with enduring humor. He was the J. F. Enders University Professor at Harvard, and was associated with the Marine Biological Laboratory at Woods Hole. Among his many honors was his election as a foreign member of the Royal Society.

A Tribute to John Nicholls

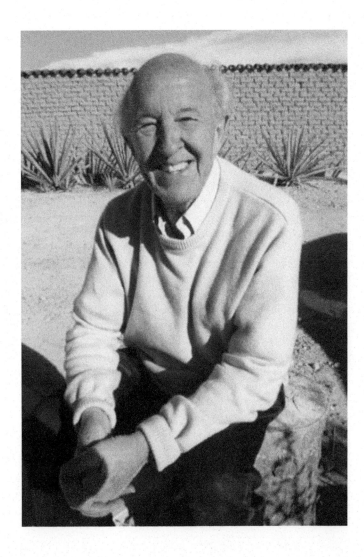

In this edition, John decided not to be an author. His decision did not surprise those of us who had the fortune to be under his supervision or to have him as a colleague and friend: John did not sign publications if he did not participate in the experiments. He was, however, essential for the sixth edition. He joined numerous planning meetings held at University College London, where his experience wisely guided and informed our discussions. Moreover, he read, discussed, and edited a number of chapters.

The long-lasting collaboration and friendship between John and Steve Kuffler, which led to the creation of *From Neuron to Brain*, started when John arrived at Harvard, being the first postdoctoral fellow of the newly created department of neurobiology. John's arrival followed his Ph.D., under Sir Bernard Katz at University College London, and an associate professorship at Oxford, under Sir Lindor Brown. With Steve Kuffler and Dick Orkand, John published classical papers on the physiology of glia. Later, Steve and John organized neurobiology courses in Cold Spring Harbor and Woods Hole. During his career, John studied the connections between individual identified central neurons and how

they regenerate after injury, and later he studied the circuitry of respiration. The quality and originality of his publications, along with his lively personality, lead him to a meteoric career at Yale, once again at Harvard, then followed by an invitation to create the Department of Neurobiology at Stanford University. Later he worked at the Biocenter of the University of Basel and in SISSA, Italy. John gave legendary courses in many countries of the five continents and inspired legions of students to follow a career in neuroscience. In recognition of his own career, John was elected a Fellow of the Royal Society, and of the Mexican Academy of Medicine. He has received numerous honorary degrees and other awards such as the Andrés Bello Medal from Venezuela, and IBRO created the John Nicholls Fellowship in his honor for students from developing countries. John Nicholls Fellowship for students after his courses. John coordinated and wrote the second to the fifth editions of *From Neuron to Brain*. We regret not having his name next to ours. Any words of recognition to John are destined to fall short. Wherever he is, the standards become higher.

Preface to the Sixth Edition

This edition follows the original idea by Steve Kuffler and John Nicholls to write a book in which each chapter tells a complete story, describing beautiful experiments, from the origins of a question to the latest advances. As with the previous editions, we start with three chapters in which vision—from a light particle striking a molecule of visual pigment to the perception of shape, color, and depth in the visual cortex—forms a continuous thread that illustrates the general workings of the nervous system. The next parts go from the way by which molecules in the cell membrane produce nerve impulse signals to how such impulses in the brain generate decisions and motor responses. Then, we discuss how the nervous system forms itself, how is it refined by experience, and its capabilities of regeneration and repair after injury. The last chapter discusses the slow progress of general interest topics, such as regeneration, disease, consciousness, and our personal perspectives on the field.

The loss of three authors from the previous edition and the incorporation of two new ones produced rearrangement of the book with the addition of two new chapters. One deals with molecular events leading to memory acquisition and consolidation at synapses. The other is about massive release of signaling molecules from the neuronal surface and how it integrates the responses of all kinds of cells to influence behavior. In addition, every chapter from the previous edition has been carefully reviewed and updated. The chapters on glia and motor systems were rewritten, and the chapter on development had a substantial increase that reflects the explosive expansion of the field since the past edition. Inevitably, this new edition has increased its volume. To keep the manageable size of the book, chapters were compacted when possible while avoiding the loss of fundamental material.

Since the previous edition in 2012, technical developments have allowed experiments that were unimaginable in previous editions. For example, ultraresolution microscopy allows one to visualize molecular assemblies; organelles can form themselves in isolation from precursor cells, and genetically manipulated neurons are stimulated and visualized in action in behaving animals. Experimental answers obtained from such developments are described throughout the book. It can also be seen by the reader, however, that substantial advances are still reachable with old classical methods, such as extracellular recording and anatomical techniques. In spite of the many advances, obvious questions about the nervous system that were open at the time of the first edition still remain *terra incognita* and neuroscience remains full of open questions, some of which can be analyzed with intuition, dedication, and relatively low budgets.

The general interest of the numerous questions that emerge so naturally from the workings of the nervous system inspired Steve and John to write the first edition of this book in 1976. Forty-five years later, the classical and new discoveries convey a similar excitement. We hope that the sixth edition will evoke in young readers the same inspiration and aesthetic pleasure that made three of us—Antonino Cattaneo, Mathew Diamond, and myself—decide on careers in neurosciences.

Francisco F. De-Miguel

Acknowledgments

First of all, we wish to express our immense gratitude to our friend John G. Nicholls. More than just helping to define the authorship for this edition, John was present in the three meetings we had at University College London to work together on the book and contributed to the chapter on motor systems. His continuous advice and reviews of many of the chapters were inspiring to keep the original idea that lead Steve Kuffler and himself to write the first edition.

Two other authors from the previous edition, David Weissblat and Paul Fuchs, were unable to contribute to this edition. Instead, we were joined by Antonino Cattaneo and Francisco De-Miguel as authors.

Some material in this edition was based on chapters from the fifth edition. In this respect we wish to thank Drs. Fuchs and Weisblat for generously allowing us to adapt and update their material for this edition. We also wish to thank those colleagues who gave us invaluable comments on the book: Drs. K. Muller, A Gibb, and W. Stuhmer read most chapters. Along with Dr. Markus Rüegg, their invaluable opinions influenced the present edition. We also wish to thank our colleagues who provided original material: L. Carrillo-Reid, E. Kravitz, K. Fuxe, L. López Mascaraque, Rebeca González, P. Noguez, F. Tecuapetla, and S. Torres Platas.

This edition, in which there was a smooth transition from Sinauer Associates to Oxford University Press, was possible thanks to the excellent editorial team, originally at Sinauer, who worked together with us with uninterrupted dedication, professionalism, and patience. Our editors, Sydney Carroll and later Jessica Fiorillo, guided us along each step of the production. Martha Lorantos, our production editor, worked with us on a daily basis reviewing each chapter. The book design and layout was created by Annette Rapier and Donna DiCarlo. Joan Gemme, the art director; Elizabeth Pierson, copyeditor; and Elizabeth Morales, the figure artist made considerable contributions to this edition. Michele Beckta was our permission manager and Mark Siddall the photo researcher. It was a great pleasure to work with each of them and to learn so much from day to day.

Digital Resources
to Accompany *From Neuron to Brain*, Sixth Edition

For the Student

From Neuron to Brain, sixth edition is available as an enhanced e-book in several different formats, including RedShelf, VitalSource, and Chegg. All major mobile devices are supported. Self-study questions at the end of each section help students assess their mastery of the content and provide them with immediate feedback, facilitating participation in the learning process, and increasing retention of the content.

Enhanced e-book: 978-1-60-535933-5

For the Instructor

Oxford Learning Link provides instructors using *From Neuron to Brain* with:

An all new test bank: The test bank consists of a broad range of questions covering all the key facts and learning objectives in each chapter. The questions are keyed to Bloom's taxonomy, aligned to learning objectives and referenced to specific textbook sections. The test bank is available in multiple formats including MS Word, TestGen, and a common cartridge for import into learning management systems.

Textbook figures and tables: All of the figures and tables from the textbook are formatted for optimal legibility when projected.

PowerPoint resources: All figures and tables from each chapter with complete captions in the notes field are provided.

Oxford Learning Link Direct: Oxford Learning Link Direct brings all of the high quality digital resources for *From Neuron to Brain* directly into your local learning management system. Instructors and their LMS administrators simply download the Oxford Learning Link Direct cartridge from Oxford Learning Link, and with the turn of a digital key, incorporate content from Oxford directly into their LMS for assigning and grading.

Oxford Learning Cloud: Oxford Learning Cloud delivers the interactive e-book and the complete test bank in an intuitive, web-based learning environment for those not using a local learning management system.

To learn more about any of these resources, or to get access, please contact your local OUP representative.

About the Authors

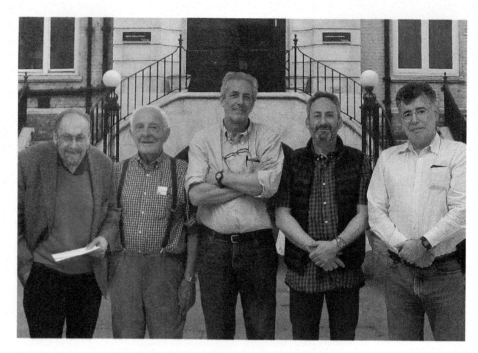

David A. Brown, A. Robert Martin, Antonino Cattaneo, Mathew E. Diamond, Francisco F. De-Miguel

A. Robert Martin is Professor Emeritus in the Department of Physiology at the University of Colorado School of Medicine. He was born in Saskatchewan in 1928 and majored in mathematics and physics at the University of Manitoba. He received a Ph.D. in Biophysics in 1955 from University College, London, where he worked on synaptic transmission in mammalian muscle under the direction of Sir Bernard Katz. From 1955 to 1957 he did postdoctoral research in the laboratory of Herbert Jasper at the Montreal Neurological Institute, studying the behavior of single cells in the motor cortex. He has taught at McGill University, the University of Utah, Yale University, and the University of Colorado Medical School, and has been a visiting professor at Monash University, Edinburgh University, and the Australian National University. His research has contributed to the understanding of synaptic transmission, including the mechanisms of transmitter release, electrical coupling at synapses, and properties of postsynaptic ion channels. He has contributed major sections to every edition of this book, except the first.

David A. Brown is a Professor in the Department of Neuroscience, Physiology and Pharmacology at University College London (UCL). He was born in London in 1936 and gained a B.Sc. in Physiology from UCL in 1957 and a Ph.D. (1961) from St. Bartholomew's Hospital Medical College ("Barts") in London (where he first met John Nicholls). He then worked as an Instructor (1965–1967) at the University of Chicago where he helped design an integrated neurobiology course for graduate medical students. After returning to London, he subsequently chaired pharmacology departments at the London School of Pharmacy and at UCL. In between he has worked in several labs in the USA and elsewhere, including three semesters (1979–1981) in the Department of Physiology and Biophysics at the University of Texas in Galveston, and a split year (1985–1986) as Fogarty Scholar-in-Residence at NIH in the labs of Mike Brownstein, Julie Axelrod, and Marshall Nirenberg. While at Galveston, he and Paul Adams (another ex-Barts colleague) discovered the M-type potassium channel as a transmitter-regulated controller of nerve cell excitability. He has since worked on the regulation of other ion channels by G protein–coupled receptors and previously on the actions and transport of GABA.

Mathew E. Diamond is Professor of Cognitive Neuroscience at the International School for Advanced Studies in Trieste, Italy (known by its Italian acronym, SISSA). He earned a Bachelor of Science degree in Engineering from the University of Virginia in 1984 and a Ph.D. in Neurobiology from the University of North Carolina in 1989. Diamond was a Postdoctoral Fellow with Ford Ebner at Brown University and then an Assistant Professor at Vanderbilt University before moving to SISSA to create the Tactile Perception and Learning Laboratory in 1996. His main interest is to specify the relationship between neuronal activity and perception. The research is carried out mostly in the tactile whisker system in rodents, but some experiments attempt to generalize the principles found in the whisker system to the processing of information in the human tactile sensory system.

Antonino Cattaneo is Professor of Physiology at the Scuola Normale Superiore in Pisa and President of the Rita Levi-Montalcini European Brain Research Institute in Rome. After obtaining his degree in biophysics at the University of Roma La Sapienza in 1976, he was a Ph.D. student under the supervision of Lamberto Maffei at Scuola Normale. In the years that followed, he was mentored by Rita Levi-Montalcini (at the National Research Council in Rome) and Cesar Milstein (at the MRC Laboratory of Molecular Biology in Cambridge, UK). From 1991 to 2008 he was Full Professor of Biophysics at the International School for Advanced Studies (SISSA) in Trieste (Italy), where he first met John Nicholls, before joining Scuola Normale himself. He spent long research periods at the MRC Laboratory of Molecular Biology (Cambridge, UK), and is a Visiting Fellow Commoner at Trinity College (Cambridge) and a Life member of Clare Hall College (Cambridge). He is a member of the EMBO (European Molecular Biology Organization), the Accademia Nazionale dei Lincei, the Accademia delle Scienze dei XL, and the Academia Europaea. His research has contributed to the understanding of the actions of neurotrophins NGF and BDNF in synaptic plasticity and in neurodegeneration. He has pioneered the subcellular targeting of recombinant antibodies to interfere with protein functions in a spatially localized way. He is currently studying the molecular mechanisms underlying the formation of memory traces in physiology and pathology.

Francisco F. De-Miguel is Professor at the Institute for Cellular Physiology at the Universidad Nacional Autónomous of México (UNAM). He was born in Mexico, in 1960 and studied biology at UNAM, followed by a Master's Degree and PhD. in neurosciences at CINVESTAV, in Mexico. From 1989 to 1992 he did postdoctoral research at the Biocenter of the University of Basel, Switzerland, in the laboratory of John G. Nicholls, studying how calcium channels redistribute during the formation of synapses. He has been Visiting Professor in the Universities of Basel, Oxford, Stanford, and Barcelona. He created the Experimenta Laboratories for Science Education, in which over 20,000 high school students have experienced scientific thinking as a tool for daily life. He has taught in Mexico; Woods Hole, Massachusetts; Pablo de Olavide University in Seville; Madrid University; University of Sao Paulo, and has organized or participated in courses in Bolivia, Brazil, Colombia, and Peru. His research concerns the non-synaptic release transmitters, and how we perceive visual art. He also coordinated the sixth edition of this book.

Brief Table of Contents

Contents

PART II ELECTRICAL PROPERTIES OF NEURONS AND GLIA 61

PART III   INTERCELLULAR COMMUNICATION   187

PART IV   INTEGRATIVE MECHANISMS   415

PART V   SENSATION   463

PART VI   DEVELOPMENT AND REGENERATION OF THE NERVOUS SYSTEM   615

PART VII   CONCLUSION   735

PART I

Introduction to the Nervous System

This introduction provides a framework for approaching chapters that deal with signaling, development, and functions of the nervous system. Readers who are curious about the brain but unfamiliar with neurobiology often face difficulties in coming to grips with the subject. Neurobiology aims to explain processes ranging from the opening of a single membrane channel to the behavior of the whole organism, so its terminology is derived from anatomy, physics, biochemistry, molecular biology, and even cognitive science. Because of the elaborate structure of the nervous system and the specialized features of neuronal signaling, the complex terminology of neurobiology is unavoidable.

Accordingly, the first three chapters in this book provide an introduction and overview of key concepts and definitions for readers who are approaching neurobiology for the first time. Chapter 1 describes the principal morphological, physiological, and molecular properties of nerve cells and their connections. As an example of a well-defined structure in which the processing of signals is largely understood, we use the retina. A major advantage is that from the outset, the electrical signals generated by retinal cells can be directly correlated to perception; this enables features of the way in which we see the world to be understood at the cellular level.

Chapters 2 and 3 return to the theme of visual processing as they follow stages of processing from the eye to the cerebral cortex. We show how the meaning of the messages becomes transformed in the cortex in a remarkable manner through precise interconnections along the pathway. The beauty and clarity of the experiments we highlight make it possible to understand the material with little background knowledge, to see where research on the brain is heading, and to appreciate why the detailed study of cellular and molecular mechanisms described in the later chapters is so interesting and important.

Our principal objective at this stage is to enable the naïve reader to think about higher functions from the outset and to see how they are dependent on and correlated to cellular mechanisms employed by nerve cells. To achieve this aim, we present the material with only essential concepts and facts, delving into more detail in later chapters.

CHAPTER 1

Principles of Signaling and Organization

The nervous system is an unresting assembly of cells that continuously receives information, analyzes it, creates percepts (that is, meaningful experiences of the surrounding world), and makes decisions. The brain then acts by producing co-ordinated, coherent muscle contractions for swimming, swallowing, or singing. Sensory information is translated to electrical signals by sensory neurons. Electrical signals are then transmitted from one nerve cell to another across specific connections. A major goal of neurobiological research is to decode the content of the information that these signals transmit. The meaning of the signals is determined by where the nerve fibers arise and where they go, as well as on the frequency and temporal pattern of the signals themselves. Signals in the optic nerve carry visual information from the retina. Similar impulses in a sensory nerve in the fingertip convey information about what is being touched. Within the brain, each individual nerve cell receives inputs from thousands of others. By integrating this information, the nerve cell creates a new message that can convey a complex meaning, such as the presence of a vertical bar of light in one's field of vision or the rough texture of sandpaper touched by one's finger. Impulses in a motor nerve, traveling to a muscle, give rise to movement.

One simplifying feature of the nervous system is that in many areas (including the retina), nerve cells with similar properties are grouped together, often in layers or clusters. Another is that the brain uses stereotyped electrical signals to transmit information. These signals consist of changes in voltage produced by electrical currents flowing across cell membranes. Neurons use only two types of electrical signals: local graded potentials, which spread over short distances, and action potentials, which are conducted rapidly over short or long distances.

Information is transmitted between one neuron and the next at specialized connections known as synapses. The signals arriving at the synapse may flow directly to adjacent neurons; alternatively, they may lead to the release of chemical transmitter molecules that bind to specific chemoreceptor molecules in the membrane of the target cell. This interaction gives rise to a local graded potential that excites or inhibits the target cell depending on the transmitter and the corresponding receptors. The efficacy of the impulse conduction and of synaptic transmission can be modified by previous activity, transmitters, hormones, and drugs.

During development, neurons depend on molecular signals derived from other cells for the generation of their own identity. These signals determine the shape and position of each neuron, its survival, its transmitter, and the targets to which it connects. Once mature, most nerve cells do not divide. Molecules in the environment of a neuron influence its capacity for repair after injury. Glial cells in the nervous system are different from neurons and contribute to neuronal signaling during development, in adulthood, and after injury.

Throughout the following chapters we attempt to explain the complex functions of the brain as a product of the underlying activity of nerve cells and their companion non-neuronal cells, the glia. A second aim is to explain the cellular and molecular mechanisms by which those signals arise. A third aim is to review how the nervous system integrates senses to generate perception. Finally, we review the way in which structures and connections that subserve functions are established during development, become modified by experience, and repair themselves after injury. As a starting point, in this chapter we summarize key concepts and essential background material.

Signaling in Simple Neuronal Circuits

Events that occur during the performance of simple reflexes can be followed and analyzed in detail. For example, when the tendon below the knee is tapped by a small hammer, thigh muscles are stretched and electrical impulses travel along sensory nerve fibers to the spinal cord. There, neurons that connect to muscles (called motoneurons because they produce movement) are excited, producing impulses and contractions in muscles. The end result is that the leg extends and the knee is straightened. Such circuits are essential for regulating muscular contractions that control movements of the body. In simple reflex behavior, in which a stimulus leads to a defined output, the roles played by the signals in just two types of cells—sensory and motor—can be readily understood.

Complex Neuronal Circuitry in Relation to Higher Functions

Analyzing signaling in complex pathways that involve many different types of neurons is far more difficult than analyzing simple reflexes. The transmission of information to the brain for perception of a sound, a touch, an odor, a visual image, or the execution of a simple voluntary movement requires the sequential activation of a multitude of cells, with thousands of neurons engaged in each stage of processing. Serious challenges in the analysis of signaling and circuitry arise from the dense packing of nerve cells, the intricacy of their connections, and the profusion of cell types. The brain, unlike an organ such as the liver, consists of heterogeneous populations of cells. Once you have discovered how one region of the liver functions, you know a great deal about the liver as a whole. Knowledge of the cerebellum, however, gives you little idea about the workings of the retina or any other part of the **central nervous system (CNS)**. Nevertheless, the retina can provide a well-defined structure for illustrating and explaining fundamental mechanisms that operate throughout the nervous system.

Despite the immense complexity of the nervous system, it is now possible to understand many aspects of the way in which neurons act as the building blocks for perception, decision making, and action. The first three chapters of this book show how one can record the activity of neurons in the pathway from the eye to the brain, following signals first in cells that specifically respond to light and then step by step through successive relays. As you read this page, signaling within the eye itself ensures that the black letters stand out from the white page in either the dim light in a room or the brilliant sunshine on a beach (not perhaps the ideal place to concentrate on this book). Specific connections in the brain create a single image in the mind's eye, even though the two eyes are situated apart on the head and have somewhat different views of the outside world. Moreover, mechanisms exist to ensure that this image stays still (even though our eyes are continually making small movements) and to provide accurate information about the distance to the book so that you can reach out to turn the page.

How do the connections of nerve cells enable such phenomena to occur? Much is now known about how these attributes of vision stem from well-defined neuronal circuits in the eye and in the initial relays in the brain, but numerous questions remain about the relation between neuronal properties and behavior. Methods such as **functional magnetic resonance imaging (fMRI)** of the human brain can reveal the locations of structures that become active as you read. But it is still not known how the neuronal signals in those regions cause you to perceive and understand the words in front of you. Moreover, while you are reading, you must maintain the posture of your body, head, and arms. The brain must further ensure that the eyeball remains moist through continuous secretion of tears, that breathing continues, and that untold other involuntary and

FIGURE 1.1 Pathways from the Eyes to the Brain. Pathways travel through the optic nerve and the optic tract. The interposed relay is the lateral geniculate nucleus. Arrows indicate how the lens reverses images and how the specific crossing of axons causes the right visual field to be represented in the left brain, and vice versa. (After S. Ramón y Cajal, 1911. *Histologie du Système Nerveux*, Vol. 2. Maloine, Paris.)

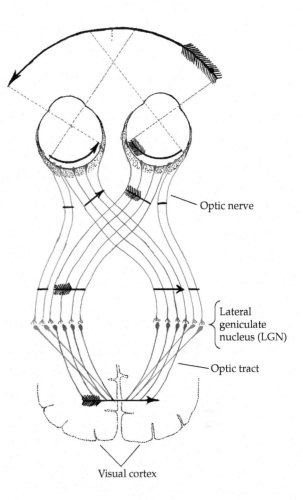

Optic nerve

Lateral geniculate nucleus (LGN)

Optic tract

Visual cortex

unconscious bodily tasks are carried out. A full description of the mechanisms underlying such integrated behavior is well beyond the scope of this book, or indeed of current knowledge. Although a full account of the nervous system processes that support reading is not realistic, the chapters to come can illustrate how shapes in front of the eye are translated into neural messages.

Organization of the Vertebrate Retina

Analysis of the visual world depends on the information coming from the retina—the initial stage of processing. Figure 1.1 shows pathways from the eye to higher centers in the brain. The optical image that falls on the retina is reversed by the lens but is otherwise a faithful representation of the external world. How can this picture be translated into our visual experience by way of electrical signals that are initiated in the retina and then travel through the optic nerves? An essential concept, applicable at every level of the nervous system, is that for function to be understood one must know the anatomy of the structure involved.

Shapes and Connections of Neurons

Figure 1.2 shows the various types of cells and their arrangement in the mammalian retina. Light entering the eye passes through the layers of transparent nerve cells and glia to reach the **photoreceptors**. Then, signals leaving the eye through the optic nerve fibers of **ganglion cells** provide the entire input for all of our vision.

The drawings of Figure 1.2 were made by Santiago Ramón y Cajal[1] before the turn of the twentieth century. Ramón y Cajal was one of the greatest students of the nervous system, selecting examples of nervous tissue from a wide range of structures and animals. He had an unfailing instinct for the essential. An important lesson from his work is that the shape and position of a neuron, as well as the origin and destination of its processes in the neural network, supply valuable clues to its function.

In Figure 1.2 it is apparent that the cells in the retina, like those elsewhere in the CNS, are densely packed. Early anatomists had to tease nervous tissue apart to see individual cells. Staining methods that impregnate every neuron are virtually useless for investigating cell shapes and connections because a structure such as the retina appears as a dark blur of intertwined cells and processes. Most of Ramón y Cajal's pictures were made with the Golgi staining method, which by a still unknown mechanism stains just a few neurons at random out of the whole population, yet stains those few cells in their entirety. The extracellular space surrounding neurons and their supporting cells is restricted to clefts only about 25 nanometers (25×10^{-9} meters) wide.

The schematic presentation in Figure 1.2 gives an idea of the orderly arrangement of the retinal neurons. It is possible to distinguish the photoreceptors, **bipolar cells** (so named because of their shape), and ganglion cells. The lines of transmission are from input to output, from photoreceptors through to ganglion cells. In addition, two other types of cells, horizontal and amacrine cells, make transverse connections linking the pathways. The Müller glial cells align parallel to the photoreceptor–ganglion cell pathway. How do the cells in Ramón y Cajal's drawings contribute to the picture of the world we see?

[1] Ramón y Cajal, S. [1909-1911] 1995. *Histology of the Nervous System*, 2 vols. Translated by Neely Swanson and Larry Swanson. Oxford University Press, New York.

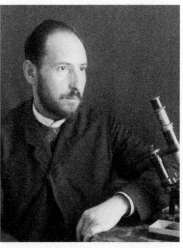

Ramón y Cajal (1852-1934)

(A)

Photoreceptors

Bipolar cells

Amacrine cells

Ganglion cells

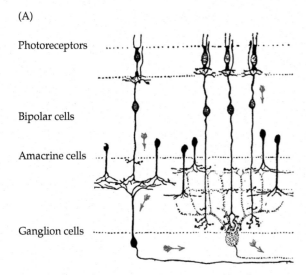

(B)

M

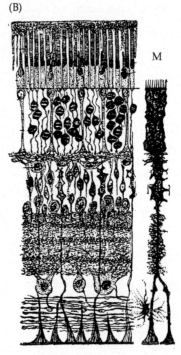

(C) Human rod and cone

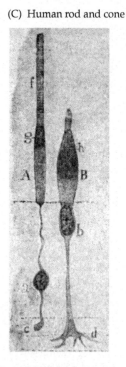

FIGURE 1.2   Structure and Connections of Cells in the Mammalian Retina. The photoreceptors (rods and cones) connect to bipolar cells. Bipolar cells in turn connect to ganglion cells, whose axons constitute the optic nerve. Horizontal cells (not shown) and amacrine cells make connections that are predominantly horizontal. (A) The scheme proposed by Ramón y Cajal for the direction taken by signals as they pass from photoreceptors to the optic nerve fibers. Arrows indicate Cajal's prediction of a through line of transmission from receptors to ganglion cells. This scheme still holds in general, but essential new pathways and feedback groups have been discovered since Ramón y Cajal's time. (B) Ramón y Cajal's depiction of the cellular elements of the retina and their orderly arrangement. The Müller (M) cell, shown on the right, is a glial cell. (C) Drawings of a human rod (left) and cone (right) isolated from the retina. Light passes through the retina (in these drawings from bottom to top) to be absorbed by the outer segment (top) of the photoreceptor. There, the light produces a signal that spreads to the terminal to influence the next cell in line. By recording electrically from each cell in the retinal circuit, one can follow signals step by step and understand how the meaning of the signals changes. (From S. Ramón y Cajal, 1911. *Histologie du Système Nerveux*, Vol. 2. Maloine, Paris.)

Cell Body, Axons, and Dendrites

The ganglion cell shown in Figure 1.3 illustrates features shared by neurons throughout the nervous system. The **cell body** (soma) of all neurons contains the nucleus and other intracellular organelles common to non-neuronal as well as neuronal cells. The long process that leaves the cell body is known as the **axon**. Its endings form connections with other neurons or cells in effector organs such as muscles and glands. The term **dendrite** (arborization) applies to branches on which incoming fibers make connections and that act as receiving stations for excitation or inhibition. It will become apparent in later chapters that the terms for describing neuronal structures, particularly dendrites, are somewhat ambiguous, but these terms are still convenient and widely used. In addition to the ganglion cell, Figure 1.3 shows other representative neurons.

Not all neurons conform to the simple plan of the cells shown in Figure 1.3. Certain nerve cells do not have an axon, while others have an axon onto which incoming connections are made. Still others have dendrites that can conduct impulses and transmit to target cells. While ganglion cells conform to the caricature of a stereotyped neuron with dendrites, a cell body, and an axon, other cells in the retina do not. For example, photoreceptors do not have an axon or obvious dendrites (see Figure 1.2C). Activity in photoreceptors does not arise through input from another neuron but from an external stimulus—light.

Techniques for Identifying Neurons and Tracing Their Connections

Although the staining technique devised by Golgi in 1873 is still used, many newer techniques have facilitated the functional identification of neurons and synaptic connections. Molecules

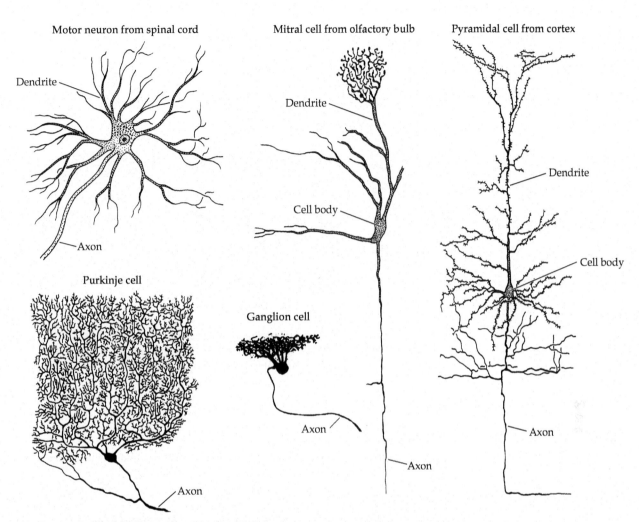

Motor neuron from spinal cord   Mitral cell from olfactory bulb   Pyramidal cell from cortex

Dendrite

Axon

Purkinje cell

Dendrite

Cell body

Ganglion cell

Axon

Axon

Dendrite

Cell body

Axon

Axon

FIGURE 1.3 Shapes and Sizes of Neurons. Neurons have branches (called dendrites), on which other neurons form synapses, and axons, which in turn make connections with other neurons. The motor neuron, drawn by the German neuroanatomist Otto Friedrich Karl Deiters in 1869, was dissected from a mammalian spinal cord. The other cells, stained by the Golgi method, were drawn by Ramón y Cajal. The pyramidal cell is from the cortex of a mouse, the mitral cell from the olfactory bulb (a relay station in the pathway concerned with smell) of a rat, the Purkinje cell from human cerebellum, and the ganglion cell from mammalian retina (animal not specified). (Motor neuron after O. Deiters. 1859. *Z. Wissenschaft Zool.* 1–12; All others after S. Ramón y Cajal, 1909, 1911. *Histologie du Système Nerveux*, Vol. 1 [purkinje and pyramidal], Vol. 2 [ganglion and mitral]. Maloine, Paris.)

that label a neuron in its entirety can be injected through a fine pipette. Fluorescent markers, such as Lucifer yellow and Tomato red, are visible as they spread through the fine processes of a living cell. Alternatively, other types of markers, such as the enzyme horseradish peroxidase or biocytin, can be injected into single neurons; after the tissue has been processed for histology, the marker in the cell appears as a dense product or bright fluorescence.

Neurons can also be stained by extracellular application of horseradish peroxidase; the enzyme is taken up by axon terminals and transported to the cell body. Fluorescent carbocyanine dyes placed close to neurons dissolve in cell membranes and diffuse over the entire surface of the cell. In recent years there has been increased use of certain viruses, such as rabies,[2] that when injected into brain tissue are absorbed by neurons, reproduce, and jump across synapses to reach other neurons. Later, the tissue is treated with fluorescent antibodies specific for the virus to make the entire infected circuit visible. These procedures are valuable for tracing the origins and destinations of axons from one region of the nervous system to another.

Antibodies have been made to characterize specific neurons, dendrites, axons, and synapses by selectively labeling intracellular or membrane components. Figure 1.4 shows

[2] Kelly, R. M., and Strick, P. L. 2000. *J. Neurosci. Methods* 103: 63–71.

FIGURE 1.4 Population of Rod Bipolar Cells Stained by an Antibody to the Enzyme Phosphokinase C. Only bipolar cells that contain the enzyme are stained. Above are photoreceptors; below are ganglion cells.

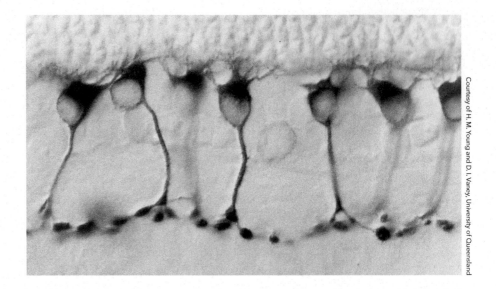

Courtesy of H. M. Young and D. I. Vaney, University of Queensland

bipolar cells that were labeled by an antibody to the enzyme phosphokinase C. Antibody techniques also provide valuable tools for following the migration and differentiation of nerve cells during development. A complementary approach for characterizing neurons is by in situ hybridization. Specific tagged probes are used to label messenger RNA that codes for a channel, receptor, transmitter, or structural element of a neuron. In animals such as fruit flies, worms, zebrafish, opossums, and mice, specific proteins, cells, or the entire nervous system can be labeled by the introduction of marker genes, driven by appropriate control element genes into the genome.

Genetic and molecular engineering are used to search for functions of particular proteins. New strains of animals with stable transgenesis can be produced by introducing a gene into an oocyte, a process referred to as gene knockin, or by eliminating a gene, referred to as gene knockout.

At the cellular level, the massive sequencing of the assortment of messenger RNA molecules (RNAsec) transcribed by a single cell or a cell population, in combination with computational analysis (a technique named **transcriptomics**), gives an account of the whole population and the amounts of messenger RNA molecules that are expressed in a developmental state or physiological condition. At the cellular level, using a technique known as RNA sequencing (RNAseq),[3] it is now possible to sequence and computationally analyze all the messenger RNA (mRNA) molecules transcribed by a single cell or cell population. The resulting profile describes the **transcriptome**: all of the mRNA transcripts, plus their relative abundances, expressed by a cell in a particular developmental state or physiological condition. Transcriptomic experiments carried out in the retina of newborn mice have distinguished 40 subtypes of ganglion cells.[4] Useful as it is for providing wide inventories of active genes, transcriptomics does not provide information about interactions between the genes or where they act in the cells. Alternative methods are necessary to answer such questions.

Non-Neuronal Cells

The distinctive cell labeled M in Figure 1.2B represents a class of non-neuronal cells present in the retina. Such cells, known as glial cells (see Chapter 10), are abundant throughout the nervous system, and greatly outnumber neurons. Unlike neurons, glial cells do not have axons or dendrites, and instead have different types of processes. Most have no specialized anatomical junctions with nerve cells. They play several roles in relation to neuronal signaling. For example, the axons of ganglion cells that run in the optic nerve conduct impulses rapidly because, once they leave the eye, the axons are surrounded by an insulating lipid sheath called **myelin**. Myelin is formed by glial cells that wrap themselves around axons during late stages of development. Retinal glial cells are known as Müller cells.

[3] Wang, Z., Gerstein, M., and Snyder, M. 2009. *Nat. Rev. Genet.* 10: 57–63.

[4] Rheaume, B.A. et al. 2018. *Nat. Comm.* 9: 2759.

Grouping of Cells According to Function

A remarkable feature of the retina is the clustering of cells according to function (see Figure 1.2). In the retina, photoreceptors and the horizontal, bipolar, amacrine, and ganglion cells all have their cell bodies and synapses situated in well-defined layers. Such layering is found in many regions of the brain. For example, the structure in which optic nerve fibers end (the lateral geniculate nucleus) consists of six readily distinguishable layers of cells. The spatial distribution of photoreceptor cells in the retina is reflected in the orderly arrangement of axons in the optic nerve. The visual map is maintained along the relays of the visual system. Similar retention of spatial order at successive stages of processing is found in other sensory modalities in other areas of the brain.

The simplified drawings of Figure 1.2 omit certain features of the organization of retinal cells. There are many distinctive types of ganglion cells, horizontal cells, bipolar cells, and amacrine cells, each with characteristic morphology, transmitters, and physiological properties. For example, the photoreceptors fall into two easily recognizable classes—**rods** and **cones**—which perform different functions. The elongated rods are extremely sensitive to small changes in illumination. As you read this page, the ambient light is too bright for the rods, which function only in dim light after a prolonged period in darkness. The cones respond to visual stimuli in bright ambient light. Moreover, the cones are further subdivided into red-, green-, or blue-sensitive photoreceptors according to which wavelengths of light most excite them. The peak responses of red-, green-, and blue-sensitive photoreceptor cells inspired engineers to create the RGB images in our computer screens and telephones. It is now common to name cones according to the peak wavelength as long (L), middle (M), or short (S) wavelength-sensitive cones. The amacrine cells provide an extreme example of cell type diversity: More than 40 types can be recognized by structural and physiological criteria. With few exceptions, the functional significance of this variety in cellular subtypes is not known. The properties and functions of the retinal cells will be described in Chapter 22.

Complexity of Connections

The arrows in Figure 1.2A indicate a through line of transmission from receptors to ganglion cells. Light falls on photoreceptors and generates electrical signals, which then influence bipolar cells. From bipolar cells, signals are conveyed to ganglion cells and then to higher centers in the brain that give rise to our perception of the outside world.

In reality, the picture is again far more complex. For example, there is a dramatic reduction in numbers from receptors to ganglion cells. More than 100 million photoreceptors provide input to just about 1 million ganglion cells, by way of interposed cells. Each individual ganglion cell therefore receives inputs from many photoreceptors (convergence). Similarly, when the axon of a single ganglion cell reaches the next relay station in the lateral geniculate nucleus, it branches extensively to supply many target cells (divergence).

In addition, other arrows could be inserted into Figure 1.2A that point sideways to indicate interactions among cells in the same layer (lateral connections) and even in the reverse direction—for example, from horizontal cells back toward photoreceptors (recurrent connections). Such convergent, divergent, lateral, and recurrent connections are consistent features of pathways elsewhere in the nervous system. Thus, the simple step-by-step processing of signals is dramatically influenced by parallel and feedback interactions.

Signaling in Nerve Cells

All nerve cells have a **resting potential**: the inside of the cell is negative with respect to the outside (extracellular) solution by less than a tenth of a volt. All electrical signals generated in nerve cells are superimposed on the resting potential. Some signals make the inside of the cell less negative (**depolarize** it); others make it more negative (**hyperpolarize** it).

Electrical signals of nerve cells fall into two main classes. The first consists of **local graded potentials**. These are generated by extrinsic physical stimuli, such as light falling on a photoreceptor in the eye, sound waves deforming a hair cell in the ear, or the pressure of an object against a tactile nerve ending in the skin, or by activity at chemical synapses. Synapses are discussed later in the chapter. Local potentials vary in amplitude, depending on the strength of the activating signal. They usually spread only a short distance from their site of origin, because the cell membrane is a poor conductor and electrical currents are lost along the fibers.

Action potentials (also referred to as nerve impulses) constitute the second major category of electrical signals. Action potentials are initiated when local graded potentials are sufficiently large to depolarize the cell membrane beyond a critical level (called the **threshold**). Once initiated, action potentials can propagate rapidly over long distances—for example, along the axons of ganglion cells in the optic nerve from the eye to the lateral geniculate nucleus on the way to the cortex, or from a motor cell in the spinal cord to a muscle in the leg. Unlike local graded potentials, action potentials are relatively fixed in amplitude and duration, like the dots in a code. Signal transmission through the retina can be summarized by the following simplified scheme:

> Light → local graded signal in photoreceptor → local graded potential in bipolar cell →
> local graded potential in ganglion cell →
> action potential in ganglion cell → conduction to higher centers

Universality of Electrical Signals

An important feature of electrical signals is that they are similar in all nerve cells, whether they (1) carry commands for movement, (2) transmit messages about colors, shapes, or painful stimuli, or (3) interconnect various portions of the brain. A second important feature of signals is that they are so similar in different animals that even a sophisticated investigator would be unable to tell with certainty whether a record of an action potential was derived from the nerve fiber of whale, mouse, monkey, worm, tarantula, or professor. In this sense, action potentials can be considered to be stereotyped units. They are the universal coins for the exchange of information in all nervous systems that have been investigated; it is the large number of neurons (on average, 86 billion in the human brain)[5] and the diversity of their connections, rather than a variety in types of signals, that account for the complexity of the tasks that can be carried out.

This idea was expressed in 1868 by the German physicist–biologist Hermann von Helmholtz. Starting from first principles, long before the facts as we know them were available, Helmholtz reasoned that:

> The nerve fibers have often been compared with telegraphic wires traversing a country, and the comparison is well fitted to illustrate the striking and important peculiarity of their mode of action. In the network of telegraphs we find everywhere the same copper or iron wires carrying the same kind of movement, a stream of electricity, but producing the most different results in the various stations according to the auxiliary apparatus with which they are connected. At one station the effect is the ringing of a bell, at another a signal is moved, at a third a recording instrument is set to work.... In short, every one of the... different actions which electricity is capable of producing may be called forth by a telegraphic wire laid to whatever spot we please, and it is always the same process in the wire itself which leads to these diverse consequences.... All the difference which is seen in the excitation of different nerves depends only upon the difference of the organs to which the nerve is united and to which it transmits the state of excitation.[6]

[5] Azevedo, F. A. et al. 2009. *J. Comp. Neurol.* 513: 532–541.

[6] Helmholtz, H. von. 1889. *Popular Scientific Lectures.* Longmans, London, UK.

Techniques for Recording Electrical Signals with Electrodes

For certain questions, it is useful to record the electrical activity from a single neuron or even a single permeable pore (a channel) in the cell membrane of a neuron; for other questions, one needs to monitor the activity in many neurons, all at the same time. In this

(A) Extracellular recording

(B) Intracellular recording

(C) Whole-cell patch recording

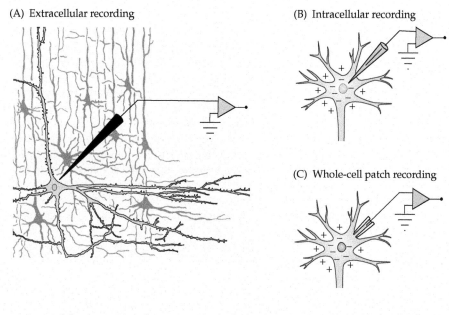

FIGURE 1.5 Electrical Recording Techniques. (A) The tip of a fine wire electrode is located close to a nerve cell in the cortex. (The wire above the tip is insulated.) Extracellular recording allows one to record from a single cell or from a group of cells. (B) Intracellular recordings are made with a fluid-filled glass capillary that has a tip of less than 1 μm in diameter, which is inserted into a neuron across the cell membrane. (C) Intracellular recordings are also made with patch electrodes. A patch electrode has a larger tip than an intracellular microelectrode, and the tip makes an extremely tight seal with the cell membrane. In whole-cell patch recording, the cell membrane ruptures, resulting in the diffusion of molecules between the pipette and the intracellular fluid, thereby creating a single electrical compartment. In cell-attached patch recording (not shown), the seal remains intact, allowing one to record currents that flow while a single ion channel in the membrane opens or closes.

section and the next we briefly summarize the key techniques for recording neuronal activity discussed throughout this book.

Recordings of action potentials were first made in the early twentieth century with fine silver wires placed on the trunk of a peripheral nerve. Currents flowing between one pair of electrodes were used to stimulate nerve fibers, while a second pair of electrodes placed some distance away recorded an extracellular voltage signal produced by the resulting nerve cell activity. The voltage signal reflected the summed action potentials of many fibers (a compound action potential).

Within the CNS, recordings from a neuron can be made with an **extracellular microelectrode**, which consists of a single wire made of metal (e.g., platinum) insulated down to an exposed conductive tip (Figure 1.5A) or a glass capillary filled with salt solution. One can also record from many individual neurons simultaneously (on the order of 100) using a **multielectrode array**. Depending on the requirements of the experiment, the array can be a large set of separate wires or a series of tiny silicon conducting points arranged within one probe, embedded in non-conducting material.[7]

Intracellular microelectrodes can be used to measure the resting membrane potential of neurons and to record local potentials and action potentials generated in the cell membrane. Such microelectrodes are usually made of glass drawn to a fine-diameter tip (0.1 micrometer [μm] or smaller) and filled with a salt solution (Figure 1.5B). The electrode is inserted through the cell membrane with the aid of a micromanipulator. The cell membrane forms a tight seal around the glass so that the integrity of the cell is not disturbed. Intracellular microelectrodes are also used for passing electrical currents across the cell membrane or for injecting molecules into the cytoplasm. At rest, there is a potential difference of about 70 millivolts (mV) between the inside and outside of a cell, the inside being negative with respect to the outside. This difference is known as the resting potential.

An alternative is to measure the membrane potential by a procedure known as **whole-cell patch recording** (Figure 1.5C). A larger pipette with a polished tip of approximately 1 μm is applied to the surface of the cell, where upon application of suction it fuses with the membrane to form a tight seal. After the membrane within the pipette tip has been ruptured, the fluid in the pipette and the intracellular fluid become a single electrical compartment. Opening and closing of individual ion channels can be detected by the cell-attached patch recording, forming a tight seal without rupturing the cell membrane.

Techniques for Imaging and Stimulating Neuronal Activity

With the use of optical recording techniques, one can follow signaling in suitable preparations. Specially fabricated dyes that bind to the cell membrane change their light

[7] Vetter, R. J. et al. 2004. *IEEE Trans. Biomed. Eng.* 51: 896-904.

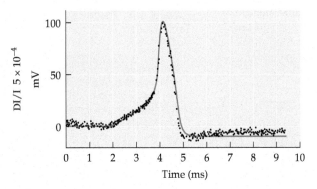

FIGURE 1.6 Comparison of Optical and Electrical Recordings. Faithful optical recording of an action potential (dots) from a squid giant axon compared with an electrical recording (solid line) with electrode. ΔI/I is a measure of the change in absorption by a voltage-sensitive merocyanine dye. ms, milliseconds. (After Y. Homma et al., 2009. *Philos. Trans. R. Soc. Lond., B* 364: 2453-2467; based on W. N. Ross et al., 1974. *Biophys. J.* 14: 983-986.)

[8] Homma, Y. et al. 2009. *Philos. Trans. R. Soc. Lond. B* 364: 2453-2467.

[9] Ji, G. et al. 2004. *J. Biol. Chem.* 279: 21461-21468.

[10] Maiti, S. et al. 1997. *Science* 275: 530-532.

[11] Ward, N. S., and Frackowiak, R. S. 2004. *Cerebrovasc. Dis.* 17 (Suppl. 3): 35-38.

[12] Bandettini, P.A. 2009. *Ann. NY Acad. Sci.* 1156: 260-293.

absorbance during changes in membrane potential. Other dyes measure changes in the level of calcium inside nerve cells.[8] Changes in light emission by fluorescent dyes provide an index of activity occurring in a single neuron or in populations of neurons. Figure 1.6 shows a recording made from a large squid axon using a voltage-sensitive dye. The optically recorded signal faithfully reproduces the voltage changes recorded by an electrode. With suitable dyes, microscopes, and cameras, one can record the ongoing activity of hundreds of nerve cells simultaneously within a discrete region of the brain. With genetic engineering, it is now possible to introduce genes whose products will give rise to optical signals based on Ca^{2+} concentration within the cell.[9] Recordings that depend on changes in emission of light by active cells are most simply made in isolated tissues maintained alive in a culture dish or in intact CNS near the surface.

Optical signals generated by deeply embedded cells are difficult to observe through overlying layers of tissue, unless one uses a laser technique known as two-photon (or multiphoton) microscopy. The technique consists of focusing a high-power, pulsed infrared laser on the sample. The intensity of the laser increases the probability that two or more photons will hit and excite simultaneously a single fluorescent molecule. Therefore, two photons of low energy arriving simultaneously can produce the effect of one single photon with twice the amount of energy, and three low-energy photons can produce the effect of a single photon that triples their energy. Moreover, the focused low-energy infrared light has better penetration of biological tissue and produces less photodamage. Multiphoton illumination can be used to excite exogenous molecules, such as calcium-sensitive dyes or fluorescent reporters; endogenous molecules such as the transmitter serotonin can be excited with two or more photons.[10]

Other noninvasive techniques are able to provide an indirect measure of activity in groups of neurons deep in the brain as well as in superficial neuronal layers. Positron emission tomography (PET) and fMRI[11] allow one to determine which regions of the awake, human brain are active in response to sensory stimulation or initiation of movements (see Chapter 25). They are particularly important in mapping brain regions involved in complex cognitive functions, such as reading, remembering, and imagining. The methods now available have a spatial resolution limited to hundreds of microns and seconds. Hence, present-day imaging methods of the human brain cannot provide information about the exact cellular location or timing of messages that are being carried by active neurons. It is realistic to hope that all this will be possible in the future since, year by year, the temporal and spatial resolution of imaging improves. The fMRI image in Figure 1.7 shows the location of activity in the visual pathway in response to a visual stimulus.

The overall activity of the eye and large portions of the brain can also be observed in the electroretinogram and electroencephalogram. These techniques collect multicellular electrical signals with electrodes placed on the eye or head, respectively. They have good time resolution but poor spatial resolution and are used to diagnose disorders of function, such as epilepsy.[12]

Stimulation of an area in the brain is now practicable by the noninvasive techniques **transcranial magnetic stimulation (TMS)** and **transcranial direct-current stimulation**

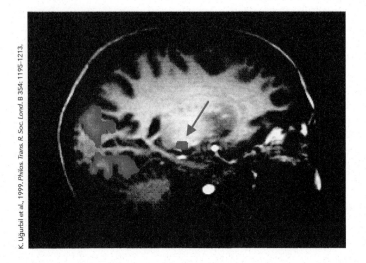

FIGURE 1.7 Magnetic Resonance Imaging of a Living Brain. The individual was presented with visual stimuli that caused activity to be generated in the lateral geniculate nucleus (red arrow), deep within the brain (see Figure 1.1 and Chapter 20), and in the visual cortex (red on left-hand side). The color represents the level of activity, red corresponding to high activity.

(**tDCS**). Stimulation of appropriate regions in conscious individuals can cause them to see lights or can induce movements. In TMS, strong magnetic fields are applied to the surface of the skull by means of an electromagnetic coil.[13] By combining imaging and stimulation techniques, one can identify brain areas involved in specific perceptual or motor tasks. For example, fMRI can be used to locate a discrete cortical region that becomes activated when a person perceives the direction of movement of dots on a computer monitor. When the same region is excited by TMS, the ability of the individual to perceive the motion is disrupted. In this way, a functional property of a specific brain region identified by imaging is confirmed by TMS. tDCS uses constant, low direct current delivered via electrodes on the head. Both TMS and tDCS are being examined for potential therapeutic uses, such as treatment of depression.

Spread of Local Graded Potentials and Passive Electrical Properties of Neurons

Implicit in the wiring diagram of Ramón y Cajal (see Figure 1.2A) is the idea that changes in illumination of the retina influence the activity of the photoreceptors and eventually the fibers leaving the eye. For this influence to take effect, signals must spread not only from cell to cell, but along a cell, from one end to the other. How, for example, does the electrical signal generated at one end of the bipolar cell (in contact with the photoreceptor) spread along its length to reach the terminal adjacent to the ganglion cell?

To answer this question, it is useful to consider the relevant structural components that carry the signals. A neuron, such as a bipolar cell, can be considered a long tube filled with a watery solution of salts (dissociated into positively and negatively charged ions) and proteins, separated from the extracellular solution by an insulating membrane. The intracellular and extracellular solutions have the same osmolarity but different ionic compositions. The cell membrane, a lipid, is relatively impermeable to the ions on either side, but ions can move through specific ion channels formed by proteins that span the membrane. Electrical and chemical signals cause the various ion channels for sodium, potassium, calcium, and chloride to open or close. Detailed information about the molecular structure of ion channels, and the way in which they allow the flow of ions, will be presented in Chapters 4 and 5.

The structure of a neuron in the retina or elsewhere limits its ability to conduct electrical signals. First, the intracellular fluid, or axoplasm, is about 10^7 times worse than a copper wire as a conductor of electricity because both the density of charge carriers (ions) and their mobility in the intracellular fluid are much lower than those of free electrons in metal. Second, the movement of currents along the axon for any great distance is hampered by the fact that the membrane is not a perfect insulator. Consequently, any current flowing along the fiber is gradually lost to the outside by leakage through ion channels in the membrane.

Passively conducted electrical signals, then, are severely attenuated and limited to a short length of nerve fiber, 1 to 2 millimeters (mm) at most. For example, a local potential generated in a small sensory fiber in the big toe will spread only about one-thousandth the distance that must be traversed for the signal to reach the spinal cord. In addition, when such a signal is brief, its time course may be severely slowed and its amplitude further attenuated by the electrical capacitance and resistance of the cell membrane. The fact that nerve fibers are extremely thin (1–20 μm in diameter in vertebrates) further reduces the amount of current they can carry.[14] Nevertheless, local graded potentials (Figure 1.8) provide the essential mechanisms for initiating propagated signals. The electrical recordings made from the neurons shown in Figure 1.8 were made from their cell bodies. The local potentials originated from synaptic actions on dendrites at a distance and spread passively to the recording site.

Spread of Potential Changes in Photoreceptors and Bipolar Cells

Because photoreceptors and bipolar cells are so short, local graded signals can spread effectively from one end of the cell to the other. The electrical signal that results from illumination of the photoreceptor is generated in the outer segment of the rod or cone. From there,

[13] Bestmann, S. et al. 2008. *Exp. Brain. Res.* 191: 383–402.

[14] Hodgkin, A. L. 1964. *The Conduction of the Nervous Impulse.* Liverpool University Press, Liverpool, UK.

it spreads passively along the cell to its terminal on the bipolar cell. Photoreceptor and bipolar cells thus constitute exceptions to the general rule that action potentials are necessary to carry information along the length of a cell. Ganglion cells, by contrast, must generate action potentials to send signals along their elongated axons in the optic nerve.

Properties of Action Potentials

The action potential is a triggered, regenerative, all-or-nothing event that is propagated along a nerve fiber. In a ganglion cell, action potentials are initiated by signals impinging on the cell from bipolar and amacrine cells, provided that these signals are sufficient to depolarize the ganglion cell to threshold. Once initiated, the amplitude and duration of the action potential are not determined by the amplitude and duration of the stimulus. Larger stimulating currents do not give rise to larger action potentials, and stimuli of longer duration do not prolong the action potential. Figure 1.9 shows that the action potential is a brief electrical pulse about 0.1 volts (V) in amplitude. At its peak, the voltage across the membrane reverses sign (i.e., the inside becomes positive). The action potential lasts for about 0.001 seconds (1 millisecond) and moves rapidly along the nerve fiber from one end to the other.

The entire action potential sequence must be completed before another action potential can be initiated at the same site. Thus, after each action potential there is a period of enforced silence, usually lasting for a few milliseconds (the refractory period). The maximal possible frequency of repeated action potentials is limited by the refractory period.

Propagation of Action Potentials along Nerve Fibers

The action potential itself causes electrical currents to spread passively ahead of it along the axon. Although the resulting depolarization falls off steeply with distance, it nevertheless exceeds threshold. Hence, the action potential provides an electrical stimulus to the next adjacent region of the axon. In this way, the impulse is reborn unchanged or "regenerated" as it propagates along the axon. The fastest action potentials in the human body travel in the largest fibers at a speed of about 120 meters/second (430 kilometers/hour, or 270 miles/hour). It takes about 10 milliseconds for a motor fiber to conduct its action potentials over 1 meter from the spinal cord to the foot.

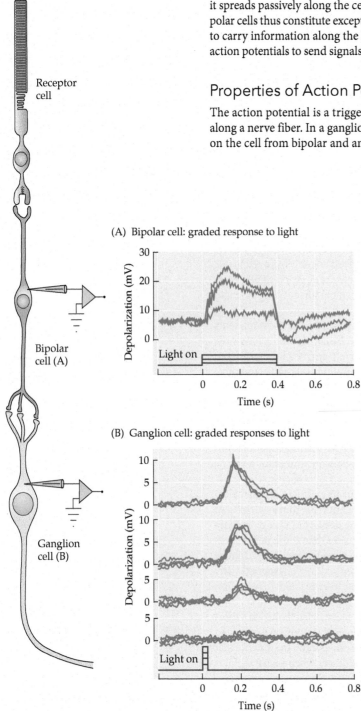

(A) Bipolar cell: graded response to light

(B) Ganglion cell: graded responses to light

FIGURE 1.8 Local Graded Potentials. Intracellular recordings were made from a bipolar cell (A) and a ganglion cell (B) with microelectrodes. The local potentials were recorded from the cell bodies and were produced by transmitters acting on the dendrites. (A) When light is absorbed by the photoreceptors, it gives rise to a signal that in turn produces a localized, graded response in the bipolar cell. The resting potential across the membrane is reduced (the trace moves in an upward direction)—an effect known as a depolarization. The size of the signal in the bipolar cell depends on the intensity of illumination, hence the term *graded*. The depolarization spreads to the far end of the bipolar cell passively. As it spreads, it becomes smaller in amplitude owing to the poor conducting properties of neurons. At the terminal of the bipolar cell, depolarization causes the release of chemical transmitter (not shown). (B) The transmitter produces a local graded potential in the ganglion cell. Because it is localized, the potential cannot spread more than 1 mm (at most) along the axon. Whereas the bipolar cell is short enough for a local potential to spread to its endings, the ganglion cell has an axon several centimeters long. s, seconds. (A after A. Kaneko and H. Hashimoto, 1969. *Vision Res.* 9: 37–55; B after D. A. Baylor and R. Fettiplace, 1979. *J. Physiol.* 288: 107–127.)

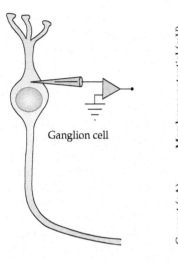

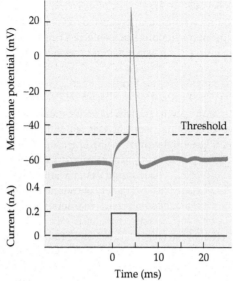

FIGURE 1.9 **Action Potential** recorded from a retinal ganglion cell with an intracellular microelectrode. When the stimulus, in this case current injected into the cell through the microelectrode, causes a depolarizing response that exceeds the threshold, the all-or-nothing action potential is initiated. During the action potential, the inside of the neuron becomes positive. The action potential propagates along the axon of the ganglion cell to its terminal, where it causes transmitter to be released. nA, nanoamperes; mV, millivolts. (After D. A. Baylor and R. Fettiplace, 1979. *J. Physiol.* 288: 107–127.)

Action Potentials as the Neural Code

Given that the action potential is fixed in amplitude, how is information about the intensity of a stimulus conveyed? Intensity is coded by frequency of firing. A more effective visual stimulus produces a greater local potential and, consequently, a higher frequency of firing in ganglion cells (Figure 1.10). The phenomenon was first described by Adrian,[15] who showed that the frequency of action potential firing in a sensory nerve in the skin is a measure of the intensity of the stimulus. In addition, Adrian observed that stronger stimuli applied to the skin give rise to activity in a larger number of sensory fibers.

The frequency of action potentials is not the only means for transmitting information—temporal patterns of firing can be critical in relaying information about external events. As a zebra finch listens to the songs of other birds in its colony, neurons in the auditory nuclei of the brain produce patterns of action potentials distributed across time. When the same song is played many times, action potentials recorded during the different repetitions are found to occur at the same instant within the tune, with a precision of a few milliseconds. The exact timing of impulses, not the overall frequency of impulses, distinguishes one song from another.[16]

Synapses: The Sites for Cell-to-Cell Communication

The structure at which one cell passes its information to the next is known as a **synapse.** As mentioned before, electrical synapses permit the direct flow of currents from one neuron to another. Chemical synapses lack continuity, and instead connect two cells by release of chemical substances. Through synaptic interactions, neurons such as ganglion cells take account of signals that arise from many photoreceptors and feed onto horizontal, bipolar, and amacrine cells, thereby creating new messages. Study of the processes underlying synaptic transmission constitutes a major theme in modern neurobiology because these mechanisms are responsible for integration and plasticity and are the targets of many therapeutic drugs.

[15] Adrian, E. D. 1946. *The Physical Background of Perception.* Clarendon, Oxford, UK.

[16] Wright, B. D. et al. 2002. In *Advances in Neural Information Processing 14*, T. G. Dietterich et al. (Eds.). MIT Press, Cambridge, MA, pp. 309–316.

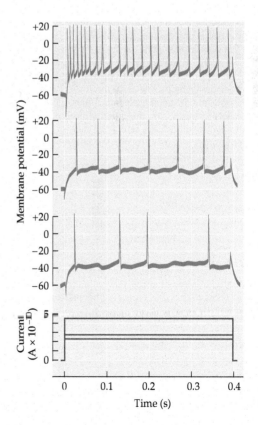

FIGURE 1.10 **Frequency as a Signal of Intensity in a Retinal Ganglion Cell.** Depolarizing current passed through the microelectrode produces action potentials. Larger currents produce more action potentials and higher frequencies of firing. (After D. A. Baylor and R. Fettiplace, 1979. *J. Physiol.* 288: 107–127.)

[17] Katz, B. 1971. *Science* 173: 123-126.
[18] Fillenz, M. 2005. *Neurosci. Biobehav. Rev.* 29: 949-962.

Chemically Mediated Synaptic Transmission

Figure 1.11 shows the highly organized structure at which a photoreceptor makes chemical synaptic connections onto a bipolar cell. The **presynaptic terminal** of the photoreceptor is separated from the **postsynaptic terminal** of the bipolar cell by a cleft that contains extracellular fluid. This space cannot be traversed by currents generated in the photoreceptor. Instead, the photoreceptor terminal releases a neurotransmitter that is stored in presynaptic vesicles. The transmitter, the amino acid glutamate in this case, diffuses across the cleft to interact with specific protein molecules, known as receptors, that are embedded in the membrane of the postsynaptic bipolar cell. (This terminology can—but should not—lead to confusion: The term **receptor**, as used here, means a **chemoreceptor molecule** and is not the same thing as a **sensory receptor** cell that responds to external physical stimuli, such as a photoreceptor.) The transmitters in a neuron and the receptors on its surface can be identified and visualized by a variety of techniques, including antibody labeling and genetic transfection of so-called reporter constructs, which lead to the production of fluorescent proteins in cells or in selected molecules.

Activation of the receptor molecules in a bipolar cell by glutamate sets up local graded potentials that spread to its terminals. As a general rule, the more presynaptic neurons activated, the more synaptic terminals release transmitter, the larger the number of activated postsynaptic receptors, and the larger the postsynaptic effect. Release of transmitter from the presynaptic terminal and its binding by receptors in postsynaptic targets occur across a timescale of only about 1 millisecond. Essential features of synaptic transmission were first revealed by Katz, Kuffler, and their colleagues.[17] These investigators used the responses of receptors in muscle as a bioassay with extremely high sensitivity and time resolution for measuring transmitter release. Modern methods for measuring the transmitter directly include voltammetry, in which special carbon fiber probes produce graded electrical signals in response to a particular transmitter (such as serotonin) as it is released from a presynaptic terminal.[18]

Excitation and Inhibition

A feature of synaptic transmission, as exemplified by the interactions between photoreceptors and bipolar cells in the retina, is that the transmitter released by a presynaptic terminal can excite or inhibit the firing of the next cell, depending on the receptors that cell possesses. For example, one class of glutamate receptors localized to certain bipolar cells reacts to glutamate by causing an excitatory signal (i.e., moving the membrane potential toward threshold). This signal spreads passively to the bipolar cell terminals at the other end of the cell, where it causes liberation of transmitter. Other classes of bipolar cells contain different glutamate receptors that produce a signal of the opposite sign when activated by glutamate (i.e., moving the membrane away from threshold). Again, the electrical signal spreads along the bipolar cell, but in this case it suppresses the release of transmitter. **Excitatory** and **inhibitory synaptic potentials** in ganglion cells are shown in Figure 1.12.

FIGURE 1.11 Structure of a Synapse. (A) The principal features of synaptic structures made by a photoreceptor on a bipolar cell. (B) Electron micrograph showing the appearance of a typical synapse in the retina of a macaque monkey. The vesicles that store transmitter are in the presynaptic terminal; a narrow cleft separates the pre- and postsynaptic membranes. The postsynaptic membrane is densely stained. Transmitter released from the presynaptic amacrine cell diffuses across the cleft to interact with receptors on the postsynaptic ganglion cell.

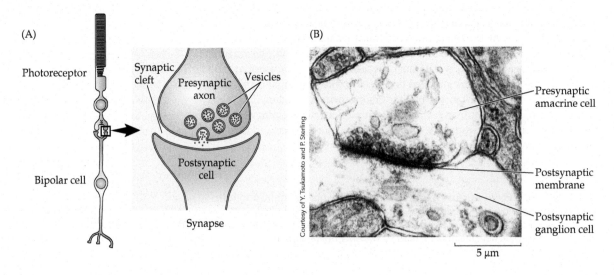

FIGURE 1.12 Excitation and Inhibition. Intracellular recordings from a ganglion cell showing excitatory and inhibitory synaptic potentials. (A) A ganglion cell is depolarized by continuous release of excitatory transmitter during retinal illumination. If the depolarizing synaptic potential is large enough, threshold is crossed and action potentials are initiated in the ganglion cell. (B) Illumination of a different group of photoreceptors causes inhibition. Hyperpolarization of the membrane makes it more difficult to initiate an action potential. (After D. A. Baylor and R. Fettiplace, 1979. *J. Physiol.* 288: 107-127.)

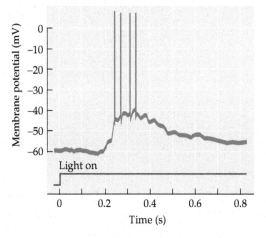

(A) Excitatory synaptic potentials

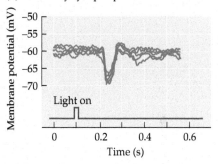

(B) Inhibitory synaptic potential

In neurons throughout the nervous system, combined excitatory and inhibitory inputs determine whether or not the threshold for initiation of an action potential will be reached. For example, a ganglion cell, as mentioned, receives both excitatory and inhibitory inputs. If excitation is sufficient to depolarize the cell membrane to threshold, then an action potential is generated and its message is transmitted to the next destination; if not, no message is sent. In motoneurons in the spinal cord, to use a different example, excitatory and inhibitory influences from different fibers determine whether or not a finger will be flexed. A motoneuron of this sort receives 10,000 or more incoming fibers (Figure 1.13). These fibers release transmitters that drive the membrane potential toward or away from the threshold for impulse initiation. An individual Purkinje cell in the cerebellum receives more than 100,000 inputs.

Artificial excitation and inhibition produced experimentally are tools for testing the contribution of any given neuron type to behavior. As foreseen by Francis Crick, a requirement for understanding brain function is "to be able to turn the firing of one or more types of neuron on or off in the alert animal in a rapid manner. The ideal signal would be light."[19] **Optogenetics** has made this idea possible.[20,21] Microbial light-sensitive molecules known as channelrhodopsins respond to illumination with blue light by exciting neurons. Genetic manipulations permit an investigator to target channelrhodopsins to selected neuronal types in the living brain. Illumination of channelrhodopsins expressed in brain regions, through an optic fiber, evokes series of action potentials that can be accurately and precisely controlled by the duration and intensity of the light. Such responses occur with a millisecond timescale. Inhibition can be obtained by illuminating other types of proteins, the halorhodopsins (or certain other types of channelrhodopsins), with yellow light. By combining both types of proteins and illuminating with corresponding light colors in freely moving animals, one can excite or inhibit specific relays in a neuronal pathway to explore its contribution to behavior.[22,23]

[19] Crick, F. H. 1979. *Sci. Am.* 241: 219-232.

[20] Zemelman, B. V. et al. 2002. *Neuron* 33: 15-22.

[21] Nagel, G. et al. 2002. *Science* 296: 2395-2398.

[22] Lima, S. Q., and Miesenboeck, G. 2005. *Cell* 121: 141-152.

[23] Boyden, E. S. et al. 2005. *Nat. Neurosci.* 8: 1263-1268.

Electrical Transmission

Although synaptic transmission between most neurons involves the release of transmitter molecules, the membranes of many cells in the retina and in the rest of the nervous system are instead linked by specialized junctions. At such synapses electrical transmission occurs. The pre- and postsynaptic membranes are closely apposed and linked by channels that connect the intracellular fluids of the two cells. This close connection allows local electrical potentials and even action potentials to spread directly from cell to cell without a chemical transmitter and without delay. Injected metabolites and dyes can also spread from cell to cell. One important example in the retina is provided by the horizontal cells, which are electrically coupled). By virtue of this property, graded depolarizing or hyperpolarizing potentials can spread

FIGURE 1.13 Multiple Connections of Individual Neurons. Approximately 10,000 presynaptic axons converge to form endings that are distributed over the surface of a motor neuron in the spinal cord. The drawing is based on a reconstruction made from electron micrographs. (From R. Poritsky, 1969. *J. Comp. Neurol.* 135: 423-452.)

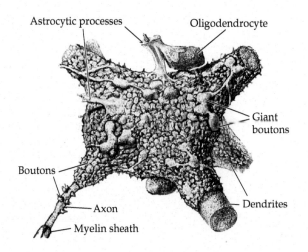

Astrocytic processes

Oligodendrocyte

Giant boutons

Boutons

Dendrites

Axon

Myelin sheath

from one horizontal cell to the next, with marked effect on the processing of visual information in the retina. Electrical synapses are found throughout the CNS of vertebrates and invertebrates. They also connect the glial cells in the nervous system and non-neuronal cells of other tissues in the body.

Modulation of Synaptic Efficacy

Chemically mediated synaptic transmission shows great plasticity. Dramatic changes occur in the amount of transmitter that is released by a signal—such as an action potential or a local potential—that invades a presynaptic terminal. The photoreceptors in the retina provide an example: The amount of the transmitter glutamate that is released by a rod or cone in response to a standard light stimulus can be increased or decreased by feedback to the terminal from horizontal cells. The horizontal cells themselves are influenced by other photoreceptors. This feedback loop plays a critical role in the way the eye adapts to different levels of illumination.

Other mechanisms that influence transmitter release depend on the history of impulse activity. During and after a train of impulses in a neuron, the amount of transmitter it releases can increase or decrease dramatically, depending on the frequency and duration of the activity. Modulation of efficacy, called **plasticity**, meaning temporary changes in synaptic efficacy, can also be postsynaptic in origin. Some changes last seconds to minutes; others may last hours to days. The long-term plastic changes in synaptic efficacy are maintained by changes in gene expression and protein synthesis. A tight molecular cross talk between synapses and the nucleus induces the synthesis of the new proteins that sustain long-term plastic changes in synaptic efficiency.

Extrasynaptic Communication by Release of Transmitters

The nervous system has the striking capacity to grade the functioning of large populations of cells in timescales ranging from seconds to hours to days through **extrasynaptic release** of transmitters—that is, release occurring from the cell body, dendrites, and axon in the absence of synaptic structures. Increases in the level of electrical activity of neurons can result in the extrasynaptic release of transmitters. Receptors in other neurons and in glial cells are targeted by these molecules. In response, they release the same or other transmitters, peptides, and small proteins. Glial cells respond by coupling blood flow to the increase of electrical activity. Extrasynaptic communication adapts the responses of the nervous system by modulating its function from sensory inputs to motor outputs.

Cellular and Molecular Biology of Neurons

Like other types of cells, neurons possess the cellular machinery for metabolic activity for synthesizing intracellular and membrane proteins, and for distributing them to precise locations in the cell. Each type of neuron synthesizes, stores, and releases its characteristic transmitter(s). The receptors for specific transmitters are located at well-defined sites on the postsynaptic cell under the presynaptic terminals. In addition, other membrane proteins, known as pumps and transporters, maintain the constancy of the internal and external milieu of the cell. The presynaptic terminals of optic nerve fibers of ganglion cells (like those of photoreceptors and bipolar cells, and indeed like all presynaptic nerve terminals) contain in their membranes specific channels through which calcium ions can flow. Calcium entry triggers the release of transmitters and can activate intracellular cascades of enzymes and regulate numerous other cellular processes.

A major specialization in the cell biology of neurons, compared with other types of cells, arises from the presence of the axon and dendrites. Axons do not have adequate machinery for synthesizing all the proteins they need. Hence, essential molecules are carried to the nerve terminals by a process known as axonal transport, often over long distances. Molecules required for maintenance of structure and function, as well as for the appropriate membrane channels, travel from the cell body in this way; similarly, molecules taken up at the ending are carried back to the cell body. In addition to protein transport, neurons use mRNA transport into axons and dendrites to synthetize proteins locally, on demand.[24] Axons of developing adult retinal ganglion cells locally translate mRNAs encoding proteins involved in synaptic transmission, synaptic plasticity, and axonal survival.[25]

Neurons are different from most other cells in that, with few exceptions, they cannot divide after differentiation. As a result, in an adult human, neurons in the CNS that have been destroyed usually cannot be replaced. An exception has been provided by the finding that neural stem cells have been isolated in two neurogenic niches of the adult mammalian brain (including the human brain). Such stem cells can give rise to differentiated neurons and glia in the adult brain.

Signals for Development of the Nervous System

The high degree of organization in a structure such as the retina poses a fascinating problem. Whereas a computer requires a brain to wire it, the brain must establish and tune its own connections. What seems so puzzling is how the proper assembly of the parts endows the brain with its extraordinary properties.

In the mature retina, each cell type is situated in the correct layer—or even sublayer—and makes the correct connections with the appropriate targets. This arrangement is a prerequisite for function. For ganglion cells to develop, for example, precursor cells must divide, migrate, differentiate into the appropriate shapes with the appropriate properties, and receive specific synapses. The axons must find their way over long distances through the optic nerve to end in the appropriate layer of the next relay station. Similar processes must occur for the various divisions of the nervous system so that complex structures required for function are formed.

Study of the mechanisms by which highly complex structures, such as the retina, are formed presents a key challenge in modern neurobiology. A good strategy to address such questions is to perform *cell fate mapping*. During the formation of the nervous system and even in the adult, neurons and glia originate from common precursor cells. One can determine how clones of neurons and glia are produced and where they migrate to. Figure 1.14 shows living neurons and glial cells in the cerebral cortex of an adult mouse. Using the StarTrack technique developed by López-Mascaraque and her colleagues,[26] one can study the origin and fate of morphologically identifiable neurons and glia. Precursor cells are labeled transgenically with engineered gene sequences that code for fluorescent proteins. A mixture of plasmids coding for different color proteins is then injected into mice brains in utero. Application of a weak current that produces transient pores in the cell membrane (electroporation) causes the genes to become incorporated into cells. The transfected genes express their proteins specifically in the precursor cells, some of which express one color and others of which may express other colors. One can then identify the neuronal or glial progeny, in embryos and newborn or adult animals, by their characteristic color emissions.

An understanding of how intricate wiring diagrams are established in development often provides clues about function and about the genesis of functional disorders. In other words, if you know how an electrical circuit has been wired, you may be able to understand what the components are doing, and consequently, you may be able to repair it. Certain molecules are essential for differentiation, outgrowth of axons, pathfinding, synapse formation, and survival of neurons. Such molecules are now being identified at an ever-increasing rate, and their mechanisms of action are being studied. Interestingly, molecular signals that give rise to the outgrowth of axons and

[24] Hafner, A. S. et al. 2019. *Science* 364: 650.

[25] Shigeoka, T. et al. 2016. *Cell* 166: 181–182.

[26] Bribián, A. et al. 2016. *Neuroscience* 323: 10-19.

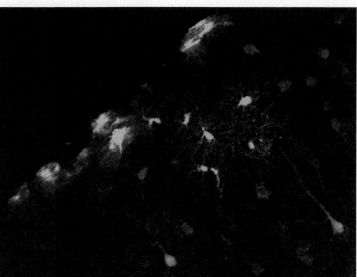

Courtesy of Drs. Laura Lopez-Mascaraque and Rebeca Sánchez-González, Instituto Cajal-CSIC

FIGURE 1.14 Clonal Tracking of Neurons and Glia Produced by Individual Precursor Cells. Image of the cortex of an adult mouse, showing clonal staining of neurons (red and pale green), astrocytes (a type of glial cell; bright blue), and NG2 (glial precursor) cells (bright green). The clones produced by individual precursor cells can be detected by their color and morphology.

(A) 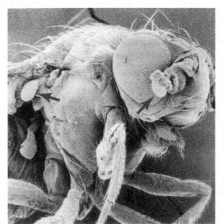 (B)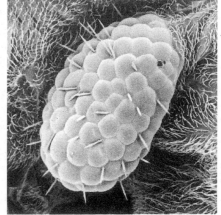

Both photos from G. Halder et al., 1995. *Science 267*: 1788-1792

FIGURE 1.15 Genetic Influences on Development of the Eye in the Fruit Fly (*Drosophila*). A gene known as *eyeless* controls development of the eye in the fruit fly. After deletion of this gene, eyes fail to appear. Overexpression leads to the development of ectopic eyes that are morphologically normal. (A) This scanning electron micrograph shows ectopic eyes on the antenna (right arrow) and wing (left arrow). (B) The wing eye shown at higher magnification.

formation of connections can be regulated by electrical signals. Activity plays a role in determining the pattern of connections.

Genetic approaches have made it possible to identify genes that control the differentiation of entire organs, such as the eye as a whole. Gehring[27] and his colleagues studied the expression of a gene in the fruit fly (*Drosophila*), known as *eyeless*, that controls the development of the eyes. After deletion of this gene in the germline, eyes fail to develop in the progeny for generation after generation. Homologous genes in mice and humans (known as *Small eye* and aniridia, respectively) share extensive sequence identity and have similar developmental functions. If the fly *eyeless* gene or the mammalian homologue of the gene is introduced and overexpressed in the fly, it develops multiple ectopic eyes over its antennae, wings, and legs (Figure 1.15). The gene can therefore orchestrate the formation of an entire eye, in a mouse or a fly, even though the eyes themselves have completely different structures and properties.

Remarkably, Sasai and his colleagues have reproduced a complex developmental eye structure from mouse or human embryonic progenitor cell aggregates from the retina maintained in isolation. Under appropriate three-dimensional culture conditions, progenitor cells divide and differentiate to form the main retinal cells, which then spontaneously and precisely stratify in layers (Figure 1.16). This remarkable finding demonstrates that the development of the optic cup and the retina in these simple three-dimensional cultures depends on an intrinsic self-organizing program.[28,29]

Regeneration of the Nervous System after Injury

Not only does the nervous system wire itself when it is developing, but it can also restore certain connections after injury (again something your computer cannot do!). For example, axons in an arm can grow back after the nerve has been injured so that function can be restored; the hand can once again be moved, and sensation returns. Similarly, in a frog, fish, or an invertebrate such as the leech, lesions in the CNS are followed by axon regeneration and functional recovery. After the optic nerve of a frog or a fish has been cut, fibers grow back to the brain and the animal can see again. However, in the adult mammalian CNS regeneration does not occur. The molecular signals that cause this failure are not yet known.

[27] Halder, G., Callaerts, P., and Gehring, W. J. 1995. *Science* 267: 1788-1792.

[28] Eiraku, M. et al. 2011. *Nature* 472: 51-56.

[29] Nakano, T. et al. 2012. *Cell Stem Cell* 10: 771-785.

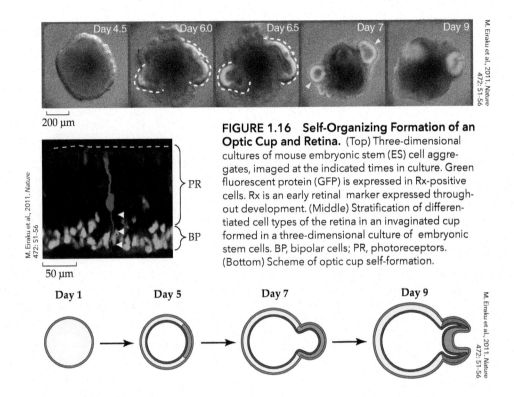

FIGURE 1.16 Self-Organizing Formation of an Optic Cup and Retina. (Top) Three-dimensional cultures of mouse embryonic stem (ES) cell aggregates, imaged at the indicated times in culture. Green fluorescent protein (GFP) is expressed in Rx-positive cells. Rx is an early retinal marker expressed throughout development. (Middle) Stratification of differentiated cell types of the retina in an invaginated cup formed in a three-dimensional culture of embryonic stem cells. BP, bipolar cells; PR, photoreceptors. (Bottom) Scheme of optic cup self-formation.

SUMMARY

- Neurons are connected to each other in a highly specific manner.
- At synapses, information is transmitted from cell to cell.
- In relatively simple circuits, such as those in the retina, it is possible to trace connections and understand the meaning of signals.
- Neurons in the eye and brain act as building blocks for perception.
- Signals in neurons are highly stereotyped and similar in all animals.
- Action potentials conduct unfailingly over long distances.

- Local graded potentials depend on passive electrical properties of nerve cells and spread only over short distances.
- Owing to the peculiar structure of neurons, specialized cellular mechanisms are required for axonal transport of proteins and organelles to and from the cell body.
- During development, neurons migrate to their final destinations and become connected to their targets.
- Molecular cues provide guidance for growing axons.

Suggested Reading

All the experiments and concepts described in this introductory chapter are treated in more detail and fully referenced in later chapters. The following sources represent key reviews that show how essential concepts of neurobiology have developed over the years.

Harder to buy new but still fascinating:

Adrian, E. D. 1946. *The Physical Background of Perception.* Clarendon, Oxford, UK.

Helmholtz, H. 1962/1927. *Helmholtz's Treatise on Physiological Optics.* J. P. C. Southhall (Ed.). Dover, New York, NY.

Hodgkin, A. L. 1964. *The Conduction of the Nervous Impulse.* Liverpool University Press, Liverpool, UK.

Katz, B. 1966. *Nerve, Muscle, and Synapse.* McGraw-Hill, New York, NY.

Ramón y Cajal, S. [1909–1911] 1995. *Histology of the Nervous System,* 2 vols. Translated by Neely Swanson and Larry Swanson. Oxford University Press, New York, NY.

Sherrington, C. S. 1906. *The Integrative Action of the Nervous System.* Reprint, Yale University Press, New Haven, CT, 1961.

CHAPTER 2

Signaling in the Visual System

The processing of signals that carry information about black-and-white images from the retina to the visual cortex is used here to illustrate how essential characteristics of the images are extracted and retained at each relay point. Neuronal signals that are evoked by light begin in the retina. They are sent by ganglion cell axons to a relay, the lateral geniculate nucleus (LGN), and then to higher centers in the visual cortex that produce our perception of scenes with objects and background, movement, shade, depth, and color. Signaling at each level is best analyzed in terms of the receptive fields of neurons. A receptive field in the visual system is defined as the area of the retinal surface (or corresponding region of the visual field) that, upon illumination, enhances or inhibits the activity of a neuron. A useful strategy for analyzing the visual system is to define the optimal pattern of illumination and the receptive field for each neuron.

The spread of visual responses carrying night vision explains how signaling acquires sophistication and complexity from one relay to another. The receptive field of most retinal ganglion cells and neurons in the LGN consists of a small circular area on the retina. The cells respond to contrast rather than diffuse illumination. Geniculate axons project to form a new map of the visual fields in the primary visual cortex. The receptive field of neurons in the primary visual cortex for the most part consists of lines, bars, or edges with a particular orientation. Cortical neurons give no response to diffuse illumination. The optimal stimulus for a simple cell is an oriented edge or bar, which may be light or dark, with a defined width, shining on a precise place in the retina. Complex cells also respond to oriented bars, but their discharges are evoked over a wider area than occurs with simple cells. End inhibition, which is a decrease in the response of a neuron as the length of an image increases, gives rise to more elaborate stimulus requirements, such as a corner or a line that stops. Most cortical cells respond to appropriate illumination of both eyes. Receptive fields of simple cells result from convergence of several geniculate afferents with adjoining field centers. The response properties of complex cells depend on inputs from simple and other cortical cells. Cortical neurons detect only the edges of white or black patterns on a background with inverse contrast.

Throughout the visual pathways, the emphasis is on contrast, color, movement, depth, and boundaries, although particular cells in the retina have intrinsic photosensitivity and detect diffuse levels of light. This distinction enables the nervous system to expand its visual sensitivity by comparing levels of light and to jettison irrelevant information in the visual fields.

This chapter describes the functional properties of neurons at successive stages in the black-and white (and also monochromatic or color-blind) visual pathway of night vision. Chapter 22 will describe the color pathway. Our aim is to show how neuronal activity is related to higher functions, such as visual perception, using as background knowledge only the basic information provided in Chapter 1. Chapter 3 will show in greater detail how structure and function are intimately related at every level.

Experiments have produced an overwhelming body of work on psychophysics, color vision, dark adaptation, retinal pigments, transduction, transmitters, and the organization of the retina (see Chapter 22). Each of these topics can form the basis of a self-contained monograph (see the Suggested Reading section at the end of the chapter). The same applies to comparative aspects of the visual system in invertebrates, lower vertebrates, and mammals. Since a comprehensive account is not possible within the scope of this book, we have selected experiments that provide a continuous thread, extending from the properties of cells in the retina to mechanisms that underlie perception.

Pathways in the Visual System

The initial step in visual processing is the formation on each retina of a sharp image of the outside world. Essential for clear vision are: (1) correct focus of the image by adjustment of the curvature of the lens of the eye (accommodation), (2) regulation of light entering the eye by the diameter of the pupil, and (3) convergence of the two eyes to ensure that matching images fall on corresponding points of both retinas. Our vision depends critically on the region of the retina that is being used (Figure 2.1). We can read small black-and-white print near the center of gaze, where light falls on the fovea, but not in the

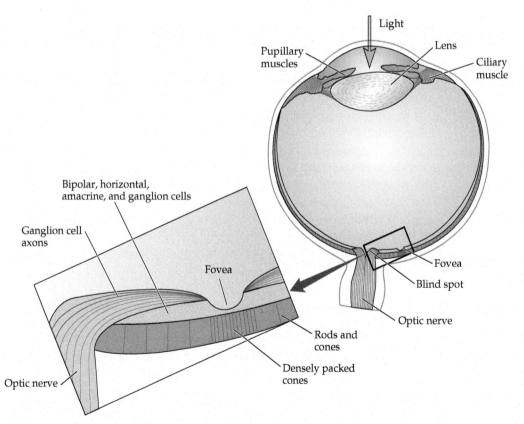

FIGURE 2.1   Pathways for Light and Arrangement of Cells in the Retina. Cross section through the human eye. Light must pass through the lens and layers of cells in order to reach the rod and cone photoreceptors. The fovea is a specialized area, containing only densely packed, slender cones. It is used for fine discrimination. In the fovea, the superficial layers of cells are spread apart, and this feature permits light to have more direct access to the photoreceptors than elsewhere in the retina. The point at which the optic nerve exits the eye has no photoreceptors and constitutes a blind spot.

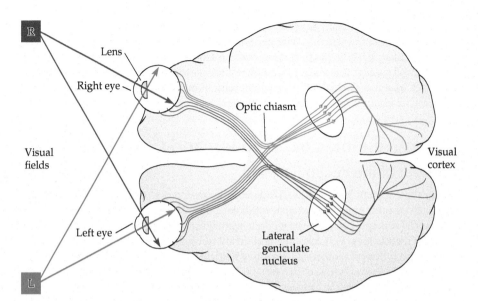

FIGURE 2.2 Visual Pathways.
the right side of each retina, shown in blue, projects to the right lateral geniculate nucleus. Thus, the right visual cortex receives information exclusively from the left half of the visual field.

peripheral field of vision. This loss of acuity arises from reduction in the density of photoreceptors in the retina (see Chapter 22), not from optical distortion outside the central region.

The pathways from the eye to the cerebral cortex in the human brain are illustrated in Figure 2.2, which depicts some of the major landmarks of the visual system; this anatomical information constitutes the bare minimum for following the electrical signals as they pass from relay to relay. The output from each retina divides in two at the optic chiasm. The right side of each retina projects to the right cerebral hemisphere. Because of optical reversal by the lens, the right side of each retina receives the image of the visual world on the left side of the head. Each cerebral hemisphere, therefore, sees the opposite side of the outside world. Accordingly, people with damage to the right cerebral hemisphere caused by trauma or disease become blind in the left visual field, and vice versa. Other pathways that branch off to the midbrain are described in Chapter 22. They are concerned primarily with regulating eye movements, pupillary responses, and circadian rhythms.

The optic nerve fibers that arise from ganglion cells in the retina end on layers of cells in a relay station of the thalamus called the lateral geniculate nucleus, or LGN (*geniculate* means "bent like a knee"). In each of the six principal layers of this structure (Figure 2.3), the outside world is represented as a coherent map of the field seen by one eye, either on the same or the opposite side. Geniculate axons in turn project through the optic radiation to the cerebral cortex. We will discuss the six layers of the visual cortex and the arrangements of maps in Chapter 3. For present purposes, it is sufficient to state that in the monkey, the optic radiation ends on a folded plate of cells about 2 mm thick. This region of the brain is known as the primary visual cortex, or visual area 1 (also called V1), and lies posteriorly in the occipital lobe. Adjacent regions of cortex are also concerned with vision. From the primary visual cortex, the progression through the brain becomes ever more complex, with no end point in sight.

Convergence and Divergence of Connections

By examining the cellular anatomy of the various structures in the visual pathway, one can exclude the possibility that information is handed on unchanged from level to level. The neurons converge and diverge extensively at every stage; that is, each cell receives many inputs and makes connections with several other cells (see Chapter 1). A neuron in the lateral geniculate nucleus

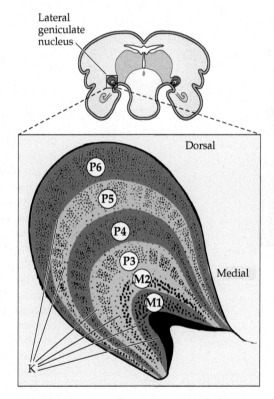

FIGURE 2.3 The Monkey Lateral Geniculate Nucleus (LGN) has six major layers designated parvocellular, or P (3, 4, 5, 6), and magnocellular, or M (1, 2), separated by the koniocellular (K) layers. In the monkey, each layer is supplied by only one eye and contains cells with specialized response properties. Red signifies input from the contralateral eye and blue from the ipsilateral eye. (After J. Szentágothai, 1973. In *Visual Centers in the Brain. Handbook of Sensory Physiology* [*Central Processing of Visual Information Part B*], Vol. 7/3/3B, Jung R. [Ed.]. Springer, Berlin.)

receives its input from many ganglion cells, and it in turn supplies many cortical neurons. Hence, as impulses travel to the cortex and within the cortex itself, there occurs a funneling and, simultaneously, a distribution of information. Converging impulses of different origin are integrated at each stage into an entirely new message that takes account of all the inputs. Moreover, except at the level of the ganglion cells, information also flows in the opposite direction, for example from cortex down to lateral geniculate nucleus.[1,2]

Receptive Fields of Ganglion and Geniculate Cells
Concept of the Receptive Field

Neurons take account of influences arriving from diverse inputs to create their own new messages with new meanings. Sherrington, who coined the word *synapse*, also revealed many of the essential concepts that permeate modern neurobiology by experiments in which he measured the contractions of muscles, before electrical recordings were possible. One such concept was **integration**;[3] another was **receptive field**, in relation to sites that when stimulated promote reflex actions (see also Chapter 21). The concept of the receptive field, later introduced to the visual system by Hartline,[4] has provided a key for understanding the significance of the signals, not only in the retina but at successive stages in the cortex. The receptive field of a neuron in the visual system can be defined as *the area of the retina from which the activity of a neuron can be influenced by light* (see also Chapter 22). Illumination outside a receptive field produces no effect on firing. The receptive field itself can be subdivided into distinct regions, some of which increase activity and others of which suppress it.

Output of the Retina

Many years before the electrical responses of photoreceptors or bipolar cells in the retina could be measured, important information was obtained by recording from ganglion cells. Thus, the first analysis of signaling in the retina was made at the output stage, the end result of synaptic interactions in the retina. It was a simplification and shortcut to go straight to the output. Kuffler[5] was the first to show that a ganglion cell responds best to a small light spot or dark spot that falls on a few receptors in a particular region of the retina. Previously investigators had used flashes of bright light in an attempt to achieve maximal stimulation of the retina. Massive stimulation of this type applied to the retina, the ear, and other sensory systems gives little information about how information is processed with fine discrimination under normal conditions.

When one records from a particular cell in the visual system, the first task is to find the location of its receptive field. Characteristically, most neurons throughout the visual system show discharges at rest even in the absence of illumination. Appropriate stimuli do not necessarily initiate activity but may modulate the resting discharge, causing either an increase or a decrease of frequency. The principal novelty in the study of the visual system was the use of discrete, circumscribed spots for stimulation of selected areas of the retina, instead of diffuse uniform illumination. A convenient way of illuminating particular portions of the retina is to anesthetize the animal and place it facing a screen or a computer, at a distance for which its eyes are properly refracted. When one then shines patterns of light onto the screen or displays computer-generated images, these will be well focused on the retinal surface (Figure 2.4).

Kuffler showed that in the cat visual system a small region of illumination gives rise to a brisk discharge of action potentials (see Figure 2.4B). A larger spot shone over the same part of the retina is far less effective: This is because an additional group of receptors arranged circumferentially around the first set also responds to the change in illumination. The action of these photoreceptors on bipolar cells gives rise to inhibition of ganglion cell firing (see Chapter 22). Summation of the excitatory effect of a small central spot and the inhibitory effect from the surrounding region causes the ganglion cell to be relatively insensitive to diffuse light. In a second major category of ganglion cells, the optimal visual stimulus consists of a small dark spot surrounded by light (see Figure 2.4C). For either cell, the spotlike center and its surround are antagonistic; therefore, if both center and surround are illuminated simultaneously, they tend to cancel each other's contribution.

[1] Conley, M., Penny, G. R., and Diamond, I. T. 1987. *J. Comp. Neurol.* 256: 71-87.

[2] Ichida, J. M., and Casagrande, V. A. 2002. *J. Comp. Neurol.* 4 54: 272-283.

[3] Hartline, H. K. 1940. *Am. J. Physiol.* 130: 690-699.

[4] Kuffler, S. W. 1953. *J. Neurophysiol.* 16: 37-68.

[5] Hubel, D. H. 1988. *Eye, Brain, and Vision.* Scientific American Library, New York.

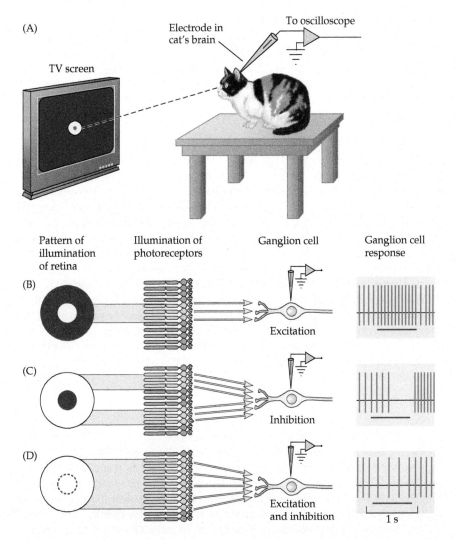

(A)

To oscilloscope

Electrode in
cat's brain

TV screen

Pattern of
illumination
of retina

Illumination of
photoreceptors

Ganglion cell

Ganglion cell
response

(B)

Excitation

(C)

Inhibition

(D)

Excitation
and inhibition

1 s

FIGURE 2.4   Receptive Fields of Ganglion Cells. (A) The eyes of an anesthetized, light-adapted cat focus on a television screen with various patterns of light generated by a computer or shone by a projector. An electrode records the responses from a single cell in the visual pathway. Light or shadow falling onto a restricted area of the screen may increase or decrease the frequency of signals given by the neuron. One can delineate the receptive field of the cell by determining the areas on the screen from which the neuron's firing is influenced. Receptive fields in ganglion cells in the retinas of cats and monkeys are grouped into two main classes: on-center fields (B) and off-center fields (C). On-center cells respond best to a spot of light shone onto the central part of the receptive field. Illumination (indicated by the red bar below records) of the surrounding area with a spot or a ring of light reduces or suppresses the discharges and causes responses when the light is turned off. Off-center cells slow down or stop signaling when the central area of their field is illuminated and accelerate when the light is turned off. Light shone onto the surround of an off-center receptive field causes excitation of the neuron. (D) Illumination of both groups of receptors causes integration of excitation and inhibition and a weak discharge of action potentials. (B–D after S. W. Kuffler, 1953. *J. Neurophysiol.* 16: 37–68.)

Figure 2.4 shows characteristic responses of the two major types of retinal ganglion cells to illumination in a lightly anesthetized cat. Ganglion cells with an "on" center, such as the one shown in Figure 2.4B, respond best to a small spot of light surrounded by darkness. The cell whose responses are shown in Figure 2.4C is an "off"center cell, which responds best to a small dark spot surrounded by light. For the on-center receptive field in Figure 2.4, light produces the most vigorous response if it completely fills the center, whereas for most effective inhibition of firing, the light must cover the entire ring-shaped area. When the inhibitory annular light is turned off, the ganglion cell gives an exuberant off discharge. An off-center field has a converse organization, with inhibition arising in the circular center. For either cell, the spotlike center and its surround are antagonistic; therefore, Figure 2.4D shows that both center and surround are illuminated simultaneously, they tend to cancel each other's contribution.

The meaning of the signal in a ganglion cell has thereby become more complex than information simply about light or dark. Instead, the action potentials report the presence of a contrasting pattern of light in a particular region of the visual field. This occurs because each ganglion cell is influenced, albeit indirectly, not by one photoreceptor but by many. For any given ganglion cell, the specific connections through bipolar, horizontal, and amacrine cells determine the pattern of light that is required for it to discharge action potentials (see Chapter 22). Hubel has succinctly put Kuffler's achievement in perspective:

> *What is especially interesting to me is the unexpectedness of the results, as reflected in the failure of anyone before Kuffler to guess that something like center–surround receptive fields could exist.*[6]

[6] D. H. Hubel, 1988. *Eye, Brain, and Vision.* Scientific American Library, New York.

Such procedures had been foreshadowed by pioneering work on the eye of a simple invertebrate, the horseshoe crab *Limulus*,[3] and on the retina of the frog.[7,8] Kuffler's initial choice of the cat was a lucky one; in the rabbit, for example, the situation would have been more complicated. Rabbit ganglion cells have elaborate receptive fields that respond to such complex features as edges or to movement in a particular direction.[9,10] Equally complex are lower vertebrates, such as frogs and salamanders.[11] A general law seems to emerge: The dumber the animal, the smarter its retina (D. A. Baylor, personal communication).

Lateral Geniculate Cell Receptive Field Organization

The responses of cells in the LGN are similar to those of retinal ganglion cells.[12] As in the retina, a small spot of light, about 0.5 mm in diameter, shone onto a part of the receptive field is far more effective than diffuse illumination in producing excitation. Furthermore, the same spot of light can have opposite effects, depending on the exact position of the stimulus within the receptive field. In one area, a small spot of light excites the cell for the duration of illumination, while simply shifting the spot by 1 mm or less across the retinal surface gives rise to inhibition. Again, as in the retina, two basic receptive field types predominate, on-center and off-center geniculate cells. The receptive fields of both types are roughly concentric.

While ganglion and geniculate cells have very similar receptive field organization, they are not identical. For example, descending connections from layer 6 of the visual cortex project to geniculate neurons to modulate their firing; there is, however, no comparable descending input to ganglion cells. In addition there are subtle differences in receptive field properties, such as even greater failure of geniculate cells to respond to diffuse illumination. It is a general problem that the precise part played by thalamic structures (including the LGN) in transferring information to the cortex is still not fully understood.[13,14]

Sizes of Receptive Fields

Neighboring cells in the visual system collect information from very similar, but not identical, areas of the retina.[15] Even a small (0.1 mm) spot of light on the retina covers the receptive fields of many ganglion and geniculate cells. Some are inhibited, others excited. Throughout the visual system, *neurons processing related information are clustered together*. In sensory systems this means that the central neurons dealing with a particular area of the surface can communicate with each other over short distances. This appears to be an economical arrangement, as it minimizes the need for long lines of communication and simplifies formation of connections (see Chapters 3 and 25). Since neighboring regions of the retina make connections with neighboring geniculate cells, the receptive fields of adjacent neurons overlap over most of their area.[15] Both the region of the cat retina with small receptive field centers, the *area centralis*, and the fovea in the monkey project onto the greater portion of each geniculate layer. A similar distribution has been found in humans by using functional magnetic resonance imaging (fMRI).[16] There are relatively few cells devoted to the peripheral retina. This extensive representation of the fovea reflects the high density of foveal receptors necessary for high-acuity vision.

Moreover, the size of the receptive field of a ganglion, geniculate, or cortical cell depends on its location in the retina (or visual field). The receptive fields of cells situated in the central areas of the retina have much smaller centers than those at the periphery; receptive fields are smallest in the fovea, where visual acuity is highest.[17] The central on or off region of such a midget ganglion cell's receptive field can be supplied by a single cone and is accordingly only about 2.5 µm in diameter. Note that receptive fields can be described either as dimensions on the retina or as degrees of arc subtended by the stimulus. In human eyes, 1 mm on the retina corresponds to about 4°. For reference, the image of the moon has a diameter of 1/8 mm on the human retina, corresponding to 0.5° or 30 minutes of arc.

There are similar gradations of receptive field size and spatial dimension in the somatosensory system. A higher-order sensory neuron in the brain, responding to a fine touch applied to the skin of the fingertip, has a much smaller receptive field than that of a neuron whose field is on the skin of the upper arm (see Chapter 25). To discern the form of an object, we use our fingertips and fovea, not the less discriminating regions with poorer resolution.

[7] Barlow, H. B. 1953. *J. Physiol.* 119: 69-88.

[8] Barlow, H. B., Hill, R. M., and Levick, W. R. 1964. *J. Physiol.* 173: 377-407.

[9] Oyster, C. W., and Barlow, H. B. 1967. *Science* 155: 841-842.

[10] Baccus, S. A. et al. 2008. *J. Neurosci.* 28: 6807-6817.

[11] Hubel, D. H., and Wiesel, T. N. 1961. *J. Physiol.* 155: 385-398.

[12] Sherman, S. M. 2007. *Curr. Opin. Neurobiol.* 17: 417-422.

[13] Guillery, R. W. 2005. *Prog. Brain Res.* 149: 235-256.

[14] Borghuis, B. G. et al. 2008. *J. Neurosci.* 28: 3178-3189.

[15] Yeh, C. I. et al. 2009. *J. Neurophysiol.* 101: 2166-2185.

[16] Kastner, S., Schneider, K. A., and Wunderlich, K. 2006. *Prog. Brain Res.* 155: 125-143.

[17] Balasubramanian, V., and Sterling, P. 2009. *J. Physiol.* 587: 2753-2767.

Classification of Ganglion and Geniculate Cells

Superimposed on the general scheme of on- or off-center receptive fields, ganglion cells in the monkey retina can be grouped into two main anatomical and physiological categories, denoted as magnocellular (M) and parvocellular (P) (see Figure 2.3).[18] P ganglion cells project to the four dorsal layers of smaller cells in the LGN (the **parvocellular division**), whereas M ganglion cells project to the larger cells in two ventral layers (the **magnocellular division**). Chapter 3 will describe how the characteristics of neurons in the M and P pathways are maintained at successive levels in the visual system. In brief, P ganglion cells have small receptive field centers, high spatial resolution, and are sensitive to color. P cells provide information about fine detail at high contrast. M cells have larger receptive fields than P cells and are more sensitive to small differences in contrast and to movement; they fire at higher frequencies and conduct impulses more rapidly along their larger-diameter axons. In the cat, which has no color vision, the classification of ganglion cells is different, with X, Y, and W groups.[15] Groups X and Y are in some respects parallel to P and M in their properties, but there are major differences and the two classifications are not interchangeable.

What Information Do Ganglion and Geniculate Cells Convey?

A striking feature of ganglion and geniculate cells with their concentric fields is that they tell a different story from that provided by primary sensory receptors. They do not convey information about absolute levels of illumination; they behave in a similar fashion at different background levels of light. They ignore much of the information of the photoreceptors, which work more like a photographic plate or a light meter. Rather, they measure differences within their receptive fields by comparing the degree of illumination between the center and the surround. They are exquisitely tuned to detect such contrast as the edge of an image crossing the opposing regions of a receptive field. By having a greater sensitivity to abrupt rather than to gradual intensity changes, ganglion cells overcome the low-range photosensitivity of receptor cells. By comparing abrupt discontinuities rather than graded changes of luminance, ganglion and geniculate cells detect contrast, which is the most relevant information of images. In the example shown in Figure 2.5, the squares labeled A and B have exactly the same luminance, but they look different owing to the relative differences with their surrounding squares. Chapter 22 describes a class of retinal ganglion cells that do respond to diffuse illumination but do not project to the visual cortex or play a part in form perception.[19]

Experiments made in the salamander retina by Baylor, Meister, and their colleagues suggest that temporal aspects of firing by ganglion cells can also contribute to spatial resolution.[20,21] Throughout the previous discussion, the trains of impulses recorded from individual neurons have been treated as separate lines from which the analysis of visual input is made by the brain. Synchrony of firing by two cells, however, may be an additional variable. Analysis of the degree of synchrony can be used by higher centers to obtain information about light falling on the retina that cannot be deduced from looking at the firing of the two ganglion cells separately.

Complexity of the Information Conveyed by Action Potentials

At a distance of only two synaptic relays beyond the retina, even more sophisticated information about the visual world is provided by the action potentials in cortical nerve cells. Hubel and Wiesel[22] showed that cortical neurons do not respond simply to concentric contrast. Instead, distinctive patterns are the required stimuli for different types of cortical cells. For example, one type of cortical cell in the visual pathway responds selectively to a bar of light with a specific orientation (vertical, oblique, or horizontal), moving in a particular direction in a

[18] Malpeli, J. G., Lee, D., and Baker, F. H. 1996. *J. Comp. Neurol.* 375: 363–377.

[19] Fu, Y. et al. 2005. *Curr. Opin. Neurobiol.* 15: 415–422.

[20] Meister, M., Lagnado, L., and Baylor, D. A. 1995. *Science* 270: 1207–1210.

[21] Gollisch, T., and Meister, M. 2008. *Science* 319: 1108–1111.

[22] Hubel, D. H., and Wiesel, T. N. 1977. *Proc. R. Soc. Lond. B, Biol. Sci.* 198: 1–59.

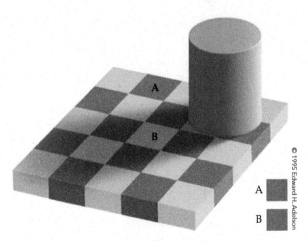

FIGURE 2.5 Visual Perception of Contrast.
Some clear and dark squares on the checkerboard are shadowed by the cylinder. The area labeled A appears darker than the area labeled B. However, they have identical luminance.

particular part of the visual field. The firing of this type of cortical cell is not influenced by diffuse light or by a bar of an inappropriate orientation or one moving in the wrong direction. Hence, its action potentials provide precise information about the visual stimulus to higher centers in the brain. This increase in the meaning attributed to a stereotyped action potential is explained by the precise connections of lower-order cells to the cortical cell, and the way in which the cortical cell integrates incoming signals by summation of localized graded potentials.

Two important conclusions about signaling in the nervous system are: (1) Nerve cells act as the building blocks for perception, and (2) the abstract significance of the message can be extremely complex, depending on the number of inputs a neuron receives. It turns out that the progressive integration of information derived from lower-order units can lead to the generation of highly complex and specific stimulus requirements for higher-order central neurons. For example, Chapter 23 will show that specific cells exist in visual association areas that respond selectively to a face. In addition, the temporal grouping and patterning of impulses can provide information about the quality of the stimulus.

Cortical Receptive Fields

Responses of cortical neurons, like those of the retinal ganglion and geniculate cells, tend to occur on a background of maintained activity. A consistent observation is that discharges of cortical neurons are not significantly influenced by diffuse illumination of the retina. The neuronal firing rate is altered only when certain demands about the position and form of the stimulus on the retina are met. Insensitivity to diffuse light is a more pronounced feature of the process already noted in the retina and the lateral geniculate nucleus; it results from equally matched antagonistic actions between the inhibitory and excitatory regions in the receptive fields of cortical cells. The receptive fields of most cortical neurons have configurations that differ from those of retinal or geniculate cells, so spots of light often have little or no effect. In his Nobel address, Hubel described the experiment in which he and Wiesel first recognized this essential property:

> Our first real discovery came about as a surprise. For three or four hours, we got absolutely nowhere. Then gradually we began to elicit some vague and inconsistent responses by stimulating somewhere in the midperiphery of the retina. We were inserting the glass slide with its black spot into the slot of the ophthalmoscope when suddenly, over the audio monitor, the cell went off like a machine gun. After some fussing and fiddling, we found out what was happening. The response had nothing to do with the black dot. As the glass slide was inserted, its edge was casting onto the retina a faint but sharp shadow, a straight dark line on a light background. That was what the cell wanted, and it wanted it, moreover, in just one narrow range of orientations. This was unheard of. It is hard now to think back and realize just how free we were from any idea of what cortical cells might be doing in an animal's daily life.[23]

By following a progression of clues, Hubel and Wiesel worked out the appropriate light stimuli for various cortical cells (Box 2.1); initially they classified the receptive fields as **simple receptive fields** or **complex receptive fields**. Each of these categories includes several subgroups and important variables that bear on perceptual mechanisms. A major difference observed from ganglion and geniculate cells is that individual simple and complex cells are, for the most part, driven by both eyes.

Responses of Simple Cells

Once again, there is a specialization for detecting differences. The spotlike contrast representation of ganglion cells has been transformed and extended into a line or an edge. Resolution has not been lost, but instead has been incorporated into a more complex pattern. As shown in Figure 2.6, the visual cortex

[23] Hubel. D. H. 1981. Nobel Lecture. www.nobelprize.org/prizes/medicine/1981/hubel/lecture/ © The Nobel Foundation.

(A)

Prestriate

Striate

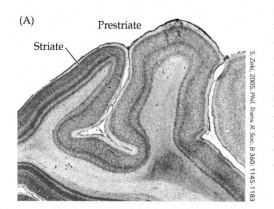

S. Zeki, 2005, Phil. Trans. R. Soc. B 360: 1145–1183

(B)

1
2
3
4A
4B
4C
5
6

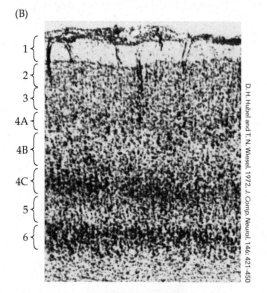

D. H. Hubel and T. N. Wiesel, 1972. J. Comp. Neurol. 146: 421–450

FIGURE 2.6 Architecture of Visual Cortex. (A) Section showing clear striation in area 17 that is absent from the adjacent prestriate area. (B) Distinct layering of cells in a section of striate cortex of the macaque monkey, stained to show cell bodies (Nissl stain). Fibers arriving from the LGN end in layers 4A, 4B, and 4C.

BOX 2.1 Strategies for Exploring the Cortex

In 1953 Stephen Kuffler pioneered the experimental analysis of the mammalian visual system by concentrating on receptive field organization and the meaning of signals in the cat optic nerve.[4] A clear, continuous thread from signaling to perception was subsequently provided through the beautiful experiments of Hubel and Wiesel and the large body of work they inspired.

The procedure used by Hubel and Wiesel, the monitoring of activity in single neurons, might seem an unprofitable way to study higher functions in which large numbers of cells take part. What chance do physiologists have of gaining insight into complex actions within the brain when they sample only one or a few of the billions of neurons in the brain, a hopelessly small fraction of the total number? A feature that simplifies the situation in the visual cortex is that the major cell types are laid out in an apparently well-ordered manner as repeating units: Adjacent points in the retina project to adjacent points on the cortical surface. Thus, the visual cortex is designed to bring an identical set of neural analyzers to bear on each tiny segment of the visual field.

The problem faced by Hubel and Wiesel in 1958 was to find out how signals denoting small, bright, dark, or colored spots in the retina could be transmuted into signals that conveyed information about the shape, size, color, movement, and depth of objects. Techniques that are routinely used now—such as optical recording, horseradish peroxidase injection, and brain scanning—had not yet been thought of. At the outset, Hubel and Wiesel faced completely unanswered questions, which they tackled by assuming that visual centers in the cortex would perform their processing according to principles similar to those in the retina, but at a more advanced level. It is worth pointing out that they started their work at a time when not only was nothing known about how neurons functioned in the visual cortex, but far worse, the field abounded with misleading or frankly wrong hypotheses derived from

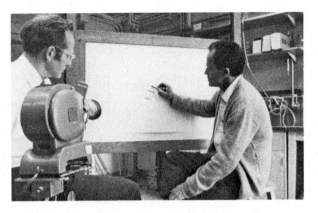

David H. Hubel (left) and Torsten N. Wiesel during an experiment, about 1969. A cat, not shown, also faces the screen.

experiments made by shining bright flashes of light into the eye or by cortical lesions. For example, neurons in the visual cortex were described in 1953 as being on, off, on-off, or Type A neurons (which did not respond to anything at all). Pioneering work that reveals brand new concepts that stand the test of time often starts not from nothing but from a wealth of confused data.

One crucial strategy in Hubel and Wiesel's analysis was the use of stimuli that mimic those occurring under natural conditions. For example, edges, contours, and simple patterns presented to the eye revealed features of its organization that could never have been detected by using bright flashes without form. Another key to the success of Hubel and Wiesel's approach lay in asking not simply what stimulus evokes a response in a particular neuron, but rather what is the *most effective* stimulus. Pursuit of this question through the various stages of the visual system has elicited many surprising and remarkable results. Their early papers demonstrated that the receptive fields of simple and complex cells in the primary visual cortex constitute initial stages of pattern recognition.

has a clear striation with six layers. Most simple cells are found in layers 4 and 6 and deep in layer 3. All these layers receive direct input from the LGN (although layer 4C is the most favored destination, as we will describe in Chapter 3). Receptive fields of simple cells can be mapped with stationary spots of light, and they exhibit several variations.[24–26] One type of simple cell has a receptive field that consists of an extended narrow central portion, flanked by two antagonistic areas. The center may be either excitatory or inhibitory. Figure 2.7 shows the receptive field of a simple cell in the striate cortex mapped out with spots of light that excited only weakly in the center (because the spots covered only a small fraction of the central on area).

The requirements of such simple cell are exacting, as illustrated in Figure 2.7C. For optimal activation, these cells need a bar of light that is not more than a certain width, that entirely fills the central area, and that is oriented at a certain angle. Illumination of the surrounding areas suppresses any ongoing activity or reduces the efficacy of a simultaneous

[24] Hubel, D. H., and Wiesel, T. N. 1959. *J. Physiol.* 148: 574–591.

[25] Hubel, D. H., and Wiesel, T. N. 1962. *J. Physiol.* 160: 106–154.

[26] Hubel, D. H., and Wiesel, T. N. 1968. *J. Physiol.* 195: 215–243.

FIGURE 2.7 Responses of a Simple Cell in Cat Striate Cortex to spots of light (A) and bars of light (C). The receptive field (B) has a narrow central on area (+) flanked by symmetrical antagonistic off areas (-). The best stimulus for this cell is a vertically oriented light bar in the center of its receptive field (see fifth record from the top in C). Other orientations are less effective or ineffective. Diffuse light does not stimulate. The red bar above each record in A and C indicates the duration of stimulation. (After D. H. Hubel and T. N. Wiesel, 1959. *J. Physiol.* 148: 574–591.)

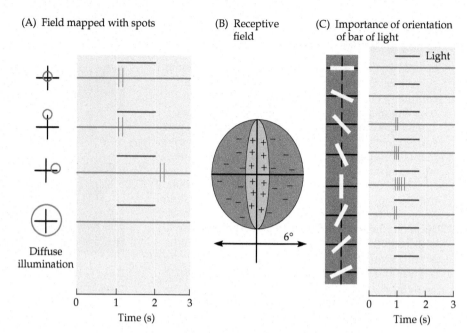

center excitation. As predicted by mapping with spots of light, a vertically oriented bar is the most effective stimulus. Even small deviations from that pattern result in a diminished response. Different orientations and positions are effective stimuli for other single cells. Altogether, single cells respond to a wide range of orientations and positions. A different population of simple cells is activated by rotating the stimulus or by shifting its position in the visual field. The distribution of inhibitory–excitatory flanks in various simple cell receptive fields may not be symmetrical, or the field may consist of two longitudinal regions facing each other—one excitatory, the other inhibitory.

Figure 2.8 shows examples of four such receptive fields, all with a common axis of orientation but with differences in the distribution of areas within the field. For the receptive field in Figure 2.8A, a narrow slit of light oriented from 1 o'clock to 7 o'clock (assuming the visual field corresponds to a clock face with 12 o'clock high) elicits the best response. A dark bar in the same place but with light flanks suppresses ongoing spontaneous activity. Cells with the field shapes shown in Figure 2.8B,C fire optimally with a dark bar in the central area. For the field shown in Figure 2.8D, an edge with light on the left and darkness on the right produces the most effective "on" response, whereas reversing the dark and light areas is best for eliciting "off" discharges. In simple cells, the optimal width of the narrow light or dark bar is comparable to the diameters of the on- or off-center regions in the doughnut-shaped receptive fields of ganglion or lateral geniculate cells. Thus, cortical cells that have fields derived from the fovea are most excited by bars narrower than those that excite cells with fields in retinal periphery. The common properties of all simple cells are (1) that they respond best to a properly oriented stimulus positioned so as not to encroach on antagonistic zones, and (2) that stationary slits or spots can be used to define on and off areas. In addition to these features, most simple cells respond to similar visual stimuli in either eye.

At the time Hubel and Wiesel made their remarkable experiments, neurons could be recorded only one by one using sharp extracellular electrodes. New multielectrode

FIGURE 2.8 Receptive Fields of Simple Cells in Cat Striate Cortex. In practice, all possible orientations are observed for each type of field. The optimal stimuli are a narrow slit or bar of light in the center for (A); a dark bar for (B) and (C); and an edge with dark on the right for (D). Considerable asymmetry can be present, as in (C). (After D. H. Hubel and T. N. Wiesel, 1962. *J. Physiol.* 160: 106–154.)

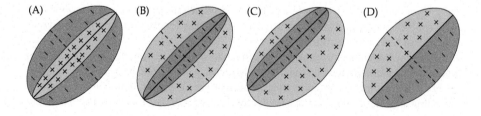

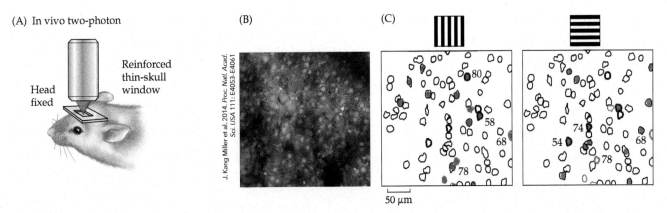

FIGURE 2.9 Selective Responses of Cortical Neurons to Visual Stimulation with Drifting-Gratings. (A) Methodology for optical recording from cortical neurons in the living mouse. Two-photon calcium imaging is made from layers 2 and 3 of primary visual cortex through a reinforced thin-skull window. The awake mouse is visually stimulated with vertical or horizontal drifting-gratings such as those shown in (C). (B) Calcium signals recorded from cell bodies of neurons that were incubated with the calcium-sensitive dye Oregon green (green spots) can be distinguished from signals produced by satellite glial cells that were selectively stained with the fluorescent dye SR101 (yellow spots). (C) Spatial maps of neurons responding selectively to the vertical (left) or horizontal (right) grafts. (A,C modified from L. Carrillo-Reid et al., 2016. *Science* 353: 691–694. Reprinted with permission from AAAS.)

techniques such as those mentioned in Chapter 1 permit recording from dozens of neurons simultaneously. Alternatively, it is possible to obtain optical recordings of neurons, for example in the visual cortex of living animals. In the experiment shown in Figure 2.9, neurons in the visual cortex of mice were incubated with calcium-sensitive dyes that emit fluorescence when neurons are electrically active and calcium goes into them. Deep optical recordings can be done with two-photon microscopy across a lowered sheet of skull. The penetration of the infrared light permits visualization of the activity of populations of neurons in layers 2 and 3. Figure 2.9 shows that illumination of the eye with drifting-gratings (a pattern of bars that pass in front of one of the mouse's eyes) produces synchronous responses in certain neurons. As expected, these responses are selective to the orientation of the bars; illumination with an orthogonal graft activates a different set of neurons.[27] (Similar results obtained in cats are discussed in Chapter 3.) The transformation of information can be simply summarized as follows:

- A signal in a photoreceptor indicates a change in light intensity in that area of the field of vision.
- A signal in a ganglion cell or lateral geniculate nucleus indicates the presence of contrast.
- A signal in a cortical neuron indicates the presence of an oriented bar or edge of light.

Binocular fusion, which is not possible in the retina or the LGN, first appears in the visual cortex. Figure 2.10 shows the binocular responses evoked in a simple cell in the cat visual cortex by a horizontally oriented bar, shone onto the same region of either the left or the right retina. Another constant and remarkable feature of simple cells is that in spite of all the different proportions of inhibitory and excitatory areas, the two contributions match exactly and cancel each other's effectiveness, so diffuse illumination of the entire receptive field produces a feeble response at best (see Figure 2.7). The off areas in cortical fields are not always able to initiate impulses in response to dark bars. Frequently (particularly in end inhibition and in the more elaborate fields we will describe shortly), illumination of the off area can be detected only as a reduction in the discharge evoked from the on area. The movement of edges or bars of the appropriate orientation is a highly effective technique for initiating impulses.

For depth perception, which is a magnocellular pathway function, there exists another binocular specialization of receptive fields in which an object out of the plane of focus casts

[27] Carrillo-Reid, L. et al. 2016. *Science* 353: 691–694.

[28] Barlow, H. B., Blakemore, C., and Pettigrew, J. D. 1967. *J. Physiol.* 193: 327–342.

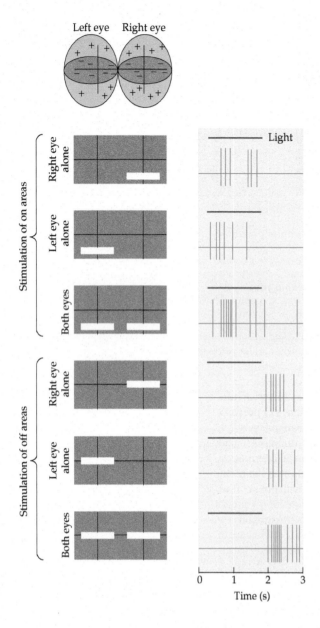

FIGURE 2.10 Binocular Activation of a Simple Cortical Neuron that has identical receptive fields in both eyes. Simultaneous illumination of corresponding on areas (+) of right and left receptive fields is more effective than stimulation of one alone (upper three records). In the same way, stimulation of off areas (–) in the two eyes reinforces off discharges (lower three records). In contrast, cells used for depth perception have receptive fields in both eyes but in disparate regions of the visual field. Such cells require that the bar be placed farther from or closer to the eye than the plane of focus. (After D. H. Hubel and T. N. Wiesel, 1959. *J. Physiol.* 148: 574-591.)

images on disparate parts of the two retinas.[23,28] Neurons with properties that fit the binocular cell's ability for depth perception have been found in primary and association visual cortex. For such cells, the best stimulus is an appropriately oriented bar in front of the plane of focus (for certain cells) or beyond it (for others). Impulses fail to be evoked by presenting the bar only to one eye or the other as well as to both eyes in the plane of focus. It is the disparity of the position on the two retinas that these cells require. Depth perception as such probably arises in higher cortical areas. For example, clusters of neurons with similar binocular disparity preferences are found in an area of visual association cortex known as V5 or middle temporal (MT; see Chapters 3 and 23).[29] The depth perception of a trained monkey was predictably altered when such a cluster was electrically stimulated.

Synthesis of the Simple Receptive Field

In 1962 Hubel and Wiesel provided a tentative hypothesis to explain the origin of cortical receptive fields.[24] Their scheme had the advantage of using known mechanisms to explain how a nerve cell can respond so selectively to a visual pattern—such as the oriented lines that excite simple cells. They suggested that in the cortex, simple cell receptive fields behave as if they are built from large numbers of geniculate fields.[24] This is illustrated in Figure 2.11, in which the fields of geniculate neurons connected to a cortical cell are lined up in such a way that a properly oriented bar of light, traversing their centers, would excite them all strongly. If the bar were widened or displaced slightly to either side, it would fall on the inhibitory surround of each cell and reduce or stop the excitatory output. Convergence of these geniculate neurons could produce a cortical cell whose optimal stimulus would be just such an oriented bar of light.

Connections such as these were postulated by Hubel and Wiesel as the simplest that could account for orientation selectivity. That is, the pattern of geniculate innervation itself determines the response characteristics of cortical neurons. This would constitute a feedforward mechanism. An alternative hypothesis was that intracortical connections and lateral inhibition were responsible for the sharpness of receptive field orientation, stemming from the suppression of excitability by laterally placed or inappropriately oriented stimuli and the insensitivity to contrast.

Tests to distinguish between the various schemes could not be made directly by Hubel and Wiesel, since they made all their recordings with extracellular electrodes. Intracellular recordings are much more difficult to make and to maintain in the brain without damaging the cell. But they have an advantage: Unlike extracellular recordings, an intracellular electrode allows one to assess the potency as well as the source of excitatory and inhibitory synapses arriving at a cell from various inputs. Thus, fibers coming to a neuron from the lateral geniculate nucleus or from the cortex can be stimulated selectively and their effects observed directly.

[29] DeAngelis, G. C., Cumming, B. G., and Newsome, W. T. 1998. *Nature* 394: 677-680.

[30] Jin, J. et al. 2011. *Nat. Neurosci.* 14: 232-238.

[31] Ferster, D., Chung, S., and Wheat, H. 1996. *Nature* 380: 249-252.

[32] Finn, I. M., Priebe, N. J., and Ferster, D. 2007. *Neuron* 54: 137-152.

[33] Priebe, N. J., and Ferster, D. 2008. *Neuron* 57: 482-497.

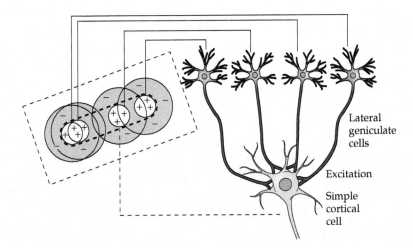

FIGURE 2.11 Synthesis of Simple Receptive Fields. Hypothesis devised by Hubel and Wiesel to explain the synthesis of simple cell receptive fields. The elongated receptive field of a simple cell is produced by the convergence of inputs from many geniculate neurons (only four are shown) whose concentric receptive fields are aligned on the retina. (After D. H. Hubel and T. N. Wiesel, 1962. *J. Physiol.* 160: 106–154.)

Ferster, Alonso, and their colleagues[30,31] achieved a major advance toward a more detailed analysis of how a receptive field is built up from its inputs. They succeeded in recording from individual simple and complex cells with intracellular microelectrodes.[29–33] Recordings made from a simple cell that responds to a vertically oriented bar with high specificity are shown in Figure 2.12. In such records, bursts of synaptic and action potentials are activated by specific visual patterns. They are produced by transmitter release from geniculate axons as well as from intracortical connections. These experiments have shown that direct geniculo-cortical excitatory potentials sum to greater amplitudes at preferred orientations, as would be expected if the arrangement illustrated in Figure 2.11 existed.

Although the pattern of geniculate inputs is sufficient for orientation tuning of simple cells in visual cortex, additional refinement is provided by both inhibitory and excitatory intracortical connections. Intracellular recordings from simple cells show that illumination of surrounding off areas produces inhibitory synaptic potentials. These can serve to

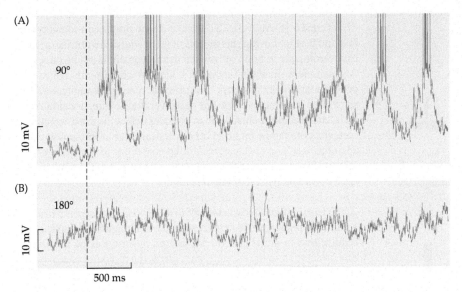

FIGURE 2.12 Intracellular Recording from a Simple Cell in Primary Visual Cortex of an Anesthetized Cat. Stimuli consisted of moving gratings and were applied at the time of the dotted line at the beginning of the traces. (A) With repeated presentations of a visual stimulus oriented vertically at 90°, the cell shows strong depolarization, clear-cut synaptic excitatory potentials, and bursts of action potentials. (B) Similar stimuli applied at right angles (i.e., horizontally) fail to depolarize or stimulate the cell. (After I. Lampl et al., 2001. *Neuron* 30: 263–274.)

(A) Importance of orientation   (B) Relative unimportance of position

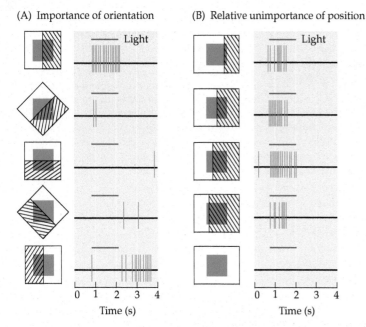

FIGURE 2.13 **Responses of a Complex Cell in Cat Striate Cortex.**
The cell responds best to a vertical edge located within its receptive field
(the blue square). (A) With light on the left and dark (hatching) on the right
(top record), there is an on response. With light on the right (bottom record), there is an off response. Orientation other than vertical is less effective. (B) The position of the border within the field is not important. Illumination of the entire receptive field (bottom record) produces no response.
(After D. H. Hubel and T. N. Wiesel, 1962. *J. Physiol.* 160: 106–154.)

[34] Priebe, N. J., and Ferster, D. 2012.
Neuron 75: 194–208.

[35] Pack, C. C. et al. 2003. *Neuron* 39:
671–680.

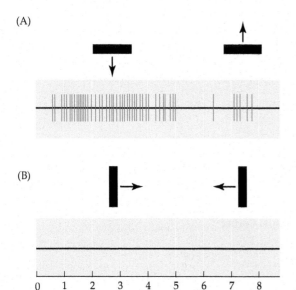

sharpen orientation selectivity and to maintain tuning
as visual contrast varies but are not, on their own, responsible for the formation of on and off areas.[34]

Responses of Complex Cells

In recordings made from individual neurons in the visual cortex, one finds, in addition to simple cells, other neurons, called complex cells, which behave quite
differently. These complex cells, which are abundant
in layers 2, 3, and 5, have two important properties in
common with simple cells: (1) Illumination of the entire field is ineffective, and (2) they require specific field
axis orientation of a dark–light boundary. The responses of a complex cell are shown in Figure 2.13. Complex
cells, like simple cells, have comparable receptive fields
in corresponding regions of both retinas. The demand,
however, for precise positioning of the stimulus, observed in simple cells, is relaxed in complex cells. In addition, there are no longer distinct on and off areas that
can be mapped with small spots of light. As long as a
properly oriented stimulus falls within the boundary of
the receptive field, most complex cells will respond, as
in the examples illustrated in Figure 2.13. In this cell,
the vertical edge causes nearly equivalent responses at
any of four locations. Other orientations are ineffective.
Extending the visual stimulus beyond the boundary of
the field has no effect. The meaning of the signals arising from complex cells, therefore, differs significantly
from that of simple cells. The simple cell localizes an
oriented bar of light to a particular position within the receptive field,
whereas the signals of a complex cell provide information about *orientation without strict reference to position.*

RESPONSES TO MOVING STIMULI   Many simple and complex cells
respond best to moving slits or bars of fixed width and precise orientation. Some cells respond only when the movement is in one direction.
An example is shown in Figure 2.14. Downward movement of the bar
evokes a far brisker response than upward movement; as Figure 2.14B
shows, the orientation of the bar remains critical. Directional sensitivity is a feature commonly found in complex cells. Still more demanding
complex cells can be found in other cortical areas (see Chapters 3 and
23). Once again, intracellular recordings enable one to explain how such
movement sensitivity is achieved in cortical neurons as the result of synaptic potentials evoked by visual stimuli.[32]

CORTICAL NEURONS THAT RESPOND TO LINES THAT STOP
An interesting feature of certain simple and complex cells is that they
require bars or edges that do not extend beyond a fixed length.[25,35]
The orientation of the stimulus and, often, the direction of movement

FIGURE 2.14   **Preferred Direction of Movement for a Complex
Cell in Cat Visual Cortex.** (A) The cell gives brisk responses to the
downward movement of a horizontal bar but only a feeble response to
upward movement. (B) A vertically oriented bar evokes no firing of action potentials in the same cell. (After D. H. Hubel and T. N. Wiesel, 1962.
J. Physiol. 160: 106–154.)

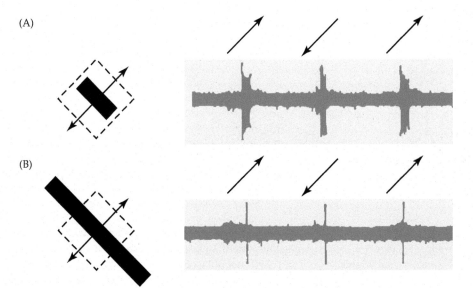

FIGURE 2.15 Action Potentials in a Complex Cell in layer 2 of cat visual cortex in response to bars of different length. (A) The neuron fires when the obliquely oriented bar is moved down or up. In this trial, the bar was short. (B) A longer bar of the same orientation and the same direction of movement elicits almost no response. Hence, this cell recognizes an edge that stops, a characteristic known as end inhibition, or end stopping. (After D. H. Hubel and T. N. Wiesel, 1968. *J. Physiol.* 195: 215-243.)

are critical. Figure 2.15 shows recordings from a cell responding best to an obliquely oriented bar of light. Stretching the bar beyond an optimal length reduced its effectiveness as a stimulus. It is as though there are additional off areas that exist on either side of the fields shown in dashed lines in Figure 2.15. Light with the appropriate pattern falling in these areas tends to suppress firing. However, diffuse illumination outside the field does not diminish the response. It is therefore not a conventional off area, as such. **End inhibition**, or **end stopping**, is the name given to this property.

Hence, for a complex cell of this sort the best stimulus is an appropriately oriented bar or edge, of a defined length, that stops at a particular place. The cell requires a discontinuity in the visual pattern if it is to respond. It is worth emphasizing what a major achievement it was for Hubel and Wiesel to show unequivocally that a particular neuron requires *this* particular stimulus for it to fire.

The properties of the neurons that require a lateral border line can provide a cue to a clinical observation in humans, known as the **completion phenomenon**, which occurs when small retinal or cortical lesions cause blind areas, or scotomas. In this condition, forms or shapes projected onto the retina appear to contain an empty region in the visual field corresponding to the site of the lesion. Yet if individuals look at striped

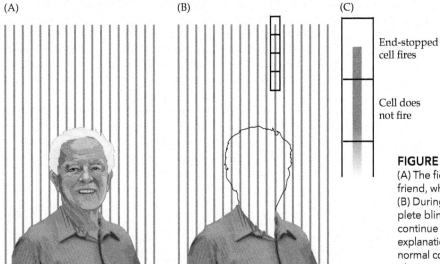

FIGURE 2.16 The Completion Phenomenon. (A) The field of a person viewing the head of his friend, who is sitting against striped wallpaper. (B) During a migraine attack, a small area of complete blindness occurs in the field, yet the stripes continue through the blind area. (C) A possible explanation for (B), at the cellular level, is that under normal conditions end-stopped neurons would be silent, except at the top and the bottom of the field where the line stops.

(A) Complex

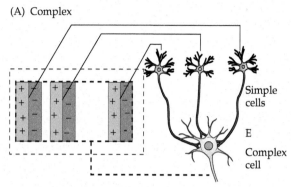

(B) Complex with end inhibition

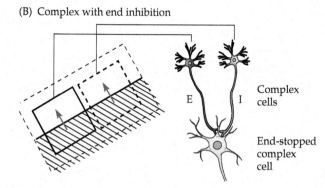

FIGURE 2.17 Synthesis of Complex Receptive Fields.
(A) Convergent input from simple cells responding best to a vertically oriented edge at slightly different positions could bring about the behavior of a complex cell that responds well to a vertically oriented edge situated anywhere within its field. (B) Each of two complex cells responds best to an obliquely oriented edge. But one cell is excitatory and the other is inhibitory to the end-stopped complex cell. Hence, an edge that covers both fields (as in the sketch) is ineffective, whereas a corner restricted to the left field would excite. E = excitation; I = inhibition. (After D. H. Hubel and T. N. Wiesel, 1962. *J. Physiol.* 160: 106-154; and 1965. *J. Neurophysiol.* 28: 229-289.)

wallpaper (Figure 2.16), a straight-line pattern, or a zebra, they see the pattern continue through the blind area.

Synthesis of the Complex Receptive Field

In the same way that the receptive field of a simple cortical cell can be built up by the convergence of geniculate afferents, so too could the receptive field of a complex cortical cell be synthesized by combining those of simple cells.[24,36] Figure 2.17 presents a hypothetical complex cell that is excited by a vertical edge stimulus that falls anywhere within the area of the receptive field. This is so because wherever the edge falls, one of the simple fields is traversed at its vertical inhibitory–excitatory boundary. The other simple fields do not respond because both of their components are either illuminated or darkened uniformly. Diffuse illumination of the entire field covers all component fields equally, and therefore none fires.

One can postulate that only one or a few of the simple cells need to fire at any one position of the stimulus to evoke a near maximal response in a complex cell. Consistent with this hypothesis, intracellular recording from complex cells reveals few monosynaptic contacts from the lateral geniculate nucleus. Instead, there is a preponderance of long-latency inputs,

[36] Hirsch, J. A., and Martinez, L.M. 2006. *Trends Neurosci.* 29: 30-39.

[37] Finn, I. M., and Ferster, D. 2007. *J. Neurosci.* 27: 9638-9648.

TABLE 2.1

Characteristics of receptive fields at successive levels of the visual system

Type of cell	Shape of field	What is best stimulus?	How good is diffuse light as a stimulus?
Photoreceptor	⊕	Light	Good
Ganglion cell		Small spot or narrow bar over center	Moderate
Geniculate		Small spot or narrow bar over center	Poor
Simple (layers 4 and 6)		Narrow bar or edge (some end-inhibited)	Ineffective
Complex (outside layer 4)		Bar or edge	Ineffective
End-inhibited complex (outside layer 4)		Line or edge that stops; corner or angle	Ineffective

presumably arising from cortical simple cells.[37] The tentative scheme for an end-stopped complex cell is illustrated in Figure 2.17B. There, two complex cells with opposing synaptic effects combine to produce the end-stopped complex cell that could detect a corner.

Receptive Fields: Units for Form Perception

Together these results lend support to the idea of hierarchical organization whereby increasing complexity in receptive field organization is produced by the orderly convergence of appropriate inputs. This feature does not mean that each receptive field of succeeding complexity is generated solely by combining inputs derived from the immediately preceding level. For instance, complex cells can receive inputs from LGN cells.[38] Moreover, numerous horizontal connections between visual neurons are prevalent throughout the cortex.[39] As mentioned previously, cortical input serves to sharpen the orientation tuning of simple cells. Nonetheless, the original working hypothesis proposed by Hubel and Wiesel in 1962 continues to provide a clear, elegant, and reasonable conceptual framework on which to design new experimental tests.

Table 2.1 summarizes some of the key characteristics of receptive fields at successive levels of the visual system. Each eye conveys to the brain information collected from regions of various sizes on the retinal surface. The emphasis is not on diffuse illumination. Rather the visual system extracts information about contrast by comparing the level of activity in cells with adjoining receptive fields. At each higher level, such neural computations define ever more elaborate spatial features.

This process can be appreciated by considering the types of signals generated by a square patch of light as shown in Figure 2.18. On-center retinal ganglion cells within the square increase their discharge (at least initially), while off-center cells are suppressed. The best-stimulated ganglion cells, however, are those subjected to the maximum contrast—that is, those having centers lying immediately adjacent to the boundary between the light and dark areas, and consequently having less activation of their inhibitory regions. Neurons in the LGN behave similarly. Cortical cells having receptive fields lying either completely within the square or outside it send no signals because diffuse illumination is not an effective stimulus. Only those simple cells with receptive fields oriented to coincide with the horizontal or vertical boundaries of the square will be stimulated.

Is orientation of stimulus important?	Are there distinct on and off areas within receptor fields?	Are cells driven by both eyes?	Can cells respond selectively to movement in one direction?
No	No	No	No
No	Yes	No	No
No	Yes	No	No
Yes	Yes	Yes (except in layer 4)	Some can
Yes	No	Yes	Some can
Yes	No	Yes	Some can

[38] Martinez, L. M., and Alonso, J. M. 2001. *Neuron* 32: 515–525.

[39] Stettler, D. D. et al. 2002. *Neuron* 36: 739–750.

FIGURE 2.18 Responses of Neurons to a Pattern.
When a square patch of light is presented to the retina, signals arise predominately from ganglion cells and lateral geniculate cells whose receptive fields lie close to the border of the square—and not from those subjected to uniform light or darkness. The cell whose fields are situated exactly at the four corners of the square will fire best of all. Simple and complex cells having receptive fields with the correct position (i.e., situated along the border or at a corner) and the correct orientation preference will also fire, while those not on the border or with an inappropriate orientation will remain silent. Activity level is indicated by the number of radiating lines around each field.

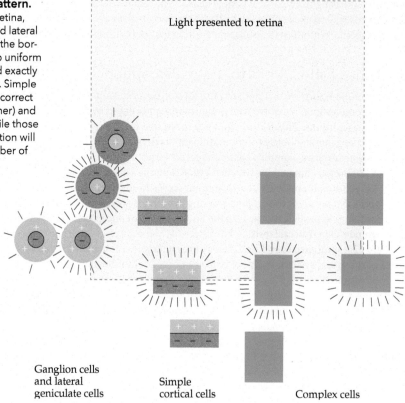

Ganglion cells and lateral geniculate cells

Simple cortical cells

Complex cells

Similar considerations apply to the stimulation of complex cells, which also require properly oriented bars or edges. End-inhibited simple or complex cells detect the corner of the square or a line that stops. There is an important difference between the two, however, which is related to the fact that the eyes continually make small saccadic eye movements. These are not perceived as motion but are essential for preventing photoreceptor adaptation as the eyes fixate. Each microsaccade causes a new population of simple cells with exactly the same orientation but with slightly different receptive field location to be thrown into action. For those complex cells that see the square, however, a boundary of appropriate orientation can be anywhere within the field. Thus, many of the same complex cells will continue to fire during eye movements, as long as the displacement is small and the pattern does not pass outside the receptive field of the cell.

If the preceding considerations are valid, the surprising conclusion is that the primary visual cortex receives little information about the absolute level of uniform illumination within the square. Signals arrive only from the cells with receptive fields situated close to the border. This hypothesis is supported by an easily replicated psychophysical experiment. A square that appears light when surrounded by a black border can be made to appear dark merely by increasing the brightness of the surround. In other words, we perceive the difference or contrast at the boundary, and it is by that standard that the brightness in the uniformly illuminated central area is judged (see Figure 2.5).

This is not to say that general luminance is entirely ignored by the nervous system. For example, we do know if a room is dark or light and that the diameter of the eye's pupil varies with ambient light intensity. Such responses depend on a particular group of ganglion cells that send their output to a region of the brain called the suprachiasmatic nucleus, which regulates the day–night circadian rhythm (see Chapters 19 and 22).

The work of Hubel and Wiesel and others has made clear that the first general step in visual analysis is to construct representations of lines or edges from the center–surround, spotlike receptive fields of the retina. In V1, the visual system begins to derive form from the retinal map. Finding these connections has given us our first glimpse into how the brain computes. But these first steps in the detection of a line or even a corner remain a long way from complete visual recognition during which shape, color, size, and motion are all combined, so that we can recognize a car, a cow, or the face of a friend. In Chapter 3 we describe how geniculate and cortical neurons are arranged spatially, in a highly orderly manner.

It is appropriate to close this chapter with a quotation from Sherrington, written long before receptive fields were mapped for single cells. Sherrington's somewhat opaque style (unlike that of Helmholtz) often makes it difficult to read his profoundly original papers and books. Yet the following paragraph reveals his poetic insight into the physiology of vision:

> *The chief wonder of all we have not touched on yet. Wonder of wonders, though familiar even to boredom. So much with us that we forget it all the time. The eye sends, as we saw, into the cell-and-fibre forest of the brain throughout the waking day continual rhythmic streams of tiny, individual evanescent, electrical potentials. This throbbing streaming crowd of electrified shifting points in the spongework of the brain bears no obvious semblance in space-pattern, and even in temporal relation resembles but a little remotely the tiny two-dimensional upside-down picture of the outside world which the eye-ball paints on the beginnings of its nerve-fibres to electrical storm. And the electrical storm so set up is one which affects a whole population of brain-cells. Electrical charges having in themselves not the faintest elements of the visual—having, for instance, nothing of "distance," "right-side-upness," no "vertical," nor "horizontal," nor "color," nor "brightness," nor "shadow," nor "roundness," nor "squareness," nor "contour," nor "transparency," nor "opacity," nor "near," nor "far," nor visual anything—yet conjure up all these. A shower of little electrical leaks conjures up for me, when I look, the landscape; the castle on the height, or when I look at him, my friend's face and how distant he is from me they tell me. Taking their word for it, I go forward and my other senses confirm that he is there.*[40]

[40] Sherrington, C. S. 1951. *Man on His Nature*. Cambridge University Press, Cambridge, UK.

SUMMARY

- The receptive field of a neuron in the visual system is the area of the retina or visual field that, upon illumination, enhances or inhibits signaling.

- An important strategy for analyzing the visual system is to define the optimal light stimulus for each neuron.

- The pathway for color blind permits the study of progressive integration steps for visual perception.

- Ganglion cells in the retina and cells in the lateral geniculate nucleus respond best to contrast in the form of small spots of light surrounded by darkness, or dark spots surrounded by light.

- Ganglion cells and lateral geniculate nucleus cells respond poorly to diffuse light.

- Simple cells in striate cortex, V1, respond to oriented light or dark bars. Their receptive fields can be mapped with spots of light, as though composed of adjoining lateral geniculate center-surround receptive fields.

- Complex cells in striate cortex also respond to oriented bars or edges. However, their receptive fields cannot be mapped with spots of light. They result from the convergence of multiple simple cells with adjoining receptive areas.

- Simple and complex cells respond to movement of bars or edges.

- End inhibition, or end stopping, results when an additional suppressive zone specifies the optimal length for a simple or complex cell. These cells provide information about where a line ends or about the position of a corner.

Suggested Reading

General Reviews

Kremkow, J., and Alonso, J. M. 2018.Thalamocortical circuits and functional architecture. *Ann. Rev. Vis. Sci.* 4: 5.1–5.23.

Guillery, R. W. 2005. Anatomical pathways that link perception and action. *Prog. Brain Res.* 149: 235–256.

Hubel, D. H., and Wiesel, T. N. 2005. *Brain and Visual Perception*. Oxford University Press, New York.

Priebe, N. J., and Ferster, D. 2012. Mechanisms of neuronal computation in mammalian visual cortex. *Neuron*. 75: 194–208

Original Papers

Finn, I. M., and Ferster, D. 2007. Computational diversity in complex cells of cat primary visual cortex. *J. Neurosci.* 27: 9638–9648.

Hubel, D. H., and Wiesel, T. N. 1959. Receptive fields of single neurones in the cat's striate cortex. *J. Physiol.* 148: 574–591.

Hubel, D. H., and Wiesel, T. N. 1968. Receptive fields and functional architecture of monkey striate cortex. *J. Physiol.* 195: 215–243.

Kuffler, S. W. 1953. Discharge patterns and functional organization of the mammalian retina. *J. Neurophysiol.* 16: 37–68.

Lampl, I., Anderson, J. S., Gillespie, D. C., and Ferster, D. 2001. Prediction of orientation selectivity from receptive field architecture in simple cells of cat visual cortex. *Neuron* 30: 263–274.

Stettler, D. D., Das, A., Bennett, J., and Gilbert, C. D. 2002. Lateral connectivity and contextual interactions in macaque primary visual cortex. *Neuron* 36: 739–750.

CHAPTER 3

Functional Architecture of the Visual Cortex

The visual cortex is characterized by vertically arranged columns of neurons with similar properties. Each column spans the depth of the cortex and receives its input from a small region of the visual field. Adjacent columns receive input from adjacent positions of the visual field, and all the columns together form a map. Maps on their own, however, do not provide a complete picture of the functional architecture of the visual cortex; for that, one needs to know how the neurons that respond to specific visual stimuli are arranged in three dimensions. Detailed information about structure turns out to be essential for understanding how visual information is processed in the brain. The six layers of the primary visual cortex (V1) have specific organizational properties: Incoming fibers from the lateral geniculate nucleus for the most part form synapses in layer 4. Neurons in upper layers (2, 3) and deeper layers (5, 6) receive their inputs from the cortex and project to other layers or areas. Neurons that are preferentially driven by the right or the left eye are grouped in ocular dominance columns. Columns of neurons fire vigorously when a border or edge of a specific angle is presented within the receptive field; these constitute orientation columns. The ocular dominance and orientation columns were first discovered by recording electrical activity, cell after cell, as electrodes traversed the cortical thickness. Ocular dominance and orientation columns are revealed directly in the living animal by optical techniques that display activated regions in the cortex. The word *column* is still used even though the arrangement consists of cortical slabs (for ocular dominance) or pinwheels (for orientation), rather than narrow columns. Each column of cortical cells functions as a module, operating on input from one location in visual space and forwarding the processed information to other areas. The location of the receptive fields of neurons in a column is the same throughout the depth of the cortex.

Neurons from the lateral geniculate nucleus with different properties supply distinct regions of the visual cortex. Magnocellular (M) axons (concerned with movement, contrast, and depth) end more superficially in layer 4 than do parvocellular (P) axons (concerned with position and color). Koniocellular (K) geniculate axons (short wavelength) project differentially to clusters outside layer 4 called blobs. Blobs were first revealed by stains for the enzyme cytochrome oxidase. Although mixing of M, P, and K streams occurs throughout the visual pathways, features such as color and motion are processed separately. This phenomenon is illustrated not only by physiological recordings but also by the fact that a lesion in a discrete region of the brain can result in selective loss of just one feature, such as color.

In Chapter 2 we followed the flow of information from the retina to the primary visual cortex and described the effects of visual stimuli on successively higher-order cortical cells. This approach provided an understanding of the cellular mechanisms for the initial analysis of form and motion at each point in the visual field. Our task now is to describe how neurons are organized spatially to subserve their functions in the visual pathways (see Figure 2.2). In this chapter we show how inputs from the two eyes arrive at the visual cortex and how cells are grouped according to their physiological functions. We next examine the evidence that motion and color are analyzed in parallel channels through the cortex. Finally, we introduce examples of higher levels of processing in visual areas beyond the primary visual cortex, a topic dealt with in detail in Chapter 25.

From Chapters 1 and 2 it is apparent that knowledge of structure is not just a dull exercise that can be skipped over. Such knowledge is essential if one is to understand how different aspects of a scene (e.g., *form, color, depth, motion*) are encoded in the cortex. A remarkable feature of the visual structure described in this chapter is that completely new and unexpected findings about how the brain is structured anatomically came first from a series of physiological recordings made from single neurons, one at a time. Hubel and Wiesel have recalled that "to attack such a three-dimensional problem with a one-dimensional weapon is a dismaying exercise in tedium, like trying to cut the back lawn with a pair of nail scissors."[1]

We will show that in visual area 1 (V1) there is point-to-point representation of the retina. Within this retinotopic map, inputs from the two eyes come together and are sorted into **ocular dominance columns**. These columns consist of vertically stacked groups of neurons that respond better either to the left eye or the right eye. In addition, there are other major functional groupings, consisting of **orientation columns** of cells (all of which respond to a specific line orientation, such as vertical, oblique, or horizontal), and still other clusters of cells devoted to colors. Like Chapter 2, this chapter makes continual reference to older experiments. The reason is that the work by Hubel and Wiesel represents a solid foundation, which has been confirmed, modified, and extended by others but not superseded.

From Lateral Geniculate Nucleus to Visual Cortex

Segregation of Retinal Inputs to the Lateral Geniculate Nucleus

Neurons in the six principal layers of the LGN are grouped according to structure and function. In primates, including humans, geniculate layers 6, 4, and 1 are supplied by the contralateral eye, while layers 5, 3, and 2 are supplied by the ipsilateral eye.[2] The complete segregation of endings from each eye into separate cell layers has been shown by microelectrode recording and a variety of anatomical techniques.[3,4] Particularly striking is the arborization of a single optic nerve fiber that has been injected with the enzyme horseradish peroxidase, as shown in Figure 3.1. The terminals are all confined to the layers supplied by that eye, with no spillover across the border.

Another major feature of the LGN is segregation according to the size of neurons, which in turn bears on their function. As described in Chapter 2, cells in the deep layers 1 and 2 of the lateral geniculate nucleus are larger than those in layers 3, 4, 5, and 6, and this gave rise to the terms **magnocellular (M) cells** (large cells with large receptive fields) and **parvocellular (P) cells** (small cells with small receptive fields) (see Figure 3.1B). In Chapter 2 we showed that the same classification holds for ganglion cells in the retina. M neurons respond preferentially to movement, depth, and contrast, while P neurons respond to position and color. Between each of the M and P layers lies a zone of small cells: the interlaminar, or koniocellular (K), layers. K cells are distinct from M and P cells and provide the visual cortex with a third channel, which is concerned primarily with information about short-wavelength color (blue light).[5,6]

Cytoarchitecture of the Visual Cortex

Visual information passes to the cortex from the LGN through the optic radiation. In the monkey, the optic radiation ends mainly (but not exclusively[7]) in V1 (also called striate cortex or area 17, terms based on anatomical criteria developed at the

[1] Hubel, D. H., and Wiesel, T. N. 1977. *Proc. R. Soc. Lond. B* 198: 1–59.

[2] Guillery, R. W. 1970. *J. Comp. Neurol.* 138: 339–368.

[3] Hubel, D. H., and Wiesel, T. N. 1972. *J. Comp. Neurol.* 146: 421–450.

[4] Callaway, E. M. 2005. *J. Physiol.* 566: 13–19.

[5] Roy, S. et al. 2009. *Eur. J. Neurosci.* 30: 1517–1526.

[6] Casagrande, V. A. et al. 2007. *Cereb. Cortex* 17: 2334–2345.

[7] Sincich, L. C. et al. 2004. *Nat. Neurosci.* 7: 1123–1128.

Lateral geniculate nucleus

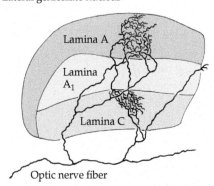

Lamina A

Lamina A₁

Lamina C

Optic nerve fiber

FIGURE 3.1 Retinal axon terminations in the Lateral Geniculate Nucleus (LGN). Termination of an optic nerve fiber in cat LGN, which has three principal layers. A single on-center axon from the contralateral eye was injected with horseradish peroxidase. Branches end in layers A and C but not in A₁. (After D. B. Bowling and C. R. Michael, 1980. *Nature* 286: 899–902.)

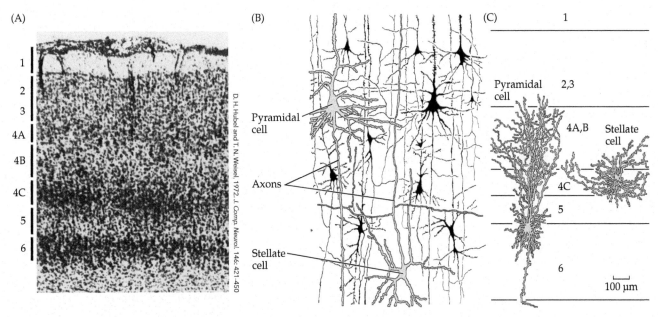

FIGURE 3.2 Architecture of Visual Cortex. (A) Distinct layering of cells in a section of striate cortex of the macaque monkey, stained to show cell bodies (Nissl stain). Fibers, arriving from the lateral geniculate nucleus, end in layers 4A, 4B, and 4C. (B) Drawing of pyramidal and stellate cells in cat visual cortex. The processes (stained with Golgi technique) for the most part run radially through the thickness of the cortex and extend for relatively short distances laterally. (C) Drawing from photographs of a pyramidal cell and a spiny stellate cell in cat cortex that had been injected with horseradish peroxidase after their activity had been recorded. Both were simple cells. (B afer S. Ramón y Cajal, 1911. *Histologie du Système Nerveux*, Vol. 2. Maloine, Paris; C from C. D. Gilbert and T. N. Wiesel, 1979. *Nature* 280: 120-125.)

beginning of the twentieth century; see Appendix C-3). V1 lies posteriorly in the occipital lobe (see Figure 3.4) and can be recognized in cross section by its characteristic appearance. In sections of V1, incoming bundles of fibers form a clear stripe that can be seen by the naked eye (hence the name *striate*) (Figure 3.2A).

In histological sections of the cortex, neurons can be classified according to their shapes.[8] The two principal groups of neurons are known as stellate cells and pyramidal cells. Examples of these cells are shown in Figure 3.2B,C.[9] The axon of the pyramidal cell is long, and descends into the white matter; the stellate cell axon tends to terminate locally. These two groups of cells exhibit other variations that bear on their functional properties—for instance, all pyramidal cells have spines on the dendrites, while some stellate cells lack spines. There are other descriptively named cortical neurons (double bouquet cells, chandelier cells, basket cells, and crescent cells) as well as neuroglial cells. Characteristically, processes of cells for the most part run vertically through the thickness of the cortex (at right angles to the surface, or *radially*). Connections between primary and higher-order visual cortices are made by axons that run in bundles through the white matter underlying the cellular layers.[10]

Other regions of cortex (V2–V5) are also concerned with vision.[11] Their exact boundaries cannot be defined by simple inspection of the brain but have been delineated by several techniques. These include imaging, molecular biology, genomics, experimental lesions, psychophysics, and physiology.[12–17] As will be shown in Chapter 25, different visual areas communicate with one another in both directions and perform different types of analyses relating to form, color, depth, and movement.

Inputs, Outputs, and Layering of Cortex

The organization of geniculate projections to the striate cortex is illustrated in Figure 3.3A. Six layers of nerve cells are evident within the gray matter of V1, as in other regions of the brain (see Figure 3.2A). The inputs are shown on the left side of Figure 3.3A. Incoming

[8] Niell, C. M. 2015. *Annu. Rev. Neurosci.* 38: 413-431.

[9] Gilbert, C. D., and Wiesel, T. N. 1979. *Nature* 280: 120-125.

[10] Zeki, S. 1990. *Disc. Neurosci.* 6: 1-64.

[11] Van Essen, D. C. 1997. *Nature* 385: 313-318.

[12] Hubel, D. H., and Wiesel, T. N. 1965. *J. Neurophysiol.* 28: 229-289.

[13] Maunsell, J. H., and Newsome, W. T. 1987. *Annu. Rev. Neurosci.* 10: 363-401.

[14] Adams, D. L., and Zeki, S. 2001. *J. Neurophysiol.* 86: 2195-2203.

[15] Orban, G. A., Van Essen, D., and Vanduffel, W. 2004. *Trends Cogn. Sci.* 8: 315-324.

[16] Tsao, D. Y. et al. 2006. *Science* 311: 670-674.

[17] Tasic, B. et al. 2018. *Nature* 563: 72-78.

FIGURE 3.3 Connections of Visual Cortex. (A) The layers are shown with their various inputs, outputs, and cell types. Note that inputs from the lateral geniculate nucleus end mainly in layer 4. Those arising from magnocellular layers end principally in 4Cα and 4B, whereas those from parvocellular layers end in 4A and 4Cβ. Koniocellular pathways end in superficial layers and in structures known as blobs, represented as colored forms in layers 2-3 (see Figure 3.10A). Simple cells are found mainly in layers 4 and 6, complex cells in layers 2, 3, 5, and 6. Cells in layers 2, 3, and 4B send axons to other cortical areas; cells in layers 5 and 6 send axons to the superior colliculus and the lateral geniculate nucleus deep in the brain. (B) Principal arborizations of geniculate axons and cortical neurons in the cat. In addition to these vertical connections, many cells have long horizontal connections running within a layer to distant regions of the cortex. (A after D. H Hubel, 1988. *Eye, Brain, and Vision*. Scientific American Library, New York; and L. C. Sincich and J. C. Horton, 2005. *Ann. Rev. Neurosci.* 28: 303-326; B after C. D. Gilbert and T. N. Wiesel, 1981. In F. O. Schmitt, F. G. Worden, and F. Dennis (eds.), *The Organization of the Cerebral Cortex*. MIT Press, Cambridge, MA.)

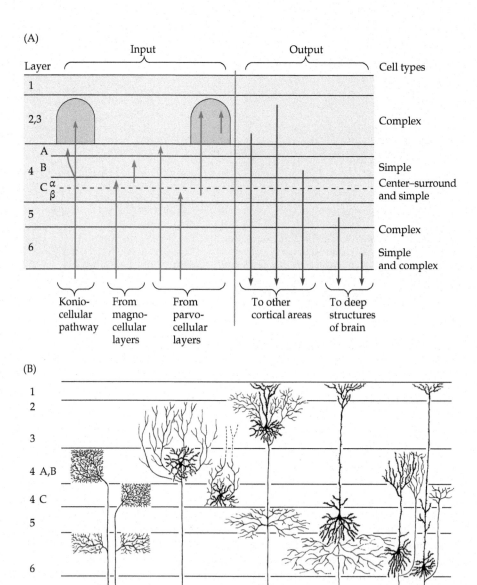

[18] Hubel, D. H. 1988. *Eye, Brain, and Vision*. Scientific American Library, New York.

[19] Hirsch, J. A. et al. 1998. *J. Neurosci.* 18: 8086-8094.

geniculate fibers for the most part end in layer 4, with some contacts also made in layer 6 (see the next paragraph).[18] Superficial layers of the cortex receive inputs from the pulvinar, a region of the thalamus. Numerous cortical cells, especially those in layer 2 and the upper portions of layers 3 and 5, receive inputs from neurons within the cortex.

The outputs from cortical layers 6, 5, 4, 3, and 2 are shown on the right side of Figure 3.3A A single cell that sends efferent signals out of the cortex can also mediate intracortical connections from one layer to another. For example, the axons of cells in layer 6, in addition to supplying the geniculate, can end in one of several other cortical layers, depending on the cell type.[19]

From this anatomy a general pattern emerges: Information from the retina is transmitted to cortical cells (mainly in layer 4) by geniculate axons, handed on from neuron to neuron through the thickness of the cortex, and then sent out to other regions of the brain by fibers looping out through white matter. The typical morphologies of these output cells are illustrated in Figure 3.3B, along with the geniculate axon termination. The radial, or vertical, organization of the cortex suggests that *columns* of neurons serve as computational units, processing some feature of the visual scene and passing it on to other cortical regions. Lateral connections also exist (i.e., parallel to the surface of the cortex); they enable neurons

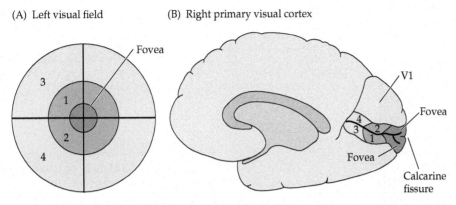

(A) Left visual field   (B) Right primary visual cortex

FIGURE 3.4   Visual Field Map of the Cortex. (A) The visual field is divided into a central zone (the fovea) and eight hemiquadrants. The left visual field maps onto the right primary visual cortex. (B) In humans, the primary visual cortex (V1) lies almost entirely on the medial surface of the occipital lobe. The foveal region is situated in the farthest posterior portion, with the peripheral zones mapping anteriorly. The fovea claims a disproportionate share of the primary visual cortex.

in neighboring areas to communicate with one another (see the section "Horizontal Intracortical Connections"). In addition, geniculate inputs project directly to areas of cortex beyond V1, for example to visual area 5 (see the section "Association Areas of Visual Cortex"), which is concerned with movement and depth perception.[7]

Retinotopic Maps

Visual processing in the cortex consists of bidirectional streams of information (to and from the input region, V1) passing through a sequence of topographically organized regions. Maps of the visual fields in adjacent areas are oriented in mirror fashion across cortical gyri (folds), a feature that facilitates communication.[11] Before the era of single-cell analysis, projection maps were made by shining light onto parts of the retina and recording with gross electrodes.[20] These maps, and those made by functional magnetic resonance imaging (fMRI), show that much more cortical area is devoted to representation of the fovea than to representation of the rest of the retina. This comes as no surprise, since form vision is served principally by the higher densities of photoreceptors in foveal and parafoveal areas and is analogous to the enlarged areas devoted to the hand and face in the primary somatosensory cortex (see Chapter 23). The retinal fovea is mapped onto the occipital pole of the cerebral cortex, while the map of the retinal periphery extends anteriorly, along the medial surface of the occipital lobe (see Figure 3.4).[21] Because of image reversal by the eye, the upper visual field appears on the lower retina and is projected to V1 below the calcarine fissure; accordingly, lower visual fields map above the calcarine fissure.

Ocular Dominance Columns

Whether we look at an object with one or both eyes, we see only one image, even though the positions of the object's projection are slightly different on the two retinas. Interestingly, well over 100 years ago Johannes Müller suggested that individual nerve fibers from the two eyes might fuse or become connected to the same cells in the brain. By this intuition, he almost exactly anticipated Hubel and Wiesel's results (see Figure 2.8).[1,22]

Hubel and Wiesel's early experiments showed cortical cells with similar properties to be aggregated together in a vertical array.[1] In any one penetration through the cortex, as the electrode was advanced from the surface through layer after layer to white matter, all cells were found to share certain common properties. Thus, as the electrode descended through the cortex, all the neurons encountered had the same receptive field position and were all excited by light stimuli given to the same eye.

[20] Daniel, P. M., and Whitteridge, D. 1961. *J. Physiol.* 159: 203–221.

[21] Van Essen, D. C., and Drury, H. A. 1997. *J. Neurosci.* 17: 7079–7102.

[22] Hubel, D. H., and Wiesel, T. N. 1959. *J. Physiol.* 148: 574–591.

(A)

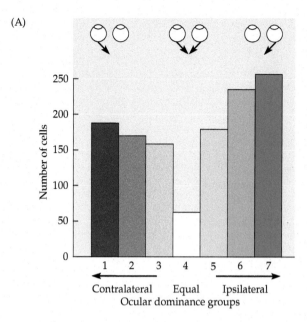

(B)

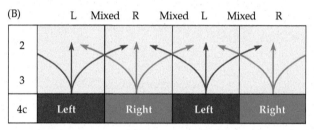

FIGURE 3.5 Physiological Demonstrations of Ocular Dominance Columns. (A) Eye preference of 1116 cells in V1 of 28 rhesus monkeys. Most cells (groups 2–6) are driven by both eyes. (B) Diagram showing how inputs from two eyes arriving in layer 4 of the cortex are combined in more superficial layers through horizontal or oblique connections to create cells with binocular fields. (A after T. Wiesel and D. H. Hubel, 1974. *J. Comp. Neurol.* 158: 307-318; B after D. H. Hubel, 1988. *Eye, Brain and Vision.* Scientific American Library, New York.)

Figure 3.5, summarizing the results of many physiological recordings, shows the variation in eye preference (or ocular dominance) of neurons in the monkey striate cortex. The cells (total of 1116) are subdivided into seven groups. In groups 2, 3, 5, and 6, the effect of one eye is stronger than that of the other, while in group 4 the effectiveness of the two eyes is equal. It is clear from the histogram that the majority of cells respond preferentially to one of the two eyes. Cells in groups 1 and 7, however, are driven exclusively by the left or the right eye, respectively. These monocularly driven cells occur mainly in layer 4, the principal receiving station for geniculate inputs. Above and below layer 4, simple, complex, and end-stopped cortical neurons (see Chapter 2) are driven by both eyes.

Ocular dominance column was the term that Hubel and Wiesel used to describe the vertical segregation of neurons through the thickness of V1 according to eye preference. Their terminology followed the original concept of cortical columns, which was introduced by Mountcastle for somatosensory cortex on the basis of skin receptive field position.[23-25] Anatomical studies on cats and monkeys confirmed that the cells in one layer of the LGN project to aggregates of target cells in layer 4 that are separate from those supplied by the other eye.[26] The aggregates appear as alternating stripes or bands of cortical cells, each supplied exclusively by one eye. As already mentioned, cells are driven by both eyes in the deeper and more superficial cortical layers, although one eye usually dominates.

One of the first techniques for demonstrating columns histologically was to destroy a small group of cells in one layer of the lateral geniculate nucleus and examine the cortex later for degenerating terminals. These terminals appeared in layer 4 in a characteristic pattern of alternating, well-demarcated regions[3] that corresponded to areas driven by the eye supplying the lesioned layer of the LGN.

Later, the ocular dominance pattern over the entire visual cortex was demonstrated by injecting radioactive amino acids, such as leucine or proline, into one eye. The amino acid was taken up by ganglion cells in the retina and incorporated into protein. In time, the labeled protein was transported from ganglion cells along the optic nerve fibers to their terminals within the lateral geniculate nucleus (it is not yet known whether or how trans-synaptic transport of protein is used physiologically). An extraordinary feature was that the label was then transferred to the geniculate cells and on to the endings of their axons in the cortex, revealing the striking ocular dominance pattern shown in Figure 3.6.[27-29]

At the cellular level, a similar pattern has been revealed in layer 4 by injection of horseradish peroxidase into individual axons of lateral geniculate neurons as they approach the cortex.[4] The axon shown in Figure 3.6C arises from an off-center geniculate fiber (see Chapter 2) that gave transient responses to dark, moving spots. It ends in two distinct clusters of processes in layer 4. The processes are separated by a blank area corresponding in size to the territory supplied by the other eye. Such morphological studies have borne out and added depth to the original description of ocular dominance columns presented by Hubel and Wiesel in 1962.

23 Mountcastle, V. B. 1957. *J. Neurophysiol.* 20: 408-434.

24 Hubel, D. H., and Wiesel, T. N. 1962. *J. Physiol.* 160: 106-154.

25 Hubel, D. H., and Wiesel, T. N. 1968. *J. Physiol.* 195: 215-243.

26 Weyand, T. 2015. *Rev. Neurosci.* 27: 135-157.

27 Specht, S., and Grafstein, B. 1973. *Exp. Neurol.* 41: 705-722.

28 LeVay, S., Hubel, D. H., and Wiesel, T. N. 1975. *J. Comp. Neurol.* 159: 559-576.

29 LeVay, S. et al. 1985. *J. Neurosci.* 5: 486-501.

(A) (B)

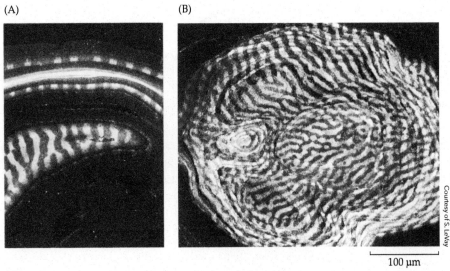

Courtesy of S. LeVay

100 µm

(C)

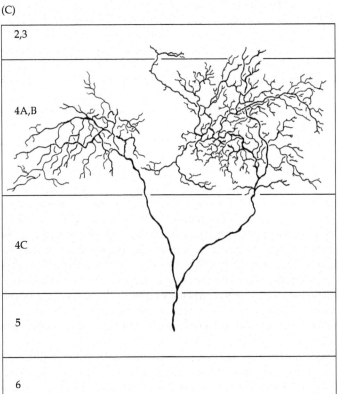

2,3

4A,B

4C

5

6

FIGURE 3.6 Ocular Dominance Columns (A,B) The disposition in layer 4 of radioactive terminals of geniculate axons supplied by the injected eye (radioactivity causes deposition of silver grains in overlaid photographic emulsion, which then appear as white areas in dark-field photographs). The labeled stripes interdigitate with unlabeled areas supplied by the noninjected eye. The center-to-center distance between ocular dominance patches for one eye is approximately 1.0 mm. (A convenient way to visualize the pattern is to imagine that layer 4 corresponds to the layer of cream in a chocolate cake, seen from above after the upper layer of cake has been removed). (C) An off-center cell in the lateral geniculate nucleus that responded best to a small dark spot. It was injected with horseradish peroxidase to show its terminals ending in layer 4 of the cat visual cortex. The terminals are grouped in two separate clusters, corresponding to columns supplied by the injected eye, separated by a vacant zone supplied by the other eye. (C after C. D. Gilbert and T. N. Wiesel, 1979. *Nature* 280: 120–125.)

Demonstration of Ocular Dominance Columns by Imaging

Ocular dominance columns in the visual cortex can be visualized directly in intact animals. Activity in a large area of cortex is monitored while visual stimuli are presented to the animal. The technique uses activity-dependent optical signals that arise from changes in tissue reflectivity or changes in fluorescence of extrinsically applied dyes.[30–32] Figure 3.7 shows ocular dominance columns detected by this kind of experiment, in which a visual stimulus was applied repeatedly to only one eye. The striped pattern is like that obtained after injection of radioactive amino acids into one eye (see Figure 3.6). The presence of these stripes through the depth of cortex confirms the concept of ocular dominance "slabs" (rather than columns) subdividing the retinotopic map. The representation of information from both

[30] Grinvald, A. et al. 1986. *Nature*. 324: 361–364.

[31] Ts'o, D. Y. et al. 1990. *Science*. 249: 417–420.

[32] Ts'o, D. Y, Zarella, M., and Burkitt, G. 2009. *J. Physiol.* 587: 2791–2805.

Courtesy of A. Grinvald

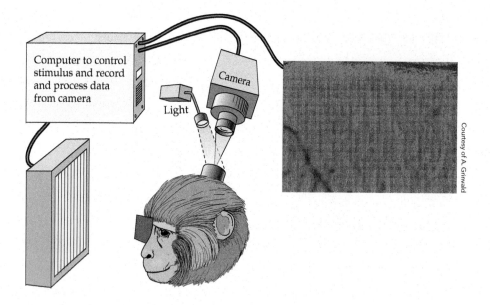

FIGURE 3.7 Display of Ocular Dominance Columns by Optical Imaging. A sensitive camera detects changes in light reflected from the monkey cortex following activity induced in just one eye. The intensity changes are color-coded so that active areas are red. The pattern of red stripes corresponds to ocular dominance columns revealed by anatomical labeling methods (see Figure 3.6). (After D. Y. Ts'o et al., 1990. *Science* 249: 417–420.)

eyes, associated with a stimulus at one position in the visual field, is integrated by neighboring cells in the visual cortex (see Figure 3.6B). The maps shown in Figure 3.7 was observed without the use of dyes; they are a reflection of altered blood flow and oxygenation in the active area. By use of a staining technique for the enzyme cytochrome oxidase (described in the section "Cell Groupings for Color"), Horton and his colleagues have mapped the complete arrangement of ocular dominance columns in postmortem human visual cortex.[33]

[33] Adams, D. L., Sincich, L. C., and Horton, J. C. 2007. *J. Neurosci.* 27: 10391–10403.

[34] Hubel, D. H., and Wiesel, T. N. 1974. *J. Comp. Neurol.* 158: 267–294.

Orientation Columns

What other functional groupings occur among cells of V1? In Chapter 2 we described the orientation preferences of simple and complex cells, so we might ask whether this feature is systematically mapped across the cortex. A sample experiment is shown in Figure 3.8 in which a microelectrode is inserted perpendicular to the surface of the cortex in V1 of the cat.[23] Each bar indicates the location of one cell and its preferred receptive field orientation in the progression through the cortical depth. Small lesions are made at significant points along the electrode track by passing current through the electrode. From these lesions and an end point (indicated by the circle at the end of each electrode track), the position of each recorded cell is reconstructed. In the left-hand track, the first 38 cells are optimally driven by bars or edges at about 0° (close to horizontal), at one position in the visual field. After the electrode has penetrated about 0.6 mm, the receptive field orientation changes to about 45°. In a second track (to the right) more tangential to the cortical surface than the first track, successive cells have slightly different receptive field positions and field orientations. In this oblique penetration, the orientation preference changes in a regular manner, as though moving through a series of columns with different preferred orientations. The orientation columns receive their input from cells with largely overlapping receptive fields on the retinal surface.

Information about how the orientation columns are spatially arranged in the visual cortex of monkeys and cats was first obtained by making tangential electrode penetrations through the cortex like that on the right side of Figure 3.8.[1,24,34] Each 50-μm advance of the electrode horizontally along the cortex was accompanied by a change in orientation preference of about 10°, sometimes in a regular sequence

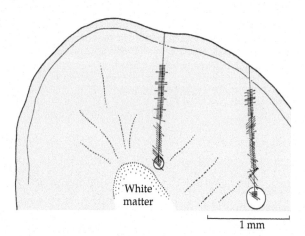

FIGURE 3.8 Axis Orientation of Receptive Fields of Neurons encountered as an electrode traverses the cortex of a cat. Cell after cell tends to have the same axis orientation, indicated by the angle of the bar to the electrode track. The penetration to the right is more oblique; consequently, the track crosses several columns and the axis orientations change frequently. The position of each cell is determined by making lesions repeatedly and at the end of the penetration (circle), and reconstructing the electrode track in serial sections of the brain. Such experiments have established that cat and monkey cells with similar axis orientation are stacked in columns running at right angles to the cortical surface. (After D. H. Hubel and T. N. Wiesel, 1962. *J. Physiol.* 160: 106–154.)

(A)

(B)

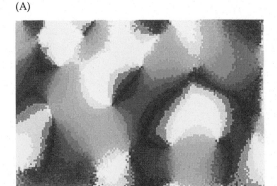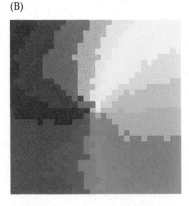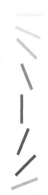

FIGURE 3.9 Detection of Orientation Columns (Pinwheels) by Optical Imaging.
The activity-dependent reflectance of visual cortex was recorded by a sensitive camera while an eye was stimulated with oriented bars. (A) Each orientation caused maximal changes in different regions; orientation contours are represented by different colors. Although the pattern seems at first disorderly, close inspection reveals centers at which all orientation contours come together in a pinwheel, as shown in (B). Note that each orientation is represented only once and that the sequence is beautifully precise. Such pinwheel centers occur at regular distances from each other. The bars on the right show eight different orientations for the visual stimuli, represented by colors (e.g., yellow represents horizontal, blue represents vertical). (After T. Bonhoeffer and A. Grinvald, 1991. *Nature* 353: 429–431.)

through 180°. The orientation columns were narrower than those for ocular dominance—20 to 50 µm wide, compared with 250 to 500 µm.

After the initial anatomical demonstration of orientation columns based on the uptake of 2-deoxyglucose by active cells,[35] the organization was studied in detail by optical imaging techniques in living animals.[30,36–38] In an example experiment, the presentation of visual stimuli in a variety of orientations produced activity in different cortical zones (Figure 3.9A). The response to each orientation is represented by a different color. What is striking is the arrangement of the orientation columns with respect to one another. At first, the organization appears disorderly. However, careful inspection reveals the presence of pinwheels*— centered on focal points at which all the orientations come together (Figure 3.9B). From the focal point, the cells responsive to a particular orientation radiate in an extraordinarily regular manner. Some pinwheels are systematically organized with a clockwise progression, others with a counterclockwise progression. Each orientation appears only once in the cycle.[39]

Cell Groupings for Color

In their initial experiments, Hubel and Wiesel worked with cats, which do not have color vision. It was therefore not expected that color-coding cells would be found in the visual cortex. However, even in monkeys, which do see color, color-coding cells were missed in early experiments on the visual cortex. In Chapter 22 we will show that in the retina of monkeys and humans, cones preferentially absorb light in long-, medium-, and short-wavelength ranges. The outputs from those cones converge onto color-coded horizontal cells, ganglion cells, and lateral geniculate cells of the parvocellular division. The color-sensitive parvo cells were at first missed in monkey cortex because they are separately aggregated in small clusters, known as patches or blobs, a name that has persisted in the literature. Blobs are roughly circular patches of cells (Figure 3.10A) mainly in layers 2 and 3 but also in 5 and 6. They were first detected by Wong-Riley, who used stains to visualize cytochrome oxidase, an enzyme associated with areas of high metabolic activity.[40] Her experiments, devoted to a completely different problem, ended up revealing fundamental aspects of cortical

[35] Sokoloff, L. 1977. *J. Neurochem.* 29: 13–26.

[36] Bonhoeffer, T., and Grinvald, A. 1991. *Nature* 353: 429–431.

[37] Hubener, M. et al. 1997. *J. Neurosci.* 17: 9270–9284.

[38] Ohki, K. et al. 2006. *Nature* 442: 925–928.

[39] Swindale, N. V., Matsubara, J. A., and Cynader, M. S. 1987. *J. Neurosci.* 7: 1414–1427.

[40] Wong-Riley, M. 1989. *Trends Neurosci.* 12: 94–101.

* Note: A pinwheel is a toy consisting of small brightly colored vanes pinned to a stick (hence the name) through their center point. The pinwheel rotates when moved by wind.

FIGURE 3.10 Blobs in Macaque Primary Visual Cortex. (A) Array of small blobs viewed in a horizontal section through layers 2 and 3. These small spots (which according to Hubel make the brain look as if it had measles) become apparent after the distribution of cytochrome oxidase has been revealed by histochemistry. (B) Diagram showing projections of M, P, and K geniculate fibers to V1 and the subsequent projection to V2. MT = middle temporal cortex. (After L. C. Sincich and J. C. Horton, 2005. *Annu. Rev. Neurosci.* 28: 303-326.)

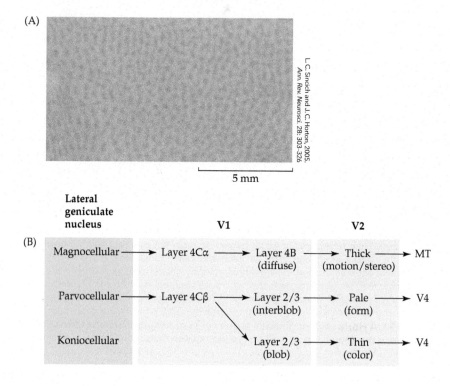

(A)

L. C. Sincich and J. C. Horton, 2005.
Ann. Rev. Neurosci. 28: 303-326

5 mm

(B)

Lateral geniculate nucleus	V1		V2	
Magnocellular →	Layer 4Cα →	Layer 4B (diffuse) →	Thick (motion/stereo) →	MT
Parvocellular →	Layer 4Cβ →	Layer 2/3 (interblob) →	Pale (form) →	V4
Koniocellular		Layer 2/3 (blob) →	Thin (color) →	V4

structure in primates, the patches of cytochrome oxidase stain are precisely arranged in parallel rows about 0.5 mm apart. Their positions correspond to the centers of ocular dominance columns.[41,42]

Recordings of neuronal firing show that many cells within the blobs are color-sensitive and have concentric fields with on and off regions.[43] These observations led to the suggestion that the cytochrome oxidase blobs represent a separate pathway for color, intermingled with the orientation and ocular dominance columns.[4,6,44,45] The blobs also receive inputs from M sublayers of layer 4C and contain neurons with M-like response properties.[46] The blob–interblob regions provide an as yet incompletely understood sorting and recombination of the M, P, and K pathways (Figure 3.10B). Important aspects of color vision, including photoreceptor pigments, retinal connections, and color constancy, are dealt with in Chapter 22.

Connections of Magnocellular and Parvocellular Pathways between V1 and V2

Visual area 2 (V2, also known as area 18) immediately surrounds V1, receives inputs from it, and projects back onto it (Figure 3.11). In V2 the striate appearance is lost, large cells are found superficially, and coarse, obliquely running myelinated fibers are seen in the deeper layers. The technique of staining for cytochrome oxidase has made it possible to study columnar organization and to trace connections of magnocellular and parvocellular systems from one visual area to another. It has also been important for displaying features of cortical architecture in postmortem human brains. As shown in Figure 3.11, staining V2 with cytochrome oxidase produces a pattern different from that seen in V1.[42] The stain in V2 appears as a series of thick and thin stripes, alternating with paler areas having less enzyme activity. These parallel stripes run at right angles to the border between V1 and V2. After horseradish peroxidase is injected into blobs (parvo) of V1, it is taken up by axon terminals and transported retrogradely, revealing that nerve cells providing input to the blobs are located in the thin stripes in V2. The connections are reciprocal: Injections of horseradish peroxidase into thin stripes label cells in V1 blobs.[40,47–50] In contrast, the interblob regions project to the pale stripes. The thick stripes receive primarily magnocellular information from layers 4B and 4Cα. Remarkably, this functional subdivision can be distinguished even at a molecular level; for instance, the monoclonal antibody Cat-301 preferentially labels magnocellular pathways throughout the monkey visual cortex.[51,52]

[41] Livingstone, M. S., and Hubel, D. H. 1984. *J. Neurosci.* 4: 309-356.

[42] Sincich, L. C., and Horton, J. C. 2005. *Ann. Rev. Neurosci.* 28: 303-326.

[43] Ts'o, D. Y., and Gilbert, C. D. 1988. *J. Neurosci.* 8: 1712-1727.

[44] Livingstone, M. S., and Hubel, D. 1988. *Science* 240: 740-749.

[45] Lu, H. D., and Roe, A. W. 2008. *Cereb. Cortex* 18: 516-533.

[46] Merigan, W. H., and Maunsell, J. H. R. 1993. *Annu. Rev. Neurosci.* 16: 369-402.

[47] Livingstone, M. S., and Hubel, D. H. 1987. *J. Neurosci.* 7: 3371-3377.

[48] Ts'o, D. Y., Roe, A. W., and Gilbert, C. D. 2001. *Vision Res.* 41: 1333-1349.

[49] Sincich, L. C., Jocson, C. M., and Horton, J. C. 2007. *Cereb. Cortex* 17: 935-941.

[50] Shmuel, A. et al. 2005. *J. Neurosci.* 25: 2117-2131.

[51] Preuss, T. M., and Coleman, G. Q. 2002. *Cereb. Cortex* 12: 671-691.

[52] Deyoe, E. A. et al. 1990. *Vis. Neurosci.* 5: 67-81.

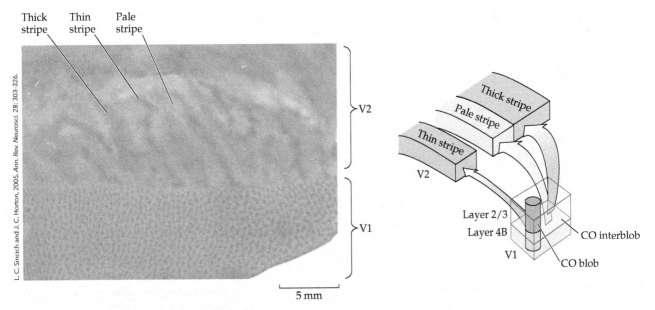

L. C. Sincich and J. C. Horton, 2005. *Ann. Rev. Neurosci.* 28: 303-326.

Thick stripe Thin stripe Pale stripe

V2

V1

5 mm

Thick stripe
Pale stripe
Thin stripe
V2

Layer 2/3
Layer 4B
V1

CO interblob
CO blob

FIGURE 3.11   A Horizontal Section through Cortex of Macaque Monkey V1 and V2 stained to reveal the distribution of cytochrome oxidase blobs (also known as patches) in V1 and stripes in V2. The border between the two areas is well defined and is in accord with characteristics of receptive field organization in V1 and V2. At the transition, the fine array of patches gives way to thick and thin stripes in repeating cycles. CO = cytochrome oxidase. (After L. C. Sincich and J. C. Horton, 2005. *Ann. Rev. Neurosci.* 28: 303-326.)

Magnocellular neurons that respond to depth or movement are abundant in V2.[12,53] An example is shown in Figure 3.12. In this experiment, a dye that changes magnitude of fluorescence in response to changes in intracellular calcium concentration was injected into V2 of a cat. Individual cells responded preferentially to movement of visual stimuli in one direction. This figure shows that resolution at the level of single cells can be achieved in living cortex (see Chapter 2).

Relations between Ocular Dominance and Orientation Columns

Ocular dominance and orientation columns represent just two functional arrangements that characterize neurons in visual cortex. Direction of movement, spatial frequency (essentially a reflection of receptive field size), and image disparity (an important determinant in depth perception)[25,53–55] also appear in columnar arrangements in the cortex. The question then arises as to how all necessary aspects of image analysis can be carried out for each point on the retinotopically mapped cortex. The intermingling of functional columns schematized in Figure 3.13 provides part of the answer. Indeed, long before optical imaging was used to observe such relationships, Hubel and Wiesel proposed a conceptual scheme they termed a hypercolumn (also known as an *ice cube*). In the hypercolumn, all possible orientations for corresponding regions of the visual field for both eyes could be represented. An adjacent hypercolumn would analyze information in the same way for an adjacent but overlapping part of the visual field and so on, until the entire retina was mapped across the cortex.

[53] Ohki, K. et al. 2005. *Nature* 433: 597–603.

[54] Barlow, H. B., Blakemore, C., and Pettigrew, J. D. 1967. *J. Physiol.* 193: 327–342.

[55] Westheimer, G. 2009. *J. Physiol.* 587: 2807–2816.

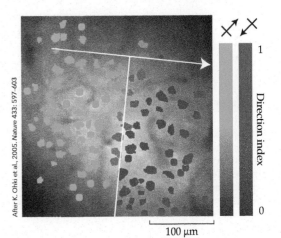

After K. Ohki et al., 2005. *Nature* 433: 597-603

Direction index

100 μm

FIGURE 3.12   Neurons Responding to Moving Stimuli imaged by calcium dye in cat visual cortex (V2). Cells colored green responded to stimuli moving obliquely upward, those colored red to movement in the opposite direction. Gray cells responded to both movements. Cells are plainly arranged in columns with high resolution.

(A) V1

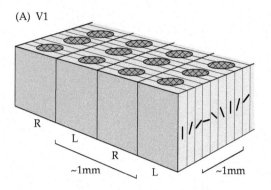

(B) V2

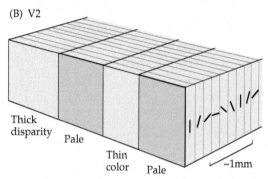

FIGURE 3.13 Scheme Proposed by Hubel and Wiesel for the Arrangement of Ocular Dominance and Orientation Columns in V1. (A) Within a cube of cortical tissue (resembling an ice cube), the sets of columns for eye preference and orientation run at right angles to one another. Blobs are represented as circles. (B) Similarly, the thick stripes and thin stripes revealed by stains for cytochrome oxidase are orthogonal to the orientation columns. (After D. Y. Ts'o et al., 2009. *J. Physiol.* 587: 2791–2805; based on M. S. Livingstone and D. H. Hubel, 1984. *J. Neurosci.* 4: 309–356 and D. H. Hubel and T. N. Wiesel, 1977. *Proc. R. Soc. Lond. B. Biol. Sci.* 198: 1–59.)

Once the pinwheel arrangements for cells with particular orientation preferences were found, it was clear that the ice-cube hypercolumn was an oversimplification.[32] When optical imaging methods are used to reveal the relationship between orientation and ocular dominance columns, a complex picture is seen. In the experiment shown in Figure 3.14, cortical activity was imaged for eye-specific stimulation and for stimulation with a series of oriented bars. In Figure 3.14A, each orientation contour is indicated by a separate color (an iso-orientation contour) and ocular dominance columns are shown by dark lines. In Figure 3.14B ocular dominance columns are tinted pale or dark. The orientation pinwheels are clearly seen as the convergence of iso-orientation contours, and a set of contour lines between pinwheels typically crosses an ocular dominance boundary at right angles (as in the original Hubel and Wiesel hypercolumn). That is, most orientation domains are split into ipsilateral and contralateral halves, and thus serve the two eyes for that region of visual space. Each pinwheel center tends to occur near the center of an ocular dominance patch.[32,37]

Horizontal Intracortical Connections

In V1 additional connections have been described that suggest principles of organization in addition to those considered thus far. Whereas classic staining techniques (see Figure 3.2), such as Golgi impregnation, revealed a preponderance of neuronal processes that run perpendicularly from layer to layer, intracellular injections of single cells have demonstrated that cortical neurons also have long horizontal processes that

(A)

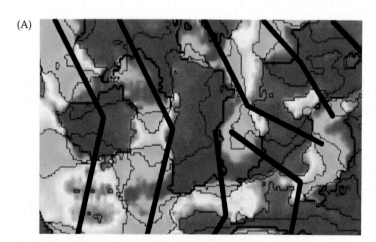

(B)

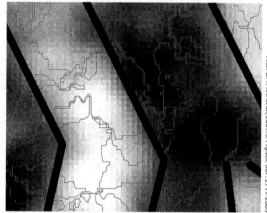

After D. Y. Ts'o et al., 2009. *J. Physiol.* 587: 2791–2805

FIGURE 3.14 Spatial Relation of Orientation and Ocular Dominance Columns in primate cortex revealed by imaging. (A) The broad, linear ocular dominance columns are separated by thick, dark lines. The orientation columns (i.e., pinwheels) are color-coded as in Figure 3.9, with yellow representing neuron populations responding to horizontally oriented visual stimuli and blue representing vertical preference. Intermediate orientations are red or green. (B) A closer view of the same area of cortex with the ocular dominance columns tinted dark (left eye) or pale (right eye). The centers of the pinwheels traced from (A) lie within the ocular dominance columns. Their contours, radiating around the clock, tend to cross the border of the ocular dominance column at right angles. While the picture is more complex than the original ice-cube model, the principles of organization remain similar.

(A)

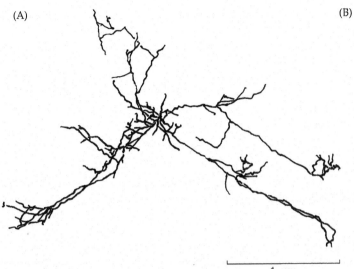

1 mm

(B)

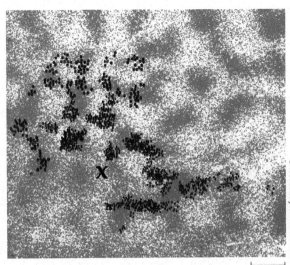

From C. D. Gilbert and T. N. Wiesel, 1989. *J. Neurosci.* 9: 2432-2442. © 1989 Society for Neuroscience

100 μm

FIGURE 3.15 Horizontal Connections in Visual Cortex.
(A) Surface view of pyramidal cell in cat V1, after labeling with horseradish peroxidase. The processes extended for nearly 3 mm across the cortical surface. Fine branches and synaptic boutons of this neuron occurred in several discrete clusters separated by 800 μm or more. (B) Labeled microspheres were injected into a region where cells had vertical orientation preference (large black "X"). The microspheres were taken up by axon terminals and transported back to the somata of cells projecting to the injection site. Vertical orientation columns were also labeled using 2-deoxy-glucose during stimulation with vertically oriented bars of light. The labeled microspheres were found in 2-deoxyglucose-labeled areas, showing that horizontal connections occurred between cells with the same orientation specificity. (A from C. D. Gilbert and T. N. Wiesel, 1983. *J. Neurosci.* 3: 1116-1133. © 1983 Society for Neuroscience.)

extend laterally from column to column (Figure 3.15).[56-58] Connections such as these contribute to the synthesis of elongated receptive fields of simple cells in layer 6 of V1: The receptive fields of layer 5 cells are combined and added end-to-end on the layer 6 simple cell by way of long horizontal axons. Many simple and complex cells are found with long horizontal projections that extend more than 8 mm, corresponding to several hypercolumns. An individual neuron can therefore integrate information over an area of retina several times larger than the receptive field measured by conventional electro-physiological techniques.

Of particular interest is the fact that connections are made only between columns that have similar orientation specificity. Evidence for such specific interconnections has been obtained by two additional methods. First, when labeled microbeads are injected into one column, they are transported to a distant hypercolumn with the same orientation preference (see Figure 3.15B). Second, the high degree of cross-correlation of the firing patterns of neurons with the same orientation preference in two widely separated columns indicates that the neurons are interconnected. Moreover, after a lesion is made in the retina, cortical cells that are deprived of input can show responses to distant stimuli that would be outside their normal receptive fields, thanks to inputs that existed previously but did not produce responses.[43]

In spite of its incompleteness, the original ice-cube scheme shown in Figure 3.13 still represents the simplest way to imagine how orientation, color, and eye preference may be combined. There remains the challenge of incorporating additional features of visual analysis, such as the perception of depth and movement, into a comprehensive scheme.

Construction of a Single, Unified Visual Field from Inputs Arising in Two Eyes

A problem arises from the fact that each half of the brain deals only with the visual field on the opposite side of the world. How are the representations in the two cortices knitted together to produce the single image of the world that we perceive? That each hemicortex is wired to build up the percept of one-half of the external world but not the other is a general property

[56] Gilbert, C. D., and Wiesel, T. N. 1989. *J. Neurosci.* 9: 2432-2442.

[57] Ts'o, D. Y., Gilbert, C. D., and Wiesel, T. N. 1986. *J. Neurosci.* 6: 1160-1170.

[58] Stettler, D. D. et al. 2002. *Neuron* 36: 739-750.

of the two hemispheres in relation to perception not just for vision, but also for sensations of touch and position. What happens at the midline? How do the two sides of our brain fuse the right world and the left world together with no hint of a seam or discontinuity?

The obvious way to preserve continuity is to join the left and the right visual fields together at the midline, in register. Such interactions would allow a complete picture to be formed with specific connections between the two hemispheres. There would, however, be little purpose in linking fields seen out of the corners of the two eyes that look on quite different parts of the world. As described in Box 3.1, highly specific connections between neurons with receptive fields exactly at the midline have been found experimentally to run from cortex to cortex through the **corpus callosum**.[59]

[59] Hubel, D. H., and Wiesel, T. N. 1967. *J. Neurophysiol.* 30: 1561-1573.

BOX 3.1 Corpus Callosum

The general question of how information is transferred between the hemispheres has been studied in humans and in monkeys by Sperry, Gazzaniga, Berlucchi, and their colleagues.[60-64] Concentrating on the coordinating role of the corpus callosum, a bundle of fibers that runs between the two hemispheres, they have shown that the fibers are involved in the transfer of information and learning from one hemisphere to the other. Thus, the fusing or knitting together of the two fields of vision is mediated by fibers in the corpus callosum. Certain cells have receptive fields that straddle the midline and receive information about both sides of the visual world. These cells lie at the boundary of V1 and V2, and they combine inputs from both hemispheres by way of the corpus callosum. Interestingly, these cells lie in layer 3, which contains neurons known to send their axons to other regions of cortex. The organization and orientation preference of two receptive fields that are brought together in this way are similar. Projections from nerve cells in one hemisphere to the other have been shown anatomically by injecting horseradish peroxidase into the cortex at the boundary of V1 and V2.[65] Enzyme taken up by terminals is transported to neuronal cell bodies situated at exactly corresponding sites in opposite hemispheres. Cutting or cooling the corpus callosum (which blocks conduction) causes the receptive field to shrink and become confined to just one side of the midline (the usual arrangement for cortical cells). Furthermore, recordings from single fibers in the callosum show that they have receptive fields close to the midline, not in the periphery.

The role of callosal fibers was clearly demonstrated in an experiment of Berlucchi and Rizzolatti.[62] They made a longitudinal cut through the optic chiasm, thereby severing all direct connections to the cortex from the contralateral eye. Yet provided the corpus callosum was intact, some cells in the cortex with fields close to the midline could still respond to appropriate visual stimulation of the contralateral eye.

The lateralization of cortical function is shown schematically in the figure. The left hand and left visual field project to the right hemisphere. The right hand and right visual field project to the left hemisphere, in which specialized language function resides.

[60] Sperry, R. W. 1970. *Proc. Res. Assoc. Nerv. Ment. Dis.* 48: 123-138.
[61] Gazzaniga, M. S. 2005. *Nat. Rev. Neurosci.* 6: 653-659.
[62] Berlucchi, G., and Rizzolatti, G. 1968. *Science* 159: 308-310.
[63] Glickstein, M., and Berlucchi, G. 2008. *Cortex* 44: 914-927.
[64] Doron, K. W., and Gazzaniga, M. S. 2008. *Cortex* 44: 1023-1029.

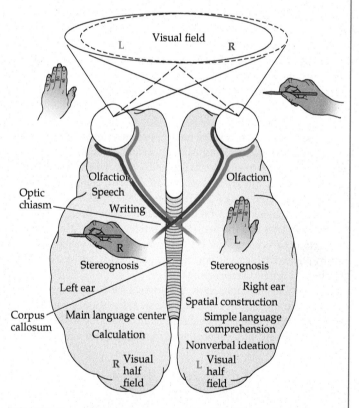

(After R. W. Sperry. 1970. In *Perception and its Disorders*, D. A. Hamburg et al., (Eds.), pp. 123-138. Williams & Wilkins, Baltimore, MD.)

Association Areas of Visual Cortex

In Chapter 25 we will describe how psychophysical measurements, electrical recordings, brain imaging, and studies of individuals with specific lesions have demonstrated the presence of physically separate brain regions beyond V1 (Figure 3.16), the visual association areas. These regions are concerned with different aspects of visual analysis, such as perception of depth, color,[66] movement, and faces.[16] We will show in Chapter 25, for example, that localized lesions of a small area (V4) lead to loss of all color vision: Individuals see everything in shades of black and white but have no defects in their memory, consciousness, or intellect.[10] Similarly, we will show that in another area, the middle temporal cortex (MT; also known as V5), neurons are clustered that respond specifically to movements in specific directions and to depth perception.

MT is of particular interest since experiments made in this area bear on a general question regarding all the studies described so far: Does a neuron that responds to a particular stimulus, say a vertical bar moving toward the left, actually take part in the perception of the event? Or is it simply a concomitant along the sensory pathway, perhaps superfluous to the precept itself? By stimulating and recording from single columns, Newsome and his colleagues have shown that individual columns and individual cells are indeed directly involved in the perception of movement in a specific direction.[67,68] Discussion of these elegant experiments requires more background knowledge and will be presented in Chapter 25.

[65] Shatz, C. J. 1977. *J. Comp. Neurol.* 173: 497–518.

[66] Zeki, S. et al. 1991. *J. Neurosci.* 11: 641–649.

[67] Cohen, M. R., and Newsome, W. T. 2004. *Curr. Opin. Neurobiol.* 14: 169–177.

[68] Cohen, M. R., and Newsome, W. T. 2009. *J. Neurosci.* 29: 6635–6648.

(A)

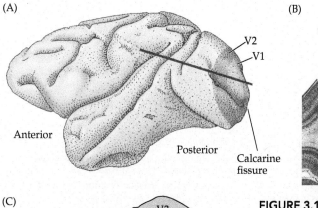

Anterior

Posterior

Calcarine fissure

V2
V1

(B)

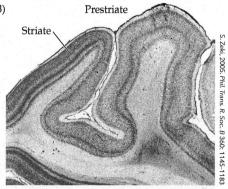

Prestriate

Striate

S. Zeki, 2005. *Phil. Trans. R. Soc. B* 360: 1145–1183

(C)

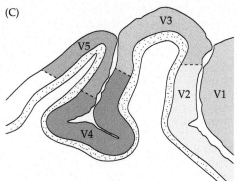

V3
V5
V4
V2
V1

FIGURE 3.16 Relation of Primary Visual Cortex (V1) to V2, V3, V4, and V5 in the Monkey. (A) The cortex and plane of section passing through V1 and V2. The boundary between V1 and V2 is unambiguous. (B,C) A section through the occipital cortex. In (B), the boundary between V1 (striate) and V2 (prestriate) occurs at the dotted line, where the striped appearance is lost. The boundaries between V2, V3, V4, and V5 are revealed by a combination of physiological and anatomical studies.

SUMMARY

- Inputs from the two eyes segregate to different layers of the lateral geniculate nucleus.

- The layers are in retinotopic register. Neurons in each layer are functionally distinct, comprising magnocellular-, parvocellular-, or koniocellular-response types.

- The six layers of primary visual cortex (V1) serve as input and output stages of cortical processing.

- Geniculate afferents from the two eyes are segregated in layer 4C of striate cortex, establishing ocular dominance columns that can be detected physiologically and anatomically.

- Magnocellular and parvocellular layers of the LGN project specifically to different sublayers of cortical layer 4C.

- Neurons in V1 are organized according to eye preference and orientation selectivity.

- Most cortical neurons receive input from corresponding points in the visual field of the two eyes.

- The layout of ocular dominance slabs and orientation pinwheels can be visualized by the imaging of activity-dependent optical signals from the brain surface.

- Iso-orientation contours tend to intersect ocular dominance domains at right angles, and each orientation domain is shared between two ocular dominance columns.

- Magnocellular, parvocellular, and koniocellular pathways form parallel channels from the retina to V1 and beyond.

- Small areas, called blobs, in the center of each ocular dominance column are revealed by cytochrome oxidase staining and code for color.

- Imaging techniques allow one to map projections to V1 and V2 as well as still more highly specialized regions concerned with the analysis of form, movement, color, and depth.

Suggested Reading

General Reviews

Callaway, E. M. 2005. Structure and function of parallel pathways in the primate early visual system. *J. Physiol.* 566: 13–19.

Cohen, M. R., and Newsome, W. T. 2004. What electrical microstimulation has revealed about the neural basis of cognition. *Curr. Opin. Neurobiol.* 14: 169–177.

Doron, K. W., and Gazzaniga, M. S. 2008. Neuroimaging techniques offer new perspectives on callosal transfer and interhemispheric communication. *Cortex* 44: 1023–1029.

Gilbert, C. D., and Wiesel, T. N. 1979. Morphology and intracortical projections of functionally characterised neurones in the cat visual cortex. *Nature* 280: 120–125.

Glickstein, M., and Berlucchi, G. 2008. Classical disconnection studies of the corpus callosum. *Cortex* 44: 914–927.

Hawkins, J., and Blakeslee, S. 2004. *On Intelligence.* Times Books, New York, NY.

Hubel, D. H., and Wiesel, T. N. 1977. Functional architecture of macaque monkey visual cortex (Ferrier Lecture). *Proc. R. Soc. Lond. B.* 198: 1–59.

Hubel, D. H., and Wiesel, T. N. 2005. *Visual Perception.* Oxford University Press, Oxford, UK. (This remarkable book contains all the papers by Hubel and Wiesel, as well as a stylish, informative, and witty commentary on how the work was done and what was found in later years by others.)

Mountcastle, V. B. 1997. The columnar organization of the neocortex. *Brain* 120: 701–722.

Sincich, L. C., and Horton, J. C. 2005. The circuitry of V1 AND V2: Integration of color, form, and motion. *Ann. Rev. Neurosci.* 28: 303–326.

Ts'o, D. Y, Zarella, M., and Burkitt, G. 2009. Whither the hypercolumn? *J. Physiol.* 587: 2791–2805.

Van Essen, D. C. 2005. Corticocortical and thalamocortical information flow in the primate visual system. *Prog. Brain Res.* 149: 173–185.

Zeki, S. (Ed.) 2005. Cerebral cartography 1905–2005. *Philos. Trans. R. Soc. Lond. B.* 360: 649–862.

Original Papers

Adams, D. L., Sincich, L. C., and Horton, J. C. 2007. Complete pattern of ocular dominance columns in human primary visual cortex. *J. Neurosci.* 27: 10391–10403.

Cohen, M. R., and Newsome, W. T. 2009. Estimates of the contribution of single neurons to perception depend on timescale and noise correlation. *J. Neurosci.* 29: 6635–6648.

Doron, K. W., and Gazzaniga, M. S. 2008. Neuroimaging techniques offer new perspectives on callosal transfer and interhemispheric communication. *Cortex* 44: 1023–1029.

Gilbert, C. D., and Wiesel, T. N. 1989. Columnar specificity of intrinsic horizontal and cortico-cortical connections in cat visual cortex. *J. Neurosci.* 9: 2432–2442.

Hubel, D. H., and Wiesel, T. N. 1959. Receptive fields of single neurones in the cat's striate cortex. *J. Physiol.* 148: 574–591.

Hubel, D. H., and Wiesel, T. N. 1968. Receptive fields and functional architecture of monkey striate cortex. *J. Physiol.* 195: 215–243.

LeVay, S., Hubel, D. H., and Wiesel, T. N. 1975. The pattern of ocular dominance columns in macaque visual cortex revealed by a reduced silver stain. *J. Comp. Neurol.* 159: 559–576.

Livingstone, M. S., and Hubel, D. 1988. Segregation of form, color, movement, and depth: Anatomy, physiology, and perception. *Science* 240: 740–749.

Ohki, K.-, Chung, S.-, Ch'ng, Y. H.-, Kara, P., and Reid, R. C. 2005. Functional imaging with cellular resolution reveals precise micro-architecture in visual cortex. *Nature* 433: 597–603.

Ohki, K., Chung, S., Kara, P., Hübener, M., Bonhoeffer, T., and Reid, R. C. 2006. Highly ordered arrangement of single neurons in orientation pinwheels. *Nature* 442: 925–928.

Tsao, D. Y., Freiwald, W. A., Tootell, R. B., and Livingstone, M. S. 2006. A cortical region consisting entirely of face-selective cells. *Science* 311: 670–674.

PART II

Electrical Properties of Neurons and Glia

This section deals with the functional and structural properties of the neuron that enable it to generate and transmit electrical signals, and sets the stage for following sections that deal with how neurons, once activated, transmit their signals from one to another in order to produce integrated behavior. We also include the general properties and functions of satellite glial cells, as a way to introduce some integrative properties of the nervous system at the cellular level.

We begin in Chapter 4 with the functional properties of ion channels in the nerve cell membrane. These channels determine the electrical characteristics of the neuron by allowing selective movement of ions into and out of the cell at rest and during signal generation. In Chapter 5 we discuss how the molecular structure of ion channels accounts for their ion selectivity and enables them to regulate ion movements in response to a variety of stimuli.

In Chapter 6 we move on to the behavior of the membrane as a whole and describe how its overall ion selectivity determines the resting membrane potential of the cell. Chapter 7 discusses in detail how selective activation of voltage-activated cation channels, principally sodium and potassium channels, leads to the generation of the action potential, which is the basis of all long-distance signaling in the nervous system. Chapter 8 describes how subthreshold "passive" signals spread in nerve fibers, and how the action potential, once initiated, is transmitted from one region of the neuron to the next.

In Chapter 9 we consider mechanisms for active transport of ions across the cell membrane, transport necessary to maintain the ionic composition of the cytoplasm in the face of constant leaks of ions into and out of the cell at rest and during electrical activity. Finally, in Chapter 10 we discuss the functional properties of glial cells and how glia and neurons interact during signal transmission.

CHAPTER 4

Ion Channels and Signaling

Electrical signals in nerve cells are all mediated by the flow of ions through pores in the nerve cell membrane. These pores are formed by transmembrane proteins called ion channels. It is possible to record and measure ion currents through single channels. In this chapter we discuss the functional properties of ion channels, such as their specificity for one ion species or another and how their activity is regulated. Most individual channels are selective for either cations or anions, and some cation channels are highly selective for a single ion species, such as sodium.

Channels fluctuate between open and closed states, often with a characteristic open time. Their contribution to the flow of ion current across the cell membrane is controlled by the relative amount of time they spend in the open state. Channel opening is regulated by a variety of mechanisms. Some of these are physical, such as changes in membrane tension, membrane potential, or temperature; others are chemical, involving the binding of activating molecules (ligands) to sites on the extracellular mouth of the channel or of particular ions or molecules to the inner mouth.

In addition to the kinetics of opening and closing, an important property of channels is the ability of an open channel to pass ion current. One way in which ions can pass through a channel is by simple diffusion; another is by interacting with internal binding sites, hopping from one to the next as the ions pass through the pore. In either case, movement through the channel is passive, driven by concentration gradients and by the electrical potential gradient across the membrane. The ability of ions to move through the open channel down their electrochemical gradients depends on the permeability of the channel to the ion species involved and to the concentration of the ions at either mouth of the channel. These two factors, permeability and concentration, determine the channel conductance.

In Chapter 1 we discussed how the transfer of information in the nervous system is mediated by two types of electrical signals in nerve cells: graded potentials, which are localized to specific regions of the nerve cell membrane, and action potentials, which may propagate along the entire length of a neuron. These signals are superimposed on a steady electrical potential across the cell membrane, called the **resting membrane potential**. Depending on cell type, nerve cells at rest have steady membrane potentials ranging from about −30 mV to almost −100 mV. The negative sign indicates that the inside of the membrane is negative with respect to the outside. Signaling in the nervous system is mediated by changes in the membrane potential. For example, in sensory receptors, an appropriate stimulus, such as touch, sound, or light, causes local **depolarization** (making the membrane potential less negative) or **hyperpolarization** (membrane potential more negative). Similarly, neurotransmitters at synapses act by depolarizing or hyperpolarizing the postsynaptic cell. **Action potentials**, which are large, brief pulses of depolarization and repolarization, propagate along axons to carry information from one place to the next in the nervous system.

Such changes in membrane potential are produced by the movement of ions across the nerve cell membrane. For example, inward movement of positively charged sodium ions reduces the net negative charge on the inner surface of the membrane, or in other words, causes depolarization. Conversely, outward movement of potassium ions results in an increase in net negative charge, causing hyperpolarization, as does inward movement of negatively charged chloride ions.

How do ions move across the cell membrane, and how is their movement regulated? The pathway for rapid movement of ions into and out of the cell is through **ion channels**, which are protein molecules that span the membrane and form pores through which ions can pass. Ion currents are regulated by controlling the rate at which these channels open and close. Thus, a variety of channel types in the membrane enable neurons to receive signals from the external world, or from other neurons, to carry signals over long distances, to modulate the activity of other neurons and effector organs, and to alter their own signaling properties in response to internal metabolic changes. All of the complexities of perception and analysis of neural signals depend ultimately on ion channel activity, as does the generation of complex motor outputs from the nervous system.

Properties of Ion Channels

The Nerve Cell Membrane

Cell membranes consist of a fluid mosaic of lipid and protein molecules. As shown in Figure 4.1A, the lipid molecules are arranged in a bilayer about 6 nm in thickness, with their polar, hydrophilic heads facing outward and their hydrophobic tails extending to the middle of the layer. The lipid is sparingly permeable to water and virtually impermeable to ions. Embedded in the lipid bilayer are protein molecules, some on the extracellular side, some facing the cytoplasm, and some spanning the membrane. Many of the membrane-spanning proteins form ion channels. Ions such as potassium, sodium, calcium, and chloride move through such channels passively, driven by concentration gradients and by the electrical potential across the membrane.

Another set of membrane-spanning proteins functions as **transport molecules** (pumps and transporters) that move substances across the membrane against their electrochemical gradients. Transport molecules maintain the ionic composition of the cytoplasm by pumping back across the cell membrane ion species that have leaked through channels into or out of the cell. They also perform the important function of carrying metabolic substances, such as glucose and amino acids, across cell membranes. Properties of transport molecules are discussed in Chapter 9.

What Does an Ion Channel Look Like?

The molecular composition of ion channels and their configuration in the cell membrane are discussed in detail in later chapters, but it is useful at this point to have some idea of the general physical features of an ion channel protein. These are illustrated in Figure 4.1B. The protein spans the membrane, with a central water-filled pore open to both the intracellular

(A)

(B)

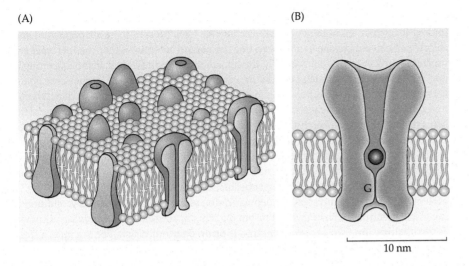

10 nm

FIGURE 4.1   Cell Membrane and Ion Channel. (A) The cell membrane is composed of a lipid bilayer embedded with proteins. Some of the proteins traverse the lipid layer, and some of these, in turn, form membrane channels. (B) Schematic representation of a membrane channel in cross section, with a central water-filled pore. The channel "gate" (G) opens and closes irregularly. Opening of the gate may be regulated by the membrane potential, the binding of a ligand to the channel, or other biophysical or biochemical conditions. A sodium ion, surrounded by a single shell of water molecules, is shown to scale in the pore for size comparison.

and extracellular spaces. On each side of the membrane, the pore widens to form a vestibule. Within the plane of the membrane, a segment of the pore is constricted and lined with a ring of negative charges to form a **selectivity filter** for cations. Conversely, a ring of positive charges would promote anion selectivity. Finally, the channel contains a **gate** that opens and closes to control ion movement through the channel. The size of the protein varies considerably from one channel type to the next, and some have additional structural features. Figure 4.1B represents a channel of medium dimensions.

Channel Selectivity

Membrane channels vary considerably in their selectivity: Some are permeable to cations, some to anions. Some cation channels are selective for a single ion species, and allow permeation of sodium, potassium, or calcium almost exclusively. Others are relatively nonspecific, allowing the passage of even small organic cations. Anion channels involved in signaling tend to have low specificity but are referred to as chloride channels, because chloride is the major permeant anion in biological solutions. There are also channels that connect adjacent cells (connexons) and allow the passage of most inorganic ions and many small organic molecules. These will be discussed in Chapter 8.

Open and Closed States

It is convenient to represent protein molecules as static structures; however, they are never still. Because of their thermal energies, all large molecules are inherently dynamic. At room temperature, chemical bonds stretch and relax, and twist and wave around their equilibrium positions. Although individual movements are only of the order of 10^{-12} meters in magnitude, with frequencies approaching 10^{13} Hz, such atomic trembling can underlie much larger and slower changes in conformation of the molecule. This is because numerous rapid motions of the atoms occasionally allow groups to slide by one another in spite of mutual repulsive interactions that would otherwise keep them in place. Such a transition, once achieved, can last for many milliseconds or even seconds. An example is hemoglobin, in which the binding sites for oxygen to the heme groups are buried inside the molecule and are not immediately accessible. Binding of oxygen, and its subsequent escape, can be accomplished only when a transient access pathway to the heme pocket is formed.[1]

In ion channel proteins, molecular transitions occur between open and closed states, with transitions between states being virtually instantaneous. If we examine the behavior of any given channel, we find that open times vary randomly—sometimes the channel opens for only a millisecond or less, sometimes for much longer (see Figure 4.5). However, each channel has its own characteristic **mean open time** (τ) around which individual open times fluctuate.

[1]Karplus, M., and Petsko, G. A. 1990. *Nature* 347: 631-639.

Some channels in the resting cell membrane open frequently; thus, the probability of finding such channels in the open state is relatively high. Most of these are potassium and chloride channels associated with the resting membrane potential. Other channel types are predominantly in the closed state, and the probability of an individual channel opening is low. When such channels are **activated** by an appropriate stimulus, the frequency of openings increases sharply. By contrast, channels that open frequently at rest may be **deactivated** by a stimulus (i.e., their frequency of opening is decreased). An important point to remember is that activation or deactivation of a channel means an increase or decrease in the frequency of channel opening, not an increase or decrease in the channel's mean open time.

In addition to activation and deactivation, there are two other conditions that regulate current flow through ion channels. The first is that certain channels can enter a conformational state in which activation no longer occurs, even though the activating stimulus is still present. In channels that respond to depolarization of the cell membrane, this condition is called **inactivation**; in channels that respond to chemical stimuli, the condition is known as **desensitization**. The second condition is **open channel block**. For example, a large molecule (such as a toxin) can bind to a channel and physically occlude the pore. Another example is the block of some cation channels by magnesium ions, which do not permeate the channel but bind in its inner mouth and prevent the permeation of other cations.

Modes of Activation

Figure 4.2 summarizes the modes of channel activation. Some channels respond specifically to physical changes in the nerve cell membrane. Prominent in this group are several voltage-activated channels. An example is the **voltage-sensitive sodium channel**, which is responsible for the regenerative depolarization that underlies the rising phase of the action potential (see Chapter 7). Also in this group are mechanically activated channels, responding, for example, to stretch of the cell membrane. These **mechanoreceptor channels** are found in a variety of cells that respond to mechanical stimulation, both inside and outside the nervous system (see Chapter 5).

Other channels are activated when chemical agonists attach to binding sites on the channel protein. These **ligand-activated channels** are further divided into two subgroups, depending on whether the binding sites are extracellular or intracellular. Those responding

(A) Channels activated by physical changes in the cell membrane

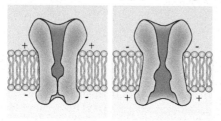 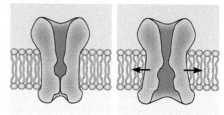

Voltage-activated   Mechanically-activated

(B) Channels activated by ligands

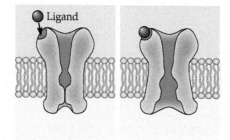 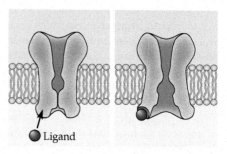

Extracellular activation   Intracellular activation

FIGURE 4.2 Modes of Channel Activation. The probability of channel opening is influenced by a variety of stimuli. (A) Some channels respond to changes in the physical state of the membrane, specifically: changes in membrane potential (voltage-activated) or mechanical distortion (mechanically activated). (B) Ligand-activated channels respond to chemical agonists, which attach to binding sites on the channel protein. Neurotransmitters, such as glycine and acetylcholine, act on extracellular binding sites. Included among a wide variety of intracellular ligands are calcium ions, subunits of G proteins, and cyclic nucleotides.

to extracellular activation include, for example, cation channels in the postsynaptic membranes of skeletal muscle that are activated by the neurotransmitter acetylcholine (ACh), released from presynaptic nerve terminals (see Chapter 11). This activation allows sodium to enter the cell, causing muscle depolarization. Channels activated intracellularly may be sensitive to local changes in concentration of a specific ion. For example, one type of potassium channel is activated by an increase in intracellular calcium concentration in the adjacent cytoplasm. In many neurons, these calcium-activated potassium channels play a role in repolarizing the membrane during termination of the action potential. Other intracellular ligands that modulate channel opening include the cyclic nucleotides: Cyclic GMP is responsible for the activation of cation channels in retinal rods, thereby playing an important role in visual transduction (see Chapter 22).

It should be noted that these classifications are not rigid: Some calcium-activated potassium channels are also voltage-sensitive, and some voltage-activated channels are sensitive to intracellular ligands.

Measurement of Single-Channel Currents

Intracellular Recording with Microelectrodes

The first experiments designed to examine the properties of membrane channels were done by measuring spontaneous fluctuations in membrane potential ("noise") during depolarization of the neuromuscular junction by the neurotransmitter acetylcholine. The membrane potential was measured using glass microelectrodes inserted into muscles at the junctional region. This method of recording membrane potential was introduced by Ling and Gerard in 1949.[2] Development of the method was a milestone as important as the introduction of patch clamp recording three decades later. The technique provided a method for accurate measurements of resting membrane potentials, action potentials, and responses to synaptic activation in muscle fibers and neurons.

The intracellular recording technique is illustrated in Figure 4.3A. A sharp glass micropipette, with a tip diameter of less than 0.5 μm and filled with a concentrated salt solution (e.g., 3*M* KCl), serves as an electrode and is connected to an amplifier to record the potential at the tip of the pipette. When the pipette is pushed against the cell membrane, penetration into the cytoplasm is

[2]Ling, G., and Gerard, R. W. 1949. *J. Cell Comp. Physiol.* 34: 383–396.

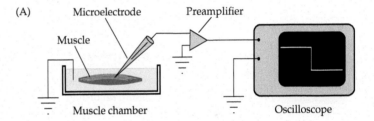

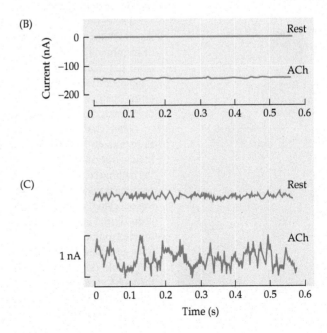

FIGURE 4.3 Intracellular Recording of Channel Noise. (A) Arrangement for recording membrane potentials of muscle fibers with a microelectrode. The electrode is connected to a preamplifier, and the signals are displayed on a computer screen. Penetration of the electrode into a fiber is marked by the sudden appearance of the resting potential (downward deflection on the screen). After penetration, changes in potential, resulting from channel activation, can be measured. (B) Intracellular records of the effect of acetylcholine (ACh). In this experiment, additional circuitry was used to record membrane current (rather than membrane potential). At rest (upper trace), there is no current across the membrane; application of ACh produces about 130 nanoamperes (nA) of inward current (lower trace). (C) Traces in (B) are shown at greater amplification. There is little fluctuation in the baseline at rest; the inward current produced by ACh shows relatively large fluctuations ("noise"), which is due to random opening and closing of ACh-activated channels. Analysis of the increased noise yields values for the single-channel current and mean open time of the channels. (Records modified from C. R. Anderson and C. F. Stevens, 1973. *J. Physiol.* 235: 665–691.)

[3]Katz, B., and Miledi, R. 1972. *J. Physiol.* 224: 665–699.

[4]Anderson, C. R., and Stevens, C. F. 1973. *J. Physiol.* 235: 665–691.

[5]Neher, E., Sakmann, B., and Steinbach, J. H. 1978. *Pflügers Arch.* 375: 219–228.

[6]Hamill, O. P. et al. 1981. *Pflügers Arch.* 391: 85–100.

signaled by the sudden appearance of the resting potential. If the penetration is successful, the membrane seals around the outer surface of the pipette, so that the cytoplasm remains isolated from the extracellular fluid.

Channel Noise

In the early 1970s, Katz and Miledi did pioneering experiments on frog muscle fibers, in which they used intracellular recording techniques to examine the characteristics of the noise produced by acetylcholine (ACh) at the neuromuscular junction.[3] At this synapse, ACh released from the presynaptic nerve terminal opens ligand-gated channels in the postsynaptic membrane. These channels allow cations to enter, thus depolarizing the muscle (see Chapter 11). Katz and Miledi applied ACh directly to the synaptic region and observed that the resulting depolarization was "noisy;" that is, during the depolarization, fluctuations in the electrical recording were larger than the normal baseline fluctuations at rest. This increase in noise was due to the random opening and closing of the ACh-activated channels. In other words, application of ACh resulted in the opening of a large number of channels, and this number fluctuated in a random way as ACh molecules bombarded the membrane.

By applying **noise analysis** techniques, Katz and Miledi were able to obtain information about the behavior of the individual channels activated by ACh. Subsequently, in similar experiments on the same preparation, Anderson and Stevens used fluctuations in membrane current to deduce the size and duration of ion currents through single channel[4] (Figure 4.3B,C).

Although noise analysis involves moderately complex algebra, the principles underlying it are straightforward. First, if the single-channel currents are relatively large, then the noise will be large as well. Second, channels that open for a relatively long time will produce only low-frequency noise; channels that open only briefly will produce higher frequency noise. Examination of the amplitude and the frequency composition of the noise produced by ACh-activated channels at the neuromuscular junction showed that about 10 million ions per second flowed through an open channel and that the mean open time (τ) of the channels was 1–2 milliseconds.

Patch Clamp Recording

Noise analysis has been supplanted by direct observation of channel currents, using **patch clamp recording** methods. These methods provide direct answers to questions of obvious physiological interest about channels. For example, how much current does a single channel carry? How long does a channel stay open? How do its open and closed times depend on voltage or on the activating molecule?

The development of the patch clamp by Erwin Neher, Bert Sakmann, and their colleagues[5,6] has made an enormous contribution to our knowledge of the functional behavior of membrane channels. Patch clamp recording methods involve sealing the tip of a small (ca. 1 μm internal diameter) glass pipette to the membrane of a cell (Figure 4.4A). Under ideal conditions, with slight suction on the pipette, a seal resistance of greater than 10^9 ohms (hence a gigaohm seal) is formed around the rim of the pipette tip between the cell membrane and the glass (Figure 4.4B).

Patch clamp methods permit several recording configurations. Having made a seal to form a **cell-attached patch**, one can then pull the patch from the cell to form an **inside-out patch** (Figure 4.4C), with the cytoplasmic face of the patch membrane facing the bathing solution. Alternatively, after forming a cell-attached patch, one can apply slight additional suction to rupture the membrane inside the patch and thereby provide access to the cell cytoplasm. In this condition, currents are recorded from the entire cell (**whole-cell recording**; Figure 4.4D). Finally, one may first obtain a whole-cell recording and then pull the electrode away from the cell to form a thin neck of membrane that separates and seals to form an **outside-out patch** (Figure 4.4E).

Whole-cell recording with a patch pipette provides a measure of macroscopic current through the cell membrane outside the patch. Recording from inside-out and outside-out patches enables detection of currents through individual membrane channels in the patch itself. Each type of patch has its own advantage, depending on the type of channels being

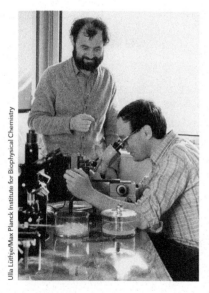

Erwin Neher and Bert Sakmann

Ulla Lüthje/Max Planck Institute for Biophysical Chemistry

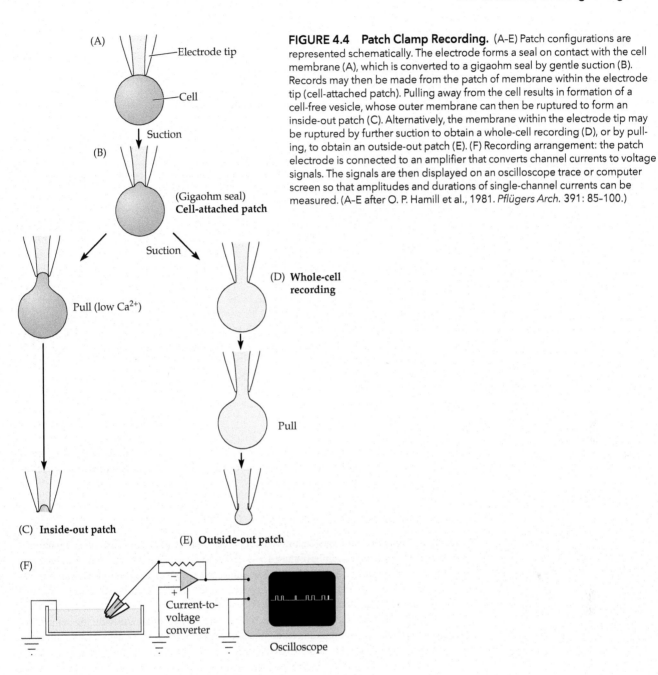

FIGURE 4.4 Patch Clamp Recording. (A–E) Patch configurations are represented schematically. The electrode forms a seal on contact with the cell membrane (A), which is converted to a gigaohm seal by gentle suction (B). Records may then be made from the patch of membrane within the electrode tip (cell-attached patch). Pulling away from the cell results in formation of a cell-free vesicle, whose outer membrane can then be ruptured to form an inside-out patch (C). Alternatively, the membrane within the electrode tip may be ruptured by further suction to obtain a whole-cell recording (D), or by pulling, to obtain an outside-out patch (E). (F) Recording arrangement: the patch electrode is connected to an amplifier that converts channel currents to voltage signals. The signals are then displayed on an oscilloscope trace or computer screen so that amplitudes and durations of single-channel currents can be measured. (A–E after O. P. Hamill et al., 1981. *Pflügers Arch.* 391: 85–100.)

studied and the kind of information one wishes to obtain. For example, if one wants to apply a variety of chemical ligands to the outer membrane of a patch, then an outside-out patch is most convenient.

One feature of whole-cell recording is that substances can move between the cell cytoplasm and the pipette. This feature (sometimes referred to as dialysis) can be useful in providing a method for changing the preexisting intracellular ion concentrations to match those in the pipette. However, particularly if the cell is small, important cytoplasmic components can be lost rapidly into the pipette solution. Such loss can be avoided by using a **perforated patch**.[7] The patch pipette is loaded with a pore-forming substance (e.g., the antibiotic nystatin) and a seal is formed to the cell. After a delay, pores are formed in the patch that allow whole-cell currents to be recorded without loss of intracellular macromolecules.

Whatever kind of patch is used, small currents across the patch membrane can be recorded by connecting the pipette to an appropriate amplifier (Figure 4.4F). The high-resistance seal ensures that such currents flow through the amplifier rather than

[7]Horn, R., and Marty, A. 1988. *J. Gen. Physiol.* 92: 145–149.

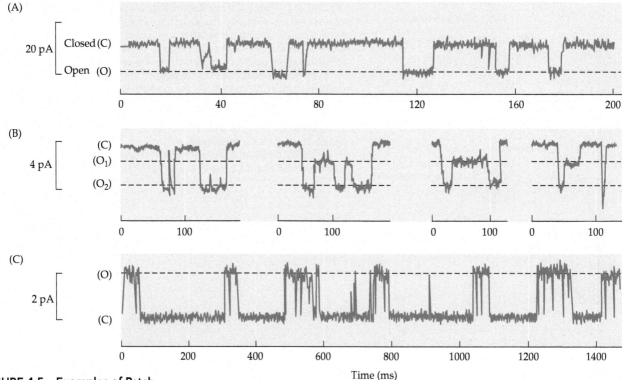

FIGURE 4.5 Examples of Patch Clamp Recordings. (A) Glutamate-activated channel currents recorded in a cell-attached patch from locust muscle occur irregularly, with a single amplitude and varied open times. Downward deflections indicate current flowing into the cell. (B) Acetylcholine-activated currents from single channels in an outside-out patch from cultured embryonic rat muscle reach a maximum amplitude of about 3 picoamperes (pA) and relax to a substate current of about 1.5 pA. Downward deflections indicate inward current. (C) Pulses of outward current through glycine-activated chloride channels in an outside-out patch from cultured chick spinal cord cells are interrupted by fast closing and reopening transitions, thereby producing bursts. (A after S. G. Cull-Candy et al., 1980. *J. Physiol.* 321: 195–210; B after O. P. Hamill and B. Sakmann, 1981. *Nature* 294: 462–464; C after A. I. McNiven and A. R. Martin, unpublished.)

escaping through the rim of the patch. The recorded events consist of rectangular pulses of current, reflecting the opening and closing of single channels. In other words, one observes in real time the activity of individual protein molecules in the membrane.

Single-Channel Currents

In their simplest form, single-channel current pulses appear irregularly, with nearly fixed amplitudes and variable durations (Figure 4.5A). However, in some cases current records are more complex. For instance, channels exhibit open states with more than one current level, as in Figure 4.5B, where the open channels often close to smaller "substate" levels. In addition, channels may display complicated kinetics, such as channel openings that occur in bursts (Figure 4.5C).

In summary, patch clamp techniques offer two advantages for studying the behavior of channels. First, the isolation of a small patch of membrane allows one to observe the activity of only a few channels, rather than the thousands that may be active in an intact cell; and second, the very high resistance of the seal enables one to record extremely small currents. As a result, one can obtain accurate measures of the amplitudes of single-channel currents and analyze the kinetic behavior of the channels.

Channel Conductance

The kinetic behavior of a channel—that is, the durations of its closed and open states—can provide information about the steps involved in channel opening and closing, and the rate constants associated with these steps. The channel current, by contrast, is a direct measure of how rapidly ions move through a channel. The current depends not only on channel properties but also on the transmembrane potential. The patch clamp recording system allows one to apply a voltage to the pipette solution and thereby produce a voltage difference across the membrane patch. Consider, for example, the outside-out membrane patch in Figure 4.6, which contains a single, spontaneously active channel that is permeable to potassium. The solutions in both the patch pipette and the bath contain 150 mM potassium. Potassium ions move in both directions through the open channel, but because the concentrations are equal, there is no net movement in either direction when no potential is applied to the pipette (see Figure 4.6B).

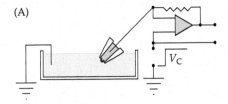

(B)

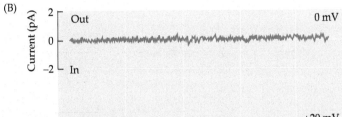

(C)

(D)

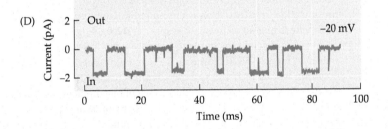

(E)

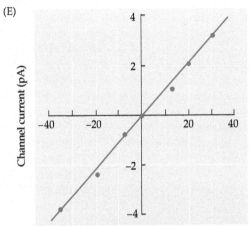

Patch potential (mV)

FIGURE 4.6 Effect of Potential on Currents through a single, spontaneously active potassium channel in an outside-out patch, with 150 mM potassium in both the electrode and the bathing solution. (A) The recording system. The output from the patch clamp amplifier is proportional to the current across the patch. A potential is applied to the electrode (and hence to the patch) by applying a command potential (V_C) to the amplifier as shown. Current flowing into the electrode is shown as negative. (B) When no potential is applied to the patch, no channel currents are seen, because there is no net flux of potassium through the channels. (C) Application of +20 mV to the electrode results in an outward current of about 2 pA through the channels. (D) A -20 mV potential results in inward channel currents of the same amplitude. (E) Channel currents as a function of applied voltage. The slope of the line indicates the channel conductance (γ). In this case γ = 110 picosiemens (pS).

When a voltage of +20 mV is applied (see Figure 4.6C), each channel opening results in a pulse of outward current, because positively charged potassium ions are driven outward through the channel by the electrical gradient between the pipette solution and the bath. However, when the inside is made negative by 20 mV (see Figure 4.6D), current flows in the other direction through the open channel into the pipette.

The effect of voltage on the size of the current is plotted in Figure 4.6E. The relationship is linear; the current (I) through the channel is proportional to the voltage applied to it:

$$I = \gamma (V - V_0)$$

Many readers will recognize this as an expression of Ohm's law. V_0 is the voltage across the membrane at which the current is zero, and ($V - V_0$) is the **driving force** for current through the channel. In this example $V_0 = 0$, but that is not always the case (see Figure 4.7). The constant of proportionality, γ, is called the **channel conductance**. It is a measure of the ability of the channel to pass current. For a particular applied voltage, a high conductance channel will carry a lot of current, while a low conductance channel will carry only a little.

The unit of conductance is the Siemens (S); 1 S = 1 ampere/volt. In nerve cells, the potential across the membrane is usually expressed in units of millivolts (1 mV = 10^{-3} V), currents through single channels in picoamperes (1 pA = 10^{-12} A), and conductances of single channels in picosiemens (1 pS = 10^{-12} S). In Figure 4.6E, a potential of +20 mV produces a current of about 2.2 pA, so the channel conductance ($\gamma = I/V$) is 2.2 pA/20 mV = 110 pS.

Conductance and Permeability

The conductance of a channel depends on two factors. The first is the ease with which ions can pass through the open channel; this is an intrinsic property of the channel known as the

channel permeability. The second is the concentration of the ions in the region of the channel. Clearly, if there are no potassium ions in the inside and outside solutions, there can be no current flow through an open potassium channel—no matter how large its permeability or how great a potential is applied. If only a few potassium ions are present, then for a given permeability and a given potential, the channel current will be smaller than when potassium ions are present in abundance. One way to think of these relationships is as follows:

> open channel → permeability
>
> permeability + ions → conductance

Equilibrium Potential

In the previous example of channel current in Figure 4.6, the concentration of potassium ions was the same on both sides of the membrane patch. What happens when we make the concentrations different? Imagine that we make an outside-out patch, as shown in Figure 4.7A, with potassium concentrations of 3 mM in the bath and 90 mM in the electrode (similar to normal extracellular and intracellular potassium concentrations for many cells). Under those conditions, potassium ions will move through the channels from the pipette to the bath down their concentration gradient, even when no potential is applied to the pipette (Figure 4.7B). If the pipette is made positive with respect to the bath, the potential gradient across the membrane will accelerate the outward potassium ion movement, and the channel current will increase (Figure 4.7C). However, if the pipette is made negative, outward movement of potassium will be retarded and the channel current will decrease (Figure 4.7D). With sufficiently large negativity, potassium ions will flow inward across the membrane against their concentration gradient (Figure 4.7E). If we make several such observations and plot channel current against applied voltage, the result is similar to that shown in Figure 4.7F.

Figure 4.7F illustrates that the potassium current through the channel depends on both the electrical potential across the membrane and on the potassium concentration gradient—that is, on the **electrochemical gradient** for potassium. Unlike the result when the potassium concentration was the same on both sides of the membrane (see Figure 4.6), the channel current is zero when the potential applied to the pipette is about –85 mV. In this condition, the concentration gradient, which would otherwise produce an outward flux of potassium through the channel, is balanced exactly by the electrical potential gradient that tends to move potassium inward. The potential that just balances the potassium concentration gradient is called the **potassium equilibrium potential**, E_K. When the membrane potential is at E_K, the driving force for potassium current is zero; at any other potential (V), the driving force is (V–E_K). The equilibrium potential depends only on the ion concentrations on either side of the membrane and not on the properties of the channel or the mechanism of ion permeation through the channel.

The Nernst Equation

Exactly how large a potential is required to balance a given potassium concentration difference across the membrane? One guess might be that E_K would be proportional simply to the difference between the inside concentration $[K]_i$ and the outside concentration $[K]_o$; however, this assumption is not quite right. It turns out instead that the required potential depends on the difference between the *logarithms* of the concentrations:

$$E_K = k\left(\ln[K]_o - \ln[K]_i\right)$$

The constant k is given by RT/zF, where R is the thermodynamic gas constant, T is the absolute temperature, z is the valence of the ion (in this case +1), and F is the Faraday (the number of coulombs of charge in one mole of monovalent ion). The answer, then, is

$$E_K = \frac{RT}{zF}\left(\ln[K]_o - \ln[K]\right)_i$$

which is the same as

$$E_K = \frac{RT}{zF} \ln \frac{[K]_o}{[K]_i}$$

This is the **Nernst equation** for potassium. RT/zF has the dimensions of volts and is equal to about 25 mV at room temperature (20°C). It is sometimes more convenient to use the logarithm to the base 10 (log) of the concentration ratio, rather than the natural logarithm (ln). Then RT/zF must be multiplied by ln (10), or 2.31, which gives a value of 58 mV.

In summary,

$$E_K = 25 \ln \frac{[K]_o}{[K]_i} = 58 \log \frac{[K]_o}{[K]_i}$$

At mammalian body temperature (37°C), 58 mV increases to about 61 mV. For the cell shown in Figure 4.7, the value of E_K (–85 mV) agrees with the given concentration ratio (1/30).

It should be noted that the rate of diffusion of an ion down a concentration gradient is not strictly related to its concentration. In all but the weakest solutions, ions are subject to interactions with one another, for example electrostatic attraction or repulsion. The result of such interactions is that the effective concentration of the ion is reduced. The effective concentration of an ion in solution is called its **activity**. In theory, the Nernst equation should be written with an activity ratio rather than a concentration ratio. However, because the total concentrations of ions inside and outside the cell are similar (see Chapter 6), the activity ratio for any particular ion is not significantly different from its concentration ratio.

Nonlinear Current-Voltage Relations

A second feature of the current–voltage relation shown in Figure 4.7F is that, unlike the one in Figure 4.6E, it is not linear. As we move away from the equilibrium potential in the depolarizing direction, the outward current increases more and more rapidly as the potential

(A)

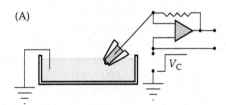

FIGURE 4.7 Reversal Potential for Potassium Currents in a hypothetical experiment using an outside-out patch with potassium concentrations of 90 mM in the recording pipette ("intracellular") and 3 mM in the bathing solution ("extracellular"). (A) Recording arrangement. (B) With no potential applied to the pipette, flux of potassium from the electrode to the bath along its concentration gradient produces outward channel currents. (C) When a potential of +20 mV is applied to the pipette, outward currents increase in amplitude. (D) Application of -50 mV to the pipette reduces outward currents. (E) At -100 mV, currents are reversed. (F) The current-voltage relation indicates zero current at -85 mV, which is the potassium equilibrium potential (E_K)

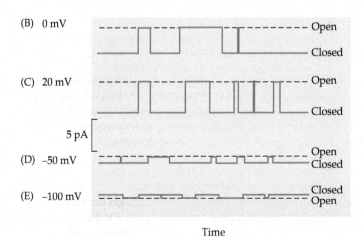

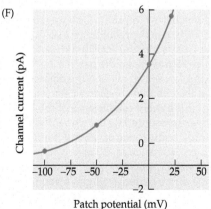

becomes more and more positive. Conversely, when the membrane is made more negative (hyperpolarized), the inward current increases more slowly with hyperpolarization. This is because of the dependence of conductance on concentration. There is a much higher potassium concentration inside the pipette than in the external solution. Consequently, there are more ions available to carry outward current than to carry inward current. The farther we move away from the equilibrium potential, the more prominent the effect becomes, so that the current–voltage relation has a marked upward curvature, even though, in this example, the channel permeability is quite independent of voltage.

Nonlinear current–voltage relations also occur in some channels because the channels themselves rectify (i.e., their permeability is voltage-dependent). One example is a voltage-sensitive potassium channel, called the **inward rectifier** channel, which allows potassium to move into the cell when the membrane potential is negative to the potassium equilibrium potential, but it permits little or no outward movement when the potential difference is reversed. Its current–voltage relation is similar to that shown in Box 4.1.

Ion Permeation through Channels

How do ions actually pass through channels? One way could be by diffusion through a water-filled pore. Diffusion formed the basis of early ideas about ion permeation, but for most channels diffusion does not provide an adequate description of the permeation process. This is because the channels themselves interact with the ions. For example, because they are charged, ions in solution are always accompanied by closely apposed water

---

BOX **4.1**   ## Measuring Channel Conductance

Investigators often state that some channel or other has a particular conductance, say 100 pS. Because conductance depends on concentration, such a statement tells us little unless we know the ionic conditions under which the measurement was made. For example, if the stated conductance is that of a potassium channel with a potassium concentration of 150 mM on either side of the membrane, then in a more physiological environment, with a potassium concentration of only 5 mM on the extracellular side, the channel conductance can be expected to be five to ten times smaller.

A second problem arises when the current-voltage relation is not linear, either because the ion concentrations on either side of the channel are not symmetrical (see Figure 4.7F), or because the channel itself is heavily rectifying. Under these circumstances, the conductance is not constant, and it is necessary to specify the potential at which it is measured. One way to define the conductance is to use the relation $\gamma = I/(V-V_0)$. In the accompanying illustration, the equilibrium potential for the current (V_0) is –75 mV. When the patch is held at V = –25 mV, the driving force is 50 mV and the channel current is 0.6 pA. Thus, the channel conductance is 0.6 pA/50 mV = 12 pS. This is the **chord conductance** of the channel at –25 mV, and is represented by the slope of the solid red line. The chord conductance at –25 mV is not the same as the chord conductance at –50 mV.

A second way of specifying conductance is to measure the slope of the current-voltage relation (dI/dV) at

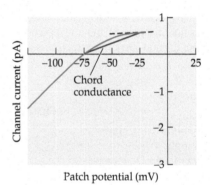

the point of interest. This is called the **slope conductance**. In this illustration, the slope of the current-voltage relation at –25 mV (dashed line) is about 3 pS. The measurement tells us that although the channel is passing a substantial current at –25 mV, it will not pass proportionally more as the driving force is increased.

In summary, the conductance characteristics of a channel can be specified precisely only by showing a complete current-voltage relation and by specifying the ionic conditions under which it was obtained. Single numbers given in the literature for channel conductance usually refer to chord conductance and, in the absence of additional information, provide only a rough indication of the channel characteristics.

molecules. In the case of cations, the water molecules are oriented so that the oxygen molecules, which carry net negative charges, lie closest to the ion. If the pore is relatively narrow, then an ion must acquire a certain amount of energy in order to escape from its associated waters of hydration and squeeze through the neck of the channel (see Chapter 5). Once in the channel, the ion may be attracted to, or repelled by, electrostatic charges lining the channel wall, or it may be bound to sites from which it must escape to continue its journey. Such interactions affect both ion selectivity and rate of ion flux through the channel. Channel models that deal with ion permeation in this way are called **Eyring rate theory** models.[8] In general, such models are more successful than simple diffusion models in describing channel selectivity and conductance.

An important point to remember is that all the ion fluxes that underlie signaling are due to ions moving passively through open channels along concentration and potential gradients. In other words, the neuron makes use of standing electrochemical gradients to generate ion movements, and hence to generate electrical signals. It is obvious that such fluxes would eventually dissipate the gradients. This does not happen, however, because cells use metabolic energy to maintain the ionic composition of the cytoplasm. Specialized mechanisms underlying the active transport of ions are discussed in Chapter 9.

[8]Johnson, F. H., Eyring, H., and Polissar, M. J. 1954. *The Kinetic Basis of Molecular Biology.* Wiley, New York.

SUMMARY

- Electrical signals in the nervous system are generated by the movement of ions across the nerve cell membrane. These ion currents flow through the aqueous pores of membrane proteins known as ion channels.

- Channels vary in their selectivity: Some cation channels allow only sodium, potassium, or calcium to pass, while others are less selective. Anion channels are relatively nonselective for smaller anions but pass mainly chloride ions because of the relative abundance of chloride in the extracellular and intracellular fluids.

- Channels fluctuate between open and closed states. Each channel has a characteristic mean open time. When channels are activated, their frequency of opening increases. Deactivation reduces opening frequency. Channels may also be inactivated or blocked.

- Channels can be classified by their mode of activation: mechanically activated, voltage-activated, and ligand-activated.

- Ions move through channels passively in response to concentration and electrical gradients across the membrane.

- The net flux of ions through a channel down a concentration gradient can be reduced by an opposing electrical gradient. The electrical potential that reduces the net flux to exactly zero is called the equilibrium potential for that ion species. The relation between equilibrium potential and the concentration gradient is given by the Nernst equation.

- The driving force for movement of an ion across the membrane is the difference between its equilibrium potential and the actual membrane potential. The flow of ion current through a channel depends on the driving force for the ion in question and on the conductance of the channel for that ion. The conductance depends, in turn, on the intrinsic ion permeability of the channel and, in addition, on the inside and outside ion concentrations.

Suggested Reading

Hamill, O. P., Marty, A., Neher, E., Sakmann, B., and Sigworth, J. 1981. Improved patch-clamp techniques for high-resolution current recording from cells and cell-free membrane patches. *Pflügers Arch.* 391: 85–100.

Hille, B. 2001. *Ion Channels in Excitable Membranes*, 3rd ed. Oxford University Press/Sinauer, Sunderland, MA. pp. 347–375.

Pun, R. Y. K., and Lecar, H. 2001. Patch clamp techniques and analysis. In N. Sperelakis (Ed.), *Cell Physiology Source Book*, 3rd ed. Academic Press, San Diego. pp. 441–453.

CHAPTER 5

Structure of Ion Channels

The molecular structure of ion channels has been resolved and related to their functional properties by a variety of experimental methods. These include biochemical isolation of channel proteins, molecular cloning to determine amino acid sequences of the proteins, site-directed mutagenesis to alter the sequences in selected locations, and expression of channel proteins in host cells to examine channel function. In addition, high-resolution electron microscopy and X-ray crystallography have revealed the three-dimensional structure of ion channels.

These combined experimental approaches have been applied most extensively to a ligand-activated channel, the nicotinic acetylcholine receptor (nAChR). The receptor is composed of five separate protein subunits, arranged around a central pore. Two of these—the α-subunits—contain receptors for the ligand. Each subunit contains a large extracellular domain, a smaller intracellular domain, and four membrane-spanning regions (M1–M4), connected by intracellular and extracellular loops. The five M2 regions line the pore and form the channel gating structure. The ACh receptor is representative of a genetic superfamily known as Cys-loop receptors, which include receptors for glycine, γ-aminobutyric acid (GABA), and 5-hydroxytryptamine (5-HT).

Voltage-activated channels form another superfamily. The voltage-activated sodium channel is a single large protein molecule with four repeating domains arranged around a central pore, each with six transmembrane segments (S1–S6). In each domain, the loop of amino acids between S5 and S6 dips into the center of the structure to contribute to the pore lining. Voltage-activated calcium channels have a similar structure. Voltage-activated potassium channels are similar in molecular configuration but with one important difference: Instead of being single molecules, they are assembled from four separate subunits.

Detailed knowledge of the molecular structure of the Cys-loop receptors and voltage-activated channels has provided a firm basis for analyzing the structure and function of other channel types.

For the nervous system to function properly, neurons must perform a widely varied repertoire of electrical behaviors. Thus, an impulse generated by one neuron may suppress the electrical activity of dozens of its neighbors, travel over long distances to excite other neuronal groups, and influence the responsiveness of still other target neurons in a variety of more subtle ways. All of these signals are mediated by the activation or deactivation of ion channels, thereby regulating the flow of ion currents across the nerve cell membranes. In this chapter we discuss experiments that have led to our current knowledge of the molecular structure of ion channels and how specific structural components are related to ion channel function.

Three experimental advances were instrumental in obtaining this information. The first was the development of techniques to isolate and sequence **complementary DNA (cDNA)** clones of channel proteins and thus obtain the corresponding amino acid sequences. These techniques also provide the opportunity to alter bases in the DNA (site-directed mutagenesis) and thereby substitute one amino acid for another at selected locations in the protein. The second advance was the development of techniques whereby messenger RNA (mRNA) derived from cDNA clones can be used to express channel proteins in host cells such as *Xenopus* oocytes. In this way, the functional properties of cloned channels can be measured. The combination of techniques makes it possible to tinker with specific regions of a channel molecule and then determine how such tinkering affects its function. For example, changing even a single amino acid can have a marked effect on the ion selectivity of a channel. Finally, refined electron microscope imaging procedures and X-ray crystallography have provided a detailed physical view of channel structure at the molecular level. These approaches have yielded remarkably detailed information about two particular channel types: ligand-activated channels, represented by the nicotinic acetylcholine receptor, and voltage-activated cation channels.

Ligand-Activated Channels

The Nicotinic Acetylcholine Receptor

The first channel to be studied in detail was the **nicotinic acetylcholine receptor (nAChR)**. Note that for ligand-activated channels, the word *receptor* rather than *channel* is used routinely; this is because characterization of such molecules has relied primarily on the binding of activating molecules (agonists), antagonists, toxins, and antibodies, rather than on the specific channel properties of the protein. Nicotinic acetylcholine receptors are expressed in postsynaptic membranes of vertebrate skeletal muscle fibers, in neurons throughout the nervous systems of invertebrates and vertebrates, and in the neuroeffector junctions of electric organs of several electric fish. The receptors are activated by ACh released from presynaptic nerve terminals, and upon activation, open to form channels through which cations can enter or leave the postsynaptic cell. They are designated *nicotinic* because the actions of ACh are mimicked by nicotine, and also to distinguish them from the very different AChRs that can be activated by muscarine. Muscarinic AChRs (see Chapter 11) do not form ion channels; instead, their activation sets in motion intracellular messenger systems that, in turn, affect ion channel activity.

Biochemical isolation and characterization of the nAChR were facilitated by the availability of a concentrated source of receptors—the remarkably dense assembly of synapses on electrocyte membranes in the electric organ of the ray *Torpedo*. The electrocytes of this and other strongly electric fish are modified muscle cells. Large numbers of them are arrayed anatomically, and when depolarized simultaneously they can produce, as a group, voltages approaching 100 volts, with currents sufficient to stun nearby prey in the surrounding water.

After extraction from the electrocyte membranes, nAChR molecules were separated from other membrane proteins by using their high affinity for α-bungarotoxin, a neurotoxin known to bind to channels with high specificity in intact electrocytes and in vertebrate muscle. Protein purification of the *Torpedo* nAChR yielded a 250-kilodalton (kD) complex, with two α-bungarotoxin binding sites. Separation on denaturing gels yielded four glycoprotein subunits (α, β, γ, and δ) of about 40, 50, 60, and 65 kD, respectively. Because toxin molecules bind to the α-subunit, and to account for the molecular weight of the intact protein, a pentameric structure (α2βγδ) was proposed.[1] The isolated nAChR was shown to retain the major functional properties of the native ion channel when reincorporated into lipid vesicles.[2]

The size and orientation of the intact channel with respect to the lipid membrane have been determined by electron imaging and by other physical techniques.[3–6] Figure 5.1 shows

[1]Raftery, M. A. et al. 1980. *Science* 208: 1454-1457.

[2]Tank, D. W. et al. 1983. *Proc. Natl. Acad. Sci. USA* 80: 5129-5133.

[3]Wise, D. S., Schoenborn, B. P., and Karlin, A. 1981. *J. Biol. Chem.* 256: 4124-4126.

[4]Unwin, N., Toyoshima, C., and Kubalek, E. 1988. *J. Cell Biol.* 107: 1123-1138.

[5]Toyoshima, C., and Unwin, N. 1988. *Nature* 336: 247-250.

[6]Unwin, N. 2005. *J. Mol. Biol.* 346: 967-989.

FIGURE 5.1 The ACh Receptor Consists of Five Subunits. There are two α-, one β-, one γ-, and one δ-subunits spaced radially in increments of about 72 degrees around a central pore. The extracellular domain extends about 8 nm above the plane of the membrane and contains a central vestibule about 2 nm in diameter, which leads into the transmembrane channel. The hatched area indicates the location of one of two binding sites on the α-subunits. The second one is on the other α-subunit, adjacent to the δ-subunit. The intracellular domain extends about 4 nm below the membrane, with five lateral openings between the subunits leading from the intracellular end of the channel to the cytoplasm. (After N. Unwin, 2005. *J. Mol. Biol.* 346: 967-989.)

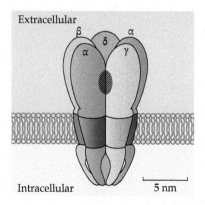

the channel's physical structure. The five subunits form a circular array around a central pore. The extracellular domain extends about 8 nm above the plane of the membrane and is about 8 nm in diameter, with a central vestibule 2 nm in diameter leading into the transmembrane channel. The hatched area indicates the location of one of two binding sites. The second one is on the other α-subunit, adjacent to the δ-subunit. The intracellular domain extends about 4 nm below the membrane, with five lateral openings between the subunits leading from the intracellular end of the channel to the cytoplasm. The pore of the open channel is about 0.7 nm in diameter, as predicted from earlier measurements of its selectivity to large cations.[7,8]

Amino Acid Sequence of AChR Subunits

The cDNA for each subunit was cloned and sequenced by S. Numa and his colleagues in 1982.[9-11] Figure 5.2 shows the corresponding amino acid sequence for the α-subunit from *Torpedo*. The sequences of the other three subunits are highly similar (homologous), with

[7] Maeno, T., Edwards, C., and Anraku, M. 1977. *J. Neurobiol.* 8: 173-184.

[8] Dwyer, T. M., Adams, D. J., and Hille, B. 1980. *J. Gen. Physiol.* 75: 469-492.

[9] Noda, M. et al. 1982. *Nature* 299: 793-797.

[10] Noda, M. et al. 1983. *Nature* 301: 251-255.

[11] Noda, M. et al. 1983. *Nature* 302: 528-532.

```
                                              Met Ile Leu Cys
 -20                        -10
Ser Tyr Trp His Val Gly Leu Val Leu Leu Leu Phe Ser Cys Cys Gly Leu Val Leu Gly

                            10                                        20
Ser Glu His Glu Thr Arg Leu Val Ala Asn Leu Leu Glu Asn Tyr Asn Lys Val Ile Arg

                            30                                        40
Pro Val Glu His His Thr His Phe Val Asp Ile Thr Val Gly Leu Gln Leu Ile Gln Leu

                            50                                        60
Ile Ser Val Asp Glu Val Asn Gln Ile Val Glu Thr Asn Val Arg Leu Arg Gln Gln Trp

                            70                                        80
Ile Asp Val Arg Leu Arg Trp Asn Pro Ala Asp Tyr Gly Gly Ile Lys Lys Ile Arg Leu

                            90                                        100
Pro Ser Asp Asp Val Trp Leu Pro Asp Leu Val Leu Tyr Asn Asn Ala Asp Gly Asp Phe

                            110                                       120
Ala Ile Val His Met Thr Lys Leu Leu Leu Asp Tyr Thr Gly Lys Ile Met Trp Thr Pro

                            130                                       140
Pro Ala Ile Phe Lys Ser Tyr Cys Glu Ile Ile Val Thr His Phe Pro Phe Asp Gln Gln

                            150                                       160
Asn Cys Thr Met Lys Leu Gly Ile Trp Thr Tyr Asp Gly Thr Lys Val Ser Ile Ser Pro

                            170                                       180
Glu Ser Asp Arg Pro Asp Leu Ser Thr Phe Met Leu Ser Gly Glu Trp Val Met Lys Asp

                            190                                       200
Tyr Arg Gly Trp Lys His Trp Val Tyr Tyr Thr Cys Cys Pro Asp Thr Pro Tyr Leu Asp

                            210                                       220
Ile Thr Tyr His Phe Ile Met Gln Arg Ile Pro Leu Tyr Phe Val Val Asn Val Ile Ile

                            230                                       240
Pro Cys Leu Leu Phe Ser Phe Leu Thr Gly Leu Val Phe Tyr Leu Pro Thr Asp Ser Gly
          M1
                            250                                       260
Glu Lys Met Thr Leu Ser Ile Ser Val Leu Leu Ser Leu Thr Val Phe Leu Leu Val Ile
                                            M2
                            270                                       280
Val Glu Leu Ile Pro Ser Thr Ser Ser Ala Val Pro Leu Ile Gly Lys Tyr Met Leu Phe

                            290                                       300
Thr Met Ile Phe Val Ile Ser Ser Ile Ile Ile Thr Val Val Val Ile Asn Thr His His
               M3
                            310                                       320
Arg Ser Pro Ser Thr His Thr Met Pro Gln Trp Val Arg Lys Ile Phe Ile Asp Thr Ile

                            330                                       340
Pro Asn Val Met Phe Phe Ser Thr Met Lys Arg Ala Ser Lys Glu Lys Gln Glu Asn Lys

                            350                                       360
Ile Phe Ala Asp Asp Ile Asp Ile Ser Asp Ile Ser Gly Lys Gln Val Thr Gly Glu Val

                            370                                       380
Ile Phe Gln Thr Pro Leu Ile Lys Asn Pro Asp Val Lys Ser Ala Ile Glu Gly Val Lys

                            390                                       400
Tyr Ile Ala Glu His Met Lys Ser Asp Glu Glu Ser Ser Asn Ala Ala Glu Glu Trp Lys
          MA
                            410                                       420
Tyr Val Ala Met Val Ile Asp His Ile Leu Leu Cys Val Phe Met Leu Ile Cys Ile Ile
                                                        M4
                            430
Gly Thr Val Ser Val Phe Ala Gly Arg Leu Ile Glu Leu Ser Gln Glu Gly
```

Met-Gly — Signal sequence

Cys — Cysteine residues linked by a disulfide bond

····· — Membrane-spanning α-helices

- - - — Helices in extracellular and intracellular spaces

MA — Helix within the cytoplasm

FIGURE 5.2 Amino Acid Sequence of the nAChR Receptor α-Subunit from Torpedo. Sequences in orange indicate membrane-spanning α-helices (M1, M2, M3, and M4); blue-labeled segments extend beyond the membrane plane into the extracellular and intracellular spaces. The helix labeled "MA" resides entirely within the cytoplasm. The underlined cysteine (Cys) residues, at positions 128 and 142, are linked by a disulfide bond, so that the intervening 13 residues form a Cys loop, characteristic of a large number of receptors. The initial underlined segment is the signal sequence. (Sequence after M. Noda et al., 1982. *Nature* 299: 793-797; designation of helical segments from N. Unwin, 2005. *J. Mol. Biol.* 346: 967-989.)

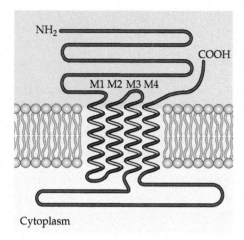

Cytoplasm

FIGURE 5.3   Model of the Tertiary Structure of an AChR Subunit, as proposed originally from amino acid sequence analysis. Regions M1 through M4 each form membrane-spanning helices, and both the carboxy terminal and the amino terminus of the peptide lie in the extracellular space.

various amino acid insertions and deletions, so that discussion of the structural configuration of any one subunit is generally applicable to the others. Sequences of subunits from human and bovine muscle are slightly different, and an additional subunit, similar to γ and designated ε, is found in fetal calf muscle.[12]

Higher Order Chemical Structure

Although the primary structure of the subunits does not provide unique information about how the polypeptide chains are arranged in the membrane, various models can be made, based on the characteristics of the amino acids in the sequence.

As with any very large protein, segments of the molecule can be expected to fold into ordered secondary structures, such as α-helices or β-sheets. These secondary structures themselves fold, producing a tertiary structure in each subunit. Finally, five subunits join together to form the complete quaternary structure (i.e., the channel). Models of the secondary and tertiary structures depend on several considerations, one being the identification of extended runs of nonpolar (and hence hydrophobic) amino acid residues in the primary sequence. Such sequences are capable of forming α-helices or other structures of sufficient length to span the membrane. In the original model proposed by Numa and his colleagues for the subunit structures,[9] four such regions were identified (M1–M4; see Figure 5.2), and the model shown in Figure 5.3 was postulated. The reader may find it useful to use the hydropathy indices (Box 5.1) of the amino acid residues in these regions to verify the validity of these conclusions.

How do we know which parts of the molecule are extracellular and which are intracellular? To begin with, the NH_2 terminus is preceded by a relatively hydrophobic region of 24 amino acids (see Figure 5.2), which is taken to be the signal sequence necessary for insertion of the protein into the membrane. Consequently, the NH_2 terminus is placed extracellularly. Consistent with this orientation is the fact that the two adjacent cysteine residues at positions 192 and 193 in the α-subunit are associated with the extracellular binding site for ACh. In addition, the initial extracellular segment constitutes about half of the entire molecule, which corresponds to the mass distribution of the intact receptor (see Figure 5.1). Given an even number of membrane crossings, the carboxylic acid (COOH) terminus is also extracellular. The general features of the model are in agreement with other observations. For example, when closely packed, AChRs aggregate in pairs (dimers) formed by disulfide bridges extending between cysteine residues near the COOH terminals of the subunits. These bridges have been shown to be extracellular.[13,14]

Other Nicotinic ACh Receptors

After the nAChR was sequenced, similar isolation and sequencing were carried out for subunits of neuronal nAChR from autonomic ganglia and from vertebrate brain. Subunits analogous to the muscle receptor α-subunit are identified by the presence of adjacent cysteine residues near the proximal end of the amino terminus (positions 192 and 193 in Figure 5.2). The remaining subunits are designated as β. Together with the subunits from electroplax and muscle, they form a family of common genetic origin.[15] To date, 12 subunits have been isolated from chicken and rat nervous systems: α_2–α_{10} and β_2–β_4. Injection into oocytes of mRNA for any one of α_2–α_6, or α_{10} with β_2, β_3, or β_4, results in the formation of heteromultimeric channels. Expression of α_7, α_8, or α_9 alone is sufficient for formation of homomultimeric channels. The existence of a large family of subunits available for channel formation enables them to combine selectively to form a diverse variety of channel isotypes with different functional properties, such as ion selectivity, conductance, and kinetics. We discuss specific examples related to functional properties of the nervous system in later chapters.

[12]Takai, T. et al. 1985. *Nature* 315: 761–764.

[13]McCrea, P. D., Popot, J.-L., and Engleman, D. M. 1987. *EMBO J.* 6: 3619–3626.

[14]DiPaola, M., Czajkowski, C., and Karlin, A. 1989. *J. Biol.Chem.* 264: 15457–15463.

[15]Millar, N. S., and Gotti, C. 2009. *Neuropharmacology* 56: 237–246.

| BOX **5.1** | Classification of Amino Acids |

Channel subunits, like all other peptides, are composed of amino acids, and it is the amino acid side chains that determine many of the local chemical and physical properties of the subunits. The 20 amino acids fall into three groups: neutral, acidic, and basic, as shown (parentheses contain three-letter and one-letter abbreviations). Acidic and basic amino acids are hydrophilic. The neutral amino acids are arranged according to hydropathy indices (numbers below each amino acid) proposed by Kyte and

Doolittle,[16] starting with the most hydrophobic (positive numbers) and progressing to the most hydrophilic (negative numbers). Sections of a peptide are candidates for membrane-spanning regions if they contain sequences of hydrophobic amino acids capable of forming an α-helix long enough to traverse the lipid bilayer (about 20 amino acid residues; see Figure 5.2).

[16]Kyte, J., and Doolittle, R. F. 1982. *J. Mol. Biol.* 157: 105–132.

NEUTRAL

| Strongly Hydrophobic | | | | | | Weakly Hydrophobic |

Isoleucine (Ile, I)	Valine (Val, V)	Leucine (Leu, L)	Phenylalanine (Phe, F)	Cysteine (Cys, C)	Methionine (Met, M)	Alanine (Ala, A)
4.5	4.2	3.8	2.8	2.5	1.9	1.8

| Weakly Hydrophilic | | | | | | Strongly Hydrophilic |

Glycine (Gly, G)	Threonine (Thr, T)	Serine (Ser, S)	Tryptophan (Trp, W)	Tyrosine (Tyr, Y)	Proline (Pro, P)	Glutamine (Gln, Q)	Asparagine (Asn, N)
−0.4	−0.7	−0.8	−0.9	−1.3	−1.6	−3.5	−3.5

| ACIDIC | | | BASIC | | |

Aspartic acid (Asp, D)	Glutamic acid (Glu, E)		Histidine (His, H)	Lysine (Lys, K)	Arginine (Arg, R)
−3.5	−3.5		−3.2	−3.9	−4.5

A Receptor Superfamily

While the amino acid sequence and chemical structure of the nAChR were being determined, it became apparent that other channel-forming receptors were similar in molecular composition. We now know that the nAChR is a member of a large **superfamily** of channel-forming receptors, known collectively as **Cys-loop receptors**, so called because all subunits in the superfamily have a pair of disulfide-bonded cysteines (Cys 128 and Cys 142 in Figure 5.2) separated by 13 amino acid residues. Other members of the superfamily include receptors for serotonin (**5-HT$_3$** and **MOD-1 receptors**), the **glycine receptor**

(**GlyR**), receptors for γ-aminobutyric acid (**GABA**$_A$ and the invertebrate **EXP-1 receptors**), an invertebrate **glutamate-gated chloride receptor (GluCl)**, and a receptor activated by ionic zinc (**ZAC**).[17]

The 5-HT$_3$ receptors form cation channels with functional properties similar to those of nAChR.[18] Similarly, the GABA-activated EXP-1 channel[19] and the ZAC channel[20] are both cation-selective. EXP-1 is found in invertebrates, and ZAC sequences have been identified in human and rat genomes. The remaining members of the superfamily form channels that are anion-selective. GABA$_A$ receptors,[21] together with GlyR,[22] subserve inhibitory synaptic transmission in vertebrate and invertebrate nervous systems (see Chapter 11). MOD-1 channels[23] and GluCl channels[24] are found only in invertebrates.

Like the nAChR, each receptor type has several subunit isotypes. For example, 16 different GABA$_A$ subunit polypeptides have been identified in vertebrates by recombinant DNA techniques: α_1–α_6, β_1–β_3, γ_1–γ_3, δ, ε, π, and θ.

Three additional ρ subunits contribute to GABA$_A$ variants, formerly specified separately as GABA$_C$ receptors.[21] Five GlyR subunits have been identified, four α and one β.[22] Two 5-HT$_3$ receptor subunits, 5-HT$_{3A}$ and 5-HT$_{3B}$, have been described, and genes for three additional homologous polypeptides (5-HT$_{3C}$–5-HT$_{3E}$) have been isolated.[25]

Receptor Structure and Function

Two techniques have been essential in determining the relations between receptor structure and function. The first, site-directed mutagenesis, involves the construction of mutant cDNAs, with mutations directed at a particular site in the receptor protein, such that selected amino acids with particular properties (e.g., positively or negatively charged, highly polar or nonpolar) are replaced by others with different properties. The second technique is the expression of mutant receptors in host cells, such as *Xenopus* oocytes, subsequent to injection of mRNA encoding the mutated nAChRs. Oocytes typically do not express nAChRs or other ligand-activated channels in their membranes. Yet after the mutant message has been injected, they not only express the protein subunits but also assemble them in the membrane to form functionally active channels.[26] In such experiments, electrical recording techniques are used to measure the characteristics of single-channel currents or whole-cell currents (representing the behavior of the entire population of inserted channels). Various mutations have been found that affect ligand binding and thereby channel activation, while other mutations affect the ion selectivity of the channels and channel conductance. Some of the mutations affecting selectivity and conductance are located on the M2 helices, suggesting that these form the lining of the open channel (see Figure 5.5).

Structure of the Pore Lining

In order to examine the idea that the M2 helices line the open channel pore, it is useful to consider in more detail their amino acid sequences. These are as follows for mouse nAChR α- and δ-subunits, going from cytoplasm (E [Glu] 241; see Figure 5.2) to extracellular fluid:

<pre>
        -1'   1'   3'   5'   7'   9'   11' 13' 15' 17' 19'
α: E K M T L S I S V L L S L T V F L L V I V E
(Intracellular)   (Extracellular)
δ: E K T S V A I S V L L A Q S V F L L L I S Q
</pre>

The primed numbering system enables comparison between M2 regions of different receptor subunits.[27] It starts at zero at the predicted cytoplasmic end of the helix and proceeds toward the extracellular region.

We might expect the hydrophilic amino acids (see Box 5.1), such as the serines (S) and threonines (T), to be exposed to the aqueous pore, whereas the more hydrophobic isoleucines (I), for example, would be nestled against the membrane lipid or other parts of the protein. In accordance with this idea, replacing the serine in the underlined positions (6') with alanine (which is weakly hydrophobic) produced a marked reduction in channel conductance.[28] In addition, the binding affinity for the molecule QX222, which binds readily

[17] Lester, H. A. et al. 2004. *Trends Neurosci.* 27: 329–336.

[18] Peters, J. A., Hales, T. G., and Lambert, J. J. 2006. *Trends Pharmacol. Sci.* 26: 587–594.

[19] Beg, A. A., and Jorgensen, E. M. 2003. *Nat. Neurosci.* 6: 1145–1152.

[20] Davies, P. A. et al. 2003. *J. Biol. Chem.* 278: 712–717.

[21] Olsen, R. W., and Sieghart, W. 2009. *Neuropharmacology* 56: 141–148.

[22] Lynch, J. W. 2009. *Neuropharmacology* 56: 303–309.

[23] Ranganathan, R., Cannon, S. C., and Horvitz, H. R. 2000. *Nature* 408: 470–475.

[24] Cully, D. S. et al. 1994. *Nature* 371: 707–711.

[25] Niesler, B. et al. 2003. *Gene* 310: 101–111.

[26] Miledi, R., Parker, I., and Sumikawa, K. 1983. *Proc. R. Soc. Lond., B., Biol. Sci.* 218: 481–484.

[27] Charnet, P. et al. 1990. *Neuron* 4: 87–95.

[28] Leonard, R. J. et al. 1988. *Science* 242: 1578–1581.

to the open channel in the native receptor, was greatly reduced. These effects are consistent with the idea that the serine residues are exposed to the aqueous channel.

Not all of the exposed amino acids are hydrophilic, however. The residues highlighted in color in the α-subunit sequence illustrated here, which include leucine and valine at positions 9′, 13′ and 16′, all appear to contribute to the pore lining. These were identified by Karlin and his colleagues with a technique known as cysteine scanning, in which residues are mutated, one at a time, to cysteine.[29] Mutant α-subunits were expressed in oocytes together with wild-type β, γ, and δ counterparts. Membrane currents produced by ACh were measured before and after exposure of the oocyte to the hydrophilic reagent methanethiosulfonate ethylammonium (MTSEA). The reagent reacts selectively with the cysteine sulfhydryl group, but it can only do so if the substituted cysteine is at a water-accessible position on the subunit (i.e., exposed to the aqueous pore). The reagent attenuated the responses to ACh only in channels with α-subunit mutations in the highlighted positions. The pattern of exposure is consistent with the idea that the identified residues reside along one side of a helical sequence.

Analogous experiments were done by Changeux and his colleagues on native nAChR by locating binding sites for chlorpromazine, a molecule that blocks ion flux through the channel.[30,31] Tritiated chlorpromazine was made to react with amino acid side chains within the open channel in response to an intense flash of ultraviolet light (photolabeling). The channel subunits were then isolated and scanned for radioactivity. Consistent with the substituted cysteine experiments, the radioactive label was present in all four subunits only on the M2 segments, and was located at positions 2′, 6′, and 9′.

High-Resolution Imaging of the nAChR

A powerful approach to the question of channel topology is the use of high-resolution electron microscopy. Unwin and his colleagues have applied this technique to nAChRs from *Torpedo* electric organs.[6] Isolated membranes from the electrocytes assemble readily into tubular vesicles, with the receptors themselves arrayed in an orderly lattice, as shown in the low-power micrographs of Figure 5.4A. Higher-magnification images reveal the general shape and orientation of the receptor in the membrane (Figure 5.4B,C).

By using very large numbers of images and combining digital averaging techniques with crystallographic analysis, Unwin and his colleagues were able to describe in detail the structure of the receptor at the molecular level with a resolution of 0.4 nm. The results are summarized in Figure 5.5, which shows a view of two of the five subunits on either side of the central pore.

The extracellular domain of each subunit is built around a sequence of β-strands and their associated connecting loops, arranged into outer (red) and inner (blue) sheets. This arrangement is closely analogous to the crystal structure of another molecule, acetylcholine-binding protein (AChBP), described in detail by Brejc and his colleagues.[32] AChBP is a soluble protein that is secreted by snail glial cells at cholinergic synapses. Like the nAChR, it is composed of five subunits, and it modulates synaptic transmission by binding ACh in the synaptic cleft.

[29] Karlin, A. 2002. *Nat. Rev. Neurosci.* 3: 102–114.

[30] Giraudat, J. et al. 1986. *Proc. Natl. Acad. Sci. USA* 83: 2719–2723.

[31] Giraudat, J. et al. 1987. *Biochemistry* 26: 2410–2418.

[32] Brejc, K. et al. 2001. *Nature* 4 11: 269–276.

(A)   (B)   (C)

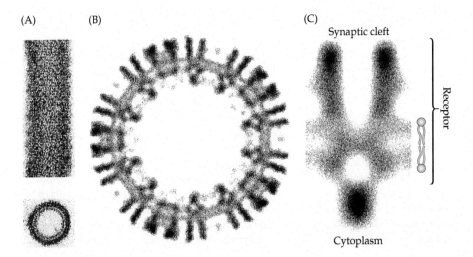

Synaptic cleft

Receptor

Cytoplasm

FIGURE 5.4 Electron Microscope Images of Acetylcholine Receptors. (A) Longitudinal and transverse images of cylindrical vesicles from postsynaptic membranes of *Torpedo*, showing closely packed ACh receptors. (B) Transverse section of the tube at higher magnification. (C) Further enlarged image of a single receptor, showing its position and size relative to the membrane bilayer. The dense blob under the receptor is an intracellular receptor-associated protein. (Courtesy of N. Unwin.)

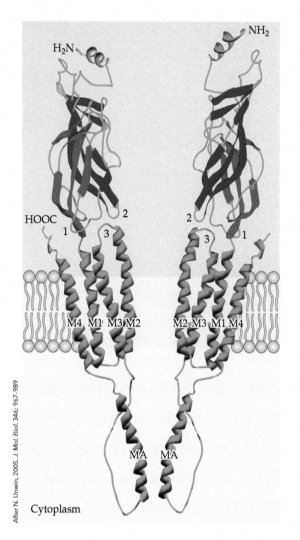

After N. Unwin, 2005. *J. Mol. Biol. 346: 967-989*

FIGURE 5.5 High-Resolution Structure of nAChR Subunits.
Schematic view of two subunits, flanking the central cavity. The extracellular domain of each subunit is built around a sequence of β-strands and their associated connecting loops, arranged into outer (red) and inner (blue) sheets. It is connected to the first membrane-spanning α-helix, M1. The second α-helix, M2, lies central to the other three, so that the complete set of five M2 helices forms the pore lining. The intracellular domain is formed by the sequence between M3 and M4, including the α-helix MA. Ligand binding to the extracellular domain causes reorientation of the inner and outer β-strands; this movement is transmitted to the pore region by interaction between one or more extracellular loops (1, 2) and the M2-M3 loop (3).

In general then, the transmembrane regions of all nAChR subunits are composed of the α-helices M1–M4 and are joined to the extracellular domains at the beginning of M1. The M2 helix lies central to the other three, so that the five M2 segments together form the pore lining. The intracellular portions are formed by the sequences between M3 and M4, including the α-helix MA.

The techniques of high-resolution imaging have provided a remarkably detailed picture of the ACh receptor and of other membrane channels. Even finer structural detail has been obtained using cryo-electron microscopy.[33]

Receptor Activation

Binding of ACh to the nAChR results in structural modification of the extracellular domains of the two α-subunits.[34,35] How this structural rearrangement leads to functional activation has been studied by Unwin and Fujiyoshi using a remarkable technique called plunge freezing.[36] Preparations of nACh receptors on microscope grids were plunged into liquid nitrogen–cooled methane within 10 ms after being sprayed with droplets containing 100 mM ACh, thereby trapping the receptors in the open-channel state. This allowed detailed study by electron crystallography of structural changes associated with channel opening. The structural rearrangements of the α-subunits were found to be transmitted non-uniformly to the adjacent subunits. The largest structural displacements were in the β- and γ-subunits, the most prominent being that transmitted from αγ to β. The δ-subunit moved the least.

The extracellular part of each subunit interacts through connecting loops with ends of the M1–M4 membrane segments, and with the M2–M3 loop (see Figure 5.5). Extracellular displacement of the β-subunit is particularly tightly coupled across the loop region, producing displacement of the membrane helices. In response to the displacement of αγ, the extracellular part of β moves outward, its base tilting away from the axis of the receptor. This tilting motion is transmitted to the underlying helices, including M2. M2 helices vary slightly in structural detail. For example, in the closed channel, δM2 and particularly αγM2 are bowed slightly inward (Figure 5.6A). Outward movement of the β-subunit (lying between αγ and δ) causes them to straighten (Figure 5.6B). The combined movements of the βM2, αγM2, and δM2 helices modulate the dimensions of the pore, allowing access to the channel gate.

Observations have been made of the X-ray structure of a family of bacterial ligand-gated membrane channels in the open and closed states.[37–39] These channels are analogous in structure to mammalian Cys-loop receptors and are activated by protons. In the closed state, the channels are constricted by a ring of hydrophobic side chains in M2, equivalent to those at L9′ and V13′ in the mammalian channel (Figure 5.6C). Upon activation, the constriction is removed by outward displacement of the M2 helices (Figure 5.6D).

The M2 peptides, when expressed alone in lipid bilayers, form channels with selectivity and conductances similar to those of native nAChR channels from *Torpedo*.[40] In addition, spontaneously occurring channel currents are recorded with mean open times similar to those of native channel currents. Thus, it appears that current flow through the open channel is regulated by spontaneous fluctuations within the channel structure itself, perhaps in the region of the hydrophobic rings or at the more constricted cytoplasmic end of the pore.

[33] Fernandez-Liero, R., and Scheres, S. H. W. 2016. *Nature* 537: 339-346.

[34] Unwin, N. 1995. *Nature* 373: 37-43.

[35] Unwin, N. et al. 2002. *J. Mol. Biol.* 319: 1165-1176.

[36] Unwin, N., and Fujiyoshi, Y. 2012. *J. Mol. Biol.* 422: 617-634.

[37] Bocquet, N. et al. 2009. *Nature* 457: 111-114.

[38] Hilf, R. J., and Dutzler, R. 2008. *Nature* 452: 375-379.

[39] Hilf, R. J., and Dutzler, R. 2009. *Nature* 457: 115-118.

[40] Montal, M. O. et al. 1993. *FEBS Lett.* 320: 261-266.

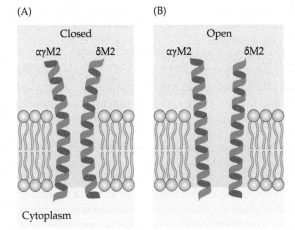

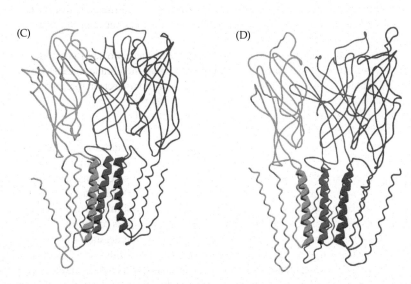

FIGURE 5.6 Receptor Channel Gating. (A,B) M2 helices from the α- and δ-subunits of the nACh receptor in the closed (A) and open (B) state. In the closed state, the helices bow inward, forming a hydrophobic constriction that is believed to function as the gate. In the open state, the helices straighten, increasing the dimensions of the pore and allowing access to the gating region. Smaller changes occur in the αδM2, βM2, and γM2 helices. (C,D) X-ray structure of an analogous bacterial ligand-gated channel, showing three of the M2 helices in the closed (C) and open (D) state. (A,B after N. Unwin and Y. Fujiyoshi, 2012. *J. Mol. Biol.* 422: 617–634; C,D after V. Tsetlin and F. Hucho, 2009. *Curr. Opin. Pharmacol.* 9: 306–310.)

Ion Selectivity and Conductance

The open channel is narrowest in the 2′ region, with a pore diameter of about 0.6 nm in anion channels and 0.8 nm in cation channels.[41] This region is therefore assumed to be critical for ion selectivity and conductance. In the nAChR, substituting the threonine at position 2′ with different residues illustrates the importance of both pore size and polarity. Polar substitutions result in higher channel conductance than do nonpolar substitutions, and for both classes, conductance decreases with increasing side chain volume of the substituted residue.[42,43]

One surprising characteristic of the Cys-loop receptors is that they include both cation- and anion-selective channels. The differences in charge selectivity are related to differences in the sign of the charged residues along the ion pathway.[41] If we examine the amino acid sequence in the M2 subunits, we find that nAChRs (and 5-HT₃ receptors) have a negatively charged residue (E⁻) at position –1′, just at the cytoplasmic surface, and another extracellularly at position 20′. Thus, the five M2 helices surround the pore with two distinct negatively charged rings that can be expected to promote cation selectivity. In glycine (and GABA) receptors, the corresponding residues at positions –1′ and 20′ are either positive or neutral (A⁰):

		−1′	1′																				19′	20′
AChR	α7	E⁻	K⁺	I	S	L	G	I	T	V	L	L	S	L	T	V	F	M	L	L	V	A⁰	E⁻
GlyR	α1	A⁰	R⁺	V	G	L	G	I	T	T	V	L	T	M	T	T	Q	S	S	G	S	R⁺	A⁰

When the M2 residues in neuronal nAChR homomultimeric α7 channels are altered to mimic those in GlyR channels, the channel selectivity is changed from cationic to anionic.[44] Conversely, the reverse mutations in the GlyR produce cation-selective channels.[45] Charge

[41] Keramidas, A. et al. 2004. *Prog. Biophys. Mol. Biol.* 86: 161–204.

[42] Imoto, K. et al. 1991. *FEBS Lett.* 289: 193–200.

[43] Villarroel, A. et al. 1991. *Proc. R. Soc. Lond., B., Biol. Sci.* 243: 69–74.

[44] Galzi, J.-L. et al. 1992. *Nature* 359: 500–505.

[45] Keramidas, A. et al. 2000. *Biophys. J.* 78: 247–259.

selectivity of GABAC and 5-HT3A channels is also reversed by similar mutations.[46,47] Thus, anion channels require positively charged residues at position $-1'$, and cation channels require negative residues in the same position.

Apart from determining charge selectivity of the channel, the charged rings have a marked effect on channel conductance.[48] In the nAChR, reducing the charge on the intracellular ring has the greatest effect, resulting in a reduction in both inward and outward current. Charge reduction in the outer ring also reduces conductance, with a greater effect on inward current. Similar observations have been made on GlyR- and GABA-activated channels.[46]

Other segments of the ion pathway also contribute to ion selectivity and conductance. In the cation-selective channels, the walls of the channel vestibules have a net excess of negative charges, while in anion-selective channels the excess is positive. The outer vestibule is about 2 nm in diameter, and the effective radius for electrostatic interaction in physiological solutions is about 1 nm, so excess charges in the vestibules might contribute considerably to accumulation of counter ions, thereby enhancing channel conductance. Of particular interest are the intracellular funnels leading laterally from the pore into the cytoplasm (see Figure 5.1). Because of their relatively small diameter (< 1 nm), they may be expected to play a role in ion permeation. Evidence for such a role has been obtained in 5-HT$_3$ receptors.[49] Homomeric 5-HT$_{3A}$ receptors, which form cation channels of very low conductance (about 1 picosiemens [pS]), have three arginine residues in each MA–M4 loop close to M4. Mutations that replace the positively charged arginines with neutral or negative residues increase the channel conductance by more than 20-fold. Furthermore, the arginine residues are absent in 5-HT$_{3B}$ subunits, and accordingly, heteromultimeric 5-HT$_3$ channels have a much larger conductance (about 16 pS) than the homomeric 5-HT$_3$A channels.

Voltage-Activated Channels

Channels activated specifically by depolarization of the cell membrane include voltage-activated sodium channels, responsible for the depolarizing phase of the nerve action potential, and voltage-activated potassium channels, associated with membrane repolarization. Also included in this group are voltage-activated calcium channels, which in some tissues are responsible for action potential generation or prolongation and subserve many other functions, such as muscle contraction and release of neurotransmitters. Each of these three families of channels has several isotypes found in different species and in different parts of the nervous system, and like the nAChR and its homologues, they constitute a superfamily of common genetic origin.

The Voltage-Activated Sodium Channel

The methods that were used to characterize the molecular structure of the nAChR were applied with equal success to the voltage-activated sodium channel. The essential steps were biochemical extraction and isolation of the protein,[50–52] followed by isolation of cDNA clones and deduction of the amino acid sequence.[53] As with the nAChR experiments, an electric fish—this time the eel *Electrophorus electricus*—provided a rich source of material, and high-affinity toxins, principally tetrodotoxin (TTX) and saxitoxin (STX), were available to facilitate isolation of the protein. Both of these molecules block ion conduction in the native channels by occluding the pore of the open channel. Subsequently, sodium channels were isolated from brain and skeletal muscle. The sodium channel purified from eel consists of a single large (260-kD) protein and is representative of a diverse family of structurally similar proteins.

In mammals the functional sodium channel consists of the primary 260-kD protein (the α-subunit) acting in combination with one or more secondary structures (β-subunits). Genes have been identified

[46] Wotring, V. E., Miller, T. S., and Weiss, D. S. 2003. *J. Physiol.* 548: 527–540.

[47] Gunthorpe, M. J., and Lummis, S. C. R. 2001. *J. Biol. Chem.* 276: 10977–10983.

[48] Imoto, K. et al. 1998. *Nature* 335: 645–648.

[49] Kelley, S. P. et al. 2003. *Nature* 424: 321–324.

[50] Miller, J., Agnew, W. S., and Levinson, S. R. 1985. *Biochemistry* 22: 462–470.

[51] Hartshorn, R. P., and Catterall, W. A. 1984. *J. Biol. Chem.* 259: 1667–1675.

[52] Barchi, R. L. 1983. *J. Neurochem.* 40: 1377–1385.

[53] Noda, M. et al. 1984. *Nature* 312: 121–127.

TABLE 5.1

Voltage-activated sodium channels

Designation	Primary localization	Human gene
Na$_v$1.1–1.3	Central nervous system	*SNC1A–3A*
Na$_v$1.4	Skeletal muscle	*SNC4A*
Na$_v$1.5	Heart muscle	*SNC5A*
Na$_v$1.6	Central and peripheral nervous systems	*SNC8A*
Na$_v$1.7–1.9	Peripheral nervous system	*SNC9A–11A*

Source: A. L. Goldin et al., 2000. *Neuron* 28: 365–368.

that encode a family of nine α-subunits (Table 5.1), designated $Na_v1.1$–$Na_v1.9$.[54] One of the isoforms, $Na_v1.4$, has been found only in skeletal muscle, and a second, $Na_v1.5$, in denervated heart muscle and skeletal muscle. Of the remainder, $Na_v1.1$–1.3 and $Na_v1.6$ are found in the central nervous system, and $Na_v1.6$–1.9 in the peripheral nervous system. Four β-subunits, $β_1$–$β_4$, are expressed in mammalian brain.[55,56] These range in size from 33 to 36 kD and have been shown to affect the sodium channel kinetics and voltage dependence.[57]

Amino Acid Sequence and Tertiary Structure of the Sodium Channel

The eel sodium channel is composed of a sequence of 1832 amino acids, containing four successive domains (I–IV) of 300 to 400 residues, with about a 50% sequence homology from one to the next. Each domain is architecturally similar to one subunit of the nAChR family of channel proteins. However, unlike nAChR subunits, the sodium channel domains are expressed together as a single protein. Within each domain are multiple hydrophobic or mixed hydrophobic and hydrophilic (amphipathic) sequences capable of forming transmembrane helices. As shown in Figure 5.7A, each domain has six such membrane-spanning segments, designated S1–S6. As with the nAChR subunits, the domains are arranged radially around the pore of the channel.

Of particular interest is the S4 region, which is highly conserved in all four domains and has a positively charged arginine or lysine residue at every third position on the transmembrane helix. This feature occurs in all voltage-sensitive channels and provides the coupling between voltage changes across the membrane and channel activation.[58]

After translation, the channel protein is heavily glycosylated. About 30% of the mass of the mature eel channel consists of carbohydrate chains containing large amounts of sialic acid. In the α-subunits of mammalian sodium channels, glycosylation is more variable: $Na_v1.1$ through $Na_v1.4$ are 15% to 30% glycosylated, whereas $Na_v1.5$ and 1.9 are only about 5% carbohydrate.[59,60] Also indicated in Figure 5.7A is the structure of the β-subunits. These have a large extracellular N-terminal domain with immunoglobulin-like folds, a single membrane-spanning region, and a shorter intracellular C-terminal segment.

Voltage-Activated Calcium Channels

The family of voltage-activated calcium channels comprises several subtypes that have been classified by their functional properties, such as sensitivity to membrane depolarization and persistence of activation.[61,62] Channel isotypes have been cloned from skeletal, cardiac, and smooth muscle and from brain. These isotypes fall into three gene families. The functional and gene classifications are summarized in Table 5.2. The amino acid sequence of the primary channel-forming subunit ($α_1$) is similar to that of the voltage-activated sodium channel.[63] In particular, the putative transmembrane regions, S1 to S6, are highly homologous with those of the sodium channel, and the tertiary structure is entirely analogous, as indicated in Figure 5.7B.

TABLE 5.2

Voltage-activated calcium channels

Type[a]	Threshold[b]	Inactivation	Designation[c]	Human gene
L	HV	Very slow	Cav 1.1, 1.2, 1.3, 1.4	*CACNA1S, 1C, 1D, 1F*
N	HV	Slow	Cav 2.2	*CACNA1B*
P/Q	HV	Slow	Cav 2.1	*CACNA1A*
R	HV	Very slow	Cav 2.3	*CACNA1E*
T	LV	Fast	Cav 3.1, 3.2, 3.3	*CACNA1G, 1H, 1I*

Source: E. A. Ertel et al. 2000. *Neuron* 25: 533-535

[a]The abbreviations T, L, and N originally meant Transient, Long-lasting, and Neither T nor L. P refers to Purkinje cells. R and Q are merely differentiators.

[b]HV and LV indicate high-voltage and low-voltage thresholds for activation.

[c]Classification according to E. A. Ertel et al., 2000. *Neuron* 25: 533-535.

[54]Goldin, A. L. et al. 2000. *Neuron* 28: 365-368.

[55]Yu, F. H., and Catterall, W. A. 2003. *Genome Biol.* 4: 207.1-207.7.

[56]Diss, J. K. J., Fraser, S. P., and Djamgoz, M. B. A. 2004. *Eur. Biophys. J.* 33: 180-195.

[57]Yu, F. H. et al. 2003. *J. Neurosci.* 23: 7577-7585.

[58]Stühmer, W. et al. 1989. *Nature* 239: 597-603.

[59]Marban, E., Yamagishi, T., and Tomaselli, G. F. 1998. *J. Physiol.* 508: 647-657.

[60]Tyrrell, L. et al. 2001. *J. Neurosci.* 21: 9629-9637.

[61]Hofmann, F., Biel, M., and Flockerzi, V. 1994. *Ann. Rev. Neurosci.* 17: 399-418.

[62]Randall, A., and Tsien, R. W. 1995. *J. Neurosci.* 15: 2995-3012.

[63]Tanabe, T. et al. 1987. *Nature* 328: 313-318.

(A) Sodium channel

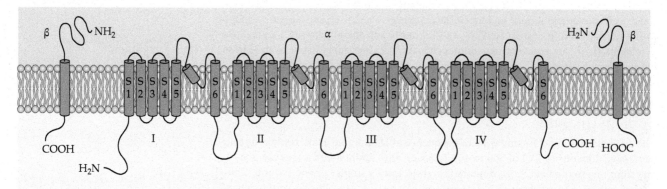

(B) Calcium channel

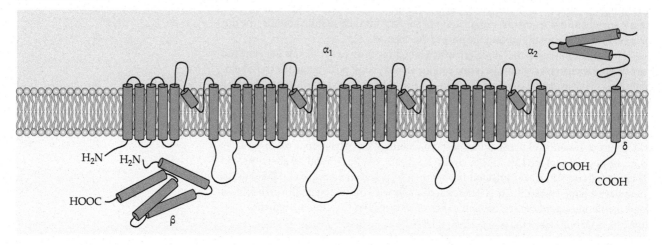

(C) Potassium channel

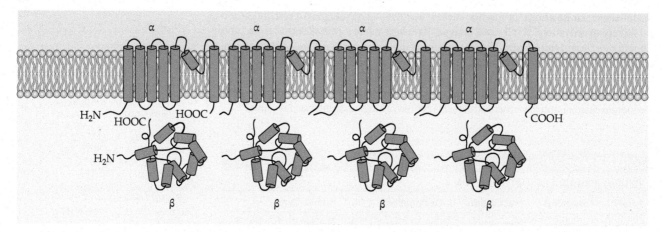

FIGURE 5.7 **Voltage-Activated Channel Structure.** (A) Primary (α) subunit of the voltage-activated sodium channel is a single protein with four domains (I–IV) connected by intracellular and extracellular loops. Each domain has six transmembrane segments (S1–S6), with a pore-forming structure (called a P-loop) between the fifth and sixth. The primary channel is accompanied by auxiliary (β) subunits. (B) The voltage-activated calcium channel α1-subunit is similar in structure and is accompanied by three auxiliary subunits: α_2, β, and δ. (C) The potassium channel comprises four separate α-subunits, corresponding to one domain of the sodium channel α-subunit. Each is associated with a cytoplasmic β-subunit. (A,B after R. J. French and G. W. Zamponi, 2005. *IEEE Trans. NanoBioscience* 4: 58–69; C after S. B. Long et al., 2005. *Science* 309: 897–903.)

Although expression of α_1-subunits alone is sufficient for formation of functional calcium channels in host cells, two accessory subunits are co-expressed in native cell membranes: α_2–δ, a dimer with the extracellular α_2 portion linked to the membrane-spanning δ portion by a disulfide bridge; β, a membrane protein located intracellularly (see Figure 5.7B). Co-expression of various subunit combinations suggests that the α_2–δ- and β-subunits influence both channel conductance and kinetics.[64,65]

Voltage-Activated Potassium Channels

Voltage-sensitive potassium channels play an important role in nerve excitation and conduction. Several distinct genetic messages give rise to a diverse family of these proteins. The first potassium channel to be sequenced was the potassium A-channel protein from *Drosophila*, named Shaker for a genetic mutant in which expression of the channel is defective.[66] When the mutant flies are anesthetized (for example, for counting), they go through a period of trembling, or *shaking*, before becoming immobile. The mutation itself provided a different approach to cloning the channel—one that did not rely on prior identification of the protein. Genetic analysis indicated the approximate location of the *Shaker* gene on the *Drosophila* genome. Overlapping genomic clones from normal and mutant flies were isolated from that region, and comparison of normal and mutant sequences led to identification of the *Shaker* gene.

An unexpected finding was that the amino acid sequence of the protein was much shorter than that of voltage-sensitive sodium and calcium channels. It contained a single domain, similar to domain IV of the eel sodium channel. Experimental evidence indicates that four of the single protein α-subunits assemble to form multimeric ion channels in the membrane (Figure 5.7C), thus mimicking the structure of the voltage-dependent sodium and calcium channels.[67]

Twelve distinct subfamilies of potassium channel proteins have been cloned. These are listed in Table 5.3. Each subfamily comprises several isotypes (e.g., K_v1.1, 1.2, 1.3, etc.). Isotypes from the same subfamily, when expressed in host cells, combine to form heteromultimeric channels, but those from different subfamilies do not.[68] Like sodium and calcium channels, voltage-activated potassium channels are expressed with accessory (β) subunits.[69] Three subfamilies have been identified: $K_v\beta1$, $K_v\beta2$, and $K_v\beta3$. When expressed with the primary subunits, the β-subunits affect the voltage-sensitivity and inactivation properties of the channels.

Pore Formation in Voltage-Activated Channels

A consistent feature of all of the voltage-activated channel sequences is a moderately hydrophobic region in the extracellular S5–S6 loop. In experiments similar to those described previously for the M2 region of the nAChR, single point mutations in this region of the sodium channel reduced the sensitivity of the channel to the blocking molecules tetrodotoxin (TTX) and saxitoxin (STX) and drastically reduced the channel conductance.[70,71] Mutations in this region of the Shaker potassium channel reduced the binding affinity for the blocking molecule tetraethylammonium (TEA) and altered the conductance properties of the channel.[72,73] It was concluded that the S5–S6 segment dips into the channel mouth to form the upper part of the pore region—a conclusion that was later confirmed by X-ray diffraction. S5–S6 is now known as the P-loop (*P* for *pore*).

When the substituted cysteine accessibility method (SCAM) was used to identify residues exposed to the pore lining, the residues were found not only on the P-loop but also on the S6 transmembrane helix, indicating that S6 helices line the pore between the P-loop and the cytoplasm.[74,75]

High-Resolution Imaging of Voltage-Activated Channels

High-resolution images of voltage-activated channels have revealed their structural organization in great detail. The structure of potassium channels from *Streptomyces lividans* ($K_{CS}A$ channels) has been examined with X-ray crystallography at a resolution at 5.2 Å.[76] These bacterial channels belong to a class of potassium

[64] Walker, D., and De Waard, M. 1998. *Trends Neurosci.* 21: 148-154.

[65] French, R. J., and Zamponi, G. W. 2005. *IEEE Trans. Nanobiosci.* 4: 58-69.

[66] Papazian, D. M. et al. 1987. *Science* 237: 749-753.

[67] Timpe, L. C. et al. 1988. *Nature* 331: 143-145.

[68] Salkoff, L. et al. 1992. *Trends Neurosci.* 15: 161-166.

[69] Hanlon, M. R., and Wallace, B. A. 2002. *Biochemistry* 41: 2886-2894.

[70] Pusch, M. et al. 1991. *Eur. Biophys. J.* 20: 127-133.

[71] Noda, M. et al. 1989. *FEBS Lett.* 259: 213-216.

[72] Yool, A. J., and Schwarz, T. L. 1991. *Nature* 349: 700-704.

[73] Yellen, G. et al. 1991. *Science* 251: 939-942.

[74] Liu, Y. et al. 1997. *Neuron* 19: 175-184.

[75] Lu, T. et al. 1999. *Neuron* 22: 571-580.

[76] Doyle, D. A. et al. 1998. *Science* 280: 69-77.

TABLE 5.3

Voltage-activated potassium channels

Subunit designation	Name	Human gene
K_v1.1–1.8	*Shaker*	*KCNA1–7, 10*
K_v2.1, 2.2	*Shab*	*KCNB1–2*
K_v3.1–3.4	*Shaw*	*KCNC1–4*
K_v4.1–4.3	*Shal*	*KCND1–3*
K_v7.1–7.5	*dKCNQ*	*KCNQ1–5*
K_v10.1, 10.2	*eag (ether-a-go-go)*	*KCNH1, 5*
K_v11.1–11.3	*erg*	*KCNH2, 6, 7*
K_v12.1–12.3	*elk*	*KCNH8, 3, 4*

FIGURE 5.8.   Structure of Potassium K$_{CS}$A Channel. Sectional view of a potassium K$_{CS}$A channel showing two of the four subunits, one on either side of the central pore. Each subunit has two membrane-spanning helices and a short helix pointing into the pore. The connections between the outer helices and the short helices form four turrets that surround the pore entrance and contain binding sites for blocking molecules. The four connections between the short helices and the inner helices combine to form the selectivity filter, which allows the permeation of potassium, cesium, and rubidium but excludes smaller cations such as sodium and lithium (see text). (After D. A. Doyle et al., 1998. *Science* 280: 69-77.)

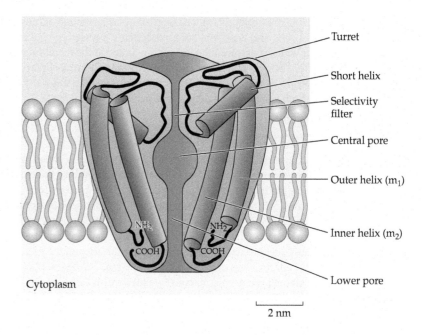

Turret

Short helix

Selectivity filter

Central pore

Outer helix (m$_1$)

Inner helix (m$_2$)

Lower pore

Cytoplasm

2 nm

channels that are only weakly voltage-sensitive and whose subunits have only two transmembrane segments rather than six. The two segments, M1 and M2, are structurally equivalent to S5 and S6 in the voltage-activated channels, and the M1–M2 link represents the P-loop. The K$_{CS}$A channel is a tetramer. Figure 5.8 is a sectional view of the channel, showing its major structural features. Near the amino terminus of each subunit is an outer helix (m$_1$) that spans the membrane from the cytoplasmic side of the membrane to the outer surface. The outer helix is followed by a short helix that points into the pore and then by an inner helix (m$_2$) that returns to the cytoplasmic side. The links between the outer and short helices form four turrets that surround the external opening of the pore and contain the binding sites for TEA and channel-blocking toxins. The link between the central end of the short helix and the inner helix contributes to the pore structure. These four inner links combine to form a restricted passage responsible for the ion selectivity of the channel—the selectivity filter. A relatively large central cavity and a smaller internal pore connect the selectivity filter with the cytoplasm.

The crystal structure of the complete Shaker voltage-dependent potassium channel is also known.[77] The arrangement of the α-subunit is shown schematically in Figure 5.9A. The molecule has two distinct regions—the voltage-sensing region, consisting of S1–S4, and the pore-forming region formed by S5 and S6.

Figure 5.9B shows a schematic view of the complete channel. The four S5 and S6 helices of the α-subunits interlace to form a boxlike structure around the pore. As in the K$_{CS}$A channel, the S6 helices line the pore, and the S5–S6 linker dips into the extracellular opening to form the selectivity filter. The voltage-sensing regions sit somewhat apart at the four corners of the central structure.

In addition to X-ray crystallography, cryo-electron microscopy has been used to obtain detailed images of voltage-sensitive sodium and calcium channels, with a resolution of about 0.4 nm.[78,79] The structural arrangements of their voltage-sensitive and pore-forming regions are entirely analogous to those of the Shaker potassium channel.

Selectivity and Conductance

Selectivity for potassium is achieved by both the size and molecular composition of the selectivity filter,[80] which in the K$_{CS}$A channel has a diameter of about 0.3 nm. The amino acids in its wall are oriented so that successive rings of four carbonyl oxygen atoms, one from each subunit, are exposed to the pore. The pore diameter is adequate to accommodate a dehydrated potassium ion (about 0.27 nm in diameter), but stripping waters of hydration from the penetrating ion requires considerable energy (see Chapter 4). This requirement is

[77] Long, S. B., Campbell, E. B., and MacKinnon, R. 2005a. *Science* 309: 897-903.

[78] Shen, H. et al. 2017. *Science* 355: eaal4326.

[79] Wu, J. et al. 2016. *Nature* 537: 191-196.

[80] Nimigean, C. M., Chappie, J. S., and Miller, C. 2005. *Biochemistry* 42: 9263-9268.

(A)

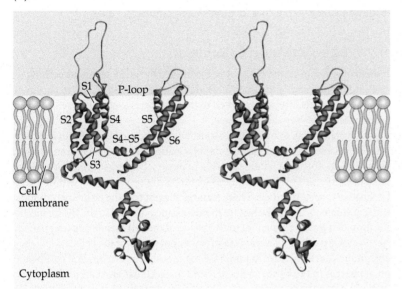

Cell
membrane

Cytoplasm

(B)

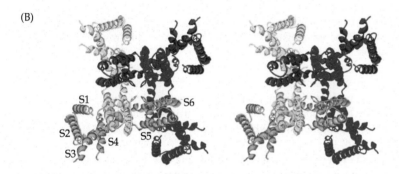

FIGURE 5.9 Stereo Images of Mammalian K$_v$1.2 Channels.* (A) A single α-subunit viewed parallel to the plane of the membrane, showing the arrangement of helices S1 to S6, the P-loop, the S4–S5 linker, and the cytoplasmic N-terminal region. (B) A complete channel, comprising four subunits, looking into the pore from the extracellular side. S5 and S6 helices interlace to form the channel, with P-loops dipping into the pore. Voltage-sensing regions S1 to S4 lie at the corners and are connected to the channel region by the S4–S5 linker. (After S. B. Long et al., 2005. *Science* 309: 897–903.)

minimized by the exposed oxygens, which provide effective substitutes for the oxygen atoms that typically surround the hydrated molecule. Smaller ions, such as sodium (diameter 0.19 nm) and lithium (0.12 nm), are excluded because they cannot make intimate contact with all four oxygens simultaneously, and so remain hydrated. Ions larger than cesium (0.33 nm diameter) cannot penetrate the pore because of their size. This structural basis for ion selectivity is in accordance with traditional ideas about ion permeation through channels.[81]

Other regions of the potassium channel contribute to its conductance properties. For example, in the K$_{CS}$A channel, replacing a neutral alanine residue with glutamate near the cytoplasmic end of M2, so as to form a ring of negative charges near the channel mouth, results in a significant increase in conductance.[75] Similarly, in K$_v$2.1 channels, conductance is increased by replacing a ring of positively charged lysines in the outer vestibule with neutral residues.[82]

In sodium and calcium channels, both selectivity and conductance are altered by mutations in the P-loop. For example, mutations in the P-loops at corresponding positions on each of the four domains can result in sodium channels acquiring the characteristics of calcium channels.[83] One prominent characteristic of the calcium channel is a ring of four negative charges around the pore, formed by glutamate residues in the loops. In sodium channels, the four corresponding residues (D⁻, E⁻, K⁺, A) form a ring with a net charge of –1. Replacement of the alanine and lysine residues with glutamate results in increased calcium permeability and block of sodium ion permeation by the presence of calcium.

---

* VIEWING STEREOGRAMS. To see a three-dimensional representation from a pair of stereo images, hold the page at a normal viewing distance (about 12") and look at the space between the images, staring *through* the page as if you were trying to focus on a distant object beyond the book. Do *not* attempt to bring the images themselves into focus. "Ghosts" of the two images will drift together to form a third, three-dimensional image, lying between the other two. After the central image is stable, you can then focus on its details.

[81] Mullins, L. J. 1975. *Biophys. J.* 15: 921–931.

[82] Consiglio, J. F., Andalib, P., and Korn, S. J. 2003. *J. Gen. Physiol.* 121: 111–124.

[83] Heinemann, S. H. et al. 1992. *Nature* 356: 441–443.

Conversely, in calcium channels, the reverse mutations at the same positions reduce calcium permeability and allow permeation of monovalent cations.[84]

Gating of Voltage-Activated Channels

Structural studies suggest that closed channels are occluded by the S6 segments coming together near the cytoplasmic end of the pore. This idea is supported by SCAM experiments in Shaker potassium channels. Probes presented to the cytoplasmic end of closed channels were able to penetrate only a very short distance.[72]

For voltage-activated gating to occur, there must be charged elements within the channel protein that are displaced by membrane depolarization. The S4 helix is an obvious candidate. As previously noted, it contains a string of positively charged lysine or arginine residues, located at every third position, and this feature is highly conserved within the superfamily of voltage-activated channels. These features suggest that the S4 helices comprise the voltage-sensing elements that link changes in membrane potential to the gating mechanism.[85] Application of a positive potential to the inside of the cell membrane (depolarization) would displace the positive charges so as to cause movement of the helix.

Several techniques have provided support for the idea that activation is accompanied by translation of charges in the S4 segments between intracellular and extracellular spaces.[86] For example, in cysteine accessibility experiments, residues at either end of the S4 helix were mutated to cysteine and the accessibility of cysteine sulfhydryl groups to hydrophilic reagents tested.[87,88] Residues inaccessible from outside the cell at rest became accessible when the membrane was depolarized. Similarly, residues accessible from the inside at rest became inaccessible upon depolarization.

We will discuss the nature of the S4 helix displacement in more detail in Chapter 7. In any event, movements of the charged S4 segments are in some way transmitted to the S6 helices in each of the four domains, thereby opening a conducting pathway from the channel pore to the cytoplasm.[89] The structural arrangement of the Shaker channel suggests that S4–S6 coupling is through interactions between the S4–S5 linker and the cytoplasmic end of S6.

A large body of evidence has accumulated showing that gating of channel currents can occur quite independently of the S4 coupled gating mechanism.[90] For example, when the voltage-activated gate in Shaker K_v channels is disabled by charge-neutralizing mutations in S4, the channel continues to pass current pulses with kinetics indistinguishable from those in the wild-type channel.[91] Other experiments suggest that current switching in P-loop channels may involve the selectivity filter. Mutations in that region of the K_v channel have been shown to affect not only channel conductance (as expected) but also the kinetics of the rapid gating transitions.[92] Similarly, mutations in the selectivity filter of inwardly rectifying channels (K_{ir}; see Table 5.4), which are constitutively active unless blocked by magnesium at their cytoplasmic end, alter the channels' gating properties.[93,94] In addition, accessibility studies on open and closed SK and CNG channels, which are ligand-activated (see Table 5.4), suggest the presence of a gate in the same region.[95,96] These kinds of observations suggest the presence of a dual gating system, with the voltage-coupled gating mechanism providing access to the channel and ion currents through the open channel being switched on and off by fluctuations in the region of the selectivity filter.

Following activation, many voltage-sensitive channels then **inactivate**. That is, they enter a state that no longer allows the passage of ions through the pore. The principal mechanism of inactivation involves cytoplasmic residues moving into the mouth of the pore, thereby blocking access to the channel. We will discuss this mechanism in detail in Chapter 7.

Mechanoreceptor Channels

There is a wide diversity of sensory cells, called mechanoreceptors, that respond to various types of mechanical stimuli, for example pressure or vibration (see Chapter 23). These cells, found both inside and outside the nervous system, generate electrical responses to mechanical disturbance of their cell membranes. Several membrane channels

[84] Yang, N. et al. 1993. *Nature* 366: 158–161.

[85] Sigworth, F. J. 1994. *Quart. Rev. Biophys.* 27: 1–40.

[86] Bezanilla, F. 2008. *Nature Rev. Mol. Cell Biol.* 9: 323–332.

[87] Yang, N., George, A. L., and Horn, R. 1996. *Neuron* 16: 113–122.

[88] Larsson, H. P. et al. 1996. *Neuron* 16: 387–397.

[89] Long, S. B., Campbell, E. B., and MacKinnon, R. 2005. *Science* 309: 903–908.

[90] Korn, S. J., and Trapani, J. G. 2005. *IEEE Trans Nanobiosci.* 4: 21–33.

[91] Bao, H. et al. 1999. *J. Gen. Physiol.* 113: 139–151.

[92] Liu, Y., and Joho, R. H. 1998. *Pflügers Arch.* 435: 654–661.

[93] Lu, T. et al. 2001. *Nature Neurosci.* 4: 239–246.

[94] So, I. et al. 2001. *J. Physiol.* 531: 37–50.

[95] Bruening-Wright, A. et al. 2002. *J. Neurosci.* 22: 6499–6506.

[96] Flynn, G. E., Johnson, J., P., Jr., and Zagotta, W. N. 2001. *Nature Rev. Neurosci.* 2: 643–652.

(A)

(B)

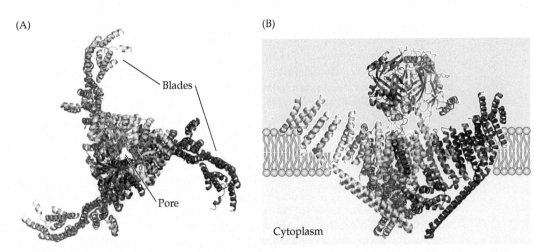

FIGURE 5.10 **Piezo Channel Structure.** (A) Looking down on the extracellular surface. Three extended structures (the blades) radiate symmetrically from a core of transmembrane helices forming the channel. (B) Looking into the plane of the membrane. The core is covered on the extracellular surface by a cap known as the C-terminal extracellular domain. (From D. Purves et al. 2018. *Neuroscience*, 6th ed. Oxford University Press/Sinauer, Sunderland, MA. After J. Ge et al., 2015. *Nature* 527: 64-69.)

have been shown to mediate responses to mechanical stimuli, for example TRP channels (see the next section, "Other Channels"), but it is only in the last decade that we have been able to define channels that respond uniquely to membrane distortion.[97]

Piezo Channels

One group of mechanoreceptor channels consists of two proteins found in mammals, Piezo 1 and Piezo 2, and a third ortholog found in *Drosophila*.[98,99] The channels are permeable to cations with conductances in the range of 25 to 30 pS. Piezo 1 is expressed predominantly in tissues exposed to changes in fluid pressure and blood flow (kidneys, red blood cells), whereas Piezo 2 is found mainly in sensory neurons and their associated mechanoreceptors (dorsal root ganglion cells, Merkel cells). Piezo 1 and 2 are very large proteins, comprising roughly 2600 amino acids, with more than 14 transmembrane domains.

Studies with cryo-electron microscopy reveal a propeller-shaped trimeric complex, with three curved blades radiating from a central core (Figure 5.10).[100] The C-terminal extracellular domain forms a cap over the core. Several models have been proposed to explain how various stimuli (membrane depression or stretch, shear flow of fluids) could lead to opening of the channels.[99]

Hair Cell Channels

Four putative mechanoreceptor channel subunit proteins have been identified in hair cells of the cochlea and vestibular apparatus (see Chapter 24): TMC (Transmembrane Channel-like Protein) 1 and 2, TMHS (Tetraspan Membrane Protein of Hair Cell Cilia), and TMIE (Transmembrane Inner Ear Protein).[97] All are essential for mechanotransduction, but whether they are actual channel components or instead serve an auxiliary role in the transduction process is not yet clear.

Mutations in the *TMC1* gene have been identified with hearing disorders in humans, and associated with deafness in mice. In addition, expression of TMC1 and 2 corresponds to the onset of mechanotransduction in the utricle and cochlea of newborn mice. However, only *TMC1*-deficient mice display deafness. Vestibular defects, by contrast, require double knockout of both genes. Hydropathy plots suggest that the TMC1 subunit consists of six transmembrane domains with intracellular N and C terminals.[101] The structure is reminiscent of that other channel-forming subunits. However, it has yet to be demonstrated that expression of TMC1 in heterologous cells can generate an ion channel, so its role in hair cell mechanotransduction remains uncertain.[102]

Both TMHS and TMIE are required for generation of hair cell mechanoreceptor currents, but their exact role, if any, in channel formation is unknown.

[97] Ranade, S. S., Syeda, R., and Patapoutian, A. 2015. *Neuron* 87: 1162-1179.

[98] Coste, B. et al. 2010. *Science* 330: 55-60.

[99] Wu, J., Lewis, A. H., and Grandi, J. 2017. *Trends in Biochem. Sci.* 42: 57-71.

[100] Zhao, Q. et al. 2018. *Nature* 554: 487-492.

[101] Labay, V. et al. 2010. *Biochemistry* 409: 8592-8598.

[102] Fettiplace, R. 2016. *Biophys. J.* 111: 3-9.

Other Channels

There is a large number of other channels important for neuronal function, with a wide variety of structural configurations. Some are assembled from subunits that have as few as two transmembrane helices each. Others are formed by a single large molecule. Some of these channels are catalogued in Table 5.4. An extensive list of channel subunits, their official names, and their gene designations can be found at the web site of The International Union of Basic and Clinical Pharmacology/British Pharmacological Society: http://www.guidetopharmacology.org.

Glutamate Receptors

Glutamate is the most prevalent excitatory neurotransmitter in the central nervous system, activating three cation channel types (see Chapter 14). The three types have distinct functional properties and are distinguished experimentally by their different sensitivities to glutamate analogues.[103] One responds selectively to *N*-methyl-D-aspartate (NMDA). The other two are activated selectively by α-amino-3-hydroxy-5-methyl-4-isoxazolepropionic acid (AMPA) and kainate. Because of this selectivity, the three chemical analogues are important experimental tools. Remember, however, that the native neurotransmitter for all three receptor types is glutamate, not one of the analogues.

[103] Dingledine, R. et al. 1999. *Pharmacol. Rev.* 51: 7–61.

TABLE 5.4

Other membrane channel types

Channel name	Ligand	Permeability	Subunits	Human genes
LIGAND ACTIVATED				
NMDA[a]	Glutamate	Cations	GluN1, 2A–D, 3A,B	*GRIN1, 2A–D, 3A,B*
AMPA[a]	Glutamate	Cations	GluA1–4	*GRIA1–4*
Kainate[a]	Glutamate	Cations	GluK1–5	*GRIK1–5*
P2X[b]	ATP	Cations	P2X1–P2X7	*P2RX1–7*
INTRACELLULAR ACTIVATION				
CNG[c,d]	cAMP, cGMP	Cations	CNGA1–4, CNGB1, B3	CNGA1–4, CNGB1, B3
BK[e]	Calcium	Potassium	KCa 1.1	KCNMA1
SK[e]	Calcium	Potassium	KCa 2.1–2.3	KCNN1–3
IK[e]	Calcium	Potassium	KCa 3.1	KCNN4
VOLTAGE-SENSITIVE				
CLC[f]	—	Chloride	CLC0, CLC1,2	*CLCN0,1,2*
Kir[g]	—	Inward potassium	Kir1.1, Kir2.1–4, Kir3.1–4, Kir4.1–2, Kir5.1, Kir6.1–2, Kir7.1	*KCNJ1, J2, 12, 4, 14, J3, 6, 9, 5, J10, 15, J16, J8, 11, J13*
(2P)[h]	—	Potassium	K_{2P} 1.1–10.1, K_{2P}12.1, 13.1, K_{2P} 15.1–18.1	*KCNK1–10, 12, 13, 15–18*
TRP CHANNELS[i]				
TRPC	Various	Cations	TRPC1–7	
TRPV	Various	Cations	TRPV1–6	
TRPM	Various	Cations	TRPM1–8	
TRPML	Various	Cations	TRPML 1–3	
TRPP	Various	Cations	TRPP1–3	
TRPA1	Various	Cations	TRPA1	

[a]G. L. Collingridge et al., 2009. *Neuropharmacology* 56: 2–5; [b]M. F. Jarvis and B. Khakh, 2009. *Neuropharmacology* 56: 208–215; [c]K. Matulef and W. Zagotta, 2003. *Annu. Rev. Cell. Dev. Biol.* 19: 23–44; [d]J. Bradley et al., 2005. *Curr. Opin. Neurobiol.* 15: 343–349; [e]A. D. Wei et al., 2005. *Pharmacol. Rev.* 57: 463–472; [f]M. Pusch and T. J. Jentsch, 2005. *IEEE Trans. Nanobiosci.* 4: 49–57; [g]Y. Kubo et al., 2005. *Pharmacol. Rev.* 57: 509–526; [h]S. A. N. Goldstein et al., 2001. *Nat. Rev. Neurosci.* 2: 175–184; [i]L.-J.Wu et al., 2010. *Pharmacol. Rev.* 62: 381–404.

So far, 16 cDNAs for glutamate receptor subunits have been identified by molecular cloning.[104] Seven of these—GluN1, GluN2A through 2D, and GluN3A and B—are involved in the formation of NMDA receptors. AMPA receptors are formed from another set, designated GluA1–4, and kainate receptors are assembled from subunits GluK1–3 combined with GluK4 or 5. Two homologous subunits, δ_1 and δ_2, remain unassigned to any particular receptor. The subunit proteins have four putative transmembrane segments. However, the second segment, rather than crossing the membrane, enters from the cytoplasmic face to form a hairpin loop contributing to the pore lining.[105] The subunits are believed to be phylogenetically related to the potassium channel family, and their structure resembles that of an upside-down potassium $K_{CS}A$ channel subunit, with an additional transmembrane segment (Figure 5.11A).[106] Unlike in nAChR subunits, the C terminus of glutamate receptors is intracellular. Both the N terminus and the M3–M4 loop contribute to the ligand binding sites. The complete receptor is a tetramer.

ATP-Activated Channels

Adenosine-5′-triphosphate (ATP) acts as a neurotransmitter in smooth muscle cells, in autonomic ganglion cells, and in neurons of the central nervous system (see Chapter 14). Because ATP is a purine, its receptor molecules are known as purinergic (P) receptors. P2X receptors form ligand-gated cation channels that subserve a wide variety of functions.[107] P2Y receptors do not form ion channels, but activate intracellular messenger systems. Seven P2X subunits (P2X1–P2X7) have been cloned.[108] Their proposed tertiary structure, with two membrane-spanning segments, is similar to that of the $K_{CS}A$ subunits and to subunits of inwardly rectifying channels (see Figure 5.11B).

Channels Activated by Cyclic Nucleotides

Receptors in the retina (see Chapter 22) and olfactory epithelium are activated by intracellular cyclic AMP or cyclic GMP. The receptors form cation channels, with varying selectivities for potassium, sodium, or calcium. They are similar in structure to voltage-sensitive cation channels, being composed of four subunits, each with six membrane-spanning regions and a P-loop between S5 and S6.[109,110] The S4 helix contains a sequence of charged residues, but these are fewer in number than found in the voltage-sensitive family (usually four rather than six or seven). Consistent with the channel being activated by intracellular ligands, most of the channel's mass is on the cytoplasmic side of the membrane. In vertebrates, six members of the cyclic nucleotide-gated (CNG) gene family have been identified. CNGA1 and CNGB1 (later designated CNGB1a) were first found in bovine rod photoreceptors. Three CNGA1 subunits combine with one CNGB1 to form the native rod channel. In cones, CNG channels composed of two other subunits, designated CNGA3 and CNGB3, expressed in a stoichiometric ratio of 2:2. Yet another pair of subunits, CNGA2 and CNGA4, is found in olfactory neurons. These combine with an alternatively spliced variant of CNGB1 (CNGB1b) to form the olfactory receptor channel, with stoichiometry $(A2)_2(A4)(B1b)$.

Calcium-Activated Potassium Channels

Calcium-activated potassium channels are activated by local changes in cytoplasmic calcium and are divided into three categories according to their potassium conductance: big (BK), small (SK), and intermediate (IK).[111,112] BK channels are also voltage-sensitive and are activated by the concerted action of membrane depolarization and increased intracellular calcium. Their conductance is over 100 pS. SK channels are voltage-insensitive and have conductances of 10 pS or less. The IK channel conductance is in the order of 50 pS.

[104] Hollman, M., Maron, C., and Heinemann, S. 1994. *Neuron* 13: 1331-1343.

[105] Lodge, D. 2009. *Neuropharmacol.* 56: 6-21.

[106] Wollmuth, L. P., and Sobolevsky, A. I. 2004. *Trends Neurosci.* 27: 321-328.

[107] Abbracchino, M. P. et al. 2009. *Trends Neurosci.* 32: 19-29.

[108] Jarvis, M. F., and Khakh, B. S. 2009. *Neuropharmacol.* 56: 208-215.

[109] Matulef, K., and Zagotta, W. N. 2003. *Annu. Rev. Cell. Dev. Biol.* 19: 23-44.

[110] Bradley, J., Reisert, J., and Frings, S. 2005. *Current Opin. Neurobiol.* 15: 343-349.

[111] Vergara, C. et al. 1998. *Curr. Opin. Neurobiol.* 8: 321-329.

[112] Falker, B., and Adelman, J. P. 2008. *Neuron* 59: 873-881.

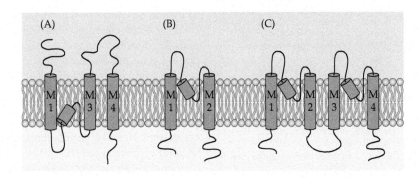

FIGURE 5.11 Other Channel Subunit Configurations. (A) The glutamate receptor subunit has three transmembrane helices with an intramembranous loop entering from the cytoplasm. (B) The inwardly rectifying potassium channel subunit is similar to the $K_{CS}A$ subunit, with two transmembrane segments and an intervening P-loop. (C) The 2P potassium channel subunit has four transmembrane segments and two P-loops. The complete channel is a dimer rather than a tetramer.

Structurally, SK and IK channel subunits share their overall transmembrane topology with voltage-activated potassium channels, but the only notable homology in amino acid sequence is in the P-loop. BK channel subunits are similar in topology but have seven, rather than six, membrane crossings, with the additional transmembrane segment (S0) carrying the amino terminus into the extracellular domain.

Voltage-Sensitive Chloride Channels

Voltage-activated chloride channels (ClCs) have the interesting property that each channel molecule contains two independent pores that are gated together.[113] The molecule consists of two identical subunits, each of which is composed of 18 α-helices and forms its own independent channel.[114] ClC-0 was first cloned from the electric organ of *Torpedo*. The channel is found in high density on the non-innervated face of the cells and provides a low-resistance pathway for currents generated by electrical activity of the innervated face. It belongs to a large family that includes at least nine mammalian homologues. ClC-0 is found in mammalian brain. ClC-1 channels in mammalian skeletal muscle fibers are major contributors to the resting membrane conductance and serve to stabilize the membrane potential at its resting level. ClC-2 appears to be associated with cell volume regulation and therefore may be stretch-sensitive. Two other isotypes, ClC-K1 and ClC-K2, are associated with chloride reabsorption in the kidney. Other branches of the family, ClC-3 to ClC-7, are predominantly found in membranes of intracellular vesicles.

Inwardly Rectifying Potassium Channels

Inwardly rectifying potassium channels (K_{ir} channels) allow the movement of potassium ions into cells when the membrane potential is negative with respect to the potassium equilibrium potential, but allow little outward potassium movement when the driving force is in the opposite direction. The absence of outward potassium flux is associated with blockade of the channels by intracellular magnesium and/or by intracellular polyamines.[115] The channel is a tetramer, with each subunit having only two membrane-spanning helices (Figure 5.11B), similar to the $K_{CS}A$ channel (see Figure 5.8). Seven subfamilies of the channel ($K_{ir}1$–$K_{ir}7$) have been cloned from brain, heart, and kidney.[116] The channels display a variety of functional properties. One family, $K_{ir}3$, forms channels that are activated by intracellular G proteins (see Chapter 12).

2P Channels

The family of 2P potassium channels is so called because each subunit contains two pore-forming loops.[117] The subunit has four transmembrane regions, M1–M4, with pore-forming loops M1–M2 and M3–M4 (Figure 5.11C). Two subunits assemble in the membrane to form the channel. 2P channels are open at normal cell resting potentials and are a major contributor to the resting potassium conductance, or "leak" pathways across cell membranes. The first 2P channel was cloned from *Drosophila*, and subsequently 16 homologous mammalian subunits have been described.

Transient Receptor Potential Channels

Transient receptor potential (TRP) channels constitute a large superfamily of cation-selective channels that are formed in the membrane by the assembly of four subunits. The first TRP channel to be identified and cloned is associated with visual transduction in *Drosophila*. Photoreceptors in mutants lacking the *trp* gene are unable to maintain a sustained response to light (Box 5.2). Instead, the receptor potential adapts rapidly (i.e., becomes transient—hence the name). More than 50 TRP subunit genes have now been identified, at least 28 of them in mammals.[118,119] The subunits are characterized by six transmembrane segments with a pore loop between the fifth and sixth segments, with extended cytoplasmic N- and C-terminal regions. Although the subunits lack charged residues in S4, some of the channels are voltage-sensitive. The channels are generally nonselective, but their calcium permeability varies over a wide range. The mammalian TRP superfamily is

[113] Miller, C., and White, M. M. 1984. *Proc. Nat. Acad. Sci. USA* 81: 2772-2775.

[114] Pusch, M., and Jentsch, T. J. 2005. *IEEE Trans. Nanobiosci.* 4: 49-57.

[115] Lu, Z. 2004. *Annu. Rev. Physiol.* 66: 103-129.

[116] Nicholls, C. G., and Lopatin, A. N. 1997. *Annu. Rev. Physiol.* 59: 171-191.

[117] Goldstein, S. A. N. et al. 2001. *Nat. Rev. Neurosci.* 2: 175-184.

[118] Nilius, B., and Voets, T. 2005. *Pflügers Arch.* 451: 1-10.

[119] Wu, L.-J. et al. 2010. *Pharmacol. Rev.* 62: 381-404.

BOX **5.2**   Channelopathies

A channelopathy may be loosely defined as a human or animal disease or pathological condition arising from the malfunction of an ion channel. The term is usually applied (as it is here) to genetically transmitted diseases resulting from mutations in ion channel genes, though it is sometimes also applied to acquired malfunctions such as myasthenia gravis, an autoimmune disease affecting muscle nicotinic acetylcholine receptors.

Hundreds of disease-producing mutations in human ion channel genes or associated proteins have been discovered (e.g., see Spillane et al., 2016[120]). Notwithstanding this, the occurrence of diseases resulting directly from mutations to a single gene is relatively rare. However, inherited mutations provide natural experiments that can provide valuable information about the normal function of ion channel species. Here we provide examples from three types of channels: a voltage-gated sodium channel (Nav1.7), the K_v7 family of voltage-gated potassium channels, and the TRP family of cation channels.

A painless sodium channel

In 2006 Cox and colleagues described several children belonging to three families "with the extraordinary phenotype of a congenital inability to perceive any form of pain, in whom all other sensory modalities were preserved and the peripheral and central nervous systems were apparently otherwise intact."[121] They called this "channelopathy-associated insensitivity to pain" and illustrated it with a ten year-old boy who performed "street-theater" by sticking knives through his arms and walking on hot coals without feeling any pain. The researchers tracked the defect down to single base mutations in the *SCN9A* gene encoding the α-subunit of the

$Na_v1.7$ sodium channel. Interestingly, while members of the three families had different point mutations, all were in the pore region of the α-subunit of the $Na_v1.7$ channel (Figure A) and resulted in loss of the ability of the channel to generate inward sodium flux in response to depolarization (Figure B).

The $Na_v1.7$ channel was already known to be expressed in pain-sensing (nociceptive) sensory neurons, but the natural experiment performed by the human mutations confirmed its functional importance. There are many other reported mutations in the SCN9A gene.[122] Interestingly, some of these are gain-of-function mutations and increase the current carried by $Na_v1.7$ channels. These lead to a burning sensation and enhanced pain from the extremities in a condition called erythromelalgia.[122]

A mutation-prone potassium channel family causing cardiac arrhythmias, epilepsy, and deafness

Much of our knowledge about potassium channel genes and channel protein composition derives from natural genetic mutations. The K_v7 family of K^+ channel subunits was discovered during studies on human genetic mutations. The family comprises five members, $K_v7.1$ through $K_v7.5$, encoded by the KCNQ1-5 genes.

(Continued)

---

[120]Spillane, J., Kullmann, D. M., and Hanna, M. G. 2016. *J. Neurol. Neurosurg. Psychiatry* 87: 37-48.

[121]Cox, J. J. et al. 2006. *Nature* 444: 894-898.

[122]Dib-Hajj, S. D. et al. 2013. *Nature Rev. Neurosci.* 14: 49-62.

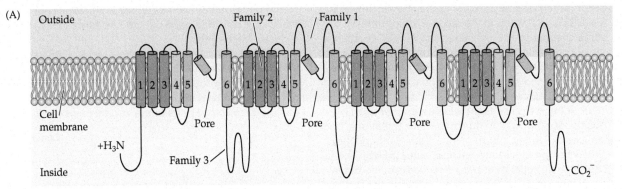

(A)

Family 1	2961 G→A	W897X
Family 2	2298 delete T	1767X
Family 3	1378 C→G	S459X

Primary structure of the α-subunit of the Nav1.7 sodium channel, showing the position of the mutations generating a congenital insensitivity to pain in three different families so afflicted. The base mutations (e.g., 2961 G→A) and consequent amino acid changes (e.g., W897X) are indicated below the diagram (X means more than one possible amino acid). The amino acid changes are nonsense changes, so the expressed protein is incomplete. (After J. J. Cox et al., 2006. *Nature* 444: 894-898.)

BOX **5.2** Channelopathies (continued)

(B)   (1) Current/time

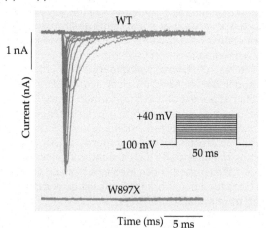

(2) Current/voltage

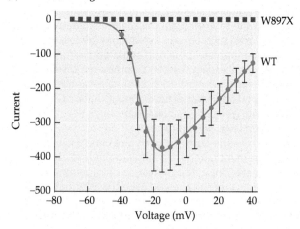

Currents generated by membrane depolarization in human embryonic kidney cells transfected with cDNA encoding normal (wild-type, WT) or mutated (W897X, corresponding to the mutation in Family 1 in Figure A) $Na_v1.7$ α-subunits, together with cDNAs for $β_1$- and $β_2$-subunits. Inward currents are plotted downward. (1) Real-time currents generated by 50-ms command steps to between –70 and + 40 mV in 5-mV increments from a holding potential of –100 mV. (2) Plots of mean peak current density (pA x pF$^{\wedge 1}$ = picoAmps /picofarad) against command potential for wild-type (WT) and mutated (W897X) channels. Note that the wild-type channel generated large inward currents, whereas the mutated channel yielded negligible currents. (B after J. J. Cox et al., 2006. *Nature* 444: 894.)

Of these five subunits, four (80%) show genetic mutations with characteristic phenotypes (see Soldovieri et al., 2011[123]).

$K_v7.1$, in combination with the β-subunit KCNE1, forms the cardiac delayed rectifier current IKs, which repolarizes the ventricular action potential. Genetic mutations that reduce $K_v7.1$ function therefore delay ventricular repolarization, thus lengthening the cardiac action potential and prolonging the interval between the QRS and T waves in the electrocardiogram.[124] In some children the cardiac effects of KCNQ1 mutations are accompanied by severe congenital deafness, which occurs because fully functional $K_v7.1$ K^+ channels are required for the secretion of cochlear endolymph by specialized epithelial cells.

$K_v7.2$ and $K_v7.3$ channels were also identified by positional cloning from human genetic mutations, from families exhibiting a form of inherited infant epilepsy called benign familial neonatal seizures (BFNS). The condition appears during the first weeks of life but in most cases spontaneously resolves during the first few weeks. $K_v7.2$ channels are expressed at nodes of Ranvier, and thus mutations of KCNQ2 can lead to peripheral nerve hyperexcitability (myokymia).[125]

Normally $K_v7.2$ and 7.3 subunits combine to form the widely expressed M-channel,[126] which acts as a brake on the excitability of a variety of neurons and their axons (see Chapter 21). A defective $K_v7.2$ subunit will therefore reduce the number of functional M-channels and hence increase neuronal excitability. In mice, pups with both KCNQ2 genes truncated (homozygotes) die within the first day after birth from respiratory failure,[127] and neurons from their embryos have no M-current at all, as expected for a nonfunctional $K_v7.2$ subunit.[128] Humans with $K_v7.2$ or 7.3 mutations normally have only one gene affected, so have a partially reduced M-current.

KCNQ4 was cloned by homology screening against a human retinal cDNA library using a partial KCNQ3 sequence.[129] The protein product ($K_v7.4$) forms a species of M-channel that is strongly concentrated in the inner ear and some other parts of the auditory and vestibular

(Continued)

[123]Soldovieri, M. V., Miceli, F., and Taglialatela, M. 2011. *Physiology* 26: 365–376.

[124]Wang, Q. et al. 1996. *Nat. Genet.* 12: 17–23.

[125]Dedek K. et al. 2001. *Proc. Natl. Acad. Sci. USA* 98: 12272–12277.

[126]Wang, H. S. et al. 1998. *Science* 282: 1890–1893.

[127]Watanabe, H. et al. 2000. *J. Neurochem.* 75: 28–33.

[128]Robbins, J. et al. 2013. *PLoS ONE* 88:e71809

[129]Kubisch, C. et al. 1999. *Cell* 96: 437–446.

BOX 5.2 Channelopathies (continued)

systems. Mutations in the human *KCNQ4* gene give rise to a form of progressive familial deafness called DFNA2, due to loss of a component of K+ current in cochlear hair cells, with their eventual degeneration. K$_v$7.4 is also concentrated in the afferent synaptic calyx endings surround vestibular hair cells. As a consequence, a proportion of individuals with DFA2 show disturbances of vestibular function.

Overall, members of the K$_v$7 family have been found to act as regulators of excitability, and guardians against overexcitability, in the heart and nervous system. They accomplish this by providing a level of potassium conductance suitable for maintaining the cell membrane potential at an appropriate level and counteracting depolarizing currents.

A blind fly lights the way to an extensive new family of cation channels

In 1969 Cosens and Manning described a mutant strain of the fruit fly *Drosophila melanogaster* that appeared to be functionally blind in certain optometric tests.[130] Instead of showing a sustained response to long light exposures, as measured by electroretinography (ERG), the mutants showed a rapidly inactivating—hence transient—response, due to their lack of the *transient receptor potential* (*trp*) gene (Figure C). The *Drosophila trp* gene was cloned and the projected TRP protein sequence determined by Montell and Rubin in 1989.[131] The protein is concentrated in the S-cone photoreceptors of the fly; its function as a Ca^{2+}-permeable ion channel generating a visual response in *Drosophila* was established by Hardie and Minke in 1992.[132]

It should be noted that the gene mutations responsible for the original blind *trp* phenotype are all null mutants, so the TRP protein is not expressed.[131] This lack of expression (see Figure D2) results in the unmasking of TRP by removal of the prolonged response shown in Figure D1. In other words, the actual TRP protein is responsible for the prolonged depolarization.

Equivalent human TRPC (C = classical) channels were subsequently isolated by homology screening of a human brain cDNA library[133] and a human embryonic kidney cell library,[134] and by 2007 the number of human homologs had been expanded to 27.[135] One channel of interest is TRPV1, the capsaicin receptor responsible for the burning sensation of hot peppers (see Chapter 23). It is highly localized to mammalian nociceptive sensory neurons and contributes to the physiological sensation of cutaneous heat, including noxious heat. When the channel opens, it admits Na$^+$ and Ca^{2+}, leading to depolarization and excitation. Ca^{2+} influx can also induce sensory nerve degeneration. The three-dimensional structure of the TRPV1 channel in its open and closed states has recently been determined by cryo-electron microscopy.[136]

[130]Cosens, D. J., and Manning, A. 1969. *Nature* 224: 285–287.
[131]Montell, C., and Rubin, G. M. 1989. *Neuron* 2: 1313–1323.
[132]Hardie, R. C., and Minke, B. 1992. *Neuron* 8: 643–651.
[133]Wes, P. D. 1995. *Proc. Natl. Acad. Sci. USA* 92: 9652–9656.
[134]Zhu, X. et al. 1995. *FEBS Lett.* 373: 193–198.
[135]Clapham, D. E. 2007. *Cell.* 129: doi: 10.1016/j.cell.2007.03.034.
[136]Henderson, R. 2013. *Nature* 504: 93–94.

(C) (1)

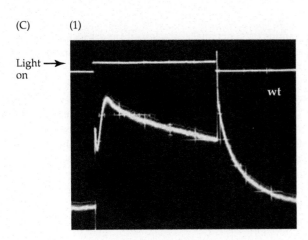

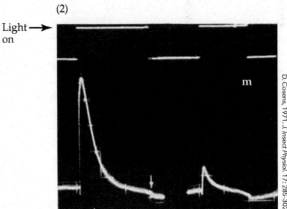

Wild-type and trp mutant fruit fly electroretinograms
Electroretinograms (ERGs) recorded from the eyes of a normal (wild-type, wt) *Drosophila* (1) and a blind *trp* mutant (m) *Drosophila* (2) in response to the light pulses indicated above the ERG records. Note that the wild-type eye shows a sustained ERG response to a 20-s light pulse, whereas the ERG response of the mutant rapidly fades even though the light pulse is stronger, and also responds poorly to a second light pulse.

divided into six groups (see Table 5.4), each with its own set of functional characteristics, which vary widely from one group to the next. Some channels respond to light, others to odorants, to mechanical stimuli, to changes in osmolarity, or to changes in temperature. For example, the TRPV family is involved in heat detection, and TRPM8 in the detection of cold (see Chapter 23). A special feature of TRPV1 channels is their ability to respond with different conductance levels to endogenous agonists that produce pain.[137]

Diversity of Subunits

A feature of channel structure is the remarkably wide diversity of subunit isotypes. Thus, there are more than a dozen nAChR subunits and an even greater number of potassium channel and glutamate receptor subunits. How does this diversity arise? Generally, each channel or channel subunit is encoded by a separate gene, but two additional mechanisms have been identified. The first is called alternative splicing. Most proteins are encoded in several different segments of DNA known as exons. In some cases, instead of combining uniquely to form mRNA for a specific subunit, transcripts of the exons enter into various alternative combinations to generate mRNA for a variety of subunit isotypes. During transcription, an unknown regulatory mechanism determines which of the alternative RNAs are to be used. The remaining RNAs are excised from the transcript and the desired RNA segments spliced together to form the final mRNA. Shaker potassium channel and voltage-gated calcium channel isotypes are generated in this way.[138]

Another method of obtaining subunit diversity is by **RNA editing**. Examples include the glutamate receptor subunits GluA2, GluK3, and GluK4. These carry either a glutamine or arginine residue within the pore. The presence of the arginine residue severely depresses the calcium permeability of the channel and alters its ion conductance properties. It turns out that the genomic DNA for all three subunits harbors a glutamine codon (CAG) for that position, even though an arginine codon (CGG) can be found in the mRNAs.[139] The change in base sequence is accomplished by RNA editing in the cell nucleus. Virtually the entire message for GluA2 is edited in this way, as well as some of the message for GluK3 and GluK4. In GluK4, additional A-G editing is found in a different region of the pore.[140] RNA editing at a single site in the glycine receptor subunit GlyRα$_3$ has been shown to underlie a marked increase in glycine sensitivity.[141]

Conclusion

The techniques used to examine the functional characteristics and structural details of the Cys-loop receptors on the one hand, and the voltage-activated cation channels on the other hand, have led to a remarkable increase in our knowledge of the detail of channel structure and function. The two channel types, although appearing to be quite different at first glance, have a similar functional organization. Both are composed of three essential parts: a signal-sensing domain, a transmembrane pore-forming domain, and a cytoplasmic domain.

In Cys-loop receptors, the sensing domain is the ligand-binding region of the molecule, located appropriately in the extracellular space. The ligand-binding region is connected to M1 and, when activated, interacts with the connecting loop between M1 and M2 to shift M2 outward, thereby opening the pore. By necessity, voltage-activated channels have their sensing region in the membrane itself, with the S4 helix being the essential sensing element. Their activation is entirely equivalent to that of the Cys-loop receptors: The voltage sensor is connected to S5 and, upon depolarization, interacts with the S5–S6 loop to move S6 out of the pore.

The cytoplasmic region of the channels has a variety of functions. In the Cys-loop receptors and voltage-activated channels, the region plays a role in ion selectivity, and in voltage-activated channels it plays a major role in inactivation. In addition, channels activated by intracellular ligands have cytoplasmic ligand-binding sites that are coupled with the transmembrane region so as to open the channel pore during activation.

As a general rule, channels that are relatively selective, such as the voltage-activated channels, are usually tetramers (one exception is the dimeric 2P channel); larger, less selective

[137] Canul-Sánchez, J. A. et al. 2018. *J. Gen. Physiol.* 150: 1735-1746.

[138] Lipscombe, D., Allen, S. E., and Toro, C. P. 2013. *Trends Neurosci.* 36: 598-609.

[139] Sommer, B. et al. 1991. *Cell* 67: 11-19.

[140] Köhler, M. et al. 1993. *Neuron* 10: 491-500.

[141] Meier, J. C. et al. 2005. *Nat. Neurosci.* 8: 736-774.

ligand-activated channels are pentamers. As an extension of this principle, the largest and least selective channels—vertebrate gap junctions—have a hexameric structure (see Chapter 8).

The techniques now at hand will enable us to build on these general principles and provide even more intimate details of how the molecular organization of a given channel affects its functional properties, and hence its role in nervous system function.

SUMMARY

- Nicotinic acetylcholine receptors (nAChRs) from the electric organ of Torpedo consist of five subunits (two α and three others designated β, γ, and δ) arranged around a central pore.

- In each subunit of the nAChR the string of amino acids folds to form four membrane-spanning helices (M1–M4) joined by intracellular and extracellular loops. The extracellular loops in the α-subunits contain the binding sites for ACh. The M2 helices form the central pore of the channel.

- Binding of ACh to the two α-subunits results in a change in configuration that is transmitted to the M2 helices, which move radially outward to widen the pore and allow ion flux through the channel.

- AChRs belong to a superfamily of Cys-loop receptors, which include receptors for γ-aminobutyric acid (GABA), glycine, and 5-hydroxytryptamine (5-HT).

- The voltage-activated sodium channel from eel electric organs is a single molecule of about 1800 amino acids within which there are four repeating domains (I–IV). The domains are arranged around the central pore and are architecturally equivalent to the subunits of other channels. Within each domain are six membrane-spanning helices (S1–S6) connected by intracellular and extracellular loops. The primary (α) subunits of mammalian sodium channels are homologous with the eel channel but are expressed in the membrane in concert with auxiliary (β) subunits.

- The family of voltage-activated calcium channel proteins is analogous in structure to the voltage-activated sodium channel. Voltage-activated potassium channels are structurally similar but with an important genetic difference—the four repeating

units are expressed as individual subunits, not as repeating domains of a single molecule. Together, the three voltage-activated channels constitute a genetic superfamily.

- The voltage-activated sodium, calcium, and potassium channels are known as P-loop channels because of a loop of amino acids that enters the membrane from the extracellular side between S5 and S6 in each of the four domains. The P-loop forms the outer part of the pore lining and plays a major role in the ion selectivity of the channel. The remainder of the pore is lined by cytoplasmic ends of the S6 helices.

- Depolarization of the membrane displaces the S4 helices (which have several positively charged residues), which in turn produces an outward movement of the S6 helices to open the pore.

- Inactivation of voltage-activated channels occurs when one of the intracellular loops of the amino acid swings into the cytoplasmic mouth of the open channel, thereby preventing ion flux through the pore.

- Mechanoreceptor channels, of which there are several types, are activated by mechanical stimuli. In particular, Piezo channels have been characterized in some detail. They are cation channels with a conductance of 25 to 30 pS. They are much larger than other channel proteins, comprising roughly 2600 amino acids, with more than 14 transmembrane domains.

- The techniques used for structural analysis of membrane channels have led to a widespread understanding of the molecular organization of several other channel types.

Suggested Reading

General Reviews

Catterall, W. A. 2014. Structure and function of voltage-gated sodium channels at atomic resolution. *Exp. Physiol.* 99: 35-51.

Lipscombe, D., Allen, S. E., and Toro, C. P. 2013. Control of neuronal voltage-gated calcium ion channels from RNA to protein. *Trends Neurosci.* 36: 598–609. doi: 10.1016/j.tins.2013.06.008. Epub 2013 Jul 30. Review.

Long, S. B., Campbell, E. B., and MacKinnon, R. 2005a. Crystal structure of a mammalian voltage-dependent *Shaker* family K⁺ channel. *Science* 309: 897–903.

Long, S., B., Campbell, E. B., and MacKinnon, R. 2005. Voltage sensor of K$_v$1.2: Structural basis of electromechanical coupling. *Science* 309: 903–908.

Miyazawa, A., Fujiyoshi, Y., and Unwin, N. 2003. Structure and gating mechanism of the acetylcholine receptor pore. *Nature* 423: 949–955.

Original Papers

Ranade, S. S., Syeda, R., and Patapoutian, A. 2015. Mechanically activated ion channels. *Neuron* 87: 1162–1179.

Shen, H., Jhou, Q., Pan, X., Wu, J., and Yan, N. 2017. Structure of a eukaryotic voltage-gated sodium channel at near-atomic resolution. *Science* 355: eaal4326. DOI:10.1126/science, aal4326.

Unwin, N. 2005. Refined structure of the nicotinic acetylcholine receptor at 4 Å resolution. *J. Mol. Biol.* 346: 967–989.

CHAPTER 6

Ionic Basis of the Resting Potential

At rest, a neuron has a stable electrical potential across its outer cell membrane, the inside being negative with respect to the outside. In the neuron, the intracellular potassium concentration is high compared with that in the extracellular fluid, whereas the intracellular concentrations of sodium and chloride are low. As a result, potassium tends to diffuse out of the cell and sodium and chloride tend to diffuse in. The tendency for potassium ions to move out of the cell and for chloride ions to move in is opposed by the membrane potential.

In this chapter we discuss the relations between concentration and potential, first for a model cell whose membrane is permeable only to potassium and chloride. In this cell, the concentration gradients and the membrane potential can be balanced exactly, so that there is no net flux of either ion across the membrane. The membrane potential is then equal to the equilibrium potential for both potassium and chloride. In the model cell, changing the extracellular potassium concentration changes the potassium equilibrium potential, and hence the membrane potential. In contrast, changing extracellular chloride concentration eventually leads to an equivalent change in intracellular chloride, so that the chloride equilibrium potential and the membrane potential are unchanged.

Real cells are also permeable to sodium. At rest, sodium ions constantly move into the cell, reducing the internal negativity of the membrane. As a result, potassium, being no longer in equilibrium, leaks out. If there were no compensation, these fluxes would lead to changes in the internal concentrations of sodium and potassium. However, the concentrations are maintained by the sodium–potassium exchange pump, which transports sodium out and potassium in across the cell membrane in a ratio of three parts sodium to two parts potassium. The resting membrane potential depends on the potassium equilibrium potential, the sodium equilibrium potential, the relative permeability of the cell membrane to the two ions, and the pump ratio. At the resting potential, the passive fluxes of sodium and potassium are exactly matched by the rates at which they are transported in the opposite direction. Because the sodium–potassium exchange pump transports more positive ions outward than inward across the membrane, it makes a direct contribution of several millivolts to the membrane potential.

The chloride equilibrium potential may be positive or negative relative to the resting membrane potential, depending on the chloride transport processes. Although the chloride distribution plays little role in determining the resting membrane potential, substantial chloride permeability is important in some cells for electrical stability.

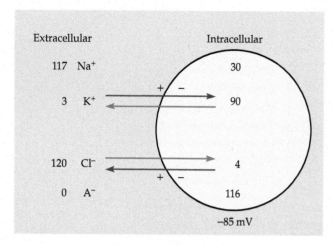

Extracellular | Intracellular

117 Na⁺ · 30

3 K⁺ · 90

120 Cl⁻ · 4

0 A⁻ · 116

−85 mV

FIGURE 6.1 Ion Distributions in a Model Cell. The cell membrane is impermeable to Na^+ and the internal anion (A^-) and permeable to K^+ and Cl^-. The concentration gradient for K^+ tends to drive it out of the cell (upper blue arrow), while the potential gradient tends to attract K^+ into the cell (upper red arrow). In a cell at rest, the two forces are exactly in balance. Concentration and electrical gradients for Cl^- are in the reverse directions. Ion concentrations are expressed in millimolar (mM).

Electrical signals are generated in nerve cells and muscle fibers primarily by changes in permeability of the cell membrane to ions such as sodium and potassium. Increases in permeability allow ions to move inward or outward across the cell membrane down their electrochemical gradients. As we discussed in Chapter 4, permeability increases are due to activation of ion channels. Ions moving through the open channels change the charge on the cell membrane, and hence change the membrane potential. In order to understand how signals are generated, it is necessary first to understand how the standing ion gradients across the cell membrane determine the resting membrane potential.

A Model Cell

It is useful to begin with the idealized model cell shown in Figure 6.1. This cell contains potassium, sodium, chloride, and a large anion species, and it is bathed in a solution of sodium and potassium chloride. Other ions present in real cells (e.g., calcium or magnesium) are ignored for the moment, as their direct contributions to the resting membrane potential are negligible. The extracellular and intracellular ion concentrations in the model cell are similar to those found in frogs. In birds and mammals, ion concentrations are somewhat higher, while in marine invertebrates (e.g., squid) they are very much higher (Table 6.1). The model cell membrane is permeable to potassium and chloride, but not to sodium or to the internal anion. There are three major requirements for a cell to remain in a stable condition:

1. The intracellular and extracellular solutions must each be electrically neutral. For example, a solution of chloride ions alone cannot exist; their negative charges must be balanced by an equal number of positive charges on cations such as sodium or potassium.

2. The cell must be in osmotic balance. Otherwise water will enter or leave the cell, causing it to swell or shrink. Osmotic balance is achieved when the total concentration of solute particles inside the cell is equal to that on the outside.

3. There must be no net movement of any particular ion into or out of the cell.

Ionic Equilibrium

How are the concentrations of the permeant ions maintained in the model cell, and what electrical potential is developed across the cell membrane? Figure 6.1 shows that the two ions are distributed in reverse ratios—potassium is more concentrated on the inside of the cell, chloride on the outside. Imagine first that the membrane is permeable only to potassium. The question that arises immediately is why potassium ions do not diffuse out of the cell until the concentrations on either side of the cell membrane are equal. The answer is that the process is self-limiting. As the potassium ions diffuse outward, positive charges accumulate on the outer surface of the membrane and excess negative charges are left on the inner surface. As a result, an electrical potential develops across the membrane, with the inside being negative with respect to the outside. The electrical gradient slows the efflux of positively charged potassium ions, and when the potential becomes sufficiently large, further net efflux of potassium is stopped. The potential at which this occurs is called the **potassium equilibrium potential (E_K)**. At E_K, the effects of the concentration gradient and the potential gradient on ion flux through the membrane balance one another exactly. Individual potassium ions still enter and leave the cell, but no *net* movement occurs. The potassium ions are in equilibrium.

The conditions for potassium to be in equilibrium across the cell membrane are the same as those described in Chapter 4 for

---

TABLE 6.1

Concentrations of ions inside and outside freshly isolated axons of squid

Ion	Concentration (mM)		
	Axoplasm	Blood	Seawater
Potassium	400	20	10
Sodium	50	440	460
Chloride	60	560	540
Calcium	0.1 μM[a]	10	10

Source: After A. L. Hodgkin, 1964. *The Conduction of the Nervous Impulse.* Liverpool University Press, Liverpool, based on A. L. Hodgkin, 1951. *Biol. Rev.* 26: 339-409.

[a] Ionized intracellular calcium from P. F. Baker et al., 1971. *J. Physiol.* 218: 709-755.

maintaining zero net flux through an individual channel in a membrane patch. There, a concentration gradient was balanced by a potential applied to the patch pipette. The important difference here is that the ion flux itself produces the required transmembrane potential. In other words, equilibrium in the model cell is automatic and inevitable. Recall from Chapter 4 that the potassium equilibrium potential is given by the Nernst equation:

$$E_K = \frac{RT}{zF} \ln \frac{[K]_o}{[K]_i} = 58 \log \frac{[K]_o}{[K]_i}$$

where $[K]_o$ and $[K]_i$ are the external and internal potassium ion concentrations, respectively. For the cell shown in Figure 6.1, at 25°C E_K is 58 log (1/30) = –85 mV. Suppose now that, in addition to potassium channels, the membrane has chloride channels. Because for an anion $z = -1$, the equilibrium potential for chloride is:

$$E_{Cl} = -58 \log \frac{[Cl]_o}{[Cl]_i}$$

or from the properties of logarithmic ratio

$$E_{Cl} = 58 \log \frac{[Cl]_i}{[Cl]_o}$$

In our model cell, the chloride concentration ratio is again 1/30 and E_{Cl} is also –85 mV. As with potassium, the membrane potential of –85 mV balances exactly the tendency for chloride to move down its concentration gradient, in this case *into* the cell.

In summary, the tendency both for potassium ions to leave the cell and for chloride ions to diffuse inward is opposed by the membrane potential. Because the concentration ratios for the two ions are of exactly the same magnitude (1:30), their equilibrium potentials are exactly the same. As potassium and chloride are the only two ions that can move across the membrane and both are in equilibrium at –85 mV, the model cell can exist indefinitely without any net gain or loss of ions.

Electrical Neutrality

The charge separation across the membrane of our model cell means there is an excess of anions inside the cell and of cations outside. This appears to violate the principle of electrical neutrality but, in fact, does not. Potassium ions diffusing outward collect as excess cations against the outer membrane surface, leaving excess anions closely attracted to the inner surface. Both the potassium ions and the counter ions they leave behind are, in effect, removed from the intracellular bulk solution, leaving it neutral. Similarly, chloride ions diffusing inward add to the collection of excess anions on the inner surface of the membrane and leave counterions in the outer charged layer, so the extracellular solution remains neutral as well. The outer layer of cations and inner layer of anions, of equal and opposite charges, are not in free solution but are held to the membrane surface by mutual attraction. Thus, the membrane acts as a capacitor, separating and storing charge. This does not mean that any given anion or cation is locked in position against the membrane. Ions in the charged layer interchange freely with those in the bulk solution. The point is that although the identities of the ions in the layer are constantly changing, their total number remains constant, and the bulk solution stays neutral.

Another question we might ask about charge separation is whether or not the number of ions accumulated in the charged layer represents a significant fraction of the total number of ions in the cell. The answer is that it does not. If we consider our model cell to have a radius of 25 μm, then at a concentration of 120 millimolar (mM) there are roughly 4×10^{12} cations and an equal number of anions in the cytoplasm. At a membrane potential of –85 mV the amount of charge separated by the membrane is about 5×10^{11} univalent ions/cm^2 (see Chapter 8). Our cell has a surface area of about 8×10^{-5} cm^2, so there are approximately 4×10^7 negative ions collected at the inner surface of the membrane, which is 1/100,000 the number in free solution.

The Effect of Extracellular Potassium and Chloride on Membrane Potential

In neurons and in many other cells, the steady-state resting membrane potential is sensitive to changes in extracellular potassium concentration but is relatively unaffected by changes in extracellular chloride. To understand how this comes about, it is useful to consider the consequences of such changes in the model cell. We will assume throughout this discussion that the volume of the extracellular fluid is infinitely large relative to the volume of the cell. Thus, movements of ions and water into or out of the cell have no significant effect on extracellular concentrations.

Figure 6.2A shows the changes in intracellular composition and membrane potential that result from increasing extracellular potassium from 3 mM to 6 mM. The extracellular sodium concentration is reduced by 3 mM to keep the osmolarity unchanged. The increase in extracellular potassium reduces the concentration gradient for outward potassium movement, while initially leaving the electrical gradient unchanged. As a result, there will be a net inward movement of potassium ions. As positive charges accumulate on its inner surface, the membrane is depolarized. This in turn means that chloride ions are no longer in equilibrium and they move into the cell as well. Potassium and chloride entry continue until a new equilibrium is established, and both ions are at a new concentration ratio consistent with the new membrane potential, in this example –68 mV.

Potassium and chloride entry is accompanied by entry of water to maintain osmotic balance, resulting in a slight increase in cell volume. When the new equilibrium is reached, intracellular potassium has increased in concentration from 90 mM to 91 mM, intracellular chloride from 4 mM to 7.9 mM, and the cell volume has increased by 3.5%.

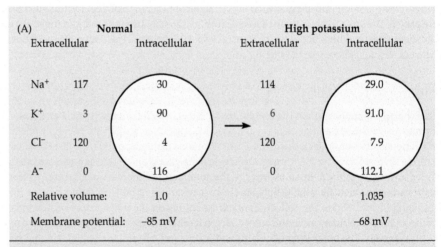

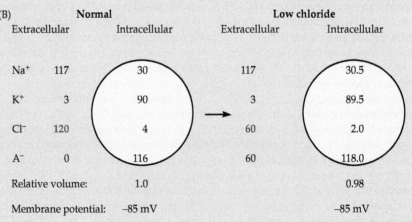

FIGURE 6.2 Effects of Changing Extracellular Ion Composition on intracellular ion concentrations and membrane potential. (A) When extracellular K$^+$ is doubled, a corresponding reduction in extracellular Na$^+$ keeps osmolarity constant. (B) Half the extracellular Cl$^-$ is replaced by an impermeant anion, A$^-$. Ion concentrations are mM, and extracellular volumes are assumed to be very large with respect to cell volumes so that fluxes into and out of the cell do not change extracellular concentrations.

At first glance it seems that more chloride than potassium has entered the cell, but think what the concentrations would be if the cell did *not* increase in volume: The concentrations of both ions would be greater than the indicated values by 3.5%. Thus, the intracellular chloride concentration would be about 8.2 mM (instead of 7.9 mM after the entry of water), and intracellular potassium would be about 94.2 mM—both being 4.2 mM higher than in the original solution. In other words, we can think first of potassium and chloride entering in equal quantities (except for the trivial difference required to change the charge on the membrane) and then of water following to achieve the final concentrations shown in the figure.

Similar considerations apply to changes in extracellular chloride concentration, but with a marked difference: When the new steady state is finally reached, the membrane potential is essentially unchanged. The consequences of a 50% reduction in extracellular chloride concentration are shown in Figure 6.2B, in which 60 mM of chloride in the solution bathing the cell is replaced by an impermeant anion. Chloride leaves the cell, depolarizing the membrane toward a new chloride equilibrium potential (–68 mV). Potassium, no longer being in equilibrium, leaves as well. As in the previous example, potassium and chloride leave the cell in equal quantities (accompanied by water). Because the intracellular concentration of potassium is high, the fractional change in concentration produced by the efflux is relatively small. However, the efflux of chloride causes a sizable fractional change in the intracellular chloride concentration, and hence in the chloride equilibrium potential. As chloride continues to leave the cell, the equilibrium potential returns toward its original value of –85 mV. The process continues until the chloride and potassium equilibrium potentials are again equal and the membrane potential is restored.

Membrane Potentials in Squid Axons

The idea that the resting membrane potential is the result of an unequal distribution of potassium ions between the extracellular and intracellular fluids was first proposed by Julius Bernstein[1] in 1902. He could not test this hypothesis directly, however, because there was no satisfactory way of measuring membrane potential. It is now possible to measure membrane potential accurately and to see whether changes in external and internal potassium concentrations produce the potential changes predicted by the Nernst relation. The first such experiments were done on giant axons that innervate the mantle of the squid. The axons are up to 1 mm in diameter,[2] and their large size permits the insertion of recording electrodes into their cytoplasm to measure transmembrane potential directly (Figure 6.3A). Furthermore,

[1]Bernstein, J. 1902. *Pflügers Arch.* 92: 521–562.

[2]Young, J. Z. 1937. *Q. J. Microsc. Sci.* 78: 367–387.

FIGURE 6.3 Recording from a Squid Axon. (A) Isolated squid giant axon with axial recording electrode inside. (B) Extrusion of axoplasm from the axon, which is then cannulated and perfused internally. (C) Comparison of recordings before perfusion ("Intact") and after perfusion ("Perfused") shows that the resting and action potentials are unaffected by removal of the axoplasm. (B and C after P. F. Baker et al., 1962. *J. Physiol.* 164: 330–354.)

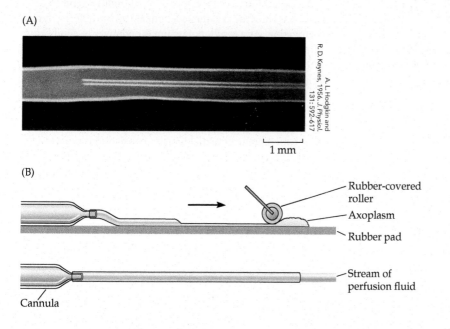

(A)

A. L. Hodgkin and R. D. Keynes, 1956. *J. Physiol.* 131: 592–617.

1 mm

(B)

Rubber-covered roller

Axoplasm

Rubber pad

Cannula

Stream of perfusion fluid

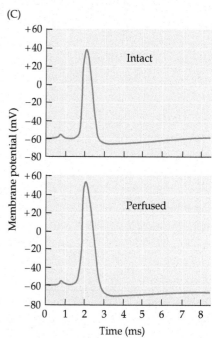

(C)

they are remarkably resilient and continue to function even when their axoplasm has been squeezed out with a rubber roller and replaced with an internal perfusate (Figure 6.3B,C)! Thus their internal as well as external ionic composition can be controlled.

The concentrations of some of the major ions in squid blood and in the axoplasm of the squid nerves are given in Table 6.1 (several ions, including magnesium and internal anions, are omitted). Experiments on isolated axons are usually done in seawater, with the ratio of intracellular to extracellular potassium concentrations being 40:1. In these conditions the membrane potential is –65 to –70 mV, considerably less negative than the potassium equilibrium potential of –93 mV, but more negative than the chloride equilibrium potential, which is about –55 mV.

Bernstein's hypothesis was tested by measuring the resting membrane potential and comparing it with the potassium equilibrium potential at various extracellular potassium concentrations. As with our model cell, these changes would not be expected to produce a significant change in internal potassium concentration. From the Nernst equation, changing the concentration ratio by a factor of ten should change the membrane potential by 58 mV at room temperature. The results of an experiment on squid axon in which the external potassium concentration was changed are shown in Figure 6.4. The external concentration is plotted on a logarithmic scale on the abscissa and the membrane potential on the ordinate. The expected slope of 58 mV per tenfold change in extracellular potassium concentration is realized only at relatively high concentrations (solid straight line), with the slope becoming less and less steep as external potassium is reduced. This result indicates that the potassium ion distribution is not the only factor contributing to the membrane potential.

The Effect of Sodium Permeability

From the experiments on squid axon we can conclude that the hypothesis put forward by Bernstein in 1902 is almost correct; the membrane potential is strongly, but not exclusively, dependent on the potassium concentration ratio. We can explain the deviation from the Nernst relation shown in Figure 6.4 simply by abandoning the notion that the membrane is impermeable to sodium. Real nerve cell membranes, in fact, have a permeability to sodium that ranges between 1% and 10% of their permeability to potassium.

To consider the effect of sodium permeability, we begin with our model cell (see Figure 6.1) and, for the moment, ignore any movement of chloride ions. The Nernst equation tells us that sodium would be in equilibrium at a membrane potential of +34 mV (E_{Na}), far from the actual membrane potential of –85 mV. So if we make the membrane permeable to sodium, both the concentration gradient and the membrane potential tend to drive sodium into the cell. As sodium ions enter the cell, they accumulate on the inner surface of the membrane, causing depolarization. As a result, potassium is no longer in equilibrium and potassium ions leave the cell. As depolarization progresses, the membrane potential moves closer to the sodium equilibrium potential and farther from the potassium equilibrium potential. As this happens, the sodium influx decreases and the potassium efflux increases. The process continues until the influx of sodium is exactly balanced by the efflux of potassium. At that point there is no further charge accumulation, and the membrane potential remains constant. In summary, the membrane potential lies between the potassium and sodium equilibrium potentials and is the potential at which the sodium and potassium currents are exactly equal and opposite.

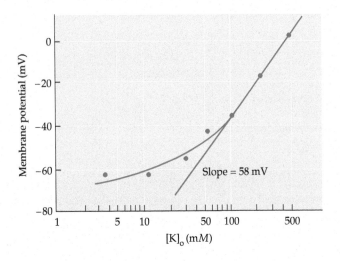

FIGURE 6.4 Membrane Potential versus External Potassium Concentration in a squid axon, plotted on a semilogarithmic scale. The straight line is drawn with a slope of 58 mV per tenfold change in extracellular potassium concentration, according to the Nernst equation. Because the membrane is also permeable to sodium, the points deviate from the straight line, especially at low potassium concentrations. (After A. L. Hodgkin and P. Horowicz, 1959. *J. Physiol.* 145: 405–432.)

Chloride ions participate in the process as well, but as we have already seen, there is ultimately an adjustment in intracellular chloride concentration in the model cell, so that the chloride equilibrium potential matches the new membrane potential. As the cation fluxes reach a balance, the intracellular chloride concentration increases until there is no net chloride flux across the membrane.

The Constant Field Equation

To determine the exact membrane potential in our model cell, we have to consider the individual ion currents across the membrane. The inward sodium current (I_{Na}) depends on the driving force for sodium, which is the difference between the membrane potential and the sodium equilibrium potential, $V_m - E_{Na}$ (see Chapter 4). The sodium current also depends on the sodium conductance of the membrane, or g_{Na}. The sodium conductance is a measure of the ease with which sodium can pass through the membrane and depends on the number of open sodium channels—the more open channels, the greater the conductance. So the sodium current is:

$$I_{Na} = g_{Na}(V_m - E_{Na})$$

The same relationship holds for potassium and chloride:

$$I_K = g_K(V_m - E_K)$$
$$I_{Cl} = g_{Cl}(V_m - E_{Cl})$$

If we assume that chloride is in equilibrium, so that $I_{Cl} = 0$, then for the membrane potential to remain constant, the potassium and sodium currents must be equal and opposite:

$$g_K(V_m - E_K) = -g_{Na}(V_m - E_{Na})$$

It is useful to examine this relationship in more detail. Suppose g_K is much larger than g_{Na}. Then, if the currents are to be equal, the driving force for potassium efflux must be much smaller than that for sodium entry. In other words, the membrane potential must be much closer to E_K than to E_{Na}. Conversely, if g_{Na} is relatively large, the membrane potential will be closer to E_{Na}.

By rearranging the equation we arrive at an expression for the membrane potential:

$$V_m = \frac{g_K E_K + g_{Na} E_{Na}}{g_K + g_{Na}}$$

If, for some reason, chloride is not at equilibrium, then chloride currents across the membrane must be considered and the equation becomes slightly more complicated:

$$V_m = \frac{g_K E_K + g_{Na} E_{Na} + g_{Cl} E_{Cl}}{g_K + g_{Na} + g_{Cl}}$$

These ideas were developed originally by Goldman,[3] and independently by Hodgkin and Katz.[4] However, instead of considering equilibrium potentials and conductances, they derived an equation for membrane potential in terms of ion concentrations outside ($[K]_o$, $[Na]_o$, $[Cl]_o$) and inside ($[K]_i$, etc.) the cell, and membrane *permeability* to each ion (p_K, p_{Na}, and p_{Cl}):

$$V_m = 58\log \frac{p_K[K]_o + p_{Na}[Na]_o + p_{Cl}[Cl]_i}{p_K[K]_i + p_{Na}[Na]_i + p_{Cl}[Cl]_o}$$

Note that the chloride ratios are reversed, as occurred previously in the Nernst equation, because the chloride valence is –1.

[3]Goldman, D. E. 1943. *J. Gen. Physiol.* 27: 37-60.

[4]Hodgkin, A. L., and Katz, B. 1949. *J. Physiol.* 108: 37-77.

As before, if chloride is in equilibrium, the chloride terms disappear. This equation is sometimes called the GHK equation for its originators, and is also known as the **constant field equation**, because one of the assumptions made in arriving at the expression was that the voltage gradient, or "field," across the membrane is uniform. The constant field equation is entirely analogous to the previous equation and makes the same predictions: When the permeability to potassium is very high relative to the sodium and chloride permeabilities, the sodium and chloride terms become negligible and the membrane potential approaches the equilibrium potential for potassium: $V_m = 58 \log ([K]_o/([K]_i)$. Increasing sodium permeability causes the membrane potential to move toward the sodium equilibrium potential.

The constant field equation provides us with a useful general principle to remember: The membrane potential depends on the relative conductances (or permeabilities) of the membrane to the major ions, and on the equilibrium potentials for those ions. In real cells the resting permeabilities to potassium and chloride are relatively high. Hence, the resting membrane potential is close to the potassium and chloride equilibrium potentials. When sodium permeability is increased, as occurs during an action potential (see Chapter 7) or an excitatory postsynaptic potential (see Chapter 11), the membrane potential moves toward the sodium equilibrium potential.

The Resting Membrane Potential

As useful as the constant field equation is, it does not provide us with an accurate description of the resting membrane potential, because the requirement for zero net current across the membrane is not, in itself, adequate. Instead, for the cell to remain in a stable condition, *each* individual ion current must be zero. As a result, under the conditions of the constant field equation, the cell would gradually fill up with sodium and chloride and lose potassium. In real cells, intracellular sodium and potassium concentrations are kept constant by a sodium–potassium exchange pump (sodium–potassium ATPase; see Chapter 9). As sodium and potassium leak into and out of the cell, the pump transports a matching amount of each ion in the opposite direction (Figure 6.5). Thus, metabolic energy is used to maintain the cell in a **steady state**.

In order to have a more complete and accurate description of the resting membrane potential, we must consider both the passive ion fluxes and the activity of the pump. Again, we first consider the currents carried by passive fluxes of sodium and potassium across the membrane:

$$I_{Na} = g_{Na}(V_m - E_{Na})$$
$$I_K = g_K(V_m - E_K)$$

We no longer assume that the sodium and potassium currents are equal and opposite, but if we know how they are related we can, as before, obtain an equation for the membrane potential in terms of the sodium and potassium equilibrium potentials and their relative conductances. The relationship between the sodium and potassium currents is given by the characteristics of the pump. Because it keeps intracellular sodium and potassium concentrations constant by transporting the ions in the ratio of 3 Na to 2 K (see Chapter 9), it follows that the passive ion fluxes must be in the same ratio: $I_{Na}:I_K = 3:2$. So we can write:

$$\frac{I_{Na}}{I_K} = \frac{g_{Na}(V_m - E_{Na})}{g_K(V_m - E_K)} = -1.5$$

The ratio is negative because the sodium and potassium currents are flowing in opposite directions. By rearranging the equation we get an expression for the membrane potential:

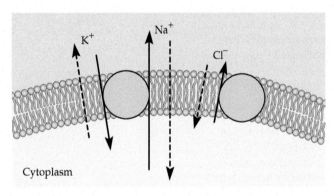

FIGURE 6.5 Passive Ion Fluxes and Pumps in a Steady State. Net passive ion movements across the membrane are indicated by dashed arrows, and transport systems by solid arrows and circles. Lengths of arrows indicate the magnitudes of net ion movements. Total flux is zero for each ion. For example, net inward leak of Na$^+$ is equal to the rate of outward transport. Na$^+$:K$^+$ transport is coupled with a ratio of 3:2. In any particular cell, Cl$^-$ transport may be outward (as shown) or inward.

$$V_\mathrm{m} = \frac{1.5 g_\mathrm{K} E_\mathrm{K} + g_\mathrm{Na} E_\mathrm{Na}}{1.5 g_\mathrm{K} + g_\mathrm{Na}}$$

[5]Mullins, L. J., and Noda, K. 1963. *J. Gen. Physiol.* 47: 117-132.

[6]Martin, A. R. 1979. Appendix to Matthews, G., and Wickelgren, W. O. *J. Physiol.* 293: 393-414.

The equation is similar to the expression derived previously for the model cell and makes the same kinds of predictions. As before, the membrane potential depends on the relative magnitudes of g_K and g_Na. The difference is that the potassium term is multiplied by a factor of 1.5. Because of this factor, the membrane potential is closer to E_K than would otherwise be the case. Thus, the driving force for sodium entry is increased and that for potassium influx reduced. As a result, the passive fluxes are in a ratio of 3 Na to 2 K rather than 1:1.

In summary, the real cell differs from the model cell in that the resting membrane potential is the potential at which the passive influx of sodium is 1.5 times the passive efflux of potassium, rather than the potential at which the two fluxes are equal and opposite. The passive inward and outward currents are determined by the equilibrium potentials and conductances for the two ions; the required ratio of 3:2 is determined by the transport characteristics of the pump.

The problem of finding an expression for the resting membrane potential of real cells, taking into account the transport activity, was first considered by Mullins and Noda,[5] who used intracellular microelectrodes to study the effects of ionic changes on membrane potential in muscle. Like Goldman, Hodgkin, and Katz, they derived an expression for membrane potential in terms of permeabilities and concentrations. The result is equivalent to the constant field equation we have just derived using conductances and equilibrium potentials:

$$V_\mathrm{m} = 58 \log \frac{r p_\mathrm{K}[\mathrm{K}]_\mathrm{o} + p_\mathrm{Na}[\mathrm{Na}]_\mathrm{o}}{r p_\mathrm{K}[\mathrm{K}]_\mathrm{i} + p_\mathrm{Na}[\mathrm{Na}]_\mathrm{i}}$$

where r is the absolute value of the transport ratio (3:2). The equation provides an accurate description of the membrane potential when the cell is at rest—that is, when all the permeant ions are in a steady state.

Chloride Distribution

How do these considerations apply to chloride? As for all other ions, there must be no net chloride current across the resting membrane. As already discussed (see Figure 6.2B), chloride is able to reach equilibrium simply by an appropriate adjustment in internal concentration, without affecting the steady-state membrane potential. In many cells, however, there are transport systems for chloride as well (see Chapter 9). In squid axon and in muscle, chloride is transported actively into the cells; in many nerve cells, active transport is outward (see Figure 6.5). The effect of inward transport is to add an increment to the equilibrium concentration such that there is an outward leak of chloride equal to the rate of transport in the opposite direction.[6] Outward transport has the reverse effect.

An Electrical Model of the Membrane

The characteristics of the nerve cell membrane endow it with the electrical properties illustrated in Figure 6.6. First, because the membrane is an insulating layer separating electrical charges on its inner and outer surfaces, it has the properties of a capacitor. In parallel with the capacitor are conductance pathways, represented by resistors that allow ion fluxes into and out of the cell. The

FIGURE 6.6 Electrical Model of the Steady-State Cell shown in Figure 6.2. E_K, E_Na, and E_Cl are the Nernst potentials for the individual ions. The individual ion conductances are represented by resistors, with a resistance of $1/g$ for each ion. The individual ion currents I_K, I_Na, and I_Cl are equal and opposite to the currents $I_\mathrm{T(K)}$, $I_\mathrm{T(Na)}$, and $I_\mathrm{T(Cl)}$ supplied by the sodium-potassium exchange pump ($T_\mathrm{Na-K}$) and the chloride pump (T_Cl), so that the net flux of each ion across the membrane is zero. The resulting membrane potential (V_m) determines the amount of charge stored on the membrane capacitor (C_m).

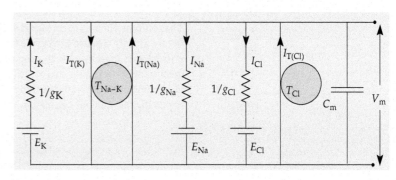

electrical resistance in each pathway is inversely related to the conductance for the ion in question: The greater the ion conductance, the lower the resistance to current flow. Passive ion currents through the resistors are driven by batteries that represent the equilibrium potentials for each of the ions. The passive currents are equal and opposite to the corresponding currents generated by the pumps, so that the net current across the membrane for each ion is zero.

Predicted Values of Membrane Potential

How do these considerations explain the relation between potassium concentration and membrane potential shown in Figure 6.4? This can be seen by using real numbers in the equations. In squid axon, the permeability constants for potassium and sodium are roughly in the ratio 1.0:0.04.[7] We can use these relative values, together with the ion concentrations given in Table 6.1, to calculate the resting membrane potential in seawater:

$$V_m = 58 \log \frac{(1.5)(10) + (0.04)(460)}{(1.5)(400) + (0.04)(50)} = -73 \, \text{mV}$$

Now we can see quantitatively why, when extracellular potassium is altered, the membrane potential fails to follow the Nernst potential for potassium. If, in the numerator of the equation, we look at the magnitude of the term involving extracellular potassium concentration ($1.5 \times 10 = 15$ mM) and the term that involves extracellular sodium concentration ($0.04 \times 460 = 18.4$ mM), we see that potassium contributes only about 45% of the total. Because of this, doubling the external potassium concentration does not double the numerator (as would happen in the Nernst equation), and as a consequence, the effect on the potential of changing extracellular potassium concentration is less than would be expected if potassium were the only permeant ion. When the external potassium concentration is raised to a high enough level (100 mM in Figure 6.4), the potassium term becomes sufficiently dominant for the current–voltage relation to approach the theoretical limit of 58 mV per tenfold change in concentration. This effect is enhanced by the fact that many potassium channels are voltage-activated (see Chapter 7). When the membrane is depolarized by increasing the extracellular potassium concentration, the voltage-activated channels open, thereby increasing the potassium permeability. As a result, the relative contribution of potassium to the membrane potential is increased still further.

In general, nerve cells have resting potentials of the order of –70 mV. In some cells, such as vertebrate skeletal muscle,[8] the resting potential can be –90 mV or larger, reflecting a low ratio of sodium-to-potassium permeability. Glial cells in particular have a very low resting permeability to sodium, so their membrane potential is nearly identical to the potassium equilibrium potential (see Chapter 10). Other cells, such as leech ganglion cells[8] and photoreceptors in the vertebrate retina,[9] have relatively high membrane permeability to sodium and resting membrane potentials as small as –40 mV.

Contribution of the Sodium-Potassium Pump to the Membrane Potential

The sodium–potassium transport system is **electrogenic** (capable of generating an electrical current) because each cycle of the pump results in the net outward transfer of one positive ion, thereby contributing to the excess negative charge on the inner face of the membrane. How large is this contribution? An easy way to find out is to calculate what the membrane potential would be if the pump were *not* electrogenic or, in other words, if $r = 1$. Repeating the previous calculation with this condition gives the following:

$$V_m = 58 \log \frac{(1.0)(10) + (0.04)(460)}{(1.0)(400) + (0.04)(50)} = -67 \, \text{mV}$$

[7]Fatt, P., and Katz, B. 1951. *J. Physiol.* 115: 320-370.

[8]Nicholls, J. G., and Baylor, D. A. 1968. *J. Neurophysiol.* 31: 740-757.

[9]Baylor, D. A., and Fuortes, M. G. F. 1970. *J. Physiol.* 207: 77-92.

The result is 6 mV less than the previous value, so the pump contributes –6 mV to the resting potential. In general, the size of the pump contribution depends on several factors, particularly the relative ion permeabilities. For a transport ratio of 3:2, the steady-state contribution to the resting membrane potential is limited to a maximum of about –11 mV.[10] If the transport process is stopped, the electrogenic contribution disappears immediately and the membrane potential then declines gradually as the cell gains sodium and loses potassium.

It is interesting that the *rate* of transport does not appear in the equation, apart from the implicit requirement that it must match the passive ion fluxes. Theoretical calculations indicate that once that requirement is met, any further increase in sodium–potassium pump activity can be expected to have very little effect on the steady-state resting membrane potential.[11] This is largely because the transport system is dependent on intracellular sodium concentration (see Chapter 9). Any increase in pump rate results in hyperpolarization and depletion of intracellular sodium. As the sodium concentration falls, the pump rate and the membrane potential return toward their previous value.

What Ion Channels Are Associated with the Resting Potential?

The resting permeabilities of membranes to sodium, potassium, and chloride have been determined in many nerve cells. Underlying these is a wide variety of membrane channels that permit the passage of anions and cations into and out of the cell. However, the precise identification of the channels underlying these ionic **leak currents** in any specific cells is difficult. A significant fraction of the resting potassium current is likely to be through 2P potassium channels (see Chapter 5), which tend to be open at the resting membrane potential.[12,13] In addition, many nerve cells have M-type potassium channels that are open at rest and closed by intracellular messengers (see Chapter 19). M-currents, together with accompanying h-currents, are responsible for most of the potassium leak in sympathetic ganglion cells.[14] H-currents are carried by HCN (hyperpolarization-activated cyclic nucleotide-gated) channels that are activated by hyperpolarization—and some of which are open at normal resting potentials.[15] HCN channels are cation channels with a sodium-to-potassium permeability ratio (p_{Na}/p_K) of about 0.25 and thus are responsible for a fraction of the sodium leak current as well. Other contributors to resting potassium permeability include channels activated by intracellular cations, namely sodium-activated and calcium-activated potassium channels. Finally, a few voltage-sensitive potassium channels associated with the action potential may be open at rest.

Apart from HCN channels, the major source of resting sodium permeability is the so-called NALCN (sodium leak channel, nonselective) channel that is open at rest.[16] NALCN channels are virtually nonselective for monovalent cations ($p_{Na}/p_K \approx 1.1$), so that at normal resting potentials the main ion movement through the channels is inward sodium flux. An additional sodium influx occurs not through channels, but rather through sodium-dependent secondary active transport systems (see Chapter 9). Finally, tetrodotoxin has been shown to block a small fraction of the resting sodium conductance,[8] indicating a contribution by voltage-activated sodium channels.

An unusual pathological leak current in skeletal muscle cells is found in a neuromuscular disease known as hypokalemic periodic paralysis. The current is unusual in that it does not involve ion movements through open channels. Instead, it is associated with cation fluxes through a normally occluded protein pore around the sodium channel S4 helix.[17] This so-called omega current (see Chapter 7) is associated with a mutation in which charge-carrying arginine residues on the helix are replaced by smaller neutral amino acids, thereby allowing cations to permeate the pore. The result is a constant inward leak of sodium into the muscle cell.

The family of chloride channels of the CLC family (ClCs; see Chapter 5) is widely distributed in nerve and muscle. The presence of ClCs is important in that they serve to stabilize the membrane potential (see the next section). The channels also interact with chloride transport systems to determine intracellular chloride concentrations.[18,19] For example, in embryonic hippocampal neurons, ClC expression is low, and E_{Cl} is positive to the resting membrane potential because of inward transport and accumulation of chloride in the cytoplasm. In adult neurons, expression of ClCs increases the chloride conductance of the membrane so that excess accumulation does not occur. In central nervous system neurons, ClCs can account for as much as 10% of the resting membrane conductance.[20]

[10]Martin, A. R., and Levinson, S. R. 1985. *Muscle Nerve* 8: 354-362.

[11]Fraser, J. A., and Huang, C. L.-H. 2004. *J. Physiol.* 559: 459-478.

[12]Brown, D. A. 2000. *Curr. Biol.* 10: R456-459.

[13]Goldstein, S. A. N. et al. 2001. *Nat. Rev. Neurosci.* 2: 175-184.

[14]Lamas, J. A. et al. 2002. *Neuroreport* 13: 585-591.

[15]Biel, M. et al. 2009. *Physiol. Rev.* 89: 847-885.

[16]Lu, B. et al. 2007. *Cell* 129: 371-383.

[17]Sokolov, S., Scheuer, T., and Catterall, W. A. 2007. *Nature* 446: 76-78.

[18]Staley, K. et al. 1997. *Neuron* 17: 543-551.

[19]Meladinić, M. et al. 1999. *Proc. R. Soc. Lond., B, Biol. Sci.* 266: 1207-1213.

[20]Gold, M. R., and Martin, A. R. 1983. *J. Physiol.* 342: 99-117.

Changes in Membrane Potential

It is important to keep in mind that this discussion of resting membrane potential is always in reference to *steady-state* conditions. For example, we have said that changing extracellular chloride concentration has little effect on membrane potential because the intracellular chloride concentration accommodates to the change. That is true in the long run, but the intracellular adjustment takes time, and while it is occurring, there is indeed a transient effect.

The steady-state potential is the baseline on which all changes in membrane potential are superimposed. How are such changes in potential produced? In general, transient changes, such as those that mediate signaling between cells in the nervous system, are the result of transient changes in membrane permeability. As we already know from the constant field equation, an increase in sodium permeability (or a decrease in potassium permeability) will move the membrane potential toward the sodium equilibrium potential, producing depolarization. Conversely, an increase in potassium permeability will produce hyperpolarization. Another ion of importance in signaling is calcium. Intracellular calcium concentration is very low, and in most cells E_{Ca} is greater than +150 mV. Thus, an increase in calcium permeability results in calcium influx and depolarization.

The role of chloride permeability in the control of membrane potential is of particular interest. As we have noted, chloride makes little contribution to the resting membrane potential. Instead, intracellular chloride concentration adjusts to the potential and is modified by whatever chloride transport mechanisms are operating in the cell membrane. The effect of a transient increase in chloride permeability can be either hyperpolarizing or depolarizing, depending on whether the chloride equilibrium potential is negative or positive to the resting potential. The equilibrium potential, in turn, depends on whether intracellular chloride is depleted or concentrated by the transport system. In either case, the change in potential is usually relatively small. Even so, an increase in chloride permeability can be important for the regulation of signaling because it tends to hold the membrane potential near the chloride equilibrium potential and thus attenuates changes in potential produced by other influences.

Stabilization of the membrane potential in this way is important for controlling the excitability of many cells, such as skeletal muscle fibers, that have a relatively high chloride permeability at rest. In such cells, a transient influx of positive ions causes less depolarization than would otherwise be the case, because it is countered by an influx of chloride through already open channels. This mechanism is of some significance, as illustrated by the fact that chloride channel mutations that reduce chloride conductance are responsible for several muscle diseases. The diseased muscles are hyperexcitable (myotonic) due to loss of the normal stabilizing influence of a high chloride conductance.[21,22]

[21]Barchi, R. L. 1997. *Neurobiol. Dis.* 4: 254-264.

[22]Cannon, S. C. 1997. *Trends. Neurosci.* 19: 3-10.

SUMMARY

- Nerve cells have high intracellular concentrations of potassium and low intracellular concentrations of sodium and chloride, so potassium tends to diffuse out of the cell and sodium and chloride tend to diffuse in. The tendency for potassium and chloride to diffuse down their concentration gradients is opposed by the electrical potential across the cell membrane.

- In a model cell that is permeable only to potassium and chloride, the concentration gradients can be balanced exactly by the membrane potential, so that there is no net flux of either ion across the membrane. The membrane potential is then equal to the equilibrium potential for both potassium and chloride.

- Changing the extracellular potassium concentration changes the potassium equilibrium potential and, hence, the membrane potential. Changing extracellular chloride concentration, by contrast, leads ultimately to a change in intracellular chloride, so that the chloride equilibrium potential and the membrane potential differ from their original values only transiently.

- In addition to being permeable to potassium and chloride, the cell membrane of real cells is permeable to sodium. As a result, there is a constant influx of sodium into the cell and an efflux of potassium. These fluxes are balanced exactly by active transport of the ions in opposite directions, in the ratio of 3 Na to 2 K. Under these circumstances, the membrane potential depends on the sodium equilibrium potential, the potassium equilibrium potential, the relative conductance of the membrane to the two ions, and the sodium-potassium exchange pump ratio.

- Because the sodium-potassium exchange pump transports more positive ions outward than inward across the membrane, it can make a direct contribution of several millivolts to the membrane potential.

- The chloride equilibrium potential may be positive or negative to the resting membrane potential, depending on chloride transport processes. Although the chloride distribution plays little role in determining the resting membrane potential, high chloride permeability is important for electrical stability.

Suggested Reading

Hodgkin, A. L., and Katz, B. 1949. The effect of sodium ions on the electrical activity of the giant axon of the squid. *J. Physiol.* 108: 37–77. (The constant field equation is derived in Appendix A of this paper.)

Mullins, L. J., and Noda, K. 1963. The influence of sodium-free solutions on membrane potential of frog muscle fibers. *J. Gen. Physiol.* 47: 117–132.

CHAPTER 7

Ionic Basis of the Action Potential

The ion mechanisms responsible for generating action potentials have been described quantitatively, largely through the use of the voltage clamp method to measure membrane currents. From such measurements, it is possible to determine which components of the currents are carried by each ion species, and to deduce the magnitude and time course of the underlying changes in ion conductances. The experiments have shown that depolarization rapidly increases sodium conductance and, more slowly, potassium conductance. The activation of sodium conductance is transient, being followed by inactivation. The increase in potassium conductance persists for as long as the depolarizing pulse is maintained. The dependence of sodium and potassium conductances on membrane potential and their sequential timing account quantitatively for the amplitude and time course of the action potential as well as for other phenomena, such as threshold and refractory period.

Other channels, in addition to the voltage-dependent sodium and potassium channels just cited, can be involved in action potential generation. In some cells, voltage-activated calcium channels are responsible for the rising phase of the action potential, and repolarization can involve currents associated with activation of several additional potassium channel types. The action potential itself can be followed by afterpotentials, which are periods of hyperpolarization or depolarization mediated by prolonged changes in membrane conductance.

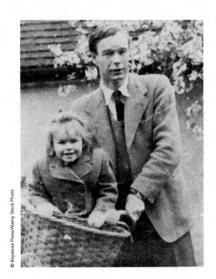

A. L. Hodgkin, 1949

In Chapter 6 we showed how the membrane potential of a nerve cell depends on its relative permeability to the major ions present in the extracellular and intracellular fluids, particularly sodium and potassium. The membrane potential of a cell at rest is near the potassium equilibrium potential (E_K) because of the relatively high permeability of its membrane for potassium. It was discovered more than 100 years ago that sodium ions were necessary for nerve and muscle cells to produce an action potential, and evidence gradually accumulated to support the idea that the mechanism underlying action potential generation was an increase in sodium permeability that drove the membrane potential toward the sodium equilibrium potential.

Critical experiments were done in the early 1950s by Hodgkin, Huxley, and Katz[1] and by Hodgkin and Huxley.[2-5] Two main features contributed to the success of their experiments: One was the availability of the giant axon of squid, and the other was a newly developed experimental tool called the **voltage clamp**. These researchers found that the rising and falling phases of the action potential were accompanied by a large, transient influx of sodium ions, followed by an efflux of potassium. They then were able to deduce the underlying changes in membrane conductance and to show that these were of the correct magnitude and time course to account exactly for the magnitude and time course of the action potential. Since that time a great number of similar experiments have been carried out on other nerve cells and on muscle cells, and many new experimental techniques have been applied to the problem. Almost 70 years later, the basic conclusions of Hodgkin, Huxley, and Katz still stand. One of their remarkable achievements was their speculation that the membrane currents passed through ion-specific channels, whose properties they predicted with surprising accuracy.

[1] Hodgkin, A. L., Huxley, A. F., and Katz, B. 1952. *J. Physiol.* 116: 424-448.

[2] Hodgkin, A. L., and Huxley, A. F. 1952a. *J. Physiol.* 116: 449-472.

[3] Hodgkin, A. L., and Huxley, A. F. 1952b. *J. Physiol.* 116: 473-496.

[4] Hodgkin, A. L., and Huxley, A. F. 1952c. *J. Physiol.* 116: 497-506.

[5] Hodgkin, A. L., and Huxley, A. F. 1952d. *J. Physiol.* 117: 500-544.

[6] Marmont, G. 1949. *J. Cell. Physiol.* 34: 351-382.

Voltage Clamp Experiments

The voltage clamp technique was devised by Cole and his colleagues[6] and developed further by Hodgkin, Huxley, and Katz.[1] The aim of the experiments was to identify the nature of the ion currents underlying the action potential and to determine their magnitude and time course. Box 7.1 describes the experimental arrangement. All we need to know to understand the experiments themselves is that the method permits one to set the membrane potential of the cell almost instantaneously to any level and hold it there (that is, "clamp" it) while at the same time record the current flowing across the membrane. Figure 7.1 shows an example of

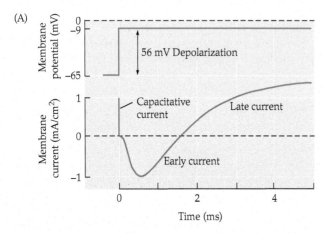

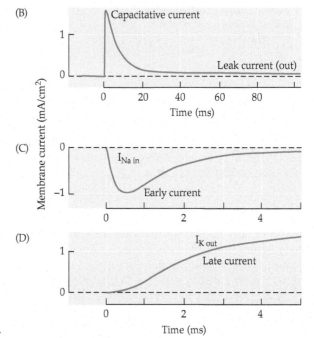

FIGURE 7.1   Membrane Currents Produced by Depolarization. (A) Currents measured by voltage clamp during a 56-mV depolarization of a squid axon membrane. The currents (lower trace) consist of a brief, positive capacitative current, an early transient phase of inward current, and a late, maintained outward current. These three currents are shown separately in B, C, and D, respectively. (B) The capacitative current lasts for only a few microseconds (note the change in timescale). The small outward leakage current is due to movement of potassium and chloride. (C) The early inward current is due to sodium entry. (D) The late outward current is due to potassium movement out of the fiber.

BOX 7.1   The Voltage Clamp

The figure shown here illustrates an experimental arrangement for voltage clamp experiments on squid axons. Two fine silver wires are inserted longitudinally into the axon, which is bathed in seawater. One of the wires provides a measure of the potential inside the fiber with respect to that of the seawater (which is grounded), or in other words, a measure of the membrane potential (V_m). It is also connected to one input of the voltage clamp amplifier. The other input is connected to a variable voltage source, which can be set by the person doing the experiment; the value to which it is set is thus known as the command potential. The voltage clamp amplifier delivers current from its output whenever there is a voltage difference between the inputs. The output current flows across the cell membrane between the second fine silver wire and the seawater (arrows); it is measured by the voltage drop across a small series resistor.

The circuit is arranged so that the output current tends to cancel any voltage difference between the two inputs (negative feedback). It works as follows: First, suppose that the resting potential of the fiber is –70 mV and the command potential is set to –70 mV as well. Because the voltages at the two inputs of the amplifier are equal, there will be no output current. If the command potential is stepped to, say, –65 mV, then because of the 5-mV difference between the inputs, the amplifier delivers positive current into the axon and across the cell membrane. The current produces a voltage drop across the membrane, driving V_m to –65 mV and removing the voltage difference between the two inputs. In this way, the membrane potential is kept equal to the command potential. If the circuitry is properly designed, the change in V_m is achieved within a few microseconds.

Now suppose that the command potential is stepped from –70 mV to –15 mV. We would expect the

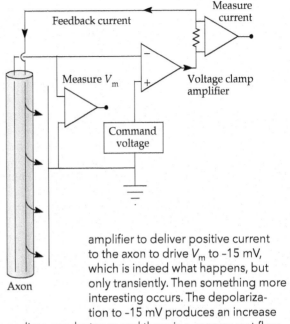

amplifier to deliver positive current to the axon to drive V_m to –15 mV, which is indeed what happens, but only transiently. Then something more interesting occurs. The depolarization to –15 mV produces an increase in sodium conductance and there is a consequent flow of sodium ions *inward*, across the membrane. In the absence of the clamp, this influx would tend to depolarize the membrane still further (i.e., toward the sodium equilibrium potential); with the clamp in place, however, the amplifier provides just the correct amount of negative current to hold the membrane potential constant. In other words, the current provided by the amplifier is exactly equal to the current flowing across the membrane. Here, then, is the great power of the voltage clamp: In addition to holding the membrane potential constant, it provides an exact measure of the membrane current required to do so. Voltage clamp measurements can now be made in small nerve cells by using the whole-cell method of patch clamp recording (see Chapter 4).

---

the currents that occur when the membrane potential is stepped suddenly from its resting value (in this example –65 mV) to a depolarized level (–9 mV). The current produced by the voltage step consists of three phases: (1) a brief outward surge lasting only a few microseconds (μs), (2) an early inward current, and (3) a late outward current.

Capacitative and Leak Currents

The initial brief surge of current is the **capacitative current**, which occurs because the step from one potential to another alters the charge on the membrane capacitance. If the clamp amplifier is capable of delivering a large amount of current, then the membrane can be charged rapidly and this current will last only a very short time. In practice, the surge of capacitative current lasts only about 20 μs and can be ignored when analyzing the subsequent ion currents.

The capacitative current is followed by a small, steady outward current known as **leak current**, which flows through the resting membrane conductances (see Figure 7.1B). Leak current is carried largely by potassium and chloride ions, varies linearly with voltage

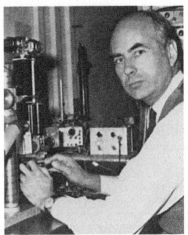

A. F. Huxley, 1974

displacement from rest in either direction, and lasts throughout the duration of the voltage step. However, during most of the response, it is obscured by the much larger ion currents associated with the action potential.

Ion Currents Carried by Sodium and Potassium

Turning now to the second and third phases of membrane current, Hodgkin and Huxley showed that these currents were due to the entry of sodium across the cell membrane, followed by the exit of potassium. In addition, they were able to deduce the relative size and time course of the separate currents. One convenient procedure was to abolish the sodium current by replacing most of the extracellular sodium with choline (an impermeant cation). With an appropriate reduction in extracellular sodium concentration, the sodium equilibrium potential could be made equal to the potential during the depolarizing step. As a result, there was no driving force for sodium entry during the step and thus no net current through the activated sodium channels. This left only the potassium current, as shown in Figure 7.1D. Subtraction of the potassium current from the total ion current (see Figure 7.1A) then revealed the magnitude and time course of the sodium current (see Figure 7.1C).

Selective Poisons for Sodium and Potassium Channels

Pharmacological methods now exist for blocking sodium and potassium currents selectively (Figure 7.2). Two toxins that have been particularly useful for inactivating sodium channels are tetrodotoxin (TTX) and its pharmacological equivalent saxitoxin (STX).[7,8] TTX is a virulent poison, concentrated in the ovaries and other organs of puffer fish. STX is synthesized by marine dinoflagellates and concentrated by filter-feeding shellfish, such as the butter clam *Saxidomus*. Its virulence competes with that of TTX—ingestion of a single clam (cooked or not) can be fatal. Sodium channels are blocked by several snail toxins (conotoxins) as well.[9]

The great advantage of TTX for neurophysiological studies is its high specificity. When a TTX-poisoned axon is subjected to a depolarizing voltage step, no inward sodium current is seen; only the delayed outward potassium current is seen (see Figure 7.2B). The potassium current is unchanged in amplitude and time course by the poison. Application of TTX to the inside of the membrane by adding it to an internal perfusing solution has no effect. The actions of STX are indistinguishable from those of TTX. Both toxins appear to bind to the same site in the outer mouth of the channel through which sodium ions move, thereby physically blocking ion current through the channel.[10]

Dependence of Ion Currents on Membrane Potential

Having established that the early and late currents were due to sodium influx followed by potassium efflux, Hodgkin and Huxley then determined how the magnitude and time course of the currents depended on membrane potential. Figure 7.3A shows the currents produced by various levels of depolarization from a holding potential of –65 mV. First of all, a step hyperpolarization to –85 mV (lowest record) produces only a small inward leak current, as would be expected from the resting properties of the membrane. As already shown in Figure 7.1, moderately depolarizing steps each produce an early inward current followed by a sustained outward current. With greater depolarizations, the early current becomes smaller, is absent at about +52 mV, and then reverses to become outward as the depolarizing step is increased still further to +65 mV.

[7] Llewellyn, L. E. 2009. *Prog. Mol. Subcell. Biol.* 46: 67-87.

[8] Watters, M. R. 2005. *Semin. Neurol.* 25: 278-289.

[9] Terlau, H., and Olivera, B. M. 2004. *Physiol. Rev.* 84: 41-68.

[10] Hille, B. 1970. *Prog. Biophys. Mol. Biol.* 21: 1-32.

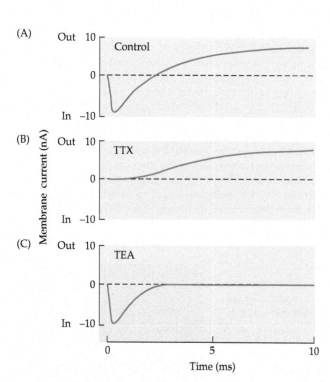

FIGURE 7.2 Pharmacological Separation of Membrane Currents into Sodium and Potassium Components. Membrane currents produced by clamping the membrane potential to 0 mV in a frog myelinated nerve. (A) A control record in normal bathing solution. (B) The addition of 300 nanomolar (n*M*) tetrodotoxin (TTX) causes the sodium current to disappear while the potassium current remains. (C) The addition of tetraethylammonium (TEA) blocks the potassium current, leaving the sodium current intact. (A and B after B. Hille, 1966. *Nature* 210: 1220-1222. C after B. Hille, 1967. *J. Gen. Physiol.* 50: 1287-1302.)

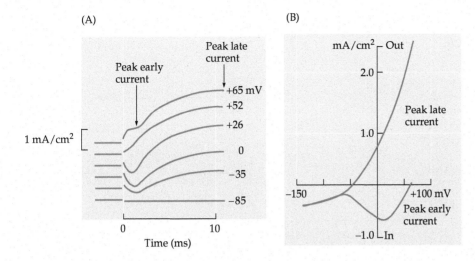

FIGURE 7.3 Dependence of Early and Late Currents on Potential. (A) Currents produced by voltage steps from a holding potential of –65 mV to a hyperpolarized level of –85 mV and then to successively increasing depolarized levels as indicated. The late potassium current increases as the depolarizing steps increase. The early sodium current first increases, then decreases with increasing depolarization, is absent at +52 mV, and reverses in sign at +65 mV. (B) Peak currents plotted against the potential to which the membrane is stepped. Late outward current increases rapidly with depolarization. Early inward current first increases in magnitude, then decreases, reversing to outward current at about +52 mV, which is the sodium equilibrium potential. (After A. L. Hodgkin et al., 1952. *J. Physiol.* 116: 424–448.)

Isolation of the currents underlying the action potential has also been aided by the discovery of several substances that block voltage-activated potassium channels. For example, in squid axons and in frog myelinated axons, Armstrong, Hille, and others have shown that voltage-activated potassium currents are blocked by tetraethylammonium (TEA) in concentrations greater than 10 mM (see Figure 7.2C).[11] In squid axons, TEA must be added to the internal solution and exerts its action at the inner mouth of the potassium channel; in other preparations, such as the frog node of Ranvier, TEA is effective when applied to the outside as well. Axons have a variety of other potassium channels that are blocked by compounds, such as 4-aminopyridine (4-AP), as well as the peptide toxins apamin, dendrotoxin, and charybdotoxin.[12]

The dependence of the two currents on membrane potential is shown in Figure 7.3B, where the peak amplitude of the early current and the steady-state amplitude of the late current are plotted against the potential to which the membrane is stepped. With hyperpolarizing voltage steps, there are no time-dependent (early and late) currents; the membrane simply responds as a passive resistor, with the expected inward current. The late current also behaves as one would expect of a resistor in the sense that depolarization produces outward current. However, as the depolarization is increased, the magnitude of the current becomes much greater than expected from the resting membrane properties. This is due to the activation of voltage-gated potassium channels. As the membrane potential becomes more positive, more and more potassium channels open, allowing additional current to flow through the membrane. The behavior of the early inward current is much more complex than that of the outward current. The early current first increases with increasing depolarization and then decreases, becoming zero at about +52 mV and then reversing in sign. The reversal potential is very near the equilibrium potential for sodium, as expected for a current carried by sodium ions.

The magnitude of the sodium current at any membrane potential depends on the sodium conductance (g_{Na}) and on the difference between membrane potential and the sodium equilibrium potential ($V_m – E_{Na}$). One might expect, therefore, that the peak inward current would *decrease* as the membrane potential step gets progressively closer to the sodium equilibrium potential, reducing the driving force for sodium entry. However, between about –50 mV and +10 mV there is a marked increase in sodium conductance due to the activation of an increasing number of voltage-gated sodium channels, which greatly outweighs the decrease in driving force. Thus, the sodium current, $i_{Na} = g_{Na}(V_m – E_{Na})$, increases. In this voltage range, the current–voltage relation is said to have a region of negative slope conductance. Beyond about +10 mV there is no further increase in conductance and the current decreases toward zero as the step potential approaches the sodium equilibrium potential.

Inactivation of the Sodium Current

The time courses of the sodium and potassium currents are markedly different. The potassium current is much delayed relative to the onset of the sodium current, but once

[11] Armstrong, C. M., and Hille, B. 1972. *J. Gen. Physiol.* 59: 388–400.
[12] Jenkinson, D. H. 2006. *Brit. J. Pharmacol.* 147: S63–S71.

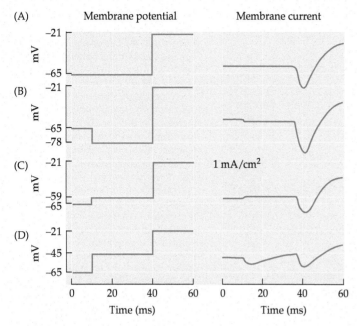

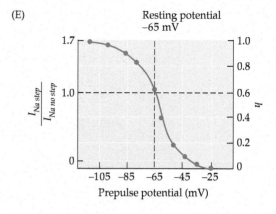

FIGURE 7.4 Effect of Membrane Potential on Sodium Currents.
(A) A depolarizing step from –65 to –21 mV produces an inward sodium current followed by outward potassium current. (B) When the depolarizing step is preceded by a 30-ms hyperpolarizing step, the sodium current is increased. (C,D) Prior depolarizing steps reduce the size of the inward current. (E) The fractional increase or reduction of the sodium current as a function of membrane potential during the preceding conditioning step is shown. Maximum current is about 1.7 times larger than the control value, with a hyperpolarizing step to –105 mV. A depolarizing step to –25 mV reduces the subsequent response to zero. Full range of the sodium current (represented with the single parameter h) is scaled from zero to 100% on the right-hand ordinate (see text). (After A. L. Hodgkin and A. F. Huxley, 1952. *J. Physiol.* 116: 497–506.)

developed, it remains high throughout the duration of the step. The sodium current, by contrast, rises much more rapidly but then decreases to zero, even though the membrane depolarization is maintained. This decline of the sodium current is called **inactivation**.

Hodgkin and Huxley had the insight to realize that activation of the sodium current and its subsequent inactivation represented two separate processes and so designed experiments to study the nature of inactivation in detail. In particular, they investigated the effect of hyperpolarizing and depolarizing prepulses on the peak amplitude of the sodium current produced by a subsequent depolarizing step.

Records from such an experiment are shown in Figure 7.4. In Figure 7.4A, the membrane is stepped from a holding potential of –65 mV to –21 mV, producing a peak sodium current of about 1 milliampere/centimeter^2 (mA/cm^2). When the step is preceded by a hyperpolarizing prepulse to –78 mV, the peak sodium current is increased (see Figure 7.4B). Depolarizing prepulses, however, cause a decrease in the sodium current (see Figure 7.4C,D). The effects of hyperpolarizing and depolarizing prepulses are time-dependent; thus, brief pulses of only a few milliseconds duration have little effect. In the experiment shown here, the prepulses are of sufficient duration (30 ms) for the effects to reach their maximum. The results are shown quantitatively in Figure 7.4E, in which the peak sodium current is plotted against the potential during the prepulse. The peak current after a prepulse is expressed as a fraction of the control current. With a depolarizing prepulse to about –25 mV, the subsequent sodium current is reduced to zero (i.e., inactivation is complete). Hyperpolarizing prepulses to –100 mV or beyond increase the sodium current by a maximum of about 70%. Hodgkin and Huxley represented this range of sodium currents from zero to their maximum value with a single parameter (h), varying from zero to 1, as indicated on the right-hand ordinate of Figure 7.4E. Note that zero means no activation (complete inactivation), and 1 means full activation (no inactivation). In these experiments, the peak sodium current reaches only about 60% of its maximum value upon depolarization from the resting potential. Subsequent experiments have shown that all neurons show some degree of sodium channel inactivation at rest.

Sodium and Potassium Conductances as Functions of Potential

Having measured the magnitude and time course of sodium and potassium currents as a function of the membrane potential (V_m) and knowing the equilibrium potentials (E_{Na} and E_K), Hodgkin and Huxley were then able to deduce the magnitude and time courses of the sodium and potassium conductance changes, using the relations:

$$g_{Na} = \frac{I_{Na}}{(V_m - E_{Na})}$$

$$g_K = \frac{I_K}{(V_m - E_K)}$$

FIGURE 7.5 Sodium and Potassium Conductances.
(A) Conductance changes produced by voltage steps from –65 mV to the indicated potentials. Peak sodium conductance and steady-state potassium conductance both increase with increasing depolarization. (B) Peak sodium conductance and steady-state potassium conductance plotted against the potential to which the membrane is stepped. Both increase steeply with depolarization between –20 and +10 mV. mS = millisiemens (A after A. L. Hodgkin and A. F. Huxley, 1952. *Proc. Roy. Soc. Lond. B* 140: 177-183, based on A. L. Hodgkin and A. F. Huxley, 1952. *J. Physiol.* 116: 449-472. B after A. L. Hodgkin and A. F. Huxley, 1952. *J. Physiol.* 116: 449-472.)

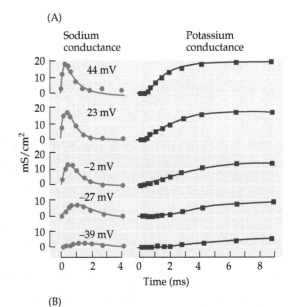

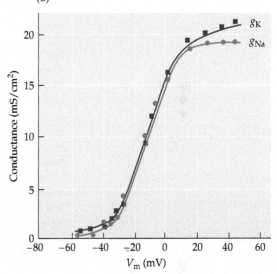

The results for five different voltage steps are shown in Figure 7.5A. Both g_{Na} and g_K increase progressively with increasing membrane depolarization. Figure 7.5B shows the relations between peak conductance and membrane potential for sodium and potassium. The curves are remarkably similar, indicating that the two gating mechanisms have similar voltage sensitivities. In summary, the results obtained by Hodgkin and Huxley indicate that depolarization of the nerve membrane leads to three distinct processes: (1) activation of a sodium conductance mechanism; (2) subsequent inactivation of that mechanism; and (3) delayed activation of a potassium conductance mechanism.

Quantitative Description of Sodium and Potassium Conductances

After obtaining these experimental results, Hodgkin and Huxley proceeded to develop a mathematical description of the precise time courses of the sodium and potassium conductance changes produced by the depolarizing voltage steps. To deal first with the potassium conductance, one might imagine that the effect of a sudden change in membrane potential would be to cause the movement of one or more charges in a voltage-sensitive potassium channel that would then lead to channel opening. If a single process were involved, then the change in the overall potassium conductance might be expected to be governed by ordinary, first-order kinetics—that is, its rise after the onset of the voltage step would be exponential. Instead the onset of the conductance change was found to be S-shaped, with a marked delay. Because of this delay and because the potassium conductance increase occurred during depolarization but not hyperpolarization (i.e., it rectified), it was called the **delayed rectifier**. Hodgkin and Huxley were able to account for the S-shaped onset of the conductance by assuming that the opening of each potassium channel required the activation of four first-order processes, for example the movement of four charged particles in the membrane. In other words, the S-shaped time course of activation could be fitted by the product of four exponential distributions. The increase in potassium conductance for a given voltage step, then, was described by the relation:

$$g_K = g_{K(max)} n^4$$

where $g_{K(max)}$ is the maximum conductance reached for the particular voltage step and n is a rising exponential function varying between zero and unity, given by $n = 1 - e^{-(t/\tau_n)}$. Raising the exponential expression to the fourth power suggests that channel activation involves cooperative action of all four potassium channel subunits (see Chapter 5).

The exponential time constant (τ_n) is also voltage-dependent, with the increase in conductance becoming more rapid with larger depolarizing steps. At 10°C, τ_n ranges from about 4 ms for small depolarizations to 1 ms for depolarization to zero mV.

The time course of the rise in sodium conductance, also S-shaped, was fitted by an exponential raised to the third power. In contrast, the fall in sodium conductance due to inactivation was consistent with a simple exponential decay process. For a given voltage step, the overall time course of the sodium conductance change was the product of the activation and inactivation processes:

$$g_{Na} = g_{Na(max)}m^3h$$

where $g_{Na(max)}$ is the maximum level to which g_{Na} would rise if there were no inactivation and $m = 1 - e-(t/\tau_m)$. The inactivation process is a falling, rather than a rising, exponential and is given by $h = e-(t/\tau_h)$. As with the potassium activation time constant, both τ_m and τ_h are voltage-dependent. The activation time constant τ_m is much shorter than that for potassium, having a value at 10°C of the order of 0.6 ms near the resting potential and decreasing to about 0.2 ms at zero potential. The inactivation time constant τ_h, by contrast, is similar to that for potassium activation.

Reconstruction of the Action Potential

Once the theoretical expressions were obtained for sodium and potassium conductances as a function of voltage and time, Hodgkin and Huxley were able to predict the entire time course of both the action potential and the underlying conductance changes. Starting with a depolarizing step to just above threshold, they used their equations to calculate what the subsequent potential changes would be at successive intervals of 0.01 ms. Thus, during the first 0.01 ms after the membrane had been depolarized to say, –45 mV, they calculated how g_{Na} and g_K would change, what increments of I_{Na} and I_K would result, and then the effect of the net current on V_m. Knowing the change in V_m at the end of the first 0.01 ms, they then repeated the calculations for the next time increment, and so on, all through the rising and falling phases of the action potential. This was a laborious exercise in the days before computers or even electronic calculators; Huxley had to make do with a slide rule.

The calculations duplicated with remarkable accuracy the naturally occurring action potential in the squid axon. In order to appreciate fully the magnitude of this accomplishment, it is necessary to keep in mind that the calculations used to duplicate the action potential were based on current measurements made under completely artificial conditions, with the membrane potential clamped first at one value and then at another. The mechanisms of action potential generation are summarized in Figure 7.6, which shows the calculated magnitude and time course of a propagated action potential in a squid axon, together with the calculated changes in sodium and potassium conductance.

Threshold and Refractory Period

In addition to describing the action potential, Hodgkin and Huxley were able to use their results to explain, in terms of ion conductance changes, many other properties of excitable axons, including the refractory period and the threshold for excitation (see Chapter 1). Furthermore, their findings are applicable to a wide variety of other excitable tissues.

How do the findings predict the threshold membrane potential at which the impulse takes off? It would seem that a discontinuity, such as that which occurs at the **threshold for excitation**, would require a discontinuity in g_{Na} or g_K, yet both vary smoothly with membrane potential. The absence of any discontinuity can be understood if we imagine passing current through the

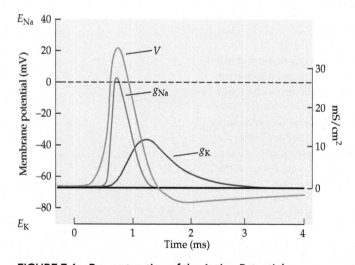

FIGURE 7.6 Reconstruction of the Action Potential.
The relation between changes in sodium and potassium conductances (g_{Na} and g_K) and the action potential (V) are calculated for a propagated action potential in a squid axon. (After A. L. Hodgkin and A. F. Huxley, 1952. *J. Physiol.* 117: 500-544.)

membrane to depolarize it just to threshold and then turning the current off. Because the membrane is depolarized, there will be an increase in outward current over that at rest (through potassium and leak channels). We will also have activated some sodium channels, increasing the inward sodium current. At threshold, the inward and outward currents are exactly equal and opposite, just as they are at rest. However, there is an important difference: The balance of currents is now unstable. If a few extra sodium ions enter the cell, the depolarization is increased, g_{Na} increases, and more sodium enters. The outward current can no longer keep up with the sodium influx, and the regenerative process explodes. If, however, a few extra potassium ions leave the cell, the depolarization is decreased, g_{Na} decreases rapidly, sodium current decreases, and the excess outward current causes repolarization. As the membrane potential approaches its resting level, the potassium current decreases until it again equals the resting inward sodium current. Depolarization above threshold results in an increase in g_{Na} sufficient for inward sodium movement to swamp outward potassium movement immediately. Subthreshold depolarization fails to increase g_{Na} sufficiently to override the resting potassium conductance.

And how is the refractory period explained? Two changes develop during an action potential that make it impossible for the nerve fiber to produce a second action potential immediately. First, inactivation of sodium channels is maximal during the falling phase of the action potential and requires several more milliseconds to be removed. During this time few, if any, channels are available to contribute to a new increase in g_{Na}. This results in an **absolute refractory period** that lasts throughout the falling phase of the action potential and during which no amount of externally applied depolarization can initiate a second regenerative response. Second, because of activation of potassium channels, g_K is very large during the falling phase of the action potential and decreases slowly back to its resting level. Thus, a very large increase in g_{Na} is required to override the residual g_K and thereby initiate a regenerative depolarization. These mechanisms combine to produce a **relative refractory period**, during which the threshold gradually returns to normal as the potassium channels close and the sodium channels recover from inactivation.

It was an extraordinary achievement for Hodgkin and Huxley to have provided rigorous quantitative explanations for such complex biophysical properties of membranes. Their findings have since been shown to be generally applicable to action potential generation in both invertebrate and vertebrate neurons. However, the characteristics of action potentials vary greatly from one cell to another. For example, their durations can range from as little as 200 μs up to many milliseconds. Associated with these differences in duration is the rate at which neurons can fire repetitively. Some manage to generate only a few action potentials per second, while others can fire at frequencies approaching 1000 per second. These differences are related to differences in the channel types underlying depolarization and repolarization.[13] For example, in central nervous system neurons with brief spikes and high-frequency capability, the voltage-gated potassium channels associated with repolarization usually belong to the K_v3 family (see Chapter 5 for potassium channel classification). These channels have a very steep voltage dependence and activate and deactivate rapidly. They thereby promote rapid repolarization and, consequently, rapid removal of sodium channel inactivation.

Further differences from the squid axon relate to the fact that in most neurons, currents through voltage-activated sodium and potassium channels are not the only contributors to the action potential. For example, inward currents through voltage-activated calcium channels can enhance and prolong depolarization. At the same time, calcium entry into the cell can generate outward potassium currents through calcium-activated potassium channels and thereby shorten the action potential. Thus, the characteristics of any given action potential depend on which types of ion channels are present in the membrane and on how currents through these channels interact.

Although our knowledge of single-channel behavior has provided a new breadth to our understanding of the molecular mechanisms underlying the action potential, by no stretch of the imagination would single-channel studies on their own—without the earlier voltage clamp experiments and insights—have been able to account for how a nerve cell generates and conducts impulses. The older work has become enriched by, rather than supplanted by, the new.

[13] Bean, B. P. 2007. *Nat. Rev. Neurosci.* 8: 451–465.

Gating Currents

Hodgkin and Huxley suggested that sodium channel activation was associated with the translocation of charged structures or particles within the membrane. Such charge movements would be expected to add to the capacitative current produced by a depolarizing voltage step. After several technical difficulties were resolved, currents of the expected magnitude and time course were finally seen.[14,15] They are known as **gating currents**.

How is the gating current separated from the usual capacitative current expected with a step change in membrane potential (e.g., as seen in Figure 7.1)? Briefly, currents associated merely with charging and discharging the membrane capacitance should be symmetrical. That is, they should be of the same magnitude for depolarizing steps as for hyperpolarizing steps. However, currents associated with sodium channel activation should appear upon a depolarization of 50 mV from a holding potential of –70 mV, but not upon 50-mV hyperpolarization. In other words, if the channels are already closed, there should be no gating current upon further hyperpolarization. Similarly, gating currents associated with channel closing might be expected at the termination of a brief depolarizing pulse but not after a hyperpolarizing pulse. One way of recording gating currents in an experiment is to sum the currents produced by two identical voltage steps of opposite polarity, as shown in Figure 7.7A. The asymmetry due to gating currents is shown in parts (a) and (b) of the figure. The current at the beginning of the depolarizing pulse is larger than that produced by the hyperpolarizing pulse because of the additional charge movement associated with gating of the sodium channel. When the two currents are added (part c), the net result is the gating current. Gating currents are also known as **asymmetry currents**. Figure 7.7B shows an example of gating current in squid axon, obtained by cancellation of the capacitative current. Voltage-sensitive potassium currents were blocked with TEA. A step depolarization of an internally perfused squid axon produced an outward gating current, followed by inward sodium current. The sodium current was much smaller than usual because the extracellular sodium concentration was reduced to 20% of normal. Figure 7.7C shows the gating current alone after tetrodotoxin was added to the solution to prevent sodium from entering the cell (note the change in scale). The evidence that asymmetry currents are, in fact, associated with sodium channel activation has been summarized by Armstrong.[16]

[14] Armstrong, C. M., and Bezanilla, F. 1974. *J. Gen. Physiol.* 63: 533-552.

[15] Keynes, R. D., and Rojas, E. 1974. *J. Physiol.* 239: 393-434.

[16] Armstrong, C. M. 1981. *Physiol. Rev.* 61: 644-683.

[17] Bezanilla, F. 2005. *IEEE Trans. Nanobiosci.* 4: 34-48.

[18] Bezanilla, F. 2008. *Nature Rev. Mol. Cell Biol.* 9: 323-332.

[19] Jiang, Y. et al. 2003. *Nature* 423: 42-84.

[20] Chanda, B. et al. 2005. *Nature* 436: 852-856.

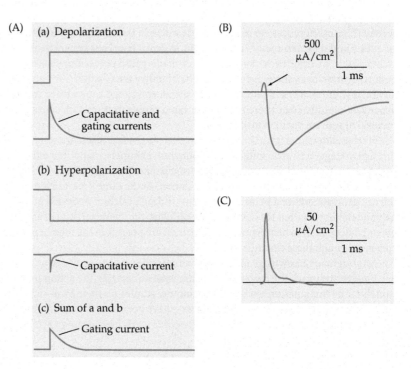

FIGURE 7.7 Sodium Gating Current. (A) Method of separating gating current from capacitative current. (a) A depolarizing pulse produces a capacitive current in the membrane, plus a gating current. (b) A hyperpolarizing pulse of the same amplitude produces a capacitative current only. (c) When the responses to a hyperpolarizing and a depolarizing pulse are summed, capacitative currents cancel out and only the gating current remains. (B) Current record from a squid axon in response to a depolarizing pulse, after cancellation of capacitative current. The inward sodium current is decreased by reducing extracellular sodium to 20% of normal. A small outward current (arrow) preceding the inward current is the sodium channel gating current. (C) Response to depolarization from the same preparation after adding TTX to the bathing solution and recording at higher amplification. Only the gating current remains. μA = microamperes. (B,C after C. M. Armstrong and F. Bezanilla, 1977. *J. Gen. Physiol.* 70: 567-590.)

Mechanisms of Activation and Inactivation

It is well established that the gating currents are associated with translocation of positively charged residues in the S4 segments of the channel protein (see Chapter 5), and the total charge transfer has been estimated in Shaker potassium channels to be about 13 unit charges per channel, or if all four S4 segments participate, about $3e_0$ per segment.[17] Various schemes have been proposed in which the S4 helix responds to depolarization by translating and/or rotating within the membrane, thereby effecting a transfer of charge between the inner and outer aqueous compartments.[18] Examples include a paddle model, in which the helix moves within the membrane to provide an outward charge translocation of about 20 Å,[19] and a rotational model with charge translation over a relatively short distance.[20] Figure 7.8 shows an example of the rotational model. When the membrane is at the resting potential, positive charges on the S4 helix are exposed to the cytoplasm by way of an aqueous crevice extending into the protein structure, and the channel opening is blocked at the cytoplasmic end by close apposition of the S6 helices (see Figure 7.8A). Upon depolarization, the change in potential causes the helix to rotate, driving the charges on S4 into the extracellular region of the crevice (see Figure 7.8B). The rotary movement is coupled to the S6 helix so as to open the pore.

Resonant energy transfer experiments with the $Na_v1.4$ sodium channel have been used to measure intramolecular distances between fixed positions in the voltage-sensitive regions of the channel and charged residues in the S4 helix.[21] The change in position of the residues upon depolarization was found to be consistent with a rotation of S4 of roughly 180°.

The idea of a crevice, or gating pore, around S4 is supported by experiments on sodium and potassium channels in which the charged arginine residues on the outer segment of the S4 helix are replaced with much shorter residues, such as alanine or serine.[22–24] These substitutions give rise to cation currents (known as omega currents) through the closed channels, presumably by way of the gating pore.

The identification of a channel structure associated with inactivation was made first on potassium A-channels from *Drosophila*. Experiments on this channel provided evidence that a particular intracellular string of amino acids is associated with inactivation, and revived the **ball-and-chain model** of sodium channel inactivation that had been proposed more than a decade earlier by Armstrong and Bezanilla.[25] In this model, a clump of amino acids (the ball) is tethered by a string of residues (the chain) to the main channel structure. Upon depolarization, the ball binds to a site in the inner vestibule of the channel, thereby blocking the pore (Figure 7.9). This model of inactivation was tested in potassium A-channels by examining the behavior of channels formed in oocytes from mutant subunits (recall that the A-channel is a tetramer rather than a single polypeptide). Mutations and deletions were made in the 80 or so amino acids between the amino terminus and the first (S1) membrane helix.[26] Channels formed by mutant subunits with deletion of residues 6–46 showed virtually no inactivation, suggesting that some or all of these residues were involved in the normal inactivation process. When a synthetic peptide matching the first 20 amino acids in the N-terminal chain was simply added to the solution bathing the cytoplasmic face of the membrane, inactivation was restored with a linear dose-dependence over the concentration range of 0 to 100 μM.[27]

This amazing observation provides unusually strong support for the idea that in potassium A-channel subunits,

[21] Kubota, K. et al. 2017. *Proc. Nat. Acad. Sci. USA* 114: E1857–E1865.

[22] Tombola, F., Pathak, M. M., and Isacoff, E. E. 2005. *Neuron* 45: 379–388.

[23] Sokolov, S., Scheuer, T., and Catterall, W. A. 2005. *Neuron* 47: 183–189.

[24] Gamal El-Din, T. M. et al. 2010. *Channels* 4: 1–8.

[25] Armstrong, C. M., and Bezanilla, F. 1977. *J. Gen. Physiol.* 70: 567–590.

[26] Hoshi, T., Zagotta, W. N., and Aldrich, R. W. 1990. *Science* 250: 533–550.

[27] Zagotta, W. N., Hoshi, T., and Aldrich, R. W. 1990. *Science* 250: 568–571.

(A) Closed channel

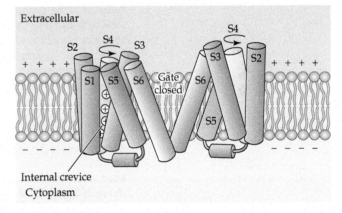

(B) Open channel

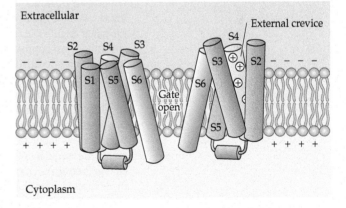

FIGURE 7.8 Proposed Scheme for Voltage Gating. The figure shows two apposed potassium channel subunits. Aqueous crevices connect S4 segments to the inner and outer solutions. (A) In the closed channel, positively charged residues on S4 are exposed to the intracellular solution via the internal crevice. S6 segments occlude the intracellular mouth of the channel. (B) Depolarization of the membrane causes rotation of S4, exposing the charges to the external crevice, and thus to the extracellular surface. S4 rotation interacts with the S6 segments to open the gate. (Based on A. Cha et al., 1999. *Nature* 402: 809–813.)

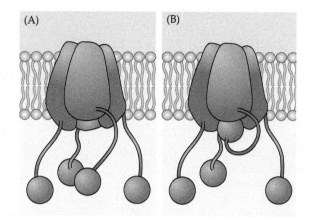

(A)   (B)

FIGURE 7.9   Ball-and-Chain Model of Inactivation of a Voltage-Activated Potassium Channel. One ball and chain element is chained to each of the four channel subunits. (A) Gating elements at the cytoplasmic end of the channel are open. (B) One of the four inactivation balls enters the open vestibule to block the open channel. The actual blocking mechanism comprises a string of about 45 amino acid residues (see text).

the first 20 or so amino acid residues constitute a blocking particle responsible for inactivation of the channel. Because it involves the N-terminal structure, this type of inactivation in potassium channels is often referred to as N-type inactivation. Some potassium channels also display a much slower C-type inactivation, originally suspected to involve the C terminus but later found to be related to structures near the outer mouth of the pore.[28,29]

Experiments with sodium channels have identified the intracellular loop between domains III and IV as being closely involved in the inactivation process. The loop is about 45 residues in length and is envisioned as a hairpin that swings into the inner vestibule of the channel to block the pore. In experiments with rat brain channels expressed in oocytes, three adjacent amino acid residues in the middle of the loop have been identified as essential for inactivation to occur.[30] When they were removed or replaced by site-directed mutagenesis, inactivation was severely attenuated or abolished. Similar experiments also identified groups of glycine and proline residues at either end of the loop involved in inactivation. These are assumed to be hinge regions that allow the hairpin to flip into the vestibule.[31]

Activation and Inactivation of Single Channels

The time course of activation and inactivation of the macroscopic sodium current shown in Figure 7.1 does not mirror the time course of current through a single channel. The responses of single channels to a depolarizing voltage step are shown in Figure 7.10. The records are from a cell-attached patch on a cultured rat muscle fiber that contained only a few active sodium channels.[32] To remove any resting inactivation of sodium channels, a steady command potential was applied to the electrode, hyperpolarizing the patch membrane to –100 mV or so. In a series of successive trials, a 40-mV depolarizing pulse was applied to the electrode for about 20 ms, as shown in Figure 7.10B trace (a). In about one-third of the trials recorded in trace (b), no sodium channels were activated. In the remainder, one or more single-channel currents appeared during the pulse, occurring most frequently near the onset of depolarization. The mean channel current was 1.6 picoamperes (pA). Assuming the sodium equilibrium potential to be +30 mV, the driving potential for sodium entry was about –90 mV; thus, the single-channel conductance was about 18 picosiemens (pS). This is comparable to sodium channel conductances measured in a variety of other cells. When 300 of the individual traces were added together, as shown in trace (c), the summed current followed the same time course as that expected from the whole-cell sodium current.

A major point of interest in Figure 7.10 is that the channel mean open time (0.7 ms) is short relative to the overall time course of the summed current. Specifically, the time constant of decay of the summed current (about 4 ms) does not reflect the length of time that individual channels remain open. Instead, it indicates a slow decay in the probability of channel opening. The processes of activation (m^3) and inactivation (h) represent first an increase, and then a decrease in the *probability* that a channel will open for a brief period. Their product (m^3h) describes the time course of the overall probability change. The probability increases rapidly near the beginning of the pulse, reaches a peak, and then decreases with time. In any given trial an individual channel may open immediately after the onset of the pulse, at any subsequent time during the pulse, or not at all.

[28] Hoshi, T., Zagotta, W. N., and Aldrich, R. W. 1991. *Neuron* 7: 547-556.

[29] Choi, K. L., Aldrich, R. W., and Yellen, G. 1991. *Proc. Natl. Acad. Sci. USA* 88: 5092-5095.

[30] Kellenberger, S. et al. 1997. *J. Gen. Physiol.* 109: 589-605.

[31] Kellenberger, S. et al. 1997. *J. Gen. Physiol.* 109: 607-617.

[32] Sigworth, F. J., and Neher, E. 1980. *Nature* 287: 447-449.

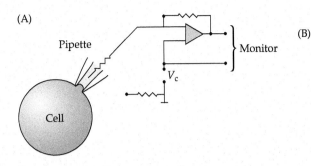

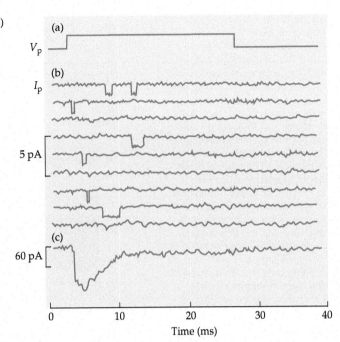

FIGURE 7.10 Sodium Channel Currents. Currents were recorded from cell-attached patch on cultured rat muscle cell. (A) Recording arrangement. (B) Repeated depolarizing voltage pulses applied to the patch, with waveform shown in (a), produce single-channel currents (downward deflections) in the nine successive records, as shown in (b). The sum of 300 such records (c) shows that channels open most often in the initial 1–2 ms after onset of the pulse, after which the probability of channel opening declines with the time constant of inactivation. (After F. J. Sigworth and E. Neher, 1980. *Nature* 287: 447–449.)

Afterpotentials

One of the characteristics of the action potential shown in Figure 7.6 is that it is followed by a transient **afterhyperpolarizing potential (AHP)** that persists for several milliseconds before the membrane potential returns to its resting level. The AHP occurs because delayed rectifier channels continue to open for a period that outlasts the action potential, and the resulting increase in potassium conductance drives the membrane toward the potassium equilibrium potential. As the channel openings gradually cease, the membrane potential returns to its resting level.

In addition to potassium channels associated with the delayed rectifier current, neurons have several potassium channel types whose activation contributes to the falling phase of the action potential and subsequent afterhyperpolarization.[33] The most prominent of these are calcium-activated potassium channels (see Chapter 5). During the action potential, calcium ions enter the cell through voltage-activated calcium channels (see next section) and produce increases in potassium conductance that contribute to both the repolarization and the subsequent hyperpolarizing potentials. Figure 7.11 illustrates this effect. In Figure 7.11A, an action potential produced in a frog spinal motoneuron by a brief depolarizing current pulse is followed by two separate phases of hyperpolarization. The first is due to the persistent activation of delayed rectifier channels. The second, slower phase is due to potassium efflux through calcium-activated potassium channels, and disappears after the preparation has been soaked in Ca^{2+}-free solution (see Figure 7.11B). The prolonged time course reflects the time taken for the cytoplasmic calcium concentration to return to its resting value. Short trains of action potentials have a cumulative effect on the size of the slow AHP, as successive impulses add additional increments to the intracellular calcium accumulation (see Figure 7.11C).

The slow AHP is mediated primarily by potassium entry through so-called small K (SK) channels (see Chapter 5). Other potassium channels, known as big K (BK), are present in many neurons as well. These open very quickly and contribute to the rapid termination of the action potential in concert with delayed rectifier channels.

Potassium ion fluxes associated with repolarization and hyperpolarization play an important role in regulating the frequency of ongoing action potential activity. An example is shown in Figure 7.11D,E. A steady current pulse applied to a vagal motoneuron depolarizes the membrane and produces a train of action potentials that gradually decreases

[33] Hille, B. 2001. *Ion Channels of Excitable Membranes*, 3rd ed. Oxford University Press/Sinauer, Sunderland, MA. pp. 136–147.

FIGURE 7.11 Hyperpolarizing Afterpotentials. (A) Action potential in a frog spinal motoneuron is followed by an afterhyperpolarization (AHP) with two phases: slow and fast. (B) After the preparation is soaked in low-calcium bathing solution, the slow AHP disappears, suggesting that it depends on calcium influx during the action potential. (C) Superimposed records of trains of action potentials in a guinea pig vagal motoneuron. The size of the slow AHP increases as the number of successive action potentials in a train is increased from one to six. (D) A steady depolarizing current produces a train of action potentials that decreases in frequency (adapts) before dying out. A longer-duration record reveals a large, slow AHP after the depolarizing current pulse is removed. (E) After block of voltage-sensitive calcium channels by the addition of cadmium to the bathing solution, the adaptation and slow AHP disappear. (A,B after E. F. Barrett and J. N. Barrett, 1976. *J. Physiol.* 255: 737–774; C–E after Y. Yarom et al., 1985. *Neuroscience* 16: 719–737.)

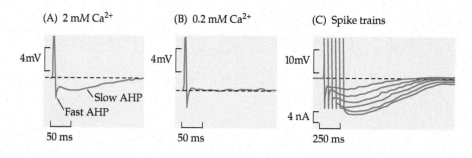

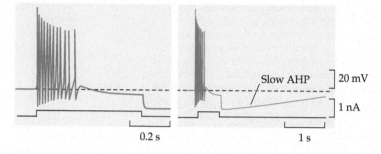

(D) Spike frequency adaptation

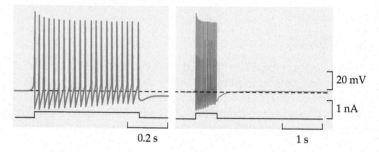

(E) Block by 5 m*M* Cd²⁺

in frequency and finally stops (see Figure 7.11D). Although not apparent in the record, the frequency adaptation and eventual cessation of activity occur because the depolarization produced by the applied current declines from its initial value, finally falling below threshold for excitation. This decrease in magnitude of the depolarization is because of a steady increase in potassium conductance produced by the ongoing increase in intracellular calcium concentration during the train. The increase in potassium conductance is apparent when the events are observed on a slower timescale—a large, slow AHP is seen to persist for several seconds after the end of the depolarizing pulse.

When the same procedure is repeated with calcium entry blocked, the frequency adaptation and the prolonged AHP both disappear (see Figure 7.11E). The frequency of the ongoing train of action potentials is now determined by the interaction between the early AHP and the depolarizing current pulse. After each action potential, the increased potassium conductance repolarizes the membrane below threshold for action potential initiation; as the potassium conductance returns toward its resting level, depolarization by the current pulse is restored and another action potential is initiated.

One additional factor can contribute to hyperpolarization and regulation of repetitive activity, namely the sodium–potassium exchange pump. The pump extrudes three sodium ions in exchange for two potassium ions and therefore contributes to the membrane potential (see Chapter 6). The rate of transport by the pump, and hence its contribution to the membrane potential, increases with increasing intracellular sodium concentration. Consequently, sodium accumulation during repetitive activity, particularly in small cells, can result in transient hyperpolarization that lasts until the excess sodium is extruded.[34,35]

[34] Jansen, J. K. S., and Nicholls, J. G. 1973. *J. Physiol.* 229: 635–655.

[35] Darbon, P. et al. 2003. *J. Neurophysiol.* 90: 3119–3129.

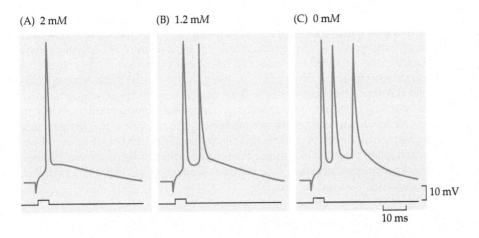

(A) 2 mM (B) 1.2 mM (C) 0 mM

10 mV

10 ms

FIGURE 7.12 Depolarizing Afterpotentials. A single action potential in a rat hippocampal pyramidal cell, produced by a brief depolarizing pulse, is followed by a sustained afterdepolarization (ADP). When the external Ca²⁺ concentration is reduced from 2 mM to 1.2 mM, the ADP becomes larger and initiates a second action potential. Reduction of the external Ca²⁺ concentration to zero results in a further increase in the ADP. (After D. Golomb et al., 2006. *J. Neurophysiol.* 96: 1912–1926.)

Some neurons, for example cerebellar Purkinje cells, exhibit prolonged depolarization following the action potential.[36,37] This **afterdepolarizing potential (ADP)** is associated with activation of a TTX-sensitive sodium current (I_{NaP}), which has a low threshold of activation and very slow inactivation.[38]

Just as calcium-activated potassium currents determine the magnitude and time course of the AHP, they also participate in regulating the ADP. After a single action potential or a short train of action potentials, the slow sodium current competes with potassium currents for control of the membrane potential. This interaction is illustrated in Figure 7.12. With normal extracellular calcium concentration (2 mM), a brief depolarization applied to a rat hippocampal pyramidal cell produces a single action potential, followed by a prolonged ADP. When calcium influx during the action potential is decreased by reducing the external calcium concentration to 1.2 mM and then to zero, calcium influx and hence the calcium-activated potassium current are also reduced and the ADP becomes larger. The increase in amplitude leads to a brief burst of action potentials in response to the single stimulus. Such bursting behavior, which is typical of a variety of cells in the central nervous system, is regulated by the interplay of sodium and potassium currents following the initial excitation.

There remains the question of how the afterdepolarizing potential is terminated, given the very slow inactivation of the sodium channels. Termination is accomplished by potassium current through voltage-activated M-channels, which activate and inactivate slowly. M-channels are open at the resting potential and further activated by depolarization (see Chapter 6). Depolarization by the prolonged sodium current increases M-channel activation, and the resulting increase in outward potassium current repolarizes the membrane until activation of the sodium channels is removed.[36]

The channel isotype responsible for the prolonged sodium current in hippocampal pyramidal cells has not been identified, but it is known that the cells contain an abundance of SCNA8 (Na_v6) channels.[39] Cerebellar Purkinje cells also exhibit prolonged sodium currents that produce ADPs and burst responses to single stimuli. These characteristics are disrupted in Purkinje cells from mutant mice in which SCNA8 channels are not expressed.[40]

The Role of Calcium in Excitation

Calcium Action Potentials

The membranes of nerve and muscle fibers contain a variety of voltage-activated calcium channels (see Chapter 5 for calcium channel classifications and properties). Calcium ions enter the cell through these channels during the action potential, and this entry plays a key role in a variety of important processes. For example, a transient increase in intracellular calcium during the action potential is responsible for secretion of chemical transmitters by neurons and for contraction of muscle fibers.

In some muscle fibers and some neurons, calcium currents become sufficiently large to contribute significantly to, or even be solely responsible for, the rising phase of the action potential. Because g_{Ca} increases with depolarization, the process is a regenerative one,

[36] Azouz, R., Jensen, M. S., and Yaari, Y. 1996. *J. Physiol.* 492: 211–223.

[37] Golomb, D., Yue, C., and Yaari, Y. 2006. *J. Neurophysiol.* 96: 1912–1926.

[38] French, C. R. et al. 1990. *J. Gen. Physiol.* 95: 1139–1157.

[39] Schaller, K. L. et al. 1995. *J. Neurosci.* 15: 3231–3242.

[40] Raman, I. M. et al. 1997. *Neuron* 19: 881–891.

entirely analogous to that discussed for sodium. Calcium action potentials were first studied in invertebrate muscle fibers by Fatt and Ginsborg[41] and subsequently by Hagiwara.[42] Calcium action potentials occur in cardiac muscle in a wide variety of invertebrate neurons and neurons in the vertebrate autonomic and central nervous systems.[43] They also occur in immature neurons during development as well as in non-neuronal cells, such as endocrine cells and some invertebrate egg cells. The voltage-dependent calcium currents can be blocked by adding millimolar concentrations of cobalt, manganese, or cadmium ions to the extracellular bathing solution. Barium can substitute for calcium as the permeant ion, whereas magnesium cannot. A particularly striking example of the coexistence of sodium and calcium action potentials in the same cell is found in mammalian cerebellar Purkinje cells, which generate sodium action potentials in their soma and calcium action potentials in the branches of their dendritic trees.[44,45]

Calcium Ions and Excitability

Calcium ions also affect excitation. For instance, a reduction in extracellular calcium increases the excitability of nerve and muscle cells; conversely, increasing extracellular calcium decreases excitability. Frankenhaeuser and Hodgkin[46] used voltage clamp experiments to examine these effects in the squid axon and found that when extracellular calcium was reduced, the voltage dependence of sodium channel activation was shifted so that smaller depolarizing pulses were required to reach threshold and to produce sodium currents equivalent to those in normal solution. The reduction in depolarizing pulse amplitudes was constant throughout the range of excitation and depended on calcium concentration. A fivefold reduction in extracellular calcium resulted in a 10-mV to 15-mV reduction in the depolarization required for action potential initiation. The magnitude of the effect in this and in other nerve and muscle cells means that normal calcium levels are essential for maintaining a margin of safety between the resting potential and the threshold for action potential initiation.

[41] Fatt, P., and Ginsborg, B. L. 1958. *J. Physiol.* 142: 516–543.

[42] Hagiwara, S., and Byerly, L. 1981. *Annu. Rev. Neurosci.* 4: 69–125.

[43] Hille, B. 2001. *Ion Channels of Excitable Membranes,* 3rd ed. Oxford University Press/Sinauer, Sunderland, MA. pp. 95–98.

[44] Llinas, R., and Sugimori, M. 1980. *J. Physiol.* 305: 197–213.

[45] Ross, W. N., Lasser-Ross, N., and Werman, R. 1990. *Proc. R. Soc. Lond., B, Biol. Sci.* 240: 173–185.

[46] Frankenhaeuser, B., and Hodgkin, A. L. 1957. *J. Physiol.* 137: 218–244.

SUMMARY

- The action potential in most nerve cell membranes is produced by a transient increase in sodium conductance that drives the membrane potential toward the sodium equilibrium potential, which is then followed by an increase in potassium conductance that returns the membrane potential to its resting level.

- The increases in conductance occur because sodium and potassium channels in the membrane are voltage-dependent; that is, their probability of opening increases with depolarization.

- Voltage clamp experiments on squid axons have provided detailed information about the voltage dependence and time course of the conductance changes. When the cell membrane is depolarized, the sodium conductance is activated rapidly and then inactivated. Potassium conductance is activated with a delay and remains high as long as the depolarization is maintained.

- The time and voltage dependence of the sodium and potassium conductance changes account precisely for the amplitude and time course of the action potential as well as for other phenomena, such as activation threshold and refractory period.

- Activation of sodium and potassium conductances by depolarization requires, in theory, charge movements within the membrane. Appropriate charge movements, called gating currents, have been measured.

- Calcium plays an important role in excitation. In some cells calcium influx, rather than sodium influx, is responsible for the rising phase of the action potential. Extracellular calcium also controls membrane excitability, which increases with decreasing calcium concentration.

Suggested Reading

General Reviews

Armstrong, C. M., and Hille, B. 1998. Voltage-gated ion channels and electrical excitability. *Neuron* 20: 371–380.

Bean, B. P. 2007. The action potential in mammalian central neurons. *Nat. Rev. Neurosci.* 8: 451–465.

Hille, B. 2001. *Ion Channels of Excitable Membranes,* 3rd ed. Oxford University Press/Sinauer, Sunderland, MA. Chapters 2–5.

Original Papers

Frankenhaeuser, B., and Hodgkin, A. L. 1957. The action of calcium on the electrical properties of squid axons. *J. Physiol.* 137: 218–244.

Hodgkin, A. L., and Huxley, A. F. 1952a. Currents carried by sodium and potassium ion through the membrane of the giant axon of *Loligo. J. Physiol.* 116: 449–472.

Hodgkin, A. L., and Huxley, A. F. 1952b. The components of the membrane conductance in the giant axon of *Loligo. J. Physiol.* 116: 473–496.

Hodgkin, A. L., and Huxley, A. F. 1952c. The dual effect of membrane potential on sodium conductance in the giant axon of *Loligo. J. Physiol.* 116: 497–506.

Hodgkin, A. L., and Huxley, A. F. 1952d. A quantitative description of membrane current and its application to conduction and excitation in nerve. *J. Physiol.* 117: 500–544.

Hodgkin, A. L., Huxley, A. F., and Katz, B. 1952. Measurement of current-voltage relations in the membrane of the giant axon of *Loligo. J. Physiol.* 116: 424–448.

CHAPTER 8

Electrical Signaling in Neurons

In order to understand how signals are transmitted from one place to another in the nervous system it is necessary to know how they are generated in individual neurons and how they spread from one region of the cell to the next. Small depolarizing or hyperpolarizing signals spread passively along a nerve axon or dendrite, decreasing in amplitude over a short distance. The amplitude attenuation depends on several factors, principally the diameter and membrane properties of the fiber. Signals spread farther along a fiber with a large diameter and high membrane resistance. The electrical capacitance of the membrane influences both the time course and spatial spread of the electrical signal. Larger depolarizations give rise to action potentials. Once initiated, action potentials are regenerative and self-propagating, traveling from their point of origin over the full length of the nerve process with no loss of amplitude.

The axons of many vertebrate nerve cells are covered by a high-resistance, low-capacitance myelin sheath. This sheath acts as an insulator and forces currents associated with the nerve impulse to flow through the membrane where the sheath is interrupted (nodes of Ranvier). This increases the conduction velocity by bringing more distant regions of the axon to threshold sooner. In addition, electrical activity can pass between neurons through specialized regions of close membrane apposition called gap junctions. Intercellular channels, called connexons, provide pathways for current flow through gap junctions.

(A)

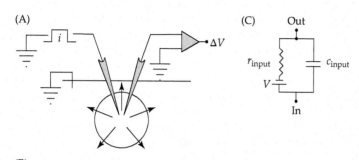

(C)

(B)

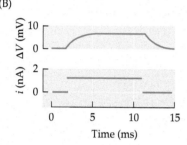

FIGURE 8.1   Response to Current Injection recorded from a spherical cell immersed in bathing solution. (A) Two electrodes are inserted into the cell, one to pass current and the other to record the resulting voltage change. Positive current injected into the cytoplasm flows outward across the cell membrane. (B) A pulse of positive current (i) produces a depolarization (ΔV) that rises gradually to its final value and then decays after the current is terminated. (C) An electrical model of the cell. r_{input} = the resistance of the cell membrane; c_{input} = membrane capacitance; V = resting membrane potential.

In this chapter we consider how electrical signals are carried along the processes of neurons. Small depolarizing or hyperpolarizing signals, generated locally in an axon or dendrite, die out over a relatively short distance. These signals occur in sensory receptors and in postsynaptic regions of neurons. If local depolarizations are sufficiently large, they produce action potentials that rise transiently to many times the amplitude of the initial signal. Action potentials are self-propagating and generally spread from their point of origin throughout the entire neuronal process without loss of amplitude. The spread of both local potentials and action potentials depends on the passive electrical properties of the cell.

We begin by considering current flow across the membrane of a simple spherical cell. In the experiment illustrated in Figure 8.1A, two microelectrodes are inserted into the cell, one to pass current across the membrane and the other to record the resulting change in membrane potential. A positive current pulse produces a depolarization that rises gradually to its final value and then dissipates after termination of the pulse (Figure 8.1B). Two questions arise from this kind of experiment: (1) What determines the size of the potential change? (2) What determines the rate of rise and fall of the potentials at the beginning and end of the current?

To answer these questions, it is useful to refer to the electrical model of the cell shown in Figure 8.1C. The **input resistance** (r_{input}) of the cell represents the pathway for current flow across the cell membrane. Input resistance is the inverse of the input conductance of the cell ($r_{input} = 1/g_{input}$), which in turn is made up of the sum of the membrane conductances to sodium, potassium, chloride, and other ions, lumped into a single pathway. The capacitor (c_{input}) represents the **input capacitance** of the cell, and is the electrical equivalent of the charged layers on the extracellular and intracellular surfaces of the lipid membrane. The membrane's capacitance is determined by the electrical insulating properties and thickness of the membrane lipid. The battery, V, represents the resting membrane potential.

In considering the size of the potential change, it is useful to recall Ohm's law: A given amount of current, i, passed through a resistor, r, produces a voltage $v = ir$ (see Appendix A). In the case of our spherical cell, the input resistance of the cell determines the maximum amplitude finally reached during the voltage change (ΔV_{max}). So, we can write:

$$\Delta V_{max} = i r_{input}$$

The rise of the change in potential is slowed because the cell membrane has an input capacitance. To understand its effect, it is necessary to recall that the charge on the capacitor, q, varies with potential, V, according to the relation $q = cV$ (see Appendix A). This means that a membrane potential change must be accompanied by a corresponding change in the charge stored in the membrane capacitance. At the beginning of the current pulse, only a fraction of the current flows across the input resistance to produce a change in potential. The remainder is diverted to the capacitor in order to alter its charge. Initially the rate of change of potential is relatively rapid and the capacitive current is relatively large. At the end of the pulse, the potential change has reached its final value, the capacitor is fully charged to the new level, and all of the current flows through the resistor. After the current pulse is terminated, the potential returns slowly to its original level as current drains off the capacitor through the resistor.

The rise of the membrane potential change follows an exponential time course, its time dependence being described by the relation $\Delta V_m = \Delta V_{max}[1 - e^{(-t/\tau)}]$, where τ is the **input time constant** of the membrane, and the time, t, is measured from the onset of the pulse. Similarly, when the current pulse is terminated, the potential change decays exponentially to zero: $\Delta V_m = \Delta V_{max} e^{(-t/\tau)}$. Both expressions give the same estimate of the τ value. The input time constant is given by the product of the input resistance and the input capacitance: $\tau = r_{input}c_{input}$.

Specific Electrical Properties of Cell Membranes

The input resistance and capacitance of the spherical cell depend not only on the resistive and capacitive properties of the cell membrane but also on the size of the cell. The **specific capacitance** of the membrane (C_m) is the capacitance of 1 square centimeter of membrane. The input capacitance of a spherical cell is given simply by the capacitance per unit of area times the surface area of the cell: $c_{input} = C_m(4\pi r^2)$. The larger the cell, the greater the input capacitance. Typically, cell membranes have capacitances of the order of 1 μF/cm^2 (1μF = 10^{-6} farads; see Appendix A for definitions of electrical constants). This means that at a resting potential of –80 mV the amount of charge stored on the inner surface of the membrane ($q = C_m V$) is $(1 \times 10^{-6}$ F$) \times (80 \times 10^{-3}$ V$) = 8 \times 10^{-8}$ coulombs/cm^2, which is 5×10^{11} univalent ions (0.8 picomole [pmol]) for each square centimeter.

Similarly, the **specific resistance** of the membrane (R_m) is the resistance of 1 square centimeter of membrane. However, its relation to input resistance is reversed: In general, a large cell has more ion channels in its membrane than a small cell, and therefore will have a lower resistance to the flow of ion current. In other words, the input resistance of a cell is inversely related to membrane area. For a spherical cell, $r_{input} = R_m/(4\pi r^2)$. For this reason, R_m has the units Ωcm^2. Measurements of the specific resistance of a variety of neuronal membranes range from less than 1,000 Ωcm^2 for membranes with a large number of active ion channels to more than 50,000 Ωcm^2 for membranes with relatively few such channels. Suppose we select a value of 2000 Ωcm^2, which is equivalent to a conductance of 5×10^8 picosiemens (pS)/cm^2. It follows that if the average open membrane channel has a conductance of 50 pS, then the number of open channels in the resting membrane at any given time would be 10^7/cm^2. The input time constant, being the product of the input resistance and the input capacitance, is independent of cell size and is equal to the time constant of the membrane: $\tau_m = R_m C_m$.

Flow of Current in a Nerve Fiber

The effects of injecting a pulse of current into a nerve fiber, such as an axon or a dendrite, are more complex than those seen in a simple spherical cell because the membrane is extended to enclose a cylinder and can no longer be represented by a single resistor and capacitor. In addition, because current injected into a fiber not only flows outward through the membrane but also spreads longitudinally along the core of the fiber, the response is affected by the electrical properties of the cytoplasm.

Figure 8.2A shows an experimental arrangement for measuring the response of a nerve fiber to current injection through a microelectrode. As with the spherical cell, a second electrode is used to measure the response, but this time it is withdrawn repeatedly and reinserted to measure the voltage change at increasing distances from the current-passing electrode. The results of such a set of measurements are shown in Figure 8.2B. The potential change near the point of current injection (0 mm from the current electrode) is relatively large and rises rapidly to its final value. As the recording electrode is moved farther and farther from the current electrode, the potentials become smaller and slower. Potentials produced in this way are known as **electrotonic potentials**.

The final amplitudes of the electrotonic potentials are plotted against distance from the current electrode in Figure 8.2C. The amplitudes fall exponentially with distance according to the relation:

$$\Delta V = \Delta V_0 e^{-x/\lambda}$$

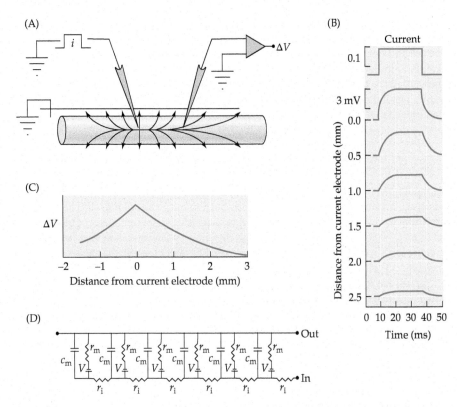

FIGURE 8.2 Response to Current Injection recorded from a nerve fiber immersed in bathing solution. (A) Two electrodes are inserted into the fiber—one to pass current and the other to record the resulting voltage change. Positive current injected into the cytoplasm flows longitudinally along the fiber and outward across the cell membrane. (B) Responses to a rectangular current pulse recorded at various distances from the current electrode. At zero electrode separation, the electrotonic potential rises rapidly to its maximum amplitude. As the recording electrode is moved to progressively increasing distances from the current source, the potentials become smaller and slower in time course. (C) Plot of response amplitude against distance from the current electrode. Decay of the response (ΔV) with distance is exponential. (D) An electrical model of the axon. V = membrane potential; r_m and c_m = membrane resistance and capacitance per unit length of axon; r_i = internal longitudinal resistance per unit length of the cytoplasm. (Records in B based on A. L. Hodgkin and W. A. H. Rushton, 1946. *Proc. R. Soc. Lond., B* 133: 444–479.)

where x is the distance from the current source and λ is the **length constant** of the fiber. The voltage change at zero separation is proportional to the size of the injected current:

$$\Delta V_0 = i r_{input}$$

where r_{input} is the input resistance of the fiber.

In summary, two factors, r_{input} and λ, determine the size of the response to current injection and how far the signal will spread along the fiber. To illustrate how these two factors depend on the properties of the fiber, it is again convenient to refer to an electrical model, shown in Figure 8.2D. The model is obtained by imagining that the fiber is cut along its length into a series of short cylinders. The membrane resistance of each cylindrical segment is represented by the resistor r_m, the capacitance by c_m, and the membrane potential by the battery V_m. The internal pathway for ionic flow along the axoplasm from the midpoint of one cylinder to the next is represented by the resistor r_i. Because nerves in a recording chamber are normally bathed in a large volume of fluid, resistance along the outside of the cylinders is represented as being zero. This approximation is not always adequate in the central nervous system (CNS), where nerve axons, dendrites, and glial cells are closely packed, thereby causing pathways for extracellular current flow to be restricted. Any length can be selected for the cylinders themselves; however, by convention, the resistances r_m and

BOX 8.1 Relation between Cable Constants and Specific Membrane Properties

The cable parameters r_m, c_m, and r_i refer to a 1-cm length of fiber. The first two parameters, r_m and c_m, depend on the specific resistance and capacitance of the fiber membrane and, in addition, on fiber diameter. The capacitance c_m has the units μF/cm. Its relation to the specific membrane capacitance (C_m, μF/cm^2) is given by $c_m = C_m(2\pi a)$, with $2\pi a$ being the surface area of a unit length of fiber of radius a. The resistance r_m, which has the units Ωcm, is related to the specific membrane resistance (R_m, Ωcm^2) by $r_m = R_m/(2\pi a)$.

The internal longitudinal resistance, r_i, is expressed as Ω/cm, and is related to the specific resistance of the cytoplasm, ρ, by $r_i = \rho/(\pi a^2)$, πa^2 being the cross-sectional area of the fiber. The specific resistance depends, in turn, on the intracellular ion concentrations and mobilities. The specific resistance of squid axoplasm is about 30 Ωcm at 20°C, or about 10^7 times that of copper. In mammals, in which the cytoplasmic ion concentration is lower, the specific resistance is

about 125 Ωcm at 37°C; in frogs, with still lower ion concentration, the specific resistance is about 250 Ωcm at 20°C.

These aforementioned relations can be used to deduce the dependence on fiber diameter of the input resistance and length constant. Thus, the input resistance is:

$$r_{input} = 0.5 \left(r_m r_i \right)^{1/2} = \left(\frac{\rho R_m}{2\pi^2 a^3} \right)^{1/2}$$

and the length constant is:

$$\lambda = \left(\frac{r_m}{r_i} \right)^{1/2} = \left(\frac{a R_m}{2\rho} \right)^{1/2}$$

So the input resistance decreases as fiber size increases, varying with the 3/2 power of the radius, and the length constant increases with the square root of the radius.

---

r_i and the capacitance c_m are specified for a 1-cm length of axon. Their relations to the specific properties of the membrane and cytoplasm are given in Box 8.1. This type of analysis was first used to examine the electrical behavior of undersea cables, and the parameters r_m, c_m, and r_i are sometimes referred to as cable properties.

Current injected into the fiber flows longitudinally along the fiber away from the tip of the electrode; as it does so, some of it is lost by outward movement through the membrane. The distance the potential spreads depends on the relative ease with which ions carrying the current escape through the cell membrane, as compared with the ease of ion movement through the cytoplasm. If the membrane resistance is low relative to that of the cytoplasm, then current will leak outward through the membrane before it can spread very far. A higher-resistance membrane, by contrast, will allow a greater portion of the current to spread along the fiber before escaping to the external solution. So the length constant increases as membrane resistance increases, and decreases when the internal longitudinal resistance increases. The exact relation is given by:

$$\lambda = \left(\frac{r_m}{r_i} \right)^{1/2}$$

The input resistance depends on the resistance encountered by current flowing from the point of injection back into the extracellular fluid. Because the pathways for current flow include both r_i and r_m, both contribute to the input resistance:

$$r_{input} = 0.5 \, (r_m r_i)^{1/2}$$

The factor 0.5 appears because the fiber extends in both directions from the point of current injection; each half has a resistance $(r_m r_i)^{1/2}$.

In general, large processes have greater length constants than small ones. This is because the membrane resistance depends on the surface area of the fiber and therefore varies inversely with fiber diameter, whereas the internal resistance depends on cross-sectional area and varies inversely with the square of the diameter. So as fiber diameter increases, r_i decreases more rapidly than r_m and the ratio r_m/r_i increases. Conversely, large processes have a lower input resistance than small processes because both the input resistance and longitudinal resistances are smaller (see Box 8.1). Other properties being equal, an excitatory synaptic potential (see Chapter 11) will be smaller in a large dendritic process (smaller r_{input}) than in a small one. However, in a larger dendrite the synaptic potential will spread farther toward the cell body (larger λ).

In axons and dendrites, the rates of rise and fall of electrotonic potentials depend on both the membrane time constant ($\tau_m = r_m c_m$) and the internal longitudinal resistance, but do not follow an exponential time course. At the onset of the pulse, current flows rapidly into nearby membrane capacitors, but then slows as an increasingly larger fraction of the current is diverted to longitudinal flow through the cytoplasm. The potentials rise much more slowly at points distant from the current electrode than at points nearby because the internal longitudinal resistance reduces the current flowing into the more distant capacitors.

Action Potential Propagation

Once generated, action potentials typically propagate along the entire length of a nerve fiber without attenuation. This propagation depends on the passive spread of current ahead of the active region to depolarize the next segment of membrane to threshold. To illustrate the nature of the current flow involved in impulse generation and propagation, we can imagine the action potential frozen at an instant in time and plot its spatial distribution along a fiber, as shown in Figure 8.3. The distance occupied depends on the duration of the action potential and the rate of conduction along the fiber. For example, if the action potential duration is 2 ms and if it is conducted at 10 m/s, or 10 mm/ms, then the potential will be spread over a 20-mm length of axon (almost an inch). Near the leading edge of the action potential, the cell membrane is depolarized by a rapid influx of sodium ions along their concentration gradient. Just as when current is injected through a microelectrode, the inward current spreads longitudinally through the axoplasm. Current spread ahead of the active region causes a new segment of membrane to be polarized toward threshold. Behind the peak of the action potential the potassium conductance is high and current flows out through potassium channels, returning the membrane potential toward its resting level.

Normally, impulses arise at one end of an axon and travel to the other. However, there is no inherent directionality to propagation. Impulses produced in the middle of a muscle fiber at a neuromuscular junction travel away from the junction in both directions toward the tendons. However, except in unusual circumstances, an action potential cannot double back on itself, reversing its direction of propagation. This is because the peak depolarization is followed by a **refractory period** during which re-excitation cannot occur (see Chapter 7). During this period, sodium channels remain inactivated, and the potassium conductance is still high, so that even if sodium channels were active, depolarization would be difficult. Because of the refractory period, the active region of the membrane, as it moves along a fiber, is followed by a refractory region that cannot be re-excited. As the membrane potential returns to its resting value, sodium channel inactivation is removed, potassium conductance returns to normal, and excitability recovers.

The rate of propagation of the action potential is influenced by both the space constant and time constant of the fiber. If the time constant is small, the membrane will depolarize to threshold quickly and the conduction velocity will be relatively high. If the space constant is large, the depolarization will spread a correspondingly large distance ahead of the active region, again speeding propagation of the signal. The result is that large fibers conduct more rapidly than small fibers because of their larger space constants. As already noted, the membrane time constant is independent of fiber size. Numerically, conduction velocity increases with the square root of fiber diameter.

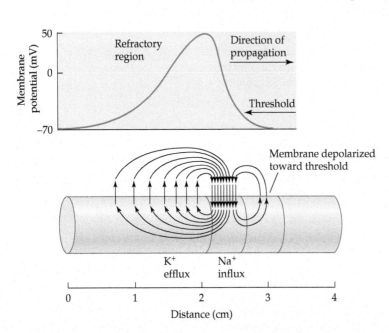

FIGURE 8.3 Current Flow during an Action Potential at an instant in time. Rapid depolarization on the rising phase of the action potential is due to influx of positively charged sodium ions. The positive current spreads ahead of the impulse, depolarizing the adjacent segment of membrane toward threshold. Efflux of potassium ions behind the peak leads to repolarization.

Myelinated Nerves and Saltatory Conduction

In the vertebrate nervous system, nerve fibers larger than about 1 μm in diameter are myelinated. Myelin is formed in the periphery by Schwann cells and in the CNS by oligodendrocytes (see Chapter 10). The cells wrap themselves tightly around axons, and with each wrap the cytoplasm in between the membrane pair is squeezed out so that the result is a spiral of tightly packed membranes. The number of wrappings (lamellae) ranges from a low of between 10 and 20 to a maximum of about 160. In this way the effective membrane resistance is greatly increased and the membrane capacitance reduced. The myelin sheath usually occupies 20% to 40% of the overall diameter of the fiber and is interrupted periodically by nodes of Ranvier, exposing narrow patches of axonal membrane.[1] The internodal distance is usually about 100 times the external diameter of the fiber and ranges from 200 μm to 2 mm.

The effect of the myelin sheath is to restrict membrane current flow largely to the nodes, because ions cannot flow easily into or out of the high-resistance internodal region, and the internodal capacitive currents are very small as well. As a result, excitation jumps from node to node, thereby greatly increasing the conduction velocity. Such impulse propagation is called saltatory conduction (from Latin *saltare*, to jump, leap or dance). Saltatory conduction does not mean that the action potential occurs in only one node at time. While excitation is jumping from one node to the next on the leading edge of the action potential, many nodes behind are still active. Myelinated axons not only conduct more rapidly than unmyelinated ones but also are capable of firing at higher frequencies for more prolonged periods of time.

Conduction velocities of myelinated fibers vary from a few meters per second up to more than 100 m/s. The world speed record is held by glial-ensheathed axons of the shrimp, which conduct at speeds in excess of 200 m/s (447 miles/hour).[2] In the vertebrate nervous system, peripheral nerves have been classified into groups according to conduction velocity and function (Box 8.2). Theoretical calculations suggest that in myelinated fibers conduction velocity should be proportional to the diameter of the fiber. In mammals, large myelinated fibers (> 11 μm in diameter) have a conduction velocity in meters per second equal to approximately six times their outside diameter in micrometers; for smaller fibers the constant of proportionality is about 4.5.[3]

Distribution of Channels in Myelinated Fibers

In myelinated fibers, voltage-sensitive sodium channels are highly concentrated in the nodes of Ranvier, with potassium channels more concentrated under the paranodal sheath.[4] The properties of the axon membrane in the paranodal regions normally covered by myelin were examined by Ritchie and his colleagues by loosening the myelin with enzyme treatment or osmotic shock.[5] Voltage clamp studies were then made of currents in the region of the node and compared with those obtained before the treatment. Previous experiments had suggested that, in rabbit nerve, nodes of Ranvier normally display only inward sodium current upon excitation. Repolarization after sodium channel inactivation appeared not to involve a transient increase in potassium conductance (as in other cells considered so far) but instead only passive current flow through a relatively large resting conductance. When the axon membrane adjacent to the nodes (the paranodal region) was exposed, excitation then produced a delayed outward potassium current, with no increase in inward current, indicating that the newly exposed membrane contained delayed rectifier channels but not sodium channels. Later immunocytochemical studies on rat myelinated nerve confirmed that delayed rectifier potassium channels (K_v1.1 and K_v1.2) were confined to the paranodal region (Figure 8.4A; see also Chapter 10).[6,7]

In the meantime, further voltage clamp experiments revealed that the potassium current underlying repolarization at intact nodes had more complex features than expected of passive ion flux through resting channels—most notably a slowly inactivating component, labeled I_{Ks}.[8,9] A clue to the nature of the slowly inactivating current was provided by the observation that mutations that impair the function of the potassium channel subunit KCNQ2 cause neuronal hyperexcitability, manifested by epileptic seizures and by involuntary muscle contractions (myokymia caused by spontaneous discharges in peripheral motor axons).[10] KCNQ2 (K_v7.2) combines with other members of the KCNQ family to form

[1] Susuki, K., and Rasband, M. N. 2008. *Curr. Opin. Cell Biol.* 20: 616-623.

[2] Xu, K., and Terakawa, S. 1999. *J. Exp. Biol.* 202: 1979-1989.

[3] Arbuthnott, E. R., Boyd, I. A., and Kalu, K. U. 1980. *J. Physiol.* 308: 125-157.

[4] Vabnick, I., and Shrager, P. 1998. *J. Neurobiol.* 37: 80-96.

[5] Chiu, S. Y., and Ritchie, J. M. 1981. *J. Physiol.* 313: 415-437.

[6] Wang, H. et al. 1993. *Nature* 365: 75-79.

[7] Rasband, M. N. et al. 1998. *J. Neurosci.* 18: 36-47.

[8] Dubois, J. M. 1983. *Prog. Biophys. Mol. Biol.* 42: 1-20.

[9] Roper, J., and Schwarz, J. R. 1989. *J. Physiol.* 416: 93-110.

[10] Dedek, K. et al. 2001. *Proc. Natl. Acad. Sci. USA* 98: 12272-12277.

BOX 8.2 Classification of Vertebrate Nerve Fibers

If we use external electrodes to stimulate all the fibers in a peripheral nerve at one end and then record its electrical response some distance away, the record will have a series of peaks. The peaks occur because of dispersion of nerve impulses that travel at different velocities in different fibers, and therefore arrive at the recording electrode at different times after the stimulus. For example, a record taken from a rat sciatic nerve with 50 mm between the stimulating and recording electrode might look like the following (the rapid deflection at the begin-

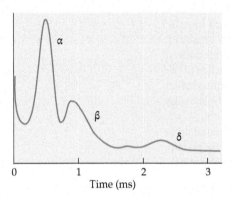

Time (ms)

ning is an artifact due to current spread from the stimulating electrode):Vertebrate nerve fibers were classified into groups on the basis of differences in conduction velocity, combined with differences in function. Unfortunately, two such classifications arose independently. In the first system, group A refers to myelinated fibers in peripheral nerve; in mammals, these conduct at velocities

ranging from 5 to 120 m/s. Group A fibers were further subdivided according to conduction velocity into α (80–120 m/s), β (30–80 m/s), and δ (5–30 m/s). These conduction velocity peaks are indicated in the record. The term γ fibers is reserved for motor nerves supplying muscle spindles (see Chapter 27), which have conduction velocities that span the β and lower part of the α range. Group B consists of myelinated fibers in the autonomic nervous system that have conduction velocities in the lower part of the A-fiber range. Group C refers to unmyelinated fibers, which conduct very slowly (less than 2 m/s).

The second nomenclature is used to classify sensory fibers arising in muscle: Group I, corresponding to Aα; Group II, corresponding to Aβ; and Group III, corresponding to Aδ. Group I afferent fibers were further classified into two subgroups, depending on whether they conveyed information from muscle spindles (Ia) or from sensory receptors in tendons (Ib) (see Chapter 27).

Fiber size affects other electrical properties of nerves in addition to conduction velocity. When a nerve trunk is stimulated with external electrodes, large fibers are excited more readily than small ones (i.e., their excitation threshold is lower). This is fortunate for clinical purposes, as it allows testing of thresholds and conduction velocity in motor nerves, for example, without exciting much smaller pain fibers. Just as larger fibers are easier to excite, they are also harder to block, for example by cooling or by local anesthetic, which means that pain fibers can be blocked without interfering with conduction in larger motor and sensory fibers. One exception to this general rule is block by localized pressure for which large axons are affected first, then smaller ones, as the pressure is increased.

---

the voltage-sensitive channels underlying the M-current (see Chapter 20). M-channels are activated by depolarization and inactivate very slowly. Their activation threshold is such that a fraction of the population is open at rest. Subsequent immunohistochemical studies confirmed that KCNQ2 subunits are expressed at nodes of Ranvier in rat sciatic nerve as well as at nodes and initial segments of myelinated CNS fibers.[11] In addition, voltage clamp studies on rat peripheral nerve fibers have shown that the I_{Ks} currents have all the biophysical and pharmacological properties of M-currents.[12] It is now apparent that M-channels are an important regulator of neuronal excitability throughout the nervous system. At nodes of Ranvier they serve to prevent spontaneous (ectopic) action potential discharges or repetitive discharges following invasion by a single action potential,[12] while at axon initial segments they regulate action potential threshold to suppress spontaneous firing.[13]

Mammalian axons that have been demyelinated chronically by exposure to diphtheria toxin can develop continuous conduction through a demyelinated region, suggesting that after demyelination, voltage-activated sodium channels appear in the exposed axon membrane.[14] Labeling of demyelinated nerves with antibodies to sodium channels shows that channels disappear from clusters in the former nodal regions and that new channels are distributed along previously myelinated regions (Figure 8.4B). Voltage-activated potassium channels are redistributed as well.[15] Upon remyelination there is restoration of normal clustering of sodium and potassium channels in newly formed nodes and paranodal regions.

[11] Devaux, J. J. et al. 2004. *J. Neurosci.* 24: 1236–1244.

[12] Schwarz, J. R. et al. 2006. *J. Physiol.* 573: 17–34.

[13] Shah, M. M. et al. 2008. *Proc. Natl. Acad. Sci. USA* 22: 7869–7874.

[14] England, J. D., Levinson, S. R., and Shrager, P. 1996. *Microsc. Res. Tech.* 34: 445–451.

[15] Bostock, H., Sears, T. A., and Sherratt, R. M. 1981. *J. Physiol.* 313: 301–315.

(A)

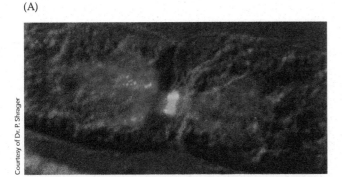

Courtesy of Dr. P. Shrager

FIGURE 8.4 Distribution of Sodium and Potassium Channels in myelinated axons. (A) In rat sciatic nerve, sodium channels (green) are tightly clustered in the node of Ranvier and potassium channels (red) are sequestered in the paranodal region. Note the sharp decrease in axon diameter within the node. (B) Disruption of sodium channel distribution after demyelination of goldfish lateral line nerve. (a) In the myelinated axon, sodium channel staining (yellow–green) is restricted to the nodal region (arrow). (b) Fourteen days after the beginning of demyelination, sodium channels appear in irregular patches. (c) At 21 days, more patches have appeared and are distributed along the length of the nerve. (A, see M. N. Rasband et al., 1998. *J. Neurosci.* 18: 36–47; B, see J. D. England et al., 1996. *Microsc. Res. Tech.* 34: 445–451.)

(B)

(a)

(b)

(c)

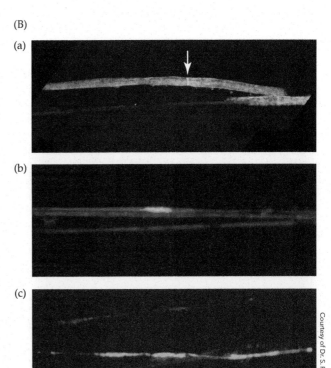

Courtesy of Dr. S. R. Levinson

Geometry and Conduction Block

A simple unmyelinated axon with uniform membrane properties is not representative of an entire neuron, with its cell body, elaborate dendritic arborization, and numerous axonal branches with terminals. The complex geometry of the neuron provides many possibilities for blocking action potential propagation. Specifically, propagation may fail wherever there is an abrupt expansion of membrane area. In such a situation the active membrane may not be able to provide enough current to depolarize the larger membrane area to threshold. For example, where an axon divides into two branches, the safety factor for propagation is reduced because current from the active segment of the single axon must contribute sufficient current to depolarize both branches to threshold. Under normal circumstances an impulse will usually propagate into both branches, but after repeated firing propagation may become blocked at the branch point. Other factors contribute to such block. For instance, in leech sensory cells, block can occur because of persistent hyperpolarization induced by increased electrogenic activity of the sodium pump (see Chapter 9) and long-lasting increases in potassium permeability, both of which increase the amount of current required for depolarization to threshold.[16,17]

In myelinated peripheral nerve the safety factor for conduction is about 5; that is, the depolarization produced at a node by excitation of a preceding node is approximately five times larger than necessary to reach threshold. Again, this safety factor is reduced where branching occurs. Similarly, when the myelin sheath terminates, for example near the end of a motor nerve, the current from the last node is then distributed over a large area of unmyelinated nerve terminal membrane and, as a consequence, provides less overall depolarization than would occur at a node. It is advantageous that the last few internodes before an unmyelinated terminal are shorter than normal, so that more nodes contribute to depolarization of the terminal.

Conduction in Dendrites

Apart from considerations of geometry, some regions of the neuron have a lower threshold for action potential initiation than others. This was first observed in spinal motoneurons

[18]Coombs, J. S., Eccles, J. C., and Fatt, P. 1955. *J. Physiol.* 130: 291-325.

[19]Kuffler, S. W., and Eyzaguirre, C. 1955. *J. Gen. Physiol.* 39: 87-119.

[20]Li, C.-L., and Jasper, H. H. 1953. *J. Physiol.* 121: 117-140.

[21]Llinás, R., and Sugimori, M. 1980. *J. Physiol.* 305: 197-213.

[22]Stuart, G., Schiller, J., and Sakmann, B. 1997. *J. Physiol.* 505: 617-632.

[23]Svoboda, K. et al. 1999. *Nat. Neurosci.* 2: 65-73.

by J. C. Eccles and his colleagues.[18] They found that upon depolarization action potentials were initiated first in the axon hillock, where the initial segment of the axon joins the cell body, and then propagated both outward along the axon and back into the soma and dendrites of the cell. At about the same time, Kuffler and Eyzaguirre found that depolarization of the dendrites in the crayfish stretch receptor initiated action potentials in or near the cell body, rather than in the dendrites themselves.[19] Observations of this kind led to the idea that dendrites were generally inexcitable and served only to transmit signals passively from dendritic synapses to the initial segment of the axon. This idea arose in spite of numerous observations to the contrary. For example, earlier extracellular recordings of electrical activity within the mammalian motor cortex by Li and Jasper gave clear indication of action potentials traveling upward along pyramidal cell dendrites from their cell bodies to the cortical surface, with a conduction velocity of about 3 m/s.[20]

Dendritic action potentials are now known to occur in a variety of neurons, and are mediated by regenerative sodium and calcium currents. Cerebellar Purkinje cells, in addition to producing sodium action potentials in their somatic region, generate calcium action potentials in their dendrites.[21] As shown in Figure 8.5A, calcium action potentials generated in a dendrite spread effectively into the soma. Somatic action potentials, by contrast, are not propagated into the dendrites but spread passively a short distance into the dendritic tree.

Like Purkinje cells, cortical pyramidal cells exhibit sodium action potentials in their somatic regions, usually arising in the initial segment of the axon. In addition, regenerative calcium potentials are observed in the distal dendrite.[22,23] Responses of a pyramidal cell to depolarization of the distal dendrite by activation of excitatory synapses (see Chapter 11) are shown in Figure 8.5B. Modest synaptic activation (see part a) produces dendritic depolarization that is attenuated as it spreads passively toward the soma. Upon arrival, the depolarization produces a somatic action potential that then spreads back into the dendrite. Stronger synaptic depolarization (see part b) results in direct activation of a dendritic calcium action potential that precedes the action potential generated in the soma.

Although there is now ample evidence of regenerative activity in dendrites, the general principle that the axon

(A)

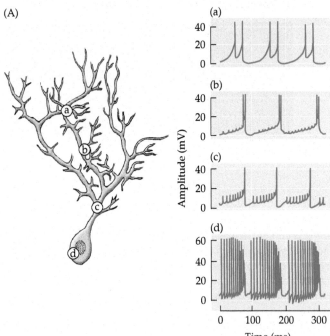

(B)

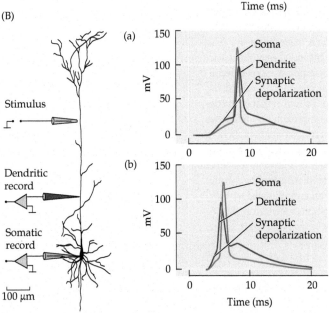

FIGURE 8.5   Spread of Action Potentials in Dendrites. (A) Records from a cerebellar Purkinje cell, obtained by impaling the cell at the indicated locations and passing a depolarizing current through the electrode. Near the end of the dendritic tree (a), depolarization produces long-duration calcium action potentials. In the cell soma (d), a steady depolarizing current produces high-frequency sodium action potentials, interrupted periodically by calcium action potentials. At intermediate locations (b,c), depolarization produces calcium action potentials in the dendrite. Accompanying sodium action potentials generated in the soma spread passively into the dendritic tree and die out after a short distance. (B) Conduction in a cortical pyramidal cell. A cortical cell dendrite is depolarized by activating distal excitatory synapses. (a) Moderate depolarization of the dendrite spreads to the soma, where it initiates an action potential (blue record). In the dendrite, the initial depolarization is larger, and is followed by an action potential that spreads back from the soma (red record). (b) Larger depolarization produces a calcium action potential in the dendrite that precedes action potential initiation in the soma. (A after R. Llinás and M. Sugimori, 1980. *J. Physiol.* 305: 197-213; B after G. Stuart et al., 1997. *J. Physiol.* 505: 617-632.)

hillock is the most excitable region of the cell still holds for most types of neurons that have been examined.[24] Propagation of electrical signals in a dendrite is clearly more complex than in an axon.[25] Dendrites are likely to contain a variety of voltage-dependent channels in addition to those associated with the action potential, and the coexistence of action potentials and synaptic potentials in the dendritic tree adds still more complexity. For example, the safety factor for backpropagation of action potentials will depend on the input resistance of the various branches; the input resistances, in turn, will depend on the extent of activity at excitatory and inhibitory synapses. Thus, whether or not backpropagation occurs depends on synaptic activity.[26–28] At the same time, synaptic channels that are voltage-dependent will behave differently from one moment to the next, depending on whether backpropagation has occurred.[29] These factors add considerable difficulty to the analysis of signal processing in dendrites.

Pathways for Current Flow between Cells

In most circumstances an action potential arriving at a nerve terminal has little or no direct electrical influence on the next cell. Currents generated by the action potential flow preferentially through the low-resistance extracellular space. Contact between cells is usually limited to a small area of apposition, and the resistances of the small areas of membrane are far too high to allow any significant current flow between the cells. Certain cells, however, exhibit **electrical coupling**. These include cardiac and smooth muscle cells, epithelial cells, gland cells, and a variety of neurons. Here we describe special intercellular structures that allow the processes of one neuron to be in electrical continuity with the next neuron, thereby allowing current flow between them. The specific properties and functional role of electrical synapses are discussed in Chapter 11.

At sites of electrical coupling the intercellular current flows through gap junctions. The gap junction is a region of close apposition of two cells that is characterized by aggregates of particles distributed in corresponding arrays in each of the adjoining membranes (Figure 8.6A,B). Each particle, called a connexon, comprises six protein subunits arranged in a circle, about 10 nm in diameter, around a central core. Identical particles in the apposing cells are exactly paired to span the 3.5-nm gap in the region of contact.

About 20 connexon subunits (connexins) have been isolated, ranging in weight from 26 to 57 kilodaltons (kD).[30,31] Each was named according to its deduced weight; for example, Cx32 (32 kD), found in rat liver, Cx40, in heart muscle, and so on. Connexons can be assembled from one type of connexin (homomeric) or more than one (heteromeric), and an intercellular channel can be formed from two identical connexons (homotypic) or two different connexons (heterotypic). The primary amino acid sequence of the connexins indicates that the molecule is composed of four transmembrane helices, M1–M4, connected by one intracellular and two extracellular loops (Figure 8.6C). This structure has been confirmed by electron crystallographic studies on Cx43.[32] A study with high-resolution (3.5Å) crystallography has provided a detailed image of the molecular structure of the entire Cx26 intercellular channel.[33] The molecule has an outer diameter of 9 nm at the cytoplasmic ends, tapering to a minimum of 5 nm in the middle of the extracellular bridge. The open pore has a diameter of 3.5 nm at each entrance, narrowing to 1.4 nm at the outer faces of the membranes and widening to 2.5 nm in the intercellular region (Figure 8.6D). In the intercellular region, the E1 and E2 loops of each connexin form a tight, double-layered ring around the channel interior with six copies of the N-terminal half of E1 lining the pore. The two rings interdigitate in the center of the cleft with an overlap of about 6 nm.

Conductance and permeability of the connexons have been studied extensively, both as hemichannels expressed in individual host cells, such as *Xenopus* oocytes, and as complete gap junction channels expressed in paired cells.[23,24] Complete channels allow passage of molecules up to about 1 nm in diameter and 1,000 Daltons in molecular mass. However, molecular selectivity and conductance vary widely depending on subunit composition.[34] For example, Cx43 channels are more than 100 times more permeable to adenosine triphosphate (ATP) and 40 times more permeable to glutamate than are Cx32 channels. Channel conductance is also highly variable, ranging from 15 pS for Cx36 channels to 300 pS for Cx43 in normal physiological solutions.

[24]Stuart, G. et al. 1997. *Trends Neurosci.* 20: 125-131.

[25]Waters, J., Schaefer, A., and Sakmann, B. 2005. *Prog. Biophys. Mol. Biol.* 87: 145-170.

[26]Tsubokawa, H., and Ross, W. N. 1996. *J. Neurophysiol.* 76: 2896-2906.

[27]Sandler, V. M., and Ross, W. N. 1999. *J. Neurophysiol.* 81: 216-224.

[28]Larkum, M. E., Zhu, J. J., and Sakmann, B. 1999. *Nature* 398: 338-341.

[29]Markram, H. et al. 1997. *Science* 275: 213-215.

[30]Sosinsky, G. E., and Nicholson, B. J. 2005. *Biochim. Biophys. Acta* 1711: 99-125.

[31]Evans, W. H., and Martin, P. E. M. 2002. *Mol. Membr. Biol.* 19: 121-136.

[32]Fleishman, S. J. et al. 2004. *Mol. Cell* 15: 879-888.

[33]Maeda, S. et al. 2009. *Nature* 458: 597-604.

[34]Ma, M., and Dahl, G. 2006. *Biophys. J.* 90: 151-163.

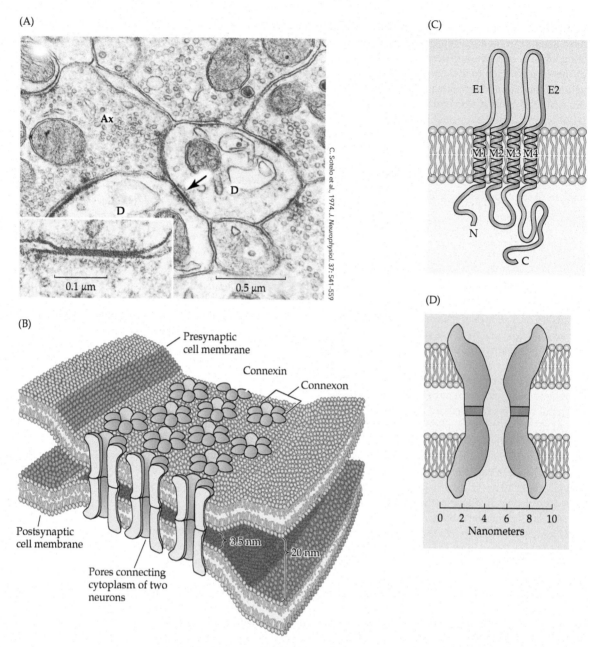

(A)

Ax

D

D

0.1 µm

0.5 µm

C. Sotelo et al., 1974. J. Neurophysiol. 37: 541–559

(C)

E1   E2

M1 M2 M3 M4

N

C

(B)

Presynaptic
cell membrane

Connexin

Connexon

Postsynaptic
cell membrane

Pores connecting
cytoplasm of two
neurons

3.5 nm

20 nm

(D)

0   2   4   6   8   10
Nanometers

FIGURE 8.6 **Gap Junctions between Neurons.** (A) Two dendrites (labeled D) in the inferior olivary nucleus of the cat are joined by a gap junction (arrow), shown at higher magnification in the inset. The usual space between the cells is almost obliterated in the contact area, which is traversed by cross bridges. (B) Schematic view of a gap junction, showing close membrane apposition bridged by a group of paired connexons–each connexon comprises six connexin subunits. (C) A connexin subunit consists of four membrane-spanning helices, M1–M4. Amino acid loops E1 and E2 project into the extracellular space. (D) Cross section through a connexon pair, showing relative dimensions and based on high-resolution images of Cx26. The open channel is 3.5 nm in diameter at each entrance, narrowing to 1.4 nm at the extracellular membrane faces. Orange band represents the region of overlap of the extracellular loops. (B after D. Purves et al., 1997. *Neuroscience*. Oxford University Press/ Sinauer: Sunderland, MA; D based on S. Maeda et al., 2009. *Nature* 458: 597-604.)

Even with the lowest single-channel conductance, individual gap junctions provide a significant pathway for current flow between cells because of the high packing density of the channels. For example, a tight junction 0.2 μm in diameter may contain more than 300 connexon pairs.[35] At 15 pS each, the total conductance through the junction would be 4.5 nanosiemens (nS). This is several thousand times greater than the conductance through two tightly apposed cell membranes with the same area and no connexons.

[35]Cantino, D., and Mugnani, E. 1975. *J. Neurocytol.* 4: 505-536.

SUMMARY

- The spread of local graded potentials in a neuron and the propagation of action potentials along a nerve fiber depend on the electrical properties of the cytoplasm and the cell membrane.

- When a steady current is injected into a cylindrical fiber, the size of a local graded potential is determined by the input resistance of the fiber (r_{input}), and the distance over which it spreads is determined by the length constant of the fiber (λ); r_{input} and λ depend, in turn, on the resistance of the fiber membrane (r_m) and the longitudinal resistance of the axoplasm (r_i).

- In addition to having a resistance, a nerve fiber membrane has a capacitance. The effect of the membrane capacitance (c_m) is to slow the rise and decay of signals. The magnitude of this effect is determined by the membrane time constant, $\tau_m = r_m c_m$.

- Propagation of an action potential along a fiber depends on the passive spread of current from the active region into the next segment of membrane.

The conduction velocity depends on the time constant and length constant of the membrane and is proportional to fiber diameter.

- Large nerve fibers in vertebrates are wrapped in myelin sheaths, with regularly spaced gaps or nodes between ensheathing glia or Schwann cells. During action potential propagation, excitation jumps from one node to the next (saltatory conduction).

- Action potential propagation is influenced by geometrical factors that produce changes in membrane area. For example, block of propagation may occur at branch points in nerve terminal arborizations, and conduction may have a preferred direction in tapered dendrites.

- Transfer of electrical signals from one cell to the next requires special low-resistance connections called gap junctions. A gap junction is formed by a collection of connexons, which are proteins that form aqueous channels between the cytoplasms of adjacent cells.

Suggested Reading

General Reviews

Evans, W. H. and Martin, P. E. M. 2002. Gap junctions: structure and function. *Mol. Membr. Biol.* 19: 121–136.

Sosinsky, G. E., and Nicholson, B. J. 2005. Structural organization of gap junction channels. *Biochim. Biophys. Acta.* 1711: 99–125.

Susuki, K. and Rasband, M. N. 2008. Molecular mechanisms of node of Ranvier formation. *Curr. Opin. Cell Biol.* 20: 616–623.

Original Papers

Maeda, S., Nakagawa, S., Suga, M., Yamashita, E., Oshima, A., Fujiyoshi, Y., and Tsukihara, T. 2009. Structure of the connexin 26 gap junction channel at 3.5Å resolution. *Nature* 458: 597–604.

Schwarz, J. R., Glassmeier, G., Cooper, E. C., Kao, T. C., Nodera, H., Tabuena, D., Kaji, R., and Bostock, H. 2006. KCNQ channels mediate IKs, a slow K+ current regulating excitability in the rat node of Ranvier. *J. Physiol.* 573: 17–34.

Vabnick, I. and Shrager, P. 1998. Ion channel redistribution and function during development of the myelinated axon. *J. Neurobiol.* 37: 80–96.

Waters, J., Schaefer, A., and Sakmann, B. 2005. Backpropagating action potentials in neurones: measurement, mechanisms and potential functions. *Prog. Biophys. Mol. Biol.* 87: 145–170.

CHAPTER 9

Ion Transport across Cell Membranes

There is a constant flux of ions across the outer cell membrane of neurons, both at rest and during electrical activity. The flux is driven by electrical and chemical concentration gradients. In the face of such movements, concentrations in the cytoplasm are kept constant by transport mechanisms that use energy to move ions back across the membrane against their electrochemical gradients. Maintenance of intracellular ion concentrations is essential to maintain both the resting membrane potential and the ability to generate electrical signals.

Primary active transport uses energy provided by the hydrolysis of adenosine triphosphate (ATP). The most prevalent transport mechanism of this kind is the sodium–potassium exchange pump. The molecule responsible for transport is an enzyme, sodium–potassium ATPase, which carries three sodium ions out of the cell and two potassium ions in, for every molecule of ATP hydrolyzed. Each cycle of the pump results in the net movement of one ionic charge across the membrane, so the pump is said to be electrogenic. Two different forms of calcium ATPase are responsible for calcium transport out of the cytoplasm: Plasma cell membrane calcium ATPase pumps calcium out of the cell, and endoplasmic and sarcoplasmic reticulum ATPases pump calcium from the cytoplasm into intracellular compartments.

Secondary active transport uses the movement of sodium down its electrochemical gradient to transport other ions across the membrane either in the same direction (cotransport) or in the opposite direction (ion exchange). An example is sodium–calcium exchange, in which the influx of three sodium ions is used to transport a single calcium ion out of the cell. Like all other secondary transport systems, this exchange system is reversible, and depending on the chemical and electrical gradients for the two ions, it can be made to run in a forward or backward direction. A second sodium–calcium exchange system, found in retinal cells, transports a single calcium ion plus one potassium ion out of the cell in exchange for four sodium ions. Sodium influx is also used to transport chloride and bicarbonate across the cell membrane. All such mechanisms provide pathways for sodium to enter the cell down its electrochemical gradient, and therefore depend on sodium–potassium ATPase to maintain that gradient.

Transport of neurotransmitters plays an important role in nervous system function. In presynaptic terminals transmitters are packaged in vesicles, ready for release. After release, they are removed from extracellular spaces by uptake mechanisms in the plasma cell membranes of neurons and glial cells. Transport into vesicles is by a hydrogen-transmitter exchange system. The hydrogen gradient is maintained, in turn, by hydrogen ATPase in the vesicle membrane. Uptake of the transmitters from extracellular spaces is by sodium cotransport systems.

Several transport ATPases and ion exchangers have been isolated and cloned, and their configurations in the membrane have been determined. All appear to have 10 to 12 transmembrane segments, and are assumed to form channel-like structures through which substances are moved by alternate exposure of binding sites to the extracellular and intracellular spaces.

At rest and during electrical activity, ions move into and out of cells along their electrochemical gradients. Clearly, if such ion movements continued without compensation the system eventually would run down and both the concentration gradients and the potential across the cell membrane would disappear. Recovery of ions that leak into or out of the cell at rest or during electrical activity is accomplished by a variety of transport mechanisms that move ions back across the membrane against their electrochemical gradients. **Primary active transport** is driven directly by metabolic energy, specifically by the hydrolysis of ATP. **Secondary active transport** uses energy provided by the flux of an ion (usually sodium) down its established electrochemical gradient to transport other ions across the cell membrane, either in the same direction (cotransport) or in the opposite direction (ion exchange).

The Sodium-Potassium Exchange Pump

Most excitable cells have resting membrane potentials in the range of –60 to –90 mV, while the equilibrium potential for sodium (E_{Na}) is usually of the order of +50 mV. Thus, there is a large electrochemical gradient tending to drive sodium into the cell, and it enters continuously through various pathways in the cell membrane. In addition, the equilibrium potential for potassium (E_K) is more negative than the resting potential, so potassium ions continually move out of the cell. In order to maintain the viability of the cell, it is necessary to transport sodium back out and potassium back in, against their electrochemical gradients. This perpetual task is carried out by the **sodium-potassium exchange pump**, which in its usual mode of operation transports three sodium ions out across the cell membrane for every two potassium ions carried inward.

Early studies of sodium–potassium exchange were done by Hodgkin and Keynes and their colleagues on the giant axon of the squid,[1,2] where it was shown clearly that the source of energy for the transport process was hydrolysis of ATP. During the same period, Skou[3] demonstrated that an ATPase isolated from crab nerve had many of the biochemical properties that would be expected of a sodium–potassium exchange pump. Specifically, just as both sodium and potassium are required for the pump to work, the enzyme was stimulated by the simultaneous presence of sodium and potassium. Moreover, both sodium–potassium exchange and activity of the enzyme were inhibited by the poisonous glycoside ouabain. These observations led to the conclusion that the enzyme, **sodium-potassium ATPase**, is itself the transport molecule. It is one of a family of P-type ATPases (so called because they form a phosphorylated intermediate) that derive energy for ion translocation from hydrolysis of ATP. Other members of the same family include calcium ATPases, which transport calcium out of the cytoplasm of cells, and vacuolar hydrogen ATPase, which transports protons into intracellular acidic vacuoles, including synaptic vesicles.

Biochemical Properties of Sodium-Potassium ATPase

The biochemical properties of sodium–potassium ATPase have been known for many years.[4,5] The stoichiometry of cation binding to the enzyme is as expected from the transport characteristics: Three sodium and two potassium ions are bound for each molecule of ATP hydrolyzed. The requirement for sodium is remarkably specific. It is the only substrate accepted for net outward transport; conversely, it is the only monovalent cation *not* accepted for inward transport. Thus, lithium, ammonium, rubidium, cesium, and thallium are all able to substitute for potassium in the external solution but not for sodium in the internal solution. The requirement for external potassium is not absolute. In its absence the pump will extrude sodium at about 10% of capacity in an uncoupled mode. The transport system is blocked specifically by digitalis glycosides (drugs used for treating congestive heart failure), particularly ouabain and strophanthidin. Although they block

[1]Hodgkin, A. L., and Keynes, R. D. 1955. *J. Physiol.* 128: 28-60.

[2]Caldwell, P. C. et al. 1960. *J. Physiol.* 152: 561-590.

[3]Skou, J. C. 1957. *Biochim. Biophys. Acta* 23: 394-401.

[4]Skou, J. C. 1988. *Methods Enzymol.* 156: 1-25.

[5]Jorgensen, P. L., Hakansson, K. O., and Karlish, S. J. D. 2003. *Annu. Rev. Physiol.* 65: 817-849.

sodium and potassium transport by ATPase, these drugs have no effect on the passive movements of sodium and potassium through membrane channels.

Experimental Evidence That the Pump Is Electrogenic

Because sodium–potassium ATPase transports unequal numbers of sodium and potassium ions, each cycle of the pump results in the outward movement of one positive charge across the membrane. For this reason the pump is said to be **electrogenic**. The electrogenic nature of the pump was tested experimentally in squid axons,[1,2,6] and in a remarkable set of experiments by Thomas, using snail neurons.[7,8] Snail neurons are sufficiently large to permit the insertion of several micropipettes through the cell membrane into the cytoplasm without damaging the cell. To examine how internal sodium concentration affected pump current and membrane potential, Thomas used two intracellular pipettes to deposit ions in the cell, one filled with sodium acetate and the other with lithium acetate (Figure 9.1A). A third

[6] Baker, P. F. et al. 1969. *J. Physiol.* 200: 459–496.

[7] Thomas, R. C. 1969. *J. Physiol.* 201: 495–514.

[8] Thomas, R. C. 1972. *J. Physiol.* 220: 55–71.

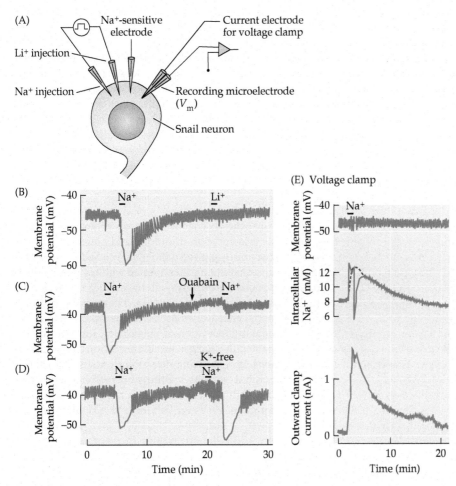

FIGURE 9.1 Effects of Sodium Injection into a snail neuron on intracellular sodium concentration, membrane potential, and membrane current. (A) Two micropipettes are used to inject either sodium or lithium; a sodium-sensitive electrode measures [Na]$_i$; another electrode measures membrane potential and is also used in combination with a current-passing electrode to hold the membrane potential steady while measuring membrane current (shown in E). (B) Hyperpolarization of the membrane following intracellular injection of sodium. Note that the small rapid deflections are spontaneously occurring action potentials, reduced in size because of the poor frequency response of the pen recorder. Injection of lithium does not produce hyperpolarization. (C) After application of ouabain (20 µg/ml), which blocks the sodium pump, hyperpolarization by sodium injection is greatly reduced. (D) Removal of potassium from the extracellular solution blocks the pump, so that sodium injection produces no hyperpolarization until potassium is restored. (E) Measurements of membrane current, with the membrane potential clamped at –47 mV. Sodium injection results in an increase in intracellular sodium concentration, and an outward current across the cell membrane. Sharp deflections on the sodium concentration record are artifacts from the injection system; the dashed line indicates the time course of the change in concentration. (After R. C. Thomas, 1969. *J. Physiol.* 201: 495–514.)

intracellular pipette was used as an electrode to record membrane potential. A fourth pipette was used as a current electrode for voltage clamp experiments (see Chapter 7), and yet a fifth, made of sodium-sensitive glass, monitored the intracellular sodium concentration! To inject sodium, the sodium-filled pipette was made positive with respect to the lithium pipette. Thus, current flow in the injection system was between the two pipettes, with none of the injected current flowing through the cell membrane.

The result of sodium injection is shown in Figure 9.1B. After a brief injection, the cell became hyperpolarized by about 15 mV, presumably because of increased pump activity. The potential recovered gradually over several minutes, as the excess sodium was extruded. Injection of lithium (by making the lithium pipette positive) produced no hyperpolarization.

Several lines of evidence showed that the potential change after sodium injection was due to the action of a sodium pump. For example, the hyperpolarization could be greatly reduced or abolished by addition of the transport inhibitor, ouabain, to the bathing solution (Figure 9.1C). Similarly, sodium injection had little effect on potential when potassium was absent from the external solution; reintroduction of potassium after sodium injection, however, resulted in immediate hyperpolarization (Figure 9.1D).

Quantitative estimates of the pump rate and the exchange ratio were obtained by voltage clamp experiments. This technique provided a means of measuring ion current across the membrane while the membrane potential was held constant (i.e., clamped). At the same time, intracellular sodium concentration was monitored. Sodium injection produced a transient rise in intracellular sodium, which was accompanied by a surge of outward current whose amplitude and duration followed the sodium concentration change (Figure 9.1E). The net charge carried out of the cell, which was calculated by measuring the area under the membrane current, amounted to only about one-third of the charge injected in the form of sodium ions. This result was consistent with the idea that for every three sodium ions pumped out of the cell, two potassium ions were carried inward.

Mechanism of Ion Translocation

The general sequence of events believed to underlie translocation of sodium and potassium by the enzyme is illustrated in Figure 9.2. Sodium and potassium binding sites, located within a channel-like structure, are exposed alternately to the intracellular and extracellular solutions. The cyclic conformational changes are driven by phosphorylation and dephosphorylation of the protein, and are accompanied by changes in binding affinity for the two ions. Inward-facing sites have a low affinity for potassium and a high affinity for sodium (see Figure 9.2A). Binding of three sodium ions causes a conformational change that leads to ATP binding, followed by phosphorylation of the enzyme (see Figure 9.2B). Phosphorylation then produces a further

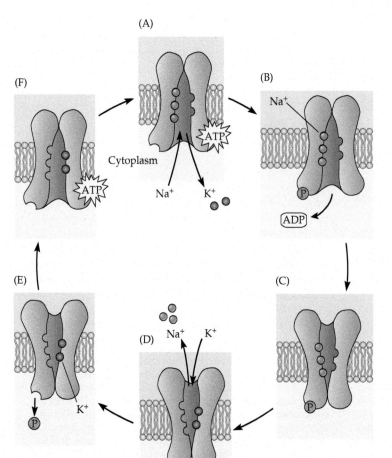

FIGURE 9.2 Alternating Access Model for Ion Translocation by Na-K ATPase. (A) Inward-facing binding sites have a high affinity for sodium, a low affinity for potassium, and bind three sodium ions. (B) Sodium binding is followed by phosphorylation of the enzyme. (C) Phosphorylated enzyme undergoes a conformational change so that binding sites face the extracellular solution. (D) Outward-facing sites have a low affinity for sodium, a high affinity for potassium, and bind two potassium ions. (E) Potassium binding leads to dephosphorylation. (F) Dephosphorylation is followed by a return to the starting conformation. (After D. J. Horisberger, 2004. *Physiology* 19: 377–387.)

conformational change so that the ion-binding sites are exposed to the extracellular solution (see Figure 9.2C). The outward-facing sites have low sodium and high potassium affinities, so that the sodium ions are replaced by two potassium ions (see Figure 9.2D). Potassium binding leads to dephosphorylation of the enzyme and a return to the starting conformation (see Figure 9.2E,F). The potassium ions are then released into the cytoplasm.

Calcium Pumps

Changes in intracellular calcium are important for many neuronal functions. For example, increases in cytoplasmic calcium concentration mediate the release of neurotransmitters at synapses, activation of ion channels in the cell membrane, and regulation of several cytoplasmic enzymes. In muscle, increased intracellular calcium initiates contraction. Because these functional roles are associated with transient increases in cytoplasmic calcium concentration, it is important that the resting concentration be kept low. Otherwise the various mechanisms would be activated continuously rather than in response to specific stimuli.

Transient increases in cytoplasmic calcium concentration are mediated either by entry of calcium through channels in the plasma cell membrane or by release from intracellular stores; return to resting concentration is achieved by activation of several transport proteins in the plasma cell membrane and in membranes of the intracellular storage compartments, principally the endoplasmic reticulum (sarcoplasmic reticulum in muscle) and mitochondria.[9,10] In most neurons cytoplasmic concentrations of free calcium range from 10 to 100 nM. The extracellular calcium concentration in vertebrate interstitial fluid is in the range of 2 to 5 mM, so outward transport across the membrane is against a substantial electrochemical gradient. Transport systems within the cell maintain high concentrations of calcium within intracellular compartments. Calcium concentrations in the endoplasmic reticulum can reach 400 μM, and in the sarcoplasmic reticulum of muscle can be as high as 10 mM. Transport of calcium out of the cytoplasm, across the plasma cell membrane, and into membrane-bound intracellular compartments is accomplished by **calcium ATPase**.[11] An additional mechanism for transport of calcium across the plasma cell membrane that does not involve enzyme activity is discussed later in this chapter.

Endoplasmic and Sarcoplasmic Reticulum Calcium ATPase

One family of calcium ATPases is concentrated in membranes of the endoplasmic reticulum of neurons and in the sarcoplasmic reticulum of muscle. These ATPases transport calcium from the cytoplasm into the membrane-bound intracellular compartments. In muscle, contraction is triggered by the release of calcium from the sarcoplasmic reticulum into the myoplasm. Rapid return of cytoplasmic calcium to its resting level, and hence prompt muscle relaxation, is accomplished by a high density of calcium ATPase in the sarcoplasmic reticulum membrane. The calcium transport cycle is analogous to that described for sodium–potassium ATPase and begins with the attachment of two calcium ions to high-affinity ($K_{m(Ca)} \approx 100$ nM) sites facing the cytoplasm. The enzyme is then phosphorylated and undergoes a conformational change, resulting in the release of the calcium ions to the reticular compartment. Release of the bound calcium is followed by dephosphorylation and return to the starting molecular configuration.

Plasma Cell Membrane Calcium ATPase

Calcium ATPase is also found in the plasma cell membrane of all cells. The plasma cell membrane enzyme is similar in structure and function to its endoplasmic and sarcoplasmic reticular counterpart but differs in some details. The intracellular binding site has a high affinity for calcium. During the transport cycle, extrusion of one calcium ion is accompanied by inward transport of two hydrogen ions, so the transport is electrically neutral.[12] This ensures that after calcium influx, recovery of intracellular calcium concentration is not influenced by membrane potential. In nerve and muscle the enzyme is only sparsely distributed in the plasma cell membrane, so its transport capacity is relatively low. Nonetheless, it is adequate to compensate for calcium influx into resting cells.

[9] MacLennan, D. H., Abu-Abed, M., and Kang, C. H. 2002. *J. Mol. Cell. Cardiol.* 34: 897-918.

[10] Rizzuto, R., and Pozzan, T. 2006. *Physiol. Rev.* 86: 369-408.

[11] Carafoli, E., and Brini, M. 2000. *Curr. Opin. Chem. Biol.* 4: 152-161.

[12] Thomas, R. C. 2009. *J. Physiol.* 87: 315-327.

Sodium-Calcium Exchange

Many ion transport mechanisms make use of an entirely different principle for the up-hill transfer of ions across the cell membrane: Instead of relying on hydrolysis of ATP, ion movement is coupled to the inward flux of sodium down its electrochemical gradient. Sodium, entering the cell down its electrochemical gradient through transport molecules, provides the energy required to carry other ions uphill against their electrochemical gradients, either into or out of the cell. A simple example is the 1:1 sodium–hydrogen exchange mechanism that contributes to the maintenance of intracellular pH. Hydrogen ions are carried out of the cell against their electrochemical gradient in exchange for inward movement of sodium. Calcium, potassium, chloride, and bicarbonate are also transported in this way. These secondary transport systems account for a measurable fraction of the sodium entry into the resting cell. Ultimately, of course, the mechanisms depend on sodium–potassium ATPase to maintain the sodium gradient by pumping sodium ions back out of the cell. In some instances, potassium ions moving out of the cell down their electrochemical gradient also contribute energy to ion transport processes.

The NCX Transport System

At least two sodium–calcium exchange systems are found in plasma cell membranes. The most widely distributed of these is the sodium–calcium exchange (NCX) system.[13,14] The transport molecule carries one calcium ion outward for every three sodium ions entering the cell. The NCX exchanger has a lower affinity for calcium ($K_{1/2Ca} \approx 1.0$ μM) than does calcium ATPase, but because the exchange molecules occur at a much higher density, their transport capacity is about 50 times greater. The exchange system is called into play in excitable cells when calcium influx during electrical activity overwhelms the transport ability of the ATPase.

The experiment shown in Figure 9.3 illustrates the operation of the sodium–calcium exchange mechanism in a squid axon. The intracellular concentration of ionized calcium was measured by luminescence of the calcium indicator, aequorin. In the steady state, the influx of calcium along its electrochemical gradient is balanced by outward transport through the ion exchanger (see Figure 9.3A). At the beginning of the experiment (see Figure 9.3B), the intracellular calcium concentration is relatively high, as the axon is bathed in high (112 mM) levels of calcium. When the extracellular calcium concentration is reduced, the passive influx decreases. As a result, the intracellular calcium concentration falls, restoring the driving force for calcium entry until the passive influx again equals the rate of extrusion. Reducing the extracellular sodium concentration, however, increases intracellular calcium concentration. This is because the reduced driving force for sodium entry reduces the rate at which the exchanger extrudes calcium.

[13] Blaustein, M. P., and Lederer, W. J. 1999. *Physiol. Rev.* 79: 763-854.

[14] Annunziato, L., Pignatoro, G., and DiRenzo, G. F. 2004. *Pharmacol. Rev.* 56: 633-654.

(A)

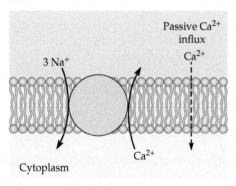

(B)

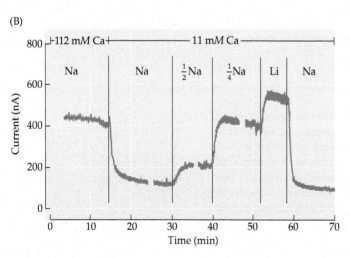

FIGURE 9.3 Transport of Calcium Ions out of a squid axon. (A) Scheme for sodium-calcium exchange. Influx of three sodium ions down their electrochemical gradient is coupled to the extrusion of one calcium ion. Calcium concentration reaches a steady state when outward transport through the exchanger is equal to the inward calcium leak. (B) Effect of changes in extracellular calcium and sodium on intracellular calcium concentration. Changes in intracellular calcium concentration are measured by changes in luminescence of injected aequorin, indicated by current from the photodetector. Increased readings mean increased intracellular free-calcium concentration. Reducing the extracellular calcium concentration from 112 mM to 11 mM reduces the intracellular concentration. Reducing extracellular sodium reduces outward calcium transport, and hence increases intracellular concentration. Lithium ions do not substitute for sodium in the transport system. (After P. F. Baker et al., 1971. *J. Physiol.* 218: 709-755.)

Intracellular calcium concentration then rises until calcium influx is reduced by the same amount. Replacement of sodium by lithium (which does not enter the exchanger) results in a further increase in intracellular calcium.

Reversal of Sodium–Calcium Exchange

Ion exchange mechanisms can be made to run backward by altering one or more of the ion gradients involved in the exchange. An interesting feature of the NCX family of exchangers is that such reversal can occur readily under physiological conditions, in which case calcium *enters* through the system and sodium is extruded. The direction of transport is determined simply by whether the energy provided by the entry of three sodium ions is greater than or less than the energy required to extrude one calcium ion. One factor determining this energy balance is the membrane potential of the cell. Such dependence on potential arises because the exchange is not electrically neutral; rather, each forward cycle of the transport molecule results in a net transfer of one positive charge inward across the membrane. As a result, forward transport is facilitated by membrane hyperpolarization and impeded, or even reversed, by depolarization.

The energy dissipated by sodium entry (or required for extrusion) is simply the product of charge moved across the membrane and the driving force for this movement; in other words, it is the charge multiplied by the difference between the sodium equilibrium potential (E_{Na}) and the membrane potential (V_m). For three sodium ions, this is $3(E_{Na} - V_m)$. Similarly, for a single (divalent) calcium ion, the energy is $2(E_{Ca} - V_m)$. At some value of membrane potential the energies will be exactly equal and no exchange will occur. If we call this point the reversal potential, V_r, then:

$$3(E_{Na} - V_r) = 2(E_{Ca} - V_r)$$

and (by rearrangement)

$$V_r = 3E_{Na} - 2E_{Ca}$$

At potentials more negative than V_r, sodium moves into the cell and calcium is transported out. At more positive potentials, the sodium and calcium fluxes are reversed.

Now suppose a nerve cell has internal sodium and calcium ion concentrations of 15 mM and 100 nM, respectively, and is bathed in a solution containing 150 mM sodium and 2 mM calcium. These concentrations are reasonable physiological values for mammalian cells. Using the Nernst equation (see Chapter 4), the equilibrium potential for sodium is +58 mV and for calcium is +124 mV. Ion movement through the exchanger is zero at a membrane potential (V_r) of –74 mV. This is in the range of resting membrane potentials for many cells so that, in any given cell, ion movements through the exchanger may be either inward or outward, depending on the exact membrane potential, and on whether or not there has been previous sodium or calcium accumulation.

Sodium–Calcium Exchange in Retinal Rods

It is evident that the NCX type of exchanger would be a poor system for calcium extrusion from cells with low resting potentials; rather than being extruded, calcium would be accumulated until a relatively high steady-state concentration was reached in the cytoplasm. An example of such a cell is the vertebrate retinal rod, which has a resting membrane potential of the order of –40 mV (see Chapter 22). These cells contain a second kind of sodium–calcium exchange molecule in the plasma cell membranes of their outer segments.[15] In addition to transporting sodium and calcium, the molecule transports potassium, and therefore is given the designation NCKX. The NCKX system is given an additional boost over the NCX exchanger by two differences in stoichiometry: (1) Four (rather than three) sodium ions enter for each calcium ion extruded, and (2) additional work is available from the extrusion of one potassium ion that, like sodium, moves down its electrochemical gradient during the exchange. The reversal potential for sodium–potassium–calcium exchange is:

$$V_r = 4E_{Na} - E_K - 2E_{Ca}$$

---

[15] Schnetkamp, P. P. M. 2004. *Pflügers Arch.* 447: 683-688.

Using the previous assumptions about E_{Na} (58 mV) and E_{Ca} (124 mV) and assuming that $E_K = -90$ mV, then $V_r = +74$ mV. Clearly, transport through the RetX exchanger is unlikely to reverse.

Another way of viewing the exchange system is to ask what the intracellular concentration of calcium would be if V_r were equal to the resting potential of the cell. Using the same assumptions about sodium and potassium, we find that when $V_r = -40$ mV, $E_{Ca} = 181$ mV. With 2 mM extracellular calcium, this is equivalent to an intracellular concentration of 1 nM. In other words, at a membrane potential of -40 mV it is energetically possible for the exchanger to reduce the cytoplasmic calcium concentration to 1 nM. However, this low concentration could not be achieved in practice because it is about two orders of magnitude smaller than the affinity of the exchange molecule for calcium.

Chloride Transport

Intracellular chloride concentration is closely regulated in all cells. Such regulation is particularly important in neurons because direct synaptic inhibition (see Chapter 11) depends on the maintenance of low intracellular chloride. Although chloride-sensitive ATPases have been demonstrated in several tissues, including the brain,[16] the bulk of chloride transport across the plasma cell membrane of nerve cells is by secondary transport mechanisms. The most important are two cation-coupled transport systems: (1) a sodium–potassium–chloride transport mechanism that moves chloride into the cell, and (2) an outward potassium–chloride cotransport. In addition, all cells have one or more chloride–bicarbonate exchange systems that are concerned primarily with intracellular pH regulation.

Inward Chloride Transport

In many cells, such as skeletal muscle fibers, tubular cells of the kidney, and squid axons, chloride is actively accumulated. Chloride accumulation is dependent on the extracellular concentrations of both sodium and potassium, and the system transports all three ions inward across the cell membrane.[17] The movement of sodium down its concentration gradient supplies the required energy. In squid axons the Na–K–Cl stoichiometry has been shown to be 2:1:3. In cells of the kidney the Na–K–Cl stoichiometry is 1:1:2, and the renal transport system operates in parallel with a second, potassium-independent mechanism that transports sodium and chloride in a 1:1 ratio (Figure 9.4A).

[16]Gerencser, G. A., and Zhang, J. 2003. *Biochim. Biophys. Acta* 1618: 133–139.

[17]Russell, J. M. 2000. *Physiol. Rev.* 80: 211–276.

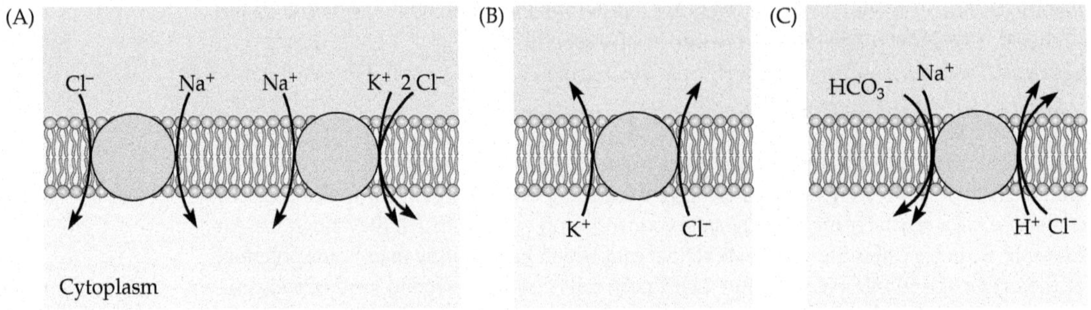

FIGURE 9.4 Mechanisms of Chloride Transport. (A) In many cells, inward chloride transport is mediated by two independent mechanisms, both using the electrochemical gradient for sodium. One is sodium-chloride cotransport. The other is sodium-potassium-chloride cotransport, with a stoichiometry of 1:1:2. (B) Potassium-chloride cotransport uses the outward electrochemical gradient for potassium to transport chloride out of the cell. (C) Sodium-dependent chloride-bicarbonate exchange uses the inward sodium gradient to move chloride out of the cell, at the same time exchanging bicarbonate with hydrogen ions. Note that all the chloride transport systems are electrically neutral.

Outward Potassium-Chloride Cotransport

A second major transport mechanism for chloride involves cotransport of chloride and potassium outward, across the cell membrane (Figure 9.4B). Potassium–chloride cotransport is best known for its role in cell volume regulation in a wide variety of tissues, but there is increasing evidence that it is important in regulating intracellular chloride concentration in neurons.[18] As ion transport by the system is insensitive to extracellular sodium concentration, the energy required for outward chloride transport is supplied solely by the outward movement of potassium down its electrochemical gradient. Both the inward and outward transport systems are blocked by the chloride transport inhibitors furosemide and bumetanide.

Chloride-Bicarbonate Exchange

Chloride–bicarbonate exchange systems, operating in parallel with sodium–hydrogen exchange, serve primarily to regulate intracellular pH.[19] Simple chloride–bicarbonate exchange is driven by the outward gradient for bicarbonate produced by alkalinization of the cytoplasm and carries bicarbonate out of the cell and chloride inward on a 1:1 basis. Quantitatively, the role of this system is minimal in regulating intracellular chloride concentration in excitable cells.

Sodium-dependent chloride–bicarbonate exchange was first studied in squid axons and in snail neurons.[20,21] Recovery from acidification of the cytoplasm, by injection of hydrochloric acid (HCl), or exposure to CO_2, was prolonged when extracellular bicarbonate concentration was reduced or when intracellular chloride was depleted. In addition, recovery was virtually abolished when sodium was removed from the extracellular bathing solution. Thus, recovery involved inward movement of sodium down its electrochemical gradient, accompanied by bicarbonate, in exchange for chloride. Because the system is electrically neutral, it is assumed to include the outward transport of hydrogen ions as well, as indicated in Figure 9.4C. The exchange mechanism is inhibited by 4-acetamido-4'-isothiocyanostilbene-2,2'-disulfonic acid (SITS) and a related compound, 4,4'-diisothiocyanostilbene-2,2'-disulfonate (DIDS).

Transport of Neurotransmitters

In addition to transporting inorganic ions, nerve cells have mechanisms for accumulating a variety of other substances, including those involved in synaptic transmission (see Chapter 11). Neurotransmitters are transported into organelles within the cytoplasm of presynaptic nerve terminals (synaptic vesicles), where they are stored ready for release. After release, transmitters, such as norepinephrine, serotonin, γ-aminobutyric acid (GABA), glycine, and glutamate, are recovered from the synaptic cleft by transporters in the plasma cell membranes of either the terminals themselves or of adjacent glial cells. All of these recovery processes involve secondary transport mechanisms that use energy from the movement of sodium, potassium, or hydrogen ions down their electrochemical gradients to power transmitter accumulation.

Transport into Vesicles

Neurotransmitters are synthesized within the cytoplasm of nerve terminals and then concentrated into vesicles at synapses and in other sites of neurons (see Chapter 18) by secondary transport mechanisms coupled to proton efflux. This transport mechanism is analogous to sodium-driven secondary transport across the plasma cell membrane, but instead of a sodium gradient the system uses a proton gradient established by the transport of hydrogen ions from the cytoplasm into the vesicle by hydrogen ATPase.[22]

Three genetic families of proton-coupled transporters, designated SLC17, SLC18, and SLC32 (*SLC* means "solute carrier"), are expressed in the lipid bilayers of secretory vesicles (Table 9.1). SLC18 has three isotypes.[23] Two of these are the monoamine transporters VMAT1 (*SLC18A1*) and VMAT2 (*SLC18A2*), which are responsible for vesicular

[18] Mercado, A., Mount, D. B., and Gamba, G. 2004. *Neurochem. Res.* 29: 17-25.

[19] Romero, M. F., Fulton, C. M., and Boron, W. F. 2004. *Pflügers Arch.* 447: 495-509.

[20] Russell, J. M., and Boron, W. F. 1976. *Nature* 264: 73-74.

[21] Thomas, R. C. 1977. *J. Physiol.* 273: 317-338.

[22] Edwards, R. H. 2007. *Neuron* 55: 835-858.

[23] Elden, L. E. et al. 2004. *Pflügers Arch.* 447: 636-640.

TABLE 9.1		
Classification of neurotransmitter transporters		
Gene family	Transporter	Substrate
VESICLE LOADING		
SLC18	VMAT1,2	Norepinephrine, dopamine, histamine, serotonin
SLC18	VAChT	Acetylcholine
SLC32	VIAAT, VGAT	Glycine, GABA
SLC17	VGLUT1,2,3	Glutamate
TRANSMITTER UPTAKE		
SLC1	EAAT1 (GLAST), EAAT2–5	Glutamate
SLC6	GAT1,2	GABA
	NET	Norepinephrine
	DAT	Dopamine
	SERT	Serotonin
	GLYT1,2	Glycine

Source: L. E. Elden et al., 2004. *Pflügers Arch. Eur. J. Physiol.* 447: 636–640; B. Gasnier, 2004. *Pflügers Arch. Eur. J. Physiol.* 447: 756–759; R. J. Reimer and R. H. Edwards, 2004. *Pflügers Arch. Eur. J. Physiol.* 447: 629–635; Y. Kanai and M. Hediger, 2004. *Pflügers Arch. Eur. J. Physiol.* 447: 469–479; N. Chen et al., 2004. *Pflügers Arch. Eur. J. Physiol.* 447: 519–531.

accumulation of norepinephrine, dopamine, histamine, and serotonin (5-HT). The third, VAChT (*SLC18A3*), is responsible for accumulation of acetylcholine (ACh). GABA and glycine are concentrated by the product of a single gene family (SLC32), referred to as the vesicular inhibitory amino acid transporter (VIAAT) or vesicular GABA transporter (VGAT).[24] Glutamate has its own transport family, SLC17, for which three isoforms have been identified: VGLUT1, 2, and 3 (*SLC17A7*, *A6*, and *A8*).[25] Glutamate transport is unusual in that it includes cotransport of chloride into the vesicle.[26] VGLUT1 and 2 are distributed separately to synapses in the brain.[27] VGLUT3 is found in various neuronal and non-neuronal structures, including non-glutamatergic synapses. It is responsible for vesicular glutamate uptake in cochlear hair cells. VGLUT3 knock-out mice are profoundly deaf because their hair cells no longer release glutamate.[28]

There is a substantial electrochemical gradient for proton efflux across the vesicle membrane. For example, in filled monoaminergic and cholinergic vesicles, the pH gradient across the vesicle membrane is about 1.4 units and the electrical gradient is about +40 mV. Figure 9.5 shows the stoichiometry for the uptake systems. Because the exchanges are not electrically neutral, all are influenced by the potential across the vesicle membrane as well as on the pH gradient.

[24] Gasnier, B. 2004. *Pflügers Arch.* 447: 756–759.

[25] Takamori, S. 2006. *Neurosci. Res.* 55: 343–351.

[26] Bellochio, E. E. et al. 2000. *Science* 289: 957–960.

[27] Fremeau, R. T. et al. 2004. *Science* 304: 1815–1819.

[28] Seal, R. P. et al. 2008. *Neuron* 24: 173–174.

FIGURE 9.5 Transport of Neurotransmitters into Synaptic Vesicles. Hydrogen ATPase transports protons into the vesicle from the cytoplasm, creating an electrochemical gradient for proton efflux. Proton efflux through the secondary transport molecule provides the energy for accumulation of the neurotransmitter (T) in the vesicle. The proposed stoichiometry is 2:1 for monoamine and acetylcholine transport (A), 1:1 for glycine and GABA (B) and for glutamate (C). Glutamate transport is accompanied by chloride entry into the vesicle.

(A) Monoamines and acetylcholine

(B) GABA and glycine

(C) Glutamate

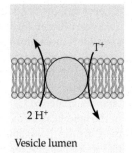
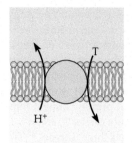
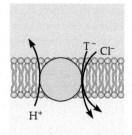

Vesicle lumen

Transmitter Uptake

After they are released, most neurotransmitters are recovered either by the neurons themselves or by adjacent glial cells (see Chapter 10). In general, such recovery serves two purposes: (1) The transmitter is removed from the extracellular space in the region of the synapse, which helps terminate its action and prevents diffusion to other synaptic regions; and (2) transmitter molecules recovered by the nerve terminal can be packaged again for rerelease. All uptake mechanisms use the electrochemical gradient for sodium to carry transmitter substances across the plasma cell membrane into the cytoplasm.

Two major transmitter uptake families are expressed in the cell membranes of neurons and glial cells.[29,30] Members of the SLC1 family mediate the uptake of glutamate and neutral amino acids, while SLC6 family members are responsible for uptake of dopamine, serotonin, norepinephrine, glycine, and GABA (see Table 9.1). Each family has several isotypes. In the SLC1 system, inward transport of one glutamate ion is coupled to the influx of two sodium ions and the efflux of one potassium ion, coupled with either the extrusion of a hydroxyl ion or influx of a proton (Figure 9.6A).[31] In the SLC6 system, uptake of each transmitter molecule is accompanied by the entry of two sodium ions and one chloride ion (Figure 9.6B).[32]

The SLC1 family includes five high-affinity glutamate transporters: excitatory amino acid transporter, or EAAT, 1, 2, 3, 4, and 5 (see Table 9.1). EAAT1, known as glial high-affinity glutamate transporter (GLAST) in humans, is found in glia and is particularly abundant in the cerebellum. It also occurs in supporting cells in the retina, and it is responsible for uptake of glutamate released by hair cells in the cochlea.[33] EAAT2 is found in astrocytes, particularly in the cerebral cortex and hippocampus. EAAT3 is expressed in neurons throughout the brain, including those in cerebral cortex, hippocampus, superior colliculus, and thalamus. EAAT4 is found primarily in cerebellar Purkinje cells on postsynaptic dendritic spines and has a substantial chloride conductance associated with substrate transport. EAAT5 occurs mainly in rod photoreceptors and bipolar cells in the retina and exhibits a prominent chloride conductance.

The SLC6 family includes transporters for GABA (GAT), norepinephrine (NET), dopamine (DAT), serotonin (SERT), and glycine (GLYT). The GABA transporter has three isoforms, GAT1, 2, and 3. GAT1 is the predominant neuronal transporter in the brain. It is found primarily along axons and around presynaptic nerve terminals. In the brain, GAT2 is found principally in meninges, ependyma, and choroid plexus and does not appear to be involved in neural signaling. GAT3 is expressed in glial cells. NET is found in noradrenergic neurons throughout the peripheral and central nervous systems and in adrenal chromaffin cells. DAT is found in dopaminergic neurons in the brain, localized around synaptic junctions. SERT is widely distributed in brain and is expressed in extrasynaptic membranes. GLYT has two isoforms. GLYT2 is the neuronal transporter, found in association with glycinergic nerve terminals. It differs from other members of the SLC6 family in that the transport stoichiometry is three sodium to one chloride to one glycine, suggesting that it is able to maintain extracellular glycine concentration at extremely low levels. GLYT1 is the predominant glial glycine transporter and has five splice variants: GLYT1a–e. Of these, GLYT1b and c are nervous system–specific, while GLYT1e and f are found only in the retina.

[29] Gether, U. et al. 2006. *Trends Pharmacol. Sci.* 27: 375-383.

[30] Torres, G. E., and Amara, S. G. 2007. *Curr. Opin. Neurobiol.* 17: 304-312.

[31] Kanai, Y., and Hediger, M. A. 2004. *Pflügers Arch.* 447: 469-479.

[32] Chen, N.-H., Reith, M. E. A., and Quick, M. W. 2004. *Pflügers Arch.* 447: 519-531.

[33] Glowatzki, E. et al. 2006. *J. Neurosci.* 26: 7659-7664.

(A) Glutamate

(B) Monoamines, GABA, glycine

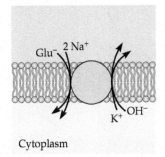

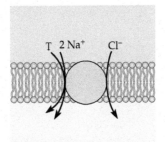

FIGURE 9.6 Uptake of Neurotransmitters. (A) Glutamate uptake is coupled to the influx of two sodium ions and the efflux of one potassium ion, and is accompanied by the extrusion of one hydroxyl (or one bicarbonate) ion. (B) In the GABA, glycine, and monoamine (norepinephrine, dopamine, and serotonin) uptake systems, recovery of the transmitter (T) is coupled to influx of two sodium ions and accompanied by the uptake of a single chloride ion. Choline from the hydrolysis of acetylcholine (not shown) is recovered into the nerve terminal with the same stoichiometry as in the GABA/glycine/monoamine systems.

[34] Iversen, L. L. et al. 2009. *Introduction to Neuropsychopharmacology.* Oxford University Press, New York, pp. 130–131.

[35] Attwell, D., Barbour, B., and Szatkowski, M. 1993. *Neuron* 11: 401–407.

[36] Cammack, J. N., and Schwartz, E. A. 1993. *J. Physiol.* 472: 81–102.

[37] Rossi, D. J., Oshima, T., and Attwell, D. 2000. *Nature* 403: 316–321.

ACh is recycled in a different way. It is synthesized in the cell cytoplasm from acetyl coenzyme A (acetyl-CoA) and choline (see Chapter 15). After ACh is released from the presynaptic terminal by exocytosis, its postsynaptic action is terminated by an enzyme (acetylcholinesterase) that hydrolyzes it to acetate and choline. Approximately half of the choline is recovered by a high-affinity (K_m 2μM) uptake mechanism and reused for ACh synthesis.[34] Like the monoamine and GABA/glycine transport systems, choline uptake is dependent on extracellular sodium and chloride concentrations.

One interesting aspect of the indirectly coupled transport mechanisms for transmitter uptake is that they are not, as a rule, electrically neutral. Thus, the direction of transport can be reversed by membrane depolarization, sometimes within the physiological range of membrane potentials.[35] Outward transport of GABA by this mechanism has been demonstrated in catfish retinal cells.[36] The transport system, then, not only mediates reuptake of the transmitter, but may also function as a mechanism for transmitter release. Reversal of transmitter uptake can have deleterious effects. After brain damage by stroke or trauma, outward transport of glutamate can lead to the accumulation of cytotoxic amounts of glutamate around neurons in the damaged area and thereby to further cell death.[37]

Molecular Structure of Transporters

So far we have dealt with functional properties of transporters with no reference to their molecular structure. As with membrane channels (see Chapter 5), each functional group is represented by a specific transport protein or, more commonly, a family of proteins. Many of these proteins have been isolated and cloned, and deductions have been made about their configurations in the membrane. In this section we summarize their structures, and examples are shown in Figure 9.7. The proteins have 9 to 12 transmembrane segments and

FIGURE 9.7 Molecular Configurations of Transport Molecules. Several transport molecules have been cloned and their structure in the membrane deduced from hydropathy analyses. (A) Sodium-potassium ATPase consists of an α-subunit with ten transmembrane segments (see text) and a smaller β-subunit spanning the membrane only once. Calcium ATPases (not shown) have a similar structure. (B) Sodium-calcium exchangers have 11 transmembrane segments. (C) Potassium-chloride cotransporters, anion exchange molecules, and sodium-potassium-chloride transporters all share the same membrane configuration, characterized by 12 transmembrane segments. (D) The monoamine uptake transporter subunit has 12 transmembrane segments. (E) The glutamate transport subunit has eight transmembrane segments and extracellular and intracellular membrane loops.

(A) Sodium–potassium ATPase

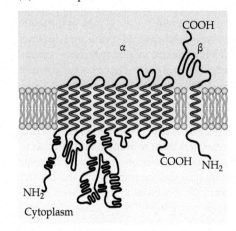

(B) Sodium–calcium exchanger

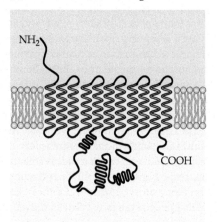

(C) Potassium–chloride cotransporter

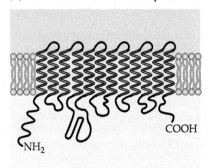

(D) Monoamine transporter

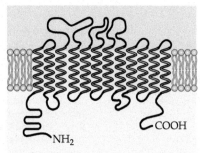

(E) Glutamate transporter

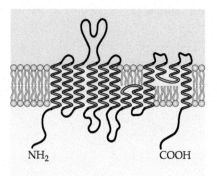

are assumed to form channel-like structures through which substances are moved by alternate exposure of binding sites to the extracellular and intracellular spaces.

ATPases

The molecular structure of sodium–potassium ATPase is known in some detail.[38,39] It is assembled from two subunits, α and β. The α-subunit, with an apparent molecular weight of about 100 kD, is responsible for the enzymatic activity of the pump and contains all the substrate binding sites. The smaller (35 kD) β-subunit has several extracellular glycosylation sites and is necessary for pump function, but its precise role is not clear. The proposed α- and β-subunit structures are shown in Figure 9.7A. The α-subunit has ten transmembrane segments, four of which (M4, M5, M6, and M8) are believed to form the transmembrane pore containing the cation-binding sites. The nucleotide binding and phosphorylation sites have been localized to the large cytoplasmic region between M4 and M5. The β-subunit contains only one putative membrane-spanning region, with the bulk of the peptide in the extracellular space. There are four α-subunit isoforms (α_1–α_4), all expressed in the nervous system. Two (β_1 and β_2) of three known β-subunit isoforms are found in nervous tissue.

Calcium ATPases consist of a single polypeptide chain of about 100 kD, analogous in structure to the α-subunit of sodium–potassium ATPase but with an extended cytoplasmic segment at the carboxyl end.[11] Unlike sodium–potassium ATPase, calcium ATPases do not require a β-subunit for enzyme activity. The sarcoplasmic and endoplasmic reticulum calcium ATPase (SERCA) family consists of three basic gene products—SERCA1, 2, and 3—each containing two alternatively spliced transcripts. The molecular structure of SERCA1a has been determined by X-ray crystallography at a resolution of 0.26 nm.[40] The family of cell membrane calcium pumps is similar in structure to the SERCA enzymes and is composed of four basic gene products (PMCA1–4). Approximately 30 additional isoforms are generated by alternative splicing.

Sodium-Calcium Exchangers

Sodium–calcium exchange molecules are widely spread throughout the animal kingdom. The NCX family of exchangers includes three mammalian homologues, NCX1–3. NCX1 is found in heart muscle, while NCX2 and 3 are found in brain.[41] The cardiac exchanger contains 938 amino acids with nine transmembrane segments (see Figure 9.7B). Homologous regions known as α-repeats are found within the molecule in segments 2, 3, and 7. The molecule has an extracellular reentry loop between segments 2 and 3, and a cytoplasmic reentry loop between segments 7 and 8. A large intracellular loop between segments 5 and 6 is the site of extensive alternative splicing. The loop contains important regulatory binding sites but is not essential for the transport process.

The NCKX1 exchanger is somewhat larger, with 1199 amino acids. Other members of the family, NCKX2–4, are smaller in size, containing 600–660 residues. All have 11 transmembrane segments and, like the NCX exchangers, have a large intracellular loop in the middle of the molecule.[15]

Chloride Transporters

The K–Cl cotransporters, KCC1–KCC4, and the Na–K–2Cl transporters, NKCC1 and NKCC2, are all members of the same genetic family of electroneutral cation-coupled transport molecules and are similar in structure.[42] The KCC proteins consist of about 1100 amino acids with intracellular amino and carboxyl terminals separated by 12 transmembrane segments (see Figure 9.7C). The NKCC molecule is slightly larger (about 1200 amino acids) with a similar topological arrangement. NKCC2 is absent from nervous tissue, being specific to kidney. KCC2 is unique in being specific to brain.

A sodium-dependent chloride–bicarbonate exchanger (NDCBE) has been cloned from human brain and also from squid axon.[43,44] The squid axon protein consists of about 1200 amino acids, with intracellular amino and carboxyl terminals separated by 14 transmembrane segments. The human exchanger is slightly smaller.

[38] Horisberger, J. D. 2004. *Physiology* 19: 377–387.

[39] Martin, D. W. 2005. *Semin. Nephrol.* 25: 282–291.

[40] Toyoshima, C. et al. 2000. *Nature* 405: 647–655.

[41] Phillipson, K. D., and Nicoll, D. A. 2000. *Annu. Rev. Physiol.* 62: 111–133.

[42] Herbert, S. C., Mount, D. B., and Gamba, G. 2004. *Pflügers Arch.* 447: 580–593.

[43] Grichtchenko, I. I. et al. 2001. *J. Biol. Chem.* 276: 8358–8363.

[44] Virkki, L. V. et al. 2003. Am. *J. Physiol.* 285: C771–C780.

Transport Molecules for Neurotransmitters

The monoamine and ACh transporters (VMAT1 and 2, and VAChT) were the first vesicular transporters to be cloned.[45] The molecules are 520 to 530 amino acids in length, and hydropathy analysis suggests that they contain 12 transmembrane segments (see Figure 9.7D).[23] VAChT is about 40% identical to VMAT1 and 2, which are about 65% identical to one another. The vesicular transport molecule for GABA and glycine has also been cloned.[46,47] Its structure is distinct from that of the monoamine and ACh transporters, with only ten putative transmembrane segments. The three members of the vesicular glutamate transport family are roughly 65 kD in mass and contain 560 to 590 amino acids, with ten potential transmembrane helices.[48]

The family of proteins associated with uptake of norepinephrine (NET), serotonin (SERT), dopamine (DAT), GABA (GAT), and glycine (GLYT) into axon terminal proteins have an apparent mass in the range of 80 to 100 kD.[49] The primary sequence of the choline transporter suggests that it may belong to the same superfamily.[50] The crystal structure of a bacterial homologue (LeuT$_{Aa}$) of the monoamine transporters has been analyzed at a resolution of 1.65 Å.[51] The molecule is a dimer with each subunit containing 12 transmembrane segments.

Five members of the family of proteins responsible for the uptake of glutamate have been isolated.[52] They are relatively small, containing 500 to 600 amino acids and having apparent masses of about 65 kD. The structure of a homologous bacterial transporter (Glt$_{Ph}$) has been resolved at a resolution of 3.5 Å.[53] Each of its three subunits has eight transmembrane segments with two hairpin loops imbedded in opposite faces of the plasma cell membrane (see Figure 9.7E).

Significance of Transport Mechanisms

Primary and secondary active ion transport molecules provide essential background mechanisms for maintaining cell homeostasis. However, their roles in nervous system function often extend well beyond such relatively mundane housekeeping duties, leading to an active role of transport in cell signaling. For example, activation of sodium–potassium ATPase by sodium accumulation during action potential activity in small nerve branches can produce a transient hyperpolarization and block conduction.

Another example is related to the effect of the neurotransmitter GABA on GABA$_A$ receptors, which when activated form chloride channels (see Chapter 11). In mature brain cells GABA causes inward chloride flux and hence hyperpolarization. However, in embryonic rat brain cells GABA produces depolarization. During postnatal development, the depolarizing response gradually disappears and eventually is replaced by hyperpolarization. This change in synaptic behavior occurs because intracellular chloride concentration is relatively high in embryonic neurons, and it decreases to the mature level during the postnatal period. The change in intracellular chloride concentration is the direct result of altered chloride transport across the cell membrane. In embryonic cells, chloride transport is dominated by the inwardly directed NKCC1 transporter, so that intracellular chloride concentration is relatively high. During postnatal development, expression of NKCC1 virtually disappears.[54] At the same time, expression of the outward chloride transporter KCC2, which is absent in embryonic cells, shows a marked increase.[55,56]

Finally, it is worth noting that monoamine transporters such as SERT are prime targets for drugs such as fluoxetine (Prozac) used in the treatment of psychiatric disorders such as depression and anxiety.[57]

In summary, it is useful to think of ion channels as mediating electrical signaling, and transport molecules as maintaining the background conditions under which such signaling occurs. We should remember, however, that the two types of molecules often interact in ways more complicated than this to regulate nervous system function.

[45] Schuldiner, S., Schirvan, A., and Linial, M. 1995. *Physiol. Rev.* 75: 369–392.

[46] McIntire, S. L. et al. 1997. *Nature* 389: 870–876.

[47] Sagne, C. et al. 1997. *FEBS Lett.* 417: 177–183.

[48] Fremeau, R. T., Jr. et al. 2002. *Proc. Natl. Acad. Sci. USA* 99: 14,488–14,493.

[49] Nelson, N., and Lill, H. 1994. *J. Exp. Biol.* 196: 213–228.

[50] Mayser, W., Schloss, P., and Betz, H. 1992. *FEBS Lett.* 305: 31–36.

[51] Yamashita, A. et al. 2005. *Nature* 437: 215–223.

[52] Palacin, M. et al. 1998. *Physiol. Rev.* 78: 969–1054.

[53] Yernool, D. et al. 2004. *Nature* 431: 811–818.

[54] Plotkin, M. D. et al. 1997. *Am. J. Physiol. Cell Physiol.* 272: C173–C183.

[55] Rivera, C. et al. 1999. *Nature* 397: 251–255.

[56] Lu, J., Karadsheh, M., and Delpire, E. 1999. *J. Neurobiol.* 39: 558–568.

[57] Iverson, L. L. et al. 2009. *Introduction to Neuropsychopharmacology.* Oxford University Press, New York, pp. 306–316.

SUMMARY

- Several membrane proteins transport substances into and out of cells. One example is sodium-potassium ATPase, which transports three sodium ions outward across the cell membrane, and two potassium ions inward, per molecule of ATP hydrolyzed. The transport system maintains intracellular sodium and potassium concentrations at constant levels in spite of steady leakage into and out of the cells.

- Calcium concentrations in the cell cytoplasm are kept low by two classes of calcium ATPases. One, cell membrane calcium ATPase, transports calcium out of the cell. The other, endoplasmic and sarcoplasmic reticulum ATPase, concentrates calcium into intracellular compartments.

- Another mechanism for calcium transport is sodium-calcium exchange: Sodium, entering the cell down its electrochemical gradient, provides energy for outward transport of calcium. This mechanism is an example of indirect transport, which relies on maintenance of the sodium gradient by sodium-potassium ATPase. In most neurons the transport molecule exchanges three sodium ions for one calcium ion. Under some physiological conditions, the exchanger can run in reverse. In retinal rods, the transport molecule carries one calcium ion and one potassium ion out of the cell in exchange for the entry of four sodium ions.

- There are two main mechanisms for extrusion of chloride from cells. One is chloride-bicarbonate exchange, which is important for intracellular pH regulation and depends on the sodium electrochemical gradient for its operation. The second is potassium-chloride cotransport, which relies on the electrochemical gradient for outward potassium movement across the cell membrane. In some cells chloride is accumulated rather than extruded. Chloride accumulation relies on the sodium electrochemical gradient and is accompanied by inward movement of potassium.

- In presynaptic vesicles, a hydrogen-transmitter exchange system transports neurotransmitters from the cytoplasm into the vesicle lumen. Neurotransmitters released from presynaptic terminals are removed from extracellular spaces by uptake systems in neuron and glial cell membranes using sodium-transmitter cotransport.

- The amino acid sequences of most transport molecules are known, and predictions have been made about their configuration in the membrane. Most have 9 to 12 transmembrane segments and are assumed to form porelike structures through which ions move by alternate exposure of binding sites to the extracellular and intracellular spaces.

Suggested Reading

Castillo, J. P. et al. 2015. Mechanism of potassium ion uptake by the Na^+/K^+-ATPase. *Nature Comm.* 6: 7622 doi: 10.1038/ncomms8622.

Carafoli, E., and Brini, M. 2000. Calcium pumps: Structural basis for and mechanisms of calcium transmembrane transport. *Curr. Opin. Chem. Biol.* 4: 152–161.

Kanai, R. et al. 2013. Crystal structure of a Na^+-bound Na^+, K^+-ATP-ase preceding the E1P state. *Nature* 502: 201–206.

Mercado, A., Mount, D. B., and Gamba, G. 2004. Electroneutral cation–chloride cotransporters in the central nervous system. *Neurochem. Res.* 29: 17–25.

Philipson, K. D., and Nicoll, D. A. 2000. Sodium–calcium exchange: A molecular perspective. *Annu. Rev. Physiol.* 62: 111–133.

Russell, J. M. 2000. Sodium–potassium–chloride cotransport. *Physiol. Rev.* 80: 211–276.

Schnetkamp, P. P. 2004. The SLC24 Na^+/Ca^{2+}-K^+ exchanger family: Vision and beyond. *Pflügers Arch.* 447: 683–688.

Torres, G. E., and Amara, S. G. 2007. Glutamate and monoamine transporters: New visions of form and function. *Curr. Opin. Neurobiol.* 17: 304–312.

CHAPTER 10

Properties and Functions of Neuroglial Cells

Nerve cells are associated with satellite cells known as neuroglial (or glial) cells, consisting of Schwann cells in the peripheral nervous system (PNS) and several types of cells in the central nervous system (CNS). In this chapter we discuss the structure and properties of the glial cells and their interactions with neurons. Their roles in development and regeneration in the nervous system and their contributions to neuronal activity and capillary blood flow are described more extensively in Chapters 18, 27, and 29.

Glial cells make up about one-half of the volume of the brain and greatly outnumber neurons. The three main types of glial cells in the CNS are oligodendrocytes, astrocytes, and radial glial cells. The fourth type, microglial cells, constitute a separate population of wandering cells. Microglial cells, unlike other glia, are of mesodermal origin. Neurons and glial cells are densely packed. Their membranes are separated from each other by narrow fluid-filled extracellular spaces that are about 20 nanometers (nm) wide. Certain glial cells contact capillaries and wrap around neurons; their processes make contacts with synaptic terminals. NG2 cells are precursors for oligodendrocytes and neurons; ependymal cells (see Chapter 18) contribute to the cerebrospinal fluid and the exchange of material with the CNS.

Glial cells have more negative resting potentials than neurons. Their cell membranes contain channels for ions, receptors for transmitters, ion transport pumps, and amino acid and transmitter transporters. The close apposition of glial and neuronal membranes permits dynamic interactions between the two types of cells. A well-established role of glia in the CNS is spatial buffering through uptake of transmitters and potassium. Neurons release potassium into narrow extracellular spaces and thereby depolarize glial membranes.

Networks of glial cells are coupled by gap junctions that permit direct passage of ions and small molecules. Adult glial cells do not generate action potentials. However, their depolarization gives rise to waves of intracellular calcium that spread rhythmically through assemblies of glial cells that are coupled by gap junctions. Activated glial cells liberate transmitters, some peptides, and proteins into extracellular space. Serine and adenosine are liberated by glia but not by neurons.

Nerve cells in the brain are intimately surrounded by satellite cells called **neuroglial cells**, **glial cells**, or **glia**. It has been estimated that they outnumber neurons by at least ten to one and make up about one-half of the bulk of the nervous system. Among the essential functions of glial cells are the following: Oligodendrocytes and Schwann cells form myelin around axons, which speeds up conduction of the nerve impulse. Both types of myelinating glial cells secrete neurotrophic molecules and guide growing axons to their targets during development. Astrocytes in the CNS cause capillaries to become impermeable to certain molecules, and thereby help create the blood–brain barrier. They also mediate the vasodilation of capillaries in regions where neuronal activity increases. Microglial cells sense the chemical and electrical environment. In the event of a lesion, microglial cells invade the region of damage or inflammation and phagocytose debris.

Historical Perspective

Glial cells were first described in 1846 by Rudolf Virchow, who thought of them as "nerve glue" and gave them their name. Excerpts from a paper by Virchow give the flavor of his thinking:

> Hitherto, considering the nervous system, I have only spoken of the really nervous part of it. But...it is important to have a knowledge of that substance...which lies between the proper nervous parts, holds them together and gives the whole its form...[this] has induced me to give it a new name, that of neuroglia...Experience shows us that this very interstitial tissue of the brain and spinal marrow is one of the most frequent sites of morbid change...Within the neuroglia run the vessels, which are therefore nearly everywhere separated from the nervous substance by a slender intervening layer, and are not in immediate contact with it.[1,2]

In subsequent years, neuroglial cells were studied intensively by neuroanatomists and pathologists, who knew them to be the most common source of tumors in the brain. This is not surprising, because certain glial cells (unlike most neurons) can still divide in the mature animal. Among early speculations about glial cell function with relation to neurons— some of which have been demonstrated with time—were the provision of nutrients, the secretion of molecules, and the prevention of "cross talk" by current spread during conduction of nerve impulses.[3–5]

Appearance and Classification of Glial Cells

A distinct structural feature of neuroglial cells compared with neurons is the absence of axons. Figure 10.1 shows representative mammalian neuroglial cells. In the vertebrate nervous system, glial cells are usually subdivided into several distinctive classes.[6,7]

Astrocytes comprise two principal subgroups: (1) fibrous astrocytes, which contain filaments and are prevalent among bundles of myelinated nerve fibers in the white matter of the brain; and (2) protoplasmic astrocytes, which contain less fibrous material and are abundant in the gray matter around nerve cell bodies, dendrites, and synapses.

Oligodendrocytes are predominant in the white matter, where they form myelin around larger axons (see Chapter 8). They appear in the CNS at the time of maximum myelinization.

Schwann cells in peripheral nerves and ganglia form myelin around the fast-conducting axons. Schwann cells also enclose smaller axons (less than 1 micrometer [μm] in diameter) without forming a myelin sheath. After a lesion they guide axons to reach their targets.

Radial glial cells play an essential role in the developing CNS. They stretch through the thickness of the spinal cord, retina, cerebellum, or cerebral cortex to the surface, forming elongated filaments along which developing neurons migrate to their final destinations. Radial glial cells may produce neurons and glial cells. In the adult CNS, radial glia are represented by Bergmann cells in the cerebellum and Müller cells in the retina. The role of radial glia during development is discussed in Chapter 27.

Microglial cells are distinct from the other glial cells in structure, properties, and lineage.[8,9] They arise from mesodermal yolk cells, become the resident cleaners of the brain,

[1] Virchow, R. 1859. *Cellular Pathology: As Based Upon Physiological and Pathological Histology.* English trans., pp. 272, 277, 279. John Churchill, London.

[2] Penfield, W. 1924. *Brain* 47: 430-452.

[3] Golgi, C. 1903. *Opera Omnia*, Vols. 1 and 2. U. Hoepli, Milan, Italy.

[4] Ramón y Cajal, S. (1909-1911) 1995. *Histology of the Nervous System*, Vol. 1. Oxford University Press, New York.

[5] Webster, H., and Aström, K. E. 2009. *Adv. Anat. Embryol. Cell Biol.* 202: 1-109.

[6] Kettenmann, H., and Ransom, B. R. (Eds.). 2005. *NeuroGlia*, 2nd ed. Oxford University Press, New York.

[7] Butt, A. M. et al. 2005. *J. Anat.* 207: 695-706.

[8] Ransohoff, R. M., and Perry, V. H. 2009. *Annu. Rev. Immunol.* 27: 119-145.

[9] Farber, K., and Kettenmann, H. 2005. *Brain Res. Brain Res. Rev.* 48: 133-143.

(A)

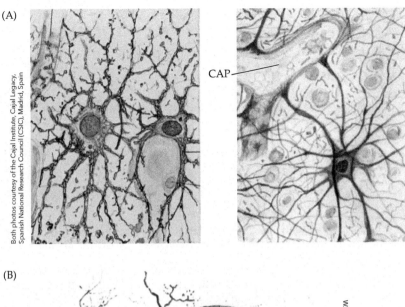

CAP

Both photos courtesy of the Cajal Institute, Cajal Legacy, Spanish National Research Council (CSIC), Madrid, Spain

FIGURE 10.1 Neuroglial Cells in Mammalian Brain. (A) Fibrous (left) and protoplasmic (right) astrocytes, stained with silver impregnation. They are closely associated with neurons. (B) Oligodendrocytes. They interact with neurons and form myelin in the central nervous system. (C) Microglial cells are small, wandering, macrophage-like cells. CAP, capillary.

(B)

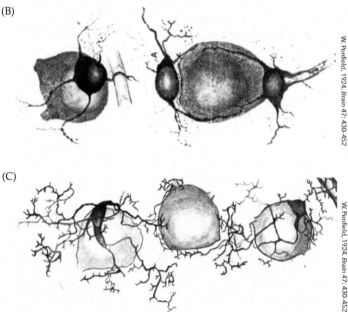

W. Penfield, 1924. *Brain* 47: 430-452

(C)

W. Penfield, 1924. *Brain* 47: 430-452

and are able to move to sites of injury. Microglial cells respond to electrical activity and chemical substances by exploring the active regions, contacting neurons and pruning synapses in the developing and adult nervous system.[10]

NG2 cells, named for expressing NG2 proteoglycan, are precursors of oligodendroglia and secondarily of astrocytes in the adult nervous system. They proliferate, migrate over short distances, and release transmitters. NG2 cells may produce action potentials. They form synaptic-like connections with neurons.[11,12]

Ependymal cells line the inner surfaces of the brain, in the ventricles, and are produced from radial glial cells by activation of a molecular cascade.[13] In the brain ventricles, the multiple cilia of ependymal cells contribute to the flow of cerebrospinal fluid, as will be discussed in Chapter 18.

Various types of glia were originally identified using the specific cytological staining methods developed by Cajal and del Río-Hortega. Glial cells were later distinguished by injecting them with labels, such as dyes in living preparations, or by immunological techniques (Figure 10.2). Antibodies have been prepared that bind specifically to each different type of glia in the CNS and PNS.[14] Fibrous astrocytes, for example, can be recognized with an antibody against a protein known as glial fibrillary acidic protein, or

[10] Salter, M. W., and Beggs, S. 2014. *Cell* 158: 15–24.

[11] Kukley, M., Capetillo-Zarate, E., and Dietrich, D. 2007. *Nat Neurosci.* 10: 311–320.

[12] Káradóttir, R. et al. 2008. *Nat Neurosci.* 11: 450–456.

[13] Kyrousi, C., Lygerou, Z., and Taraviras, S. 2017. *Glia* 65: 1032–1042.

[14] Zuo, Y. et al. 2004. *J. Neurosci.* 24: 10999–11009.

(A)   (B)

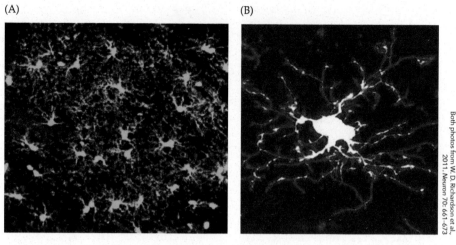

Both photos from W. D. Richardson et al., 2011. *Neuron* 70: 661–673

FIGURE 10.2   Distribution and Morphology of NG2 Cells. (A) Fluorescence image of the cerebral cortex of a transgenic mouse showing a uniform distribution of NG2 cells. (B) Two-photon fluorescence image of an NG2 cell in the cerebellum. The cell was filled with fluorescent dye through a micropipette.

[15] Bignami, A., and Dahl, D. 1974.
    J. Comp. Neurol. 153: 27–38.

[16] Zhu, X., Bergles, D. E., and Nishiyama,
    A. 2008a. *Development* 135: 145–157.

[17] Zhu, X., Hill, R. A., and Nishiyama, A.
    2008b. *Neuron Glia Biol.* 4: 19–26.

[18] Stent, G. S., and Weisblat, D. A. 1985.
    Annu. Rev. Neurosci. 8: 45–70.

[19] Lewis, K. E., and Eisen, J. S. 2003.
    Prog. Neurobiol. 69: 419–449.

[20] Luskin, M. B. 1998. *J. Neurobiol.*
    36: 221–233.

[21] Figueres-Oñate, M., García-Marqués,
    J., and López-Mascaraque, L. 2016.
    Sci Rep. 6: 33896.

[22] De Biase, L. M. et al. 2010.
    J. Neurosci. 30: 3600–3611.

[23] Viganò, F., and Dimou, L. 2016. *Brain
    Res.* 1638: 129–137.

[24] Kuffler, S.W., and Potter, D. D.1964.
    J. Neurophysiol. 27: 290–320.

[25] Scemes, E., et al. 2007. *Neuron Glia
    Biol.* 3: 199–208.

GFAP;[15] NG2 precursors are selectively identified with antibodies raised against NG2 proteoglycan (see Figure 10.2B).[16,17]

Like the neurons in the CNS and PNS, the central glial cells and Schwann cells have different embryological origins. The central glia (except for microglia) derive from precursor cells that line the neural tube, whereas Schwann cells arise from the neural crest (see Chapter 25). On the other hand, lineage tracing experiments in embryos have confirmed the original observation of del Río-Hortega that microglia derive from mesodermal precursors that leave the yolk sac and enter the neural tube via the bloodstream.

In animals such as the leech[18] and zebrafish,[19] glial cell development can be observed directly in the living embryo. Precursor cells can be labeled by injection of a marker or by infection at an early stage with a virus encoding a labeled gene that is handed on to the descendants.[20] Plasmids encoding for specific glia promoters and fluorescent proteins with different colors can be injected in the ventricles of living mouse embryos, where precursors accumulate. As we showed in Chapter 1 with the StarTrack technique, individual labeled precursors and their progeny can be tracked by fluorescent microscopy. In this way one can follow cell lineages and pinpoint the stages at which glial cells diverge from neurons during development or in the adult nervous system.[21]

Structural Relations between Neurons, Glia, and Capillaries

A glance at electron micrographs of brain tissue brings home the close packing of neurons and glia. Figure 10.3 shows an example from the cerebellum of a rat. The section is filled with neurons and glia, which can be distinguished by several criteria. Glial processes tend to be thin, at times less than 1 mm thick. Larger volumes of cytoplasm appear only around the glial nuclei. The extracellular space is restricted to narrow clefts, about 20 nm wide, that separate all cell boundaries. As will be seen in Chapter 18, astrocytes interact with capillaries by linking the activity of neurons with the capillary blood flow to increase the availability of oxygen. These integrative actions explain the origin of the oxygen increases that are detected by functional magnetic resonance imaging (fMRI) in active areas of the nervous system.

During development, occasional structures resembling synapses have been observed between glial precursors and neurons,[22] as happens after birth between NG2 precursors and neurons.[23] Electrical synapses do, however, link glial cells to one another through gap junctions (Figure 10.4) (see Chapter 8).[24,25] The relation between glial cells, neurons, and capillaries is diagrammed in Figure 10.5.

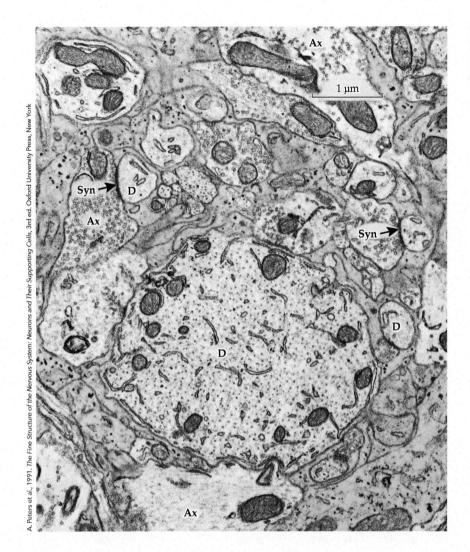

A. Peters et al, 1991. *The Fine Structure of the Nervous System: Neurons and Their Supporting Cells*, 3rd ed. Oxford University Press, New York

FIGURE 10.3   Neurons and Glial Processes in Rat Cerebellum. The glial contribution is lightly colored. The neural elements are dendrites (D) and axons (Ax). Two synapses (Syn) are marked by arrows.

Physiological Properties of Neuroglial Cell Membranes

For technical reasons, Kuffler and Potter[24] used the CNS of the leech to record from glial cells, at a time when nothing was known about their membrane properties. The glial cells in a leech ganglion are large and transparent. They appear under the dissecting microscope as spaces between nerve cells and can be recorded from with sharp microelectrodes or by patch electrodes.[26] Once its physiological properties have been established, the glial cell can be injected with a fluorescent marker, such as Lucifer yellow, and its form observed in the living preparation.

Leech glial cells have resting potentials greater (more negative) than those of neurons. The largest membrane potentials recorded from neurons are about –75 mV, whereas the values for glial cells approach –90 mV. The glial membrane behaves like a potassium electrode; that is, its behavior follows the Nernst equation in solutions containing different

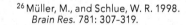

[26] Müller, M., and Schlue, W. R. 1998. *Brain Res.* 781: 307-319.

FIGURE 10.4   Neurons and Glia. Neuronal-glial and glial-glial relationships. Whereas neurons are always separated from glia by continuous clefts of extracellular space, the interiors of glial cells are linked by gap junctions. (After S. W. Kuffler and J. G. Nicholls, 1966. *Ergeb. Physiol.* 57: 1-90.)

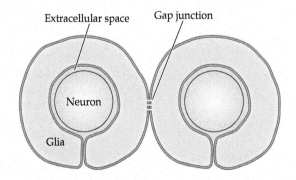

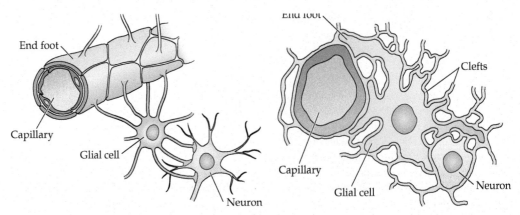

FIGURE 10.5 Neurons, Glia, and Capillaries. Relations of capillaries, glia, and neurons as seen by light and electron microscopy. The pathway for diffusion from the capillary to the neuron is through the aqueous intercellular clefts. Cell dimensions are not in proportion. (After S. W. Kuffler and J. G. Nicholls, 1966. *Ergeb. Physiol.* 57: 1–90.)

27 Kuffler, S. W., Nicholls, J. G., and Orkand, R. K. 1966. *J. Neurophysiol.* 29: 768–787.

28 Ransom, B. R., and Sontheimer, H. 1992. *J. Clin. Neurophysiol.* 9: 224–251.

29 Kuffler, S. W., and Nicholls, J. G. 1966. *Ergeb. Physiol.* 57: 1–90.

30 Rose, C. R., Ransom, B. R., and Waxman, S. G. 1997. *J. Neurophysiol.* 78: 3249–3258.

31 Ritchie, J. M. 1987. *J. Physiol.* (*Paris*) 82: 248–257.

32 Ziskin, J. L. et al. 2007. *Nat. Neurosci.* 10: 321–330.

33 Káradóttir, R. et al. 2008. *Nat. Neurosci.* 11: 450–456.

34 De Biase, L. M., Nishiyama, A., and Bergles, D. E. 2010. *J. Neurosci.* 30: 3600–3611.

35 Nielsen, S. et al. 1997. *J. Neurosci.* 17: 171–180.

36 Nagelhus, E. A., and Ottersen, O. P. 2013. Physiological roles of aquaporin-4 in brain. *Physiol. Rev.* 93: 1543–1562.

37 Blaustein, M. P. et al. 2002. *Ann. NY Acad. Sci.* 976: 356–366.

38 Marcaggi, P., and Attwell, D. 2004. *Glia* 47: 217–225.

39 Karadottir, R. et al. 2005. *Nature* 438: 1162–1166.

40 Verkhratsky, A., Krishtal, O. A., and Burnstock, G. 2009. *Mol. Neurobiol.* 39: 190–208.

41 Loewenstein, W. R. 1999. *The Touchstone of Life.* Oxford University Press, New York.

42 Iglesias, R. et al. 2009. *J. Neurosci.* 29: 7092–7097.

43 Lapato, A. S., and Tiwari-Woodruff, S. K. 2018. *J. Neurosci. Res.* 96: 31–44.

potassium concentrations (see Chapter 6). Sodium and chloride make only a small contribution to the resting membrane potential.[27]

Once leech glial cells had been described, it became practicable to record from and label amphibian and mammalian glial cells,[28] which were found to share many key properties with the leech glia. Far from being a roundabout approach, use of the leech turned out to be a shortcut to the study of glia in the vertebrate CNS.[29]

Ion Channels, Pumps, and Receptors in Glial Cell Membranes

Glial cells display a variety of ion channels and pumps in their membranes. Although potassium conductances predominate,[27] voltage-activated sodium and calcium channels are present in the membranes of astrocytes, retinal Müller cells, and Schwann cells.[30] In Müller cells, the overall ratio of potassium to sodium permeability is approximately 100:1. Patch clamp recordings have also revealed the presence of chloride channels in Schwann cells and astrocytes.[31] However, precursor glial cells, like NG2 cells, may produce action potentials and respond to vesicular release of glutamate from axons[32] by use of AMPA receptors, which are characteristic of synapses.[33,34]

The membranes of astrocytes that make contact with capillaries and with the pia concentrate the water-conducting channel aquaporin-4 (AQP4).[35] The end feet of glial processes surrounding synapses also contain AQP4 channels. In these fine processes, AQP4 channels help arrest the shrinking of the extracellular space that follows an increase in neuronal activity.[36]

Ion pumps for transport of sodium and potassium as well as of bicarbonate and protons exist in glial cells.[37] Moreover, transporters for transmitters such as glutamate, g-aminobutyric acid (GABA), and glycine are abundant: They take up transmitter liberated by neurons.[38] Most glial cells also display receptors for transmitters.[39,40]

Coupling between Glial Cells

Electrical coupling between glial cells[24,25] permits the exchange of ions and small molecules directly between cells, without passing through the extracellular space; such interconnections reduce concentration gradients.[25,29,41,42] Optical measurements of intracellular calcium show that waves and brief spikes of increased concentration occurring in activated glia spread to the adjacent glial cells (see the later section "Potassium and Calcium Movement through Glial Cells").[43]

Networks of astrocytes are coupled by connexons. Gap junctions facilitate the removal of extracellular glutamate and potassium during synaptic activity. The intracellular flow of substances from one astrocyte to another across connexons allows their intracellular concentrations of glutamate and potassium to remain low. This favors their continuous uptake following a concentration gradient from outside to inside. Elimination of connexins in transgenic mice produces accumulation of extracellular potassium and glutamate in extracellular spaces. In the hippocampus this accumulation leads to neuronal hyperexcitability, increased glutamate release, and incorporation of postsynaptic AMPA receptors.[44]

Coupling between Glia and Neurons

Electrical coupling may connect glia with neurons. In the nematode *Caenorhabditis elegans*, calcium waves generated in glial cells flow to GABAergic neurons across gap junctions. This coupling regulates the formation of axons; pharmacological uncoupling of gap junctions causes accumulation of axonal markers in neurites that would normally not produce axons. Moreover, the microtubules in those neurites are similar to those of normal axons. In vertebrate noradrenergic neurons, the low-molecular-weight marker neurobiotin injected into glial cells flows to neurons.[46] This coupling can be blocked by the gap junction blocker carbenoxolone, and antibodies against connexin recognize gap junctions that connect glia and neurons. Depolarization of glia by increasing the glutamate transport produces an increase in the neuronal firing.[45] The function of these connections remains to be understood.

Functions of Glial Cells

Over the years, almost every nervous system task for which no other obvious explanation has been found has been attributed to glial cells. In the following sections we first discuss well-established functions of glial cells and then intriguing questions about their functional role that require further elucidation. We also discuss some examples of behaviors for which no solid physiological explanation exists yet.

Generalities of Glial Cells in Development and Repair

Essential aspects of development and repair that involve glial cells are described in Chapters 25 and 27. Here we list certain key features of the functional roles played by glia:

- Glial cells secrete molecules that promote the outgrowth of neurites. [46,47]
- Certain proteins produced by glial cells inhibit neurite outgrowth.[48,49]
- Glial cells outline the aggregation of neurons into well-defined nuclei at early stages.[50,51]
- Radial glia act as stem cells for neurogenesis.[52–54]
- NG2 cells produce oligodendrocytes and astrocytes in the adult CNS.[55]
- Microglial cells migrate to the sites of lesion and remove debris.
- Schwann cells are pathways for outgrowth in peripheral nerves.[56–59]

Myelin and the Role of Glia in Axonal Conduction

One major function of oligodendrocytes and Schwann cells is to produce the myelin sheath around axons—a high-resistance covering akin to the insulating material around wires (see Chapter 8). The myelin is interrupted at the nodes of Ranvier (Figure 10.6), which occur at regular intervals.[60] Since the ion current associated with the conducted nerve impulse cannot flow across the myelin, ions can move in and out only at the nodes. As a result, the conduction velocity is increased. At nodes within the CNS, a characteristic feature is the presence of astrocytic processes that contact the axon.[61] There are differences in the mechanisms by which oligodendrocytes and Schwann cells myelinate axons. For example, one oligodendrocyte can myelinate several segments of the same axon; Schwann cells myelinate only a single segment.

For the formation of the myelin sheath and the nodes of Ranvier during development, complex and precise interactions occur between axons and glial cells, with some molecular steps being different between the CNS and PNS.[62] Rapid conduction depends on the spacing of the nodes, the seals between the glia and the axon at the paranodal areas (regions where axons and the myelin sheaths make contact), and the distribution of sodium and potassium channels at the nodes.

Oligodendrocytes have an intrinsically strong myelinating capacity: They can myelinate fixed axons, and amazingly, also certain synthetic fibers. This myelinating superpower

[44] Pannasch, U. et al. 2011. *Proc. Natl. Acad. Sci. USA* 108: 8467-8472.

[45] Alvarez-Maubecin, V. et al. 2000. *J. Neurosci.* 20 : 4091-4098.

[46] Yu, W. M., Yu, H., and Chen, Z. L. 2007. *Mol. Neurobiol.* 35: 288-297.

[47] Bampton, E. T., and Taylor, J. S. 2005. *J. Neurobiol.* 63: 29-48.

[48] Caroni, P., and Schwab, M. E. 1988. *J. Cell Biol.* 106: 1281-1288.

[49] Schwab, M. E. 2004. *Curr. Opin. Neurobiol.* 14: 118-1124.

[50] Faissner, A., and Steindler, D. 1995. *Glia* 13: 233-254.

[51] Steindler, D. A. et al. 1989. *Dev. Biol.* 131: 243-260.

[52] Hansen, D. V. et al. 2010. *Nature* 464: 554-561.

[53] Rakic, P. 2003. *Glia* 43: 19-32.

[54] Gotz, M., and Barde, Y. A. 2005. *Neuron* 46: 369-372.

[55] Nishiyama, A. et al. 2016. *Brain Res.* 1638: 116-128.

[56] Son, Y. J., and Thompson, W. J. 1995. *Neuron* 14: 125-132.

[57] Son, Y. J., and Thompson, W. J. 1995. *Neuron* 14: 133-141.

[58] Son, Y. J., Trachtenberg, J. T., and Thompson, W. J. 1996. *Trends Neurosci.* 19: 280-285.

[59] Love, F. M., Son, Y. J., and Thompson, W. J. 2003. *J. Neurobiol.* 54: 566-576.

[60] Bunge, R. P. 1968. *Physiol. Rev.* 48: 197-251.

[61] Black, J. A., and Waxman, S. G. 1988. *Glia* 1: 169-183.

[62] Eshed-Eisenbach, Y., and Peles, E. 2013. *Curr. Opin. Neurobiol.* 23: 1049-1056.

(A) Schematic diagram of arrangement of myelin

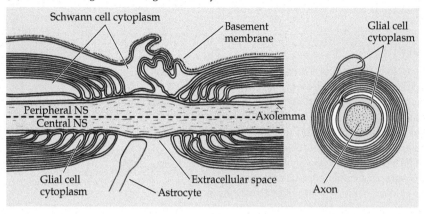

(B)

(C)

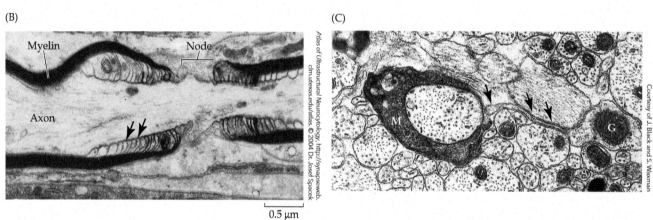

0.5 μm

Atlas of Ultrastructural Neurocytology. http://synapseweb. cln.utexas.edu/atlas. © 2004 Dr. Josef Spacek

T. J. Sims et al. 1985. Brain Res. 337: 321-331. Courtesy of J. Black and S. Waxman

FIGURE 10.6   Myelin and Nodes of Ranvier. Oligodendrocytes and Schwann cells form the wrapping of myelin around axons. (A) At the nodes of Ranvier, like the one shown here on the left, the myelin is interrupted and the axon is exposed. The upper half of the nodal region, with a loose covering of processes, is typical of the arrangement in peripheral nerves. The lower part is representative of a node in the CNS. Here an astrocytic finger comes into close apposition with the nodal membrane. To the right is a transverse section through a myelin-covered axon. (B) Electron micrograph of a nodal region in a myelinated fiber in rat CNS. At the edge of the node is a specialized close-contact area between the membrane of the axon (Axon) and the membrane of the myelin wrapping (arrows). (C) Cross section of a myelinated axon at a node that is contacted by a process (marked with arrows) from a perinodal astrocyte (G). Myelin (M) is absent at the site of contact between the astrocyte and the node. (A after R. P. Bunge, 1968. *Physiol. Rev.* 48: 197-251; A. Peters, 1960. *J. Biophys. Biochem. Cytol.* 7: 121-126.)

is downregulated during the accurate formation of the nodes. The transmembrane protein JAM2, synthesized by neurons, inhibits myelination. In experiments made in culture, the overexpression of JAM2 reduces myelination; however, in transgenic mice lacking JAM2, oligodendroglia massively invade the axons and cell bodies of neurons.[63] It is suggested that vesicular release of ATP and glutamate during axonal electrical activity enhances myelination. By contrast, silence of axonal electrical activity causes demyelinization.

The dynamic interactions between neurons and the peripheral Schwann cells have been analyzed by experiments made in living fish embryos and in tissue culture,[64–66] under conditions that parallel the development, myelination, and remyelination of axons that occur in vivo. Key proteins that play a part in Schwann cell–axon interactions have been identified. For example, Shooter and his colleagues have shown that when Schwann cells are cultured in a dish on their own, they synthesize a myelin protein known as PMP22.[67] Turnover of PMP22 is rapid, and it is degraded in the endoplasmic reticulum. When neurons are added to the culture, as illustrated in Figure 10.7, the fate of the protein changes. After contact with Schwann cells and axons, PMP22 is translocated to the Schwann cell membrane. This

[63] Redmond, S. A. et al. 2016. *Neuron.* 91: 824-836.

[64] Buckley, C. E. et al. 2010. *Glia* 58: 802-812.

[65] Liu, N. et al. 2005. *J. Neurosci. Res.* 79: 310-317.

[66] Nave, K. A., and Trapp, B. D. 2008. *Annu. Rev. Neurosci.* 31: 535-561.

[67] Pareek, S. et al. 1997. *J. Neurosci.* 17: 7754-7762.

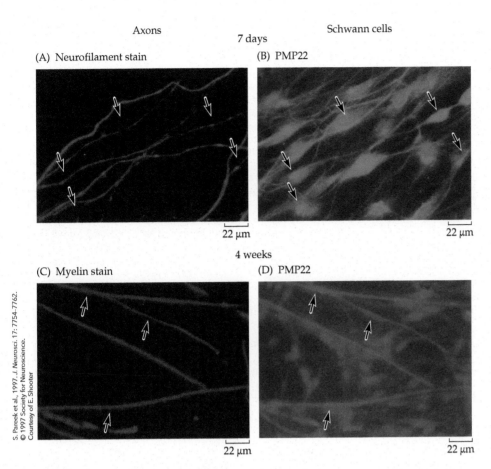

Axons

7 days

Schwann cells

(A) Neurofilament stain

(B) PMP22

22 μm

22 μm

4 weeks

(C) Myelin stain

(D) PMP22

22 μm

22 μm

S. Pareek et al., 1997. *J. Neurosci.* 17: 7754–7762.
© 1997 Society for Neuroscience.
Courtesy of E. Shooter

FIGURE 10.7   Localization of Myelin Protein PMP22 in short- and long-term myelinating cultures of axons and Schwann cells. The images show changes in the distribution of myelin protein PMP22 induced by co-culture of axons with Schwann cells. (A,B) A 1-week-old co-culture of neuronal axons (A) and Schwann cells (B) that are doubly stained with monoclonal anti-neurofilament and polyclonal PMP22 antiserum. Arrows point to Schwann cells that are in contact with neuronal processes. At this early stage the glial and neuronal proteins have different distributions, with PMP22 mainly in Schwann cell bodies. (C,D) After 4 weeks in medium that promotes myelination, PMP22 becomes co-localized with myelin segments (stained by antibody P0). Arrows point to axons (C) and to the cell bodies of elongated Schwann cells (D), with uniform PMP22 staining over the cell membrane.

is an essential step for myelin to be formed. The signals that pass between neurons and Schwann cells are not yet known, but it has been shown that a potent neurotrophin, a nerve growth factor (see Chapter 27), can regulate myelin formation.[68,69]

The exact amount of PMP22 that is produced is critical for proper myelination; with over- or underexpression of PMP22, disorders occur. Figure 10.8 shows that a change in a single amino acid of PMP22 (from leucine to proline) results in "trembler" mice, which exhibit deficient myelination and serious neurological defects. Hereditary human neuropathies arise in families with the same mutation.

Several experiments have provided evidence that glial cells can influence the clustering of sodium channels in the node of myelinated nerve fibers. Changes occur in the

[68] Chan, J. R. et al. 2004. *Neuron* 43: 183–191.

[69] Xiao, J., Kilpatrick, T. J., and Murray, S. S. 2009. *Neurosignals* 17: 265–276.

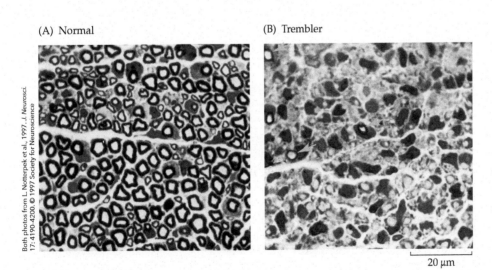

(A) Normal

(B) Trembler

20 μm

Both photos from L. Notterpek et al., 1997. *J. Neurosci.* 17: 4190–4200. © 1997 Society for Neuroscience

FIGURE 10.8   Deficient Myelination in "Trembler" Mutant Mice with a genetic defect in a myelin protein, PMP22. Morphological appearance of sciatic nerves in normal (A) and mutant (B) trembler mice, aged 10 days. Note the marked differences in axon caliber and myelin thickness between normal and trembler mice (indicated by arrows in B) in microscopic sections at equivalent magnifications. Also note the severity of demyelinization. A single amino acid mutation from leucine to proline produces trembler neuropathy in mice and in humans.

(A)

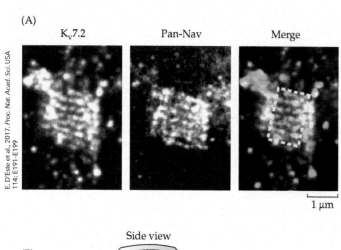

K$_v$7.2   Pan-Nav   Merge

E. D'Este et al., 2017. *Proc. Nat. Acad. Sci. USA*
114: E191–E199

1 µm

FIGURE 10.9 Molecules Contributing to the Peripheral Nodes of Ranvier. (A) Potassium KV7.2 channels intercalate with sodium (Pan-Nav) channels. The use of a specific antibody against each type of ion channel demonstrates that the channels occur in an alternating pattern. (B,C) Molecular organization of peripheral nodes of Ranvier. (B) Molecular organization of the three different compartments (node, paranode, and the region of the axon that is covered by the myelin sheath, called juxtaparanode), seen from the side. (C) The same compartments, seen from the top, showing an overlay of the axonal and glial proteins. Actin, spectrin, and ankyrin G (Ank B) form a continuous ~190-nm periodic axonal scaffold onto which channels and adhesion molecules assemble (not shown). AnkB, ankyrin B; AnkG, ankyrin G; βIIspec, βIVspec, betalV spectrin; NF155, neurofascin-155; NF186, neurofascin-186. (A,B from E. D'Este et al., 2017. *Proc. Nat. Acad. Sci.* USA 114: E191–E199.)

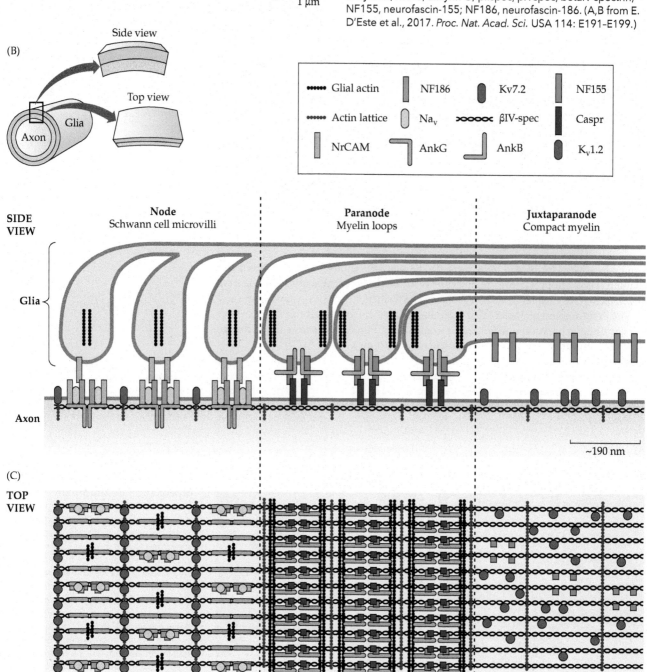

distribution of ion channels in nodes, paranodal areas, and internodes as axons become myelinated, demyelinated, and remyelinated.[70,71]

The formation of the nodes of Ranvier provides an example of cooperation between neurons and glia.[72] Their assembly starts with contact of the neuronal axon by the glial myelin sheath; the myelin sheath binds to the axonal protein ankyrin B. The clustering of the axonal protein neurofascin-186 (NF186) triggers the accumulation of a second kind of ankyrin (ankyrin G) that promotes clustering of sodium channels by binding an intracellular domain of their α-subunit[62] (see Chapter 5). Intracellularly, the complex stabilizes by its binding to the actin network of the axon. Figure 10.9 shows the molecular interactions that assemble the nodes, as studied with STED (stimulated emission depletion) optics, which have higher resolution than regular microscopy. Double staining procedures with antibodies against different combinations of pairs of 12 different proteins in the node, including sodium and potassium channels, ankyrin, and others, have permitted researchers to reconstruct the molecular arrangement of the node. There are similarities and differences in the molecular interactions giving rise to CNS and PNS nodes. Binding proteins such as ankyrins and sodium channels are common; others are specific for each type of node.

In PNS nodes, processes of Schwann cells approach the nodes and contribute to their stabilization by secreting proteins such as gliomedin, which is a ligand for the axonal cell adhesion molecules neurofascin and NrCAM. The protein that binds to the cell adhesion molecules, NF186, is contributed by the axon. The whole complex associates with sodium and potassium channels.[73]

In CNS nodes, another glial type comes into play: Astrocytic fingers approaching the nodal region show intense labeling with saxitoxin (a toxin that binds to sodium channels; see Chapter 5), indicating a high density of sodium channels in the glial membrane.[74]

Effects of Neuronal Activity on Glial Cells

Potassium Accumulation in Extracellular Space

Glial cells regulate their potassium concentration in intercellular clefts, a process known as **spatial buffering** (see Figure 10.12).[29,76,77] According to this concept, glial cells act as conduits for uptake of potassium from the clefts to preserve the constancy of the environment.[78] The release of potassium during nerve activity can depolarize glial cells. The recordings in Figure 10.10 were made from a glial cell in the optic nerve of the mud puppy

[70] Susuki, K., and Rasband, M. N. 2008. *Curr. Opin. Cell Biol.* 20: 616–623.

[71] Feinberg, K. et al. 2010. *Neuron* 65: 490–502.

[72] Herbert, A. L., and Monk, K. R. 2017. *Curr. Opin. Neurobiol.* 42: 53–60.

[73] Feinberg, K. et al. 2010. *Neuron* 65: 490–502.

[74] Ritchie, J. M. et al. 1990. *Proc. Natl. Acad. Sci. USA* 87: 9290–9294.

[75] Shrager, P., Chiu, S. Y., and Ritchie, J. M. 1985. *Proc. Natl. Acad. Sci. USA* 82: 948–952.

[76] Kofuji, P., and Newman, E. A. 2004. *Neuroscience* 129: 1045–1056.

[77] Bellot-Saez, A. Kékesi, O., Morley, J. W., and Buskila. Y. 2017. *Neurosci. Biobehav. Rev.* 77: 87–97.

[78] Kofuji, P. et al. 2000. *J. Neurosci.* 20: 5733–5740.

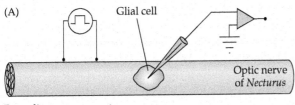

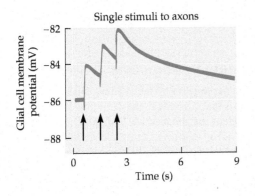

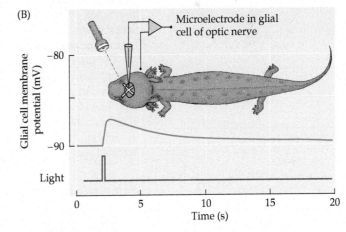

FIGURE 10.10   Effect of Action Potentials on Glial Cells in mud puppy optic nerve. (A) Synchronous impulses evoked by electrical stimulation of nerve fibers cause glial cells to become depolarized. The amplitude of the potentials depends on the number of axons activated and on the frequency of stimulation. (B) Illumination of the eye with a 0.1-second flash of light causes depolarization of a glial cell in the optic nerve of an anesthetized mud puppy with intact circulation. The lower trace monitors light stimulus. (After R. K. Orkand et al., 1966. *J. Neurophysiol.* 29: 788–806.)

FIGURE 10.11 **Responses to Potassium of a Müller Glial Cell** isolated from salamander retina. Recordings were made with an intracellular electrode while potassium was applied to different sites. A is the end foot, and G is the distal part of the cell. The sensitivity to potassium is much greater at the end foot, suggesting a higher concentration of potassium channels in that region. (After E. A. Newman, 1987. *J. Neurosci.* 7: 2423-2432. © 1987 Society for Neuroscience.)

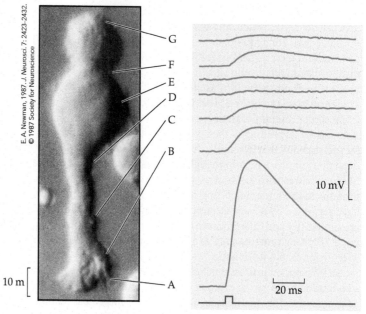

(*Necturus*). Action potentials that are initiated in the nerve fibers by electrical stimulation or by flashes of light travel past the impaled glial cell, which becomes depolarized.[79] Similarly, in the mammalian cortex, glial cells become depolarized depending on the number of nerve fibers activated and on the frequency of neuronal impulses.[80] The frequency of their activation is induced by stimulation of neural tracts, peripheral nerves, the surface of the cortex, or sensory input.[81] Astrocytes within an orientation column of the visual cortex are depolarized by visual stimuli of the appropriate orientation.[82,83]

The cause of glial depolarization is potassium efflux from axons. When potassium accumulates in the intercellular clefts, it changes the $[K]_o/[K]_i$ ratio and alters the membrane potential of glial cells (see Chapter 6). The changes in membrane potential in glial cells are proportional to the level of impulse traffic in their environment. In addition, glial cells have a differential distribution of potassium channels in their membrane. This has been tested by Newman by applying potassium to different parts of an isolated glial cell, while recording its membrane potential with an intracellular electrode. Figure 10.11 shows that the end foot of the cell is more permeable to potassium, suggesting that region has a higher density of potassium channels.[83] Neurons exposed to increased external potassium concentrations become less depolarized than glia because the neuronal membrane deviates from the Nernst equation in the physiological range (see Chapter 6). The intracellular activity of potassium changes of glial cells in response to nerve stimulation have been recorded using ion-sensitive microelectrodes. Glial cells in the olfactory cortex of guinea pig become depolarized by potassium entry through ion channels when the olfactory tract is stimulated with repetitive stimulation. Recovery of the internal potassium concentration takes minutes and is due to the activation of a Na^+/K^+ ATPase.[84] This long recovery reflects the spread of potassium through networks of coupled glial cells,[85] as we explain next.

Potassium and Calcium Movement through Glial Cells

As we discussed in Chapter 8, ion currents in nerve cells flow between regions of a cell that are at different potentials. Figure 10.12 shows that currents in the axon flow between the region that is occupied by an impulse and regions that are inactive. Since glial cells are coupled to each other by low-resistance connections,[24] the conducting properties of the glial assembly approach those of a single elongated cell. Consequently, if one glial cell becomes depolarized, a potassium inward current spreads to other regions of the cell, and through gap junctions to other glial cells. Currents generated by glial cells contribute to recordings made from the eye or the skull with extracellular electrodes. Such recordings, known as

[79] Orkand, R. K., Nicholls, J. G., and Kuffler, S. W. 1966. *J. Neurophysiol.* 29: 788-806.

[80] Ransom, B. R., and Goldring, S. 1973. *J. Neurophysiol.* 36: 869-878.

[81] Van Essen, D, and Kelly, J. 1973. *Nature* 241: 403-405.

[82] Schummers, J., Yu, H., and Sur, M. 2008. *Science* 320: 1638-1643.

[83] Newman, E. A. 1987. *J Neurosci.* 7: 2423-2432.

[84] Ballanyi, K., Grafe, P., and ten Bruggencate, G. 1987. *J. Physiol.* 382: 159-174.

[85] Dietzel, I., Heinemann, U., and Lux, H.D. 1989. *Glia* 2: 25-44.

(A)

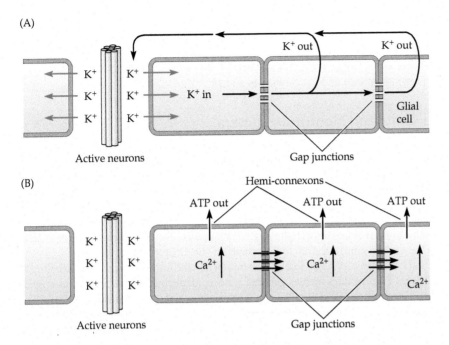

Used with permission from E. A. Newman, unpublished

FIGURE 10.12 Potassium Currents in Glial Cells. (A) The glial cells in the diagram are linked by gap junctions. Potassium released by active axons in one region depolarizes the glial cell and enters it, causing current flow and outward movement of potassium through potassium channels elsewhere in the glial tissue. The concept of spatial buffering of potassium has been postulated as a mechanism for influencing neuronal function by glial cells. (B) Depolarization of the glial cell can cause calcium waves that spread through the network. The raised intracellular calcium concentration allows ATP to leak out from the glia through hemichannels (see Chapter 8).

electroretinograms (ERGs) and electroencephalograms (EEGs), respectively, are valuable for the clinical diagnosis of pathological conditions.

In networks of glial cells in culture or in situ, transient increases in cytoplasmic calcium concentration arise by release from intracellular stores. Using fluorescent indicators, one can observe such oscillatory waves of increased calcium concentration as they propagate from glial cell to glial cell through the gap junctions[86] (Figure 10.13). Calcium waves occur spontaneously[87] or can be triggered by the depolarization produced by extracellular accumulation of potassium when neurons are active and by transmitters

[86] Metea, M. R., and Newman, E. A. 2006. *Glia* 54: 650–655.

[87] Kurth-Nelson, Z. L., Mishra, A., and Newman, E. A. 2009. *J. Neurosci.* 29: 11339–11346.

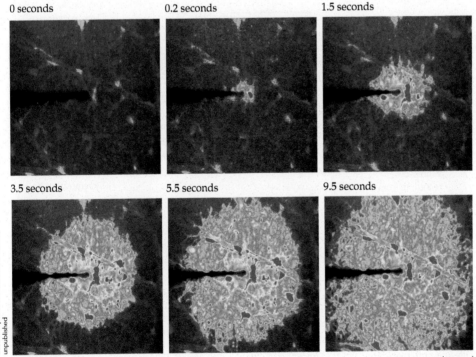

FIGURE 10.13 Calcium Wave Propagated through Retinal Glial Cells. Pseudocolor images of Ca^{2+} fluorescence within astrocytes (larger cells) and Müller cells (smaller spots) at the vitreal surface of the retina. Red represents the highest intensity, blue the lowest. The Ca^{2+} wave is evoked by a mechanical stimulus to a single astrocyte. The wave is initiated at the stimulated cell (top panel, middle) and propagates outward through neighboring astrocytes and Müller cells. Elapsed times following stimulation are noted at the top of each image.

such as glutamate or ATP.[40] Pannexin or connexin hemichannels permeable to ATP are present in extrajunctional glial cell membranes. As a result of calcium waves, hemichannels open and ATP leaks out of activated glial cells into extracellular space[42] (see Figure 10.12B; see also Chapter 17). Extracellularly, ATP exerts several functions[88] discussed in the following sections and in Chapters 14 and 18.

Glial Cells and Neurotransmitters

Transmitters such as GABA, glutamate, glycine, purines, and acetylcholine produce depolarizing or hyperpolarizing responses on glial membranes.[6,39,40,89,90] The glial receptors are similar to those of neurons in many respects. Glial membranes contain receptors for ATP and glutamate, which depolarize, allow calcium to enter, and initiate calcium waves. Many receptors in glial membranes are metabotropic. Their activation increases the intracellular calcium concentration by activation of the G protein cascade that stimulates phospholipase C. The newly formed inositol triphosphate (IP_3) opens IP_3 channels that liberate calcium from the endoplasmic reticulum to the cytoplasm (see Chapter 14).

Glial cells also play a key role in transmitter uptake under normal and pathological conditions. Transmitters such as glutamate, norepinephrine, glycine, and serotonin are taken up by neurons and glial cells.[91–93] As in neurons, glutamate transport in glial cells is coupled to inward movement of sodium along its electrochemical gradient (see Chapter 9). In the absence of a removal mechanism, excessively high levels of external glutamate can activate N-methyl-D-aspartate (NMDA) receptors in neurons, which in turn can lead to calcium entry and cell death. Quantitative estimates indicate that glial cell transport plays a key role in preventing such excessive rises in extracellular glutamate concentration.

Release of Transmitters by Glial Cells

If glial cells themselves become depolarized by raised extracellular potassium or by glutamate, or if intracellular sodium concentration is increased, their membranes transport transmitters out of the glial cell into the extracellular space.[94,95] This mechanism is similar to that for reversed transport described in Chapter 9. Transmitters released in

[88] Cheung, G. Chever, O., and Rouach, N. 2014. *Front. Cell Neurosci* 8: 348.

[89] D'Antoni, S. et al. 2008. *Neurochem. Res.* 33: 2436-2443.

[90] Qian, H. et al. 1996. *Proc. R. Soc. Lond., B, Biol. Sci.* 263: 791-796.

[91] Furness, D. N. et al. 2008. *Neuroscience* 157: 80-94.

[92] Takeda, H., Inazu, M., and Matsumiya, T. 2002. *Naunyn Schmiedebergs Arch Pharmacol.* 366: 620-623.

[93] Gomeza, J. et al. 2003. *Neuron* 40: 785-796.

[94] Billups, B., and Attwell, D. 1996. *Nature* 379: 171-174.

[95] Henneberger, C. et al. 2010. *Nature* 463: 232-236.

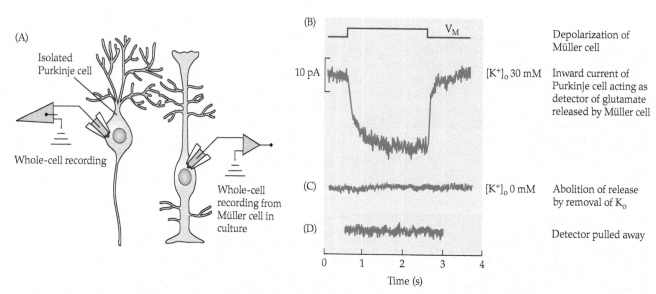

FIGURE 10.14 Release of Glutamate by Glial Cells.
Release of glutamate generated by reversal of the glutamate uptake carrier in a Müller cell. (A) Depolarization-induced release of glutamate from a Müller cell (right) is monitored by recording glutamate-elicited currents from an adjacent Purkinje cell (left). The Purkinje cell acts as a detector with high sensitivity and time resolution. (B) Depolarization of the Müller cell from −60 to +20 mV (top trace) elicits an inward current in the nearby Purkinje cell. The Purkinje cell current is generated by activation of its glutamate receptors. The response to glutamate disappears when extracellular K⁺ is omitted (in fluid containing 0 mM K⁺, reverse glutamate transport by the Müller cell is blocked) (C) or when the Purkinje cell is moved away from the Müller cell (D). (After B. Billups and D. Attwell, 1996. *Nature* 379: 171-174.)

this manner include glutamate, D-serine, ATP, adenosine, and GABA. Figure 10.14 illustrates an experiment showing currents associated with glutamate release by glial cells. This type of outward transport can exacerbate the deleterious effects of brain injury. Injured and dying nerve cells release glutamate and K^+ and depolarize glial cells, which in turn release more glutamate.

A well-established demonstration of transmitter release by glia occurs during regeneration in the PNS. At denervated motor end plates, Schwann cells come to occupy the sites vacated by motor nerve terminals. There they release multimolecular packages of acetylcholine (ACh), giving rise to miniature potentials in muscle.[96] Evidence that transmitter is released by exocytosis from astrocytes is accumulating, and its functional consequences are the subject of numerous studies. Evidence points, for example, to effects on transmitter exocytosis from astrocytes as a way of regulating EEG waves,[97] and to the buffering of glutamate as a way of regulating circadian rhythms.[98]

Messengers such as tumor necrosis factor α (TNF-α), prostaglandins, and certain proteins can also be released from glia. Experiments in culture have shown that astrocytes can release basic fibroblast growth factor and neurotrophin-3. In response, co-cultured neurons express a higher density of sodium channels.[99] Early observations of granules in glial cells suggested their role as secretory cells. Experiments have now demonstrated that astrocytes and NG2 precursor cells release substances by exocytosis. Glial cells synthesize the molecules for filling vesicles with transmitters and also the components of the fusion complex discussed in Chapter 7.

Another transmitter that is secreted by glial cells is ATP.[100] The mechanism for secreting ATP, however, is different from that used for glutamate. As in neurons, release of ATP from glial cells occurs through pannexin or connexin hemichannels[101] that open during the spread of calcium waves from one glial cell to the next.[33] Secretion of ATP by astrocytes has been implicated in the control of respiration by raised CO_2[102] levels, in increasing the frequency of AMPA receptor currents in cortical neurons,[103] in influencing circadian rhythms of suprachiasmatic nucleus in culture.[104] Elegant evidence that links the release of ATP from glial cells in response to visual stimulation, with the increase in blood flow, is presented in Chapter 18.

Immediate Effects of Glial Cells on Synaptic Transmission

A natural question that arises concerns the role of transmitters liberated from glial cells in the adult CNS. Does transmitter and peptide release by glia produce clear-cut, reproducible, and quantitatively measurable effects, for example in synaptic transmission? This question is presently being investigated in several different systems.[105–107] Evidence discussed in Chapter 17 shows that glia release transmitters and peptides in response to transmitters being liberated by neurons. Glial release bridges the activity of neurons with that in other neurons and with the flow of blood in the regions of increased activity. Such studies present major difficulties for the interpretation of the data, since recordings of synaptic events are made distantly from the sites of connections and therefore are hard to interpret.

Transfer of Metabolites from Glial Cells to Neurons

Several lines of evidence indicate that glial cells supply lactate to nerve cells. It has been proposed that lactate, rather than glucose, is taken up by active neurons to provide their prime source of energy.[108,109] The demonstration of such transfer in invertebrates and vertebrate neurons in culture has suggested a similar role for glial cells in the intact CNS under conditions of high neuronal activity or anoxia. The lactate hypothesis, although appealing, does not seem to be universal. In intact animals it is a major task to make direct measurements of the amount of lactate liberated, the increase in concentration, and the timing of release and uptake in relation to neuronal activity[110–115] (see review by Fillenz[116]). However, experiments stimulating electrical activity in hippocampal slices have shown that glucose is the main energy source of neurons.[115] Moreover, certain neurons, such as those in the leech, contain vast deposits of glycogen that suggest that glucose is their main source of energy.

[96] Reiser, G., and Miledi, R. 1988. *Pflügers Arch.* 412: 22-28.

[97] Lee, H. S. et al. 2014. *Proc. Natl. Acad. Sci. USA* 111: E3343-E3352.

[98] Brancaccio, M. et al. 2017. *Neuron* 93:1420-1435.

[99] Igelhorst, B. A. et al. 2015. *Philos. Trans. R. Soc. Lond., B, Biol. Sci.* 370: 20140194.

[100] Pangrsic, T. et al. 2007. *J. Biol. Chem.* 282: 28749-28758.

[101] Chever, O., Lee, C. Y., and Rouach, N. 2014. *J. Neurosci.* 34:11228-32.

[102] Gourine, A. V. et al. 2010. *Science* 329: 571-575.

[103] Fiacco, A., and McCarthy, K. D. 2004. *J. Neurosci.* 24: 722-732.

[104] Womac, A. D. et al. 2009. *Eur. J. Neurosci.* 30: 869-876.

[105] Halassa, M. M., and Haydon, P. G. 2010. *Annu. Rev. Physiol.* 72: 335-355.

[106] Henneberger, C. et al. 2010. *Nature* 463: 232-236.

[107] Perea, G., and Araque, A. 2010. *Brain Res.* Rev. 63: 93-102.

[108] Brown, A. M., and Ransom, B. R. 2007. *Glia* 55: 1263-1271.

[109] Magistretti, P. J. 2009. *Am. J. Clin. Nutr.* 90: 875-880.

[110] Aubert, A. et al. 2005. *Proc. Natl. Acad. Sci USA* 102: 16448-16453.

[111] Saab, A. et al. 2016. *Neuron* 91: 119-132.

[112] Beirowski, B. et al. 2014. *Nat. Neurosci.* 17: 1351-1361.

[113] Pooya, S. et al. 2015. *Nat. Commun.* 5: 1-15.

[114] Lee, Y. et al. 2012.*Nature* 487: 443-448.

[115] Díaz-García, C. M., et al. 2017. *Cell Metab.* 26: 361-374.

[116] Fillenz, M. 2005. *Neurochem. Int.* 47: 413-417.

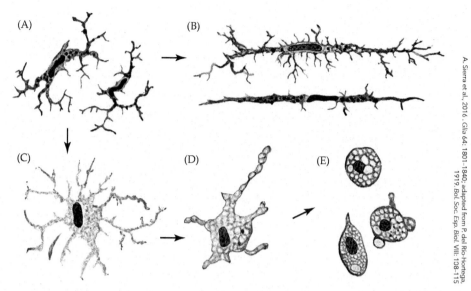

A. Sierra et al., 2016. *Glia* 64: 1801–1840; adapted from P. del Río-Hortega, 1919. *Bol. Soc. Esp. Biol.* VIII: 108–115

FIGURE 10.15 Morphological Transitions of Microglial Cells under Pathological Conditions. The drawings were made from cells that had been stained with silver carbonate. (A) Microglia in the normal brain. (B) Rod-shaped cells characteristic of diseased human brain. (C-E) Transitions of microglia in response to injury. (C) Star-shaped cell. (D) Globular shape. (E) Granuloadipose bodies with phagocytic activity, characteristic of the site of the lesion.

[117] Slobodov, U. et al. 2009. *J. Mol. Neurosci.* 39: 99–103.

[118] Sierra, A. et al. 2016. *Glia* 64: 1801–1840.

[119] Chen, A. et al. 2000. *J. Neurosci.* 20: 1036–1043.

[120] del Río-Hortega, P. 1920. *Trab. Lab. Invest. Biol. Madrid* 18: 37–82.

[121] Duan, Y., Sahley, C. L., and Muller, K. J. 2009. *Dev. Neurobiol.* 69: 60–72.

[122] Samuels, S. E. et al. 2010. *J. Gen. Physiol.* 36: 425–442.

[123] Dibaj, P. et al. 2010. *Glia* 58: 1133–1144.

[124] Nimmerjahn, A., Kirchhoff, F., and Helmchen. F. 2005. *Science* 308: 1314–1318.

[125] Sierra, A., et al. 2016. *Glia* 64: 1801–1840.

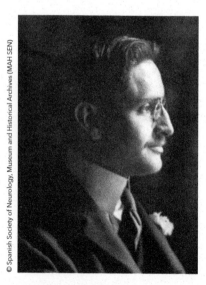

Pío del Río-Hortega circa 1919.

Microglial Cells in CNS Repair

Astrocytes, microglia, and Schwann cells react to neuronal injury by replication. They participate in the removal of debris and in scar formation (see also Chapter 29).[8,9,117] As a first step, resident microglial cells and macrophages, which invade damaged CNS from blood at the site of an injury, divide and scavenge debris from dying cells.

The early studies by del Río-Hortega showed that microglial cells are polymorphic in pathological states. Figure 10.15 shows the morphological transitions of microglia in response to injury.[118] Elongated forms (see Figure 10.15B) are frequent during their migration along nerve tracts. Moreover, in response to injury, microglial cells migrate to the sites of the lesion,2where they gradually acquire a "granuloadipose" shape indicative of their phagocytic function. The detailed mechanism that leads to these morphological changes remains unknown.

By contrast, the mechanism of migration has been carefully studied by Müller and his colleagues, taking advantage of the excellent control of variables offered by the isolated nervous system of the leech.[119] (As an aside, it may be mentioned that it was in the CNS of the leech that some of the first demonstrations of such wandering cells were made by del Río-Hortega.[120]) Normally microglial cells are evenly distributed in leech ganglia and in the bundles of axons that link them (Figure 10.16). Immediately after damage to the CNS, microglial cells migrate to the site of the lesion, at a rate of about 100 mm/hour. There they accumulate, phagocytose damaged tissue, and produce laminin—a molecule that promotes neurite outgrowth (see Chapter 27). Several lines of evidence show that microglia become activated to move by extracellular accumulation of ATP, which is released after injury. At the same time, attraction toward the lesion, as opposed to random movement, is mediated by the gas nitric oxide (NO).[121,122] In mice, as in leeches, nitric oxide activates the migration of microglial cells toward spinal cord lesions.[123]

One may wonder how universal an experiment using an animal such as the leech may be. In experiments made by Kettenmann and his colleagues visualizing fluorescent transgenically engineered microglia with two-photon microscopy, a lesion of a blood microvessel in the mouse brain produced migration of microglial cells to the site of the laser ablation. Microglial processes then covered the damaged site of the vessel (Figure 10.17).[124] Again, the early observations by Del Rio Hortega showed that microglia send processes rapidly to sites of injury.[125] These responses can be mimicked by the local

(A) 5 minutes

(B) 3 hours

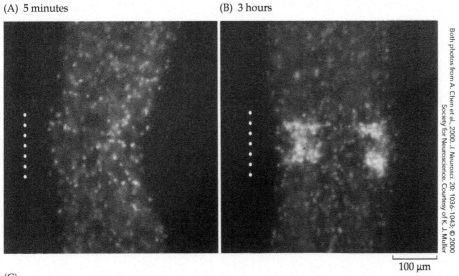

Both photos from A. Chen et al., 2000. *J. Neurosci.* 20: 1036–1043; © 2000 Society for Neuroscience. Courtesy of K. J. Muller

100 µm

(C)

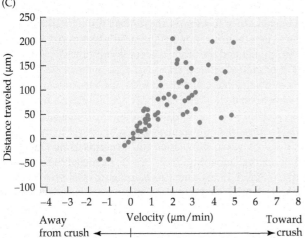

FIGURE 10.16 Migration of Microglial Cells in Injured CNS. (A) Microglia in the leech CNS were stained with a fluorescent nuclear dye (Hoechst 33342). The bundle of axons linking ganglia had been crushed 5 minutes earlier. The extent of the crush is indicated by the dotted line. The nuclei of microglial cells were still evenly distributed at this time. (B) Three hours after the injury, microglial cells had accumulated at the crush site and had produced the growth-promoting molecule laminin. (C) Velocities and distances traveled by microglial cells as they moved toward a lesion in leech CNS. Microglial cells were tracked by video-microscopy at 10-minute intervals in injured leech preparations. In uninjured preparations (not shown), microglial cells make only short, random movements. (C after E. McGlade-McCulloh et al., 1989. *Proc. Natl. Acad. Sci. USA.* 86: 1093–1097.)

(A)

(B)

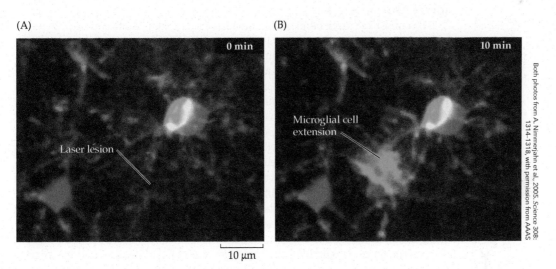

Both photos from A. Nimmerjahn et al., 2005. *Science* 308: 1314–1318, with permission from AAAS

10 µm

FIGURE 10.17 Activated Microglial Processes Cover a Lesion in a Blood Vessel. Microglia (green) and astrocytes (red) imaged with two-photon microscopy in the intact cortex of a rodent brain right before a laser injury to a microvessel (A) and 10 minutes after the laser ablation (B). Processes extended by the microglial cell covered the site of the lesion.

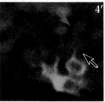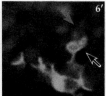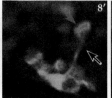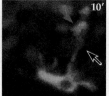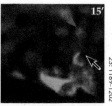

Y. Li et al., 2012. *Dev. Cell* 23: 1189-1202

FIGURE 10.18 Electrical Activity by Neurons Mobilizes Microglial Cells. The time series of multiphoton images show that microglia (green) extend processes that contact the somata (gray) of tectal visual neurons in a zebrafish larva. Neurons are visualized by the fluorescence of the dye OGB-AM. The arrows point to two somata that were subsequently contacted by a process from the same microglial cell. Labels on the top right indicate the time after irradiation.

application of ATP or can be inhibited by blocking G protein-coupled purinergic receptors and connexin channels.[126]

Responses of Microglial Cells to Electrical Activity

Once the origin of microglial cells and their function as the resident phagocytic cells in the CNS were established, it seemed that their function had been fully uncovered. Then the development of new optical techniques and the production of fluorescent microglial cell stripes in transgenic animals[127] permitted researchers to visualize in detail the behavior of individual cells in the brain of living mice. Contrary to what had been previously supposed, microglial cells in the adult brain do not rest. They continuously extend and retract fine processes[124] by which they scan their surroundings, including small contacts between neurons. For example, in larvae of zebrafish in which microglial cells have been transfected with green fluorescent protein (GFP), visual stimulation with patterns of bars produces neuronal electrical activity and microglia motility. Processes of microglial cells elongate and contact the neuronal somata (Figure 10.18). Glutamate uncaging by ultraviolet (UV) flashes succeeds in reproducing such microglial responses. In other series of experiments done with mice, microglial motility was triggered by the release of ATP through openings of pannexin channels by neurons.[126] An attractive hypothesis emerging from such observations is that transient contact by microglia guards neurons electrically, and by doing so, regulates their electrical activity and plasticity.

Microglia and Immune Responses of the CNS

In the past it was generally accepted that the tissues of the CNS were not patrolled by the surveillance mechanisms of the immune system. The blood–brain barrier (Box 10.1), the absence of a lymphatic system, and the comparative ease with which grafts can be accepted all suggest the absence of immune responses to foreign antigens. Thus, CNS functions are not disrupted by the massive allergic reactions to a bee sting or poison ivy. Astrocytes in culture and in situ, however, react with T lymphocytes, whose activity they can either stimulate or suppress. Evidence has now accumulated showing that microglia share properties with immune cells. For example, in addition to expressing receptors for neurotransmitters, microglial cells express characteristic receptors of immune cells, such as cytokine receptors. Glia and activated T lymphocytes do enter the brain and can mediate acute inflammation of brain tissue.[128-130] By using diverse signaling pathways, microglia can communicate with other glia, neurons, and immune cells. Microglial cells can release inflammatory signals. It is now being discussed that these inflammatory molecules are detrimental for the diseased brain.

An experiment that exemplifies the convergence of the immune and nervous systems to integrate function has been done, again, in the visual system. In newborn mammals the visual inputs from the retina and lateral geniculate nucleus generated in both eyes arrive at the same postsynaptic targets (see Chapter 22). The onset of vision triggers an activity-dependent elimination of the projections arriving from the ipsilateral

[126] Davalos, D. et al. 2005. *Nat. Neurosci.* 8: 752-758.

[127] Jung, S. et al. 2000. *Mol. Cell Biol.* 20: 4106-4114.

[128] Kaur, G. et al. 2010. *Neurosurg. Clin. N. Am.* 21: 43-51.

[129] Perry, V. H., Nicoll, J. A., and Holmes, C. 2010. *Nat. Rev. Neurol.* 6: 193-201.

[130] Rotshenker, S. 2009. *J. Mol. Neurosci.* 39: 99-103.

BOX 10.1   The Blood-Brain Barrier

A homeostatic system controls the fluid environment in the brain and prevents fluctuations in its composition. This constancy seems particularly important in a system in which the activity of so many cells is integrated and small variations may upset the balance of delicately poised excitatory and inhibitory influences.[131,132] Within the brain there are three fluid compartments: (1) the blood supplied to the brain through a dense network of capillaries, (2) the cerebrospinal fluid that surrounds the bulk of the nervous system and is contained in the internal cavities (ventricles), and (3) the fluid in the intercellular clefts (Figure 1).

The close anatomical arrangement of glial cells, capillaries, and neurons in the brain suggests that glial cells contribute to form a permeability barrier that regulates the flow of substances between the blood and the brain, the **blood-brain barrier**. The blood-brain barrier is located at the junctions of specialized endothelial cells that line the brain capillaries[133,134] and depends on specialized properties of the endothelial cells, which are far less permeable than those supplying organs in the periphery.[134,135] The junctions, which completely occlude the intercellular spaces between endothelial cells, account for the impermeability of brain capillaries. Molecules must go through, rather than between, endothelial cells. Conversely, the presence of endothelial cells from brain capillaries in culture causes distinctive assemblies of membrane particles to appear in astrocytes. Proteins, ions, and hydrophilic molecules cannot pass through the blood-brain barrier, while lipophilic molecules (such as alcohol) and gases can.

A second essential component of the blood-brain barrier is the choroid plexus: Specialized epithelial cells surround the choroid plexus capillaries and secrete cerebrospinal fluid.[136] The cerebrospinal fluid itself is almost devoid of protein, containing only about 1/200 of the amount present in blood plasma. Proteins, electrolytes, transmitters, and a variety of drugs, including penicillin, injected directly into the bloodstream act rapidly on peripheral tissues such as muscle, heart, or glands—but they have little or no effect on the CNS. When administered by way of the cerebrospinal fluid, however, the same substances exert a prompt and strong action.

Within the brain, ions and small particles reach neurons by passing through the narrow 20-nm intercellular clefts and not through glia. In Figure 2A, after injection of microperoxidase into cerebrospinal fluid, electron-dense molecules deposited by peroxidase reaction are lined up in clefts and fill extracellular spaces. This result shows that large molecules can pass between the ependymal cells that line the ventricles and through intercellular clefts. In contrast, the junctions between endothelial cells lining

---

[131] Abbott, N. J. et al. 2010. *Neurobiol. Dis.* 37: 13-25.

[132] Saunders, N. R. et al. 2008. *Trends Neurosci.* 31: 279-286.

[133] Brightman, M. W., and Reese, T. S. 1969. *J. Cell Biol.* 40: 668-677.

[134] Wolburg, H. et al. 2009. *Cell Tissue Res.* 335: 75-96.

[135] Tao-Cheng, J. H., Nagy, Z., and Brightman, M. W. 1987. *J. Neurosci.* 7: 3293-3299

[136] Wolburg, H., and Paulus, W. 2010. *Acta. Neuropathol.* 119: 75-88.

(A)

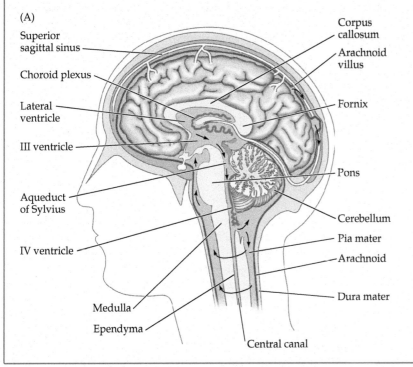

Superior sagittal sinus

Choroid plexus

Lateral ventricle

III ventricle

Aqueduct of Sylvius

IV ventricle

Medulla

Ependyma

Central canal

Corpus callosum

Arachnoid villus

Fornix

Pons

Cerebellum

Pia mater

Arachnoid

Dura mater

(B)

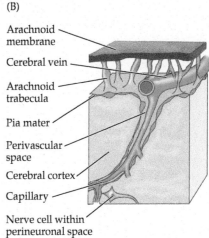

Arachnoid membrane

Cerebral vein

Arachnoid trabecula

Pia mater

Perivascular space

Cerebral cortex

Capillary

Nerve cell within perineuronal space

FIGURE 1   Distribution of Cerebrospinal Fluid and its relation to larger blood vessels and to structures surrounding the brain. (A) All spaces containing cerebrospinal fluid (CSF) communicate with each other. (B) CSF is drained into the venous system through the arachnoid villi.

| BOX **10.1** | **The Blood-Brain Barrier** (continued) |

the blood capillaries in the brain provide a barrier. Tracers injected into cerebrospinal fluid do not enter the capillaries. Figure 2B shows the opposite result. When enzyme was injected into the circulation, brain capillaries filled with enzyme but none entered the intercellular spaces. During development the barrier is already present, but the range of substances that can enter the cerebrospinal fluid is qualitatively and quantitatively different.[137] Knowledge of blood-brain barrier properties is important for understanding pharmacological actions of drugs and their effects on the body.

[137] Johansson, P. A. et al. 2008. *Bioessays* 30: 237-248.

(A)

(B)

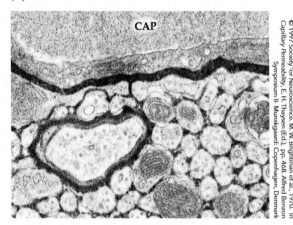

© 1997 Society for Neuroscience. M. W. Brightman et al., 1970. In *Capillary Permeability*, E. H. Thaysen (Ed.), pp. 468. Alfred Benzon Symposium II: Munksgaard: Copenhagen, Denmark

T. S. Reese and M. J. Karnovsky, 1967. *J. Cell Biol.* 34: 207-217.

FIGURE 2   Pathways for Diffusion in the Brain. (A) Demonstration in the mouse that the enzyme microperoxidase diffuses freely from cerebrospinal fluid into the intercellular spaces of the brain, which are filled with the dark reaction product. No enzyme is seen in the capillary (CAP). (B) When injected into the circulation, the enzyme fills the capillary but is prevented by the capillary endothelium from escaping into the intercellular spaces.

[138] LeVay, S., Hubel, D. H., and Wiesel, T. N. 1975. *J. Comp. Neurol.* 159: 559-576.

[139] Schafer D. P., Lehrman E. K., and Stevens, B. 2013. *Glia* 61: 24-36.

eye.[138,139] Microglial cells eliminate supernumerary synapses by a retinotopical engulfment of the inappropriate synapses. This pruning process fails in transgenic mice lacking the immunological complement receptor 3 (CR3), which in the brain is exclusively expressed by microglial cells.

SUMMARY

- Glial cells in the CNS and Schwann cells in the CNS and PNS surround and support neurons.

- Oligodendrocytes have short processes and myelinate axon segments of different cells.

- The blood-brain barrier depends on interactions of astrocytes, capillary and endothelial cells.

- Glial cells have more negative resting potentials than neurons and do not produce action potentials.

- Glial cells are electrically coupled to each other.

- Glial cell membranes contain ion channels for sodium, potassium, and calcium as well as receptors, pumps, and transporters.

- Waves of increased cytoplasmic calcium concentration, evoked in glial cells by depolarization or ATP, cause release of ATP and other transmitters.

- Glial cells play roles in development, regeneration, and homeostatic control of the fluid environment of neurons.

- Microglial cells move to sites of lesion, remove debris, and are involved in inflammatory response.

- The role of glial cells at synapses is a field of active investigation.

Suggested Reading

General Reviews

Brown, A. M., and Ransom, B. R. 2007. Astrocyte glycogen and brain energy metabolism. *Glia* 55: 1263–1271.

Clarke, L. E. and Barres, B. A. 2013. Emerging roles of astrocytes in neural circuit development. *Nat. Rev. Neurosci.* 14: 311–321. doi: 10.1038/nrn3484

Herbert, A. L. and Monk, K. R. 2017. Advances in myelinating glial cell development. *Curr. Opin. Neurobiol.* 42: 53–60. Published online 2016 Dec 6. doi: 10.1016/j.conb.2016.11.003.

Kuffler, S. W., and Nicholls, J. G. 1966. The physiology of neuroglial cells. *Ergeb. Physiol.* 57: 1–90.

Lapato, A. S. and Tiwari-Woodruff, S. K. 2018. Connexins and pannexins: At the junction of neuro-glial homeostasis and disease. *J. Neurosci. Res.* 96: 31–44. doi: 10.1002/jnr.24088.

Newman, E. A. 2004. A dialogue between glia and neurons in the retina: Modulation of neuronal excitability. *Neuron Glia Biol.* 1: 245–252.

Nishiyama, A., Boshans, L., Goncalves, C. M., Wegrzyn, J., and Patel, K. D. 2016. Lineage, fate, and fate potential of NG2-glia. *Brain Res.* 1638: 116–128.

Rakic, P. 2003. Developmental and evolutionary adaptations of cortical radial glia. *Cereb. Cortex* 13: 541–549.

Richardson, W. D., Young, K. M., Tripathi, R. B., McKenzie, I. 2011. NG2-glia as multipotent neural stem cells: Fact or fantasy? *Neuron* 70: 661–673. doi: 10.1016/j.neuron.2011.05.013.

Salter, M. W., Beggs, S. 2014. Sublime microglia: Expanding roles for the guardians of the CNS. *Cell.* 158: 15–24. doi: 10.1016/j.cell.2014.06.008.

Schwab, M. E. 2004. Nogo and axon regeneration. *Curr. Opin. Neurobiol.* 14: 118–124.

Sierra, A., de Castro, F., del Río-Hortega, J., Rafael Iglesias-Rozas, J., Garrosa, M., and Kettenmann, H. 2016. The "Big-Bang" for modern glial biology: Translation and comments on Pío del Río-Hortega 1919 series of papers on microglia. *Glia.* 64: 1801–1840. doi: 10.1002/glia.23046.

Webster, H., and Aström, K. E. 2009. Gliogenesis: Historical perspectives, 1839–1985. *Adv. Anat. Embryol. Cell. Biol.* 202: 1–109.

Wolf, S.A., Boddeke, H.W., and Kettenmann, H. 2007. Microglia in physiology and disease. *Annu. Rev. Physiol.* 79: 619–643. doi: 10.1146/annurev-physiol-022516-034406. Epub 2016 Dec 7.

Original Papers

Buckley, C. E., Marguerie, A., Alderton, W. K., and Franklin, R. J. 2010. Temporal dynamics of myelination in the zebrafish spinal cord. *Glia* 58: 802–812.

Duan, Y., Sahley, C. L., and Muller, K. J. 2009. ATP and NO dually control migration of microglia to nerve lesions. *Dev. Neurobiol.* 69: 60–72.

Fillenz, M. 2005. The role of lactate in brain metabolism. *Neurochem. Int.* 47: 413–417.

Girouard, H., Bonev, A. D., Hannah, R. M., Meredith, A., Aldrich, R. W., and Nelson, M. T. 2010. Astrocytic endfoot Ca^{2+} and BK channels determine both arteriolar dilation and constriction. *Proc. Natl. Acad. Sci. USA* 107: 3811–3816.

Hamilton, N. B., and Attwell, D. 2010. Do astrocytes really exocytose neurotransmitters? *Nat. Rev. Neurosci.* 11: 227–238.

Hansen, D. V., Lui, J. H., Parker, P. R., and Kriegstein, A. R. 2010. Neurogenic radial glia in the outer subventricular zone of human neocortex. *Nature* 464: 554–561.

Iglesias, R., Dahl, G., Qiu, F., Spray, D. C., and Scemes, E. 2009. Pannexin 1: The molecular substrate of astrocyte "hemichannels." *J. Neurosci.* 29: 7092–7097.

Johansson, P. A., Dziegielewska, K. M., Liddelow, S. A., and Saunders, N. R. 2008. The blood-CSF barrier explained: when development is not immaturity. *Bioessays* 30: 237–248.

Kuffler, S. W. and Potter, D. D. 1964. Glia in the leech central nervous system: Physiological properties and neuron-glia relationship. *J. Neurophysiol.* 27: 290–320.

Kurth-Nelson, Z. L., Mishra, A., and Newman, E. A. 2009. Spontaneous glial calcium waves in the retina develop over early adulthood. *J. Neurosci.* 29: 11339–11146.

Love, F. M., Son, Y. J., and Thompson, W. J. 2003. Activity alters muscle reinnervation and terminal sprouting by reducing the number of Schwann cell pathways that grow to link synaptic sites. *J. Neurobiol.* 54: 566–576.

Marcaggi, P. and Attwell, D. 2004. Role of glial amino acid transporters in synaptic transmission and brain energetics. *Glia* 47: 217–225.

Metea, M. R. and Newman, E. A. 2006. Calcium signaling in specialized glial cells. *Glia* 54: 650–655.

Newman, E. A. 2003. Glial cell inhibition of neurons by release of ATP. *J. Neurosci.* 23: 1659–1666.

Nimmerjahn, A., Kirchhoff, F., and Helmchen, F. 2005. Resting microglial cells are highly dynamic surveillants of brain parenchyma in vivo. *Science* 308: 1314–1318.

Rotshenker, S. 2009. The role of Galectin-3/MAC-2 in the activation of the innate-immune function of phagocytosis in microglia in injury and disease. *J. Mol. Neurosci.* 39: 99–103.

Verkhratsky, A., Krishtal, O. A., and Burnstock, G. 2009. Purinoceptors on neuroglia. *Mol. Neurobiol.* 39: 190–208.

Zuo, Y., Lubischer, J. L., Kang, H., Tian, L., Mikesh, M., Marks, A., Scofield, V. L., Maika, S., Newman, C., Krieg, P., and Thompson, W. J. 2004. Fluorescent proteins expressed in mouse transgenic lines mark subsets of glia, neurons, macrophages, and dendritic cells for vital examination. *J. Neurosci.* 24: 10999–11009.

PART III

Intercellular Communication

In Part II we described how ion and electrical gradients are maintained across a nerve cell membrane, how these gradients are used to generate electrical impulses (action potentials), and how these impulses are conducted along the processes of the nerve cell (the axons). Now we have to consider what happens when the impulse gets to the end of the axon: How is this information transmitted to another neuron or to an effector cell such as a muscle cell?

In most cases the information is transmitted across specialized contact zones called synapses. The process is termed synaptic transmission. In some instances the presynaptic action potential is conducted electrotonically across the synapse to directly depolarize the postsynaptic neuron—electrical transmission. More commonly, however, the presynaptic action potential induces the release of a chemical transmitter substance that binds to specialized target proteins (receptors) on the postsynaptic membrane. This process is called chemical transmission.

In Chapters 11 and 12 we describe two forms of chemical transmission—one in which the transmitter substance actually binds to, and opens, an ion channel, producing a very rapid, brief postsynaptic response (direct transmission), and one in which the transmitter binds to a different type of receptor and produces a slow, long-lasting postsynaptic effect by inducing a cascade of intracellular changes (indirect transmission). Then in Chapter 13 we go back to the presynaptic nerve endings and discuss how the transmitter is stored in them and how it is released by the presynaptic action potential.

There are a large number of different chemical transmitter substances in the nervous system, which makes it possible to selectively modify transmission at some synapses and not at others using specific chemicals. The pathways using the different transmitters and some of their actions on individual neurons and on overall brain function are summarized in Chapter 14. Chapter 15 gives information about the synthesis, storage, and inactivation of these transmitters. Chapters 16 and 17 deal with how the efficiency of transmission across synapses can show increases or decreases (synaptic plasticity) depending on the amount of synaptic traffic. In Chapter 17 we examine one particular and much-studied form of plasticity called long-term potentiation (LTP), thought by some to be the neurophysiological substrate of some forms of memory.

Finally, Chapter 18 explores how neurons communicate through the release of signaling molecules outside synapses, from the soma, dendrites, and axon varicosities. This mode of release is called extrasynaptic transmission. Its effects can be slow and long-lasting and may incorporate the activation of neurons, glial cells, and blood vessels.

CHAPTER 11

Mechanisms of Direct Synaptic Transmission

Synapses are points of contact between nerve cells and their targets where signals are handed on from one cell to the next. This process of synaptic transmission may be mediated through the release of a chemical neurotransmitter substance from the nerve terminal by the incoming action potential (chemical transmission) or, at certain junctions, by the direct spread of electrical current from the presynaptic neuron to the postsynaptic cell (electrical transmission).

At direct chemical synapses, the transmitter binds to receptors in the membrane of the postsynaptic cell. In this case receptors are themselves ion channels (ionotropic receptors). As a result, the conformation of the receptor changes, the channel opens, ions flow through the channel and across the membrane, and the membrane potential changes—all within a millisecond or so. A slower process, indirect chemical transmission, involving additional, intermediary steps, is described in Chapter 12.

The channels opened at excitatory synapses allow cations to enter, driving the membrane potential toward the action potential threshold. At inhibitory synapses, transmitters open channels that are permeable to anions, tending to keep the membrane potential negative to threshold. At both excitatory and inhibitory synapses, the direction of current flow is determined by the electrochemical balance of the permeant ions, as we discussed in Chapter 6.

Synapses between motor nerves and skeletal muscle fibers provide important preparations for understanding the mechanisms of direct chemical synaptic transmission. In the mammalian central nervous system (CNS), directly mediated excitation occurs at synapses where the transmitter (usually glutamate) activates excitatory ionotropic receptors. Inhibitory synaptic transmission in the CNS is mediated by release of transmitters (usually γ-aminobutyric acid [GABA] or glycine) that activate inhibitory ionotropic receptors.

More than one type of transmitter may be released at a single chemical synapse, and many transmitters act both rapidly, by binding to and opening ion channels directly, and more slowly, through indirect mechanisms. In another process known as presynaptic inhibition, a chemical transmitter acts on the presynaptic nerve ending to reduce the amount of neurotransmitter released. Electrical transmission occurs at synapses specialized for very fast reflex responses and also in the mammalian CNS, where it helps coordinate nerve cell activity.

Synaptic Transmission

Action potentials carry signals along axons from one location in the nervous system to another at speeds of up to 120 meters per second and frequencies of up to 200 impulses per second. When they arrive at the axon terminal, the information they carry is passed along to the next cell in line at specialized junctions called **synapses**. Transmission at synapses is very rapid. The recipient (postsynaptic) cell can respond in less than a millisecond to the arrival of an action potential in the presynaptic terminal. For a long time there was disagreement about how such rapid transmission occurred (Box 11.1). One possibility, widely held until the early 1950s, was that the presynaptic current spread into the postsynaptic cell (electrical transmission; Figure 11.1A). An alternative view was that transmission was mediated by release of a chemical transmitter substance from the presynaptic terminal onto the postsynaptic cell (chemical transmission; Figure 11.1B).

It is now clear that chemical transmission is the prevalent mode of synaptic communication in the vertebrate CNS and peripheral nervous system (PNS). However, electrical transmission is used at certain invertebrate and vertebrate synapses specialized for very fast responses, and is also widely used in the mammalian CNS as a mechanism for coordinating the electrical activity of groups of neurons. In this chapter we start by discussing chemical transmission, then consider examples of electrical transmission.

Chemical Synaptic Transmission

Certain obvious questions arise when one considers the elaborate scheme necessary for **chemical synaptic transmission**, which entails the secretion of a specific chemical by a nerve terminal and its interaction with specific postsynaptic receptors (see Figure 11.1B). How does the terminal liberate the chemical? Is there a special feature of the action potential mechanism that causes secretion? How is the interaction of a transmitter with its postsynaptic receptor rapidly converted into excitation or inhibition? The release process will be considered in detail in Chapter 13; here we discuss the question of how transmitters act on the postsynaptic cell at direct chemical synapses.

Many of the pioneering studies of chemical synaptic transmission were done on relatively simple preparations, such as the skeletal neuromuscular junction of the frog. At the time, this particular preparation had the advantage that the neurotransmitter acetylcholine (ACh) had been definitively identified, while the transmitters at synapses in the CNS were completely unknown (see Chapter 15). In addition, the responses to transmitter release could be reliably recorded from the postsynaptic region of the muscle cell.

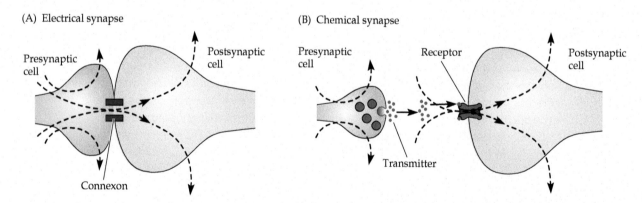

FIGURE 11.1 Electrical and Chemical Synaptic Transmission. (A) At electrical synapses, current flows directly from one cell to another through connexons (intercellular channels that cluster to form gap junctions). (B) At chemical synapses, depolarization of the presynaptic nerve terminal triggers the release of neurotransmitter molecules, which open ion channel receptors on the postsynaptic membrane, causing excitation or inhibition. Dashed lines show the direction of positive current flow.

BOX 11.1 Electrical or Chemical Transmission?

In the second half of the nineteenth century there was vigorous debate between proponents of the cell theory, who considered that neurons were independent units, and those who thought that nerve cells were a **syncytium** interconnected by protoplasmic bridges. Not until the late nineteenth century did it become generally accepted that nerve cells are independent units. This disagreement about synaptic structure was accompanied by a parallel disagreement about function. In 1843, Du Bois-Reymond showed that flow of electrical current was involved in both muscle contraction and nerve conduction, and it required only a small extension of this idea to conclude that transmission of excitation from nerve to muscle was also due to current flow (see Figure 11.1A).[1] Du Bois-Reymond himself favored an alternative explanation: the secretion by the nerve terminal of an excitatory substance that then caused muscle contraction (see Figure 11.1B). However, the idea of animal electricity had such a potent hold on people's thinking that it was more than 100 years before contrary evidence finally overcame the assumption of electrical transmission between nerve and muscle and, by extension, between nerve cells in general.

One reason why the idea of chemical synaptic transmission seemed unattractive is the speed of signaling between nerve cells or between nerve and muscle. The fraction of a second that intervenes between stimulation of a motor axon and contraction of the corresponding muscle did not appear to provide sufficient time for a chemical neurotransmitter to be released from the nerve terminal and interact with receptors on the postsynaptic target to cause excitation. This difficulty did not exist in the autonomic nervous system, which controls glands and blood vessels, where the effects of nerve stimulation are slow and prolonged (see Chapter 17). Thus, the first explicit suggestion of chemical transmission came from experiments on the sympathetic nervous system by T. R. Elliott in 1904.[2] He noted that an extract from the adrenal gland, adrenaline (epinephrine), mimicked the action of sympathetic nerve stimulation when applied directly to the target tissues and concluded with the words "Adrenalin might then be the chemical stimulant liberated on each occasion when the impulse arrives at the periphery." This

was not pursued further at that time, but instead, in 1921 Otto Loewi did a direct and simple experiment that established the chemical nature of transmission at autonomic synapses between the vagus nerve and the heart.[3] He perfused the heart of a frog and stimulated the vagus nerve, thereby slowing the heartbeat. When the fluid from the inhibited heart was transferred to a second unstimulated heart, it too began to beat more slowly. Apparently, stimulation of the vagus nerve had caused an inhibitory substance to be released into the perfusate. In subsequent experiments, Loewi and his colleagues demonstrated that the substance was mimicked in every way by acetylcholine (ACh).

It is an amusing sidelight that Loewi had the idea for his experiment in a dream, wrote it down in the middle of the night, but could not decipher his writing the next morning. Fortunately, the dream returned, and this time Loewi took no chances; he rushed to the laboratory and performed the experiment. Later he reflected:

On mature consideration, in the cold light of morning, I would not have done it. After all, it was an unlikely enough assumption that the vagus should secrete an inhibitory substance; it was still more unlikely that a chemical substance that was supposed to be effective at very close range between nerve terminal and muscle be secreted in such large amounts that it would spill over and, after being diluted by the perfusion fluid, still be able to inhibit another heart.[3]

Subsequently, in the early 1930s the role of ACh in synaptic transmission in **ganglia** in the autonomic nervous system was firmly established by Feldberg and his colleagues.[4] Highlights of such experiments and ideas from the beginning of the twentieth century are contained in the writings of Dale, who for several decades was one of the leading figures in British physiology and pharmacology.[5] Among his many contributions are the clarification of the action of acetylcholine at synapses in autonomic ganglia and the establishment of its role in **neuromuscular transmission**. Thus, in 1936 Dale and his colleagues demonstrated that acetylcholine was released by stimulating the motor nerves supplying skeletal muscle,[6] and then that application of ACh to the muscle caused contraction and that

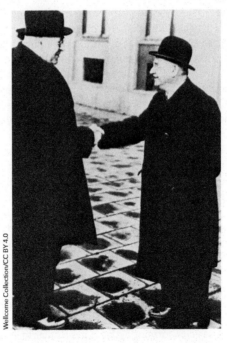

Henry Dale (left) and Otto Loewi, mid-1930s.

(Continued)

BOX 11.1 Electrical or Chemical Transmission? (continued)

the effects of both ACh and motor nerve stimulation were blocked by curare (see Boxes 11.2 and 11.3).[5]

The idea of chemical transmission between one nerve cell and another, particularly in the mammalian CNS, took rather longer to become accepted. There were several reasons for this. First, there were no model synapses to study that were comparable to the frog neuromuscular junction (see the next section). Second, the chemical transmitters in the CNS were not known (acetylcholine is not the main transmitter), so there were no good pharmacological tools to use. Third, neuron-to-neuron transmission could only be studied using electrical recording techniques, which (one suspects) might have led the investigators to think in terms of electrical current flow. One of the most ardent proponents of the electrical transmission theory was J. C. Eccles. However, he became converted to the chemical hypothesis when he and his colleagues first used microelectrodes to record from inside a motor neuron in the spinal cord of an anesthetized cat. There, they found that stimulation of excitatory or inhibitory afferent nerves produced changes in the membrane potential of the motor neuron in *opposite* directions.[7] (The nature of these potentials is described in more detail in the section Direct Synaptic Inhibition). They could not explain the opposite polarity of the inhibitory response with their previous electrical hypothesis, so they wrote:

It may therefore be concluded that inhibitory synaptic action is mediated by a specific transmitter substance that is liberated from the inhibitory synaptic knobs and causes an increase in polarization of the subjacent membrane of the motoneurone.[7]

Interestingly, not long after chemical transmission was firmly established as the accepted form of synaptic activation, in 1959 Furshpan and Potter found electrical transmission of excitation between giant axons in the crayfish.[8] Then, in 1963, electrical synaptic transmission was reported in the avian ciliary ganglion.[9] Examples of electrical transmission have multiplied manyfold since then, and we now we know that both chemical and electrical synapses are abundant in both vertebrate and invertebrate nervous systems.

---

[1] Du Bois-Reymond, E. 1848. *Untersuchungen über thierische Electricität.* Reimer, Berlin, Germany.

[2] Elliott, T. R. 1904. *J. Physiol.* 31: (Proc.) xx-xxi.

[3] Loewi, O. 1921. *Pflügers Arch.* 189: 239-242.

[4] Feldberg, W. 1945. *Physiol. Rev.* 25: 596-642.

[5] Dale, H. H. 1953. *Adventures in Physiology.* Pergamon, London.

[6] Dale, H. H., Feldberg, W., and Vogt, M. 1936. *J. Physiol.* 86: 353-380.

[7] Brock, L. G., Coombs, J. S., and Eccles, J. C. 1952. *J. Physiol.* 117: 431-460.

[8] Furshpan, E. J., and Potter, D. D. 1959. *J. Physiol.* 145: 289-325.

[9] Martin, A. R., and Pilar, G. 1963. *J. Physiol.* 168: 443-463.

Synaptic Structure

As always, knowledge of structure is a prerequisite for understanding function. Figure 11.2 illustrates the principal morphological features of the neuromuscular junction of the frog. Individual axons branch from the incoming motor nerve, lose their myelin sheath, and give off terminal branches that run in shallow grooves on the surface of the muscle. The **synaptic cleft** between the terminal and the muscle membrane is about 30 nanometers (nm) wide. Within the cleft is the **basal lamina**, which follows the contours of the muscle fiber surface. On the muscle, **postjunctional folds** radiate into the muscle fiber from the cleft at regular intervals. The grooves and folds are peculiar to skeletal muscle and are not a general feature of chemical synapses. In skeletal muscle, the region of postsynaptic specialization is known as the **motor end plate**. Schwann cell lamellae cover the nerve terminal, sending fingerlike processes around it at regularly spaced intervals.

Within the cytoplasm of the terminal, clusters of **synaptic vesicles** are abundant, with some vesicles directly in contact with electron-dense material attached to the presynaptic membrane, forming **active zones**. Synaptic vesicles are sites of ACh storage; upon excitation of the axon terminal, they fuse with the presynaptic membrane at the active zone to spill their contents into the synaptic cleft by **exocytosis** (see Chapter 13).

Synapses on nerve cells are usually made by nerve terminal swellings called **boutons**, which are separated from the postsynaptic membrane by the synaptic cleft. The presynaptic membrane of the bouton displays electron-dense regions with associated clusters of synaptic vesicles, forming active zones similar to, but smaller than, those seen in skeletal muscle (see Figure 11.2C). At nerve–nerve synapses the postsynaptic membrane often appears thickened and has electron-dense material associated with it.

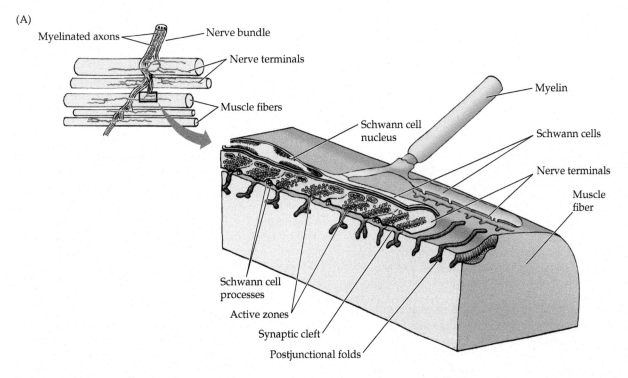

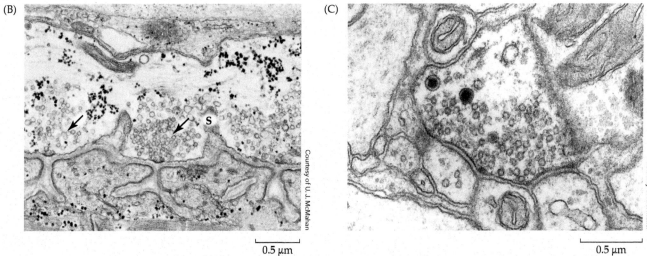

FIGURE 11.2   Structure of Chemical Synapses. (A) A three-dimensional sketch of part of the terminal arbor of a motor axon at the frog skeletal neuromuscular junction. The inset shows a camera lucida drawing of several skeletal muscle fibers and their innervation (motor nerve terminals are in red). Synaptic vesicles are clustered in the nerve terminal in special regions opposite the openings of the postjunctional folds. These regions, called active zones, are the sites of transmitter release into the synaptic cleft. Fingerlike processes of Schwann cells extend between the terminal and the postsynaptic membrane, separating active zones. (B) Electron micrograph of a longitudinal section through a portion of the neuromuscular junction. In the nerve terminal, clusters of vesicles lie over thickenings in the presynaptic membrane—the active zones (arrows). Schwann cell processes (S) separate the clusters. In the muscle, postjunctional folds open into the synaptic cleft directly under the active zone. The band of fuzzy material in the cleft, which follows the contours of the postjunctional folds, is the synaptic basal lamina. (C) Electron micrograph of synapses in the CNS of the leech. As at the frog neuromuscular junction, clusters of synaptic vesicles are focused on dense regions of the presynaptic membrane, forming active zones, and are juxtaposed with postsynaptic densities.

Synaptic Potentials at the Neuromuscular Junction

Early studies by Eccles, Katz, and Kuffler used extracellular recording techniques to study the **end plate potential (EPP)** in muscle.[10–12] The EPP is the depolarization of the end-plate region of the muscle fiber following motor nerve excitation, produced by acetylcholine

[10]Eccles, J. C., and O'Connor, W. J. 1939. *J. Physiol.* 97: 44-102.

[11]Eccles, J. C., Katz, B., and Kuffler, S. W. 1941. *J. Neurophysiol.* 4: 362-387.

[12]Eccles, J. C., Katz, B., and Kuffler, S. W. 1942. *J. Neurophysiol.* 5: 211-230.

released from the presynaptic nerve terminals. Synaptic potentials similar to these are seen in nerve cells. A synaptic potential that excites a postsynaptic cell is usually referred to as an **excitatory postsynaptic potential (EPSP)**, and one that inhibits is called an **inhibitory postsynaptic potential (IPSP)**.

Normally the amplitude of the end plate potential in a skeletal muscle fiber is much greater than that needed to initiate an action potential. The amplitude can be reduced by adding curare, a blocker of the postsynaptic receptors, to the bathing solution (Boxes 11.2 and 11.3).

BOX 11.2   Drugs and Toxins Acting at the Neuromuscular Junction

Agonists, antagonists, and potentiators

Drugs have frequently been used to increase our understanding of neuromuscular transmission. These drugs fall into two classes: those that act directly on the acetylcholine receptors and those that inhibit the enzyme acetylcholinesterase, which is responsible for the hydrolysis and inactivation of acetylcholine (see Appendix B).

Drugs acting on acetylcholine receptors

There are two types of these drugs: **agonists**, which stimulate the receptors and open the nicotinic channels; and **antagonists**, which bind to the receptors but do not open the ion channels, and so block the action of acetylcholine. Agonists include acetylcholine itself (1), the natural agonist; some synthetic choline esters, such as carbamoylcholine (carbachol); and the plant alkaloid nicotine (2), from which the receptors get their name. Antagonists include tubocurarine (3), a component of curare (a mixture of alkaloids extracted from the South American plants *Strychnos toxifera* and *Chondrodendron tomentosum*, which was used as an arrow poison to paralyze prey); and α-bungarotoxin, a component of the venom of the Taiwanese banded krait (*Bungarus multicinctus*). Tubocurarine is a reversible blocking agent (see Box 11.3). Drugs with a similar mechanism of action are used to relax skeletal muscles during surgery. Bungarotoxin binds irreversibly to the ACh receptors and is used experimentally to count or see the receptors (as shown in Figure 11.7).

Drugs that inhibit acetylcholinesterase (anticholinesterases)

Anticholinesterases potentiate cholinergic transmission. They include neostigmine (4) and physostigmine (also called eserine) (5). At the neuromuscular junction they do not alter the peak amplitude of the end plate currents but rather slow their decay rate by about three times.[13,14] This is because the released acetylcholine is not hydrolyzed and so stays longer in the synaptic cleft, until it is cleared by diffusion; this allows the acetylcholine that is released by a single nerve impulse to stimulate the nicotinic receptors several times. Anticholinesterases have much more effect on the response of the end plate to ACh in the bathing solution, because a high proportion of the acetylcholine is normally hydrolyzed by the cholinesterase in the neuromuscular junction before it can access the receptors. The drugs can be used to reverse the blocking effect of tubocurarine or to improve the muscle response in diseases in which neuromuscular transmission is defective, such as myasthenia gravis.

Anticholinesterase drugs have a more dramatic effect on both the amplitude and duration of the slow synaptic responses mediated by **muscarinic acetylcholine receptors (mAChRs)**[15] (see Chapters 12 and 14). The reasons are that the muscarinic receptors are farther away from the presynaptic nerve endings than the nicotinic receptors are, so more of the released ACh is hydrolyzed before it reaches the receptors. In addition, the muscarinic receptors are 100 to 1000 times more sensitive than nicotinic receptors to acetylcholine, so a low concentration of residual unhydrolyzed acetylcholine has a large effect. This underlies the limited use of some anticholinesterase drugs of muscarinic receptors in treating Alzheimer's disease (see Chapter 14).

---

[13] Katz, B., and Miledi, R. 1973. *J. Physiol.* 231: 549–574.
[14] Magleby, K. L., and Terrar, D. A. 1975. *J. Physiol.* 244: 467–495.
[15] Brown, D. A., and Selyanko, A. A. 1985. *J. Physiol.* 365: 335–364.

Agonists

(1) Acetylcholine

(2) Nicotine

Antagonist

(3) Tubocurarine

Potentiators – cholinesterase inhibitors

(4) Neostigmine

(5) Physostigmine (eserine)

BOX **11.3**   Action of Tubocurarine at the Motor End Plate

Reversible competitive antagonism

Tubocurarine acts as a *reversible competitive antagonist* of acetylcholine at the motor end plate (see Box 11.2), which means that it readily dissociates from the acetylcholine receptors and that its blocking action can be overcome by increasing the concentration of acetylcholine. Competition occurs because both molecules bind only transiently to the receptors. So when an ACh molecule detaches from the receptors, a tubocurarine molecule may take its place; and conversely, when the tubocurarine dissociates, ACh may take its place. The probability of one or the other substance occupying the

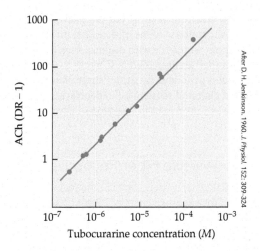

After D. H. Jenkinson. 1960. *J. Physiol.* 152: 309–324.

receptor then depends on: (1) the relative number of molecules of each substance available (i.e., on their relative concentrations) and (2) on the relative times for which they occupy the receptor. Thus, tubocurarine binds to the receptor about 100 times longer than acetylcholine; so for equal concentrations, the competition is weighted in favor of tubocurarine, but this would be equalized if the concentration of ACh were 100 times greater. This competition can be quantified as shown below.

Take a simple reversible reaction between agonist (A) and receptor (R):

$$A + R \leftrightarrow AR$$

$$K_A$$

where K_A is the equilibrium dissociation constant. Then the proportion of receptors occupied by the

agonist at equilibrium (P_{AR}) in the absence of antagonist may be given by:

$$P_{AR} = [A]/\{[A] + K_A\}$$

where [A] = concentration of A.

When the antagonist B is also present, the new receptor that is occupied by the agonist ($P_{AR(B)}$) is now given by:

$$P_{AR(B)} = [A]/\{[A] + K_A(1 + [B]/K_B)\}$$

where [B] is the concentration of B and K_B is the equilibrium dissociation constant for the reaction B + R ↔ BR. This is called the Gaddum equation[16] (see Jenkinson 2011[17] for a full derivation). Thus, to get the same response to the agonist in the presence of the antagonist as that seen before adding the antagonist, the concentration of agonist must be increased from A to A_B such that $A_B/A = \{1 + [B]/K_B\}$. The term A_B/A is frequently called the *dose ratio*, or DR, and the relationship

$$DR - 1 = [B]/K_B$$

is known as the Schild equation.[18]

In a classic piece of work, Donald Jenkinson[19] tested this for tubocurarine antagonism of acetylcholine in frog muscle. He measured the depolarization produced by ACh in the presence of increasing concentrations of tubocurarine and then plotted DR – 1 against the concentration of tubocurarine ([B]) on a double-logarithmic scale. As shown in the adjacent figure, this followed a linear relation over a 1000-fold range of tubocurarine concentrations. This provides convincing evidence for true competitive inhibition. Subsequent work[20] revealed that tubocurarine could also block the nicotinic receptor's ion channels. However, this only becomes significant at more hyperpolarized membrane potentials (–120 mV) than those in Jenkinson's experiments or those in muscle fibers in vivo.

---

[16] Gaddum, J. H. 1943. *Trans. Faraday Soc.* 39: 323–332.

[17] Jenkinson, D. H. 2011. In *Textbook of Receptor Pharmacology*, 3rd ed. CRC Press, London, U.K.

[18] Arunlakshana, O., and Schild, H. O. 1959. *Brit. J. Pharmacol. Chemother.* 14: 48–58.

[19] Jenkinson, D. H. 1960. *J. Physiol.* 152: 309–324.

[20] Colquhoun, D., Dreyer, F., and Sheridan, R. E. 1979. *J. Physiol.* 293: 247–284.

With sufficient curare (about 1 μM), the amplitude of the end plate potential is reduced to below threshold, so that it is no longer obscured by the action potential (Figure 11.3).

The intracellular microelectrode[21] was used by Fatt and Katz[22,23] to study in detail the time course and spatial distribution of the end plate potential in muscle fibers treated with curare. They stimulated the motor nerve and recorded the end plate potential intracellularly at various distances from the end plate (Figure 11.4). At the end plate the depolarization rose rapidly to a peak and then declined slowly over the next 10 to 20 ms. As they

[21] Ling, G., and Gerard, R. W. 1949. *J. Cell Comp. Physiol.* 34: 383–396.

[22] Fatt, P., and Katz, B. 1951. *J. Physiol.* 115: 320–370.

[23] Nicholls, J. G. 2007. *J. Physiol.* 578: 621–622.

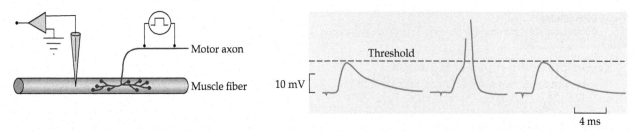

FIGURE 11.3 Synaptic Potentials Recorded with an Intracellular Microelectrode from a mammalian neuromuscular junction treated with curare. The curare concentration in the bathing solution was adjusted so that the amplitude of the synaptic potential was near threshold, and hence on occasion evoked an action potential in the muscle fiber. (After I. A. Boyd and A. R. Martin, 1956. *J. Physiol.* 132: 74–91.)

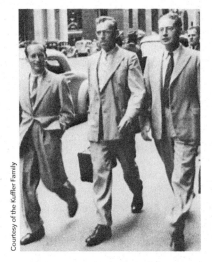

Stephen Kuffler, John Eccles, and Bernard Katz (left to right) in Australia, about 1941.

moved the recording microelectrode farther and farther away from the end plate, the end plate potential amplitude became progressively smaller and its time to peak progressively longer. Fatt and Katz showed that after reaching its peak, the end plate potential decayed at a rate that was consistent with the time constant of the muscle fiber membrane, and that the decrement in end plate potential peak amplitude with distance from the end plate was predicted by the muscle fiber cable properties described in Chapter 8. Accordingly, they concluded that the end plate potential is generated by a brief surge of current that flows into the muscle fiber locally at the end plate and causes a rapid depolarization. The potential then spreads passively beyond the end plate in both directions, becoming smaller and slower with increasing distance.

Mapping the Region of the Muscle Fiber Receptive to ACh

The existence of special properties of skeletal muscle fibers in the region of innervation has been known since the beginning of the twentieth century. Langley[24] assumed the presence of a "receptive substance" around motor nerve terminals, based on the finding that this region of the muscle fiber was particularly sensitive to various chemical agents, such as nicotine. This conclusion showed amazing insight since it was inconceivable that nicotine, which is not produced by animals, could play a physiological role at neuromuscular junctions. After the introduction of the glass microelectrode for intracellular recording, microelectrodes were also used for discrete application of ACh (and later other drugs as well) to the end plate region of muscle.[25] The technique is illustrated in Figure 11.5A.

A microelectrode is inserted into the end plate of a muscle fiber for recording membrane potentials, while an ACh-filled micropipette is held just outside the fiber. To apply ACh, a brief positive voltage pulse is applied to the top of the pipette, causing a spurt of positively charged ACh ions to leave the pipette tip. This method of ejecting charged molecules from pipettes is known as **ionophoresis**.[25] Using this method of application, del Castillo and Katz showed that ACh depolarizes the muscle fiber only at the end plate region and only when applied to the outside of the fiber.[26] When the ACh-filled pipette is placed in close apposition to the end plate

[24] Langley, J. N. 1907. *J. Physiol.* 36: 347–384.

[25] Nastuk, W. L. 1953. *Fed. Proc.* 12: 102.

[26] del Castillo, J., and Katz, B. 1955. *J. Physiol.* 128: 157–181.

FIGURE 11.4 Decay of Synaptic Potentials with Distance from the End Plate Region of a Muscle Fiber. As the distance from the end plate increases, synaptic potentials recorded by an intracellular electrode decrease in size and rise more slowly. (After P. Fatt and B. Katz, 1951. *J. Physiol.* 115: 320–370.)

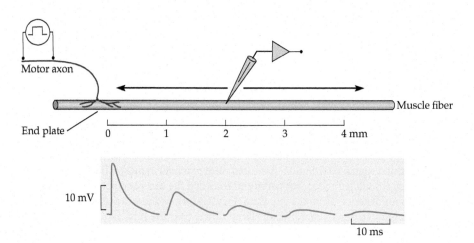

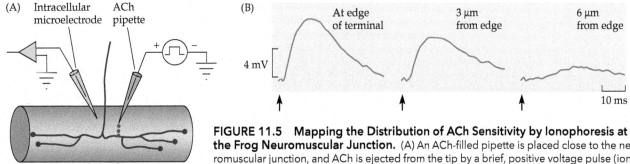

FIGURE 11.5 **Mapping the Distribution of ACh Sensitivity by Ionophoresis at the Frog Neuromuscular Junction.** (A) An ACh-filled pipette is placed close to the neuromuscular junction, and ACh is ejected from the tip by a brief, positive voltage pulse (ionophoresis). An intracellular microelectrode is used to record the response from the muscle fiber. (B) Responses to small ionophoretic pulses of ACh applied at different distances from the axon terminal (indicated by the blue dots in [A]). The amplitude and rate of rise of the response decrease rapidly as ACh is applied farther from the terminal. (After K. Peper and U. J. McMahan, 1972. *Proc. R. Soc. Lond., B* 181: 431–440.)

region, the response to ionophoresis is rapid (Figure 11.5B). Movement of the pipette by only a few micrometers results in a reduction in amplitude and slowing of the response.

The receptive substance postulated by Langley is now known to be the nicotinic ACh receptor, or nAChR (see Chapter 5). The technique of ionophoresis made it possible to map with high accuracy the distribution of these receptors in muscle fibers[27] and nerve cells.[28] This method is particularly useful with thin preparations in which the presynaptic and postsynaptic structures can be resolved with interference contrast optics,[29] and the position of the ionophoretic pipette in relation to the synapse can be determined with precision.

One such preparation is the neuromuscular junction of the snake, shown in Figure 11.6. The end plates in snake muscle are about 50 micrometers (μm) in diameter, resembling in

[27] Miledi, R. 1960. *J. Physiol.* 151: 24–30.

[28] Dennis, M. J., Harris, A. J., and Kuffler, S. W. 1971. *Proc. R. Soc. Lond., B* 177: 509–539.

[29] McMahan, U. J., Spitzer, N. C., and Peper, K. 1972. *Proc. R. Soc. Lond., B* 181: 421–430.

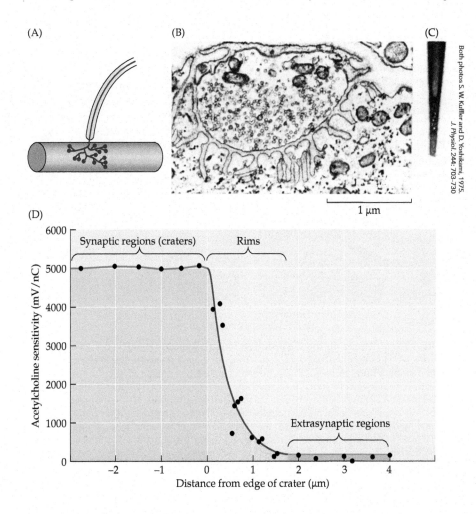

Both photos S. W. Kuffler and D. Yoshikami, 1975. *J. Physiol. 244: 703–730.*

FIGURE 11.6 **Acetylcholine Receptor Distribution at the Skeletal Neuromuscular Junction of the Snake.** (A) An end plate on a skeletal muscle of a snake. The axon terminates in a cluster of boutons. (B) Electron micrograph of a cross section through a bouton. Synaptic vesicles, which mediate ACh release from the nerve terminal, are 50 nanometers (nm) in diameter. (C) Electron micrograph of the tip of a micropipette used for ionophoresis of ACh, shown at the same magnification as (B). The pipette has an outer diameter of 100 nm and an opening of about 50 nm. (D) ACh was applied by ionophoresis across the postsynaptic crater left after the nerve terminal was removed with collagenase. The craters have a uniformly high sensitivity to ACh (5000 mV/nC), with the sensitivity declining steeply at the rims of the craters. Extrasynaptic regions have a uniformly low ACh sensitivity (100 mV/nC). (After S. W. Kuffler and D. Yoshikami, 1975. *J. Physiol.* 244: 703–730.)

their compactness those seen in mammals. Each axon terminal consists of 50 to 70 terminal swellings, analogous to synaptic boutons, from which transmitter is released. The swellings rest in craters sunk into the surface of the muscle fiber. Figure 11.6B shows an electron micrograph of such a synapse. Figure11.6C shows an electron micrograph of a typical iono-phoretic micropipette. The opening is about 50 nm, similar in size to a synaptic vesicle. In this preparation, the motor nerve terminals can be removed by bathing the muscle in a solution of the enzyme collagenase, which frees the terminal without damaging the muscle fiber.[30,31] Each of the nerve terminals then leaves behind a circumscribed crater lined with the exposed postsynaptic membrane, so that the ACh-filled micropipette can be placed directly on the postsynaptic membrane. Then 1 picocoulomb (pC) of charge passed through the pipette releases enough ACh to cause, on average, a 5-mV depolarization. The sensitivity of the membrane is then said to be 5000 mV/nanocoulomb (nC) (see Figure 11.6D). In contrast, at a distance of about 2 μm, just outside the crater, the same amount of ACh produces a response that is 50 to 100 times smaller. Along the rims of the craters, the sensitivity fluctuates over a wide range. Therefore, the conclusion from physiological mapping is that the nicotinic ACh receptors are highly concentrated in the region of the synapse.

Morphological Demonstration of the Distribution of ACh Receptors

Another way to determine the distribution of ACh receptors is to use α-bungarotoxin, the snake toxin that binds highly selectively and irreversibly to nicotinic ACh receptors. The distribution of bound toxin can be visualized using histochemical techniques. For example, fluorescent markers can be attached to α-bungarotoxin and the distribution of receptors visualized by fluorescence microscopy (Figure 11.7A); or the enzyme horseradish peroxidase (HRP) can be linked to α-bungarotoxin and its dense reaction product visualized in the

[30] Betz, W. J., and Sakmann, B. 1973. *J. Physiol.* 230: 673–688.

[31] Kuffler, S. W., and Yoshikami, D. 1975. *J. Physiol.* 244: 703–730.

[32] Burden, S. J., Sargent, P. B., and McMahan, U. J. 1979. *J. Cell Biol.* 82: 412–425.

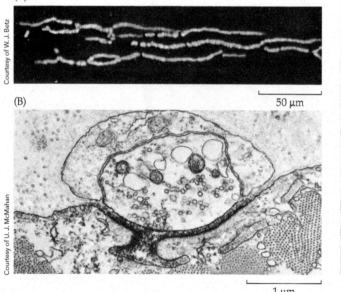
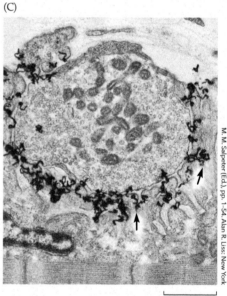

FIGURE 11.7 Visualizing the Distribution of ACh Receptors at the Neuromuscular Junction. (A) Fluorescence micrograph of a frog cutaneous pectoris muscle fiber stained with rhodamine α-bungarotoxin. (B) Electron micrograph of a cross section of a frog cutaneous pectoris neuromuscular junction labeled with horseradish peroxidase-α-bungarotoxin. A dense reaction product fills the synaptic cleft. (C) Autoradiograph of a neuromuscular junction in a lizard intercostal muscle labeled with [^{125}I]α-bungarotoxin. Silver grains (arrows) show that receptors are concentrated at the tops and along the upper third of the junctional folds. (C from M. M. Salpeter, 1987. Vertebrate neuromuscular junctions: General morphology, molecular organization, and functional consequences. In M. M. Salpeter [Ed.], *The Vertebrate Neuromuscular Junction.* Alan R. Liss, New York, pp. 1–54.)

electron microscope (Figure 11.7B).[32] Such techniques confirm that receptors are highly restricted to the membrane immediately beneath the axon terminal. Even more precise quantitative estimates of the concentration of ACh receptors than these can be obtained using radioactive α-bungarotoxin and autoradiography (Figure 11.7C).[33] By counting the number of silver grains exposed in the emulsion, the density of receptors can be determined. In muscle the density is highest along the crests and upper third of the junctional folds (about $10^4/\mu m^2$); the density in extrasynaptic regions is much lower (about $5/\mu m^2$).[34] Transmitter receptors are highly concentrated in the postsynaptic membrane at synapses throughout the CNS and PNS.

Measurement of Ion Currents Produced by ACh

How does ACh produce an inward current at the end plate? Experiments by Fatt and Katz led them to conclude that ACh produces a marked, nonspecific increase in permeability of the postsynaptic membrane to small ions.[22] Two techniques were subsequently used to assess the permeability changes produced by ACh. One involved the use of radioactive isotopes, which showed that the permeability of the postsynaptic membrane was increased to sodium, potassium, and calcium but not to chloride.[35] This experiment provided convincing evidence concerning the ion species involved but did not reveal the details of the conductance changes, their timing, or their voltage dependence. Precise information was provided by voltage clamp experiments, first performed by A. and N. Takeuchi, who used two microelectrodes to voltage clamp the end plate region of muscle fibers.[36] Figure 11.8A shows the experimental arrangement. Two microelectrodes were inserted into the end plate region of a frog muscle fiber—one for recording membrane potential (V_m), the other for injecting current to clamp the membrane potential at the desired level. The nerve was then stimulated to release ACh, or in later experiments ACh was applied directly by ionophoresis. Subsequently, similar experiments were carried out by Magleby and Stevens[37] in muscle fibers treated with hypertonic glycerol. This stops the muscle fibers from contracting, though leaving the fibers in an artificially depolarized state.

Figure 11.8B illustrates results from such a glycerol-treated muscle fiber. With the muscle membrane potential clamped at –40 mV, nerve stimulation produced an inward current,

[33]Fertuck, H. C., and Salpeter, M. M. 1974. *Proc. Natl. Acad. Sci. USA* 71: 1376-1378.

[34]Salpeter, M. M. 1987. In *The Vertebrate Neuromuscular Junction*. Alan R. Liss, New York, pp. 1-54.

[35]Jenkinson, D. H., and Nicholls, J. G. 1961. *J. Physiol.* 159: 111-127.

[36]Takeuchi, A., and Takeuchi, N. 1959. *J. Neurophysiol.* 22: 395-411.

[37]Magleby, K. L., and Stevens, C. F. 1972. *J. Physiol.* 223: 151-171.

(A)

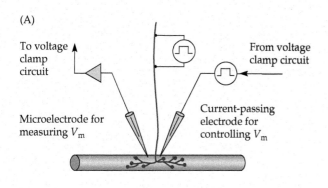

To voltage clamp circuit

From voltage clamp circuit

Microelectrode for measuring V_m

Current-passing electrode for controlling V_m

FIGURE 11.8 Reversal Potential for Synaptic Currents Measured by Voltage Clamp Recording. (A) Scheme for voltage clamp recording at the motor end plate. (B) Synaptic currents recorded from a glycerol-treated muscle fiber at membrane potentials between -120 and +38 mV. When the muscle membrane potential is clamped below 0 mV, synaptic current flows into the muscle. Such inward current would depolarize the muscle if it were not voltage clamped. When the end plate potential is clamped above 0 mV, synaptic current flows out of the cell. (C) Plot of peak end plate current as a function of membrane potential. The relation is nearly linear, with the reversal potential close to 0 mV. (B after K. L. Magleby and C. F. Stevens, 1972. *J. Physiol.* 223: 151-171; C after K. L. Magleby and C. F. Stevens, 1972. *J. Physiol.* 223: 173-197.)

(B)

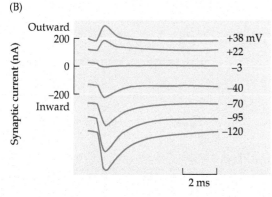

(C)

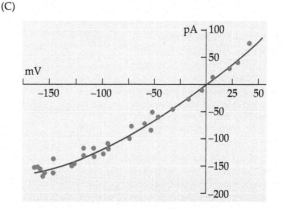

which would have caused a depolarization if the fiber had not been voltage clamped. At more negative holding potentials, the end plate current increased in amplitude. When the membrane was depolarized, the end plate current decreased in amplitude. With further depolarization, the current reversed direction and was outward.

Figure 11.8C shows a plot of the peak amplitude of the end plate current as a function of holding potential. The current changed from inward to outward near zero membrane potential. This is called the **reversal potential**, V_r (see Chapter 9). In earlier experiments on intact muscle fibers, A. and N. Takeuchi estimated the reversal potential to be about –15 mV.

Significance of the Reversal Potential

The reversal potential for the end plate current provides information about the ion currents flowing through the channels activated by ACh in the postsynaptic membrane. For example, if the channels were permeable exclusively to sodium, then current through the channels would be zero at the sodium equilibrium potential (about +50 mV). The other major ions, potassium and chloride, have equilibrium potentials near –90 mV, which is the normal resting membrane potential (see Chapter 6). The calcium equilibrium potential is equal to or greater than +120 mV. None of the ions has an equilibrium potential in the range of 0 to –15 mV. What ions, then, are involved in the response? Consistent with the results of radioactive tracer experiments,[35] A. and N. Takeuchi showed that changing the concentrations of sodium, potassium, or calcium in the bathing solution resulted in changes in the reversal potential, but changes in extracellular chloride did not.[38] They concluded that the effect of ACh was to produce a general increase in *cation* permeability.

Relative Contributions of Sodium, Potassium, and Calcium to the End Plate Potential

ACh opens channels that, at the normal resting potential, allow sodium and calcium ions to leak inward and potassium ions to leak outward along their electrochemical gradients. Because the calcium conductance of the channels is small, the contribution of calcium to the overall synaptic current can be ignored, as can that of other cations such as magnesium. (It should be noted that the low calcium *conductance* is due to its low extracellular and intracellular concentrations; the calcium *permeability* is about 20% of the sodium permeability.)

[38]Takeuchi, A., and Takeuchi, N. 1960. *J. Physiol.* 154: 52-67.

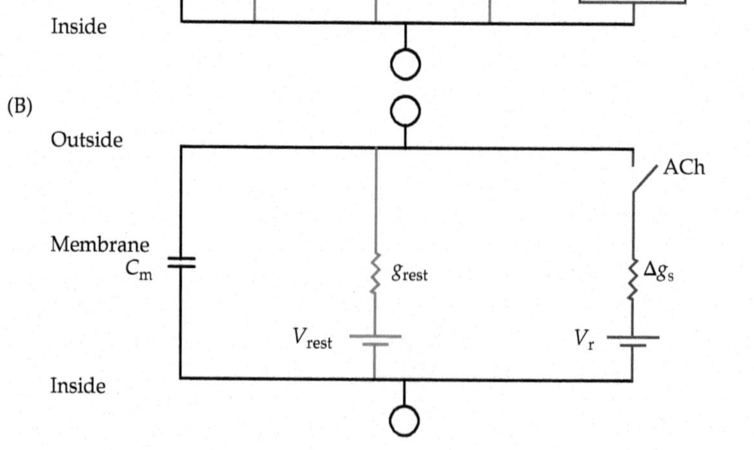

FIGURE 11.9 **Electrical Model of the Postsynaptic Membrane.** Channels activated by ACh are in parallel with the resting membrane channels and with the membrane capacitance, C_m. (A) The synaptic channel opened by ACh is electrically equivalent to two independent pathways for sodium and potassium. The resting membrane has channels for potassium, chloride, and sodium. (B) The synaptic channel can be represented as a single pathway with conductance Δg_s and a battery equal to the reversal potential V_r. The resting membrane can be represented as a single pathway with conductance g_{rest} and a battery equal to V_{rest}.

The equivalent electrical circuit is shown in Figure 11.9A. The resting membrane consists of the usual sodium, potassium, and chloride channels. It is in parallel with ACh-activated channels for sodium and potassium, Δg_{Na} and Δg_K. The Takeuchis calculated that for a reversal potential $V_r = -15$ mV, the ratio of the sodium to potassium conductance changes, $\Delta g_{Na}/\Delta g_K$, is about 1.3 (Box 11.4). The channel opened by ACh is, in fact, nearly equally permeable to sodium and potassium.[39,40] However, taking the extracellular and intracellular solutions together, there are more sodium than potassium ions available to move through the channels (see Chapter 6). Thus, for the same permeability change, the sodium conductance change is slightly larger (see Chapter 4).

Resting Membrane Conductance and Synaptic Potential Amplitude

The electrical circuit shown in Figure 11.9A can be simplified by representing the resting membrane as a single conductance, g_{rest} (equal to the sum of all the ion conductances), and a single battery, V_{rest} (equal to the resting membrane potential). Likewise, the synaptic membrane can be represented by a single conductance, Δg_s, and a battery whose voltage is equal to the reversal potential, V_r (Figure 11.9B). A feature of this electrical circuit is that the amplitude of a synaptic potential depends on both Δg_s and g_{rest}.

[39] Takeuchi, N. 1963. *J. Physiol.* 167: 128-140.

[40] Adams, D. J., Dwyer, T. M., and Hille, B. 1980. *J. Gen. Physiol.* 75: 493-510.

BOX 11.4   Electrical Model of the Motor End Plate

How did A. and N. Takeuchi calculate the ratio of sodium to potassium conductance for the channels opened by acetylcholine (ACh)? They proposed an electrical model of the muscle cell membrane similar to that shown in Figure 11.9A. Although ACh receptors do not form separate pathways for sodium and potassium, the two ions move through the channel independently. Therefore, the synaptic conductance and reversal potential can be represented by separate conductances (Δg_{Na} and Δg_K) and driving potentials (E_{Na} and E_K) for sodium and potassium. Accordingly, separate expressions can be written for the sodium and potassium currents (ΔI_{Na} and ΔI_K):

$$\Delta INa = \Delta gNa(Vm - ENa)$$

$$\Delta IK = \Delta gK(Vm - EK)$$

These equations provide a means of determining the relative conductance changes to sodium and potassium produced by ACh once the reversal potential (V_r) is determined. Since the Takeuchis considered only *changes* in current resulting from the action of ACh, they could ignore the resting membrane channels. The net synaptic current is zero at the reversal potential; therefore, at this potential the inward sodium current is exactly equal and opposite to the outward potassium current. So when $V_m = V_r$,

$$\Delta gNa(Vr - ENa) = -\Delta gK(Vr - EK)$$

It follows that

$$\frac{\Delta g_{Na}}{\Delta g_K} = \frac{-(V_r - E_K)}{-(V_r - E_{Na})}$$

We can rearrange the equations regarding synaptic sodium and potassium currents to predict the reversal potential when the relative conductances are known:

$$V_r = \frac{g_{Na}E_{Na} + \Delta g_K E_K}{(\Delta g_{Na} + \Delta g_K)}$$

Thus, the reversal potential is simply the average of the individual equilibrium potentials, weighted by the relative conductance changes. This relationship can be extended to include any number or variety of ions, so it is applicable at any synapse where transmitters produce a change in conductance of the postsynaptic membrane to one or more ions. This relationship was found to predict how changes in E_{Na} and E_K, produced by changes in extracellular concentrations of sodium and potassium, affected the reversal potential at the neuromuscular junction.[30]

Such predictions were accurate only for small changes in extracellular sodium and potassium, however, because channel conductance is determined in part by ion concentration (see Chapters 4 and 6). Therefore, the effect of a large change in sodium, potassium, or calcium concentration on reversal potential is predicted accurately only if the resulting change in conductance is taken into account. Alternatively, the analysis can be made in terms of permeabilities, using the constant field equation developed by Goldman, Hodgkin, and Katz (see Chapter 6).

For simplicity, consider the steady-state membrane potential that would develop if the synaptic conductance were activated for a long period of time. If Δg_s were much larger than g_{rest}, then the membrane potential would approach V_r. However, if Δg_s were equal to g_{rest}, then the change in membrane potential produced by activating the synaptic conductance would be only one-half as great. Thus, the amplitude of a synaptic potential can be increased by either increasing the synaptic conductance (i.e., activating more synaptic channels) or by decreasing the resting conductance. Indeed, a reduction in membrane conductance is an important mechanism for modulating synaptic strength. For example, certain inputs to autonomic ganglion cells in the bullfrog can *close* potassium channels, thereby increasing the amplitude of excitatory synaptic potentials produced by other inputs to the cell (see Chapter 19). Similarly, an excitatory current of a given amplitude will give rise to a larger depolarization in a small neuron than in a large one that has a lower input resistance (see Chapter 8).

Kinetics of Currents through Single ACh Receptor Channels

To what extent does the time course of the end plate current reflect the behavior of individual ACh channels? For example, do individual channels open and close repetitively during the end plate current, with the probability of channel opening declining with time? Or do individual channels open only once, so that the time course of the current is determined by how long channels remain open?

Definitive answers to such questions came only with the advent of patch clamp techniques, by which the behavior of individual channels could be observed directly (see Chapter 4).[41] When ACh was applied continuously, ACh channels were shown to open instantaneously, in an all-or-nothing fashion, and then close at a rate that matched exactly the rate of decay of the end plate current.[42,43] These observations can be interpreted according to the following scheme for the interaction between the transmitter molecule A (for agonist) and the postsynaptic receptor molecule R (for receptor):

$$A+R \underset{k_{-1}}{\overset{k_1}{\longleftrightarrow}} AR+A \underset{k_{-2}}{\overset{k_2}{\longleftrightarrow}} A_2R \underset{\alpha}{\overset{\beta}{\longleftrightarrow}} A_2R^*$$
$$\textit{shut} \qquad\quad \textit{shut} \qquad\quad \textit{shut} \qquad\quad \textit{open}$$

In this scheme, two ACh molecules sequentially combine with the channel (one on each α-subunit; see Chapter 5). With only one ACh molecule bound, the channel does not open (or opens very rarely). However, when the second ACh molecule binds, the channel undergoes a very fast (microseconds[44]) change in conformation from the closed (A_2R) to the open (A_2R^*) state. The transitions between the open and closed states are characterized by the rate constants α and β, as indicated. Now consider the total time course of the end plate current, as illustrated in Figure 11.10. ACh arriving at the postsynaptic membrane opens a large number of channels almost simultaneously. Because ACh is lost rapidly from the synaptic cleft (through hydrolysis by the enzyme cholinesterase and by diffusion), each receptor is activated only once. As the channels close, the synaptic current declines. Thus, the time course of decay of the end plate current reflects the rate at which individual ACh channels close. Channels close at the rate $\alpha[A_2R^*]$; that is, many channels close very quickly, and fewer and fewer channels close at longer and longer times. As with all independent or random events,

[41] Neher, E., and Sakmann, B. 1976. *Nature* 260: 799–802.

[42] Dionne, V. E., and Leibowitz, M. D. 1982. *Biophys. J.* 39: 253–261.

[43] Sakmann, B. 1992. *Neuron* 8: 613–629.

[44] Sivilotti, L., and Colquhoun, D. 2016. *J. Gen. Physiol.* 148: 79–88.

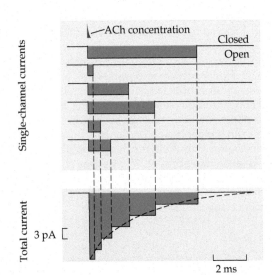

FIGURE 11.10 Total End Plate Current Is the Sum of Individual Channel Currents. Current flow through six individual channels is depicted in the top panel. Channels open instantaneously in response to ACh (added at the red marker point). ACh is rapidly hydrolyzed, so its concentration falls quickly (red marker), preventing any further channel openings. Channel open times are distributed exponentially. The individual channel currents sum to give the total end plate current (lower panel). The time constant of the decay of the total current is equal to the mean open time of the individual channels.

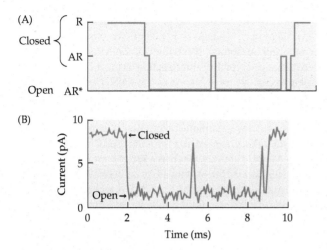

(A)

Closed { R / AR

Open   AR*

(B)

FIGURE 11.11   End Plate Nicotinic Acetylcholine Receptors Open in Bursts. (A) Predicted burst of three openings (AR*) assuming the fastest possible binding rate (5 × 10⁸ moles⁻¹ s⁻¹). The channel flips briefly to the ACh-bound state but returns to the shut (AR) state twice before the acetylcholine dissociates and the channel reverts to the R state. (B) High-resolution recording of an equivalent three-opening burst with two brief closures from a frog end plate receptor activated by the nicotinic agonist suberyldicholine. (Adapted from D. Colquhoun, 2007. *J. Physiol.* 581: 425-427; D. Colquhoun and B. Sakmann, 1985. *J. Physiol.* 369: 501-557.)

the open times are distributed exponentially, and the mean open time (τ) is equal to the time constant of the exponential decay of the end plate current, ($1/\alpha$).

With improved time resolution, it was discovered that many of these apparent single-channel openings were interrupted by one or more brief closures.[45,46] In other words, instead of having just a single opening, the ACh-bound channel can give a short burst of two or more openings (Figure 11.11). This may be explained by supposing that when the channel has reverted to the shut (A_2R) state, instead of just going back to the mono-liganded shut state AR, it can flicker back and forth a few times to the open state A_2R^* before an ACh molecule dissociates. The reason for this is that the conformational opening rate constant β is similar to the dissociation rate constant k_{-2}. This means that the original open channel lifetime (as depicted in Figure 11.11) is actually the mean burst length. This is clearly longer than the duration of a single channel opening by an amount which depends on the values of the rate constants for the open-closed channel conformational states (α,β)[47] and the rate constant for biliganded ACh-receptor unbinding (k_{-2}):

$$\tau_{(burst)} = \frac{1}{\alpha}\left(1 + \frac{\beta}{2k_{-2}}\right) + \frac{1}{\beta + 2k_{-2}}\left(\frac{\beta}{2k_{-2}}\right)$$

It is worth noting that an ACh receptor channel open for a millisecond at –70 mV will conduct about 20,000 cations into the cell—10,000 ions for each ACh molecule that binds to the receptor, which is an enormous signal amplification.

The properties of ACh receptors change during development. There is a fetal form of the ACh receptor, which has a low conductance and a long and variable open time, and an adult form, which has a higher conductance and shorter open time.[48] The switch from embryonic to adult receptors is caused by a change in subunit composition (see Chapter 5), and splice variants of one of the embryonic subunits may account for variation in channel mean open time early in development.[49] The change in properties is well adapted to the need for adequate current to stimulate the larger, fully developed muscle fibers.

Excitatory Synaptic Potentials in the CNS

The principles of synaptic excitation in the CNS follow those elucidated so beautifully at the neuromuscular junction: A pulse of transmitter released from the presynaptic bouton opens cation-selective channel receptors in the postsynaptic membrane. These receptors generate an inward **excitatory postsynaptic current (EPSC)**, which in turn depolarizes the postsynaptic membrane to produce an excitatory postsynaptic potential (EPSP).

However, there are important differences between neuromuscular and CNS synapses. The first essential difference is that the principal excitatory transmitter in the CNS is L-glutamate, not acetylcholine. Second, glutamate activates three different types of ionotropic glutamate receptors (so named after its selective agonists); kainate

[45] Colquhoun, D., and Sakmann, B. 1981. *Nature* 294: 464-466.

[46] Colquhoun, D., and Sakmann, B. 1985. *J. Physiol.* 369: 501-557.

[47] Colquhoun, D. and Hawkes, A. G. 1981. *Proc. R. Soc. Lond. B* 211: 205-235.

[48] Mishina, M. et al. 1986. *Nature* 321: 406-411.

[49] Herlitze, S. et al. 1996. *J. Physiol.* 492: 775-787.

[50] Watkins, J. C., and Evans, R. H. 1981. *Annu. Rev. Pharmacol. Toxicol.* 21: 165-204.

[51] Sah, P., Hestrin, S., and Nicoll, R. A. 1990. *J. Physiol.* 430: 605-616.

[52] Wollmuth, L. P., and Sobolevsky, A. I. 2004. *Trends Neurosci.* 27: 321-328.

[53] Edmonds, B., Gibb, A. J., and Colquhoun, D. 1995. *Annu. Rev. Physiol.* 57: 495-519.

[54] Hansen K. B, et al. 2018. *J Gen Physiol.* 150: 1081-1105.

[55] Johnson, J. W., and Ascher, P. 1987. *Nature.* 325: 529-531.

[56] Papouin, T. et al. 2012. *Cell* 150: 633-646.

[57] Nowak, L. et al. 1984. *Nature* 307: 462-465.

[58] Mayer, M. L., Westbrook, G. L., and Guthrie, P. B. 1984. *Nature* 309: 261-263.

receptors, α-amino-3-hydroxy-5-methyl-4-isoxazolepropionic acid (AMPA) receptors, and *N*-methyl-D-aspartate (NMDA) receptors[50,51] (Figure 11.12). These receptors are not structurally homologous with the nicotinic receptor.[52] Nevertheless, the AMPA receptor has similar permeability characteristics and serves the same function as the nicotinic receptor, which is to mediate fast transient excitatory transmission in the CNS. Thus, fast synaptic potentials evoked by glutamate can be reconstructed from the kinetics of AMPA receptor channels,[53] just as with end plate nicotinic channels.

The NMDA glutamate receptor has several unique properties. It is composed of two GluN1 subunits and two GluN2 subunits, arranged as a tetramer (see Chapter 5).[54] The transmitter glutamate binds to the GluN2 subunits, whereas a second amino acid, glycine or D-serine, binds to the GluN1 subunits acting as obligatory co-agonists.[55,56] Another unusual feature is that, at the normal resting potential, the NMDA receptor is tonically blocked by magnesium ions from the extracellular fluid,[57,58] which means that, even when it is activated, no current flows until the cell is depolarized from the normal resting potential toward zero (see Figure 11.12). The reason is that the positive Mg^{2+} ions bind tightly in the channel when pulled into it by the normal transmembrane electrical gradient; however, this pull is reduced and the Mg^{2+} ions dissociate when the electrical gradient is reduced. This confers a form of **rectification** to the current–voltage curve, the inward (cation) current diminishing as the membrane potential becomes progressively more inside-negative.[57] Figure 11.13 shows that the affinity of the channel for Mg^{2+} ions, and hence the degree of

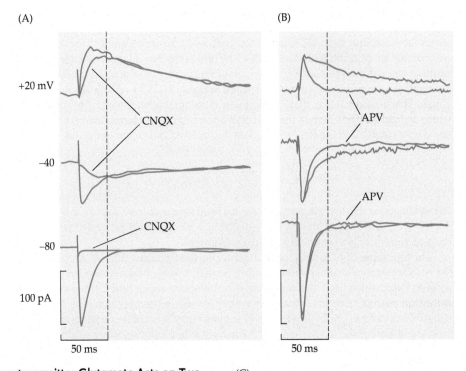

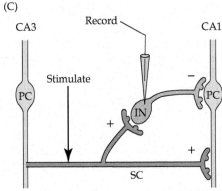

FIGURE 11.12   The Excitatory Neurotransmitter Glutamate Acts on Two Different Receptors to Produce Two Excitatory Postsynaptic Currents (EPSCs). EPSCs were recorded with a patch electrode from an interneuron in the CA1 region of a rat hippocampal slice preparation. The synaptic potentials were produced by stimulating the glutamate-releasing afferent fibers in the Schaffer collaterals. The interneuron membrane potential was held at three different values, -80, -40, and +20 mV. (A) The traces show the effect of blocking the AMPA receptors with CNQX. This suppressed all of the EPSC at -80 mV but only the first part at +20 mV, leaving a large, slower component. The latter was due to the simultaneous activation of voltage-dependent NMDA receptors, since blocking the NMDA receptors with APV. (B) left a pure, fast AMPA receptor-mediated EPSC. (C) Schematic of recording. PC = pyramidal cells; IN = interneuron; SC = Schaffer collaterals; excitation (+); inhibition (-). (A,B after P. Sah et al., 1990. *J. Physiol.* 430: 605-616.)

rectification, varies with the nature of the GluN2 subunit,[59] which has also been shown by individual subunit genetic deletion.[60]

The natural form of depolarization for unblocking the NMDA channel would be a train of preceding AMPA receptor–mediated synaptic potentials. This voltage sensitivity also means that the NMDA receptor contributes very little to normal fast signaling between brain cells—only the AMPA receptor does this. Furthermore, the NMDA channels gate rather slowly,[53] which means they open more during high-frequency synaptic activity. Also, their open time is much longer than in the AMPA receptors. As with the rectification, the duration for which the channels stay open depends on the nature of the GluN2 subunit.[59] Finally, the NMDA receptors have an unusually high permeability to calcium ions[61] and can thereby generate large increases in intracellular calcium concentration; this has several downstream messenger effects on neuronal function (see Chapter 14). All of these properties confer on the NMDA glutamate receptor a special role in synaptic development and plasticity (see Chapters 16 and 27).

In the CNS, the majority of excitatory synapses are located on the dendrites of the neurons. Synaptic potentials spread down the dendrites and through the soma to the normal site of action potential initiation at the axon hillock or axon initial segment.[62] In almost all neurons, a single synaptic EPSP is far too small to initiate an action potential; to reach threshold, the individual EPSPs have to be summated and integrated in the somato-dendritic region. In many neurons, such as the pyramidal cells of the hippocampus and cerebral cortex, and the Purkinje cells of the cerebellum, the excitatory synapses are

[59] Monyer, H. et al. 1994. *Neuron* 12: 529–540.

[60] Zhang, Y. et al. 2012. *PLoS ONE* 7: e41908.

[61] Burnashev, N. 1996. *Curr. Opin. Neurobiol.* 6: 311–317.

[62] Coombs, J. S., Curtis, D. R., and Eccles, J. C. 1957. *J. Physiol.* 139: 232–249.

[63] Spruston, N. 2008. *Nat. Rev. Neurosci.* 9: 206–221.

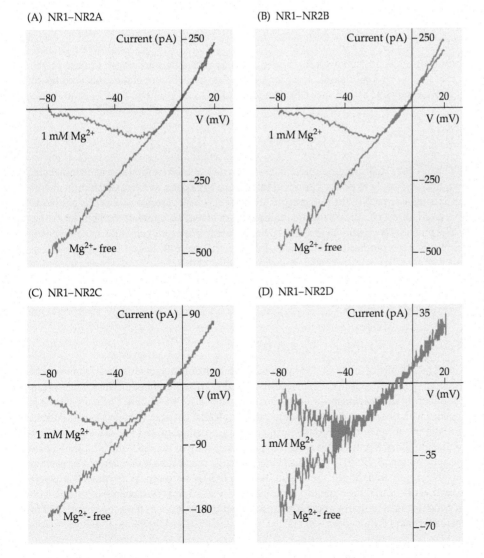

FIGURE 11.13   Mg²⁺-Dependent Rectification of Current-Voltage Curves for Recombinant NMDA Receptors. Receptors were expressed in human embryonic kidney (HEK) cells by transfecting cDNA for the GluN1 subunit together with cDNA for the following GluN2 subunits: (A) GluN2A; (B) GluN2B; (C) GluN2C; (D) GluN2D. The HEK cells were then patched with a whole-cell patch pipette to record currents through the expressed channels. Records show currents (ordinates, pA) generated by changing the membrane potential (abscissae) between –80 and +20 mV, in the presence and absence of 1 mM external Mg²⁺. Note that the currents are linearly dependent on membrane voltage in the absence of external Mg²⁺ but strongly rectify at negative potentials in the presence of Mg²⁺. Note also that current scales are smaller in (C) and (D). (After H. Monyer et al., 1994. *Neuron* 12: 529-540.)

FIGURE 11.14 Dendritic Spines and Excitatory Spine Synapses in Hippocampal Pyramidal Neurons. (A) Dendrites labeled with red Alexa 594 and counterstained for green fluorescent protein (GFP)-labeled actin-binding protein. The latter is concentrated in the dendritic spines (white arrows). (B) Electron micrographs of vesicle-filled synaptic boutons contacting dendritic spines. The red arrows mark the postsynaptic spine apparatus projecting toward the punctum adherens (point of pre- and postsynaptic membrane adhesion). (A after K. Zito et al., 2004. *Neuron* 44: 321–334; B after J. Spacek and K. M. Harris, 1998. *J. Comp. Neurol.* 393: 58–68.)

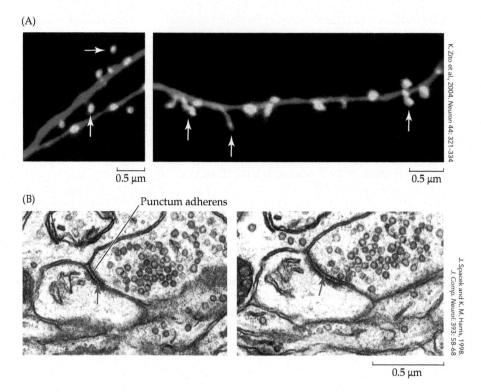

(A)

0.5 μm   0.5 μm

K. Zito et al., 2004. *Neuron* 44: 321–334

(B)

Punctum adherens

0.5 μm

J. Spacek and K. M. Harris, 1998. *J. Comp. Neurol.* 393: 58–68

located on small projections from the dendrites termed dendritic spines[63] (Figure 11.14). These spines play a special role in the long-term changes in brain function that accompany and follow synaptic activity (see Chapters 16 and 17).

Direct Chemical Synaptic Inhibition

The principles that underlie direct chemical synaptic excitation at the neuromuscular junction also apply to **direct chemical inhibitory synapses**. Whereas excitation occurs by opening channels in the postsynaptic membrane whose reversal potential is *positive* to threshold, direct chemical synaptic inhibition is achieved by opening channels whose reversal potential is *negative* to threshold. Direct chemical synaptic inhibition occurs by activating channels permeable to chloride—an anion that typically has an equilibrium potential at or near the resting potential. Pioneering studies of direct chemical synaptic inhibition were made on the crustacean neuromuscular junction,[64,65] the crayfish stretch receptor,[66] and spinal motoneurons of the cat, at which γ-aminobutyric acid (GABA) and glycine are the principal transmitters.[67]

Reversal of Inhibitory Potentials

Spinal motoneurons are inhibited by sensory inputs from antagonistic muscles, by way of inhibitory interneurons in the spinal cord. The effect of activation of inhibitory inputs can be studied by an experiment similar to that illustrated in Figure 11.15A. The motoneuron is impaled with two micropipettes—one to record potential changes, the other to pass current through the cell membrane. At the normal resting potential (about –75 mV), stimulation of the inhibitory inputs causes a slight hyperpolarization of the cell—the inhibitory postsynaptic potential (IPSP) (Figure 11.15B). When the membrane is depolarized by passing positive current into the cell, the amplitude of the IPSP is increased. When the cell is hyperpolarized to –82 mV, the inhibitory potential is very small and reversed in sign, and at –100 mV the reversed inhibitory potential is increased in amplitude. The reversal potential in this experiment is thus about –80 mV.

[64] Dudel, J., and Kuffler, S. W. 1961. *J. Physiol.* 155: 543–562.

[65] Takeuchi, A., and Takeuchi, N. 1967. *J. Physiol.* 191: 575–590.

[66] Kuffler, S. W., and Eyzaguirre, C. 1955. *J. Gen. Physiol.* 39: 155–184.

[67] Coombs, J. S., Eccles, J. C., and Fatt, P. 1955. *J. Physiol.* 130: 326–373.

[68] Hille, B. 2001. *Ion Channels of Excitable Membranes*, 3rd ed. Oxford University Press/Sinauer, Sunderland, MA.

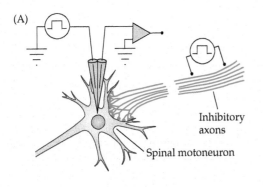

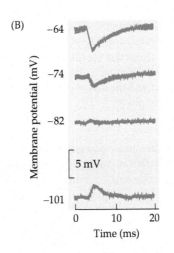

FIGURE 11.15   Direct Inhibitory Chemical Synaptic Transmission. (A) Scheme for intracellular recording from a cat spinal motoneuron and stimulation of inhibitory synaptic inputs. The membrane potential of the motoneuron is set to different levels by passing current through a second intracellular microelectrode. (B) Intracellular records of inhibitory postsynaptic potentials evoked at membrane potentials between –64 and –101 mV. The reversal potential is between –74 and –82 mV. (After J. S. Coombs et al., 1955. *J. Physiol.* 130: 326-373.)

Inhibitory channels are permeable to anions, with permeabilities roughly correlated with the hydrated radius of the penetrating ion.[68] In physiological circumstances, the only small anion present in any quantity is chloride. Thus, in spinal motoneurons injection of chloride into the cell from a micropipette shifts the chloride equilibrium potential, and hence the reversal potential for the inhibitory synaptic potential, toward zero (i.e., in the positive direction). In other preparations, changes in extracellular chloride have been shown to produce corresponding changes in the chloride equilibrium potential and the IPSP reversal potential, but such experiments often give ambiguous results. This is because changes in extracellular chloride concentration lead eventually to proportionate changes in intracellular concentration as well (see Chapter 6), so any change in chloride equilibrium potential is only transient.

One way around this difficulty is to remove chloride entirely, as shown in Figure 11.16. The records are from a reticulospinal cell in the brainstem of the lamprey, in which inhibitory synaptic transmission is mediated by glycine.[69] Membrane potential was recorded with an intracellular microelectrode. A second electrode was used to pass brief hyperpolarizing current pulses into the cell; the resulting changes in potential provided a measure of the cell's input resistance. Finally, a third micropipette was used to apply glycine to the cell close to an inhibitory synapse, using brief pressure pulses. Glycine application resulted in a slight hyperpolarization, with a marked reduction in input resistance (see Figure 11.16A), as would be expected if glycine activated a large number of chloride channels. To test this idea, chloride was removed from the bathing solution and replaced by the impermeant ion isethionate. As a result, intracellular chloride was also removed by efflux through chloride channels open at rest. After 20 minutes, glycine application produced no detectable change in membrane potential or input resistance (see Figure 11.16B), indicating that no ions other than chloride

[69]Gold, M. R., and Martin, A. R. 1983. *J. Physiol.* 342: 99-117.

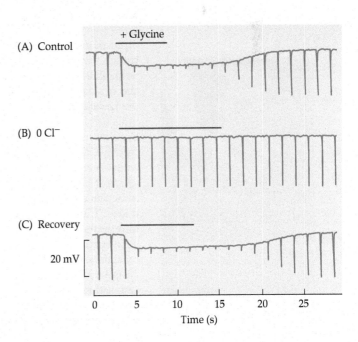

FIGURE 11.16   Inhibitory Response to Glycine Depends on Chloride. Intracellular microelectrode recordings from a neuron in the brainstem of the lamprey. (A) Resting membrane potential is –63 mV. Brief downward voltage deflections are produced by 10-nA current pulses from a second intracellular microelectrode; their amplitude indicates membrane resistance. On application of glycine (red bar), the cell is hyperpolarized by about 7 mV, and membrane resistance is reduced drastically. (B) After 20 minutes in chloride-free bathing solution, the response to glycine is abolished. (C) Five minutes after return to normal chloride solution, the response has recovered. (After M. R. Gold and A. R. Martin, 1983. *J. Physiol.* 342: 99-117.)

pass through the inhibitory channels. The restoration of normal extracellular chloride concentration (see Figure 11.16C) resulted in restoration of the response.

Given that the inhibitory response involves an increase in chloride permeability, the reversal potential for the inhibitory current will be equal to the chloride equilibrium potential (E_{Cl}), and the magnitude of the current will be given by:

$$\Delta_{\text{inhibitory}} = \Delta I_{Cl} = \Delta g_{Cl}(V_m - E_{Cl})$$

At membrane potentials positive to E_{Cl}, the current is outward, resulting in membrane hyperpolarization. In this case outward current is carried by an influx of negatively charged chloride ions. At membrane potentials negative to E_{Cl}, inhibition causes an efflux of chloride ions, resulting in depolarization.

Early in postnatal development of the mammalian CNS, GABA and glycine paradoxically depolarize and thereby excite neurons in the CNS.[70] This effect is due not to differences in the properties of the channels opened by GABA and glycine, but to a difference in the nature of a transporter that regulates the intracellular chloride concentration[71] (see Chapter 9). In embryonic neurons, chloride is transported into the neuron by a sodium–potassium–2-chloride cotransporter (NKCC), thereby generating a high intracellular chloride concentration. Because E_{Cl} is positive to V_m, activation of chloride channels by GABA or glycine then results in outward movement of chloride and hence depolarization. At birth and during early postnatal development, another transporter, a potassium–chloride cotransporter (KCC2), becomes expressed. This extrudes chloride from the neuron. E_{Cl} then becomes negative to E_m, so GABA or glycine will now hyperpolarize the cell. This chloride switch is important in brain development because GABA-releasing synapses develop earlier than glutamate-releasing synapses in the brain, so the ability of GABA to depolarize and excite embryonic neurons (and thereby to increase intracellular calcium) is thought to be crucial for the proper embryonic development of synapses and circuits.[70] However, the postnatal switch from depolarization to hyperpolarization is essential for the normal function of inhibitory circuits after birth. Thus, mice in which both genes for the outward chloride transporter KCC2 have been deleted (and so do not express any KCC2 protein) die shortly after birth because their normal central respiratory circuits do not work (see Chapter 26) and they cannot breathe.[72] The chloride transporters are capable of maintaining different intracellular chloride concentrations in neuronal processes from those in the soma.[73–75] However, in mammalian peripheral neurons and nerve fibers (which have GABA receptors but no GABAergic synapses), E_{Cl} is always depolarized to E_m, even in adult animals.[76,77]

Presynaptic Inhibition

So far we have defined excitatory and inhibitory synapses on the basis of the effect of the transmitter on the postsynaptic membrane—that is, based on whether the postsynaptic permeability change is to cations or to anions. However, several early experiments indicated that in some instances it was difficult to account for inhibition in terms of postsynaptic permeability changes alone.[78,79] The paradox was resolved by the discovery of an additional inhibitory mechanism, **presynaptic inhibition**,[80] described in the mammalian spinal cord by Frank and Fuortes[79] and by Eccles and his colleagues,[81] and at the crustacean neuromuscular junction by Dudel and Kuffler.[64] Presynaptic inhibition results in a reduction in the amount of transmitter released from excitatory nerve terminals.[82]

As shown in Figure 11.17, the action of the inhibitory nerve at the crustacean neuromuscular junction is exerted not only on the muscle fibers, but also on the excitatory terminals. The presynaptic effect is brief, reaching a peak in a few milliseconds and declining to zero after a total of 6 to 7 ms. For the maximum inhibitory effect to occur, the impulse must arrive in the inhibitory presynaptic terminal several milliseconds before the action potential arrives in the excitatory terminal. Timing is important, as shown in Figure 11.17. Parts A and B of the figure show the excitatory and inhibitory potentials following separate stimulation of the corresponding nerves. In part C, both nerves are stimulated, but the action potential in the inhibitory nerve follows that in the excitatory nerve by 1.5 ms, arriving too late to exert any effect. In Figure 11.17D, by contrast, the action potential in the inhibitory nerve precedes that in the excitatory nerve and now strongly reduces the excitatory

[70] Ben-Ari, Y. et al. 2007. *Physiol. Rev.* 87: 1215–1284.

[71] Payne, J. A. et al. 2003. *Trends Neurosci.* 26: 199–206.

[72] Hübner, C. A. et al. 2001. *Neuron* 30: 515–524.

[73] Price, G. D., and Trussell, L. O. 2006. *J. Neurosci.* 26: 11432–11436.

[74] Khirug, S. et al. 2008. *J. Neurosci.* 28: 4635–4639.

[75] Trigo, F. F., Marty, A., and Stell, B. M. 2008. *Eur. J. Neurosci.* 28: 841–848.

[76] Adams, P. R., and Brown, D. A. 1975. *J. Physiol.* 250: 85–120.

[77] Gallagher, J. P., Higashi, H., and Nishi, S. 1978. *J. Physiol.* 275: 263–282.

[78] Fatt, P., and Katz, B. 1953. *J. Physiol.* 121: 374–389.

[79] Frank, K., and Fuortes, M. G. F. 1957. *Fed. Proc.* 16: 39–40.

[80] Rudomin, P. 2009. *Exp. Brain Res.* 196: 139–151.

[81] Eccles, J. C., Eccles, R. M., and Magni, F. 1961. *J. Physiol.* 159: 147–166.

[82] Kuno, M. 1964. *J. Physiol.* 175: 100–112.

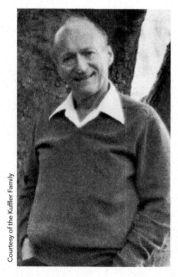

Courtesy of the Kuffler Family

Stephen W. Kuffler in 1975

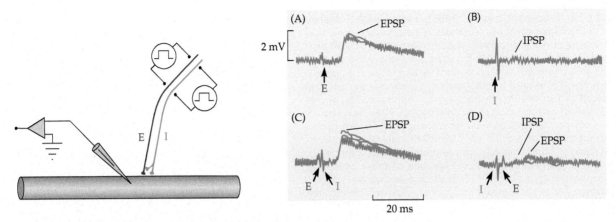

FIGURE 11.17 Presynaptic Inhibition in a Crustacean Muscle Fiber Innervated by One Excitatory and One Inhibitory Axon. (A) Stimulation of the excitatory axon (E) produces a 2-mV EPSP. (B) Stimulation of the inhibitory axon (I) produces a depolarizing IPSP of about 0.2 mV. (C) If the inhibitory stimulus follows the excitatory one by a short interval, there is no effect on the EPSP. (D) If the inhibitory stimulus precedes the excitatory one by a few milliseconds, the EPSP is almost abolished. The importance of precise timing indicates that the inhibitory nerve is having a presynaptic effect, reducing the amount of excitatory neurotransmitter that is released. (After J. Dudel and S. W. Kuffler, 1961. *J. Physiol.* 155: 543-562.)

postsynaptic potential. The presynaptic effect, like that on the postsynaptic membrane, is mediated by GABA, and is associated with a marked increase in chloride permeability in the presynaptic terminals.[83,84]

In the nervous system in general, presynaptic and postsynaptic inhibition serve quite different functions. Postsynaptic inhibition reduces the excitability of the entire cell, rendering it relatively less responsive to all excitatory inputs. Presynaptic inhibition is much more specific, aimed at a particular input and leaving the postsynaptic cell free to go about its business of integrating information from other sources.[85] Presynaptic inhibition implies that inhibitory axons make synaptic contact with axon terminals. Such axo–axonic synapses have been demonstrated directly by electron microscopy at the crustacean neuromuscular junction[86] and at numerous locations in the mammalian CNS.[87] Moreover, inhibitory nerve terminals themselves can be influenced presynaptically;[88] the requisite ultrastructural arrangement has been reported at inhibitory synapses on crayfish stretch receptors.[89]

Finally, there is an additional, quite different form of presynaptic inhibition in the mammalian nervous system that does not require the presence of specific presynaptic axo–axonal synapses, and can affect the release of transmitters from both excitatory and inhibitory terminals. This is due to the ability of transmitters (including glutamate[90] and GABA) to spill over from the synaptic cleft, back onto the presynaptic terminals where they activate metabotropic (G protein-coupled) receptors. These receptors, in turn, suppress calcium entry into the terminals and thereby reduce transmitter release (see Chapter 13). An example of this type of feedback inhibition (also called auto-inhibition) at a GABA-releasing synapse in the hippocampus is shown in Figure 11.18. Here, the authors[91] recorded the monosynaptic inhibitory postsynaptic currents from a hippocampal CA1 pyramidal neuron produced by GABA that is released by stimulating fibers in the nearby stratum radiatum. A second stimulus, given 100 ms after the first, produced a much smaller current (a phenomenon called paired-pulse depression; see Figure 11.18A). This depression was due to the spread of the released GABA to the presynaptic terminals, where it activated the metabotropic GABA_B receptor (see Figure 14.5) and so reduced the amount of transmitter released by the second stimulus, as shown schematically in Figure 11.18B. The paired-pulse depression was much reduced when the GABA_B receptors were selectively blocked with the compound 2-hydroxy-saclofen or by CGP 35348. Presynaptic inhibition mediated by metabotropic receptors is slower in onset but lasts much longer than that mediated by ionotropic receptors (shown in Figure 11.17). It needs a minimal interval between the two stimuli of 20 to

[83] Takeuchi, A., and Takeuchi, N. 1966. *J. Physiol.* 183: 433-449.

[84] Fuchs, P. A., and Getting, P. A. 1980. *J. Neurophysiol.* 43: 1547-1557.

[85] Lomeli, J. et al. 1998. *Nature* 395: 600-604.

[86] Atwood, H. L., and Morin, W. A. 1970. *J. Ultrastruct. Res.* 32: 351-369.

[87] Schmidt, R. F. 1971. *Ergeb. Physiol.* 63: 20-101.

[88] Nicholls, J. G., and Wallace, B. G. 1978. *J. Physiol.* 281: 157-170.

[89] Nakajima, Y., Tisdale, A. D., and Henkart, M. P. 1973. *Proc. Natl. Acad. Sci. USA* 70: 2462-2466.

[90] Pinheiro, P. S., and Mulle, C. 2008. *Nat. Rev. Neurosci.* 9: 423-436.

[91] Davies, C. H., and Collingridge, G. L. 1993. *J. Physiol.* 472: 245-265.

FIGURE 11.18 Presynaptic Auto-Inhibition at a GABA-Releasing Synapse in the Hippocampus. (A) Inhibitory synaptic currents (IPSCs) in a pyramidal neuron of a hippocampal slice preparation produced by two successive stimuli, delivered 100 ms apart, to inhibitory fibers in the adjacent stratum oriens. Excitatory currents were blocked with glutamate antagonists. The IPSC evoked by the second stimulus is much smaller than that produced by the first stimulus (paired-pulse depression). This depression was largely due to activation of the presynaptic GABA$_B$ receptors, since it was reduced by blocking these receptors with GABA$_B$ antagonists (0.2 mM 2-hydroxy-saclofen or 0.2 mM CGP 35348; right-hand panels). (B) GABA released from the presynaptic terminal activates chloride-conducting GABA$_A$ receptors on the postsynaptic membrane, producing an inhibitory postsynaptic current (IPSC). It also activates metabotropic GABA$_B$ receptors on the presynaptic ending that inhibit calcium channels and reduce transmitter release. (A after C. H. Davies and G. L. Collingridge, 1993. *J. Physiol.* 472: 245–265.)

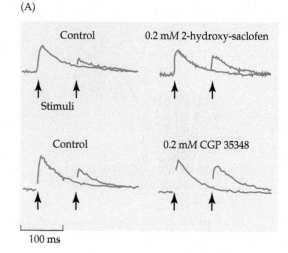

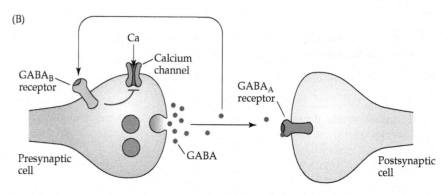

30 ms to take effect, is maximal at around 100 ms, and lasts up to a second or more. The delayed onset reflects the time it takes for the receptor to activate a G protein and inhibit the calcium channels, while the slow offset is due to the slow kinetics of G protein recovery, as we will discuss in Chapter 12.

Transmitter Receptor Localization

Figures 11.6 and 11.7 show that the acetylcholine receptors (AChRs) are highly concentrated at the motor end plate. This is because they are aggregated into a specialized postsynaptic apparatus formed by cytoskeletal, membrane, and membrane-associated proteins (Figure 11.19).[92,93] At the mammalian neuromuscular junction the acetylcholine receptors are retained in the postsynaptic complex for several days (half-time 4.7 days);[94] by contrast, the residence half-time of the extrasynaptic receptors is about a day, which is similar to the turnover time of most membrane proteins. Within the postsynaptic apparatus, a 43-kilodalton (kD) AChR-associated protein called rapsyn and components of the dystrophin complex play a key role in AChR localization. The dystrophin complex, which links together the myofiber cytoskeleton, membrane, and surrounding extracellular matrix, also provides structural support for the muscle cell.[95] Mutations in components of this complex give rise to Duchenne muscular dystrophy, in which muscle fibers are damaged and degenerate.[96] The dystrophin complex is also involved in the maintenance of some synapses in the CNS and in the localization of aquaporin water channels, so its disruption can cause a variety of nervous system disorders.[97] When a motor nerve is cut and allowed to degenerate (see Chapter 30), the AChR clustering mechanism at the end plate is disrupted such that the receptor lifetime is shortened.[98] At the same time, the number of extrajunctional receptors increases, causing denervation supersensitivity,[99] and their subunit composition reverts to the embryonic type as a result of a change in transcription.[100]

[92] Sanes, J. R., and Lichtman, J. W. 2001. *Nat. Rev. Neurosci.* 2: 791–805.

[93] Banks, G. B. et al. 2003. *J. Neurocytol.* 32: 709–726.

[94] Akaaboune, M. et al. 2002. *Neuron* 34: 865–876.

[95] Blake, D. J. et al. 2003. *Physiol. Rev.* 82: 291–329.

[96] Davies, K. E., and Nowak, K. J. 2006. *Nat. Rev. Mol. Cell Biol.* 7: 762–773.

[97] Waite, A. et al. 2009. *Ann. Med.* 41: 344–359.

[98] Loring, R. H., and Salpeter, M. M. 1980. *Proc. Natl. Acad. Sci. USA* 77: 2293–2297.

[99] Axelsson, J., and Thesleff, S. 1959. *J. Physiol.* 147: 178–193.

[100] Witzemann, V., Brenner, H. R., and Sakmann, B. 1991. *J. Cell Biol.* 114: 125–141.

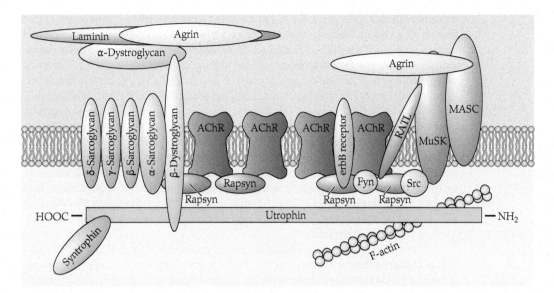

FIGURE 11.19   Postsynaptic Components of AChR-Rich Regions at the Vertebrate Skeletal Neuromuscular Junction. The dystrophin glycoprotein complex (utrophin, α- and β-dystroglycan, and the sarcoglycans) links together the actin cytoskeleton, the membrane, and the extracellular matrix. Agrin, secreted by the motor nerves, binds to laminin and α-dystroglycan; it signals, through the receptor tyrosine kinase MuSK, to trigger formation of the postsynaptic apparatus during development (see Chapter 25). Rapsyn plays a key role in linking MuSK and AChRs to the cytoskeleton. RATL and MASC are as yet unidentified components that mediate interaction of MuSK with rapsyn and agrin, respectively. Src, Fyn and ErbB are tyrosine kinases. For further details, see Figure 27.12, and J. R. Sanes and J. W. Lichtman, 2001. *Nat. Rev. Neurosci.* 2: 791–805. (After G. B. Banks et al., 2003. *J. Neurocytol.* 32: 709–726.)

The postsynaptic apparatus at excitatory synapses in the CNS is also a complex structure, containing more than 200 proteins as determined by mass spectrometry.[101,102] Three families of these proteins interact with glutamate receptors in the postsynaptic density (Figure 11.20).[103] Proteins in each of the families have one or more PDZ domains, which are conserved regions that mediate protein–protein interactions. PDZ is an acronym for three

[101] Collins, M. O. et al. 2006. *J. Neurochem.* 97: 16–23.

[102] Cheng, D. et al. 2006. *Mol. Cell. Proteomics* 5: 1158–1170.

[103] Kim, E., and Sheng, M. 2004. *Nat. Rev. Neurosci.* 5: 771–781.

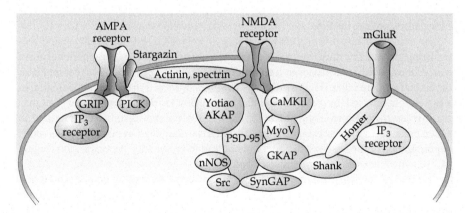

FIGURE 11.20   Glutamate Receptors Are Linked to a Postsynaptic Scaffold that includes proteins involved in intracellular signaling cascades. Metabotropic glutamate receptors, mGluRs, are described in Chapter 12. Stargazin is an ancillary protein that is required for normal trafficking and function of AMPA receptors (A. C. Jackson and R. A. Nicoll, 2011. *Neuron* 70: 178–199.). GRIP, PICK, PSD-95, and Homer are PDZ-containing proteins that bind directly to the receptors. Actinin and Shank are proteins that bind to the cytoskeletal protein F-actin.

Yotiao AKAP, GKAP, and synaptic Ras GTPases (SynGAP) are scaffold proteins that anchor and activate enzymes: AKAP binds protein kinases A and C and the protein phosphatase calcineurin; GKAP binds guanylate kinase; and SynGAP binds and activates the small GTPase Ras. nNOS = neuronal nitric oxide synthase; IP_3 = inositol trisphosphate; CaMKII = calmodulin (CaM) kinase II; Src is a small GTPase protein; MyoV (myosin-V) is a actin-based motor protein. (After E. Kim and M. Sheng, 2004. *Nat. Rev. Neurosci.* 5: 771–781.)

proteins with this common domain: *Postsynaptic density-95* (PSD-95); *Drosophila disc protein* (DlgA); and *Zonula occludens-1 protein* (zo-1). NMDA-type glutamate receptors bind to proteins of the PSD-95 family, which are major components of the postsynaptic density. AMPA-type glutamate receptors bind to proteins of the GRIP and PICK families, and metabotropic glutamate receptors bind to members of the Homer protein family. Although AMPA receptors, they bind to scaffolding proteins that localize them to subsynaptic sites, they turn over quite rapidly, and they are free to move in and out of the postsynaptic density (as is necessary for the rapid changes required for synaptic plasticity; see Chapter 17). More important, they recruit important intracellular signaling proteins that modify glutamate receptor function, dendritic architecture, and gene transcription after activation. These signaling proteins include nitric oxide synthase, calmodulin (CaM) kinase II, receptor tyrosine kinases, a guanosine triphosphate (GTP)ase-activating protein for small synaptic Ras GTPases (SynGAP), inositol trisphosphate (IP_3) receptors, and Ras-like small GTPases. Thus, these proteins determine not only receptor location, but also the consequences of receptor activation.

Localization of glycine and GABA receptors at inhibitory synapses in the CNS also requires ancillary subsynaptic proteins.[104,105] Postsynaptic clustering of glycine receptors requires the 93-kD subsynaptic protein gephyrin, which binds to the receptors and connects them to tubulin in the microtubules.[106,107] Thus, clustering is prevented when gephyrin synthesis is inhibited with an antisense nucleotide.[108] Gephyrin also is essential for localization of some $GABA_A$ receptors in postsynaptic membranes, although direct interactions between gephyrin and $GABA_A$ receptor subunits have not been demonstrated.[106] Gephyrin interacts with several intracellular components that mediate responses to activity and trophic factors.[104] Such interactions are thought to play a central role in the assembly and stabilization of postsynaptic specializations at inhibitory synapses.

Electrical Synaptic Transmission

Identification and Characterization of Electrical Synapses

In addition to the chemical transmission seen at most vertebrate synapses, there are places where electrical transmission does occur. Typical places are synapses where electrical transmission assists in coordinating or amplifying the activity of groups of neurons. Others are on reflex pathways where a particularly fast response is necessary (in the retina and the CNS). One characteristic of electrically mediated synaptic transmission is that the current spreads instantaneously from one cell to the next. At chemical synapses, there is a pause of approximately 1 ms between the arrival of an impulse in the presynaptic terminal and the appearance of an electrical potential in the postsynaptic cell. The **synaptic delay** in chemical synapses is due to the time taken for the terminal to release transmitter (see Chapter 13).

An example of fast electrical transmission was provided in 1959 by Furshpan and Potter. Using intracellular microelectrodes to record from nerve fibers in the abdominal nerve cord of the crayfish, they discovered an **electrical synapse** between axons that mediates the animal's escape reflex (Figure 11.21A).[8] They demonstrated that an action potential in a lateral giant fiber led (by direct intercellular current flow) to depolarization of a giant motor fiber leaving the cord (Figure 11.21B). The depolarization was sufficient to initiate an action potential in the postsynaptic fiber. The electrical coupling was in one direction only; depolarization of the postsynaptic fiber did not lead to presynaptic depolarization (Figure 11.21C). In other words, the synapse rectified.

Unlike the crayfish giant motor synapse, many electrical synapses do not exhibit rectification, but conduct equally well in both directions. The morphological specialization for electrical coupling at the crayfish giant motor synapse and other electrical synapses is the **gap junction**[109,110] (see Chapter 8). Gap junctions in vertebrates are formed by an assembly of **connexons**, each composed of six transmembrane connexin molecules that dock with another connexon in the adjacent cell to make a gap junction.[111,112] In invertebrates, gap junctions are formed by non-homologous but structurally somewhat similar innexons[113] comprising eight innexin subunits.[114] It is striking, however, that different molecule families forming gap junctions in vertebrates and invertebrates account for similar functions in both animal groups.

[104] Moss, S. J., and Smart, T. G. 2001. *Nat. Rev. Neurosci.* 2: 240-250.

[105] Kneussel, M., and Loebrich, S. 2007. *Biol. Cell* 99: 297-309.

[106] Sheng, M., and Lee, S. H. 2000. *Nat. Neurosci.* 3: 633-635.

[107] Fritschy, J. M., Harvey, R. J., and Schwarz, G. 2008. *Trends Neurosci.* 31: 257-264.

[108] Kirsch, J. et al. 1993. *Nature* 366: 745-748.

[109] Loewenstein, W. 1981. *Physiol. Rev.* 61: 829-913.

[110] Bennett, M. V. 1997. *J. Neurocytol.* 26: 349-366.

[111] Saez, J. C. et al. 2003. *Physiol. Rev.* 83: 1359-1400.

[112] Söhl, G., Maxeiner, S., and Willecke, K. 2005. *Nat. Rev. Neurosci.* 6: 191-200.

[113] Phelan, P. et al. 1998. *Trends Genet.* 14: 348-349.

[114] Oshima, A. et al. 2016. *J. Mol. Biol.* 428: 1227-1236.

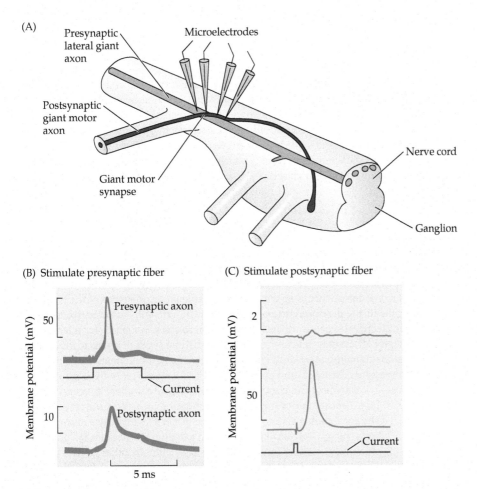

(A)

Presynaptic lateral giant axon

Microelectrodes

Postsynaptic giant motor axon

Giant motor synapse

Nerve cord

Ganglion

(B) Stimulate presynaptic fiber

Presynaptic axon

Membrane potential (mV)

50

Current

10

Postsynaptic axon

5 ms

(C) Stimulate postsynaptic fiber

Membrane potential (mV)

2

50

Current

FIGURE 11.21 Electrical Synaptic Transmission at a Giant Motor Synapse in the Crayfish Central Nervous System. (A) The experimental preparation. The presynaptic lateral giant axon makes an electrical synapse with the postsynaptic giant motor axon in the abdominal nerve cord. (B) Depolarization of the presynaptic axon spreads immediately to the postsynaptic fiber. In this case each cell reaches threshold and fires an action potential. (C) When the postsynaptic axon is stimulated directly to produce an action potential, depolarization spreads poorly from the postsynaptic to the presynaptic axon. The synapse is said to rectify. (After E. J. Furshpan and D. D. Potter, 1959. *J. Physiol.* 145: 289–325.)

The connexons (or innexons) in the membranes of the two connected neurons line up to form a conducting pathway that allows current to pass from the interior of one cell to the next. Rectification probably results from the contributions of different connexins or innexins to the pre- or postsynaptic components of the gap junction.[115,116] In the leech,[117] electrical coupling between pairs of touch sensory neurons has the remarkable property that depolarization spreads readily from either cell to the other, but hyperpolarization spreads poorly; that is, the electrical connections are doubly rectifying (see also Acklin 1988[118]). This may result from the functional contribution of a rectifying innexon to a homomeric assembly of innexin molecules in both pre- and postsynaptic membranes.[119]

Many connexins (especially connexin-36, Cx36) are strongly expressed in the vertebrate CNS,[110,120] and electrical transmission has now been demonstrated at a wide variety of central synapses.[121] Electrical connections are particularly prominent between inhibitory GABA-releasing interneurons in the hippocampus,[121] cerebral cortex,[122] and cerebellum.[123] In the rat somatosensory cortex, a single interneuron may be electrically coupled with up to 10 other interneurons at distances up to 200 μm away, forming mini-networks of 10 to 40 neurons.[124] Their effect is to synchronize interneuronal activity and contribute to some of the synchronized oscillations of electrical activity that can be recorded in these parts of the brain.[125] There is also a particularly rich network of electrical synapses in the retina.[126] The functions of these retinal electrical synapses are diverse. For example, those between horizontal cells greatly extend the cells' receptive fields and enhance the signal/noise ratio for light detection under low-light conditions, while those between amacrine cells and bipolar cells are necessary for rod input to ON bipolar cells (see Chapter 22).

The degree of electrical coupling between cells is usually expressed as a **coupling ratio**. A ratio of 1:4 means that one-fourth of the presynaptic voltage change appears in the postsynaptic cell. For cells to be strongly coupled, the resistance of the junction between the cells must be low. Efficient coupling depends not only on the number of docked connexons

[115]Phelan, P. et al. 2008. *Curr. Biol.* 18: 1955–1960.

[116]Werner, R. et al. 1989. *Proc. Natl. Acad. Sci. USA* 86: 5380–5384.

[117]Baylor, D. A., and Nicholls, J. G. 1969. *J. Physiol.* 203: 591–609.

[118]Acklin, S. E. 1988. *J. Exp. Biol.* 137: 1–11.

[119]Dykes, I. M. et al. 2004. *J. Neurosci.* 24: 886–894.

[120]Bennett, M. V., and Zukin, R. S. 2004. *Neuron* 41: 495–511.

[121]Connors, B. W., and Long, M. A. 2004. *Annu. Rev. Neurosci.* 27: 393–418.

[122]Hestrin S., and Galarreta, M. 2005. *Trends Neurosci.* 28: 304–309.

[123]Dugué, G. P. et al. 2009. *Neuron* 61: 126–139.

[124]Amitai, Y. et al. 2002. *J. Neurosci.* 22: 4142–4152.

[125]Whittington, M. A., and Traub, R. D. 2003. *Trends Neurosci.* 26: 676–682.

[126]Bloomfield, S. A., and Völgyi, B. 2009. *Nat. Rev. Neurosci.* 10: 495–506.

but also on their probability of opening. Thus, the channels can be closed more time (low population conductance) when they are phosphorylated by cyclic adenosine monophosphate (cAMP)-dependent protein kinase. This means that electrical connectivity mediated by gap junctions can be altered by neurotransmitters that affect intracellular calcium or cAMP (see Chapter 12). This occurs in the retina, where light stimulates the release of dopamine from amacrine cells. This increases cAMP in horizontal cells, which in turn activates cAMP-dependent protein kinase. Through the action of the enzyme, the gap junction connexins become phosphorylated, resulting in a decrease in the junctional conductance. As a result, the receptive field of the horizontal cell shrinks. Conversely, reduced dopamine release at night has the opposite effect of increasing the horizontal cell's receptive field and enhancing the detection of dim objects.[126]

Comparison of Electrical and Chemical Transmission

Electrical and chemical transmission often coexist at a single synapse. Such combined electrical and chemical synapses were first found in cells of the avian ciliary ganglion, where a chemical synaptic potential (produced by ACh) is preceded by an electrical coupling potential (Figure 11.22).[9] Similar synapses occur widely in vertebrates—for example, onto spinal interneurons of the lamprey,[127] spinal motoneurons of the frog, and inhibitory cells in the cerebral cortex.[128] Postsynaptic cells may also receive separate chemical and electrical synaptic inputs from different sources. For example, in leech ganglia (see Chapter 20), motor neurons receive three distinct types of synaptic input from sensory neurons signaling three different modalities: One input is chemical, one electrical, and one combined electrical and chemical.[129]

Chemical and electrical synapses are not redundant but complementary. An example of how electrical coupling influences the responses to chemical inputs also comes from the leech. The dendrites of the pair of serotonergic Retzius neurons in each ganglion are electrically coupled. A chemical excitatory input near the gap junction in either neuron permits the flow of synaptic potentials from one neuron to another, thus expanding the dendritic field of both neurons. In addition, the leak of the synaptic current that builds up the EPSP to the coupled neurites reduces the amplitude of the EPSP in proportion to the degree of coupling. Summation of smaller EPSPs when the electrical coupling is high produces a lower basal firing frequency in both neurons than the summation of larger EPSPs when the coupling is low.[130]

The presence of both electrical and chemical transmission at the same synapse provides a convenient means of comparing the two modes of transmission. This is illustrated in Figure 11.22, which shows intracellular records from a cell in the ciliary ganglion of the chick. Stimulation of the preganglionic nerve leads to an action potential in the postsynaptic cell, with very short latency (see Figure 11.22A). When the cell is hyperpolarized slightly (see Figure 11.22B), the action potential arises at a later time,

[127]Rovainen, C. M. 1967. *J. Neurophysiol.* 30: 1024–1042.

[128]Shapovalov, A. I., and Shiriaev, B. I. 1980. *J. Physiol.* 306: 1–15.

[129]Nicholls, J. G., and Purves, D. 1972. *J. Physiol.* 225: 637–656.

[130]Tovar, A. de la Rosa, Mishra, P. K. and De Miguel, F. F. 2016. *Front. Cell. Neurosci.*10: 198.

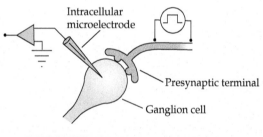

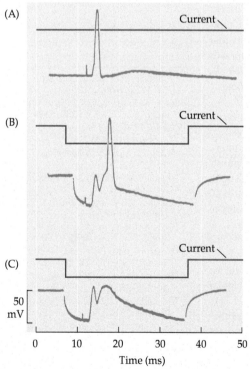

FIGURE 11.22 Electrical and Chemical Synaptic Transmission in a Chick Ciliary Ganglion Cell. (A) Stimulation of the preganglionic nerve produces an action potential in the ganglion cell (blue trace, recorded with an intracellular microelectrode). (B) When the ganglion cell is hyperpolarized by passing current through the recording electrode (red trace), the cell reaches threshold later, revealing an earlier, transient depolarization (blue trace). This depolarization is an electrical synaptic potential (coupling potential), caused by current flow into the ganglion cell from the presynaptic terminal. In (A), the electrical synaptic potential depolarized the ganglion cell to threshold, initiating an action potential. (C) Slightly greater hyperpolarization prevents the ganglion cell from reaching threshold, exposing a slower chemical synaptic potential. The chemical synaptic potential follows the coupling potential with a synaptic delay of about 2 ms at room temperature. (After A. R. Martin and G. Pilar, 1963. *J. Physiol.* 168: 443–463.)

revealing an early, brief depolarization that is now subthreshold because the cell has been hyperpolarized. This depolarization is an electrical coupling potential, produced by current flow from the presynaptic nerve terminal into the cell. Further hyperpolarization (see Figure 11.22C) blocks the initiation of the action potential altogether, revealing the underlying chemical synaptic potential. These cells then have the property that, under normal conditions, initiation of a postsynaptic action potential by chemical transmission is preempted by electrical coupling. In this example the coupling potential precedes the chemical synaptic potential by about 2 ms, providing a direct measure of the synaptic delay. Additional experiments on these cells have shown that the electrical coupling is bidirectional; that is, the synapses do not rectify.

There are several advantages to electrical transmission. One is that electrical synapses are more reliable than chemical synapses; transmission is less likely to fail because of synaptic depression or to be blocked by neurotoxins. A second advantage is the greater speed of electrical transmission. Speed is important in rapid reflexes involving escape reactions, in which the saving of a millisecond may be crucial for surviving an attack by a predator. Other functions include the synchronization of electrical activity of groups of cells[120,121] and intercellular transfer of key molecules, such as calcium, adenosine triphosphate (ATP), and cAMP.[109] Connexons have quite wide pores (12–14 Å),[111] which allow large molecules up to 1 kD to pass through. These include dyes such as Lucifer yellow and neurobiotin, which can be used to visualize electrical coupling between neurons.[109,110,123] In the brain and retina, connexons are especially abundant during embryonic and early postnatal development and may play an important role in generating the rhythmic electrical activity necessary for neural development.[131] Finally, connexons are subject to biochemical and neurotransmitter regulation, in the retina (as previously noted) and elsewhere.[132,133] Thus, gap junctions do not function merely as passive connections but can be dynamic components of neuronal circuits.

[131] Peinado, A., Juste, R., and Kayz, L. C. 1993. *Neuron* 10: 103–114.

[132] O'Donnell, P., and Grace, A. A. 1993. *J. Neurosci.* 13: 3456–3471.

[133] Halliwell, J. V., and Horne, A. L. 1998. *J. Physiol.* 506: 175–194.

SUMMARY

- Signaling between nerve cells and their targets can occur by chemical or electrical synaptic transmission. Most synapses use chemical transmission.

- At chemical synapses a neurotransmitter released from the presynaptic terminal activates receptors in the postsynaptic membrane. The time required for transmitter release imposes a minimum synaptic delay of approximately 1 ms.

- Direct chemical synaptic transmission occurs when the postsynaptic receptor activated by a neurotransmitter is itself an ion channel. Such ligand-activated ion channels are called ionotropic transmitter receptors.

- At direct excitatory synapses, such as the vertebrate skeletal neuromuscular junction, the neurotransmitter (in this case acetylcholine) opens cation-selective channels, allowing sodium, potassium, and calcium ions to flow down their electrochemical gradients.

- The relative permeability of a channel for various ions determines the reversal potential. At excitatory synapses, the reversal potential is more depolarized than the threshold for action potential initiation.

- Direct chemical synaptic inhibition occurs when a neurotransmitter opens anion-selective channels, which allow chloride ions to flow down their electrochemical gradient. The reversal potential for

such currents is the chloride equilibrium potential (ECl); inhibition occurs if ECl is more negative than threshold.

- The intracellular chloride concentration is set by inward or outward chloride transporters. During early development the chloride transport is inward so the channels opened by the inhibitory transmitter allow an outward flow of chloride ions, producing a depolarization.

- Receptors for inhibitory transmitters may also be present on presynaptic terminals, where their activation reduces transmitter release.

- Receptors for excitatory and inhibitory transmitters are aggregated into specialized regions of the postsynaptic membrane by an array of scaffolding proteins.

- Electrical synaptic transmission is mediated by the direct flow of current from cell to cell, through ion channels called connexons in vertebrates, or innexons in invertebrates, that span the apposed membranes to make a gap junction. Electrical transmission is very rapid and used at specialized synapses mediating very fast reflexes. It is also used in the retina and brain to coordinate the activity of groups of neurons.

Suggested Reading

General Reviews

Bennett, M. V., and Zukin, R. S. 2004. Electrical coupling and neuronal synchronization in the mammalian brain. *Neuron* 41: 495–511.

Edmonds, B., Gibb, A. J., and Colquhoun, D. 1995. Mechanisms of activation of muscle nicotinic acetylcholine receptors and the time course of endplate currents. *Annu. Rev. Physiol.* 57: 469–493.

Engelman, H. S., and MacDermott, A. B. 2004. Presynaptic ionotropic receptors and control of transmitter release. *Nat. Rev. Neurosci.* 5: 135–145.

Hille, B. 2001. *Ion Channels of Excitable Membranes*, 3rd ed. Sinauer, Sunderland, MA, pp.169–199.

Hirsch, N. P. 2007. Neuromuscular junction in health and disease. *Brit. J. Anaesth.* 99: 132–138.

Katz, B. 1981. Electrical exploration of acetylcholine receptors. *Postgrad. Med. J.* 57(Suppl. 1): 84–88.

Kim, E., and Sheng, M. 2004. PDZ domain proteins of synapses. *Nat. Rev. Neurosci.* 5: 771–781.

Kneussel, M., and Loebrich, S. 2007. Trafficking and synaptic anchoring of ionotropic inhibitory neurotransmitter receptors. *Biol. Cell* 99: 297–309.

Moss, S. J., and Smart, T. G. 2001. Constructing inhibitory synapses. *Nat. Rev. Neurosci.* 2: 240–250.

Nicholls, J. G. 2007. How acetylcholine gives rise to current at the motor end-plate. *J. Physiol.* 578: 621–622.

Sakmann, B. 1992. Elementary steps in synaptic transmission revealed by currents through single ion channels. *Neuron* 8: 613–629.

Sanes, J. R., and Lichtman, J. W. 2001. Induction, assembly, maturation and maintenance of a postsynaptic apparatus. *Nat. Rev. Neurosci.* 2: 791–805.

Todman, D. 2008. John Eccles (1903–1997) and the experiment that proved chemical synaptic transmission in the central nervous system. *J. Clin. Neurosci.* 15: 972–977.

Original Papers

Akaaboune, M., Grady, R. M., Turney, S., Sanes, J. R., and Lichtman, J. W. 2002. Neurotransmitter receptor dynamics studied in vivo by reversible photo-unbinding of fluorescent ligands. *Neuron* 34: 865–876.

Coombs, J. S., Eccles, J. C., and Fatt, P. 1955. The specific ionic conductances and the ionic movements across the motoneuronal membrane that produce the inhibitory post-synaptic potential. *J. Physiol.* 130: 326–373.

del Castillo, J., and Katz, B. 1955. On the localization of end-plate receptors. *J. Physiol.* 128: 157–181.

Dudel, J., and Kuffler, S. W. 1961. Presynaptic inhibition at the crayfish neuromuscular junction. *J. Physiol.* 155: 543–562.

Fatt, P., and Katz, B. 1951. An analysis of the end-plate potential recorded with an intra-cellular electrode. *J. Physiol.* 115: 320–370.

Furshpan, E. J., and Potter, D. D. 1959. Transmission at the giant motor synapses of the crayfish. *J. Physiol.* 145: 289–325.

Jackson, A. C. and Nicoll, R. A. 2011. The expanding social network of ionotropic glutamate receptor: TARPs and other transmembrane auxiliary subunits. *Neuron* 70: 178–199.

Kirsch, J., Wolters, I., Triller, A., and Betz, H. 1993. Gephyrin antisense oligonucleotides prevent glycine receptor clustering in spinal neurons. *Nature* 366: 745–748.

Kuffler, S. W., and Yoshikami, D. 1975. The distribution of acetylcholine sensitivity at the postsynaptic membrane of vertebrate skeletal twitch muscles: Iontophoretic mapping in the micron range. *J. Physiol.* 244: 703–730.

Magleby, K. L., and Stevens, C. F. 1972. A quantitative description of end-plate currents. *J. Physiol.* 223: 171–197.

Martin, A. R., and Pilar, G. 1963. Dual mode of synaptic transmission in the avian ciliary ganglion. *J. Physiol.* 168: 443–463.

Neher, E., Sakmann, B., and Steinbach, J. H. 1978. The extracellular patch clamp: A method for resolving currents through individual open channels in biological membranes. *Pflügers Arch.* 375: 219–228.

Sah, P., Hestrin, S., and Nicoll, R. A. 1990. Properties of excitatory postsynaptic currents recorded in vitro from rat hippocampal interneurones. *J. Physiol.* 430: 605–616.

Takeuchi, A., and Takeuchi, N. 1960. On the permeability of the end-plate membrane during the action of transmitter. *J. Physiol.* 154: 52–67.

Takeuchi, A., and Takeuchi, N. 1966. On the permeability of the presynaptic terminal of the crayfish neuromuscular junction during synaptic inhibition and the action of γ-aminobutyric acid. *J. Physiol.* 183: 433–449.

Takeuchi, A., and Takeuchi, N. 1967. Anion permeability of the inhibitory post-synaptic membrane of the crayfish neuromuscular junction. *J. Physiol.* 191: 575–590.

CHAPTER 12

Indirect Mechanisms of Synaptic Transmission

In addition to opening ion channels, neurotransmitters bind to other membrane receptors, known as metabotropic receptors. Metabotropic receptors influence ion channels indirectly through membrane-associated or cytoplasmic second messengers. At many synapses in the central and autonomic nervous systems, excitatory and inhibitory transmission occurs solely by these indirect mechanisms. At other locations, indirect mechanisms serve to modulate direct transmission.

Most metabotropic receptors (G protein-coupled receptors) produce their effects by first interacting with G proteins in the cell membrane. G proteins, so called because they bind guanine nucleotides, are trimers of three subunits: α, β, and γ. When a G protein is activated by its receptor, the α- and βγ-subunits dissociate. The free subunits can diffuse, and then bind to and modulate the activity of intracellular targets. Some G protein subunits bind to ion channels, producing relatively brief effects. For example, when acetylcholine (ACh) binds to its muscarinic receptors in the heart atrium, a G protein is activated and the freed βγ-subunit then opens a potassium channel, thereby slowing the heart. A second mechanism of G protein action is through activation of enzymes that produce intracellular second messengers. An example is the activation of β-adrenergic receptors in the heart by norepinephrine. The α-subunit of the dissociated G protein stimulates the enzyme adenylate cyclase. The resulting increase in intracellular cyclic adenosine monophosphate (AMP), or cAMP, activates another enzyme, cAMP-dependent protein kinase, which modifies the activity of channels and enzymes through phosphorylation. Such responses may last for seconds, minutes, or hours—often persisting long after the transmitter interaction with the receptors has stopped. These mechanisms provide both amplification and radiation of signals.

Potassium and calcium channels are prime targets for such indirect transmitter action. Indirect action can cause channels to open, close, or change their voltage sensitivity. Thus, indirectly acting transmitters open $K_{ir}3$ potassium channels in heart atrial cells; inhibit N-type ($Ca_V2.2$) calcium channels and M-type (K_V7) potassium channels in sympathetic neurons; and increase the probability that Ca_V1 calcium channels will open in response to depolarization in cardiac muscle cells. Changes in channel activation in axon terminals modify transmitter release. In postsynaptic cells, such changes alter spontaneous activity and the responses to synaptic inputs.

In addition, there are tertiary messengers, which are generated by some forms of synaptic activation. These include endocannabinoids (lipid messengers) and a gas, nitric oxide (NO). These molecules diffuse freely and so have effects outside the synapse or cell in which they are made. Calcium ions constitute another messenger and produce both short-term and long-term changes in neuron excitability and synaptic function. The long-term changes include effects on gene transcription and synaptic wiring.

Direct versus Indirect Transmission

In Chapter 11 we described the process of direct chemical transmission. In this process, a neurotransmitter released from a presynaptic ending binds to and, within a millisecond, opens ion channels (ionotropic receptors) in the postsynaptic membrane (Figure 12.1A). Thus, direct transmission is extremely fast and is required for high-speed, integrated motor performance, such as playing a trill on the piano, or for discriminating different notes at frequencies up to several kilohertz.

However, many of the essential human functions require a more gradual and longer-lasting form of communication. For example, when we are excited or frightened, our sympathetic nervous system is stimulated (see Chapter 19), and as a result, our heart rate gradually increases over many seconds. This action does not require ultrafast transmission from the sympathetic nerves to the heart but instead requires a careful adjustment to the endogenous cardiac rhythm. This form of slow modulatory transmission is also an essential component of synaptic activity in the central nervous system (CNS), where it is superimposed on the faster type of transmission mediated by the ionotropic receptors. There it serves to adjust the efficiency of synaptic transmission, and the excitability of the neuron, over seconds or minutes (or even longer).

Slow modulatory transmission uses a completely different type of membrane receptor than the ionotropic receptors responsible for fast transmission. Slow transmission uses **metabotropic receptors**. These receptors are not ion channels and do not directly excite or inhibit a neuron. Instead, they interact with other membrane proteins to initiate a sequence of steps leading to a change in ion channel activity or other metabolic processes within the neuron (Figure 12.1B). For this reason, this form of transmission is referred to as **indirect transmission**. For the vast majority of metabotropic receptors, the first target protein with which they interact is another membrane protein, called a **G protein**; hence, metabotropic receptors of this type are termed **G protein-coupled receptors** (**GPCRs**).

In the rest of this chapter we describe G proteins and G protein-coupled receptors; give examples of how they modify ion channels, both directly and indirectly, through subsequent enzymatic cascades; and describe some effects of other downstream messengers of receptor activation, such as nitric oxide (NO), endocannabinoids, and calcium ions.

(A) Direct transmitter action

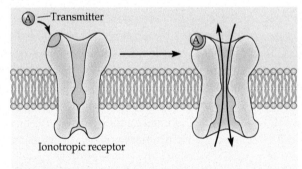

Ionotropic receptor

(B) Indirect transmitter action

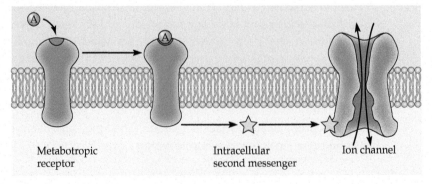

Metabotropic receptor   Intracellular second messenger   Ion channel

FIGURE 12.1 Direct and Indirect Transmitter Action. (A) At direct chemical synapses, the transmitter molecule A binds to an ionotropic receptor. Ionotropic receptors are ligand-activated ion channels. (B) Indirectly acting transmitters bind to metabotropic receptors. Metabotropic receptors are not themselves ion channels but rather activate intracellular second-messenger signaling pathways that influence the opening and closing of ion channels.

G Protein-Coupled Metabotropic Receptors and G Proteins

Structure of G Protein-Coupled Receptors

GPCRs make up a superfamily of membrane proteins characterized by seven transmembrane domains, with an extracellular amino terminus and an intracellular carboxy terminus (Figure 12.2).[1-3] For this reason, they are sometimes called 7-transmembrane (7TM) or heptahelical receptors. More than 1000 different GPCRs have been identified (Box 12.1). Those activated by ACh are called muscarinic receptors; those that bind norepinephrine are known as adrenergic receptors. Others respond to γ-aminobutyric acid (GABA), serotonin (5-HT), dopamine, glutamate, purines, or peptides; and some are activated by light (rhodopsin; see Chapter 22), odorants (see Chapter 21), or proteases.

Biochemical, structural, and molecular genetic experiments have indicated several distinct modes of ligand binding, each of which ultimately produces a similar rearrangement of the α-helical regions that form the transmembrane core of the receptor (see Figure 12.2). Portions of the second and third cytoplasmic loops, together with the membrane proximal region of the carboxy tail, mediate binding to and activation of the appropriate G protein.[1,3]

G Proteins

G proteins link the GPCR to its immediate effector protein. They are membrane proteins, so named because they bind guanine nucleotides. Each G protein is a trimer made up of three subunits: α, β, and γ (Figure 12.3).[3] There are many isoforms of each G protein subunit (21 for γ, 6 for β, 12 for γ), providing a large number of potential trimer permutations. G proteins are grouped into three main classes according to the structure and targets of their α-subunits: G_s stimulates the enzyme adenylate cyclase; G_i inhibits adenylate cyclase (and also activates

[1] Rosenbaum, D. M., Rasmussen, S. G. F., and Kobilka, B. 2009. *Nature* 459: 356–363.

[2] Ji, T. H., Grossmann, M., and Ji, I. 1998. *J. Biol. Chem.* 273: 17299–17302.

[3] Oldham, W. H., and Hamm, H. E. 2008. *Nat. Rev. Mol. Cell Biol.* 9: 60–71.

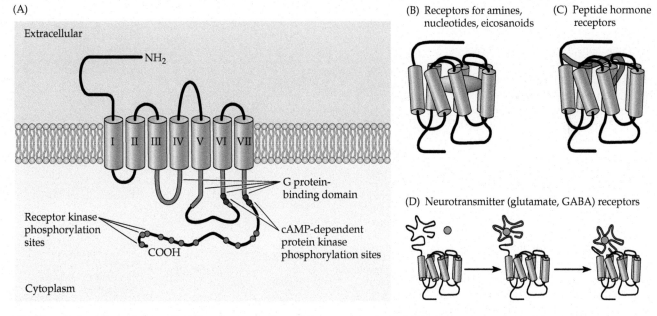

FIGURE 12.2   G Protein-Coupled Metabotropic Transmitter Receptors. (A) G protein-coupled receptors have seven transmembrane domains, an extracellular amino terminus, and an intracellular carboxy terminus. The second and third cytoplasmic loops, together with the amino terminal region of the intracellular tail, mediate binding to the appropriate G protein. Phosphorylation of sites on the carboxy terminus by G protein receptor kinases (GRKs), such as β-adrenergic receptor kinase (βARK), causes receptor desensitization, binding of the protein arrestin, and termination of the response. (B) Portions of the transmembrane domains form the ligand-binding sites of G protein-coupled receptors that bind amines, nucleotides, and eicosanoids. (C) Ligands bind to the outer portions of the transmembrane domains of peptide hormone receptors. (D) The amino terminal tail forms the ligand-binding domain of metabotropic receptors for glutamate and γ-aminobutyric acid (GABA). (After T. H. Ji et al., 1998. *J. Biol. Chem.* 273: 17299–17302, based in part on B. F. O'Dowd et al., 1989. *Annu. Rev. Neurosci.* 12: 67–83.)

FIGURE 12.3 Indirectly Coupled Transmitter Receptors Act through G Proteins. G proteins are trimers of α-, β-, and γ-subunits. Activation of a G protein-coupled metabotropic receptor by agonist binding promotes the exchange of guanosine triphosphate (GTP) for guanosine diphosphate (GDP) on the α-subunit of the G protein. This action activates the α-subunit and the βγ-complex, causing them to dissociate from the receptor and from one another. The free activated α-GTP subunit and βγ-complex each interact with target proteins. Hydrolysis of GTP to GDP and inorganic phosphate (Pi) by the endogenous GTPase activity of the α-subunit leads to reassociation of the αβγ-complex, terminating the response.

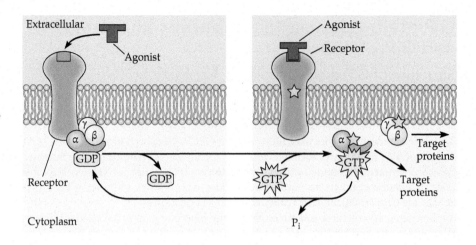

potassium channels); and G_q couples to the enzyme phospholipase C (PLC). The G_i class also includes G_t (transducin), which activates cyclic guanosine monophosphate (cGMP) phosphodiesterase (see Chapter 19), and G_o, which interacts with calcium ion channels.

The prime binding site for the receptor is the C terminus of the α-subunit, and the main determinant that specifies which G protein a receptor activates is the amino acid sequence

---

<table>
<tr><td>BOX 12.1</td><td colspan="4">Receptors, G Proteins, and Effectors: Convergence and Divergence in G Protein Signaling</td></tr>
</table>

There are more than 200 different metabotropic receptors that can couple to G proteins but a much smaller number of different G proteins. The primary receptor interaction site on the G protein is the C terminus of the α-subunit. Hence, as viewed by the receptor, there are only three families of common G proteins: G_s, G_q, and G_i/G_o. Although each family contains several members, their C-terminal sequences cannot be distinguished by the receptor. This means there is substantial convergence of different transmitters or hormones, acting through different receptors, onto the same G protein. On the output side, while some G proteins have rather specific effects (e.g., G_o selectively interacts with certain types of neuronal calcium channels), others—particularly those that activate enzymes to produce second messengers, such as cyclic AMP—can produce multiple effects on any given cell, providing divergent signaling. G_s, G_q, and G_i are present in nearly all cells, and G_o is abundant in all nerve cells. In most cells, G protein molecules are about ten times more plentiful than receptor molecules, so different recep-

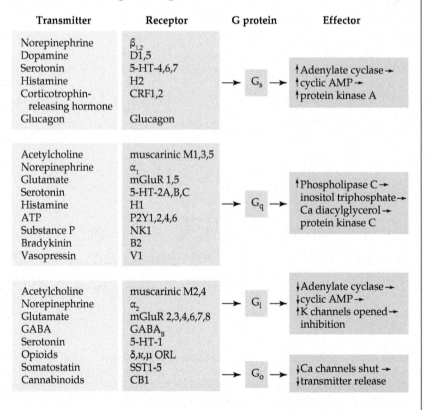

Transmitter	Receptor	G protein	Effector
Norepinephrine Dopamine Serotonin Histamine Corticotrophin- releasing hormone Glucagon	$\beta_{1,2}$ D1,5 5-HT-4,6,7 H2 CRF1,2 Glucagon	G_s	↑Adenylate cyclase → ↑cyclic AMP → ↑protein kinase A
Acetylcholine Norepinephrine Glutamate Serotonin Histamine ATP Substance P Bradykinin Vasopressin	muscarinic M1,3,5 α_1 mGluR 1,5 5-HT-2A,B,C H1 P2Y1,2,4,6 NK1 B2 V1	G_q	↑Phospholipase C → inositol triphosphate → Ca diacylglycerol → protein kinase C
Acetylcholine Norepinephrine Glutamate GABA Serotonin Opioids Somatostatin	muscarinic M2,4 α_2 mGluR 2,3,4,6,7,8 GABA$_B$ 5-HT-1 δ,κ,μ ORL SST1-5	G_i	↓Adenylate cyclase → ↓cyclic AMP → ↑K channels opened → inhibition
Cannabinoids	CB1	G_o	↓Ca channels shut → ↓transmitter release

tors do not necessarily compete for the same G protein molecules. Possible ways in which selectivity of a cell's response to different transmitters acting on the same G protein may occur are discussed in the text.

of this C terminus (although interactions with other subunits may facilitate binding). This sequence differs among the different classes of G protein (G_s, G_q, and $G_{i/o}$) but is identical or very similar among different members of each class. Hence, while some receptors are promiscuous and can couple to more than one class of G proteins, most metabotropic neurotransmitter receptors show a preferential interaction with members of one or other of the three common classes of G proteins, as shown in Box 12.1.

THE G PROTEIN CYCLE   Figure 12.3 illustrates how the G protein works. In the resting state, guanosine diphosphate (GDP) is bound to the α-subunit, and the three subunits are associated as a trimer. Interaction with an activated receptor allows guanosine triphosphate (GTP) to replace GDP on the α-subunit, resulting in dissociation of the α- and βγ-subunits. (The β- and γ-subunits remain together under physiological conditions.) The free α- and βγ-subunits then diffuse, and bind to and modulate the activity of target proteins.[3–5] The free α-subunit has intrinsic GTPase activity that results in hydrolysis of the bound GTP to GDP. This permits the reassociation of the α- and βγ-subunits into the G protein complex and terminates their activity.

The lifetime of the activated G protein subunits is modulated by proteins called GTPase-activating proteins, or GAPs, which influence the rate at which GTP, bound to the α-subunit, is hydrolyzed.[6] One family of GAPs, the RGS proteins (*Regulators of G protein Signaling*), plays an important role in determining the time course of transmitter action.[7] The details of the interactions of the G protein subunits with each other and with their receptors and targets have been explored using biomolecular X-ray crystallography[1,3] and live-cell imaging[8,9] techniques. In addition, probes have been developed for identifying responses mediated by G proteins (Box 12.2).

[4] Dascal, N. 2001. *Trends Endocrinol. Metab.* 12: 391–398.

[5] Clapham, D. E., and Neer, E. J. 1997. *Annu. Rev. Pharmacol. Toxicol.* 37: 167–203.

[6] Berman, D. M., and Gilman, A. G. 1998. *J. Biol. Chem.* 273: 1269–1272.

[7] Doupnik, C. et al. 1997. *Proc. Natl. Acad. Sci. USA* 94: 10461–10466.

[8] Hein, P. et al. 2005. *EMBO J.* 24: 4106–4114.

[9] Raveh, A., Riven, I., and Reuvenny, E. 2009. *J. Physiol.* 587: 5331–5335.

BOX 12.2   Identifying Responses Mediated by G Proteins

Several tests can be used to identify responses mediated by G proteins. For example, activation of the α-subunit requires that bound GDP be replaced by GTP. Accordingly, G protein-mediated events have an absolute requirement for cytoplasmic GTP and will be blocked by intracellular perfusion with solutions lacking GTP. Two analogues of GTP–GTPγS and Gpp(NH)p–are useful because they cannot be hydrolyzed by the endogenous GTPase activity of the α-subunit. Like GTP, they can replace GDP on the α-subunit and activate it. However, because they cannot be hydrolyzed, these analogues activate the α-subunit permanently. Thus, intracellular perfusion with either of these analogues enhances and greatly prolongs agonist-induced activation of G protein-mediated responses and may even initiate responses in the absence of agonist. However, GDPβS, an analogue of GDP, binds strongly to the GDP site on the α-subunit and resists replacement by GTP. Thus, GDPβS inhibits G protein-mediated responses by maintaining the αβγ-complex in the inactive state.

Two bacterial toxins are useful for characterizing G protein-mediated processes. Each is an enzyme that catalyzes the covalent attachment of ADP-ribose to an arginine residue on the α-subunit. Cholera toxin acts on α_s, irreversibly activating G_S; pertussis toxin acts on members of the G_i family, irreversibly blocking the activation of their α-subunit and so inhibiting responses mediated by the corresponding G proteins G_i, G_o and G_t.

GTP
Guanosine 5′-triphosphate

GDP
Guanosine 5′-diphosphate

GTPγS
Guanosine 5′-*O*-[γ-thio] triphosphate

Gpp(NH)p
Guanosine 5′- [β,γ-imido] triphosphate

GDPβS
Guanosine 5′-*O*-[β-thio] diphosphate

Modulation of Ion Channel Function by Receptor-Activated G Proteins: Direct Actions

G proteins affect ion channels in two different ways. In one way, a subunit of the activated G protein (usually the βγ-complex) may interact *directly* with the ion channel; alternatively, the G protein (usually the GTP-bound α-subunit) may activate one or more enzymes to alter ion channel function *indirectly* through one or more **second messengers**.

G Protein Activation of Potassium Channels

Much of our knowledge about the direct interaction of G proteins with ion channels comes from experiments concerning how stimulation of the vagus nerve slows or stops the heartbeat. As first shown by Loewi (see Box 11.1), this is due to the release of ACh from the vagus nerve endings. The ACh then binds to a G protein-coupled receptor—the M2 **muscarinic acetylcholine receptor, M2-mAChR** (see Box 12.1)—so called because it is selectively activated by the drug muscarine,[10] an alkaloid in the fly agaric (*Amanita muscaria*) mushroom. Figure 12.4 illustrates what happens when ACh is applied to the sinoatrial node of the rabbit heart. In Figure 12.4A a brief application of ACh causes a temporary cessation of spontaneous action potentials and a hyperpolarization of the heart muscle cell (as first shown by Burgen and Terroux[11] and Hutter and Trautwein[12]). This hyperpolarization is due to the opening of potassium channels,[13] generating the outward potassium current seen in Figure 12.4B.

The role of G proteins in coupling the muscarinic receptors to these ion channels was established in a series of experiments by Breitwieser, Szabo, Pfaffinger, Trautwein, Hille, and their colleagues. They found that intracellular GTP is required;[14] that activation of potassium channels by muscarinic agonists is greatly prolonged by intracellular application of the non-hydrolyzable analogue of GTP, known as Gpp(NH)p;[15] and that muscarinic activation of potassium channels is blocked by pertussis toxin,[14] which inactivates G_i proteins (see Box 12.2). An important advance came from experiments by David Clapham and his colleagues using inside-out excised membrane patches (Figure 12.5). They showed that the cardiac potassium channels were opened when pure recombinant βγ-subunit was applied to the intracellular side of the patch.[16] This demonstrated that the βγ-subunit, rather than the α-subunit, is responsible for potassium channel activation. Subsequent experiments with a cloned muscarinic potassium channel

[10]Dale, H. H. 1914. *J. Pharmac. Exp. Ther.* 6: 147-190.

[11]Burgen, A. S. V., and Terroux, K. G. 1953. *J. Physiol.* 120: 449-464.

[12]Hutter, O. F., and Trautwein, W. 1956. *J. Gen. Physiol.* 39: 715-733.

[13]Sakmann, B., Noma, A., and Trautwein, W. 1983. *Nature* 303: 250-253.

[14]Pfaffinger, P. J. et al. 1985. *Nature* 317: 536-538.

[15]Breitwieser, G. E., and Szabo, G. 1985. *Nature* 317: 538-540.

[16]Wickman, K. D. et al. 1994. *Nature* 368: 255-257.

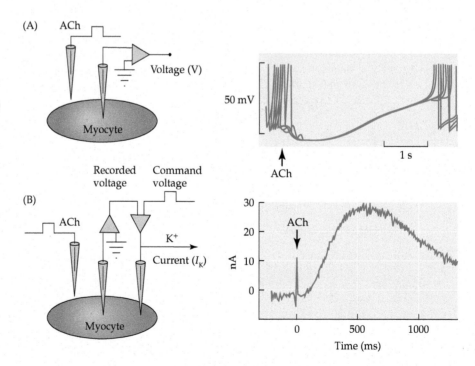

FIGURE 12.4 Acetylcholine (ACh) Opens Potassium Channels in Sinoatrial Cells of the Rabbit Heart. (A) A brief ionophoretic ejection of ACh from a micropipette transiently hyperpolarizes the cell membrane and inhibits spontaneous action potentials for about 3 seconds. (B) When membrane current is recorded using voltage clamp (see Box 7.1), a similar ACh application produces an outward K^+ current, I_K which starts after about 50 milliseconds and lasts about 1.5 seconds. (A after W. Trautwein et al., 1982. *Pflügers Arch.* 392: 307-314; B after W. Trautwein et al., 1981. In *Drug Receptors and Their Effectors*. N. J. M. Birdsall [Ed.], London: Macmillan, pp. 5-22.)

(A)

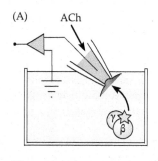

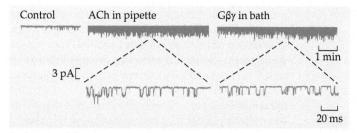

(B)

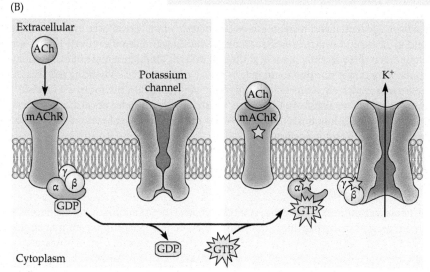

FIGURE 12.5 Direct Modulation of Channel Function by G Proteins. (A) Application of the Gβγ complex to the intracellular surface of an isolated patch of membrane from a rat atrial muscle cell (Gβγ in bath) results in an increase in potassium channel activity similar to that seen when acetylcholine (ACh) is added to the extracellular side of the patch (ACh in pipette). (B) Schematic representation of events in an intact cell. Binding of ACh to muscarinic receptors (mAChR) activates a G protein (indicated by a star); activated βγ-complex binds directly to and opens a potassium channel. (A after K. D. Wickman et al., 1994. *Nature* 368: 255–257.)

(originally named GIRK1, for G protein-activated inwardly rectifying K^+ channel, but later renamed $K_{ir}3.1$) indicated that the βγ-subunit interacts directly with potassium channels (see Figure 12.5B).[17,18]

Using muscle cells dissociated from the atrium of the heart, Soejima and Noma found that potassium channel activity in cell-attached patches was increased when muscarinic agonists were added to the patch pipette solution, but not when agonists were added to the bath (Figure 12.6).[19] Thus, activated βγ-subunits appear to be unable to traverse the region of the pipette–membrane seal to influence channels outside the patch. This so-called membrane-delimited mechanism of G protein action reflects the limited range of distance over which βγ-subunits can act. In fact, some evidence suggests that the G protein GTPase-activating protein RGS4[20] and GIRK channel are closely associated and may form a G protein–GIRK channel complex.[9,21]

[17]Reuveny, E. et al. 1994. *Nature* 370: 143–146.

[18]Huang, C.-L. et al. 1995. *Neuron* 15: 1133–1143.

[19]Soejima, M., and Noma, A. 1984. *Pflügers Arch.* 400: 424–431.

[20]Fowler, C. E. et al. 2007. *J. Physiol.* 580: 51–65.

[21]Benians, A. et al. 2005. *J. Biol. Chem.* 280: 13383–13394.

(A)

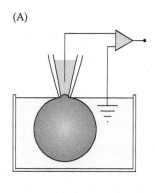

(B)

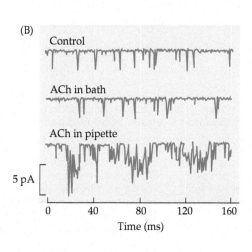

FIGURE 12.6 Direct, or Membrane-Delimited, Effects of G Proteins Operate over Short Distances. (A) Effects of acetylcholine (ACh) were assayed by cell-attached, patch clamp recording. ACh could be perfused into either the patch pipette or the bath. (B) Recordings of single-channel currents before and during addition of ACh. Channel activity increased only when ACh was added to the patch pipette. (After M. Soejima and A. Noma, 1984. *Pflügers Arch.* 400: 424–431.)

Similar G protein-activated inwardly rectifying potassium channels (GIRK channels)[22] are present in many nerve cells. There they can be activated by several different neurotransmitters through receptors coupled to Gi/Go proteins—for example, ACh, norepinephrine, GABA, and dopamine.[23] Their activation induces a postsynaptic hyperpolarization (inhibitory synaptic potential) very similar to the cardiac response to vagal stimulation. Figure 12.7 shows an example from an experiment on bullfrog ganglion cells.[24] When the nicotinic receptors in the ganglion had been blocked with curare, a few electrical stimuli, applied to the preganglionic sympathetic nerves in the descending lumbar sympathetic chain, generated a hyperpolarization of the small neurons in the lumbar sympathetic ganglia. The hyperpolarization was closely replicated by local ionophoresis of ACh onto the neurons (see Figure 12.7B). Further tests showed that both the inhibitory synaptic potential and response to ACh reversed when the cell was hyperpolarized beyond –102 mV in normal Ringer solution (containing 2 millimolar [mM] K+). It was also found that this reversal potential shifted 58 mV per tenfold increase in extracellular [K+], showing that it was due to an increased K+ conductance. When the cell was induced to fire repetitively, a short (1 second) burst of preganglionic stimulation reversibly suppressed firing (see Figure 12.7C)—very much like the response of cardiac sinoatrial cells to vagal stimulation. Indeed, the molecular mechanism for this action on ganglion cells is analogous to that in the heart.[25]

G Protein Inhibition of Calcium Channels Involved in Transmitter Release

Many neurotransmitters (including ACh, glutamate, GABA, monoamines such as norepinephrine, and many peptides) not only stimulate postsynaptic receptors but also

[22] Bichet, D., Haase, F. A., and Jan, L. Y. 2003. *Nat. Rev. Neurosci.* 4: 957-967.

[23] North, R. A. et al. 1987. *Proc. Natl. Acad. Sci. USA* 84: 5487-5491.

[24] Dodd, J., and Horn, J. P. 1983. *J. Physiol.* 334: 271-291.

[25] Fernandez-Fernandez, J. M. et al. 2001. *Eur. J. Neurosci.* 14: 283-292.

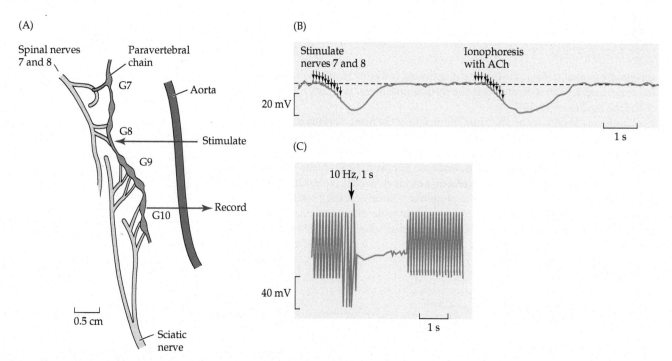

(A)

(B)

(C)

FIGURE 12.7 Cholinergic Synaptic Inhibition in the Nervous System Results from the Opening of Potassium Channels. (A) Drawing of the bullfrog lumbar sympathetic nervous system. Neurons in the ninth and tenth sympathetic ganglia (G9, G10) are innervated by descending cholinergic preganglionic fibers in spinal nerves 7 and 8 and send their postganglionic axons out in the sciatic nerve. (B) Intracellular recordings from a small neuron in the ninth sympathetic ganglion. A series of stimuli to the descending preganglionic fibers produces a slow hyperpolarization, which is imitated by electrophoretically applying acetylcholine to the neuron through a micropipette. This action results from stimulating muscarinic receptors because the nicotinic receptors were blocked using tubocurarine. (C) Preganglionic stimulation also suppresses action potential discharges of the postganglionic neuron. The neuron was made to fire repetitively by 4 minutes of preganglionic stimulation at 60 impulses per minute. This releases luteinizing hormone-releasing hormone (LHRH; see Chapter 19), which depolarizes the cell because it produces a prolonged inhibition of the M-current. (A after J. Dodd and J. P. Horn, 1983. *J. Physiol.* 334: 255-269; B,C after J. Dodd and J. P. Horn, 1983. *J. Physiol.* 334: 271-291.)

FIGURE 12.8 Presynaptic Autoreceptors Reduce Transmitter Release. (A) Norepinephrine (NE) released from sympathetic neurons combines with α_2-adrenergic receptors (called autoreceptors) in the terminal membrane, activating a G protein. The activated $\beta\gamma$-complex binds to calcium channels, decreasing calcium influx and so limiting further transmitter release. (B) Norepinephrine reduces the release of transmitter from sympathetic ganglia. Ganglia were loaded with radioactive norepinephrine and then enclosed in a perfusion chamber. Transmitter release was evoked by depolarization with a solution containing 50 mM potassium (green bars). Addition of 30 μM unlabeled norepinephrine to the perfusion solution (red bar) reduced the amount of radiolabeled transmitter released in response to potassium-induced depolarization. (B after D. Lipscombe et al., 1989. *Nature* 340: 639–642.)

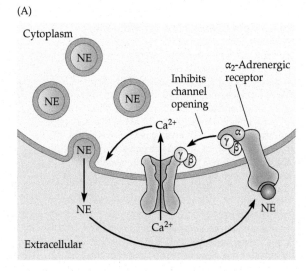

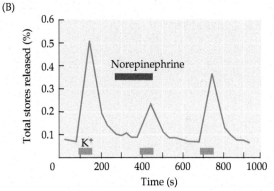

activate metabotropic receptors on the presynaptic terminals to reduce their own release (see Chapter 11). An example of this feedback inhibition (or auto-inhibition) of the release of norepinephrine from nerve terminals in frog sympathetic ganglia[26] is illustrated in Figure 12.8. As shown schematically in Figure 12.8A, the transmitter acts not only on postsynaptic target cells but also on the nerve terminals themselves. Figure 12.8B shows the release of radioactively tagged norepinephrine from the terminals in response to depolarization by elevated external potassium. Addition of norepinephrine to the bathing solution produced a marked reduction of transmitter release from the terminals.

This decrease in release is due to activation of presynaptic metabotropic α_2-adrenergic receptors (see Box 12.1). These activate G_o proteins, which in turn directly inhibit activation of N-type ($Ca_V2.2$) calcium channels (see Chapter 5). This effect is shown in the records of Figure 12.9. Single-channel calcium currents from a cell-attached patch, produced by membrane depolarization, are reduced in frequency when norepinephrine is added to the patch solution. As with the effect of ACh on potassium channels (see Figure 12.6), there was no response of the channels to the application of norepinephrine outside the patch (the response is membrane-delimited), suggesting again a close association between the G proteins and the channels.

Results of experiments in which α- or $\beta\gamma$-subunits or $\beta\gamma$-sequestering peptides were overexpressed or injected into cells indicated that it is the $\beta\gamma$-subunit that inhibits N-type calcium channels.[27–29] This is illustrated in Figure 12.10A. The inward calcium current produced by depolarizing a sympathetic ganglion cell (see part a of the figure) was reduced strongly by adding norepinephrine to the bathing solution. A similar effect was observed when a non-hydrolysable GTP analogue was added to the bath (see part b) or when $\beta\gamma$-subunits were overexpressed in the cell by prior injection of their cDNAs (see part c). The $\beta\gamma$-subunits bind directly to the calcium channel α-subunit, primarily at the intracellular linker between domains I and II[30] (see Figure 5.7B).

This interaction is voltage-dependent, with inhibition being reduced by depolarization; hence, inhibition diminishes as the depolarizing pulse is maintained.[31,32] In Figure 12.10A, this voltage dependence appears as a slowing of the calcium

[26] Lipscombe, D., Kongsamut, S., and Tsien, R. W. 1989. *Nature* 340: 639–642.

[27] Ikeda, S. R. 1996. *Nature* 380: 255–258.

[28] Herlitze, S. et al. 1996. *Nature* 380: 258–262.

[29] Delmas, P. et al. 1998. *J. Physiol.* 506: 319–329.

[30] De Waard, M. et al. 2005. *Trends Pharmacol. Sci.* 26: 427–436.

[31] Tsunoo, A., Yoshii, M., and Narahashi, T. 1986. *Proc. Natl. Acad. Sci. USA* 83: 9832–9836.

[32] Grassi, F., and Lux, H. D. 1989. *Neurosci. Lett.* 105: 113–119.

FIGURE 12.9 Norepinephrine Inhibits Calcium Channel Activity. Single-channel currents were recorded in cell-attached patches; channels were activated with a depolarizing pulse (top trace). When 30 μM norepinephrine was included in the patch electrode, the unitary currents did not change in size, but channel openings were less frequent and of shorter duration. (After D. Lipscombe et al., 1989. *Nature* 340: 639–642.)

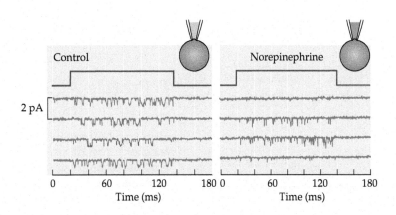

FIGURE 12.10 G Protein Regulation of Calcium Currents in a Sympathetic Neuron. Records show N-type (Ca$_V$2.2) calcium currents recorded from a rat sympathetic neuron with a whole-cell patch pipette on stepping from –80 to +10 mV. (A) Norepinephrine (NE; 10 μM) inhibits the current and slows its activation (a). This effect is imitated by adding 500 μM of the non-hydrolyzable GTP analogue Gpp(NH)p (see Box 12.2) to the pipette solution (b), or when free G protein $\beta\gamma$-subunits are overexpressed by prior cDNA injection (c). Calibration bars: 0.5 nA (vertical), 20 ms (horizontal). (B) The inhibitory actions of both norepinephrine (a) and G$\beta\gamma$ (b) are temporarily reversed by strongly depolarizing the neuron to +80 mV for 50 ms. This is because the depolarization promotes the dissociation of the G$\beta\gamma$-subunits from the calcium channel. (After S. R. Ikeda, 1996. *Nature* 380: 255–258.)

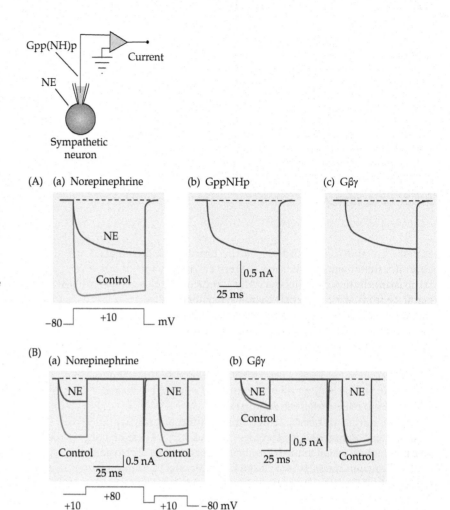

current; this suggests that the channels have been converted from their normal "willing to open" state to a "reluctant to open" state.[33] The voltage dependence is shown in another way in Figure 12.10B, by delivering a large depolarization for 50 ms between two calcium current test pulses. This accelerates the dissociation of the G protein $\beta\gamma$-subunit so that the inhibition produced by norepinephrine (see part a of the figure) or by the expressed $\beta\gamma$-subunits (see part b), seen during the first test pulse, is completely reversed when the second test pulse is given. On repolarization, channel inhibition is restored quite quickly, over 100 ms or so (not shown), as the released G$\beta\gamma$-subunits reassociate with the channel, suggesting that they have not moved far away. It has been calculated that the receptor, G protein, and channel must all be within less than 1 μm distance.[34] Recent experiments have shown that the primary response of the G protein-coupled receptor to a transmitter is also sensitive to membrane voltage[35,36] and that this property may also modify the receptors' effect on neurotransmitter release.[37]

[33] Bean, B. P. 1989. *Nature* 340: 153–157.

[34] Zhou, J., Shapiro, M. S., and Hille, B. 1997. *J. Neurophysiol.* 77: 2040–2048.

[35] Parnas, H., and Parnas, I. 2007. *Trends Neurosci.* 30: 54–61.

[36] Mahaut-Smith, M. P., Martinez-Pinna, J., and Gurung, I. S. 2008. *Trends Pharmacol. Sci.* 29: 421–429.

[37] Kupchik, Y. M. et al. 2008. *Proc. Natl. Acad. Sci. USA* 105: 4435–4440.

G Protein Activation of Cytoplasmic Second-Messenger Systems

Many G proteins do not bind directly to ion channels. Instead they modulate the activity of enzymes involved in cytoplasmic **second-messenger systems**: adenylate cyclase, phospholipase C, phospholipase A2, phosphodiesterase, and phosphatidylinositol 3-kinase. The products of these enzymes, in turn, affect targets that influence the activity of ion channels and other cellular processes. In contrast to the rapid localized responses produced by

FIGURE 12.11   Activation of β-Adrenergic Receptors in Cardiac Muscle Increases Calcium Current. (A) The increase in calcium current produced by activation of β-adrenergic receptors, in this case by the addition of 10^{-6} M norepinephrine, increases action potential amplitude and duration and the contractile tension produced by cardiac muscle cells. (B) The current-voltage relation of calcium current in a myocardial cell is measured under voltage clamp conditions in the absence and presence of 0.5 μM epinephrine—a β-adrenergic receptor agonist. (A,B after H. Reuter, 1974. *J. Physiol.* 242: 429–451.)

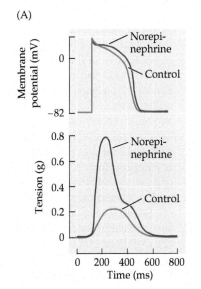

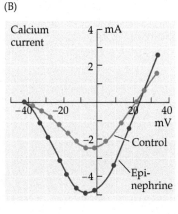

direct interaction of G protein subunits with membrane channels, the effects produced by G proteins that activate cytoplasmic second-messenger systems are slower and more widespread. They include contractions of smooth and cardiac muscles, and glandular secretion, among other effects.

β-Adrenergic Receptors Activate Calcium Channels via a G Protein—The Adenylate Cyclase Pathway

One of the most thoroughly studied examples of indirect synaptic transmission mediated by an intracellular second messenger is the activation of β-adrenergic receptors in cardiac muscle cells by norepinephrine.[38,39] This produces an increase in the rate and force of contraction of the heart, which follows an increase in the amplitude and duration of the cardiac action potential (Figure 12.11A). Voltage clamp studies by Reuter, Trautwein, Tsien, and others indicate that these effects are due to a marked increase in the calcium current associated with the action potential (Figure 12.11B). This increased calcium current is responsible for the increased size of the action potential and the increased calcium influx then triggers the marked increase in contraction.

Single-channel recording from cardiac muscle cells, using the cell-attached mode of the patch clamp technique, confirms that stimulation with a β-adrenergic receptor agonist, such as norepinephrine or isoproterenol, produces an increase in calcium channel activity (Figure 12.12). Moreover, it is not necessary that the agonist be added to the pipette

[38] Tsien, R. W. 1987. In L. K. Kaczmarek and I. B. Levitan (Eds.) *Neuromodulation: The Biochemical Control of Neuronal Excitability.* Oxford University Press, New York, pp. 206–242.

[39] McDonald, T. F. et al. 1994. *Physiol. Rev.* 74: 365–507.

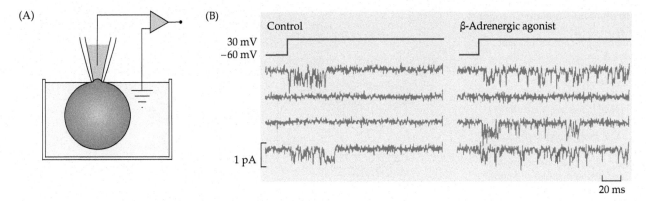

FIGURE 12.12   β-Adrenergic Agonists Cause an Increase in Calcium Channel Activity during a depolarizing pulse. (A) Recordings are from a voltage clamped cell-attached patch. (B) Consecutive records of the activity of a patch containing two calcium channels. Addition of 14 μM isoproterenol, a β-adrenergic agonist, to the bath causes an increase in calcium channel activity during depolarization. (After R. W. Tsien, 1987. *In Neuromodulation: The Biochemical Control of Neuronal Excitability*, L. K. Kaczmarek and I. B. Levitan [Eds.], pp. 206–242. Oxford University Press: New York.)

solution to observe the response. Adding isoproterenol to the medium bathing the cell causes an increase in activity of calcium channels *within* the patch—a diagnostic test for responses mediated by diffusible cytoplasmic second messengers.[38]

Activation of β-adrenergic receptors is coupled to the increase in calcium conductance through the intracellular second messenger cyclic AMP (cAMP) (Box 12.3). As illustrated in Figure 12.13, binding of norepinephrine to β-adrenergic receptors on heart cells activates a G protein, G_s. The α-subunit of G_s then binds to and activates the enzyme adenylate cyclase. Adenylate cyclase converts ATP to cAMP, a readily diffusible intracellular second messenger that activates another enzyme, cAMP-dependent protein kinase (protein kinase A or PKA). The catalytic subunits of this protein kinase mediate the transfer of phosphate from ATP to the hydroxyl groups of serine and threonine residues in a variety of enzymes and channels, thereby modifying their activity. In this case, phosphorylation of cardiac calcium channels increases their probability of opening.

Several lines of evidence are consistent with this scheme, as outlined in Box 12.3. For example, calcium channel activity is increased by forskolin, by membrane-permeable derivatives of cAMP, by inhibitors of phosphodiesterase, and by direct intracellular injection of cAMP itself. Similarly, intracellular injection of the catalytic subunit of cAMP-dependent protein kinase leads to an increase in calcium current, while injection of excess regulatory subunit or inhibitors of protein kinase blocks adrenergic stimulation of calcium currents. ATPγS, an analogue of ATP, augments adrenergic activation of calcium channels by forming stably phosphorylated proteins, while intracellular injection of protein phosphatases prevents or reverses adrenergic stimulation of calcium currents by rapidly removing protein phosphate residues.

Subsequent experiments established that the increased channel activity produced by protein kinase A resulted from the phosphorylation of the calcium channels themselves.[40,41] Phosphorylation and enhancement of cardiac calcium channel activity are facilitated by a scaffold protein called an A-kinase anchoring protein, AKAP79,[42] which binds to protein kinase A and targets it to the ion channel. Modulation of the activity of the same L-type (Ca_V1) calcium channels by other hormones is also mediated by channel phosphorylation, either through effects on adenylate cyclase and cAMP-dependent protein kinase or through different second messenger–protein kinase signaling pathways.[39]

The two-step enzymatic cascade involving adenylate cyclase and cAMP-dependent protein kinase provides significant amplification compared with direct opening or closing

[40] Curtis, B. M., and Catterall, W. A. 1986. *Biochemistry* 25: 3077-3083.

[41] Flockerzi, V. et al. 1986. *Nature* 323: 66-68.

[42] Gao, T. et al. 1997. *Neuron* 19: 185-196.

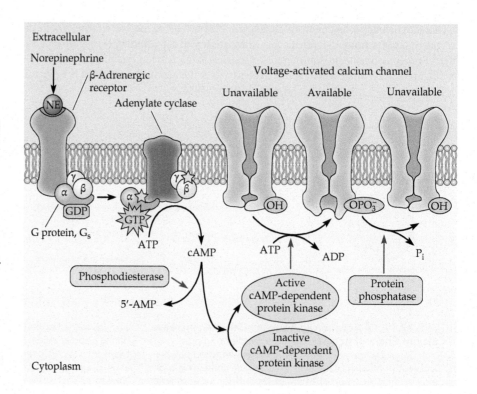

FIGURE 12.13 β-Adrenergic Receptors Act through the Intracellular Second Messenger Cyclic AMP to Increase Calcium Channel Activity. Binding of norepinephrine to β-adrenergic receptors activates, through a G protein, the enzyme adenylate cyclase. adenylate cyclase catalyzes the conversion of ATP to cyclic AMP (cAMP). As the concentration of cAMP increases, it activates cAMP-dependent protein kinase, an enzyme that phosphorylates proteins on serine and threonine residues (-OH). The response to norepinephrine is terminated by the hydrolysis of cAMP to 5′-AMP and the removal of protein phosphate residues by protein phosphatases. In cardiac muscle cells, norepinephrine causes phosphorylation of voltage-activated calcium channels, converting them to a form that can be opened by depolarization (available).

BOX **12.3** Cyclic AMP as a Second Messenger

Experiments by Sutherland, Krebs, Walsh, Rodbell, Gilman, and their colleagues, initially aimed at understanding how the hormones epinephrine and glucagon elicit breakdown of glycogen in the liver, led to the discovery of cyclic AMP (cAMP) and the concept of intracellular second messengers.[43-45] They showed that binding of the hormone to its receptor activates a G protein, which in turn stimulates the enzyme adenylate cyclase. Adenylate cyclase catalyzes the synthesis of cAMP from ATP. The increase in cAMP concentration activates cAMP-dependent protein kinase (also known as protein kinase A, or PKA), an enzyme that phosphorylates its target proteins on serine and threonine residues. The cAMP is subsequently degraded by phosphodiesterase to AMP, and the phosphate residues on the target proteins are removed by protein phosphatases (see Figure 12.13).

Some tests used to determine if the response to a transmitter or hormone is mediated by cAMP depend on activating adenylate cyclase or elevating cAMP directly. For example, intracellular injection of cAMP and addition of membrane-permeable derivatives of cAMP, such as 8-bromo-cAMP or dibutyryl-cAMP, mimic cAMP-mediated responses. Similarly, direct activation of adenylate cyclase by forskolin mimics the response. Inhibitors of

phosphodiesterase, such as the methylxanthines, theophylline, and caffeine, either mimic or enhance the response, depending on the endogenous level of cyclase activity. Other procedures test the involvement of cAMP-dependent protein kinase. This enzyme is composed of two regulatory and two catalytic subunits. In the absence of cAMP, the four subunits exist as a complex, with the regulatory subunits blocking the activity of the catalytic subunits. When cAMP binds to the regulatory subunits, the complex dissociates, freeing active catalytic subunits. Thus, intracellular injection of purified catalytic subunit will mimic responses mediated by increased cAMP, while injection of excess regulatory subunits will be inhibitory. Additional inhibitors of this enzyme have been developed, including H-8 (which also inhibits several other protein serine kinases), specific peptide inhibitors, and derivatives of ATP that cannot be used by the kinase as a source for phosphate residues. These inhibitors block responses mediated by cAMP.

By contrast, treatments that inhibit protein phosphatases augment and prolong responses mediated by cAMP. These include injection of specific phosphatase inhibitors and of ATPS, an analogue of ATP that can be used as a co-substrate by cAMP-dependent protein kinase, forming phosphoproteins with thiophosphate linkages, which are resistant to hydrolysis by protein phosphatases.

[43]Sutherland, E. W. 1972. *Science* 177: 401–408.
[44]Schramm, M., and Selinger, Z. 1984. *Science* 225: 1350–1356.
[45]Gilman, A. G. 1987. *Ann. Rev. Biochem.* 56: 615–649.

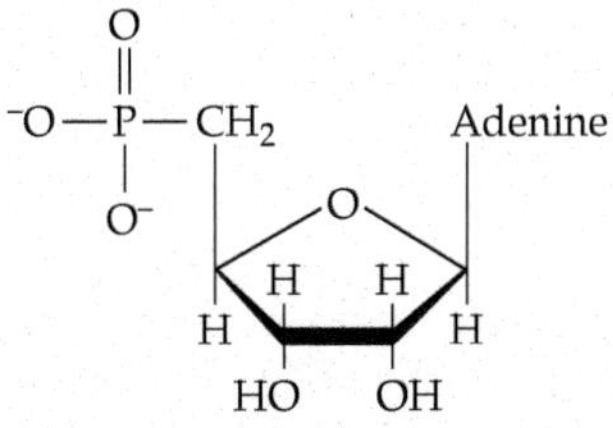

AMP
Adenosine 5′-monophosphate

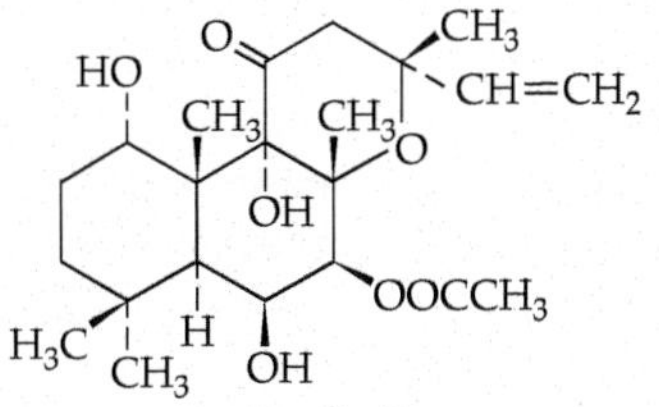

Forskolin

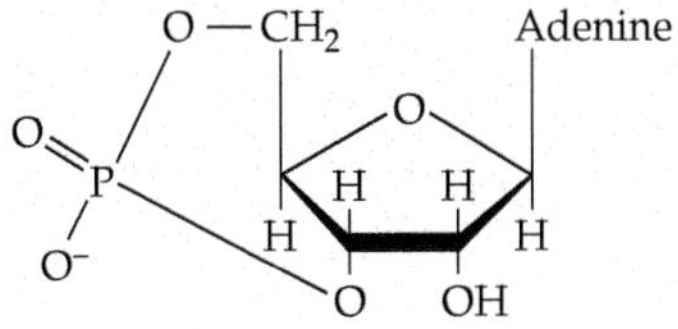

Cyclic AMP (cAMP)
Adenosine 3′, 5′-monophosphate

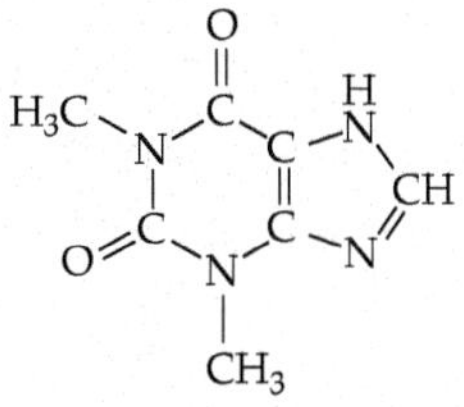

Theophylline
1, 3-Dimethylxanthine

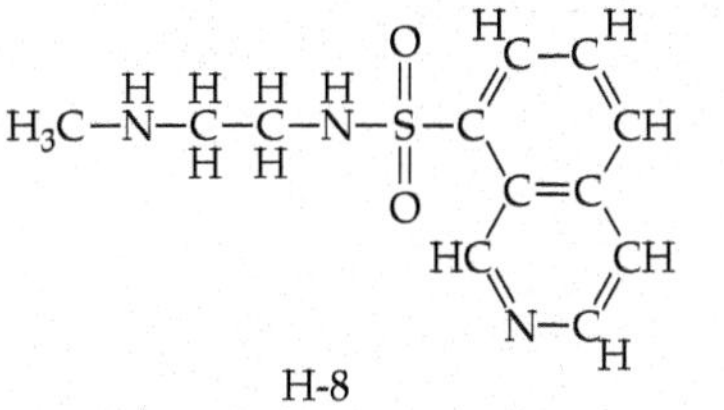

H-8
N-2-[(methylamino)ethyl]-5-isoquinolinesulfonamide

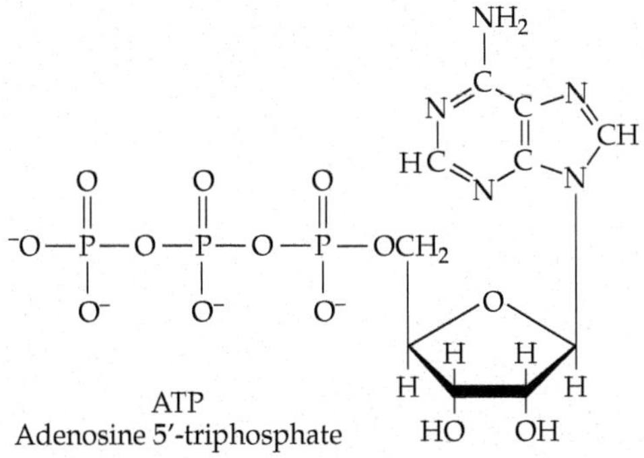

ATP
Adenosine 5′-triphosphate

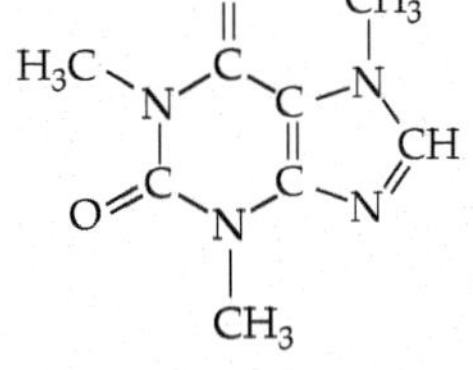

Caffeine
1, 3, 7-Trimethylxanthine

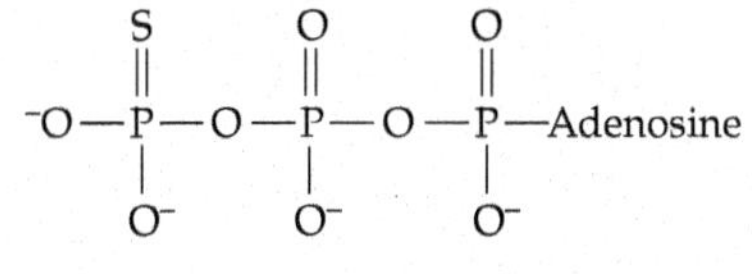

ATPγS
Adenosine 5′-O-[γ-thio]
triphosphate

of channels by activated G proteins. Each activated adenylate cyclase molecule can catalyze the synthesis of many molecules of cAMP and thereby activate many protein kinase molecules—and each activated kinase molecule can phosphorylate many more proteins. Thus, the activity of many molecules of a target protein at widespread sites may be modulated by the occupation of a few receptors. Moreover, cAMP-dependent protein kinase can phosphorylate a variety of proteins and so modulate a broad spectrum of cellular processes. However, all of this takes time. Thus, in frog atrial muscle fibers, it takes about 5 seconds after activating the β-adrenergic receptors before the calcium current begins to increase. Most of this is taken up by the time needed to generate sufficient cAMP. In experiments in which a sudden increase in cAMP was generated by flash photolysis of the precursor o-nitrobenzyl cAMP, an increase in calcium current was seen within 150 ms.[46]

Once generated, cAMP is metabolized to AMP by cyclic nucleotide phosphodiesterase (PDE) enzymes (Box 12.4). Phosphodiesterase activity plays a crucial role in determining the duration of cAMP action and in limiting the spread of cAMP from its site of generation; this has the effect of compartmentalizing the response of cardiac cell calcium channels to nearby β-receptor stimulation.[47]

[46]Nargeot, J. et al. 1983. *Proc. Natl. Acad. Sci. USA* 80: 2385-2399.

[47]Fischmeister, R. et al. 2006. *Circ. Res.* 99: 816-828.

BOX 12.4 — Phosphatidylinositol-4,5-bisphosphate (PIP$_2$) and the Phosphoinositide Cycle

Phosphatidylinositol-4,5-bisphosphate (PIP$_2$) makes up only about 1% of the phospholipids in neuronal cell membranes[48] but plays an important role in transmitter action. It is rapidly hydrolyzed through activation of the enzyme phospholipase C (PLC) when G$_q$-coupled receptors are stimulated. PIP$_2$ itself, and the two products of its hydrolysis, inositol-1,4,5-triphosphate (IP$_3$) and diacylglycerol (DAG), then act as second messengers that alter ion channel function and nerve cell activity (see Figure 12.15).

Most of the PIP$_2$ resides in the inner leaflet of the outer cell membrane.[48] It is composed of two fatty acyl chains (arachidonic acid and a fatty acid) which insert in the membrane, linked through the 1-phosphate to IP$_3$, which is negatively charged and hydrophilic, so projects into the cytoplasm.

Synthesis of PIP$_2$ starts from inositol (in the cytosol) and phosphatidic acid (in the membrane), which are combined to form phosphatidylinositol (PI). This is then sequentially phosphorylated at the 4 and 5 positions on the inositol ring by PI4-kinase and PI5-kinase, respectively, to yield PIP$_2$. PLC cleaves off the inositol ring with its three phosphates in the 1, 4, and 5 positions to give IP$_3$, which goes into the cytoplasm, leaving DAG in the membrane. PLC works very slowly at rest but is strongly activated by the GTP-bound α-subunit of G$_q$, and hence by metabotropic receptors that activate G$_q$. IP$_3$ is dephosphorylated by inositol phosphatase, eventually to inositol, while DAG is phosphorylated by DAG kinase to generate phosphatidic acid—thus, completing the PI cycle.

[48]Gamper, N. S., and Shapiro, M. S. 2007. *Nat. Rev. Neurosci.* 8: 1-14.

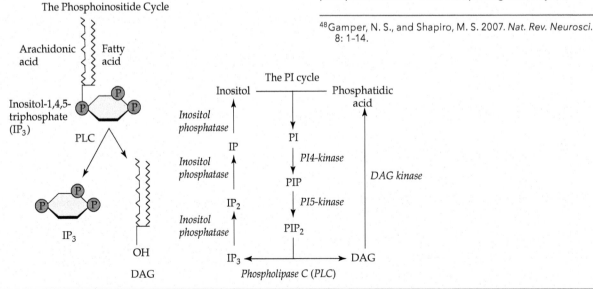

The Phosphoinositide Cycle

CYCLIC AMP DOES MORE THAN ACTIVATE ADENYLATE CYCLASE   Not all of the effects of cAMP result from activation of adenylate cyclase. Thus, the increase in heart rate produced by norepinephrine is due to a direct action of the cAMP on the channels responsible for the pacemaker current in the sinoatrial node (which is where the cardiac rhythm in the mammalian heart is generated).[49],[50] This is an inward current through cation-permeant, hyperpolarization-activated cyclic nucleotide-gated (HCN) channels that are opened by membrane hyperpolarization.[51] Thus, as shown in Figure 12.14A, HCN channels open during the hyperpolarization after an action potential in the cardiac sinoatrial node, and the resulting depolarization (the pacemaker potential) triggers the next action potential. An adrenergic agonist (in this case isoproterenol) causes an increase in the rate of pacemaker depolarization, and hence an increase in action potential frequency (see part a of the figure). This is because of an increase in the magnitude of the pacemaker current (see part b). The graph in part c shows that the increased current is due to a shift in voltage sensitivity: In isoproterenol, less hyperpolarization is required to activate the current. Records from a membrane patch show that a similar increase in pacemaker current is produced by cAMP but not by protein kinase A (Figure 12.14B). Thus, cAMP increases the current by acting directly on the channels rather than by phosphorylation. HCN channels are also present in many neurons. In some of these, they generate pacemaker currents like those in the heart, but they also have other functions.[52] Because of differences in channel subunit composition, not all of these neuronal HCN channels are affected by cAMP.[52]

[49] Brown, H. F., DiFrancesco, D., and Noble, D. 1979. *Nature* 280: 235-236.

[50] DiFrancesco, D., and Tortura, D. P. 1991. *Nature* 351: 145-147.

[51] Accili, E. A. et al. 2002. *News Physiol. Sci.* 17: 32-37.

[52] Wahl-Schott, C., and Biel, M. 2009. *Cell. Mol. Life Sci.* 66: 470-494.

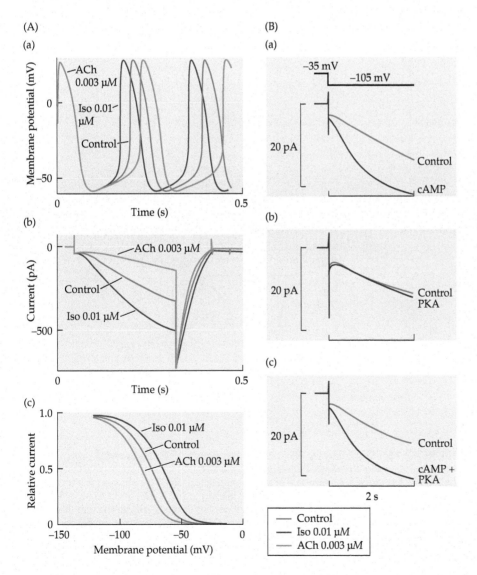

FIGURE 12.14   The Sinoatrial (SA) Node Heart Rate Is Regulated by β-Receptors through a Direct Effect of cAMP on the SA Pacemaker Current I_h. (A). Recordings from an intact rabbit SA node fiber. (a) The β-receptor agonist isoproterenol (Iso) increases the rate of spontaneous action potentials (red trace), whereas acetylcholine (ACh) reduces it (green trace). (b). ACh and Iso have opposite effects on the inward pacemaker current I_h (activated by stepping to –85 mV). (c) ACh and Iso shift the activation curves for I_h in opposite directions. Thus, HCN-channels open more readily with hyperpolarization in Iso solution, giving the faster-rising pacemaker current seen in (a), while ACh has the opposite effect. (B) Pacemaker h-current recorded in an excised inside-out SA node membrane patch with a 2-second step from –35 to –105 mV. Current is increased by cAMP (a) but not by the catalytic subunit of protein kinase A (PKA) (b), and PKA has no further effect after cAMP (c). (A after E. A. Accili et al., 2002. *News Physiol. Sci.* 17: 32-37; B after D. DiFrancesco and D. P. Tortura, 1991. *Nature* 351: 145-147.)

SOME RECEPTORS INHIBIT ADENYLATE CYCLASE   An important property of adenylate cyclase is that it is subject to **inhibition** by transmitters that act on those metabotropic receptors that couple to the inhibitory G protein Gi (i = inhibitory). Thus, in the heart, the activation of Gi by ACh (via M2 muscarinic receptors) inhibits the activation of adenylate cyclase by β-adrenoceptor stimulation. This action prevents the increase in cAMP and so inhibits the increase in calcium current amplitude produced by activating the β-receptors with isoproterenol.[53] By lowering cAMP, acetylcholine also has the opposite effect of β-adrenoceptor stimulation on the cardiac pacemaker current and action potential frequency, as shown in Figure 12.14A. This probably accounts for the opposing effects of sympathetic and vagal nerve activity on the heart rate at normal physiological rates of stimulation.[51]

G Protein Activation of Phospholipase C

Activation of phospholipase C (PLC) is the first step in another important G protein signaling pathway. This enzyme is preferentially activated by metabotropic receptors that couple to the G protein G_q (see Box 12.1). PLC catalyzes the hydrolysis of the membrane phospholipid phosphatidylinositol-4,5-bisphosphate (PIP_2). This yields two potential second messengers: inositol-1,4,5-triphosphate (IP_3), which is water-soluble and enters the cytoplasm; and diacylglycerol (DAG), which stays in the membrane (Figure 12.15; see also Box 12.4). IP_3 releases calcium ions from the endoplasmic reticulum and hence contributes to various Ca^{2+}-dependent processes (see "Calcium as an Intracellular Second Messenger," later in this chapter). DAG remains in the membrane where it activates protein kinase C (PKC) to phosphorylate a variety of target molecules, including some

[53]Fischmeister, R., and Hartzell, H. C. 1986. *J. Physiol.* 376: 183–202.

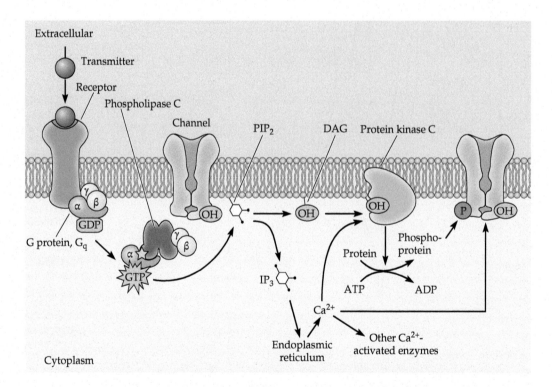

FIGURE 12.15   Signaling by PIP₂ and by Products of PIP₂ Hydrolysis. When a transmitter stimulates a receptor coupled to G$_q$, the GTP-bound G$_q$ protein activates phospholipase C to induce the hydrolysis of phosphatidylinositol-4,5-bisphosphate (PIP₂). This releases two intracellular second messengers: diacylglycerol (DAG) and inositol-1,4,5-triphosphate (IP₃). IP₃ releases calcium from the endoplasmic reticulum into the cytoplasm. DAG and calcium together activate protein kinase C (PKC). PKC catalyzes increased protein phosphorylation. Ion channel function may be modified by loss of PIP₂, by PKC-induced phosphorylation (direct or indirect), or by an effect of calcium (direct or indirect).

ion channels. One important role for PKC is to phosphorylate the ion channels in sensory nerve endings responsible for sensing burning pain; this effect contributes to the thermal hyperalgesia produced by the local inflammatory mediator bradykinin (see Chapter 21).[54] Finally, PIP$_2$ itself is a signaling molecule, so hydrolysis of PIP$_2$ can have functional consequences of its own.

Direct Actions of PIP$_2$

PIP$_2$ is required for the proper function of many membrane proteins, including several ion channels.[48] One such PIP$_2$-regulated ion channel is the **M-channel**, which is a voltage-gated K$^+$ channel that regulates the excitability of many central and peripheral neurons.[55] M-channel currents were first described in sympathetic neurons.[56] In these cells, activation of muscarinic receptors results in closure of M-channels and membrane depolarization (see Chapter 19). Channel closure following stimulation of muscarinic receptors is tightly coupled to the hydrolysis of PIP$_2$. This effect was shown using a fluorescent probe that binds to PIP$_2$ in the membrane (Figure 12.16). When a sympathetic neuron expressing the probe is challenged with a muscarinic agonist, the probe leaves the membrane and moves into the cytoplasm at the same time as the M-current is reduced. It then moves back to the membrane as the M-current recovers.[57] This particular probe—the pleckstrin-homology (PH) domain of phospholipase Cδ, tagged with the jellyfish green fluorescent protein (GFP) so that it can be seen—binds to both PIP$_2$ and to its hydrolysis product IP$_3$. Hence, translocation might result from the loss of PIP$_2$ from the membrane or gain of IP$_3$ in the cytoplasm. However, other evidence shows that channel closure results from the loss of PIP$_2$, not the formation of IP$_3$. Hence, current inhibition is reduced when the amount of PIP$_2$ in the membrane is increased, so that it is more difficult to deplete as a consequence of overexpressing its synthetic enzyme phosphatidylinositol-4-phosphate-5-kinase.[57,58] Similarly, a probe that binds to PIP$_2$ but not to IP$_3$ also shows a dissociation from the membrane.[59]

[54] Cesare, P., and McNaughton, P. A. 1996. *Proc. Natl. Acad. Sci. USA* 93: 15435-15439.

[55] Brown, D. A., and Passmore, G. M. 2009. *Brit. J. Pharmacol.* 156: 1185-1195.

[56] Brown, D. A., and Adams, P. R. 1980. *Nature* 283: 673-676.

[57] Winks, J. S. et al. 2005. *J. Neurosci.* 25: 3400-3413.

[58] Suh, B. C. et al. 2006. *Science* 314: 1454-1457.

[59] Hughes, S. et al. 2007. *Pflügers Arch.* 455: 115-124.

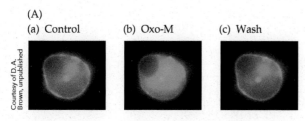

(A)
(a) Control   (b) Oxo-M   (c) Wash

Courtesy of D. A. Brown, unpublished

(B) Cytoplasmic fluorescence

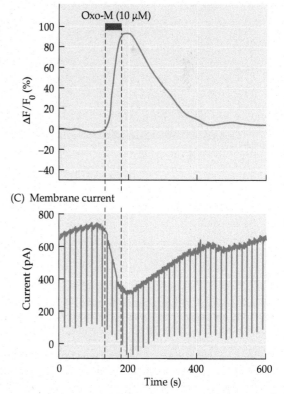

Oxo-M (10 μM)

FIGURE 12.16   Hydrolysis of Phosphatidylinositol-4,5-bisphosphate (PIP$_2$). PIP$_2$ hydrolysis accompanies cholinergic inhibition of M-current in an isolated rat sympathetic neuron. (A) The GFP-tagged PH domain of phospholipase C (GFP-PLCδ-PH) is used as a fluorescent probe to observe PIP$_2$ hydrolysis. At rest (a), the probe binds to PIP$_2$ in the membrane. The muscarinic agonist oxotremorine-M (Oxo-M) (b) stimulates PIP$_2$ hydrolysis and membrane PIP$_2$ falls, so the probe leaves the membrane and goes into the cytoplasm where it binds to free inositol-1,4,5-triphosphate (IP$_3$). On washing out the Oxo-M (c), PIP$_2$ is resynthesized so the probe returns to the membrane. (B) The time course of GFP-PLCδ-PH movement, registered as the change of fluorescence in a region of the cytoplasm. Fluorescence is expressed as fractional increase over original baseline, $\Delta F/F_0$. (C) The time course of M-current inhibition and recovery, recorded as the loss and recovery of outward K$^+$ current at -20 mV. The membrane was hyperpolarized to -50 mV for 2 seconds every 15 seconds to check the change of conductance (given by downward current deflections). Note that the change of M-current closely follows the fluorescence change. (B,C after J. S. Winks et al., 2005. *J. Neurosci.* 25: 3400-3413. © 2005 Society for Neuroscience.)

(C) Membrane current

[60]Wang, H.-S. et al. 1998. *Science* 282: 1890-1893.

[61]Li, Y. et al. 2005. *J. Neurosci.* 25: 9825-9835.

[62]Suh, B. C. et al. 2004. *J. Gen. Physiol.* 123: 663-683.

[63]Falkenburger, B. H., Jensen, J. B., and Hille, B. 2010. *J. Gen. Physiol.* 135: 81-97.

[64]Falkenburger, B. H., Jensen, J. B., and Hille, B. 2010. *J. Gen. Physiol.* 135: 99-114.

[65]Shen, W. et al. 2005. *J. Neurosci.* 25: 7449-7458.

[66]Bazan, N. G. 2006. In G. J. Siegel et al. (Eds.) *Basic Neurochemistry: Molecular, Cellular and Medical Aspects,* 7th ed. Lippincott-Raven, Philadelphia, pp. 731-741.

[67]Meves, H. 2008. *Brit. J. Pharmacol.* 155: 4-16.

[68]Majewski, H., and Iannazzo, L. 1998. *Prog. Neurobiol.* 55: 463-476.

[69]Piomelli, D. 2001. *Trends Neurosci.* 22: 17-19.

[70]Piomelli, D. et al. 1987. *Nature* 328: 38-43.

[71]Buttner, N., Siegelbaum, S. A., and Volterra, A. 1989. *Nature* 342: 553-555.

The direct effect of PIP_2 on M-channel activity is illustrated in Figure 12.17. The constituent potassium channel subunits that make up M-channels ($K_v7.2$ and $K_v7.3$;[60] see Chapter 5) were expressed in Chinese hamster ovary (CHO) cells.[61] When the membrane potential in a cell-attached patch electrode was set to 0 mV, there was modest channel activity. After pulling the patch from the cell, thereby exposing the inner membrane surface to the bathing solution, activity declined but was restored by adding a PIP_2 analogue to the bathing solution. Using this expression system, the kinetics of all of the steps linking the muscarinic receptor to the closure of M-channels have now been examined in detail by B. Hille and his colleagues.[62–64]

A similar signaling pathway appears to be responsible for the muscarinic cholinergic inhibition of M-current (and consequent increased excitability) in mammalian central neurons.[65] Indeed, loss of PIP_2 contributes to the inhibition of a wide variety of PIP_2-dependent ion channels by muscarinic (and other) receptors that stimulate its hydrolysis, including inwardly rectifying K^+ channels, twin-pore K^+ channels, Ca^{2+} channels, and TRP channels.[48]

G Protein Activation of Phospholipase A2

Another target of G protein action is phospholipase A2. This enzyme acts on DAG and on certain membrane phospholipids, such as PIP_2, to release the fatty acid arachidonic acid.[66] Arachidonic acid modulates neuronal signaling by direct effects on ion channels,[67] indirectly through activation of protein kinase C,[68] and through the actions of its metabolites.[69] In *Aplysia* sensory neurons, for example, arachidonic acid is produced in response to receptor activation by the peptide Phe-Met-Arg-Phe-NH2 (FMRFamide) and is metabolized to 12-hydroperoxy-5,8,10,14-eicosatetraenoic acid (12-HPETE). 12-HPETE, in turn, acts to open S-current potassium channels.[70,71]

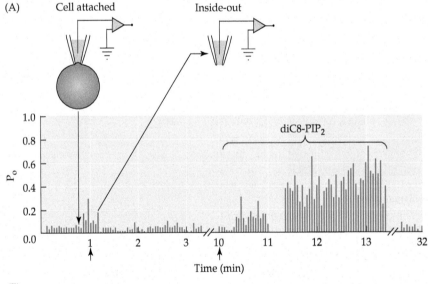

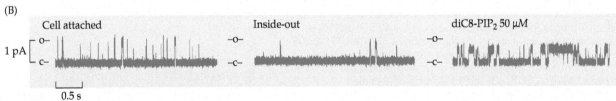

FIGURE 12.17 Phosphatidylinositol-4,5-bisphosphate (PIP₂) Is Necessary to Keep Kᵥ7.2 and 7.3 (M-Type) Potassium Channels Open. $K_v7.2$ and $K_v7.3$ mRNAs were co-expressed in a Chinese hamster ovary (CHO) cell and single-channel activity recorded using a cell-attached pipette set to 0 mV membrane potential. With the pipette on-cell, the channel showed a modest open probability (P_o) of 0.1-0.2. When the membrane patch was excised into inside-out mode (inside surface facing the bathing solution), channel activity was lost. Addition of 50 μM dioctanoyl-phosphatidylinositol-4,5-bisphosphate (diC8-PIP₂) to the bathing solution restored and increased activity. (A) Continuous time-plot of open probability recorded in 3-second runs. (B) Sample currents at a faster speed. o, open; c, closed. (After Y. Li et al., 2005. *J. Neurosci.* 25: 9825-9835. © 2005 Society for Neuroscience.)

Convergence and Divergence of Signals Generated by Indirectly Coupled Receptors

As noted earlier (see Box 12.1), a large number of different G protein-coupled receptors converge on a much smaller number of G proteins. Accordingly, they can all potentially produce the same effects on a neuron. Conversely, activation of one type of G protein can, through various pathways, potentially affect several different ion channels and other proteins in the cell. For example, the activity of a single rat superior cervical sympathetic neuron can be modulated by at least nine transmitters acting through five G protein-coupled pathways that influence two calcium channels and at least one potassium channel,[72] while in different guinea pig sympathetic neurons, muscarinic receptors can affect five different potassium currents.[73]

Selectivity and variation in the cell's response depend on: (1) what receptors are present in that particular cell; (2) which transmitters or hormones the cell actually sees; (3) what effectors are present; and (4) how the receptors, G proteins, and effectors are arranged in the cell membrane. As an example of selectivity in response, GABA (acting on $GABA_B$ receptors) can activate both G_i and G_o proteins, so as to cause potassium channels to open and calcium channels to close. Both effects occur postsynaptically, but only calcium channel inhibition is seen presynaptically. The reason is that the presynaptic nerve endings do not possess the necessary G protein-activated potassium channels.[74]

Signaling Microdomains

An example of selectivity between similar receptors is provided again by the sympathetic ganglion. In mammals, each sympathetic neuron contains both M2 and M4 muscarinic acetylcholine receptors, each of which can potentially activate both G_i and G_o proteins. However, in the rat, only the M4 receptor activates G_o (to inhibit calcium channels), while only the M2 receptor activates G_i (to open potassium channels).[25,75] These cells also show segregation between different receptors that couple to G_q and hydrolyze PIP_2. Thus, the hydrolysis resulting from activation of bradykinin receptors is accompanied by an increase in IP_3 and the release of calcium from the endoplasmic reticulum,[76] whereas no release of calcium occurs after stimulating the muscarinic ACh receptors even though they hydrolyze just as much PIP_2 and produce as much IP_3.[57,59,76] This difference is because the bradykinin receptor is held in very close association with the inositol triphosphate receptor through the actin cytoskeleton, to form what may be termed a signaling microdomain.[77] The assembly of receptors, G proteins, and their immediate effectors into multiprotein complexes—aided by cytoskeletal or scaffolding proteins—seems to be a common feature of signaling through G protein-coupled receptors.[78] Likewise, ion channels are frequently assembled with signaling protein complexes.[79,80] Such complexes serve both to increase signaling efficiency and to segregate different receptor and ion channel signaling pathways.

Divergence of G protein signaling enables a transmitter to generate an integrated response of a neuron or an effector cell to stimulation of a metabotropic receptor. For example, sympathetic nerve stimulation releases norepinephrine, which acts on β-adrenergic receptors in the heart and activates adenylate cyclase (see the earlier discussion in this chapter). This not only modifies the calcium channels to promote an increased entry of calcium during each heartbeat; it also affects various processes involved in the intracellular storage and release of calcium, and in the contractile mechanism itself, to produce a fully coordinated response of the heart to fear or excitement.[39] In the long term, with persistent or repeated stimulation, responses to metabotropic receptor stimulation can extend to changes in gene transcription, to produce long-lasting structural and functional changes in the innervated neurons or effectors.

Retrograde Signaling via Endocannabinoids

Endocannabinoids (Box 12.5) are further products of phospholipid metabolism in nerve cell membranes. They are of obvious interest in view of widespread recreational use of cannabis but—more important for our purposes—are now known to mediate a widespread form of physiological inhibition in the CNS.[81] This contributes to several aspects of CNS function,

[72] Hille, B. 1994. *Trends Neurosci.* 17: 531–536.

[73] Cassell, J. F., and McLachlan, E. M. 1987. *Brit. J. Pharmacol.* 91: 259–261.

[74] Takahashi, T., Kajikawa, Y., and Tsujimoto, T. 1998. *J. Neurosci.* 18: 3138–3146.

[75] Fernandez-Fernandez, J. M. et al. 1999. *J. Physiol.* 515: 631–637.

[76] Delmas, P. et al. 2002. *Neuron* 34: 209–220.

[77] Delmas, P., Crest, M., and Brown, D. A. 2004. *Trends Neurosci.* 27: 41–47.

[78] Bockaert, J. et al. 2010. *Annu. Rev. Pharmacol. Toxicol.* 50: 89–109.

[79] Levitan, I. B. 2006. *Nat. Neurosci.* 9: 305–310.

[80] Zhang, J. et al. 2016. *Neuron* 92: 461–478.

[81] Hashimotodani, Y., Ohno-Shosaku, T., and Kano, M. 2007. *Neuroscientist* 13: 127–137.

BOX **12.5** Formation and Metabolism of Endocannabinoids

Two endocannabinoids are known—anandamide and 2-arachidonoyl glycerol (2-AG). They both contain arachidonic acid (see Box 12.4) linked to ethanolamine and glycerol, respectively, and yield arachidonic acid upon metabolism by fatty acid amide hydrolase or monoacylglycerol lipase (MGL). They are formed from Ca^{2+}-dependent hydrolysis of membrane phospholipids (N-arachidonoyl phosphatidylethanolamine or phosphatidylinositol) by phospholipase D or phospholipase C, respectively.

The principal endocannabinoid in the mammalian nervous system is 2-AG. It is released into the interstitial space where it can act on CB1 cannabinoid receptors. These are G protein-coupled receptors that preferentially couple to the G proteins G_i and G_o. As a result, they can inhibit adenylate cyclase, activate GIRK (K_v3) potassium channels, and inhibit Ca_V2.2 calcium channels. Effects of endocannabinoids are replicated by Δ^9-tetrahydrocannabinol (the active principle of cannabis or marijuana) and the synthetic water-soluble compound WIN 55,212-2, and are antagonized by rimonabant.

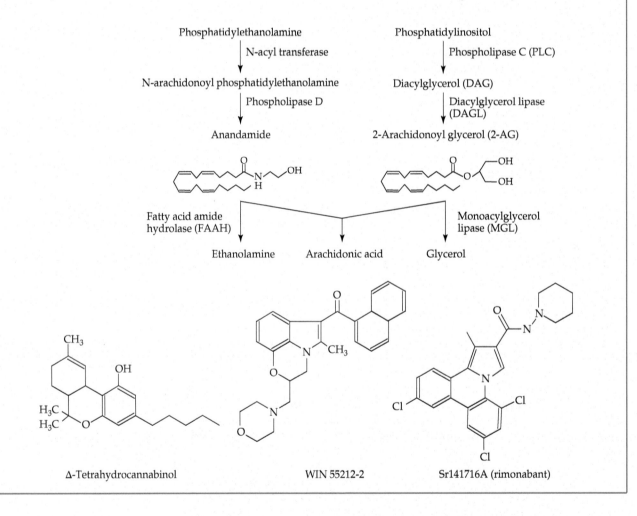

including the sensitization to sensory stimulation that occurs in chronic or neuropathic pain,[82] and forms the basis for the therapeutic applications of cannabinoid drugs.[83]

Unlike diacylglycerol (DAG) or inositol triphosphate, endocannabinoids are released from nerve cells into the extracellular space following stimuli that increase intracellular calcium (including action potentials) or activate phospholipase C (such as G_q-coupled metabotropic receptors). When released in the brain they induce retrograde inhibition of transmitter release by stimulating CB1 cannabinoid receptors (see Box 12.5) on presynaptic nerve terminals.[84,85] Thus, endocannabinoids introduce two new concepts: **retrograde synaptic signaling**, and the release of a transmitter-like messenger that is not stored in synaptic vesicles but is synthesized on demand.

[82] Pernia-Andrade, A. J. et al. 2009. *Science* 325: 760-764.

[83] Iversen, L. 2003. *Brain* 126: 1252-1270.

[84] Wilson, R. I., and Nicoll, R. A. 2002. *Science* 296: 678-682.

[85] Kano, M. et al. 2009. *Physiol. Rev.* 89: 309-380.

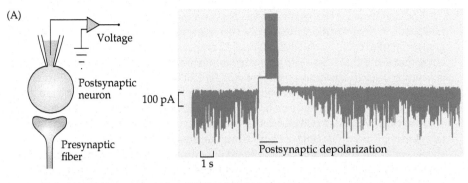

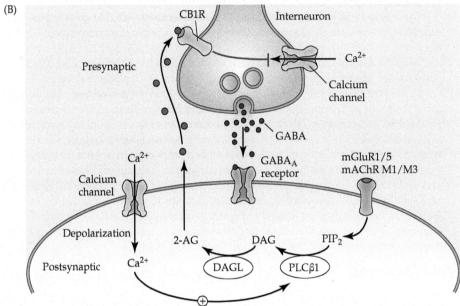

FIGURE 12.18   An Endocannabinoid Acts as a Retrograde Messenger for Depolarization-Induced Suppression of Inhibition (DSI). (A) Recording of spontaneous GABA-mediated inhibitory postsynaptic currents (IPSCs; downward deflections) in a hippocampal pyramidal neuron held at –80 mV. The cell was depolarized for 1 second to induce a train of action potentials, which transiently suppressed the IPSCs. This effect is called depolarization-induced suppression of inhibition, or DSI. (B) Suggested explanation for hippocampal DSI. Postsynaptic depolarization (or action potential activity) opens Ca^{2+} channels to produce an influx of Ca^{2+} ions. This activates phospholipase Cβ1 (PLCβ1) to hydrolyze phosphatidylinositol-4,5-bisphosphate (PIP$_2$), yielding diacylglycerol (DAG). DAG is converted to 2-arachidonoyl glycerol (2-AG) by diacylglycerol lipase (DAGL). 2-AG is then released into the interstitial space and activates the CB1 cannabinoid receptor (CB1R) on the presynaptic terminals. CB1R activates G$_i$ and G$_o$ proteins, and their βγ-subunits then inhibit Ca^{2+} entry through presynaptic Ca^{2+} channels; they may also inhibit synaptic vesicle fusion. Metabotropic glutamate receptors (mGluR1 or mGluR5) or M1 or M3 muscarinic acetylcholine receptors can also independently activate phospholipase C via the G protein G$_q$, to generate 2-AG through the same biochemical pathway. (A after A. Pitler and B. E. Alger, 1992. *J. Neurosci.* 12: 4122-4132. © 1992 Society for Neuroscience.; B after Y. Hashimotodani et al., 2007. *Neuroscientist* 13: 127-137.)

Figure 12.18A illustrates this retrograde synaptic signaling in a hippocampal pyramidal cell.[86] The records show ongoing inhibitory synaptic currents due to spontaneous release of GABA from the presynaptic terminals. Following a train of action potentials in the cell, the spontaneous inhibitory activity is almost totally suppressed, and takes several seconds to recover. Two additional features characterize this phenomenon, which is known as **depolarization-induced suppression of inhibition (DSI)**. First, the postsynaptic response to extrinsically applied GABA is unaffected, so the inhibition of transmission is presynaptic in origin. Second, the response is suppressed by injecting an intracellular calcium buffer, showing that the effect depends on elevation of calcium concentration in the cytosol. It has been suggested that the retrograde effect is initiated by calcium entry into the cell through cell's voltage-sensitive calcium channels. A similar retrograde inhibition of both inhibitory and excitatory transmission, depolarization-induced suppression of excitation (DSE), has been described in cerebellar Purkinje cells.[87,88]

[86] Pitler, T. A., and Alger, B. E. 1992. *J. Neurosci.* 12: 4122-4132.

[87] Llano, I., Leresche, N., and Marty, A. 1991. *Neuron* 6: 564-674.

[88] Kreitzer, A. C., and Regehr, W. G. 2001. *Neuron* 29: 717-727.

[89] Ohno-Shosaku, T., Maejima, T., and Kano, A. 2001. *Neuron* 29: 729–738.

[90] Wilson, R. I., and Nicoll, R. A. 2001. *Nature* 410: 588–592.

[91] Varma, N. et al. 2001. *J. Neurosci.* 21: RC188 (1–5).

[92] Matsuda, L. et al. 1990. *Nature* 346: 561–564.

[93] MacKie, K., and Hille, B. 1992. *Proc. Natl. Acad. Sci. USA* 89: 3825–3829.

[94] Caulfield, M. P., and Brown, D. A. 1992. *Brit. J. Pharmacol.* 106: 231–232.

[95] Kushmerick, C. et al. 2004. *J. Neurosci.* 24: 5955–5965.

[96] Bacci, A. et al. 2004. *Nature* 431: 312–316.

[97] Hashimotodani, Y. et al. 2007. *Neuron* 45: 257–268.

[98] Katona, I. et al. 2000. *NeuroScience* 100: 797–804.

[99] Brown, S. P., Brenowitz, S. D., and Regehr, W. D. 2003. *Nat. Neurosci.* 10: 1047–1058.

[100] Navarrete, M., and Araque, A. 2010. *Neuron* 68: 113–126.

[101] Ignarro, J. 1990. *Ann. Rev. Physiol.* 30: 535–560.

[102] Furchgott, R. F., and Zawadzki, J. V. 1980. *Nature* 288: 373–376.

[103] Palmer, R. M. J., Ferrige, J., and Moncada, S. 1987. *Nature* 324: 524–526.

The identity of the retrograde messenger as an endocannabinoid was resolved by three independent groups working on different central synapses.[89–91] It was found that retrograde inhibition could be imitated by applying cannabinoids and blocked by CB1 receptor antagonists, and that it was also prevented in mice in which the CB1 receptor has been genetically deleted. The mechanism proposed for DSI in the hippocampus is summarized in Figure 12.18B. Calcium entry enhances the activity of PLCβ1, which in turn leads to hydrolysis of PIP$_2$ and sequential generation of DAG and 2-AG (see Box 12.5). 2-AG released from the cell then binds to CB1 receptors[92] on the presynaptic terminal to inhibit transmitter release. CB1 receptors interact with G$_i$ and G$_o$ proteins to cause inhibition of calcium channels.[93–95] Because calcium influx into the presynaptic terminals is reduced, transmitter release is attenuated.[95] Postsynaptically, activation of CB1 receptors may inhibit excitability by opening G protein-activated inwardly rectifying potassium (GIRK) channels.[96]

The release of the endocannabinoid 2-AG is also increased when PLCβ1 is activated by stimulating postsynaptic G$_q$-coupled metabotropic M1 muscarinic or metabotropic glutamate receptors 1 and 5,[85] through IP$_3$-induced calcium release. Since stimulation of these receptors reinforces the effect of Ca^{2+} channel opening, the simultaneous occurrences of both forms of postsynaptic response reinforce each other, providing a form of "coincidence detection."[97]

2-AG is synthesized and released from any part of the nerve cell membrane that detects a rise in Ca^{2+} or PLC stimulation. Thus, it can exert diffuse effects. In the hippocampus, for example, depolarization of one pyramidal neuron can suppress inhibitory synapses on a neighboring neuron.[90] This effect occurs primarily on inhibitory terminals, where CB1 receptors are most concentrated, rather than on excitatory terminals.[98] In contrast, in the cerebellum, retrograde inhibition of excitatory transmission is normally confined to the activated synapses, because the postsynaptic calcium signals in the Purkinje cell dendrites are highly localized.[99] A more diffuse effect may occur during intense stimulation or when synaptic excitation is coupled with postsynaptic activation of metabotropic receptors.[85] Endocannabinoids may also affect transmission at distant synapses through activation of CB receptors on neuroglial cells, with consequent release of glutamate.[100]

Signaling via Nitric Oxide and Carbon Monoxide

Nitric oxide (NO), a water- and lipid-soluble gas produced from arginine by NO synthase (NOS), acts as a transmitter by diffusing from the cytoplasm of one cell into neighboring cells and activating guanylate cyclase.[101] NO was first characterized as an important regulator of blood pressure, mediating the vasodilation caused by acetylcholine.[102,103] Production of NO is initiated by the interaction of ACh with muscarinic receptors on vascular endothelial cells, which in turn leads to activation of phosphatidylinositide-specific phospholipase C, formation of IP$_3$, and release of calcium from intracellular stores (Figure 12.19). Calcium combines with calmodulin and activates NOS, producing NO. NO diffuses into neighboring smooth muscle cells and stimulates the soluble form of guanylate cyclase, causing an increase in cyclic guanosine monophosphate (cGMP). The cGMP, in turn, activates a cGMP-dependent protein kinase. The resulting increases in protein phosphorylation modulate the activity of potassium and calcium channels and calcium pumps, leading to a decrease in intracellular

FIGURE 12.19 Paracrine Signaling by Release of Nitric Oxide. ACh binds to muscarinic receptors (mAChR) on vascular endothelial cells, activating phosphatidylinositide-specific phospholipase C (PI-PLC). PI-PLC forms inositol-1,4,5-triphosphate (IP$_3$), which releases calcium from intracellular stores. Calcium, together with calmodulin, activates nitric oxide synthase (NOS), producing nitric oxide (NO). NO diffuses into neighboring smooth muscle cells and stimulates guanylate cyclase (GC), increasing cGMP. cGMP activates cGMP-dependent protein kinase (PKG). The resulting increases in protein phosphorylation lead to a decrease in intracellular calcium concentration, causing relaxation. NO is rapidly degraded, so that it affects only nearby cells—hence the term paracrine.

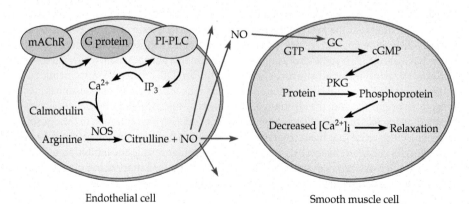

Endothelial cell　　　　Smooth muscle cell

calcium concentration and reduced Ca^{2+} sensitivity of the contractile proteins, which causes relaxation. NO is inactivated within seconds by reaction with superoxides and by formation of complexes with heme-containing proteins such as hemoglobin. The role of NO in relaxing blood vessel smooth muscles explains the vasodilator and hypotensive action of glyceryl trinitrate and other nitro-compounds, which release free NO and so act as NO donors. It also explains why phosphodiesterase-5 (PDE-5) inhibitors such as sildenafil enhance and prolong penile erections: Erection results from NO-induced cGMP-mediated penile vasodilation, and cGMP is selectively degraded to 5′-GMP by PDE-5, so PDE-5 inhibitors reduce the rate of cGMP inactivation.

The role of NO as a neurotransmitter was first established in the peripheral autonomic nervous system,[104,105] where it is released from **non-adrenergic, non-cholinergic (NANC)** fibers to relax smooth muscle in the same manner as NO released from endothelial cells. In this case, however, the stimulus for NOS is Ca^{2+} entry into the nerve terminals during the presynaptic action potential. A role in brain function was first suggested from experiments on the cerebellum, in which NO was shown to be responsible for the increase in cGMP produced by stimulating the NMDA-type ionotropic glutamate receptors (see Chapter 5).[106,107] The NMDA receptor in cerebellar granule cells is closely associated with NOS, so that the enzyme is activated by Ca^{2+} ions entering through the NMDA channels. The released NO then stimulates guanylate cyclase in the Purkinje cells or in adjacent astroglial cells.[108] In Purkinje cells, the cGMP thus formed activates the cGMP-dependent protein kinase, leading to phosphorylation and endocytosis of the postsynaptic AMPA receptor that subserves normal excitatory transmission from the parallel fibers, thereby complementing the effect of endocannabinoid in suppressing transmitter release from the presynaptic terminals. Conversely, in the hippocampus, postsynaptically generated NO may act as a retrograde messenger that contributes to long-term potentiation of excitatory transmission.[108] Because it is a freely diffusible gas, NO formed in one neuron can affect the function of neighboring neurons and synapses, up to distances of 100 μm away.[109]

As with cAMP, not all of the effects of cGMP are due to activation of cGMP-dependent protein kinase. For example, the cGMP formed in the retina following the release of NO from the illuminated retina directly opens cyclic nucleotide-gated (CNG) cation channels in cone photoreceptors; the influx of calcium through these cation channels then increases glutamate release from the cone cells.[110] Also, NO itself may produce other effects than stimulation of guanylate cyclase, such as S-nitrosylation of certain ion channel proteins.[111] Thus, NO-mediated S-nitrosylation inhibits K_v7 potassium channels in sensory neurons, leading to sensory hyperexcitability.[112]

Another endogenously produced gas with properties similar to those of NO is carbon monoxide (CO).[113] CO is formed from the degradation of heme by the enzyme heme oxygenase and, like NO, can activate guanylate cyclase to produce cGMP. In the intestinal nervous system, release of CO seems to cooperate with NO in generating the NANC relaxation of intestinal smooth muscle, since relaxation produced by stimulating the enteric neurons is equally reduced in mice lacking NO synthase or heme oxygenase. CO may also have a role in signaling in the CNS, since inhibition of heme oxygenase (like inhibition of NOS) can prevent or reverse the induction of long-term potentiation in the hippocampus.[114,115]

Like the endocannabinoids, NO and CO cannot be stored in synaptic vesicles, but are synthesized on demand and immediately released. They then diffuse indiscriminately from the site at which they are produced into neighboring cells, their spread being limited only by their short life span. Together with the exocytosis of transmitters and peptides from outside synaptic terminals discussed in Chapter 18, this type of diffuse signaling has been termed **paracrine transmission** or, in the brain, **volume transmission**. Clearly, specificity in the effects of such signals depends on the distribution and properties of enzymes activated or inhibited by NO and CO.

Calcium as an Intracellular Second Messenger

Calcium is a ubiquitous second messenger.[116–118] The concentration of free Ca^{2+} ions in the cytoplasm at rest is around 100 nM (i.e., about 1/10,000th of that in the extracellular fluid). One reason for this low concentration of free calcium ions is that most of the cytoplasmic calcium is reversibly bound to (buffered by) calcium-binding proteins. Around 98% to 99.8% of the total calcium in the cytoplasm is buffered in this way.[119–121] Cytoplasmic calcium is in

[104] Gillespie, J. S., Liu, X. R., and Martin, W. 1989. *Brit. J. Pharmacol.* 98: 1080–1082.

[105] Bult, H. et al. 1990. *Nature* 345: 346–347.

[106] Garthwaite, J., Charles, S. L., and Chess-Williams, R. 1988. *Nature* 336: 385–388.

[107] Bredt, D. S., and Snyder, S. H. 1989. *Proc. Natl. Acad. Sci. USA* 86: 9030–9033.

[108] Garthwaite, J. 2008. *Eur. J. Neurosci.* 27: 2783–2802.

[109] Steinert, J. R. et al. 2008. *Neuron* 60: 642–656.

[110] Savchenko, A., Barnes, S., and Kramer, R. H. 1997. *Nature* 390: 694–698.

[111] Ahern, P., Klyachko, V. A., and Jackson, M. B. 2002. *Trends Neurosci.* 25: 510–517.

[112] Gamper, N., and Ooi, L. 2015. *Antioxid. Redox Signal.* 22: 486–504.

[113] Snyder, S. H., Jaffrey, S. R., and Zakhary, R. 1998. *Brain Res. Brain Res. Rev.* 26: 167–175.

[114] Stevens, C. F., and Wang, Y. 1993. *Nature* 364: 147–149.

[115] Zhuo, M. et al. 1993. *Science* 260: 1946–1950.

[116] Ghosh, A., and Greenberg, M. E. 1995. *Science* 268: 239–247.

[117] Berridge M. J., Lipp, P., and Bootman, M. D. 2000. *Nat. Rev. Mol. Cell Biol.* 1: 11–21.

[118] Clapham, D. E. 2007. *Cell* 131: 1047–1058.

[119] Neher, E., and Augustine, G. J. 1992. *J. Physiol.* 450: 273–301.

[120] Trouslard, J., Marsh, S. J., and Brown, D. A. 1993. *J. Physiol.* 481: 251–271.

[121] Fierro, L., and Llano, I. 1996. *J. Physiol.* 496: 617–625.

dynamic equilibrium with extracellular calcium, and with intracellular calcium stores, principally within the endoplasmic reticulum (ER) and mitochondria. The different mechanisms for regulating cytoplasmic calcium concentration are summarized in Figure 12.20.

Since the intracellular concentration of Ca^{2+} ions is so low, there is plenty of scope for increasing it. From the viewpoint of transmitter action, two mechanisms are predominant. First, the high transmembrane Ca^{2+} gradient generates a large Ca^{2+} influx when calcium-permeable ionotropic receptors are stimulated. These include the NMDA-type ionotropic glutamate

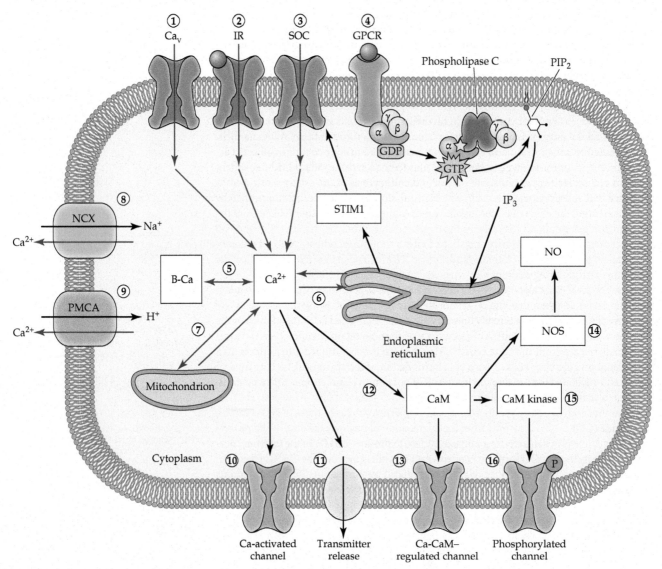

FIGURE 12.20 Calcium as an Intracellular Second Messenger. Intracellular Ca^{2+} ions in neurons are increased by (1) entry through voltage-gated calcium channels (Ca_V) during electrical activity; (2) activation of calcium-permeable ionotropic receptors (IR) by neurotransmitters such as glutamate and acetylcholine; (3) opening of store-operated calcium (SOC) channels; and (4) activation of G protein-coupled receptors (GPCR) that stimulate phospholipase C (PLC) and generate inositol-1,4,5-triphosphate (IP$_3$; see Figure 12.15). The IP$_3$ releases calcium from the endoplasmic reticulum (ER). Depletion of the ER calcium stores by IP$_3$ releases another signaling molecule, STIM1, that couples to SOC channels (principally Orai) in the outer membrane (4) to generate a second wave of calcium entry. (5) Most of the Ca^{2+} ions (98%-99%) are rapidly but reversibly buffered by calcium buffers (B-Ca). Cytosolic [Ca^{2+}] is subsequently restored by uptake into intracellular organelles—the ER (6) and, at high calcium loads, mitochondria (7)—and by extrusion via (8) the cell membrane sodium-calcium exchange pump (NCX) or (9) the cell membrane calcium ATPase (PMCA). Messenger functions include: (10) direct activation of calcium-dependent potassium, chloride, and cation channels; (11) stimulation of vesicular transmitter and hormone release; and (12) binding to and activation of calmodulin (CaM). Ca-CaM may (13) modulate other ion channels (e.g., activation of small [SK] calcium-dependent potassium channels) and activate several enzymes. These activated enzymes include (14) nitric oxide synthase (NOS) to generate another messenger, nitric oxide (NO; see Figure 12.19), and (15) calcium-calmodulin-dependent protein kinases (CaM kinase). This can phosphorylate ion channels (16) and many other molecules, to produce a variety of long-term changes in nerve cell function.

receptors[122] and nicotinic ACh receptors, especially those containing α_7- or α_9-subunits.[123] Second, metabotropic receptors that couple to G_q generate IP_3, which acts on ionotropic IP_3 receptors[124] to release Ca^{2+} from the endoplasmic reticulum (see Figure 12.20).[125]

Optical methods for imaging Ca^{2+} transients using fluorescent Ca^{2+}-binding compounds (Box 12.6) have revealed other properties of the Ca^{2+} transients produced by nerve activity and transmitter action. For example, increases in $[Ca^{2+}]$ are often confined to particular small regions of the neuron, creating calcium microdomains.[126-129] This results, in part, from the very slow diffusion of Ca^{2+} ions in the cytoplasm (about 1/50th of that in free solution[130]) because of binding to buffers and intracellular uptake. Thus, following synaptic activation of glutamate receptors, postsynaptic calcium transients may be confined for some time to individual dendrites[131] or even to a single dendritic spine.[132]

Calcium signals in these microdomains often appear as elementary events (variously called sparks, puffs, syntillas, etc.), reflecting the opening of single calcium-carrying channels or clusters of channels in the membrane or ER.[133] Though most frequently studied in non-neural cells, such events have also been seen in neurons.[134,135] Indeed, even before calcium imaging, they were detected in sympathetic neurons as spontaneous miniature outward currents (SMOCs), signifying the release of packets of calcium from the submembrane ER and consequent opening of calcium-activated potassium channels.[136] Rises in calcium concentration may also appear as oscillations or traveling waves.[117] The latter result from regenerative calcium-induced calcium release from intracellular stores. In neuronal dendrites, the calcium wave can appear as the discontinuous (saltatory) propagation of a calcium spike, rather like (but much slower than) the conduction of an action potential along a myelinated nerve fiber, as the calcium jumps from one cluster of IP_3 receptors to the next.[137]

Actions of Calcium

A rise in intracellular calcium has many effects on neuronal activity and function, as indicated in Figure 12.20. A widely studied function is to couple electrical activity with exocytosis in neurons and gland cells, as we will discuss in Chapters 13 and 18. Another direct effect is the activation of calcium-dependent potassium channels. An interesting example of this is the inhibition of cochlear hair cells by efferent cholinergic fibers in the auditory nerves (see also Chapters 21 and 24).[138] Cholinergic activation would ordinarily be excitatory, as at the neuromuscular junction. However, calcium entering through the ACh-activated channels opens adjacent calcium-activated potassium channels, thereby producing inhibition (Figure 12.21A).

[122] Burnashev, N. et al. 1995. *J. Physiol.* 485: 403-418.

[123] Fucile, S. 2004. *Cell Calcium* 35: 1-8.

[124] Mikoshiba, K. 2007. *J. Neurochem.* 102: 1426-1446.

[125] Streb, H. et al. 1983. *Nature* 306: 67-69.

[126] Ross, W. N., Arechiga, H., and Nicholls, J. G. 1988. *Proc. Natl. Acad. Sci. USA* 85: 4075-4078.

[127] Llinás, R., Sugimori, M., and Silver, R. B. 1992. *Science* 256: 677-679.

[128] Oheim, M., Kirchhoff, F., and Stühmer, W. 2006. *Cell Calcium* 40: 423-439.

[129] Parekh, A. B. 2008. *J. Physiol.* 586: 3043-3054.

[130] Hodgkin, A. L., and Keynes, R. D. 1957. *J. Physiol.* 138: 253-281.

[131] Eilers, J., Plant, T., and Konnerth, A. 1996. *Cell Calcium* 20: 215-226.

[132] Denk, W., Sugimori, M., and Llinas, R. 1995. *Proc. Natl. Acad. Sci. USA* 92: 8279-8282.

[133] Cheng, H., and Lederer, W. J. 2008. *Physiol. Revs.* 88: 1491-1545.

[134] Ouyang, K. et al. 2005. *Proc. Natl. Acad. Sci. USA* 102: 12259-12264.

[135] Manita, S., and Ross, W. N. 2009. *J. Neurosci.* 29: 7833-7845.

[136] Brown, D. A., Constanti, A., and Adams, P. R. 1983. *Cell Calcium* 4: 407-420.

[137] Fitzpatrick, J. S. et al. 2009. *J. Physiol.* 587: 1439-1459.

[138] Fuchs, P. A., and Murrow, B. W. 1992. *J. Neurosci.* 12: 800-809.

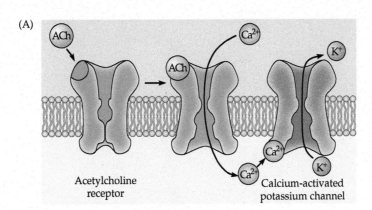
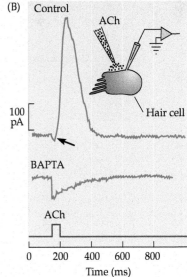

FIGURE 12.21 Inhibition by ACh-Activated Cation Channels. (A) In chick cochlear hair cells, ACh binds to nicotinic ionotropic receptors that allow cations, including calcium, to flow into the cell. Intracellular calcium causes calcium-activated potassium channels to open, leading to outward potassium current and hyperpolarization. (B) In a whole-cell recording (inset and upper record), application of ACh near the base of a hair cell produces a small, transient inward current (arrow) followed by a large outward current. In the intact cell, the outward current would be inhibitory. If the calcium chelator BAPTA is added to the recording electrode, and hence to the cell cytoplasm, ACh application produces only inward current (lower record). No outward current is seen because incoming calcium ions are chelated and so prevented from activating potassium channels. (Records provided by P. A. Fuchs.)

BOX **12.6**   Measuring Intracellular Calcium

Changes in the concentration of intracellular calcium ions are usually measured using luminescent or fluorescent calcium-binding compounds. One of the first such compounds was the luminescent jellyfish protein aequorin.[139] This comprises a 22-kD apo-aequorin (APO) protein attached via oxygen to a fluorophore coelenterazine. On binding three Ca^{2+} ions, coelenterazine is converted to the amide and the complex splits, giving off a blue light (peak 460 nm).

Because it binds three Ca^{2+} ions, aequorin responds to a wide range of Ca^{2+} concentrations (from 0.1 to >100 μM) but suffers from the disadvantage that it is broken down after binding Ca^{2+}, so the concentration rapidly declines. However, because apo-aequorin is a protein, it can be expressed in cells from its complementary DNA (cDNA) by transfection. Cells readily take up coelenterazine, and can form aequorin from the expressed apo-aequorin. Then, by adding a targeting sequence to the cDNA, the aequorin can be expressed, and Ca^{2+} monitored in subcellular organelles such as the endoplasmic reticulum.[140]

Two widely used calcium indicators are Fura-2 and Indo-1, derived from the calcium chelator 1,2-bis(o-aminophenoxy)ethane-N,N,N,N-tetraacetic acid (BAPTA) by Roger Tsien and his colleagues.[141] Fura-2 and Indo-1 are excited by ultraviolet light and show a shift in their excitation (Fura-2) or emission (Indo-1) spectrum when they bind Ca^{2+} ions. This is useful, since

the concentration of Ca^{2+} can be calculated from the change in the ratio of the fluorescence at two excitation or emission wavelengths. This ratiometric method avoids artifacts arising from changes in concentration or fluorescence quenching.

Individually, these indicators cover a narrower range of calcium concentrations than aequorin, but many different fluorescent indicators are available to cover different ranges of [Ca^{2+}]. They are not proteins, so they cannot be expressed or directed to specific subcellular organelles. Instead, for this Roger Tsien has devised another type of protein-based calcium reporter termed a cameleon.[142] Cameleons use calmodulin as the calcium sensor, coupled to a calmodulin-binding protein and two different fluorescent proteins from a jellyfish (based on green fluorescent protein, GFP) with different emission wavelengths. When the calmodulin binds calcium, it induces a conformational change in the calmodulin-binding protein, which brings the two GFP derivatives closer together so that their fluorescences interact (Förster resonance energy transfer, or FRET). FRET can be recorded using two different emission wavelengths to calculate the concentration of Ca^{2+} ions.

[139] Shimomura, O., and Johnson, F. H. 1970. *Nature* 227: 1356-1357.

[140] Montero, M. et al. 1995. *EMBO J.* 14: 5467-5475.

[141] Grynkiewicz, G., Poenie, M., and Tsien, R. Y. 1985. *J. Biol. Chem.* 260: 3440-3450.

[142] Miyawaki, A. et al. 1997. *Nature* 388: 882-887.

Coelenterazine   Aequorin   Coelenteramide

Fura-2

Fura-2 excitation spectrum

After G. Grynkiewicz et al., 1985, *J. Biol Chem.* 260: 3440-3450.

As shown in Figure 12.21B, direct application of a brief pulse of ACh produces a small transient inward current, which is due to activation of nicotinic receptors and is followed by a much larger outward current due to activation of potassium channels. After the calcium chelator 1,2-bis(o-aminophenoxy)ethane-N,N,N,N-tetraacetic acid (BAPTA) has been added to the bathing solution, activation of the potassium channels is blocked and only the inward synaptic current is seen. This mechanism is particularly effective because the cochlear nicotinic receptors are composed of α_9- and α_{10}-subunits,[143] which have an unusually high calcium permeability.[123] A similar mechanism of inhibition may occur in some neurons in the brain.[144] In both brain and cochlea,[145,146] the responsive potassium channels belong to the small-conductance (SK, $K_{Ca}2$) family; for these channels, the calcium is not sensed by the channel protein itself but by closely associated calmodulin molecules.[147] Other calcium-activated channels that participate in second-messenger-mediated responses include calcium-activated chloride channels, which contribute to olfactory sensing,[148] and cation channels that are activated by calcium-releasing metabotropic receptors,[149] which may be members of the TRP family of cation channels (see Chapter 5).

The principal molecular transducer of calcium actions is the calcium-binding protein calmodulin.[118] Calmodulin can bind four calcium ions. This induces a conformational change in the calmodulin molecule, which allows it to activate or inhibit other proteins. These include ion channels, such as the SK type of calcium-dependent potassium channel just mentioned and the IP_3-activated endoplasmic reticulum calcium channels, but the main targets of calcium-calmodulin (Ca-CaM) are enzymes, such as calcium-calmodulin-dependent protein kinases (CaM kinases), calcineurin (a protein phosphatase), and NO synthase (NOS). Activation of NOS produces the tertiary messenger NO (see Figure 12.19). CaM kinases can phosphorylate several ion channels[150] and play a major role in promoting long-term changes in nerve cell function such as long-term potentiation (see Chapter 15) and inducing changes in transcription.[116,151] Calcium also activates important calcium-binding enzymes independently of calmodulin, such as phospholipases, protein kinase C, and proteases such as calpain.

Prolonged Time Course of Indirect Transmitter Action

Synaptic interactions mediated by indirect mechanisms typically develop more slowly and last much longer than those mediated by direct mechanisms (see also Chapter 18). At the skeletal neuromuscular junction, only 1 to 2 milliseconds are required for ACh to be released, diffuse across the synaptic cleft, and bind to and open ionotropic ACh receptors. These events are much too fast to be mediated by enzymes such as adenylate cyclase or phospholipase C, which take many milliseconds to catalyze the synthesis of a single molecule of cAMP, or the hydrolysis of a membrane lipid. Even activation of a membrane channel by binding of a G protein subunit to the channel itself tends to have a time course of hundreds of milliseconds, reflecting the lifetime of the activated α-subunit. Responses mediated by enzymatic production of diffusible cytoplasmic second messengers such as cAMP or IP_3 are slower still, lasting seconds to minutes and reflecting the slow time course of changes in second-messenger concentration.

Yet experience tells us that changes in signaling in the nervous system can last a lifetime (for example, the instant recollection in old age of a childhood memory). How can such long-lasting changes in synaptic efficacy be produced? One answer comes from the properties of several of the protein kinases discussed in this chapter. These enzymes are themselves targets for phosphorylation. For example, when activated by calcium, CaM kinase II phosphorylates itself.[151] It can then become constitutively active and no longer requires the presence of the calcium-calmodulin complex for activity. This mechanism is one way by which a transient increase in calcium concentration can be translated into long-lasting activation of the kinase, which in turn can cause sustained changes in the activity of its other target proteins. Activated CaM kinase may be highly restricted in its location, to a single synapse or dendritic spine (see Chapter 17).[152]

[143] Lustig, L. R. 2006. *Anat. Rec.* 288A: 424-234.

[144] Gulledge, A. T., and Stuart, G. J. 2005. *J. Neurosci.* 28: 10305-10320.

[145] Oliver, D. et al. 2000. *Neuron* 26: 595-601.

[146] Kong, J.-H., Adelman, J. P., and Fuchs, P. A. 2008. *J. Physiol.* 586: 5471-5485.

[147] Maylie, J. et al. 2004. *J. Physiol.* 554: 255-261.

[148] Stephan, A. B. et al. 2009. *Proc. Natl. Acad. Sci. USA* 106: 10776-10781.

[149] Congar, P. et al. 1997. *J. Neurosci.* 17: 5366-5379.

[150] Levitan, I. B. 1994. *Annu. Rev. Physiol.* 56: 193-212.

[151] Soderling, T. 2000. *Curr. Opin. Neurobiol.* 10: 375-380.

[152] Lee, S. J. et al. 2009. *Nature* 458: 299-304.

For changes to persist for days or longer, protein synthesis is usually required. Many of the second-messenger systems described in this chapter have been shown to produce changes in protein synthesis.[153] Such changes typically occur as a result of activation of one or more protein phosphorylation signaling cascades, which lead to phosphorylation of transcription factors and, consequently, altered gene expression. The most rapid effects that have been measured occur in expression of immediate early genes, such as *c-fos*, which encodes the inducible transcription factor Fos. Upon translation, this protein enters the nucleus, where it regulates further gene expression, ultimately producing metabolic or structural changes that permanently alter the response of the cell.[154] The final translational step from messenger RNA (mRNA) to protein may then be restricted to individual synapses,[154] allowing such changes to be confined to specific neural pathways or patterns of neural activity.

[153] Flavell, S. W., and Greenberg, M. E. 2008. *Annu. Rev. Neurosci.* 31: 563–590.

[154] Wang, D. O. et al. 2009. *Science* 324: 1536–1540.

SUMMARY

- Neurotransmitters activate metabotropic receptors that are not themselves ion channels, but instead modify the activity of ion channels, ion pumps, or other receptor proteins by indirect mechanisms.

- Examples of metabotropic receptors include muscarinic ACh receptors; α- and β-adrenergic receptors; some of the receptors for GABA, 5-HT, dopamine, and glutamate; and receptors for neuropeptides, light, and odorants. They produce their effects through G proteins.

- G proteins are αβγ-heterotrimers. In the resting state, GDP is bound to the α-subunit, and the three subunits are associated as a trimer. When activated by a metabotropic receptor, GDP is replaced with GTP, the α- and βγ-subunits dissociate, and the free subunits activate one or more intracellular targets. The activity of G protein subunits is terminated by hydrolysis of GTP to GDP by the endogenous GTPase activity of the α-subunit followed by the recombination of the α- and βγ-subunits into a trimer.

- Some G protein βγ-subunits bind directly to ion channels and stimulate or inhibit their activity. Other G protein α- or βγ-subunits activate adenylate cyclase, phospholipase C, or phospholipase A2, generating intracellular second messengers that can have widespread effects. Changes in membrane phospholipids that result from phospholipase C activation also affect ion channel function.

- Indirectly acting transmitters influence the activity of potassium and calcium channels. The changes in potassium and calcium channel activity in turn influence the resting potential, spontaneous activity, response to other inputs, or amount of calcium entering during an action potential—and thereby, the amount of transmitter release.

- Endocannabinoids act as tertiary messengers. They are synthesized and released in response to a rise in intracellular calcium. They serve as retrograde messengers, inhibiting transmitter release from presynaptic endings.

- NO also acts as a tertiary messenger that is synthesized and released in response to a rise in calcium. It stimulates cGMP formation to affect ion channels in the same or neighboring neurons.

- Changes in intracellular calcium or calcium-calmodulin concentration regulate ion channels, phospholipases C and A2, protein kinase C, calpain, adenylate cyclase, cyclic nucleotide phosphodiesterase, and NO synthase.

- Both the distribution of changes in intracellular calcium, which can be highly localized, and their dynamics (calcium waves and oscillations) are important determinants of calcium action.

- Transmitter actions mediated by indirect mechanisms have time courses that vary from milliseconds to years. Rapid effects are produced by direct changes in ion channel activity, effects of intermediate duration by activation and phosphorylation of enzymes and other proteins, and very long-lasting effects by regulation of protein synthesis.

Suggested Reading

General Reviews

Clapham, D. E. 2007. Calcium signaling. *Cell* 131: 1047–1058.

Delmas, P., and Brown, D. A. 2005. Pathways modulating neural KCNQ/M (K$_v$7) potassium channels. *Nat. Rev. Neurosci.* 6: 850–862.

Evans, R. M., and Zamponi, G. W. 2006. Presynaptic Ca^{2+} channels—integration centers for neuronal signaling pathways. *Trends Neurosci.* 29: 617–624.

Gamper, N. S., and Shapiro, M. S. 2007. Regulation of ion transport proteins by membrane phosphoinositides. *Nat. Rev. Neurosci.* 8: 1–14.

Garthwaite, J. 2008. Concepts of neural nitric oxide-mediated transmission. *Eur. J. Neurosci.* 27: 2783–2802.

Hille, B., Dickson, E., Kruse, M., and Falkenburger, B. 2014. Dynamic metabolic control of an ion channel. *Prog Mol Biol Transl Sci.* 123: 219-247.

Kano, M., Ohno-Shosaku, T., Hashimotodani, Y., Uchigashima, M., and Watanabe, M. 2009. Endocannabinoid-mediated control of synaptic transmission. *Physiol. Rev.* 89: 309–380.

Meves, H. 2008. Arachidonic acid and ion channels: An update. *Brit. J. Pharmacol.* 155: 4–16.

Oldham, W. H., and Hamm, H. E. 2008. Heterotrimeric G protein activation by G-protein-coupled receptors. *Nat. Rev. Mol. Cell Biol.* 9: 60–71.

Parekh, A. B. 2008. Ca^{2+} microdomains near plasma membrane Ca^{2+} channels: impact on cell function. *J. Physiol.* 586: 3043–3054.

Wayman, G. A., Lee, Y. S., Tokumitsu, H., Silva, A. J., and Soderling, T. R. 2008. Calmodulin-kinases: Modulators of neuronal development and plasticity. *Neuron* 59: 914–931.

Wettschureck, N., and Offermanns, S. 2005. Mammalian G proteins and their cell type specific functions. *Physiol. Rev.* 85:1 159–1204.

Original Papers

DiFrancesco, D., and Tortura, D. P. 1991. Direct activation of cardiac pacemaker channels by intracellular cyclic AMP. *Nature* 351: 145–147.

Doupnik, C. A., Davidson, N., Lester, H. A., and Kofuji, P. 1997. RGS proteins reconstitute the rapid gating kinetics of gbetagamma-activated inwardly rectifying K$^+$ channels. *Proc. Natl. Acad. Sci. USA* 94: 10461–10466.

Fuchs, P. A., and Murrow, B. W. 1992. Cholinergic inhibition of short (outer) hair cells of the chick's cochlea. *J. Neurosci.* 12: 800–809.

Ikeda, S. R. 1996. Voltage-dependent modulation of N-type calcium channels by G-protein beta gamma subunits. *Nature* 380: 255–258.

Lipscombe, D., Kongsamut, S., and Tsien, R. W. 1989. β-Adrenergic inhibition of sympathetic neurotransmitter release mediated by modulation of N-type calcium-channel gating. *Nature* 340: 639–642.

Steinert, J. R., Kopp-Scheinpflug, C., Baker, C., Challiss, R. A., Mistry, R., Haustein, M. D., Griffin, S. J., Tong, H., Graham, B. P., and Forsythe, I. D. 2008. Nitric oxide is a volume transmitter regulating postsynaptic excitability at a glutamatergic synapse. *Neuron* 60: 642–656.

Wickman, K. D., Iñiguez-Lluhi, J. A., Davenport, P. A., Taussig, R., Krapivinsky, G. B., Linder, M. E., Gilman, A. G., and Clapham, D. E. 1994. Recombinant G-protein-subunits activate the muscarinic-gated atrial potassium channel. *Nature* 368: 255–257.

Wilson, R. I., and Nicoll, R. A. 2001. Endogenous cannabinoids mediate retrograde signaling at hippocampal synapses. *Nature* 410: 588–592.

Winks, J. S., Hughes, S., Filippov, A. K., Tatulian, L., Abogadie, F. C., Brown, D. A., and Marsh, S. J. 2005. Relationship between membrane phosphatidylinositol-4,5-bisphosphate and receptor-mediated inhibition of native neuronal M channels. *J. Neurosci.* 25: 3400–3413.

Zhang, J., Carver, C. M., Choveau, F. S. and Shapiro, M. S. 2016. Clustering and functional coupling of diverse ion channels and signaling proteins revealed by super-resolution STORM microscopy in neurons. *Neuron* 92: 461–478.

CHAPTER 13

Release of Neurotransmitters at Synapses

The stimulus for neurotransmitter release is depolarization of the nerve terminal. Release occurs as a result of calcium entry into the terminal through voltage-activated calcium channels. Invariably a delay of about 0.5 milliseconds intervenes between presynaptic depolarization and transmitter release. Part of the delay is due to the time taken for calcium channels to open; the remainder is due to the time required for calcium to cause transmitter release.

Transmitter is secreted in multimolecular packets (quanta), each containing several thousand transmitter molecules. In response to an action potential, anywhere from 1 to as many as 300 quanta are released almost synchronously from the nerve terminal, depending on the type of synapse. At rest, nerve terminals release quanta spontaneously at a slow rate, giving rise to spontaneous miniature synaptic potentials. At rest there is also a continuous, nonquantal leak of transmitter from nerve terminals.

One quantum of transmitter corresponds to the contents of one synaptic vesicle and comprises several thousand molecules of a low-molecular-weight transmitter. Vesicles rest at so-called active zones in the nerve terminal. In response to calcium entry, they release their contents by the process of exocytosis, during which the vesicle membrane fuses with, and collapses into, the presynaptic membrane, spilling the contents into the synaptic cleft. The components of the vesicle membrane are then retrieved by endocytosis, sorted in endosomes, and recycled into new synaptic vesicles.

Several questions arise concerning how presynaptic neurons release transmitter. Experimental answers to such questions require a highly sensitive, quantitative, and reliable measurement of the amount of transmitter released, with a time resolution in the millisecond range. In many of the experiments described in this chapter, this measurement is obtained by recording changes in the membrane potential of the postsynaptic cell. As we discussed in Chapter 11, the vertebrate neuromuscular junction, where the transmitter is known to be acetylcholine (ACh), offers many advantages. However, to obtain more complete information about the release process, it is useful to be able to record from the presynaptic endings as well. For example, such recordings are needed to establish how calcium and membrane potential affect transmitter release. The presynaptic terminals at vertebrate skeletal neuromuscular junctions are typically too small for electrophysiological recording (but see Morita and Barrett, 1990[1]); however, this can be done at several synapses, such as the giant fiber synapse in the stellate ganglion of the squid,[2] giant terminals of goldfish retinal bipolar cells,[3] and calyciform synapses in the avian ciliary ganglion[4] and the rodent brainstem.[5] Moreover, new techniques allow transmitter release to be monitored by means that do not require electrical recording from the postsynaptic cell. In this chapter we discuss electrophysiological and morphological experiments that characterize the release process.

Characteristics of Transmitter Release

Axon Terminal Depolarization and Release

The stellate ganglion of the squid was used by Katz and Miledi to determine the precise relation between presynaptic membrane depolarization and the amount of transmitter released.[6] Simultaneous records were made of the action potential in the presynaptic terminal and the response of the postsynaptic fiber, as shown in Figure 13.1A. When tetrodotoxin

[1] Morita, K., and Barrett, E. F. 1990. *J. Neurosci.* 10: 2614-2625.

[2] Bullock, T. H., and Hagiwara, S. 1957. *J. Gen. Physiol.* 40: 565-577.

[3] Heidelberger, R., and Matthews, G. 1992. *J. Physiol.* 447: 235-256.

[4] Martin, A. R., and Pilar, G. 1963. *J. Physiol.* 168: 443-463.

[5] Borst, J. G. G., and Sakmann, B. 1996. *Nature* 383: 431-434.

[6] Katz, B., and Miledi, R. 1967. *J. Physiol.* 192: 407-436.

(A) Stellate ganglion of squid

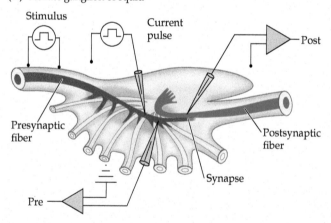

(B) Tetrodotoxin (TTX) paralysis

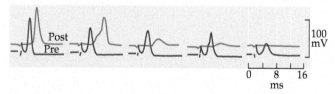

(C) Pre- and postsynaptic potential changes

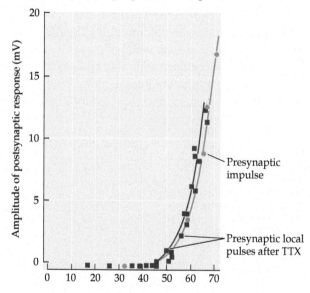

FIGURE 13.1 Presynaptic Impulse and Postsynaptic Response at a squid giant synapse. (A) Sketch of the stellate ganglion of the squid, illustrating the two large axons that form a chemical synapse. Pre- and postsynaptic axons are impaled with microelectrodes to record membrane potential, and an additional microelectrode is used to pass depolarizing current into the presynaptic terminal. (B) Simultaneous recordings from the presynaptic axons (red records) and postsynaptic axon (blue records) during the development of conduction block by tetrodotoxin (TTX). As the amplitude of the presynaptic action potential decreases, so does the size of the postsynaptic potential. Note that the two largest presynaptic action potentials evoke postsynaptic action potentials. (C) The relation between the amplitude of the presynaptic action potential and the postsynaptic potential. Green circles represent results in B; red squares represent results obtained by applying depolarizing current pulses to the presynaptic terminals after complete TTX block. (A after T. H. Bullock and S. Hagiwara, 1957. *J. Gen. Physiol.* 40: 565-577; B,C after B. Katz and R. Miledi, 1967. *J. Physiol.* 192: 407-436.)

(TTX) was applied to the preparation, the presynaptic action potential gradually decreased in amplitude over the next 15 minutes (Figure 13.1B). The postsynaptic action potential also decreased in amplitude, but then abruptly disappeared because the excitatory postsynaptic potential (EPSP) failed to reach threshold. From this point on, the size of the synaptic potential could be used as a measure of the amount of transmitter released.

When the amplitude of the EPSP is plotted against the amplitude of the failing presynaptic impulse, as in Figure 13.1C (green circles), the synaptic potential decreases rapidly as the presynaptic action potential amplitude falls below about 75 mV, and at amplitudes less than about 45 mV there are no postsynaptic responses. TTX has no effect on the sensitivity of the postsynaptic membrane to transmitter, so the fall in synaptic potential amplitude indicates a reduction in the amount of transmitter released from the presynaptic terminal. Thus, there is a threshold for transmitter release at about 45 mV depolarization, after which the amount released, and hence the EPSP amplitude, increases rapidly with presynaptic action potential amplitude.

Katz and Miledi used an additional procedure to explore further the relation between the potential amplitude and transmitter release. They placed a second electrode in the presynaptic terminal, through which they applied brief (1- to 2-ms) depolarizing current pulses, thereby mimicking a presynaptic action potential. The relation between the amplitude of the artificial action potential and that of the synaptic potential was the same as the relation obtained with the failing action potential during TTX poisoning (see Figure 13.1C, red squares). This result indicates that the normal fluxes of sodium and potassium ions responsible for the action potential are not necessary for transmitter release; only depolarization is required.

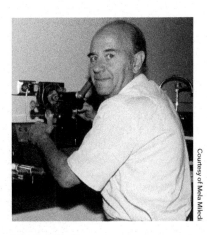

Ricardo Miledi

[7] Katz, B., and Miledi, R. 1965. *J. Physiol.* 181: 656–670.

Synaptic Delay

One characteristic of the transmitter release process evident in Figure 13.1B is that there is a lag time between the onset of the presynaptic action potential and the beginning of the synaptic potential. This lag time is known as the **synaptic delay** (see Chapter 11). In these experiments on the squid giant synapse, which were done at about 10°C, the delay was 3 to 4 ms. Detailed measurements at the frog neuromuscular junction show a synaptic delay of 0.5 ms at room temperature (about 20°C; Figure 13.2).[7] The time is too long to be accounted for by diffusion of ACh across the synaptic cleft (a distance of 50

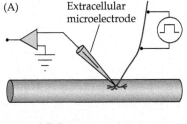

(A) Extracellular microelectrode

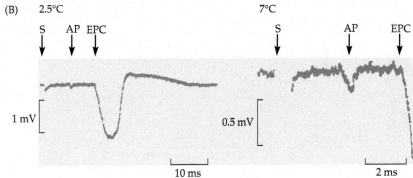

(B) 2.5°C   7°C

S   AP   EPC   S   AP   EPC

1 mV   0.5 mV

10 ms   2 ms

FIGURE 13.2 Synaptic Delay at a Chemical Synapse. (A) The motor nerve is stimulated while recording with an extracellular microelectrode at the frog neuromuscular junction. With this recording arrangement, current flowing into the nerve terminal or the muscle fiber is recorded as a negative potential. (B) Extracellular recordings of the stimulus artifact (S), the axon terminal action potential (AP), and the end plate current (EPC) at 2.5°C and 7°C. The synaptic delay is the time between the action potential in the nerve terminal and the beginning of the end plate current. (C) A plot of synaptic delay as a function of temperature, showing the decrease in synaptic delay with increasing temperature. (After B. Katz and R. Miledi, 1965. *J. Physiol.* 181: 656–670.)

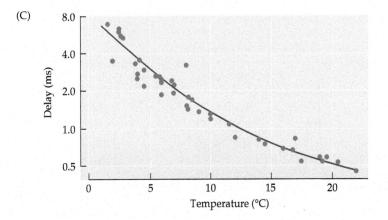

(C)

nanometers [nm]), which should take no longer than about 50 microseconds (μs). When ACh is applied to the junction ionophoretically from a micropipette, delays of as little as 150 μs can be achieved, even though the pipette is much farther from the postsynaptic receptors than are the nerve terminals. Furthermore, synaptic delay is much more sensitive to temperature than would be expected if it were due to diffusion. Cooling the frog nerve–muscle preparation to 2.5°C increases the delay to as long as 7 ms (see Figure 13.2B), whereas the delay in the response to ionophoretically applied ACh is not perceptibly altered. Thus, the delay is largely in the transmitter release mechanism.

Evidence That Calcium Is Required for Release

Calcium has long been known as an essential link in the process of synaptic transmission. When its concentration in the extracellular fluid is decreased, release of ACh at the neuromuscular junction is reduced and eventually abolished.[8,9] The importance of calcium for release has been established at synapses in general, irrespective of the nature of the transmitter. (One exception is the release of GABA from horizontal cells in the fish retina.[10]) The role of calcium has been generalized further to other secretory processes, such as the release of transmitters from axons, somata, and dendrites (extrasynaptic release; see Chapter 18), and the liberation of hormones by gland cells.[11,12] As we discuss in the next section, evoked transmitter release is preceded by calcium entry into the terminal and is antagonized by ions that block calcium entry, such as magnesium, cadmium, nickel, manganese, and cobalt. Transmitter release can be reduced, then, either by removing calcium from the bathing solution or by adding a blocking ion. For transmitter release to occur, calcium must be present in the bathing solution at the time of depolarization of the presynaptic terminal.[13]

[8] del Castillo, J., and Stark, L. 1952. *J. Physiol.* 116: 507–515.

[9] Dodge, F. A., Jr., and Rahamimoff, R. 1967. *J. Physiol.* 193: 419–432.

[10] Schwartz, E. A. 1987. *Science* 238: 350–355.

[11] Penner, R., and Neher, E. 1988. *J. Exp. Biol.* 139: 329–345.

[12] Kasai, H. 1999. *Trends Neurosci.* 22: 88–93.

[13] Katz, B., and Miledi, R. 1967. *J. Physiol.* 189: 535–544.

Measurement of Calcium Entry into Presynaptic Nerve Terminals

Entry of calcium into the nerve terminal is through voltage-sensitive calcium channels of the Ca_V2 family (see Chapter 5) that are activated upon depolarization by the presynaptic action potential. Using voltage clamp techniques, Llinás and his colleagues measured the magnitude and time course of the calcium current produced by presynaptic depolarization at the squid giant synapse. An example is shown in Figure 13.3A. The sodium and

(A)

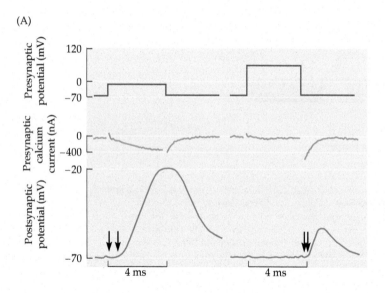

(B)

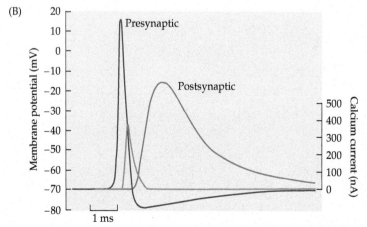

FIGURE 13.3 Presynaptic Calcium and Transmitter Release at the Squid Giant Synapse. The presynaptic terminal is voltage clamped and treated with TTX and TEA to abolish voltage-activated sodium and potassium currents. (A) Records show potentials applied to the presynaptic fiber (red upper trace), presynaptic calcium current (green middle trace), and EPSP in the postsynaptic fiber (blue lower trace). A voltage pulse from -70 to -18 mV (left panel) results in a slow inward calcium current and, after a delay of about 1 ms (arrows), an EPSP. A larger depolarization, to +60 mV (right panel), suppresses calcium entry. At the end of the pulse, a surge of calcium current is followed within about 0.2 ms (arrows) by an EPSP. (B) If a voltage change identical in shape to a normal action potential is produced by the voltage clamp (Presynaptic), then the EPSP is indistinguishable from that seen normally (Postsynaptic). The green curve gives the magnitude and time course of the calcium current. The synaptic delay between the beginning of the presynaptic depolarization and the beginning of the postsynaptic response is due in part to the time required to open calcium channels and in part to the time for calcium entry to trigger transmitter release. (After R. Llinás et al., 1982. *Sci. Am.* 247: 56–65.)

potassium conductances associated with the action potential were blocked by TTX and tetraethylammonium (TEA) so that only the voltage-activated calcium channels remained. Depolarizing the presynaptic terminal to –18 mV (upper trace, left panel) produced an inward calcium current in the terminal that increased slowly in magnitude to about 400 nA (middle trace, left panel), and a large synaptic potential in the postsynaptic cell (lower trace, left panel). When the terminal was depolarized to +60 mV (right panel), approximating the calcium equilibrium potential, the calcium current was suppressed during the pulse and no synaptic potential was seen. This demonstrates that depolarization of the terminal is not sufficient on its own to trigger release; calcium entry must also occur. On repolarization there was a brief, inward calcium current through channels remaining open after the depolarization, accompanied by a small postsynaptic potential.

The effect of an artificial action potential is shown in Figure 13.3B. A presynaptic action potential, recorded before addition of TTX and TEA to the preparation, was played back through the voltage clamp circuit to produce exactly the same voltage change in the terminal. The postsynaptic potential is indistinguishable from that produced by a normal presynaptic action potential, confirming that the sodium and potassium currents that normally accompany the action potential are not necessary for transmitter release.

The experiment shown in Figure 13.3B also enabled Llinás and his colleagues to measure the magnitude and time course of the calcium current produced by the artificial action potential (green curve). The calcium current begins about 0.5 ms after the beginning of the presynaptic depolarization, and the postsynaptic potential begins about 0.5 ms later. Thus, the time required for the presynaptic terminal to depolarize and the calcium channels to open accounts for the first half of the synaptic delay; the time required for the calcium concentration to rise within the terminal and evoke transmitter release accounts for the remainder.

An experimental technique important for characterizing the role of calcium transmitter release is the use of calcium indicator dyes to estimate intracellular calcium concentrations (see Box 12.6).[14,15] These are synthetic compounds that change their fluorescence in the presence of calcium, based on calcium chelators such as ethylene glycol-bis[2-aminoethyl ether]-N,N,N′,N′-tetraacetic acid (EGTA). An example of the use of luminescent dye to reveal changes in presynaptic calcium concentration is shown Figure 13.4. Aequorin injected into the resting presynaptic terminal of the squid giant synapse revealed discrete microdomains (see the next section) of free calcium, some with relatively high concentrations (see Figure 13.4A). After a brief train of presynaptic action potentials, the intracellular calcium concentration reached 100 to 200 μM (see Figure 13.4B).

[14] Tsien, R. Y. 1989. *Annu. Rev. Neurosci.* 12: 227–253.

[15] Rudolf, R. et al. 2003. *Nat. Rev. Mol. Cell Biol.* 4: 579–586.

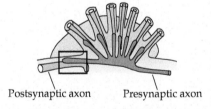

Postsynaptic axon   Presynaptic axon

FIGURE 13.4 Microdomains of Calcium within the Presynaptic Terminal at the Squid Giant Synapse. The box in the illustration shows the region imaged. (A) Distribution of calcium within the presynaptic axon terminal at rest, determined by intracellular injection of a calcium-sensitive dye. (B) A brief train of presynaptic action potentials results in the appearance of microdomains of high calcium concentration within the axon terminal. Scale indicates the calcium concentration in micromolar. (After R. Llinás et al., 1992. *Science* 256: 677–679.)

(A)

(B)

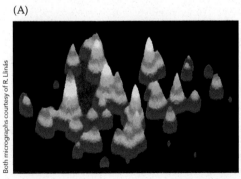

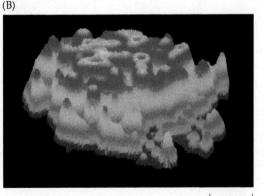

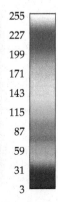

255
227
199
171
143
115
87
59
31
3

5 µm

Localization of Calcium Entry Sites

Figure 13.4 illustrates an important point about the distribution of free calcium in the cytoplasm, namely that it is not at all uniform.[16] Calcium entering the terminal through a single channel collects briefly in a small **nanodomain**, with the concentration falling rapidly over a radius of a few tens of nanometers from the channel as the ions diffuse into the bulk solution or are bound by intrinsic calcium chelators. Calcium entering through a group of closely apposed channels occupies a **microdomain** that can spread over a distance of a few hundred nanometers from the channel cluster. Because of the restricted spread of incoming ions, the spatial relation between calcium channels and their associated transmitter release sites is of critical importance.

Experiments on the squid giant synapse using calcium buffers have provided information about the proximity of calcium channels to the sites of transmitter secretion.[17] In these experiments, injection of 1,2-bis(o-aminophenoxy)ethane-N,N,N,N-tetraacetic acid (BAPTA), a potent calcium buffer, into the presynaptic terminal resulted in a severe attenuation of transmitter release, without affecting the presynaptic action potential (Figure 13.5A). However, EGTA, a calcium buffer of equal potency, had little effect on release (Figure 13.5C). This disparity is due to the fact that calcium is bound hundreds of times faster by BAPTA than by EGTA. Thus, calcium ions have little opportunity to diffuse from their site of entry before being bound by BAPTA, but can traverse some distance before being captured by EGTA (Figure 13.5B,D). From the rates of calcium diffusion and

[16] Llinás, M., Sugimori, M., and Silver, R. B. 1992 *Science* 256: 677–679.

[17] Adler, E. M. et al. 1991. *J. Neurosci.* 11: 1496–1507.

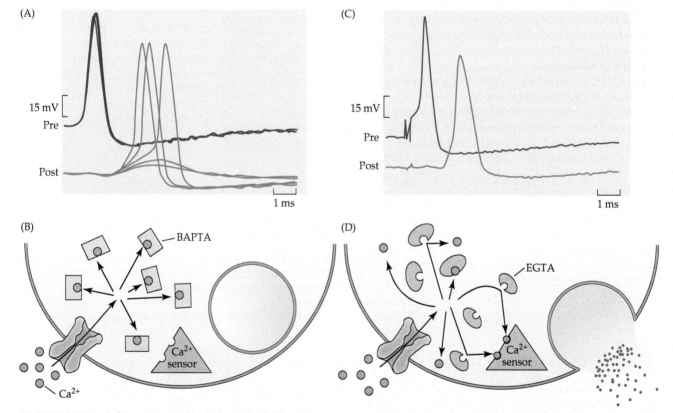

FIGURE 13.5 Calcium Enters Near the Site of Transmitter Release at the squid giant synapse. (A) Intracellular recordings from the presynaptic (Pre) and postsynaptic (Post) axons following injection of the fast calcium chelator 1,2-bis(o-aminophenoxy) ethane-N,N,N,N-tetraacetic acid (BAPTA). Superimposed traces show the reduction in the EPSP during a 4-minute BAPTA injection. (B) Calcium is bound to BAPTA before it has time to reach the calcium sensor that triggers transmitter release. (C) Superimposed intracellular recordings during a 4-minute injection of ethylene glycol-bis[2-aminoethyl ether]-N,N,N',N'-tetraacetic acid (EGTA), a chelator that binds calcium more slowly. No change in EPSP amplitude is seen. (D) Calcium reaches the sensor that triggers release faster than it becomes bound to EGTA, indicating that the site of calcium entry must be within 100 nm of the site at which calcium triggers transmitter release. (A,C after E. M. Adler et al., 1991. *J. Neurosci.* 11: 1496–1507. © 1991 Society for Neuroscience.)

binding to EGTA, it can be calculated that the calcium-binding site associated with the release process must lie within 100 nm of the site of calcium entry. However, similar experiments at some neuronal synapses have shown an effect of EGTA on release, suggesting that in these cells calcium may diffuse some distance from calcium channels to sites that trigger or modulate release.[5]

Transmitter Release by Intracellular Concentration Jumps

Another important technique for exploring the role of calcium in transmitter release is the use of photolabile calcium chelators, which release bound, or "caged," calcium upon illumination.[18,19] This provides a means of producing a transient increase in intracellular calcium in the presynaptic terminal, divorced from any change in membrane potential. An example is shown in Figure 13.6, from a glutaminergic synapse in a brain slice from the medial nucleus of the trapezoid body of the rat.[20] This synapse features a unique presynaptic structure—the calyx of Held, which is sufficiently large to allow the attachment of a patch clamp electrode for electrical recording.[21] In addition, simultaneous patch clamp records can be obtained from the postsynaptic cell.[22]

A whole-cell patch pipette was used to load the calyx with caged calcium and a low-affinity calcium indicator dye. A second patch pipette recorded postsynaptic currents, and electrodes were placed on the slice for presynaptic nerve stimulation. As shown in Figure 13.6, a brief calcium transient of appropriate amplitude and time course could produce an excitatory postsynaptic current that was indistinguishable from that produced by presynaptic nerve stimulation. Thus, a transient increase in cytoplasmic calcium concentration can account completely for the magnitude and time course of transmitter release.

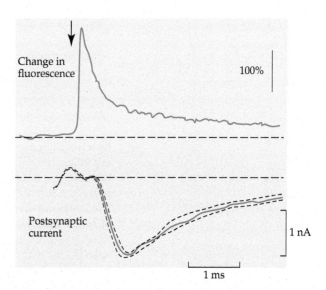

FIGURE 13.6 Change in Presynaptic Calcium Concentration and Excitatory Postsynaptic Currents at a synapse in the trapezoid body of the rat. The presynaptic alyx of Held was loaded with both caged calcium and a calcium indicator dye. Upper trace: fluorescent signal indicating a transient increase in presynaptic calcium concentration, evoked by photolysis of caged calcium with a laser flash (arrow). Lower traces: postsynaptic currents produced by the calcium transient (solid curve) and by presynaptic stimulation (dashed curves). The postsynaptic currents are identical in time course. (After J. H. Bollman and B. Sakmann, 2005. *Nat. Neurosci.* 8: 426-434.)

Other Factors Regulating Transmitter Release

From the evidence presented so far, we can conclude that the sole factor responsible for evoked transmitter release is an increase in intracellular calcium concentration, brought about by depolarization of the presynaptic terminal and opening of voltage-activated calcium channels. However, it has been demonstrated that at neuromuscular junctions of the mouse and crayfish, release may be regulated in addition by presynaptic autoreceptors (see Chapter 12).[23,24] These are G protein-coupled receptors on the presynaptic terminals which, when activated by released transmitter, act in turn to inhibit further release. In the mouse, presynaptic muscarinic cholinergic (M2) receptors are continually exposed to a resting concentration of ACh in the range of 10 to 20 nanomolar (nM), a concentration sufficient to produce tonic inhibition of the release mechanism. An additional feature of the M2 receptors is that their ACh binding affinity is voltage-dependent.[25] Given these two observations, depolarization of the nerve terminal is thought to reduce the binding affinity of the M2 receptors, thereby relieving tonic inhibition release. Upon repolarization, the inhibitory action of the M2 receptors is restored, so that the release is terminated even though the calcium concentration in the region may still be elevated. The exact nature of the coupling between the voltage-sensitive autoreceptor and the release machinery is not known. Similar observations on the crayfish neuromuscular junction, which is glutamatergic, suggest that the proposed mechanism may have general applicability. However, it does not contribute to the release process at the calyx of Held synapse, where depolarization has no effect on transmitter release triggered by uncaged calcium.[26] As shown in Figure 13.6, the time course of evoked transmitter release can be mimicked by a transient increase in cytoplasmic calcium with no accompanying depolarization.

[18] Adam, S. R. et al. 1988. *J. Am. Chem. Soc.* 110: 3212-3220.

[19] Ellis-Davies, G. C. R. 2008. *Chem. Rev.* 108: 1603-1613.

[20] Bollman, J. H., and Sakmann, B. 2005. *Nat. Neurosci.* 8: 426-434.

[21] Forsythe, I. D. 1994. *J. Physiol.* 479: 381-387.

[22] Borst, J. G. G., Helmchen, F., and Sakmann, B. 1995. *J. Physiol.* 489: 825-840.

[23] Kupchik, Y. M. et al. 2008. *Proc. Natl. Acad. Sci. USA* 105: 4435-4440.

[24] Parnas, I., and Parnas, H. 2010. *Pflügers Arch.* 460: 975-990.

[25] Ben-Chaim, Y. et al. 2006. *Nature* 444: 106-109.

[26] Felmy, F., Neher, E., and Schneggenberger, R. 2003. *Proc. Natl. Acad. Sci. USA* 100: 15200-15205.

Quantal Release

So far, the general scheme for transmitter release can be summarized as follows:

Presynaptic depolarization → calcium entry → transmitter release

Now that this general framework has been established, it remains to be shown how transmitter is secreted from the terminals. In experiments on the frog neuromuscular junction, Fatt and Katz showed that ACh can be released from terminals in multimolecular packets, which they called **quanta** (singular: *quantum*).[27] Later experiments by Kuffler and Yoshikami showed that each quantum corresponds to approximately 7000 molecules of ACh.[28] Quantal release, then, means that any response to stimulation will consist of roughly 7000 molecules, or 14,000 and so on, but not 4250 or 10,776. At any given synapse, the number of quanta released from the nerve terminal in response to an action potential (the **quantum content** of the synaptic potential) may vary considerably from trial to trial, but the mean number of molecules in each quantum (**quantal size**) is fixed (with a variance of about 10%).

Spontaneous Release of Multimolecular Quanta

The first evidence for packaging of ACh in multimolecular quanta was the observation by Fatt and Katz[27] that at the motor end plate, but not elsewhere in the muscle fiber, spontaneous depolarizations of about 1 mV occurred irregularly (Figure 13.7). These depolarizations had the same time course as the potentials evoked by nerve stimulation. The spontaneous miniature end plate potentials (MEPPs) were decreased in amplitude and eventually abolished by increasing concentrations of the ACh receptor antagonist curare, and were increased in amplitude and time course by acetylcholinesterase inhibitors, such as prostigmine (see Figure 13.7C). These two pharmacological tests indicated that the potentials were produced by the spontaneous release of discrete amounts of ACh from the nerve terminal and ruled out the possibility that they might be due to single ACh molecules. Subsequently, patch electrode recordings demonstrated directly that the

[27] Fatt, P., and Katz, B. 1952. *J. Physiol.* 117: 109-128.

[28] Kuffler, S. W., and Yoshikami, D. 1975. *J. Physiol.* 251: 465-482.

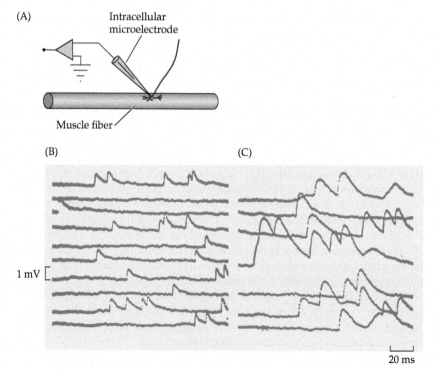

FIGURE 13.7 Miniature End Plate Potentials at the Frog Neuromuscular Junction. (A) Intracellular recording from a muscle fiber in the region of the motor end plate. (B) Miniature end plate potentials (MEPPs), about 1 mV in amplitude, occur spontaneously and are confined to the end plate region of the muscle fiber. (C) After addition of prostigmine, which prevents acetylcholinesterase from hydrolyzing ACh, MEPPs are increased in amplitude and duration, but the frequency at which they occur is unchanged. This observation indicates that each MEPP is due to a quantal packet of ACh, rather than to a single ACh molecule. (After P. Fatt and B. Katz, 1952. *J. Physiol.* 117: 109-128.)

amount of current that flows through an individual ACh receptor will produce a potential change in the muscle fiber of approximately 1 μV. Thus, an MEPP is produced by the opening of about 1300 ACh receptors. Additional evidence confirmed, in a variety of different ways, that the MEPPs are indeed due to multimolecular packets of ACh liberated by the nerve terminal. For example, depolarization of the nerve terminal by passing a steady current through it causes an increase in frequency of the spontaneous activity, whereas muscle depolarization has no effect on frequency.[29] Botulinum toxin, which blocks release of ACh in response to nerve stimuli, also abolishes the spontaneous activity.[30] Shortly after denervation of a muscle, as the motor nerve terminal degenerates, the MEPPs disappear.[31] Surprisingly, after an interim period, spontaneous potentials reappear in denervated frog muscle; these arise because of ACh released from Schwann cells that have engulfed segments of the degenerating nerve terminals by phagocytosis.[32]

Fluctuations in the End Plate Potential

A typical synaptic potential at the skeletal neuromuscular junction depolarizes the postsynaptic membrane by 50 mV to 70 mV, many times greater than the depolarization produced by a single quantum. In order to find out how this response to stimulation was related to the spontaneously released quanta, Fatt and Katz reduced the amplitude of the evoked synaptic potential by lowering the extracellular calcium and adding extracellular magnesium. Under these conditions the responses fluctuated in a stepwise manner, as shown in Figure 13.8A. Some stimuli produced no response at all—a failure of transmission. Some stimuli produced a response of about 1 mV in amplitude, similar in size and shape to an MEPP; others evoked responses that appeared to be two, three, or four times larger.

This remarkable observation led Fatt and Katz to propose the **quantum hypothesis:** that the single quantal events observed to occur spontaneously also represent the building blocks for the synaptic potentials evoked by stimulation. Normally the end plate potential is made up of about 200 quantal units, and variations in its size are not obvious. In low calcium concentrations, the quantal *size* remains the same, but the quantum *content*

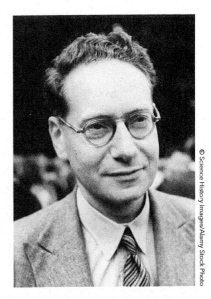

Bernard Katz, 1950

[29] del Castillo, J., and Katz, B. 1954. *J. Physiol.* 124: 586-604.

[30] Brooks, V. B. 1956. *J. Physiol.* 134: 264-277.

[31] Birks, R., Katz, B., and Miledi, R. 1960. *J. Physiol.* 150: 145-168.

[32] Reiser, G., and Miledi, R. 1989. *Brain Res.* 479: 83-97.

(A)

(B)

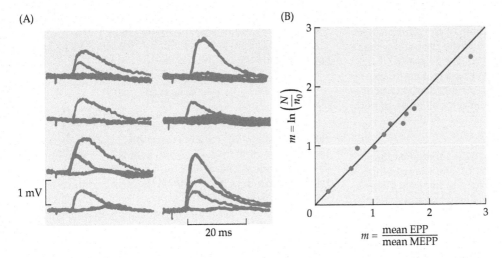

$$m = \ln\left(\frac{N}{n_0}\right)$$

$$m = \frac{\text{mean EPP}}{\text{mean MEPP}}$$

1 mV

20 ms

FIGURE 13.8   The End Plate Potential Is Composed of Quantal Units that correspond to spontaneous miniature potentials. Presynaptic release of ACh at a frog neuromuscular junction was reduced by lowering the calcium concentration in the bathing solution. (A) Sets of intracellular records, each showing two to four superimposed responses to nerve stimulation. The amplitude of the end plate potential (EPP) varies in a stepwise fashion; the smallest response corresponds in amplitude to a spontaneous miniature end plate potential (MEPP). (B) Comparison of the mean quantal content (*m*) of the EPP determined in two ways: by applying the Poisson distribution, $m = \ln(N/n_0)$ (ordinate), and by dividing the mean EPP amplitude by the mean MEPP amplitude (abscissa). Agreement of the two estimates supports the hypothesis that the EPP is composed of quantal units that correspond to spontaneous MEPPs. (A after P. Fatt and B. Katz, 1952. *J. Physiol.* 117: 109-128; B after J. del Castillo and B. Katz, 1954. *J. Physiol.* 124: 560-573.)

is small—perhaps 1 to 3 quanta—and fluctuates randomly from trial to trial, resulting in stepwise fluctuations in the amplitude of the end plate potential.

Statistical Analysis of the End Plate Potential

Del Castillo and Katz realized that to test the quantum hypothesis adequately would require a statistical analysis.[33] Accordingly, they proposed that the motor nerve terminal contains a very large number of quantal packets of ACh (n), each of which has a probability (p) of being released in response to a nerve impulse, and that quanta are released independently—that is, the release of one has no influence on the probability of release of the next. Then, in a large number of trials, the mean number of quanta released per trial (m) would be given by np, and the number of times the response consisted of 0, 1, 2, 3, 4 ...., or x quanta would be given by the **binomial distribution** (Box 13.1). However, del Castillo and Katz could not test their expectation of a binomial distribution experimentally because they had had no way of measuring n or p. The only available measure was m. In order to deal with this difficulty, they reasoned as follows:

[33] del Castillo, J., and Katz, B. 1954a. *J. Physiol.* 124: 560-573.

BOX 13.1 Statistical Fluctuation in Quantal Release

When del Castillo and Katz saw fluctuations in the quantum content of the end plate potential, they proposed that the release was a statistical process and that, consequently, it would be possible to predict the variations from one trial to the next by the binomial distribution. How does a statistical process lead to fluctuations, and how is it that these are described by the binomial equation? It is useful to look at a simple numerical example.

Suppose that a nerve terminal contains 3 quanta (a, b, and c), each with a 10% chance of being released upon arrival of an action potential, and suppose further that each time any one is released it is immediately replaced. If we call the number of available quanta n, and the release probability p, then in our example $n = 3$, $p = 0.1$. We will also define q as the probability that a quantum will *not* be released. So, $q = 1 - p = 0.9$.

In any trial, what is the likelihood that no quantum is released? We will call this p_0. The probability of one not being released is $q = 0.9$; and for all three to not be released, it is

$$p_0 = q^3 = 0.729$$

To see a single response requires that one quantum be released and the other two not. The chance of this is pq^2, and there are three ways for it to happen: Either a, b, or c is released, and the remaining two are not. So

$$p_1 = 3pq^2 = 0.243$$

By similar reasoning,

$$p_2 = 3p^2q = 0.027$$

and

$$p_3 = p^3 = 0.001$$

The sum of all the probabilities ($q^3 + 3pq^2 + 3p^2q + p^3$) is 1.0, which means that we have accounted correctly for all possible release combinations.

In 1000 trials, then, we would expect to see 729 failures, 243 single releases, 27 doubles (yielding 54

quanta), and one response with 3 quanta, for a total of 300 quanta.

The average number of quanta released per trial, which we will call m, is 300/1000 = 0.3.

So

$$m = np$$

The distribution is called a binomial distribution because $q^3 + 3q^2p + 3qp^2 + p^3$ are the terms we get when we multiply out the binomial (two-variable) expression $(q + p)^3$.

If there are n quanta in the terminal, instead of 3, then the probabilities of seeing 0, 1, 2, ... releases are given by the successive terms of the expansion of $(q + p)^n$.

The probability that x quanta will be released (p_x) is given by the relation

$$p_x = \frac{p^x q^{n-x}(n!)}{(n-x)!\,x!}$$

The Poisson distribution is based on completely different reasoning. It simply describes how the occurrences of random (independent) events in time depend on their average over time, (i.e., on m). When the quantal release probability, p, is small (for practical purposes < 0.1), binomial predictions are not significantly different from those of the Poisson distribution, in which

$$p_x = \frac{e^{-m}(m^x)}{x!}$$

It should be noted that while results that conform to the Poisson distribution support the hypothesis of a binomial distribution, they do not confirm it. However, experiments have shown that when the release probability is relatively high, the fluctuations in quantum content are indeed described by the binomial equation.

Under normal conditions, p may be assumed to be relatively large, that is a fairly large part of the synaptic population responds to an impulse. However, as we reduce the Ca and increase the Mg concentration, the chances of responding are diminished and we observe mostly complete failures with an occasional response of one or two units. Under these conditions, when p is very small, the number of units x which make up the e.p.p. in a large series of observations should be distributed in the characteristic manner described by Poisson's law.[33]

The **Poisson distribution** approximates the binomial distribution when p is very small. The crucial difference is that to predict a Poisson distribution it is necessary to know only m, the mean number of quanta released per trial. In practice, this means measuring the average response amplitude and the average miniature potential amplitude. Then:

$$m = \frac{\text{mean amplitude of evoked potentials}}{\text{mean amplitude of miniature potentials}}$$

For a Poisson distribution, in N trials the expected number of responses containing x quanta is given by

$$n_x = (N)\frac{e^{-m}(m^x)}{x!}$$

One can also determine m from the number of failures, n_0. When $x = 0$ in the Poisson equation, $n_0 = Ne^{-m}$ (since both m^0 and $0! = 1$). Rearranging this result gives

$$m = \ln\left(\frac{N}{n_0}\right)$$

Del Castillo and Katz bathed a neuromuscular junction in a solution containing low calcium and high magnesium concentrations and recorded a large number of end plate potentials evoked by nerve stimulation, as well as a large number of MEPPs. When they calculated m in these two entirely different ways, they found the estimates in excellent agreement, providing strong support for the idea of a Poisson distribution (Figure 13.8B).

A more stringent test of the applicability of the Poisson equation is to predict the entire distribution of response amplitudes, using only m and the mean amplitude of the unit potential (Figure 13.9). To do this, m is calculated from the ratio of the mean evoked potential amplitude to that of the mean MEPPs, as before. Then the number of expected responses containing 0, 1, 2, 3, ... units is calculated. To account for the slight variation in size of the unit, the expected number of responses containing 1 unit is distributed about the mean unit

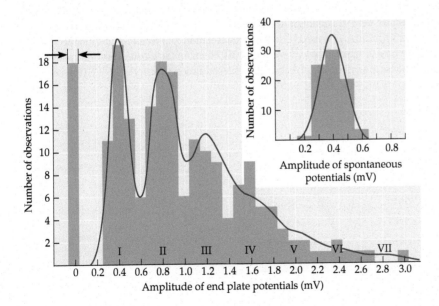

FIGURE 13.9 Amplitude Distribution of End Plate Potentials at a mammalian neuromuscular junction in high (12.5 mM) magnesium solution. The histogram shows the number of end plate potentials observed at each amplitude. The peaks of the histogram occur at 0 mV (failures) and at one, two, three, and four times the mean amplitude of the spontaneous MEPPs (inset), indicating responses comprising 1, 2, 3, and 4 quanta. The solid line represents the theoretical distribution of end plate potential amplitudes calculated according to the Poisson equation and allowing for the spread in amplitude of the quantal size. The arrows indicate the predicted number of failures. (After I. A. Boyd and A. R. Martin, 1956. *J. Physiol.* 132: 74–91.)

size, with the same variance as the spontaneous events (see Figure 13.9, inset). Similarly, the predicted number of responses containing 2, 3, or more units is distributed about their means with proportionately increasing variances. The individual distributions are then summed to give the theoretical distribution shown by the continuous curve. The agreement with the experimentally observed distribution (bars) provides additional support for the hypothesis.

At many synapses, the probability of transmitter release is sufficiently high that it is not necessary to rely on the Poisson distribution to test the quantum hypothesis. Under such conditions, the binomial distribution can be tested directly. As before, if we assume that the terminal contains n units, each with an average probability (p) of being released by a nerve stimulus, then the relative occurrence of multiple events predicted by the binomial distribution is

$$n_x = (N)\frac{p^x q^{n-x}(n!)}{(n-x)!\,x!}$$

where n_x is the number of responses containing x quanta, N is the number of trials, and $q = 1 - p$. Adherence of the release process to binomial statistics was first demonstrated at the crayfish neuromuscular junction.[34]

In summary, there is now ample evidence that transmitter is released in packets, or quanta. When the release probability (p) is very low, as in a low-calcium medium, the Poisson distribution provides a useful means of analyzing fluctuations. The applicability of the binomial hypothesis has been confirmed when the probability of release is high. In addition, binomial statistics can provide information as to whether changes in the amount of transmitter released arise from changes in the number of available quanta or in the probability of their release.

Quantum Content at Neuronal Synapse

One striking feature of the vertebrate nervous system is the reduction in mean quantum content as one moves from the neuromuscular junction, where there is little integration ($m = 200$–300), to autonomic ganglia ($m = 2$–20),[35,36] to synapses in the central nervous system (CNS; at which m can be as low as 1),[37,38] where postsynaptic cells are concerned with integrating myriad incoming signals. At the synapse between a primary afferent fiber from a muscle spindle and a spinal motoneuron, for example, the mean quantum content is about 1.[39] This does not mean, however, that transmission fails most of the time, as would be expected for a Poisson distribution. Rather, release conforms to binomial statistics, with a high probability (p ~0.9) and a low number of available quanta (n ~1).

Number of Molecules in a Quantum

Although it was clear from the experiments of Katz, Fatt, and del Castillo that at the neuromuscular junction one quantum contained more than one ACh molecule, the question of how many molecules were in a quantum remained. The first accurate determination was made by Kuffler and Yoshikami, who used very fine pipettes for ionophoresis of ACh onto the postsynaptic membrane of snake muscle.[29] By careful placement of the pipette, they were able to produce a response to a brief pulse of ACh that mimicked almost exactly the MEPP (Figure 13.10).

[34] Johnson, E. W., and Wernig, A. 1971. *J. Physiol.* 218: 757-767.

[35] Blackman, J. G., and Purves, R. D. 1969. *J. Physiol.* 203: 173-198.

[36] Martin, A. R., and Pilar, G. 1964. *J. Physiol.* 175: 1-16.

[37] Redman, S. 1990. *Physiol. Rev.* 70: 165-198.

[38] Edwards, F. A., Konnerth, A., and Sakmann, B. 1990. *J. Physiol.* 430: 213-249.

[39] Kuno, M. 1964. *J. Physiol.* 175: 81-99.

FIGURE 13.10 The Number of ACh Molecules in a Quantum, determined by mimicking an MEPP with an ionophoretic pulse of ACh. (A) An intracellular microelectrode records spontaneous MEPPs and the response to ionophoretic application of ACh. (B) An MEPP is mimicked almost exactly by an ionophoretic pulse of ACh. The rate of rise of the ionophoretic ACh pulse is slightly slower because the ACh pipette is farther from the postsynaptic membrane than is the nerve terminal. (B after S. W. Kuffler and D. Yoshikami, 1975. *J. Physiol.* 251: 465-482.)

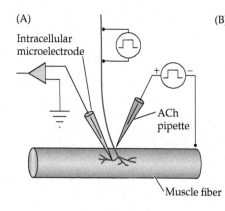

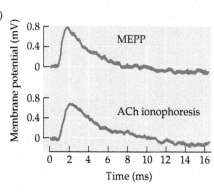

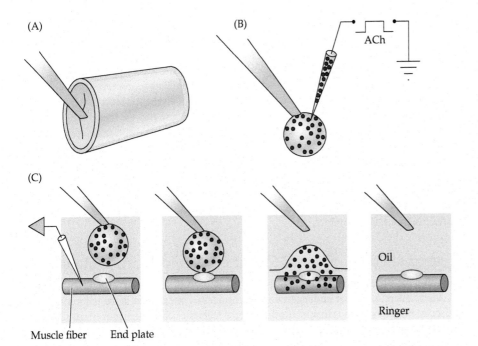

FIGURE 13.11 Assay of ACh Ejected from a Micropipette by Ionophoresis. (A) A droplet of fluid is removed from the dispensing capillary under oil. (B) ACh is injected into the droplet by a series of ionophoretic pulses, each identical to that used to mimic a spontaneous MEPP (see Figure 13.10B). (C) After its volume is measured, the ACh-loaded droplet is touched against the oil-ringer interface at the end plate of a snake muscle, discharging its contents into the aqueous phase. The depolarization of the end plate is measured (not shown) and compared with that produced by droplets with known ACh concentration. Once the concentration in the test droplet is determined, the amount of ACh released per pulse from the electrode can be calculated. (After S. W. Kuffler and D. Yoshikami, 1975. *J. Physiol.* 251: 465–482.)

To measure the number of molecules released by the pipette, ACh was released by repetitive pulses into a small (about 0.5 μl) droplet of saline under oil (Figure 13.11). The droplet was then applied to the end plate of a snake muscle fiber and the resulting depolarization measured. The response was compared with responses to droplets of exactly the same size containing known concentrations of ACh. In this way, the concentration of ACh in the test droplet was determined and the number of ACh molecules released per pulse was calculated. The pulse of ACh required to mimic an MEPP contained approximately 7000 molecules.

As we discuss later in this chapter, transmitter molecules are stored in vesicles in the presynaptic terminal, and each quantum represents the discharge of a single vesicle. Chemical measurements of the glutamate content of synaptic vesicles in the CNS estimate the number of molecules per quantum to be of the order of 4000,[40] which is the same order of magnitude as the number of ACh molecules in vesicles at the neuromuscular junction.

Number of Channels Activated by a Quantum

Given that a quantum of ACh consists of about 7000 molecules, one might expect that only a few thousand of these would actually combine with postsynaptic receptors at the neuromuscular junction—the remainder being lost to diffusion out of the cleft or hydrolysis by cholinesterases. This expectation is correct. The number of receptors activated by a quantum can be determined by comparing the conductance change that occurs during a miniature potential with that produced by a single ACh-activated channel.[41] Measurements of miniature end plate currents by voltage clamp in frog muscle indicate a peak conductance change on the order of 40 nanosiemens (nS). A single frog ACh receptor has a conductance of about 30 picosiemens (pS). Thus, an MEPP is produced by about 1300 open channels. (This corresponds to 2600 molecules of ACh, since it takes two molecules of ACh to open a channel; see Chapters 5 and 11.) This is similar to the number calculated by Katz and Miledi, who estimated the contribution of a single channel to the end plate potential from noise measurements.[42] A similar value for the number of channels opened by a quantum of transmitter was obtained at glycine-mediated inhibitory synapses in lamprey brainstem cells.[43] Lower values are observed at other synapses. For example, at synapses on hippocampal cells, a quantal response corresponds to activation of 15 to 65 channels.[39,44]

Why are there such differences among synapses? A little thought leads to the conclusion that the number of postsynaptic receptors activated by a quantum of transmitter released from a single presynaptic bouton must be tailored to the size of the cell. In large cells with low input resistances, such as skeletal muscle fibers or lamprey Müller cells, a large number of receptors

[40] Villanueva, S., Fiedler, J., and Orrego, F. 1990. *Neuroscience* 37: 2-30.

[41] Magleby, K. L., and Weinstock, M. M., 1980. *J. Physiol.* 299: 203-218.

[42] Katz, B., and Miledi, R. 1972. *J. Physiol.* 244: 665-699.

[43] Gold, M. R., and Martin, A. R. 1983. *J. Physiol.* 342: 85-98.

[44] Jonas, P., Major, G., and Sakmann, B. 1993. *J. Physiol.* 472: 615-663.

must be activated for the effect of a quantum to be significant. Activation of the same number of receptors on a much smaller cell in the CNS would overwhelm all other conductances, depolarizing the cell to a potential near zero if the synapse were excitatory, or locking its membrane potential firmly at the chloride equilibrium potential if the effect were inhibitory.

It appears that the match between cell size and the number of receptors activated by a quantum is achieved simply by matching the number of postsynaptic receptors to the size of the cell. Smaller cells have fewer receptors than larger cells, so that the size of the synaptic response is limited by receptor availability. For example, at the neuromuscular junction, receptors are packed at high density ($\sim$10,000/μm^2) throughout a large expanse of postsynaptic membrane, providing an essentially limitless sea of receptors for each quantum of transmitter. At a typical hippocampal synapse, however, the estimated postsynaptic receptor density is much lower ($\sim$2800/μm^2),[45] and the area occupied by postsynaptic membrane is very small (0.04 μm^2).[46] Thus, fewer than 100 postsynaptic receptors may be available for activation by a single quantum.

Changes in Mean Quantal Size at the Neuromuscular Junction

Although the size of miniature synaptic potentials at any particular synapse tends to remain constant, exceptions occur under certain circumstances. For example, at the tadpole neuromuscular junction, various treatments that induce high rates of spontaneous transmitter release are followed by the appearance of small-mode MEPPs, which are a fraction of the normal quantal size.[47] At neuromuscular junctions in neonatal mice, a dominant fraction of the overall MEPP amplitude distribution consists of small-mode MEPPs, so that the overall distribution is heavily skewed toward the baseline, with no discernable quantal peaks.[48] Similar skewed amplitude distributions are seen during regeneration of nerve terminals following denervation.[49] The origin of these subminiature potentials is not clear. They may occur because of incomplete filling or emptying of synaptic vesicles (see the next section).

Conversely, spontaneous synaptic potentials, larger than the usual miniature potentials, are seen occasionally.[50] In some instances these appear to be due to the spontaneous release of two or more quanta simultaneously; in other instances their size shows no clear relation to normal quantal amplitude. Finally, in some myoneural diseases that afflict humans, such as myasthenia gravis, spontaneous miniature and evoked synaptic potentials are reduced in amplitude owing to a reduction in the number of receptors in the postsynaptic membrane.[51]

Nonquantal Release

In addition to being released by the motor nerve terminal in the form of individual quanta, ACh leaks continuously from the cytoplasm into the extracellular fluid. In other words, there is a steady nonquantal "ooze" of ACh from the presynaptic terminal.[52] Indeed, the amount of ACh that leaks from the nerve terminal in this way is about 100 times greater than that released in the form of spontaneous quanta. The magnitude of the leak can be determined by comparing the total amount of ACh released from a muscle, measured biochemically, to the amount released as quanta, which is calculated from MEPP frequency and the total number of end plates in the muscle.

Under normal circumstances, the slow dribble of ACh from the presynaptic terminal does not produce a postsynaptic response; the amount of cholinesterase in the synaptic cleft is sufficient to hydrolyze most of the ACh, so that the concentration in the synaptic cleft is not more than a few tens of nanomolars. Its postsynaptic effect can be detected only when cholinesterase is inhibited. In contrast, the simultaneous release of 7000 molecules of ACh in a quantum locally overwhelms the enzyme, allowing ACh to reach its postsynaptic receptors and cause an MEPP.

Vesicles and Transmitter Release

Shortly after Katz and his colleagues demonstrated by electrophysiological methods that transmitter release was quantal, the first electron micrographs of the neuromuscular junction revealed that axon terminals contain many small membrane-bound synaptic vesicles

[45] Harris, K. M., and Landis, D. M. M. 1986. *Neuroscience* 19: 857-872.

[46] Schikorski, T., and Stevens, C. F. 1997. *J. Neurosci.* 17: 5858-5867.

[47] Kriebel, M. E., and Gross, C. E. 1974. *J. Gen. Physiol.* 64: 85-103.

[48] Erxleben, C., and Kriebel, M. E. 1988. *J. Physiol.* 400: 659-676.

[49] Denis, M. J., and Miledi, R. 1974. *J. Physiol.* 239: 571-594.

[50] Vautrin, J., and Kriebel, M. E. 1991. *Neuroscience* 41: 71-88.

[51] Drachman, D. B. 1994. *New England J. Med.* 330: 1797-1810.

[52] Vyskocil, F., Malomouzh, A. I., and Nikolsky, E. E. 2009. *Physiol. Res.* 58: 763-784.

(Figure 13.12; see also Figure 11.2).[53,54] Thus, it was suggested that a quantum of transmitter corresponds to the contents of one vesicle and that release occurs by a process of **exocytosis**, in which a vesicle fuses with the presynaptic plasma membrane and releases its contents into the synaptic cleft.[55]

Ultrastructure of Nerve Terminals

A conventional transmission electron micrograph of a horizontal section through an active zone of the neuromuscular junction is shown in Figure 13.12A. Within the cytoplasm of the presynaptic terminal are synaptic vesicles, two rows of which are lined up on either margin of density in the presynaptic membrane known as the **active zone (AZ)**. A postjunctional fold invaginates into the muscle fiber under the active zone, and Schwann cell processes penetrate into the synaptic cleft.

Figure 13.12B shows a segment of the presynaptic membrane as it might appear if split open by the technique of freeze-fracturing. Vesicles are lined up on the cytoplasmic face of the presynaptic membrane along active zones. Along the active zones, intramembranous particles protrude from the exposed fracture face of the cytoplasmic leaflet, and matching pits are seen on the fracture face of the outer leaflet. Sites of vesicle exocytosis are visualized as large indentations in the cytoplasmic portion of the membrane and as fractured vesicle stalks in the outer portion.

As described earlier, electrophysiological experiments in which calcium buffers were injected into presynaptic terminals indicated a close association between calcium channels and release sites. Thus, at least some of the pits seen in Figure 13.12B might correspond to the voltage-activated calcium channels that trigger exocytosis. Results obtained with toxin-binding studies at the neuromuscular junction of the frog and the mouse are consistent with this idea.[56-58] Omega-conotoxin, which blocks neuromuscular transmission

[53] Reger, J. F. 1958. *Anat. Rec.* 130: 7–23.

[54] Birks, R., Huxley, H. E., and Katz, B. 1960. *J. Physiol.* 150: 134–144.

[55] del Castillo, J., and Katz, B. 1956. *Prog. Biophys.* 6: 121–170.

[56] Robitaille, R., Adler, E. M., and Charlton, M. P. 1990. *Neuron* 5: 773–779.

[57] Cohen, M. W., Jones, O. T., and Angelides, K. J. 1991. *J. Neurosci.* 11: 1032–1039.

[58] Sugiura, Y. et al. 1995. *J. Neurocytol.* 24: 15–27.

(A)

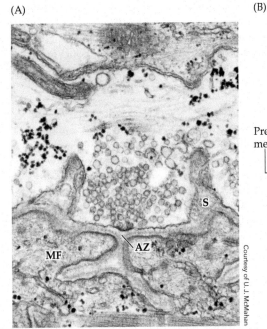

Courtesy of U. J. McMahan

(B)

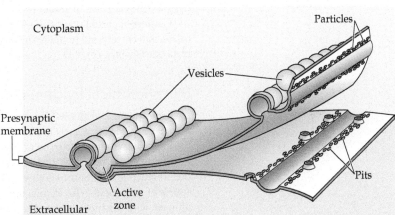

FIGURE 13.12 Synaptic Structure at the Frog Neuromuscular Junction. (A) Transmission electron micrograph of a longitudinal section through a portion of the nerve terminal. In the active zone (AZ), two vesicles lie on either side of a presynaptic membrane density. Directly under the active zone, the postsynaptic membrane invaginates into the muscle fiber (MF) to form a postjunctional fold. Schwann cell processes (S) invade the synaptic cleft to wrap around the nerve terminal. (B) Three-dimensional view of a presynaptic membrane split along its intramembranous plane as might occur in freeze-fracture. Two rows of vesicles lie along the margins of the active zones (yellow). In the split region, particles protrude from the cytoplasmic half of the membrane along the active zone, and corresponding pits are seen on the fracture face of the outer membrane leaflet. Some are represented in the process of exocytosis. Vesicles fusing with the presynaptic membrane give rise to pores and protrusions on the two fracture faces. (B after illustration by U. J. McMahan.)

(A)

(B)

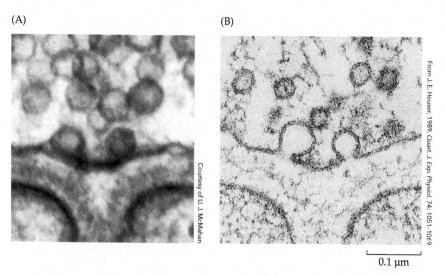

Courtesy of U. J. McMahan

From J. E. Heuser, 1989. *Quart. J. Exp. Physiol.* 74: 1051-1069

0.1 μm

FIGURE 13.13   Release of Neurotransmitter by Synaptic Vesicle Exocytosis.
High-power electron micrographs of frog neuromuscular junctions. (A) A cluster of synaptic vesicles within the presynaptic terminal contacts an electron-dense region of the presynaptic membrane, forming an active zone. (B) A single stimulus was applied to the motor nerve in the presence of 4-aminopyridine, a drug that greatly increases transmitter release by prolonging the action potential, and the tissue was frozen within milliseconds. Vesicles docked at the active zone have fused with the presynaptic membrane and released their contents into the synaptic cleft by exocytosis.

irreversibly by binding to presynaptic calcium channels,[59] was coupled to a fluorescent molecule. Upon microscopic examination, the fluorescence was found to be concentrated in narrow bands at 1-μm intervals, the same spacing as that of the active zones in the terminal.

Clusters of particles are also seen along the sides of the postjunctional folds. These are believed to correspond to the ACh receptors that are concentrated in this region of the end plate (see Chapter 11).[60-62]

Morphological Evidence for Exocytosis

An important experimental innovation developed by Heuser and Reese and their colleagues enabled frog muscle to be quick-frozen within milliseconds after a single shock to the motor nerve and then to be prepared for freeze-fracture.[63] With such an experiment it was possible to obtain electron micrographs of vesicles caught in the act of fusing with the presynaptic membrane (Figure 13.13) and to determine, with some accuracy, the time course of such fusion. To do this, the muscle is mounted on the undersurface of a falling plunger, with the motor nerve attached to stimulating electrodes. As the plunger falls, a stimulator is triggered, shocking the nerve at a selected interval before the muscle smashes into a copper block that is cooled to 4° kelvin (K) (–269°C) with liquid helium. An essential part of the experiment is that the duration of the presynaptic action potential is increased by addition of 4-aminopyridine (4-AP) to the bathing solution. This treatment greatly increases the magnitude and duration of quantal release evoked by a single shock and hence the number of vesicle openings seen in the electron micrographs (Figure 13.14A,B).

Two important observations were made. First, the maximum number of vesicle openings occurred when stimulation preceded freezing by 3 to 5 ms, which corresponded to the peak of the postsynaptic current recorded from curarized, 4-AP-treated muscles in separate experiments. In other words, the maximum number of vesicle openings coincided in time with the peak postsynaptic conductance change determined physiologically. Second, the number of vesicle openings increased with 4-AP concentration, and the increase was related linearly to the estimated increase in quantum content of the end plate potentials by 4-AP—again, obtained from separate physiological experiments (Figure 13.14C). Thus, vesicle openings were correlated both in number and in time course with quantal release.

[59] Olivera, B. M. et al. 1994. *Annu. Rev. Biochem.* 63: 823-867.

[60] Heuser, J. E., Reese, T. S., and Landis, D. M. D. 1974. *J. Neurocytol.* 3: 109-131.

[61] Peper, K. et al. 1974. *Cell Tissue Res.* 149: 437-455.

[62] Porter, C. W., and Barnard, E. A. 1975. *J. Membr. Biol.* 20: 31-49.

[63] Heuser, J. E. et al. 1979. *J. Cell Biol.* 81: 275-300.

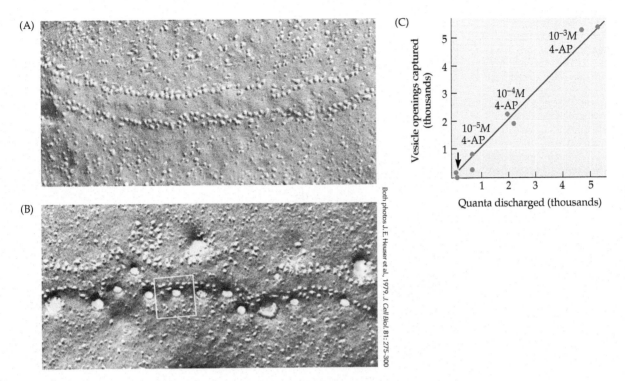

(A)

(B)

Both photos J. E. Heuser et al., 1979. *J. Cell Biol.* 81: 275–300.

(C)

Vesicle openings captured (thousands)

10⁻³M 4-AP

10⁻⁴M 4-AP

10⁻⁵M 4-AP

Quanta discharged (thousands)

FIGURE 13.14 Vesicle Exocytosis Corresponds to Quantal Release. (A) Freeze-fracture electron micrograph of the cytoplasmic half of the presynaptic membrane in a frog nerve terminal (as if observed from the synaptic cleft). The region of the active zone appears as a slight ridge delineated by membrane particles (about 10 nm in diameter). (B) Similar view of a terminal that was frozen just at the time the nerve began to discharge large numbers of quanta (5 ms after stimulation). Holes (box) are sites of vesicle fusion. (C) Comparison of the number of vesicle openings (counted in freeze-fracture images) and the number of quanta released (determined from electrophysiological recordings). The diagonal line is the 1:1 relationship expected if each vesicle that opened released 1 quantum of transmitter. Transmitter release was varied by adding different concentrations of 4-AP (arrow indicates control, without 4-AP). (C from J. E. Heuser et al., 1979. *J. Cell Biol.* 81: 275–300.)

In later experiments, Heuser and Reese characterized the time course of vesicle openings in greater detail, showing that openings first increase during a 3- to 6-ms period after stimulation and then decrease over the next 40 ms.[64] These experiments also provided a detailed picture of the progressive formation of a fusion pore and its subsequent collapse as the vesicle fused with the nerve terminal membrane (Figure 13.15).

Release of Vesicle Contents by Exocytosis

A prediction of the hypothesis that neurotransmitter release occurs by vesicle exocytosis is that stimulation will release the total soluble contents of synaptic vesicles. This prediction was first tested not in neurons but in adrenal medullary cells, from which chromaffin granules could be purified and their contents analyzed.[65] Chromaffin granules are organelles analogous to but much larger than synaptic vesicles; they contain epinephrine, norepinephrine, ATP, the synthetic enzyme dopamine β-hydroxylase, and proteins called chromogranins. All of these components are released in response to stimulation of the adrenal medulla, and they appear in the perfusate in exactly the same proportions as are found in the purified granules.

There is also good correspondence in neurons between vesicle contents and release, although it is difficult to isolate pure populations of synaptic vesicles from nerve terminals in order to determine their contents. For example, small synaptic vesicles in sympathetic neurons contain norepinephrine and ATP; the larger dense-core vesicles contain, in addition, dopamine β-hydroxylase and chromogranin A. Stimulation of sympathetic

[64] Heuser, J. E., and Reese, T. S. 1981. *J. Cell Biol.* 88: 564–580.

[65] Kirshner, N. 1969. *Adv. Biochem. Psychopharmacol.* 1: 71–89.

FIGURE 13.15 Sequence of Vesicle Fusion Reconstructed from Cryosections. The sequence of vesicle fusion reconstructed from a sequence of images after quick-freezing and cryofracture of the neuromuscular junction. The large particles in the vesicles are transmembrane proteins. The aligned particles outside the vesicles are most likely calcium channels. (A–C) Formation and expansion of the fusion pore. (D–F) Vesicle collapse during full fusion.

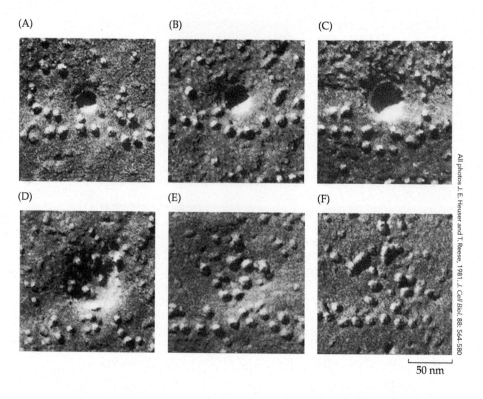

(A)   (B)   (C)

(D)   (E)   (F)

50 nm

All photos J. E. Heuser and T. Reese, 1981. *J. Cell Biol.* 88: 564–580

[66] Smith, A. D. et al. 1970. *Tissue Cell* 2: 547–568.

[67] Silinsky, E. M., and Redman, R. S. 1996. *J. Physiol.* 492: 815–822.

[68] Wagner, J. A., Carlson, S. S., and Kelly, R. B. 1978. *Biochemistry* 17: 1199–1206.

[69] Bruns, D. Riedel, D., Klingauf, J., and Jahn, R. 2000. *Neuron* 28: 205–220.

[70] Cammack, J. N., and Schwartz, E. A. 1993. *J. Physiol.* 472: 81–102.

[71] Cammack, J. N., Rakhilin, S. V., and Schwartz, E. A. 1994. *Neuron* 13: 949–960.

[72] Penner, R., and Neher, E. 1989. *Trends Neurosci.* 12: 159–163.

[73] Angleson, J. K., and Betz, W. J. 1997. *Trends Neurosci.* 20: 281–287.

[74] Lang, T. et al. 1997. *Neuron* 18: 857–863.

[75] Steyer, J. A., Horstmann, H., and Almers, W. 1997. *Nature* 388: 474–478.

[76] Albillos, A. et al. 1997. *Nature* 389: 509–512.

axons results in the release of all of these vesicle constituents.[66] Similarly, vesicles isolated from cholinergic neurons contain ATP as well as ACh, and both are released by stimulation of cholinergic nerves.[67]

The idea that one quantum of transmitter corresponds to the contents of one synaptic vesicle has been examined quantitatively for cholinergic neurons. Vesicles purified from the terminals of the cholinergic electromotor neurons in the electric organ of the marine ray *Narcine brasiliensis* (a relative of *Torpedo californica*) were found to contain about 47,000 molecules of ACh.[68] If synaptic vesicles at the frog neuromuscular junction had the same intravesicular ACh concentration, then, making allowance for their smaller size, they would contain 7000 molecules of ACh. This is in excellent agreement with electrophysiological estimates of the number of ACh molecules in a quantum.[28] A similar result was obtained when the contents of serotonin in clear (4000 molecules) and electron-dense (90,000 molecules) vesicles from leech neurons were compared.[69]

In summary, there is now much evidence that synaptic vesicles are the morphological correlate of the quantum of transmitter, each vesicle containing a few thousand transmitter molecules. Vesicles can release their contents by exocytosis both spontaneously at a low rate (producing miniature synaptic potentials) and in response to presynaptic depolarization. There is evidence that at some specialized synapses in the retina, depolarization can release transmitter through transport proteins in the presynaptic membrane, a mechanism that is nonquantal, not mediated by vesicle exocytosis, and not dependent on calcium influx.[70,71]

Monitoring Exocytosis and Endocytosis in Living Cells

The first quantitative studies of exocytosis were made on dissociated non-neuronal secretory cells, such as mast cells and chromaffin cells, in which the discharge of large, dense-cored secretory granules could be followed with a variety of techniques. These techniques included light microscopy of granules labeled with fluorescent dye, measurement of the increase in membrane capacitance produced by incorporation of vesicle membrane into the plasma membrane of the cell, and amperometry, which detects the amines released in response to stimulation.[72,73] Figure 13.16 illustrates one such experiment. Exocytosis was observed directly in cultured chromaffin cells by evanescent-wave microscopy, a fluorescence microscopy technique that greatly reduces background fluorescence by exciting only a 300-nm-thick layer of cytosol. Chromaffin granules within the cells were

FIGURE 13.16 Exocytosis Observed in Living Cells.
(A) Chromaffin cells growing on a glass cover slip in cell culture were labeled with a fluorescent dye, which becomes concentrated in chromaffin vesicles. Individual vesicles docked at the plasma membrane were visualized by evanescent-wave microscopy. At the same time, release of catecholamines was detected by amperometry. (B) High-power images of a single chromaffin vesicle at 2-second intervals after the cell was stimulated with high potassium. The spot disappears abruptly and permanently as the vesicle undergoes exocytosis and releases its fluorescent contents. (C) The time course of exocytosis in response to an increase in extracellular potassium concentration, as recorded by amperometric detection of catecholamine release and the disappearance of fluorescent spots. Note the coincidence of release and spot disappearance (the arrows mark one example). More events are recorded by amperometry than by fluorescence because the amperometric electrode detects exocytosis over a large part of the cell, while only a small portion of the cell surface is imaged by evanescent-wave microscopy. (After J. A. Steyer et al., 1997. *Nature* 388: 474–478.)

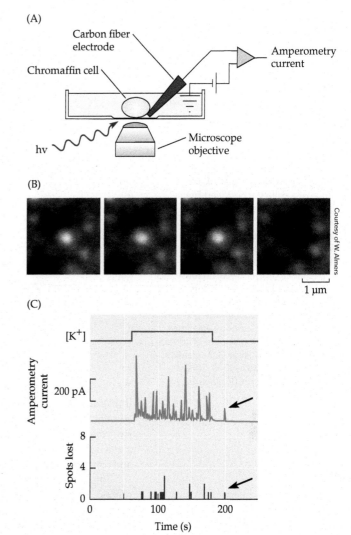

labeled with a fluorescent dye. The release of catecholamines was measured by amperometry—a very sensitive method in which a carbon fiber microelectrode is used to detect transmitters by the current they produce when they are oxidized by the voltage applied to the fiber. With evanescent-wave microscopy, individual fluorescent vesicles could be seen to dock at the plasma membrane and then disappear as they released their fluorescent contents by exocytosis.[74,75] Each time a fluorescent vesicle disappeared, the release of a quantum of transmitter was detected by amperometry.

The experiment shown in Figure 13.17 illustrates the use of capacitance measurements to monitor exocytosis. A cell-attached patch is made on a chromaffin cell, and inside the patch pipette a carbon fiber electrode detects catecholamine release. A sinusoidal signal applied to the bathing solution is used to measure changes in capacitance across the patch. Catecholamine release by exocytosis is accompanied by stepwise increases in capacitance arising from the addition of the granule membrane to the surface of the patch.[76]

Dye release and capacitance increases associated with exocytosis of vesicles have been made in CNS nerve terminals as well.

FIGURE 13.17 Coincident Increases in Membrane Capacitance and Release of Catecholamines from chromaffin cells. (A) A carbon fiber electrode inside the patch pipette measures catecholamine release by amperometry, while at the same time the electrode is used to measure capacitance within the patch. (B) Simultaneous recording of catecholamine release (top trace) and capacitance (bottom trace). All exocytotic events detected by catecholamine release coincide with increases in capacitance. Capacitance units are in femtofarads (1 fF = 10^-15 farads). (After A. Albillos et al., 1997. *Nature* 389: 509–512.)

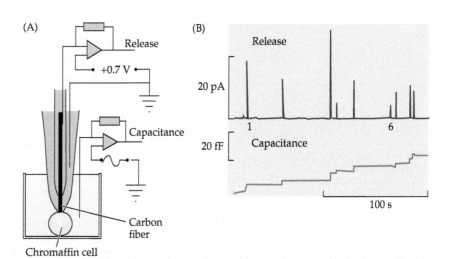

FIGURE 13.18 Release of Synaptic Vesicles from Presynaptic Nerve Terminals, monitored by loss of fluorescent dye (A) and increase in membrane capacitance (B). (A) Fluorescence records from four terminal boutons on a cultured hippocampal neuron. Vesicles in the bouton had been loaded previously with a fluorescent lipid marker. Stimulation of the presynaptic nerve (dots) caused stepwise drops in fluorescence, signaling single vesicle discharges. (B) Capacitance of a cell-attached membrane patch on the transmitter-releasing face of a calyx of Held. The patch was depolarized by perfusing the electrode with 25 m*M* KCl, starting at the beginning of the record. (a) Membrane capacitance (upper trace) increased as vesicle membranes were incorporated into the patch. (b) A magnified record of the segment between the two vertical lines in (a) shows stepwise jumps. Capacitance calibration is in attofarads (1 aF = 10^{-18} F). (A after D. A. Richards, 2009. *J. Physiol.* 587: 5073–5080; B after L. He et al., 2006. *Nature* 444: 102–105.)

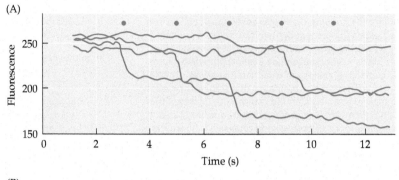

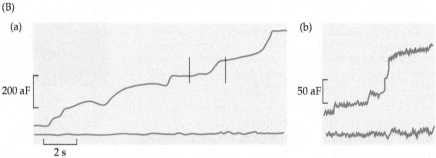

Two examples are shown in Figure 13.18. Figure 13.18A shows records of dye release from individual boutons on cultured hippocampal neurons in response to presynaptic nerve stimulation.[77] Vesicles were first loaded with a fluorescent lipid marker, with roughly five vesicles per bouton being stained. Stimulation of the presynaptic nerve resulted in stepwise drops in bouton fluorescence, indicating the exocytosis of individual vesicles and consequent dispersal of the dye.

The capacitance records in Figure 13.18B are from a different experiment on a calyx of Held.[78] The calyx was pulled away from its postsynaptic neuron so that a cell-attached patch could be made on the transmitter-releasing face. Depolarization of the patch, by perfusing the electrode with a solution containing 25 m*M* KCl in order to produce transmitter release, resulted in a steady increase in capacitance as vesicle membranes were added to the patch (see part a of the figure). The inset in part b shows stepwise jumps in more detail. A step increase of 100 attofarads (aF) corresponds to incorporation into the patch membrane of a synaptic vesicle about 50 nm in diameter.

Mechanism of Exocytosis

Exocytosis of synaptic vesicles involves the cooperative action of several intracellular proteins in the active zone. Proteins carried by the tethered vesicles bind to others in the plasma membrane and the active zone material to form a dynamic "fusion complex." At least 11 proteins participate in the process. **SNARE** (Soluble *N*-ethylmaleimide-sensitive factor *A*ttachment protein *RE*ceptor) proteins are universal components of the complex, one of which is attached to the vesicle membrane (v-SNARE) and two to the target region of the nerve terminal membrane (t-SNAREs).[79]

The interactions between the vesicle and membrane SNARE proteins that lead to exocytosis are illustrated in Figure 13.19.[80] Attached to the vesicle membrane is the SNARE protein synaptobrevin, together with a calcium sensor, synaptotagmin. Two SNARE proteins are attached to the synaptic membrane: syntaxin and SNAP-25. Figure 13.19A shows the vesicle in the docked position over the active zone. The t-SNARE syntaxin is held in a closed state by the regulatory protein Munc 18-1, and in that configuration is unable to interact with other SNARE proteins.[81] Docking is followed by a priming stage (see Figure 13.19B) in which Munc 13 interacts with the Munc 18-1/syntaxin complex to allow syntaxin to enter its open state; Munc 13 also forms a bridge between the vesicle and plasma membranes. Syntaxin then assembles with synaptobrevin and SNAP-25 to form

[77] Richards, D. A. 2009. *J. Physiol.* 587: 5073–5080.

[78] He, L. et al. 2006. *Nature* 444: 102.

[79] Südhof, T. C. 2013. *Neuron* 80: 675–690.

[80] Rizo, J. 2018. *Protein Sci.* 27: 1364–1391.

[81] Han, G. A. et al. 2010. *J. Neurochem.* 115: 1–10.

FIGURE 13.19 Mechanism of Exocytosis. (A) Docked vesicle. The vesicle membrane contains the SNARE protein synaptobrevin and the calcium sensor synaptotagmin. Two additional SNARE proteins, syntaxin and SNAP-25, are anchored to the nerve terminal plasma membrane at the active zone. Syntaxin is held in a folded, inactive configuration by Munc 18-1. (B) Vesicle in the primed position. Munc 13 forms a bridge between the vesicle and the plasma membrane and has facilitated the entry of syntaxin into its open configuration. The open syntaxin forms a ternary SNARE complex with synaptobrevin and the two arms of SNAP-25. The complex is stabilized by the presence of complexin. Calcium channels are close to the SNARE complex. (C) Calcium binds to synaptotagmin, which in turn binds to the SNARE complex, displacing complexin and inducing pore formation. (After J. Tang et al., 2006. *Cell* 126: 1175-1187; J. Rizo, 2018. *Protein Sci.* 27: 1364-1391.)

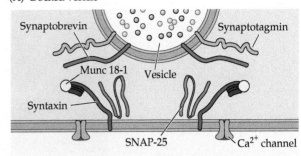

(A) Docked vesicle

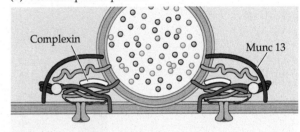

(B) Vesicle in primed position

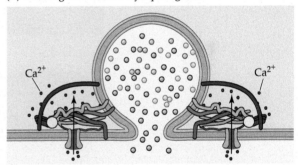

(C) Entering Ca^{2+} binds to synaptotagmin

a four-helix bundle that binds the vesicle in close contact with the plasma membrane. Attached to the bundle is the cytoplasmic regulatory protein complexin, which serves to stabilize the interaction between the synaptobrevin and syntaxin helices. Upon an action potential, calcium entering the nerve terminal through voltage-activated calcium channels binds to synaptotagmin (see Figure 13.19C), which in turn binds to the SNARE complex, displacing complexin and initiating pore formation.

High-Resolution Structure of Synaptic Vesicle Attachments

In a remarkable series of experiments using three-dimensional electron microscopy (electron tomography),[82] U. J. McMahan and his colleagues have examined the detailed structure of the active zone material (AZM) at the frog's neuromuscular junction.[83] Their studies show a highly organized array of macromolecules that connect docked vesicles to the presynaptic membrane. Figure 13.20 shows images of these structures. A central *beam* runs along the active zone in the presynaptic terminal, flanked by two rows of vesicles. Each vesicle is connected to the beam by two to four *ribs*. Other, more detailed, images have shown that the beams are separated from the presynaptic membrane by a narrow (~5 nm) gap and are connected to the membrane by one or two *pegs*. The rib–beam assemblies are closely aligned with the row of macromolecular bumps seen in freeze-fracture images of the active zone (see panel H), which form the attachment points for pegs (see panel I).

Further experiments have revealed even more complex details of the molecular structure.[84] Each docked vesicle is connected to three distinct classes of AZM macromolecules, each class lying at different depths vertical to the presynaptic membrane (Figure 13.21A,B). Accordingly, three or four ribs lie near the presynaptic membrane, two **spars** are deep to the ribs, and five to seven **booms** are deep to the spars. Whereas the peripheral ends of the ribs, spars, and booms are connected to distinct domains on the membrane of docked vesicles,[85] the central ends of each class are attached to distinct classes of macromolecules in a vertical assembly at the midline of the AZM, thus: ribs to beams, spars to **steps**, and booms to **masts**. Another class of macromolecules, the **topmasts**, links some of the nearby undocked vesicles to the masts, and pins connect the vesicle membrane to the presynaptic membrane away from the main body of the AZM.

When the neuromuscular junctions are fixed while the axons are being electrically stimulated at high frequency (10 Hz), different stages of vesicle recycling can be captured. Thus, is it possible to see vesicles in various stages of merging with the presynaptic membrane,[85] and undocked vesicles in stages of replacing previously docked vesicles. The varied reconstructions suggest a sequence of events like that shown in Figure 13.21C. After calcium entry, pins get shorter, and vesicles hemifuse [86] and then

[82] Chen, X. et al. 2002. *Neuron* 33: 397–409.

[83] Harlow, M. L. et al. 2001. *Nature* 409: 479–484.

[84] Szule, J. A., Harlow, M. L., Jung, J. H. et al. 2012. *PLOS ONE* 7: e33333.

[85] Szule, J. A., Jung, J. H., and McMahan, U. J. 2015. *Phil. Trans. R. Soc. B* 370: 20140189.

[86] Jung, J. H. et al. *Proc. Natl.Acad. Sci. USA* 113: e1098-1107.

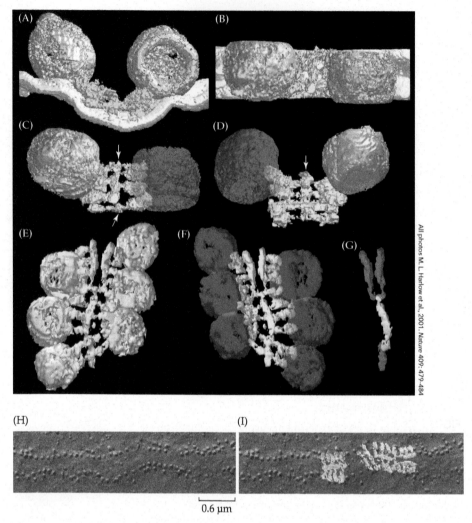

All photos M. L. Harlow et al., 2001; *Nature* 409: 479–484

0.6 μm

FIGURE 13.20 Organization of Active Zone Material at the frog neuromuscular junction. Three-dimensional images obtained by electron microscope tomography. (A,B) Transverse and horizontal views of a short section of an active zone, showing two vesicles (blue) and active zone material (yellow). (C-F): Additional views with the presynaptic membrane removed. Active zone material is organized into central ribs, with a series of transverse beams connecting them to the vesicles. Vesicles in (C) and (D) are made transparent to reveal the points of beam attachment. Not visible are pegs that connect the beams to macromolecules in the presynaptic membrane. (G) Only the beams are shown. (H,I) Size and spacing of the rib–beam structure closely match macromolecular bumps seen in a freeze-fracture replica of an active zone.

fuse with the presynaptic membrane while still associated with the AZM (see part a of Figure 13.21C). As the fused vesicles flatten into the presynaptic membrane, they first dissociate from the booms, then the spars, and finally the ribs (see parts b–e). Undocked vesicles that come to occupy the vacated docking sites on the presynaptic membrane initially form associations with the booms, then the spars, and finally the ribs and pins before contacting the presynaptic membrane.[85]

Correlation between the protein molecules involved in docking and fusion and the AZM structures involved in vesicle attachment has been difficult to establish. Spatial considerations suggest that the SNARE complex, formed by synaptobrevin, synaptotagmin, syntaxin, and SNAP-25, might be a structural component of the pins and ribs (compare Figures 13.19C and 13.21A).[87] Other structures may involve Rab proteins, a family of GTPases that participate in several cytoplasmic functions, including targeting synaptic vesicles to appropriate membrane sites.[88]

[87] Sharuna, N. et al. 2009. *J. Comp. Neurol.* 513: 457–468.

[88] Binotti, B., Jahn, R., and Chua, J. 2016. *Cells* 5: 7.

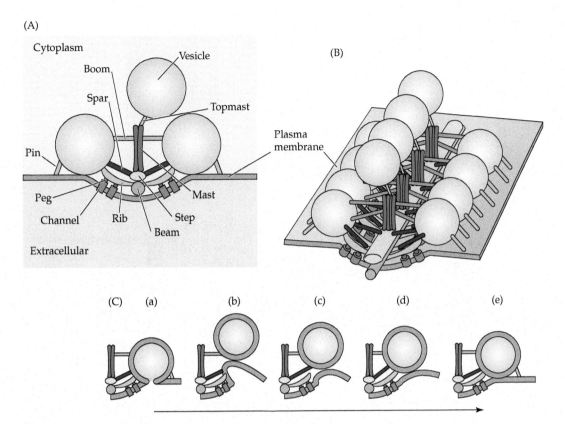

FIGURE 13.21 Schematic Representation of Macromolecules in the Active Zone at the neuromuscular junction of the frog. (A) Cross section though the active zone. A beam runs longitudinally along the active zone membrane and is connected laterally to adjacent docked synaptic vesicles by ribs. Ribs are connected to channels in the presynaptic membrane by short pegs. At the next level, a step gives rise to spars that extend out to the vesicles. Above the step, a multimolecular mast extends into the cytoplasm and is connected to the docked vesicles by booms. A topmast tethers an undocked vesicle to the mast. Lateral to the active zone the vesicles are connected to the presynaptic membrane by pins. (B) Three-dimensional view of the components in (A), showing the multiplicity of molecular attachments. (C) Scheme for replacement of docked vesicles after exocytosis. (a) Vesicle fuses with the membrane and releases transmitter while still associated with the active zone material. (b-e) As the fused vesicle collapses into the postsynaptic membrane, it dissociates first from the pins, then the booms, spars, and ribs, while the replacement vesicle associates first with booms, then spars, ribs, and pins. (From J. A. Szule et al., 2012. *PLOS ONE* 7: e33333/CC BY 4.0.)

Transmitter Release without Full Vesicle Fusion

Several lines of evidence suggest that pore formation is not followed by full vesicle fusion, but rather by closure of the pore before complete release of the vesicle contents. For example, dye releases often exhibit smaller than average jumps.[77] This process, known as **kiss-and-run**, is well established as a mode of exocytosis and, in some secretory cells, may underlie a substantial fraction of release.[89] Its role in release from nerve terminals is less clear, and the molecular mechanisms underlying the phenomenon are unknown.[90,91]

The amperometric recordings of serotonin release in Figure 13.22 provide examples of release both with and without full vesicle fusion. In some events the release produces a "foot" in the amperomeric current, followed by a fast spike, indicating full fusion and completion of the quantal release (see Figure 13.22B). In other events the spike is absent after the foot, suggesting that the pore opens and closes before full fusion (see Figure 13.22C); this kiss-and-run process permits only a subquantal release. In some cases, however, the pore remains locked open for tens of milliseconds, allowing the leak of the whole quantum without full fusion of the vesicle (see Figure 13.22D). Figure 13.22E shows the estimated average number of 5-HT molecules released in each condition.

[89] Alabi, A. A., and Tsien, R. W. 2013. *Annu. Rev. Physiol.* 785: 393–422.

[90] Rizzo, S. O. 2014. *EMBO Journal* 33: 788–822.

[91] He, L., and Wu, L.-G. 2007. *Trends Neurosci.* 30: 447–455.

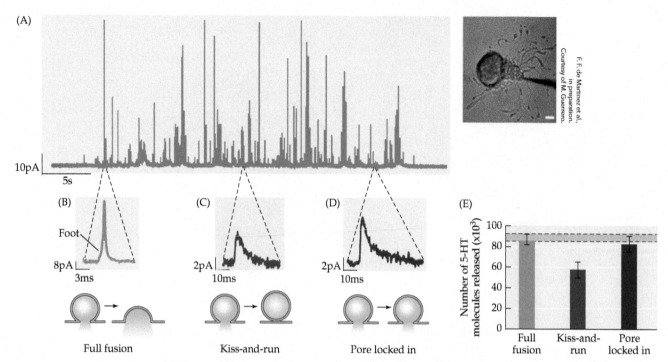

FIGURE 13.22 Amperometric Records of Serotonin Exocytosis from Electron-Dense Vesicles. Stimulation in a leech Retzius neuron in culture evokes ongoing exocytosis from the axon terminal. (A) An amperometric fiber apposed to the plasma membrane (seen as a black shadow on the image) records each exocytotic pulse. (B) Most traces (green) have a "foot," produced by the release of serotonin through the fusion pore, then a fast spike produced following full vesicle fusion. (C) Smaller spikes (red) during kiss-and-run release. (D) Other small spikes (purple) last tens of milliseconds, indicating release through a pore that remains locked in an open state without full fusion. (E) The number of molecules in each spike can be estimated from the integral of the current. The horizontal gray dashed lines are the average and error number of molecules in a quantum. (Courtesy of Francisco F. De-Miguel.)

Ribbon Synapses

Short sensory receptors (see Chapter 21), and some second-order sensory cells such as bipolar cells in the retina (see Chapter 22), do not generate action potentials. So transmitter release from these cells is ongoing, rather than occurring intermittently in response to action potential activity, and is modulated by graded changes in membrane potential that codify the intensity of the stimulus. For example, photoreceptors and bipolar cells in the retina secrete glutamate continuously by exocytosis, at rates that vary with changes in illumination (see Chapter 23). Similarly, release of glutamate by hair cells in the auditory and vestibular systems is graded with polarity and intensity of the stimulus (see Chapter 22). Both systems are able to transmit graded information accurately and continuously over a wide range of stimulus intensities, often at very high rates of vesicular release.

This ongoing release of transmitter is associated with specialized machinery not seen at phasic synapses—the **synaptic ribbon**,[92] an intracellular organelle that tethers large numbers of vesicles near the presynaptic active zone (see Chapter 23). The ribbon itself is composed largely of the protein RIBEYE. Its structure varies considerably from one type of synapse to another, but in general it is anchored to the active zone and extends from the synaptic membrane into the cytoplasm (Figure 13.23A).

The mechanisms of vesicle fusion at ribbon synapses are similar in principle to those at conventional synapses, with several differences in detail. The intracellular machinery consists of many of the same components as in non-ribbon synapses, but uses different isoforms of some proteins associated with vesicle exocytosis and recovery.[93] Calcium entry is mediated by $Ca_V1.3$ and $Ca_V1.4$ channels (known generically as **L-type channels** for their *L*ong openings with little or no inactivation) in hair cells and retinal cells, respectively,

[92] Matthews, G., and Fuchs, P. 2010. *Nat. Rev. Neurosci.* 11: 812–822.

[93] Zanazzi, G., and Matthews, G. 2009. *Mol. Neurobiol.* 39: 130.

(A)

(B)

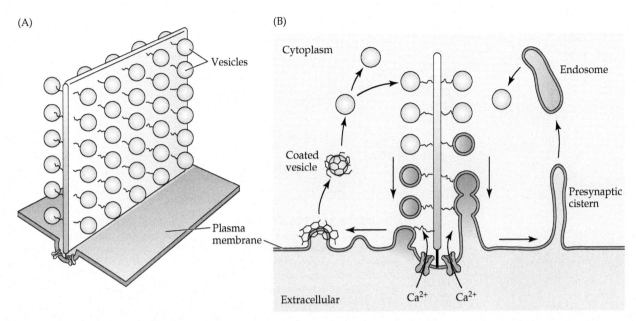

Vesicles

Plasma
membrane

Cytoplasm

Coated
vesicle

Extracellular

Ca²⁺   Ca²⁺

Endosome

Presynaptic
cistern

FIGURE 13.23 **Schematic Representation of a Synaptic Ribbon.** (A) The ribbon is anchored along the active zone of the presynaptic membrane and extends into the cytoplasm. Vesicles are tethered to the ribbon in vertical rows. (B) Possible modes of vesicle discharge and recovery. Calcium entering through channels at the base of the ribbon triggers release of single vesicles (left side of diagram), which are recovered by clathrin-mediated endocytosis. Vesicles move down the queue as release continues. Upon losing their coats, vesicles either remain in the cytoplasm or reattach to the ribbon. Alternatively (right side), several vesicles may discharge en masse by fusing serially with one another and with the membrane. Recovery may be through large endosomes and presynaptic cisterns. (B after G. Zanazzi and G. Matthews, 2009. *Mol. Neurobiol.* 39: 130–148.)

rather than the $Ca_V2.1$ (P/Q) channels or $Ca_V2.2$ (N) channels that predominate in conventional synapses. L channels allow sustained calcium influx during sustained depolarization, in contrast to N and P channels, which inactivate rapidly. The calcium channels are concentrated in the active zone near the base of the ribbon.

The role of the ribbon in relation to the release process and vesicle recycling has not yet been defined precisely. Figure 13.23B summarizes proposed schemes for the sequence of events during vesicle fusion and recovery in ribbon synapses.

Reuptake of Synaptic Vesicles

At neuromuscular, ganglionic, and CNS synapses, periods of intense stimulation have been shown to deplete synaptic vesicles and increase the surface area of the axon terminal, indicating that after releasing their contents, empty vesicles flatten out and become part of the terminal membrane.[94–96] An example is shown in Figure 13.24. At the resting synapse (see Figure 13.24A), synaptic vesicles are clustered over a presynaptic membrane thickening (release site). In a specimen fixed after prolonged stimulation (see Figure 13.24B), release sites are devoid of vesicles. When fixation is delayed for an hour after stimulation (see Figure 13.24C), synapses have recovered their initial morphological features.

How is the vesicle population restored? Heuser and Reese found that components of the vesicle membrane are retrieved and recycled into new synaptic vesicles.[97] They studied recycling of vesicles in frog motor nerve terminals by stimulating nerve–muscle preparations in the presence of horseradish peroxidase (HRP), an enzyme that catalyzes the formation of an electron-dense reaction product. When electron micrographs of terminals fixed after short periods of electrical stimulation were examined, HRP was found primarily in coated vesicles around the outer margins of the synaptic region, suggesting that these vesicles had been formed from the terminal membrane by endocytosis

[94] Ceccarelli, B., and Hurlbut, W. P. 1980. *Physiol. Rev.* 60: 396–441.

[95] Dickinson-Nelson, A., and Reese, T. S. 1983. *J. Neurosci.* 3: 42–52.

[96] Wickelgren, W. O. et al. 1985. *J. Neurosci.* 5: 1188–1201.

[97] Heuser, J. E., and Reese, T. S. 1973. *J. Cell Biol.* 57: 315–344.

(A)

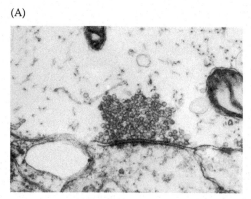

(B)

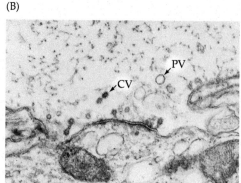

(C)

1 μm

FIGURE 13.24 Stimulation Causes a Reversible Depletion of Synaptic Vesicles in lamprey giant axons. (A) Control synapse fixed after 15 minutes in saline. Synaptic vesicles are clustered at the presynaptic membrane. (B) Synapse fixed after stimulation of the spinal cord for 15 minutes at 20 Hz. Note the depletion of synaptic vesicles, the presence of coated vesicles (CV), pleomorphic vesicles (PV), and the expanded presynaptic membrane. (C) Synapse fixed 60 minutes after cessation of stimulation. Note similarities to the control synapse in (A).

and, in the process, had captured HRP from the extracellular space (Figure 13.25A). HRP also appeared, after a delay, in synaptic vesicles (Figure 13.25B). Synaptic vesicles loaded in this way with HRP could then be depleted of the enzyme by a second period of stimulation in HRP-free medium (Figure 13.25C), thus supporting the idea that the previously recaptured membrane and enclosed HRP had been recycled into the vesicle population from which release occurs.

Vesicle Recycling Pathways

Endocytotic pathways for vesicle recycling are illustrated in Figure 13.26.[98] Recovery of the vesicle membrane and its associated proteins after exocytosis can occur through four different pathways. In kiss-and-run, the vesicle is retrieved completely (during *run*) with no change in morphology or molecular composition.[89] After complete exocytosis, some membrane components of flattened vesicles are retrieved directly as coated vesicles by endocytosis of clathrin-coated pits.[99] In addition to clathrin, other proteins serve to identify the appropriate constituents for recycling. Alternatively, flattened vesicles can be recovered rapidly into endosomes and budded off by clathrin coating ("ultrafast endocytosis"). After particularly intense stimulation, clathrin-coated vesicles are budded off from large, uncoated pits and cisterns ("bulk endocytosis"). Presumably the cisterns result from the infolding of excess terminal membrane, produced by the inability of clathrin-mediated endocytosis to keep up with vesicle membrane incorporation during exocytosis.[100] After retrieval, vesicles lose their coats and are loaded with transmitter molecules from the cytoplasm by proton-dependent transport systems in the vesicle membranes (see Figure 9.5).

Vesicle Pools

One way to follow the sequence of events during recycling is by monitoring the uptake of highly fluorescent dyes to mark recycled vesicles. This technique, developed by W. J. Betz and his colleagues,[101] offers the advantage that vesicle recycling can be observed in living preparations by monitoring the stimulation-dependent accumulation and subsequent release of dye (Figure 13.27).

[98] Chanaday, N. L., and Kavalali, E. T. 2017. *F1000Research* 6: 1734.

[99] Doherty, G. J., and McMahon, H. T. 2009. *Annu. Rev. Biochem.* 78: 815-902

[100] Wu, W., and Wu, L.-G. 2007 *Proc. Natl. Acad. Sci. USA* 104: 10234-10239.

[101] Cochilla, A. J., Angleson, J. K., and Betz, W. 1999. *Annu. Rev. Neurosci.* 22: 1-10.

(A)

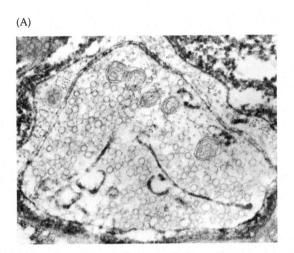

(B)

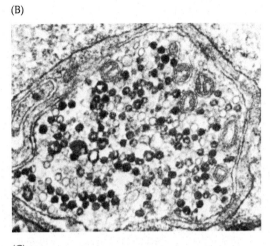

(C)

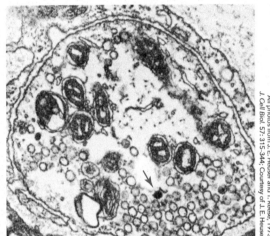

FIGURE 13.25   Recycling of Synaptic Vesicle Membrane. Electron micrographs of cross sections of frog neuromuscular junctions stained with horseradish peroxidase (HRP). (A) The nerve was stimulated for 1 minute in saline containing HRP; electron-dense reaction product can be seen in the extracellular space and in cisterns and coated vesicles. (B) The nerve was stimulated for 15 minutes in HRP, then allowed to recover for 1 hour while the HRP was washed out of the muscle. Many synaptic vesicles contain HRP reaction product, indicating that they were formed from membrane retrieved by endocytosis. (C) The axon terminal was loaded with HRP and allowed to rest, as in (B), then stimulated a second time and allowed to recover an additional hour. Few vesicles are labeled (arrow), indicating that the previously recaptured membrane and enclosed HRP had been recycled into the vesicle population from which release occurs.

Experiments of this nature have led to the designation of three distinct vesicle pools in the nerve terminal.[102] One, the readily releasable pool, contains the first vesicles to be released upon stimulation, and is depleted rapidly by high-frequency stimulation. The second, the recycling pool, recycles continuously to feed the readily releasable pool and thereby maintain a constant lower level of release. Finally the reserve pool comes into play when the recycling pool is depleted.

The existence of multiple pools is supported by a variety of other evidence. For example, in the electric organ of the marine ray *Torpedo* it was found that during stimulation, newly synthesized ACh was not spread uniformly among synaptic vesicles, but was localized to those vesicles recently formed by recycling.[103,104] Studies on mammalian motor and sympathetic axon terminals have shown that newly synthesized transmitter molecules are preferentially released.[105,106] Such results suggest that a subpopulation of vesicles recycles rapidly, while most of the vesicles are held in reserve.

The time courses of vesicle recycling vary widely from one synapse to the next. At the neuromuscular junction, the readily releasable pool is able to refill in about 1 minute through the clathrin-mediated cycle, while the reserve pool takes about 15 minutes to recover from depletion and appears to refill through surface membrane infoldings and cisterns.[92] In contrast, endocytosis in retinal bipolar cells occurs in two separate phases with time constants of 1 to 2 seconds and 10 to 15 seconds.[107] The slower component has been shown to be clathrin-dependent. The fast component is consistent with kiss-and-run recycling. Direct observation of individual vesicles with high-resolution imaging techniques has indicated that in these cells vesicle fusion is always accompanied by complete loss of FM dye,[108] and the vesicle can merge completely into the surface membrane and retract with a time constant of 1 second.[109]

[102] Riozzoli, S. O., and Betz, W. J. 2005. *Nature Rev. Neurosci.* 6: 57–69.

[103] Zimmermann, H., and Denston, C. R. 1977. *Neuroscience* 2: 695–714.

[104] Zimmermann, H., and Denston, C. R. 1977. *Neuroscience* 2: 715–730.

[105] Potter, L. T. 1970. *J. Physiol.* 206: 145–166.

[106] Kopin, I. J. et al. 1968. *J. Pharmacol. Exp. Ther.* 161: 271–278.

[107] Richards, D. A. et al. 2003. *Neuron* 39: 529–5541.

[108] Zenisesek, D. et al. 2002. *Neuron* 1085–1097.

[109] Llobet, A., Beaumont, V., and Lagnado, L. 2003. *Neuron* 40: 1075–1086.

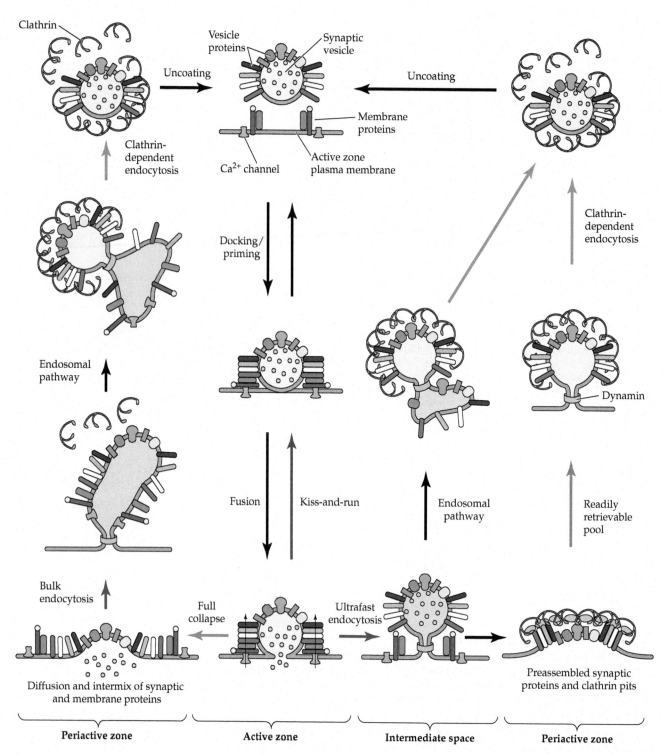

FIGURE 13.26 Four Pathways for Vesicle Recycling. After fusion, vesicles can be retrived by four possible pathways: (1) vesicles can be rapidly retrieved without morphological or molecular changes by kiss-and-run (red arrow), or (2) can fully collapse and intermix components with the plasma membrane (light blue arrow) followed by the bulk endocytosis and the endosomal pathway. (3) Proteins can be retrieved from the plasma membrane via the ultrafast endocytosis pathway (bottom right, blue arrow). (4) Synaptic vesicles are regenerated from the endosomes via a clathrin-dependent mechanism (bottom right sides, orange arrow), which would be endocytosed upon electrical activity. All possible endocytic pathways end with vesicles ready to dock and prime (black arrows at the center). (From N. L. Chanaday and E. T. Kavalali, 2017. *F1000Research* 6: 1734/CC BY 4.0.)

(A)

(B)

(C)

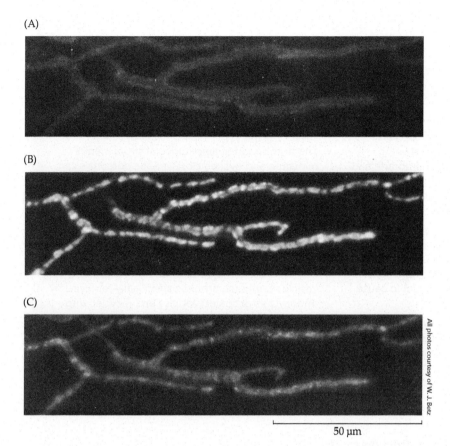

All photos courtesy of W. J. Betz

50 μm

FIGURE 13.27 Stimulation-Dependent Uptake and Release of Fluorescent Dye by Axon Terminals at the Frog Neuromuscular Junction. Fluorescence micrographs of axon terminals in a cutaneous pectoris muscle. (A) Muscle was bathed for 5 minutes in fluorescent dye (2 μ*M* FM1-43) and washed for 30 minutes. Only small amounts of dye remain associated with the terminal membrane. (B) The same muscle was then bathed in dye for 5 minutes while the nerve was stimulated (10 Hz) and washed for 30 minutes. The fluorescent patches are clusters of synaptic vesicles that were filled with dye during recycling. (C) The same muscle was then stimulated at 10 Hz for 5 minutes and washed for 30 minutes. Stimulation released most of the dye.

In synaptic terminals on cultured hippocampal neurons, the major component of refilling has a time constant of the order of 15 seconds.[110–112] A faster component, attributed to kiss-and-run, had a recovery time of about 500 milliseconds.[110] At these synapses, pH-sensitive fluorescent markers reveal brief exposures of the vesicle lumen to the extracellular space during exocytosis, suggestive of kiss-and-run exocytosis, as well as complete washout.[113]

At the calyx of Held, endocytosis has three components.[107] The first has a time constant of a few seconds and the second about 20 seconds. After intense stimulation, a third, rapid component is activated with a time constant of 1 to 2 seconds. The first component can be attributed to kiss-and-run, on the basis that transient capacitance flickers lasting a few hundred milliseconds are relatively common in the terminals.[77] The second component is consistent with clathrin-mediated endocytosis, and the third appears to involve bulk membrane recovery.

At ribbon synapses, dye-labeled vesicles have been shown to recycle selectively to the ribbons, suggesting that the attached vesicles represent the readily releasable pool. At synapses in the retina, good agreement has been found between the readily releasable pool size and the estimated total number of vesicles attached to the ribbons. Vesicles in the cytoplasm are highly mobile and presumably constitute the reserve pool.

[110] Sankaranarayanan, S., and Ryan, T. A. 2000. *Nat. Cell Biol.* 2: 197–204.

[111] Gandhi, S. P., and Stevens, C. F. 2003. *Nature* 423: 607–613.

[112] Granseth, B. et al. 2006. *Neuron* 51: 773–786.

[113] Zhang, Q., Li, Y., and Tsien, R.W. 2009. *Science* 323: 1449–1453.

SUMMARY

- When an axon terminal is depolarized, voltage-activated calcium channels open, increase the intracellular calcium concentration, and cause transmitter release.

- Transmitter is released in multimolecular packets, or quanta, that arise when transmitter-containing synaptic vesicles fuse with the plasma membrane and release their contents by exocytosis. There is also a continuous, nonquantal leak of transmitter from axon terminals at rest.

- The synaptic delay between the beginning of the presynaptic depolarization and the beginning of the postsynaptic potential is due to the time required for the nerve terminal to depolarize, calcium channels to open, and increased intracellular calcium to cause exocytosis.

- In response to an action potential, anywhere from 1 to 300 quanta are released nearly simultaneously, depending on the synapse. When the nerve terminal is at rest, single quanta are released spontaneously at a low rate, producing miniature synaptic potentials.

- Synaptic vesicles contain several thousand molecules of transmitter. The number of postsynaptic receptors activated by a quantum of transmitter varies considerably, from about 15 to 1500, depending on the synapse.

- The distribution of amplitudes of spontaneous miniature and evoked postsynaptic potentials can be analyzed by statistical methods to determine the quantal size and quantum content of the response. Neuromodulatory influences that act presynaptically tend to influence quantum content; those that act postsynaptically tend to influence quantal size.

- After exocytosis, synaptic vesicles may flatten out into the plasma membrane. Components of the vesicle membrane are then specifically retrieved by endocytosis of coated vesicles and recycled into new synaptic vesicles. Under certain circumstances, vesicles may pinch back off without ever becoming incorporated into the surface membrane.

Suggested Reading

General Reviews

Cochilla, A. J., Angleson, J. K., and Betz, W. J. 1999. Monitoring secretory membrane with FM1-43 fluorescence. *Annu. Rev. Neurosci.* 22: 1–10.

Doherty, G. J., and McMahon, H. T. 2009. Mechanisms of endocytosis. *Annu. Rev. Biochem.* 78: 815–902.

He, L., and Wu, L-G. 2007. The debate on the kiss-and-run fusion at synapses. *Trends Neurosci.* 30: 447–455.

Katz, B. 2003. Neural transmitter release: From quantal secretion to exocytosis and beyond. *J. Neurocytol.* 32: 437–446.

Kononenko, N., and Haucke, V. 2015. Molecular Mechanisms of Presynaptic Membrane Retrieval and Synaptic Vesicle Reformation. *Neuron* 85: 484–496.

Rizo, J. 2018. Mechanism of transmitter release coming into focus. *Protein Sci.* doi: 10.1002/pro.3445. PMID 29893445.

Szule, J. A., Jung, J. H., and McMahan, U. J. 2015. The structure and function of "active zone material" at synapses. *Phil Trans. R. Soc. B.* 370:2014018. doi: 10.1098/rstb.2014.0189

Vyskočil, F., Malomouzh, A. I., and Nikolsky, E. E. 2009. Non-quantal acetylcholine release at the neuromuscular junction. *Physiol. Res.* 58: 763–784.

Original Papers

Albillos, A., Dernick, G., Horstmann, H., Almers, W., Alvarez de Toledo, G., and Lindau, M. 1997. The exocytotic event in chromaffin cells revealed by patch amperometry. *Nature* 389: 509–512.

Boyd, I. A., and Martin, A. R. 1956. The end-plate potential in mammalian muscle. *J. Physiol.* 132: 74–91.

del Castillo, J., and Katz, B. 1954. Quantal components of the end-plate potential. *J. Physiol.* 124: 560–573.

Edwards, F. A., Konnerth, A., and Sakmann, B. 1990. Quantal analysis of inhibitory synaptic transmission in the dentate gyrus of rat hippocampal slices: A patch-clamp study. *J. Physiol.* 430: 213–249.

Fatt, P., and Katz, B. 1952. Spontaneous subthreshold potentials at motor nerve endings. *J. Physiol.* 117: 109–128.

Heuser, J. E., Reese, T. S., Dennis, M. J., Jan, Y., Jan, L., and Evans, L. 1979. Synaptic vesicle exocytosis captured by quick freezing and correlated with quantal transmitter release. *J. Cell Biol.* 81: 275–300.

Katz, B., and Miledi, R. 1967a. The timing of calcium action during neuromuscular transmission. *J. Physiol.* 189: 535–544.

Katz, B., and Miledi, R. 1967b. A study of synaptic transmission in the absence of nerve impulses. *J. Physiol.* 192: 407–436.

Kuffler, S. W., and Yoshikami, D. 1975b. The number of transmitter molecules in a quantum: An estimate from ionophoretic application of acetylcholine at the neuromuscular synapse. *J. Physiol.* 251: 465–482.

Llinás, R., Sugimori, M., and Silver, R. B. 1992. Microdomains of high calcium concentration in a presynaptic terminal. *Science* 256: 677–679.

Matthews, G., and Fuchs, P. 2010. The diverse roles of ribbon synapses in sensory neurotransmission. *Nat. Rev. Neurosci.* 11: 812–822.

Miller, T. M., and Heuser, J. E. 1984. Endocytosis of synaptic vesicle membrane at the frog neuromuscular junction. *J. Cell Biol.* 98: 685–698.

Ryan, T. A., Reuter, H., and Smith, S. J. 1997. Optical detection of a quantal presynaptic membrane turnover. *Nature* 388: 478–482.

Sudhof, T. C. 2013. Neurotransmitter release: the last millisecond in the lie of a synaptic vesicle. *Neuron* 80: 675–690.

Wu, L-G., Ryan, T. A., and Lagnado, L. 2007. Modes of synaptic vesicle retrieval at ribbon synapses, calyx-type synapses, and small central synapses. *J. Neurosci.* 27: 11793–11802.

Zhang, Q., Li, Y., and Tsien, R.W. 2009. The dynamic control of kiss-and-run and vesicle reuse probed with single nanoparticles. *Science* 323: 1449–1453.

CHAPTER 14

Neurotransmitters in the Central Nervous System

A large number of different chemical substances act as neurotransmitters in the nervous system. Each transmitter subserves one or more particular functions in the brain; since we cannot discuss all of them in detail, we have selected certain of the major transmitters and describe their particular roles in generating and modulating the activity of the central nervous system (CNS) and behavior.

In Chapter 11 we described the events underlying direct (or fast) synaptic transmission. In the vertebrate CNS, direct excitatory transmission is mediated by the amino acid glutamate, which acts on ionotropic glutamate receptors to open cation-permeable channels. Two other amino acids, γ-aminobutyric acid (GABA) and glycine, act as fast inhibitory neurotransmitters. They activate anion-permeable ionotropic $GABA_A$ and glycine receptors.

Superimposed on the fast action of these amino acids are the slower, modulatory actions of a wide range of transmitters and chemical messengers, mediated primarily through the activation of the metabotropic G protein-coupled receptors (see Chapter 12). The amino acids glutamate and GABA are included as modulatory transmitters, because as well as activating ionotropic receptors, they also interact with metabotropic $GABA_B$ receptors and metabotropic glutamate (mGluR) receptors. Other important modulatory transmitters include acetylcholine (ACh); the monoamines norepinephrine, dopamine, 5-hydroxytryptamine (5-HT, or serotonin), and histamine; and adenosine triphosphate (ATP) and its dephosphorylated product, adenosine. ACh, 5-HT, and ATP also activate separate subsets of ionotropic receptors. However, these ionotropic receptors are mostly located on presynaptic nerve endings, not at postsynaptic sites, so (except for 5-HT) they rarely contribute to postsynaptic responses.

Neurons that secrete norepinephrine, dopamine, 5-HT, histamine, and ACh are for the most part confined to special nuclei in the midbrain and brainstem and are relatively few in number. Nevertheless, their axons innervate wide areas of the brain and spinal cord, so these transmitters regulate important global functions of the brain, such as alertness, arousal, sleep–wake patterns, and memory recall; their loss contributes to the symptoms of some neurodegenerative diseases such as Alzheimer's disease and Parkinson's disease.

Finally, the CNS contains a wide variety of neuropeptide transmitters and hormones, all of which seem to act exclusively on metabotropic receptors. These are generally confined to particular neural pathways. As examples we discuss substance P and the opioid peptides and their role in controlling pain; the orexin (hypocretin) system and its function in sleep and feeding behavior; and the hypothalamic peptides vasopressin and oxytocin and their influence on social interaction.

Chemical Transmission in the CNS

The most fully investigated example of chemical transmission in the vertebrate nervous system is that between motor nerves and the skeletal muscle end plate described in Chapter 11. At this synapse, acetylcholine (ACh) is the transmitter substance and the motor nerves that release it are termed **cholinergic**. ACh is also the excitatory transmitter at synapses between preganglionic and postganglionic neurons in the ganglia of the autonomic nervous system (see Chapter 19). Hence, it is not surprising that, in seeking excitatory transmitters in the CNS, investigators' first thoughts turned to ACh—especially since it was well known that ACh, choline acetyltransferase, and acetylcholinesterase were all abundant in the brain.[1] Indeed, early work by Eccles and his colleagues did identify one such ganglion-like cholinergic synapse that lies between recurrent collateral branches of the cholinergic motor axons and inhibitory interneurons (or Renshaw cells) in the spinal cord.[2] However, this (plus a few other localized central synapses) proved the exception rather than the rule—even at the Renshaw cell, ACh has to share transmitter duties with another fast transmitter, glutamate.[3] (Acetylcholine *is* an important transmitter in the brain, but it has a different function from that at the neuromuscular junction, as we describe later in this chapter.)

Instead, the role of ACh as the direct excitatory transmitter in the vertebrate CNS is replaced by the amino acid **glutamate**, while two other amino acids, **γ-aminobutyric acid (GABA)** and **glycine**, act as direct inhibitory central transmitters (see Chapter 11). For these transmitters, the model synapses are not those in the vertebrate peripheral nervous system (PNS) but instead those in invertebrates such as the crustacean neuromuscular junction and stretch receptor or the insect neuromuscular junction (Box 14.1). It is as though, by some curious evolutionary change, the excitatory and inhibitory control mechanisms undertaken in the PNS of invertebrates has been brought inboard into the CNS in vertebrates.

The effects of direct excitatory and inhibitory transmission are modulated by a wide range of **indirect transmitters** (see Chapter 12) that enhance or reduce transmission through the synaptic pathways in the CNS. These indirect transmitters include both small molecules, such as ACh, ATP, and the monoamines (i.e., norepinephrine, dopamine, 5-HT, and histamine), and also a variety of neuropeptides. All of these modulators act on G protein-coupled receptors as indirect transmitters, though some (ACh, ATP, and 5-HT) also activate ligand-gated ion channels at specific loci. In many cases the action of these transmitters on their receptors occurs at a distance from the release sites (see Chapter 18). Many of these modulators were first identified as transmitters or local messengers in the PNS. The enteric nervous system (in the gut wall) has been a particularly rich source of information, especially about peptide transmitters[4] (Box.14.2). Most of these modulatory transmitters can act on several different subtypes of G protein-coupled receptors (see Chapter 12), so their postsynaptic effects on different neurons can vary and can be quite subtle and complex. Hence, it is difficult to predict their overall contribution to brain function from actions at individual synapses—their functions are often first inferred from the overall behavioral effects of pharmacologically blocking their receptors or by deleting the genes required for the synthesis of the transmitter or its receptors.

[1] Feldberg, W. 1950. *Br. Med. Bull.* 6: 312–321.

[2] Eccles, J. C., Fatt, P., and Koketsu, K. 1954. *J. Physiol.* 126: 524–562.

[3] d'Incamps, B. L., and Ascher, P. 2008. *J. Neurosci.* 28: 14121–14131.

[4] Furness, J. B. et al.1992. *Trends Neurosci.* 15: 66–71.

FIGURE 14.1   Methods for Identifying Neurotransmitters in the CNS. Labeled antibodies or nucleotide probes can be used to detect the expression of enzymes involved in synthetic and degradative pathways in the presynaptic neuron. The neurotransmitter itself can be detected by chemical reaction or by antibodies to a conjugated form of the transmitter. Specific uptake of radiolabeled transmitter can identify some neurons. Ligands or antibodies to postsynaptic receptors as well as nucleotide probes for receptor mRNA provide means to identify cells sensitive to a particular transmitter.

Mapping Neurotransmitter Pathways

An aid to understanding the physiological role of individual neurotransmitters in the CNS is to identify the particular neurons, nerve fibers, and synapses that contain them. Identification can be achieved using a variety of histochemical or immunohistochemical methods (Figure 14.1).

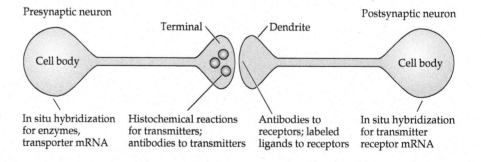

Presynaptic neuron / Terminal / Dendrite / Postsynaptic neuron

Cell body / Cell body

In situ hybridization for enzymes, transporter mRNA | Histochemical reactions for transmitters; antibodies to transmitters | Antibodies to receptors; labeled ligands to receptors | In situ hybridization for transmitter receptor mRNA

| BOX **14.1** | The Discovery of Central Transmitters: I. The Amino Acids |

γ-Aminobutyric Acid (GABA)

Although GABA was originally discovered in the mammalian brain,[5-7] its inhibitory transmitter function was first established in the peripheral nervous system (PNS) of the crayfish. In this and other crustacea there are separate, identifiable inhibitory nerves that, when stimulated, inhibit the muscle fibers and the sensory stretch receptors by increasing their chloride conductance (see Chapter 11). In 1954 Ernst Florey[8] found that an inhibitory factor (Factor I) he extracted from brain could block the discharges of the stretch receptor, and he subsequently identified GABA as the main inhibitory ingredient.[9] Two sets of researchers, Kuffler and Edwards[10] and Boistel and Fatt,[11] then showed that GABA precisely imitated the action of inhibitory nerve stimulation, respectively, on the stretch receptor and the muscle. Through much painstaking work, Kravitz and his colleagues[12] showed that GABA was highly concentrated in crustacean inhibitory axons and (crucially) could be released from them when stimulated in sufficient amounts to be a transmitter.

It took longer to establish the role of GABA in the mammalian central nervous system (CNS). One reason is that there are no discrete inhibitory fiber bundles like those in the crayfish PNS. One approach used by Curtis and his colleagues[13] was to eject GABA ionophoretically around a neuron in the CNS while stimulating excitatory and inhibitory inputs. However, they concluded that GABA was not the inhibitory transmitter but instead had a general depressant action on the somatodendritic membrane of all central neurons, irrespective of their innervation. Using the same techniques, Krnjevic[14] and his colleagues took a more optimistic view. Using intracellular recordings, they subsequently showed that GABA hyperpolarized cortical neurons and increased their membrane conductance, just like stimulating inhibitory afferents,[15] and that both effects were due to an increase in chloride conductance.[15,16] One reason why Curtis and his colleagues rejected a role for GABA in spinal cord inhibition was that its action was not antagonized by strychnine,[17] which was known to block spinal cord inhibitory postsynaptic potentials (IPSPs). Spinal inhibition was not blocked by strychnine because the principal inhibitory transmitter there is glycine, as subsequently shown by Werman and his colleagues.[18]

Glutamate

It took even longer for glutamate to be recognized as the main excitatory transmitter in the CNS. There were several reasons why. Although it is abundant in the brain, glutamate is not unique to the brain (unlike GABA); it

excited every central neuron tested; its action was replicated by other dicarboxylic amino acids;[19] and there were no antagonists of synaptic excitation to help identify the transmitter. Again, the strongest evidence came from experiments on invertebrates, particularly those of Takeuchi and Takeuchi[20] on lobster muscle, in which they found glutamate-sensitive hotspots that coincided with the excitatory postsynaptic potentials (EPSPs) initiated by motor nerve stimulation. As they stated, *"the receptors which respond to L-glutamate are identical with normal neuroreceptors."*[20] Glutamate eventually gained acceptance as the major excitatory transmitter in the mammalian CNS through demonstration of its calcium-dependent release from neurons, the development of specific blocking agents, the cloning of the receptors, and the identification of glutamate-containing synaptic vesicles.[21]

Inactivation of amino acid transmitters

One initial obstacle to the acceptance of amino acids as transmitters was that there seemed to be no enzyme like acetylcholinesterase that was capable of rapidly inactivating the transmitters. This issue was resolved with the discovery by Iversen[22] and others that there are special uptake systems by which the released amino acids (GABA, glutamate, and glycine) are rapidly reaccumulated into the nerves that release them as well as into neighboring neuroglial cells (see Chapters 10 and 15).

---

[5] Awapara, J. et al. 1950. *J. Biol. Chem.* 187: 35–39.

[6] Roberts, E., and Frankel, S. 1950. *J. Biol. Chem.* 187: 55–63.

[7] Udenfriend, S. 1950. *J. Biol. Chem.* 187: 65–69.

[8] Florey, E. 1954. *Arch. Int. Physiol.* 62: 33–53.

[9] Bazemore, A., Elliott, K. A., and Florey, E. 1956. *Nature* 178: 1052–1053.

[10] Kuffler, S. W., and Edwards, C. 1958. *J. Neurophysiol.* 21: 589–610.

[11] Boistel, J., and Fatt, P. 1958. *J. Physiol.* 144: 176–191.

[12] Otsuka, M. et al. 1966. *Proc. Natl. Acad. Sci. USA* 56: 1110–1115.

[13] Curtis, D. R., and Phillis, J. W. 1958. *Nature* 182: 323.

[14] Krnjevic, K., and Phillis, J. W. 1963. *J. Physiol.* 165: 274–304.

[15] Krnjevic, K., and Schwartz, S. 1967. *Exp. Brain Res.* 3: 320–336.

[16] Obata, K. et al. 1967. *Exp. Brain Res.* 4: 43–57.

[17] Curtis, D. R., Phillis, J. W., and Watkins, J. C. 1959. *J. Physiol.* 146: 185–203.

[18] Werman, R., Davidoff, R. A., and Aprison, M. H. 1968. *J. Neurophysiol.* 31: 81–95.

[19] Curtis, D. R., Phillis, J. W., and Watkins, J. C. 1960. *J. Physiol.* 150: 656–682.

[20] Takeuchi, A., and Takeuchi, N. 1964. *J. Physiol.* 170: 296–317.

[21] Lodge, D. 2009. *Neuropharmacology* 56: 6–21.

[22] Iversen, L. L. 1971. *Br. J. Pharmacol.* 41: 571–591.

For example, the distribution of neurons and fibers containing norepinephrine, dopamine, and 5-HT can be individually mapped using a fluorescent method devised by Hillarp and Falck,[23] in which each of these monoamines emits light of a characteristic wavelength under ultraviolet illumination after condensation with formaldehyde and consequent formation of isoquinolines (Figure 14.2). For cholinergic neurons, George Koelle and his

[23] Falck, B. et al. 1962. *J. Histochem. Cytochem.* 10: 348–354.

24 Koelle, G. B., and Friedenwald, J. S. 1949. *Proc. Soc. Exp. Biol. Med.* 70: 617–622.

25 Lewis, P. R., and Shute, C. C. 1967. *Brain* 90: 521–540.

26 Wainer, B. H. et al. 1984. *Neurochem. Int.* 6: 163–182.

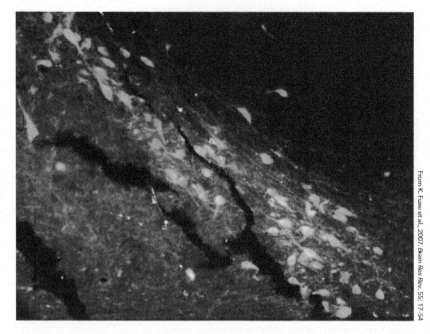

From K. Fuxe et al., 2007. *Brain Res Rev.* 55: 17-54

FIGURE 14.2 Green Fluorescent Dopaminergic Nerve Cells in the zona compacta of the rat substantia nigra revealed using the Falck–Hillarp formaldehyde fluorescent technique.[23] See A. Dahlstrum and K. Fuxe, 1964. *Axta. Physiol. Scand* 60: 293-294 for technical details.

colleagues[24] introduced a histochemical method for staining cholinesterase, the enzyme that hydrolyzes ACh. This method was used to map the distribution of cholinergic fibers in the brain[25] but was subsequently replaced by a more specific immunohistochemical method for localizing the synthetic enzyme, choline acetyltransferase (ChAT).[26]

Immunohistochemical methods have now become the method of choice for localizing most transmitters and their receptors. By using fluorescently tagged secondary antibodies, neurons and fibers containing transmitter-related proteins (such as synthetic enzymes or membrane transporters, or in the case of peptides, the transmitter itself or its precursor) can be readily seen and co-localization with other transmitters detected using different wavelength fluorophores on the secondary antibodies. Figure 14.3A shows an example in which

FIGURE 14.3 Visualization of Corticotrophin-Releasing Factor (CRF) co-localized with a marker for glutamate in synaptic terminals in the dorsal raphe nucleus. (A) The immunofluorescent localization of antibodies against CRF and the vesicular glutamate transporter VGLUT2 in synaptic terminals taken at low power. The CRF antibody was counterstained with a green fluorescent secondary antibody, and VGLUT2 antibody was counterstained with a red secondary antibody. The arrows point to three terminals that stain for both antibodies. (B) A high-power electron micrograph of one terminal that contains both antibodies and makes a synapse on a dendrite. The secondary antibody to CRF was coupled to 1-nm gold particles (arrows), while the secondary antibody to VGLUT2 was coupled to horseradish peroxidise, giving a brown deposit around the small synaptic vesicles. (From M. Waselus and E. J. Van Bockstaele, 2007. *Brain Res.* 1174: 53–65.)

(A)

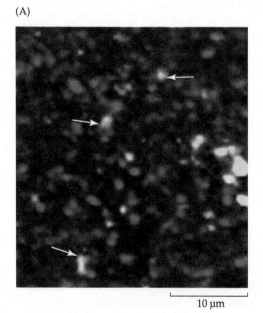

10 μm

(B)

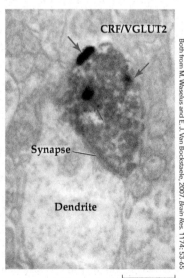

CRF/VGLUT2

Synapse

Dendrite

Both from M. Waselus and E. J. Van Bockstaele, 2007. *Brain Res.* 1174: 53-65

0.5 μm

BOX 14.2 — The Discovery of Central Transmitters: II. Neuropeptides

The first neuropeptides in the brain to be identified and sequenced were the hypothalamic hormones oxytocin and vasopressin, in 1955.[27] Since then, more than 60 other central neuropeptides have been identified.[28] How were they all discovered? The classic approach is to find an appropriate assay, test extracts from brain, and then purify and sequence the active peptides. The modern approach is to go for the gene or its messenger RNA (mRNA) product. These two approaches are well illustrated by the discovery of the **enkephalins** and the **orexins**, respectively.

The enkephalins

Enkephalins are two pentapeptides (five amino acids) that are naturally released stimulants of opiate (morphine) receptors. They were discovered by John Hughes, Hans Kosterlitz, and their colleagues in 1975.[29] Morphine itself is a plant alkaloid that comes from the opium poppy *Papaver somniferum*; the idea that there might be a morphine-like substance in the mammalian brain stemmed from the fact that morphine seemed to act on specific receptors. So there must be an endogenous ligand for them. In order to find this ligand, Hughes used the mouse vas deferens as a bioassay tissue. This tissue contracts when its afferent sympathetic nerves are stimulated; morphine reduces this contraction by inhibiting the release of norepinephrine. Using this tissue, Hughes[30] detected morphine-like activity in mammalian brain extracts, which seemed to be due to a peptide because it was abrogated by peptidases. The amino acid composition of the peptide was determined by chemical methods.[30] This showed that there were actually two peptides: one with the sequence Tyr-Gly-Gly-Phe-*Met*, which they termed met-enkephalin, the other with the sequence Tyr-Gly-Gly-Phe-*Leu*, which was called leu-enkephalin. Both were shown to replicate the effect of morphine on the vas deferens and to be antagonized by naloxone, a known morphine antagonist.

The orexins

Orexins are peptides that are released from nerves of hypothalamic origin, stimulate wakefulness, and enhance appetite; their absence causes the human sleep disorder narcolepsy. They were discovered independently by two groups of scientists starting from what are termed orphan genes—that is, genes or gene products that have no known function. One group began with the gene for the transmitter itself, the other with the gene for its receptor.

The first group (de Lecea and colleagues[31]) constructed a complementary DNA (cDNA) library from the rat hypothalamus and then made a systematic survey of which mRNA products of these cDNAs were selectively concentrated in the hypothalamus. The cDNA derived from one of these mRNA products (clone 35) encoded two peptides that were concentrated in neurons and synapses in the dorsolateral hypothalamus. These peptides excited hypothalamic neurons when applied to them.[32] The researchers called the peptides hypocretins because they were similar to the gut hormone secretin (*hypo*thalamic *secretin*).

The second group (Sakurai and colleagues[33]) started with the genes for orphan G protein-coupled receptors. They expressed the receptors in cell lines and then looked for substances in brain extracts that stimulated them and increased the cells' intracellular calcium. Again, they purified and sequenced two active proteins, and termed them orexin-A and orexin-B (because they had an appetite-stimulating, or *orexigenic*, action in rats). The researchers also determined the amino acid sequences of the responsive receptors, which they called OX1 and OX2. This work shows the power of studying orphan receptors. There are many such receptors, and they have led to the identification of several other neurotransmitters.[34,35]

[27] Du Vigneaud, V. 1955. *Harvey Lect.* 50: 1–26.

[28] Salio, C. et al. 2006. *Cell Tissue Res.* 326: 583–598.

[29] Hughes, J. et al. 1975. *Nature* 258: 577–580.

[30] Hughes, J. 1975. *Brain Res.* 88: 295–308.

[31] Gautvik, K. M. et al. 1998. *Proc. Natl. Acad. Sci. USA* 93: 8733–8738.

[32] De Lecea, L. et al. 1998. *Proc. Natl. Acad. Sci. USA* 95: 322–327.

[33] Sakurai, T. et al. 1998. *Cell* 92: 573–585.

[34] Wise, A. Jupe, S. C., and Rees, S. 2004. *Annu. Rev. Pharmacol. Toxicol.* 44: 43–66.

[35] Civelli, O. et al. 2006. *Pharmacol. Ther.* 110: 525–532.

nerve terminals in the dorsal raphe nucleus are tagged with an antibody against the vesicular glutamate transporter VGLUT2 (indicating that the vesicles contain—and presumably release—glutamate) and counterstained with a red fluorescent secondary antibody, while an antibody tagging the peptide neurotransmitter corticotrophin-releasing factor (CRF) is counterstained with a green fluorescent secondary antibody. Terminals where both are present then show up as yellow.

Immunohistochemical techniques can also be applied at the level of the electron microscope, to see which transmitter or transmitter-specific marker protein is present in individual synapses or synaptic vesicles. Thus, the vesicular glutamate transporter VGLUT2 in the glutamate-containing synaptic terminals shown in Figure 14.3A can be seen under the electron microscope in Figure 14.3B by using a secondary antibody coupled to the enzyme immuno-peroxidase, which gives a brown deposit. The presence of CRF immunoreactivity can then be marked separately using another secondary antibody coupled to electron-dense gold particles.

Visualizing Transmitter-Specific Neurons in Living Brain Tissue

Certain neurons that contain a transmitter of interest can be color-coded in vivo by using transgenic methods. This can be very helpful for subsequent electrophysiological experiments, especially for neurons that are not very numerous. For example, dopamine-releasing (dopaminergic) neurons in the mesencephalon can be color-coded with the jellyfish green fluorescent protein (GFP; see Box 12.6) by tagging the GFP cDNA onto the cDNA that codes for the promoter region of the synthesizing enzyme tyrosine hydroxylase, then expressing it in mice using transgenic techniques.[36] Subsequently, when the mesencephalon is dissected and the cells are isolated and cultured, the dopamine-secreting cells are easily identifiable by their green fluorescence, even though they contribute only a minority of cells in the mixed-cell culture.

A similar approach has been used to express a fluorescently tagged, light-activated, cation-conducting protein, channelrhodopsin-2, in the dopaminergic neurons[37] (Figure 14.4A). Then, dopaminergic neurons in an isolated midbrain slice can be stimulated selectively by a brief flash of blue light, which opens the channelrhodopsin channels to depolarize the neuron (Figure 14.4B). Selectively expressed channelrhodopsins and related proteins are now widely used as a means of stimulating (or inhibiting) neurons,[38] particularly for analyzing neural circuits in vivo,[39] since light stimulation is easier and more versatile than electrical stimulation of individual neurons through microelectrodes. This field of research has been dubbed *optogenetics*.[40,41]

[36] Jomphe, C. et al. 2005. *J. Neurosci. Methods* 146: 1-12.

[37] Stuber, G. D. et al. 2010. *J. Neurosci.* 30: 8229-8233.

[38] Gradinaru, V. et al. 2010. *Cell* 141: 154-165.

[39] Kravitz, A. V. et al. 2010. *Nature* 466: 622-626.

[40] Pastrana, E. 2011. *Nat. Methods* 8: 24-25.

[41] Diesseroth, K. 2011. *Nat. Methods* 8: 26-29.

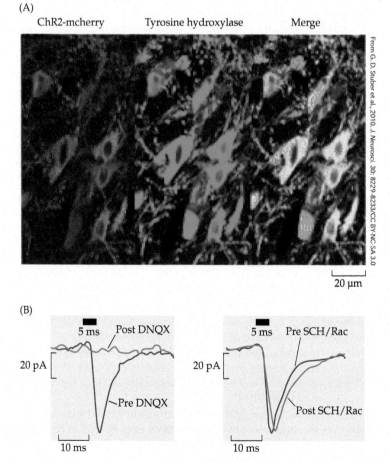

FIGURE 14.4 Transgenic Insertion of a Photo-Activatable Ion Channel that allows the selective stimulation of dopaminergic neurons and their processes. The light-sensitive cation channel, channelrhodopsin-2, tagged with the red fluorescent protein mcherry (ChR2-mcherry) was transgenically expressed from its cDNA in dopaminergic neurons in the mouse brain under the control of the promoter for the dopamine transporter. (A) Dopaminergic neurons in the ventral tegmental area (VTA) of the midbrain expressing the red ChR2-mcherry (left) and an antibody to the dopamine synthetic enzyme tyrosine hydroxylase (TH), counterstained with a green fluorescent secondary antibody (middle). The image on the right shows the left and middle pictures merged, and indicates that ChR2 is restricted to TH-positive neurons. (B) Records made from a neuron in the nucleus accumbens (which is innervated by dopaminergic fibers from the VTA) in a slice of the midbrain taken from a ChR2-expressing mouse brain. They show short-latency excitatory postsynaptic currents generated when the presynaptic fibers are stimulated by activating the ChR2 with a 5-millisecond (ms) pulse of blue light. The current was inhibited by the glutamate antagonist (DNQX, left side, blue line) but not by the dopamine antagonists SCH23390 and raclopride (SCH/Rac, right side, blue line). This means that the postsynaptic current did not result from the release of dopamine itself, but from the release of glutamate that is stored in the same nerve endings as the dopamine and that activates ionotropic glutamate receptors. (From G. D. Stuber et al., 2010. *J. Neurosci.* 30: 8229-8233/CC BY-NC-SA 3.0.)

Key Transmitters

In this section we highlight some properties and functions of a selection of the transmitters previously referred to in Boxes 14.1 and 14.2. Details of chemical structures and metabolic pathways of the small-molecule transmitters are summarized in Appendix B. More detailed information can be obtained in the book by Cooper et al.[42]

Glutamate

Glutamate is the fast excitatory transmitter that is released from neurons throughout the CNS. It activates two types of postsynaptic ionotropic receptors: fast-opening α-amino-3-hydroxy-5-methyl-4-isoxazolepropionic acid (AMPA) receptors and slower opening N-methyl-D-aspartate (NMDA) receptors (see Figure 11.12) The AMPA receptors are responsible for normal fast transmission. They are made up of GluA1–4 subunits (see Chapter 5). The speed and duration of the evoked synaptic currents vary substantially among different synapses, depending on the subunit composition of the channel and on the splice variant (*flip* or *flop*[43]) of the subunits.[44] The presence or absence of the GluA2 subunit, and the extent of its mRNA editing,[45] also affect the calcium permeability of the AMPA receptors.[46] A special group of ionotropic glutamate receptors termed GluK1–5 have a high affinity for kainic acid, a neuroexcitatory compound extracted from seaweed. Unlike AMPA receptors, these kainite receptors do not participate directly in glutamatergic fast excitatory transmission; instead they serve to modulate transmission, primarily (but not exclusively) by modifying glutamate release.[47]

One important feature of AMPA receptors is that they are not held in the postsynaptic membrane as tightly as are the nicotinic receptors at the neuromuscular junction, but are highly mobile.[48] The lifetime of individual AMPA receptors has been estimated at 10 to 30 minutes as the receptors recycle between the cell surface and the subsynaptic apparatus.[49] Several auxiliary synaptic proteins regulate this trafficking,[50] which allows for rapid changes in the numbers and subunit composition of synaptic receptors during neural activity, providing the basis for some forms of synaptic plasticity (see Chapter 17).

The NMDA receptors are made up of GluN1–3 subunits (see Chapter 5). They differ from AMPA receptors in three main respects: The channels open more slowly; they are blocked by Mg^{2+} ions and only allow ions to pass when the membrane is depolarized (see Figure 11.13); and they have a much higher permeability to Ca^+ ions than do most AMPA channels (see Chapter 11). Their voltage dependence means that they act as coincidence detectors, only allowing current to pass when the neuron is simultaneously depolarized by, for example, high-frequency activation of AMPA channels, ongoing action potential activity, or co-activation of metabotropic glutamate receptors (see next paragraph). The consequent entry of Ca^{2+} ions then induces a variety of downstream effects (see Figure 12.20)—most notably, the induction of long-term potentiation (see Chapter 17). However, there is also a downside, which is that excessive Ca^{2+} entry through NMDA channels is also neurotoxic (excitotoxic, to use the original term) and can cause neurodegeneration and ischemic neuron death (stroke).[51] NMDA receptor induction of burst-firing in neurons of the lateral habenula nucleus is suggested to contribute to depressive illness: Blockade of these NMDA receptor channels accounts for the antidepressant effect of the drug ketamine.[52]

Glutamate also activates a distinctive class of G protein-coupled receptors called **metabotropic glutamate receptors (mGluRs)**.[53] There are eight of these receptors, mGluR1–8, which are divided into three groups: group I (mGluR1,5), group II (mGluR2,3), and group III (mGluR4,6,7,8). The group I receptors are the main postsynaptic receptors. They couple to the G protein G_q and hence to the phospholipase C–phosphoinositide pathway (see Figure 12.15). Their activation causes a membrane depolarization and increased excitability, mainly by inhibiting Ca^{2+}-activated and M-type voltage-gated potassium currents. They also release calcium ions from intracellular stores by producing IP_3. IP_3 synergizes with NMDA receptor activation in inducing long-term potentiation. Thus, mice in which the gene for mGluR1 has been deleted[54] show defects in long-term potentiation and learning behavior, while mGluR5 gene-deleted mice show deficits in various forms of learning and habituation.[55] In contrast, mGluR2, 3, and 4 receptors are more strongly

[42] Cooper, J. R., Bloom, F. E., and Roth, R. H. 2003. *The Biochemical Basis of Neuropharmacology*, 8th ed. Oxford University Press, New York.

[43] Hollman, M., and Heinemann, S. 1994. *Annu. Rev. Neurosci.* 17: 31-108.

[44] Geiger, J. R. et al. 1997. *Neuron* 18: 1009-1023.

[45] Seeburg, P. H., and Hartner, J. 2003. *Curr. Opin. Neurobiol.* 13: 279-283.

[46] Cull-Candy, S., Kelly, L. and Farrant, M. 2007. *Curr. Opin. Neurobiol.* 17: 277-280.

[47] Contractor, A., Mulle, C., and Swanson, G. T. 2011. *Trends Neurosci.* 34: 154-163.

[48] Tardin, C. et al. 2003. *EMBO J.* 22: 4656-4665.

[49] Choquet, D., and Trille, A. 2003. *Nat. Rev. Neurosci.* 4: 251-265.

[50] Nicoll, R. A., Tomita, S., and Bredt, D. S. 2006. *Science* 311: 1253-1256.

[51] Papardia, S., and Hardingham, G. E. 2007. *Neuroscientist* 13: 572-579.

[52] Howe, W. M., and Kenny, P. J. 2018. *Nature*, 554: 304-305.

[53] Niswender, C., and Conn, P. J. 2010. *Ann. Rev. Pharmacol. Toxicol.* 50: 295-322.

[54] Aiba, A. et al. 1994. *Cell* 79: 365-375.

[55] Bird, M. K., and Lawrence, A. J. 2009. *Trends Pharmacol. Sci.* 30: 617-623.

(though not solely) represented in presynaptic glutamatergic fiber terminals. There, they couple to the G protein G_o, thus inhibiting the Ca_V2 Ca^{2+} channels, and reducing transmitter release. In this way they mediate a negative feedback control of glutamate release, much like the feedback inhibition of GABA release by presynaptic $GABA_B$ receptors (see Figure 11.18). When present postsynaptically, the mGluR2, 3, and 4 receptors activate inwardly rectifying potassium channels, hyperpolarizing the neuron—the opposite effect to that of stimulating mGluR1 or 5 receptors. The mGluR6 receptor hyperpolarizes retinal bipolar cells in a different way: It stimulates cGMP phosphodiesterase, producing a fall in cGMP and closure of cyclic nucleotide-gated cation channels (see Chapter 22).

GABA (γ-Aminobutyric Acid) and Glycine

GABA and glycine are the two main inhibitory neurotransmitters in the CNS. They activate chloride-conducting ionotropic GABA or glycine receptors (see Chapter 5) to produce an inhibitory postsynaptic potential (IPSP) in the postsynaptic neuron (see Chapter 11). The increase in chloride conductance tends to inhibit the generation of action potentials by the excitatory postsynaptic potentials (EPSPs). GABA is the predominant inhibitory transmitter released by neurons in the cortex and midbrain, whereas glycine plays a prominent role in the brainstem and spinal cord. Some neurons have receptors for both transmitters, which act on separate and distinguishable chloride channels,[56] and both transmitters can sometimes be released from the same neuron.[57]

GABA and glycine are concentrated in interneurons. Their primary function is to control the output of the principal excitatory neurons by negative feedback through recurrent inhibitory collaterals from the axons of these neurons. This prevents excessive excitatory discharges from the principal neurons. One example (already mentioned) is the negative feedback inhibition of motoneuron discharges by recurrent axons that innervate glycinergic interneurons (Renshaw cells) in the spinal cord.[3] The importance of inhibitory interneurons in the brain is illustrated by the fact that blocking the inhibitory GABA or glycine receptors (with bicuculline or strychnine, respectively) produces convulsions. However, inhibitory interneurons in the cortex also have more subtle functions. Because each interneuron innervates several principal neurons, they serve to coordinate the output of the principal neurons and to synchronize activity within networks of neurons.[58–60] In addition to receiving recurrent collaterals from principal neuron axons, these GABAergic interneurons also receive a direct input from collaterals of the afferent fibers to principal neurons, producing what is termed feedforward inhibition.[61] This helps set the timing of principal neurons' responses to afferent stimuli.[62]

RECEPTORS FOR GABA AND GLYCINE   Ionotropic $GABA_A$ and glycine receptors are pentameric (five-subunit) receptors homologous with nicotinic ACh receptors but with the difference that their structure favors permeation of the anion chloride instead of cations (see Chapter 5). The glycine receptor is made up of two α-subunits and three β-subunits, arranged as a ring in the order α-β-β-α-β, with four binding sites for glycine at the α–β interfaces.[63] Three genetic variants of the α-subunit are known ($α_1$–$α_3$), but only one form of the β-subunit ($β_1$). Sivilotti eloquently discusses the mechanism whereby glycine opens these channels, as deduced from single-channel analysis.[64]

The GABA receptor has a more complex structure and repertoire of subunits. There are 19 different subunits: 6 α-subunits, 3 β and 3 γ, one each of δ, ε, π, and θ, and three variants of a special ρ-subunit.[65] The most common combinations at inhibitory synapses are $α_1β_2γ_2$ (60%), $α_2β_3γ_2$ (15%–20%), and $α_3β_nγ_2$ (10%–15%).[66] Because different combinations differ in rates of activation, deactivation, and desensitization, their expression is tuned to the optimum requirements for inhibition at different synapses.[67] GABA receptors containing the δ-subunit are particularly interesting because they do not desensitize and are activated by unusually low (sub-micromolar) concentrations of GABA.[67] These δ-subunits, along with $α_6$-subunits, are present in receptors on cerebellar and hippocampal dentate gyrus granule cells. They are tonically activated by resting interstitial GABA concentrations (estimated at 300–600 nanomolar [nM]) and so produce a steady component of resting membrane current.[68] The ρ-subunits, assembled as a homomeric pentamer, make up another unique type of $GABA_A$ receptor present in the retina.

[56] Gold, M. R., and Martin, A. R. 1984. *Nature* 308: 639-641.

[57] Jonas, P., Bischofberger, J., and Sandkühler, J. 1998. *Science* 281: 419-424.

[58] Cobb, S. R. et al. 1995. *Nature* 378: 75-78.

[59] Whittington, M. A., and Traub, R. D. 2003. *Trends Neurosci.* 26: 676-682.

[60] Klausberger, T., and Somogyi, P. 2008. *Science* 321: 53-57.

[61] Buszaki, G. 1984. *Prog. Neurobiol.* 22: 131-153.

[62] Pouille, F., and Scanziani, M. 2001. *Science* 293: 1159-1163.

[63] Betz, H., and Laube, B. 2006. *J. Neurochem.* 97: 1600-1610.

[64] Sivilotti, L. 2010. *J. Physiol.* 588: 45-58.

[65] Olsen, R. W., and Sieghart, W. 2008. *Pharmacol. Rev.* 60: 243-260.

[66] Möhler, H. 2006. *Cell Tissue Res.* 326: 505-516.

[67] Brown, N. et al. 2002. *Brit. J. Pharmacol.* 136: 965-974.

[68] Farrant, M., and Nusser, Z. 2005. *Nat. Rev. Neurosci.* 6: 215-229.

The GABA$_A$ receptor is also the prime target for several important drugs that act allosterically to enhance GABA-mediated currents and IPSPs. These include benzodiazepine compounds, barbiturates, and certain anesthetics such as propofol, etomidate, and the steroid anesthetic alphaxalone.[67,69] These three groups of drugs bind at different sites on the receptor and have different actions. For example, barbiturates [70,71] and alphaxalone[72] prolong the postsynaptic current, by slowing the closure of the channels,[73] whereas benzodiazepines increase the sensitivity of the channels to GABA (by slowing dissociation) without changing open time.[74] Enhancement of GABA$_A$ receptor currents is also responsible for some of the effects of ethanol,[75,76] which is why one should not mix alcohol with benzodiazepines. Naturally occurring regulators of GABA$_A$ receptor activity in the brain include endogenous neurosteroids[77,78] and zinc ions.[79] Recent structural analysis has revealed distinct binding sites for facilitatory and inhibitory neurosteroids at the GABA$_A$ α-subunit.[80]

GABA$_B$ RECEPTORS   Like glutamate, GABA can also activate a G protein-coupled receptor. This is termed the GABA$_B$ receptor. It was discovered by Norman Bowery and his colleagues in 1980.[81] They found that GABA reduced the release of transmitters from peripheral and central neurons by activating a receptor that was not antagonized by GABA$_A$ receptor antagonists but could be selectively activated by the GABA analogue baclofen (β-chlorophenyl-GABA). They subsequently identified it as a G protein-coupled receptor because (among other properties) its action was suppressed by pertussis toxin. In fact, it turned out to be a very unusual receptor because the active receptor is a dimer of two closely similar receptors termed GABA$_{B1}$ and GABA$_{B2}$, conjoined through their intracellular C termini[82,83] (Figure 14.5). The B1-subunit has the binding site for GABA, whereas the B2-subunit is necessary to activate the G protein. Hence, both subunits have to be expressed and assembled to make a functional receptor.[84]

GABA$_B$ receptors are located both postsynaptically and presynaptically, and have different effects at the two sites.[85] Activation of *postsynaptic* receptors opens inwardly

[69] Franks, N. P. 2008. *Nat. Rev. Neurosci.* 9: 370–386.

[70] Nicoll, R. A. et al. 1975. *Nature* 258: 625–627.

[71] Scholfield, C. N. 1978. *J. Physiol.* 275: 559–566.

[72] Scholfield, C. N. 1980. *Pflügers Arch.* 383: 249–255.

[73] Steinbach, J. H., and Akk, G. 2001. *J. Physiol.* 537: 715–733.

[74] Bianchi, M. T. et al. 2009. *Epilepsy Res.* 85: 212–220.

[75] Wallner, M., Hanchar, H. J., and Olsen, R. W. 2003. *Proc. Natl. Acad. Sci. USA* 100: 15218–15223.

[76] Kumar, S. et al. 2009. *Psychopharmacology (Berl.)* 205: 529–564.

[77] Hosie, A. M. et al. 2006. *Nature* 444: 486–489.

[78] Mitchell, E. A. et al. 2008. *Neurochem. Int.* 52: 588–595.

[79] Smart, T. G., Hosie, A. M., and Miller, P. 2004. *Neuroscientist* 10: 432–442.

[80] Laverty, D. et al. 2017. *Nat. Struct. Biol.* 24: 977–984.

[81] Bowery, N. G. et al. 1980. *Nature* 283: 92–94.

[82] Couve, A., Moss, S. J., and Pangalos, M. N. 2000. *Mol. Cell. Neurosci.* 16: 296–312.

[83] Bettler, B. et al. 2004. *Physiol. Rev.* 84: 835–867.

[84] Filippov, A. K. et al. 2000. *J. Neurosci.* 20: 2867–2874.

[85] Nicoll, R. A. 2004. *Biochem. Pharmacol.* 68: 1667–1674.

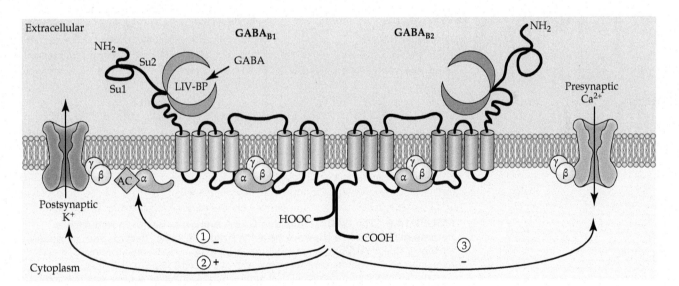

FIGURE 14.5   Schematic Diagram of the GABA$_B$ Receptor Dimer. The functional receptor is a dimer composed of GABA$_{B1}$ and GABA$_{B2}$ monomers joined through a coiled-coil domain at their C termini. Su1 and Su2 are Sushi domains. GABA binds to a part of the extracellular domain of the B1 monomer at a region homologous with the bacterial periplasmic leucine-isoleucine-valine binding protein (LIV-BP). The B2 monomer responds by activating the G proteins G$_i$ and G$_o$. The α, β and γ subunits of the G protein attached to the receptor subunits are labelled. The α-subunit of G$_i$ inhibits adenylate cyclase (pathway 1), while the βγ-subunit activates the postsynaptic G protein-gated inwardly rectifying channel (pathway 2). The βγ-subunit of G$_o$ also inhibits the Ca$_V$2 class of calcium channels in the presynaptic terminals (pathway 3). (After A. Couve et al., 2000. *Mol. Cell. Neuroscience* 16: 296–312.)

[86] Gähwiler, B. H., and Brown, D. A. 1985. *Proc. Natl. Acad. Sci. USA* 82: 1558–1562.

[87] Scanziani, M. 2000. *Neuron* 25: 673–681.

[88] Takahashi, T., Kajikawa, Y., and Tsujimoto, T. 1998. *J. Neurosci.* 18: 3138–3146.

[89] Wu, L. G., and Saggau, P. 1997. *Trends Neurosci.* 20: 204–212.

[90] Blackmer, T. et al. 2005. *Nat. Neurosci.* 8: 421–425.

[91] Woolf, N. J. 1991. *Prog. Neurobiol.* 37: 475–524.

rectifying G protein-gated potassium channels[86] (Figure 14.6), which produces a membrane hyperpolarization and delayed postsynaptic inhibition.[86] These postsynaptic $GABA_B$ receptors are located around the periphery of the synapse (perisynaptically) and do not readily respond to GABA released by a single afferent stimulus; instead, they are activated by spillover GABA escaping from the synapse during repetitive stimulation or following simultaneous activation of several GABAergic inputs.[87]

Presynaptic $GABA_B$ receptors inhibit voltage-gated calcium channels in the nerve terminal and thereby reduce transmitter release. When GABA is released, it may act on receptors on its own terminal (autoinhibition; see Figure 11.18) or on adjacent terminals that release GABA or another transmitter (i.e., heterosynaptic inhibition). Inhibition of the presynaptic calcium current and its consequent effect on transmitter release are illustrated in the experiment on calyx of Held terminals shown in Figure 14.7A. These terminals, located in the medial nucleus of the trapezoid body, are large enough to be patch clamped.[88] When the presynaptic terminal was depolarized by injecting current through the patch electrode, application of baclofen reduced both the resulting inward calcium current and the EPSP (Figure 14.7B). The reduced EPSP could be explained solely by the reduced calcium current since the relationship between inward current and EPSP amplitude was unaltered (Figure 14.7C). However, at some other synapses there may be an additional effect of the $GABA_B$-released G protein βγ-subunit on the transmitter release mechanism itself.[89,90]

Acetylcholine

Cholinergic neurons are present throughout the brainstem, midbrain, and telencephalon and provide a widespread innervation to diverse areas of the brain.[91] An important source of cholinergic axons to the cerebral cortex and hippocampus is provided by groups of neurons in

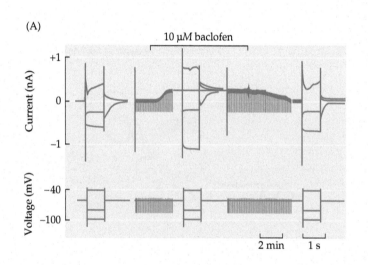

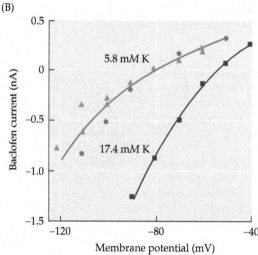

FIGURE 14.6 The GABA_B-Selective GABA Analogue Baclofen Activates a Potassium Current in a Hippocampal Pyramidal Neuron. Records from an experiment on a slice of rat hippocampus cultured in vitro for 3 weeks. (A) A continuous record of membrane current recorded at -61 mV, with one-second steps to -81 mV applied every 5 seconds (downward deflections). Just before, during, and after application of baclofen, three voltage steps, to -41, -81, and -101 mV, were applied and the currents recorded at a faster speed. Baclofen produced an outward current at -61 mV and increased the membrane conductance as shown by the increased response to the voltage steps. (B) The extra current produced by baclofen (after subtracting the resting current) recorded from this cell in 5.8- and 17.4-mM external [K⁺]. The currents were measured at the end of 1-second steps from -61 mV to the voltages shown. The current reversal potential (i.e., the potential at which the current-voltage curve crossed the zero-current line) shifted +26 mV on increasing [K⁺] threefold, which is near that (+29 mV) expected for a K⁺ current (see Chapters 6 and 11). Note that the curve shows inward rectification—that is, the current is larger at potentials negative to the reversal potential (when the direction of net K⁺ flow is into the cell) than at potentials more positive to the reversal potential, when it is outward. (After B. H. Gähwiler and D. A. Brown, 1985. *Proc. Natl. Acad. Sci. USA* 82: 1558–1562.)

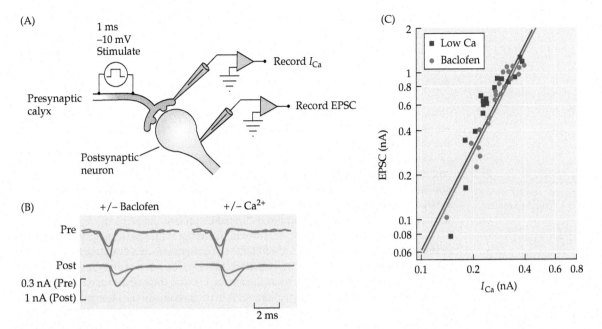

(A)

1 ms
–10 mV
Stimulate

Record I_{Ca}

Record EPSC

Presynaptic
calyx

Postsynaptic
neuron

(B)

+/– Baclofen   +/– Ca^{2+}

Pre

Post

0.3 nA (Pre)
1 nA (Post)

2 ms

(C)

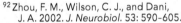

FIGURE 14.7   Presynaptic GABA$_B$ Receptors Reduce Transmitter Release by reducing terminal Ca^{2+} current. (A) The experiments were performed by simultaneously recording from the presynaptic calyx of Held in the medial nucleus of the trapezoid body and the innervated postsynaptic neuron. A 1-ms step from –70 mV to –10 mV was delivered to the calyx, and the resultant presynaptic Ca^{2+} current (I_{Ca}) and glutamatergic excitatory postsynaptic current (EPSC) were recorded. (B) Both presynaptic I_{Ca} (Pre) and postsynaptic EPSC (Post) were reduced by the GABA$_B$ receptor stimulant, baclofen (20 M), or by reducing external Ca^{2+} (replaced with Mg^{2+}). (C) EPSC amplitude plotted against presynaptic I_{Ca} in the presence of different concentrations of baclofen or Ca^{2+}. Note that baclofen did not alter the relation between Ca^{2+} current and transmitter release as measured by the EPSC, implying that its effect on transmitter release at this terminal can be explained wholly by the inhibition of the Ca^{2+} current. (After T. Takahashi et al., 1998. *J. Neurosci.* 18: 3138-3146. © 1998 Society for Neuroscience.)

the nucleus basalis and nuclei of the medial septum of the basal forebrain (Figure 14.8). Neurons in the tegmental area provide a second source of cholinergic axons to the thalamus and midbrain dopaminergic areas. These projections are broad and diffuse, and are composed of unmyelinated fibers. A third, more clearly defined tract, composed of myelinated fibers, is the habenulo–interpeduncular tract from the medial habenular nucleus to the interpeduncular nucleus. A fourth important group is formed by cholinergic interneurons in the striatum, which provide a substantial innervation within the striatum and in the olfactory tubercle.[92]

One important difference between the central and peripheral cholinergic systems concerns the sites at which ACh is released from the cholinergic fibers. Thus, while some of the cholinergic axons to the cortex end at morphologically defined synapses onto pyramidal cell dendrites,[93] akin to those described in Chapter 11, most release sites in the cortex consist of swellings (or varicosities) along the axons that do not make direct contact with the postsynaptic neuron.[94] Therefore, release is extrasynaptic (see Chapter 18). Localized release of ACh from these varicosities has been recorded in tissue culture.[95] The release process is as rapid as at true synapses but may

[92] Zhou, F. M., Wilson, C. J., and Dani, J. A. 2002. *J. Neurobiol.* 53: 590–605.

[93] Turrini, P. et al. 2001. *Neuroscience* 105: 277–285.

[94] Umbriaco, D. et al. 1994. *J. Comp. Neurol.* 348: 351–373.

[95] Allen, T. G., and Brown, D. A. 1996. *J. Physiol.* 492: 453–466.

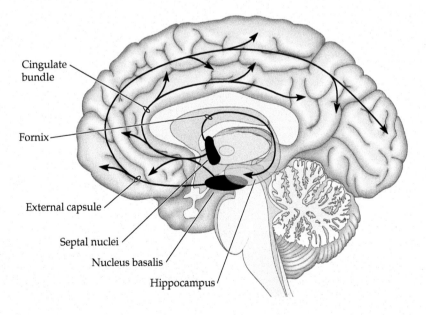

Cingulate
bundle

Fornix

External capsule

Septal nuclei

Nucleus basalis

Hippocampus

FIGURE 14.8   Cholinergic Innervation of the Cerebral Cortex and Hippocampus by neurons in the nuclei of the medial septum (the septal nuclei) and nucleus basalis.

occur some distance from the target receptors, so ACh acts diffusely, rather like a local hormone.[96] This action is also true for most of the other transmitters described in the rest of this chapter and is sometimes referred to as volume transmission[97] or (less flatteringly) the soup theory of transmission.[98] Once released, the ACh can then act on both ionotropic nicotinic and G protein-coupled muscarinic receptors.

NICOTINIC RECEPTORS AND THEIR FUNCTIONS   Neuronal nicotinic receptors[99,100] are structurally homologous with those at the neuromuscular synapse, but the pentamer is made up of only two types of subunits, α and β. There are nine neuronal α-subunits (2–10) and three β-subunits (2–4). The different combinations vary in sensitivity to ACh and in their rates of desensitization.[101] The main types in the brain are $\alpha_4\beta_2$-heteromers and homomers of α_7, but there are many others, with varying α:β stoichiometries.[102] The α_7-channels are important because they have a high permeability to Ca^{2+} ions; they are also the only neuronal channels blocked by α-bungarotoxin (see Chapter 11).

Although there are a few synapses where the receptors are in the postsynaptic membrane and generate a true EPSP (including the spinal Renshaw cells discussed earlier), these are exceptional: The vast majority of the receptors are on presynaptic axons and terminals.[101,102] Here they serve to increase the release of other transmitters such as glutamate. This effect has been clearly shown at synapses between fibers in the interpeduncular tract and neurons in the interpeduncular nucleus (Figure 14.9).[103] At this synapse, synaptic transmission is mediated by glutamate,[104] even though the fibers themselves contain ACh. Nicotine increases both the glutamatergic EPSC following afferent stimulation and the frequency of spontaneous EPSCs. These effects are due to an increase in Ca^{2+} entry into the interpeduncular fibers. They are blocked by α-bungarotoxin, indicating that the Ca^{2+} entry is mediated by α_7-nicotinic receptors.

Nicotinic ACh receptors were so called because they are activated by nicotine. The question then arises: Do the effects of inhaling nicotine result from activating these presynaptic nicotinic receptors? The answer seems to be yes. Thus, nicotine increases glutamate release from excitatory afferent fibers innervating dopaminergic neurons in the ventral tegmental area.[105] This causes a persistent increase in the activity of these neurons and increased release of dopamine from their terminals in the nucleus accumbens and prefrontal cortex; this release of dopamine is thought to be responsible for the pleasurable (rewarding) aspect of nicotine's action[106] (see the section "Dopamine"). The $\alpha_4\beta_2$-containing nicotinic receptors are particularly involved in some of the effects of nicotine,[107] and a partial agonist of these receptors, varenicline,[108] is used to treat nicotine addiction.

[96] Descarries, L., Gisiger, V., and Steriade, M. 1997. *Prog. Neurobiol.* 53: 603-625.

[97] Lendvai, B., and Vizi, E. S. 2008. *Physiol. Rev.* 88: 333-349.

[98] Sivilotti, L., and Colquhoun, D. 1995. *Science* 269: 1681-1682.

[99] Sargent, P. B. 1993. *Annu. Rev. Neurosci.* 16: 403-443.

[100] Dani, J. A., and Bertrand, D. 2007. *Annu. Rev. Pharmacol. Toxicol.* 47: 699-729.

[101] Role, L. W., and Berg, D. K. 1996. *Neuron* 16: 1077-1085.

[102] Millar, N. S., and Gotti, C. 2009. *Neuropharmacology* 56: 237-246.

[103] McGehee, D. S. et al. 1995. *Science* 269: 1692-1696.

[104] Brown, D. A., Docherty, R. J., and Halliwell, J. V. 1983. *J. Physiol.* 341: 655-670.

[105] Mansvelder, H. D., Keath, J. R., and McGehee, D. S. 2002. *Neuron* 33: 905-919.

[106] Livingstone, P. D., and Wonnacott, S. 2009. *Biochem. Pharmacol.* 78: 744-755.

[107] Xiao, C. et al. 2009. *J. Neurosci.* 29: 12428-12439.

[108] Rollema, H. et al. 2007. *Trends Pharmacol. Sci.* 28: 316-325.

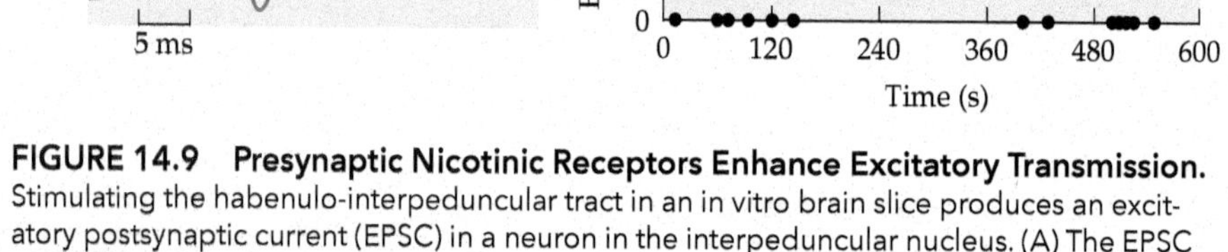

(A)   (B)

FIGURE 14.9   **Presynaptic Nicotinic Receptors Enhance Excitatory Transmission.** Stimulating the habenulo-interpeduncular tract in an in vitro brain slice produces an excitatory postsynaptic current (EPSC) in a neuron in the interpeduncular nucleus. (A) The EPSC results from the release of glutamate, since it is suppressed by a glutamate antagonist (CNQX). Nicotine (100 nM) increases the amplitude of the EPSC. (B) Other tests show that this effect is due to enhanced release of glutamate, resulting from the entry of Ca^{2+} ions through activated presynaptic α_7-containing nicotinic receptors and consequent rise in the intracellular Ca^{2+} concentration. (After D. S. McGehee et al., 1995. *Science* 269: 1692-1696.)

MUSCARINIC RECEPTORS AND THEIR EFFECTS   Most of the effects of ACh released from the cholinergic nerves to the cerebral cortex and hippocampus, as depicted in Figure 14.8, are mediated by muscarinic receptors.[109] There are five subtypes of this receptor, M1–5. The odd-numbered ones (mainly M1 and M3) link to the G protein G_q; their immediate effect is to stimulate hydrolysis of the membrane phospholipid phosphatidylinositol-4,5-bisphosphate (PIP_2). They are predominantly postsynaptic, and their principal effect is to produce a form of postsynaptic excitation. The receptors are not actually located within the subsynaptic membrane itself but just outside the synapse,[110] and they respond to diffusely released ACh, as we discussed earlier. The even-numbered receptors (M2 and M4) link to the G proteins G_o and G_i. They are primarily presynaptic where they inhibit transmitter release, but some are postsynaptic and cause a form of postsynaptic inhibition.

- *Postsynaptic excitation*   A characteristic form of muscarinic excitation is that seen in hippocampal pyramidal neurons after stimulating cholinergic afferents from the medial septum (Figure 14.10). This consists of a slow depolarization and enhanced action potential discharges.[111] It results from the inhibition of two types of K+ channels: (1) a calcium-activated K+ channel that normally generates a long-lasting ("slow") afterhyperpolarization following an action potential[112] and (2) the M-channel[113,114] (see Figures 12.16 and 19.3). Inhibition of the slow afterhyperpolarization increases the frequency and duration of action potential discharges; inhibition of the M-channel causes depolarization and enhances excitability by lowering the threshold for action potential generation in the axon initial segment.[115,116] Similar effects are seen in cerebral cortical pyramidal neurons[117,118] (innervated from the basal forebrain); inhibition of the M-current also accounts for the cholinergic excitation of medium spiny neurons in the striatum.[119] Cholinergic afferents also excite inhibitory interneurons in the hippocampus and cortex that indirectly inhibit the principal neurons. This has a strong influence on cortical network behavior.[120]

[109] Brown, D. A. 2010. *J. Mol. Neurosci.* 41: 340–346.

[110] Yamasaki, M., Matsui, M., and Watanabe, M. 2010. *J. Neurosci.* 30: 4408–4418.

[111] Cole, A. E., and Nicoll, R. A. 1984. *J. Physiol.* 352: 173–188.

[112] Madison, D. V., Lancaster, B., and Nicoll, R. A. 1987. *J. Neurosci.* 7: 733–741.

[113] Halliwell, J. V., and Adams, P. R. 1982. *Brain Res.* 250: 71–92.

[114] Gähwiler, B. H., and Brown, D. A. 1985. *Nature* 313: 577–579.

[115] Shah, M. M. et al. 2008. *Proc. Natl. Acad. Sci. USA* 105: 7869–7874.

[116] Martinello, K. et al. 2015. *Neuron* 85: 346–363.

[117] McCormick, D. A., and Williamson, A. 1989. *Proc. Natl. Acad. Sci. USA* 86: 8098–8102.

[118] Benardo, L. S. 1993. *Neuroscience* 53: 11–22.

[119] Shen, W. et al. 2005. *J. Neurosci.* 25: 7449–7458.

[120] Lawrence, J. J. 2008. *Trends Neurosci.* 31: 317–327.

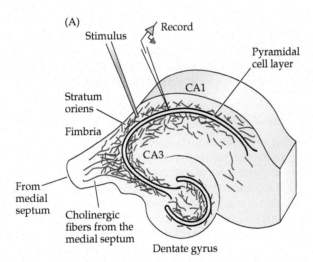

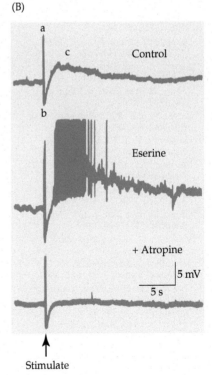

FIGURE 14.10   Stimulation of Cholinergic Fibers from the Medial Septum Excites Hippocampal Pyramidal Cells. (A) Drawing of a transverse hippocampal slice. Cholinergic fibers from the medial septum enter the slice through the fimbria and course through the stratum oriens. A stimulating electrode is placed in the stratum oriens, and an intracellular pipette is used to record from a neuron in the pyramidal cell layer. (B) Stratum oriens stimulation for 5 seconds at 20 Hz produces: (a) summed fast excitatory postsynaptic potentials due to glutamate release (probably from the cholinergic fibers); (b) summed inhibitory synaptic potentials due to GABA release from interneurons; and (c) a slow excitatory postsynaptic potential. The last is enhanced by the anticholinesterase eserine (physostigmine) and suppressed by the muscarinic receptor antagonist atropine. This effect of atropine shows that the slow excitatory postsynaptic potential results from activation of muscarinic acetylcholine receptors. (A after R. A. Nicoll, 1985. *Trends Neurosci.* 8: 533–536; B after A. E. Cole and R. A. Nicoll, 1984. *J. Physiol.* 352: 173–188.)

- *Postsynaptic inhibition* Activation of muscarinic receptors directly inhibits some cortical neurons. There are two ways in which this can happen. First, in some cortical pyramidal cells, activation of postsynaptic M1 receptors can produce inhibition, probably by releasing Ca^{2+} from intracellular stores, which in turn activates calcium-dependent K^+ channels.[121] Second, a minority of neurons have postsynaptic G_i-coupled M2 or M4 receptors that hyperpolarize neurons by activating inwardly rectifying (K_{ir}) K^+ channels[122] (see Figure 12.7).

- *Presynaptic inhibition* The release of ACh from cholinergic fibers is subject to profound feedback inhibition by presynaptically located M2 and M4 receptors. Dudar and Szerb[123] first noted this phenomenon in 1969 when they were measuring the release of ACh from the surface of the cat cerebral cortex following activation of the ascending reticular formation. They found that the amount of ACh collected was increased threefold when the muscarinic antagonist atropine was added to the collecting cup (Figure 14.11A). The mechanism responsible for this effect cannot be easily studied in the brain itself but has been explored in tissue-cultured cholinergic basal forebrain neurons, where the release of ACh from individual varicosities along their axons can be recorded with a nicotinic receptor detector patch (Figure 14.11B). The muscarinic agonist muscarine dramatically reduces this release.[96] This effect is due to the activation of M4 receptors and probably results from the inhibition of the axonal calcium current by the activated G protein.[124] These presynaptic M2 and M4 receptors are widely distributed in the nervous system. For example, they inhibit ACh release from cholinergic nerve endings in the hippocampus and striatum.[125]

OVERALL CONTRIBUTIONS TO BRAIN FUNCTION The ascending cholinergic system to the cortex and hippocampus plays a crucial role in attention[126] and memory.[127] In the cortex, ACh focuses attention to sensory information by selectively augmenting the responses of cortical neurons to a specific stimulus without increasing their background activity.[128–130] Importantly, degeneration of the basal forebrain cholinergic neurons and of their cortical and hippocampal terminals is the earliest and most profound neurodegenerative change seen in Alzheimer's disease, and it makes a major contribution to the cognitive deficits that occur in this condition.[131,132] The cholinergic interneurons in the basal ganglia have a different role in regulating motor output. Thus, muscarinic receptor antagonists were once used to reduce the tremor in Parkinson's disease before being replaced by more effective dopaminergic agonists (see the section "Dopamine").

Biogenic Amines

Biogenic amines include norepinephrine, 5-HT, dopamine, and histamine. They are notable for the fact that they are restricted to a very few neurons contained in discrete loci. However, from these nuclei, ramifying unmyelinated axons project to innervate large areas of the brain, through which they influence many states of brain function such as attention, arousal, sleep, and mood. In most cases, these axons do not terminate at discrete synapses (see Chapter 18); instead, like ACh, the transmitters are released from the somata, dendrites, and varicosities along the course of the axons and act in a diffuse manner called volume transmission.[133] These actions correlate with the fact that, with the one exception of 5-HT, their target receptors are all indirect G protein-coupled receptors that are adapted to respond to relatively low concentrations of transmitter on a slow timescale (see Chapter 12). Furthermore, there are often many subtypes of receptors for each amine capable of affecting several different ion channels, so their effects on neuronal activity can be complex and varied.

NOREPINEPHRINE The noradrenergic neurons are concentrated in a nucleus in the dorsal part of the pons called the **locus coeruleus** (or blue spot, the blue being from melanin).[134–136] In the rat, each locus (either side of the midline) contains only about 1500 neurons (in humans, about 12,000); however, the axons of these neurons innervate wide areas of the CNS, including large parts of the cerebral cortex (via the medial forebrain bundle), hippocampus, hypothalamus, and amygdala, and they even run down the spinal cord[137] (Figure 14.12).

[121] Gulledge, A. T. et al. 2009. *J. Neurosci.* 29: 9888-9902.

[122] Eggermann, E., and Feldmeyer, D. 2009. *Proc. Natl. Acad. Sci. USA* 106: 11753-11758.

[123] Dudar, J. D., and Szerb, J. C. 1969. *J. Physiol.* 203: 741-762.

[124] Allen, T. G., and Brown, D. A. 1993. *J. Physiol.* 466: 173-189.

[125] Zhang, W. et al. 2002. *J. Neurosci.* 22: 1709-1717.

[126] Sarter, M. et al. 2005. *Brain Res. Brain Res. Rev.* 48: 98-111.

[127] Hasselmo, M. E. 2006. *Curr. Opin. Neurobiol.* 16: 710-715.

[128] Murphy, P. C., and Sillitoe, A. M. 1991. *Neuroscience* 40: 13-20.

[129] Herrero, J. L. et al. 2008. *Nature* 454: 1110-1114.

[130] Goard, M., and Dan, Y. 2009. *Nat. Neurosci.* 12: 1444-1449.

[131] Mesulam, M. 2004. *Learn. Mem.* 11: 43-49.

[132] Schliebs, R., and Arendt, T. 2006. *J. Neural Transm.* 113: 1625-1644.

[133] Fuxe, K. et al. 2010. *Prog. Neurobiol.* 90: 82-100.

[134] Dahlstrom, A., and Fuxe, K. 1964. *Acta Physiol. Scand. Suppl.* 232: 1-55.

[135] Foote, S. L, Bloom, F. E., and Aston-Jones, G. 1983. *Physiol. Rev.* 63: 844-914.

[136] Berridge, C. W., and Waterhouse, B. D. 2003. *Brain Res. Brain Res. Rev.* 42: 33-84.

[137] Ungerstedt, U. 1971. *Acta Physiol. Scand. Suppl.* 367: 1-49.

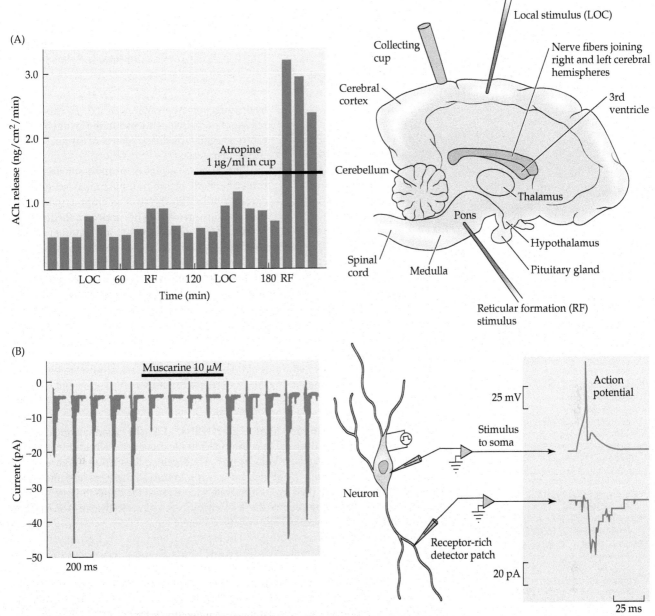

FIGURE 14.11 Muscarinic Autoreceptors Inhibit Acetylcholine Release from Cholinergic Forebrain Afferents. (A) Acetylcholine (ACh) released from the surface of the parietal cortex of an anesthetized cat was collected into a cortical cup every 10 minutes and subsequently assayed. Local stimulation (LOC) of cholinergic afferent fibers and stimulation of midbrain reticular formation (RF) are shown. The muscarinic receptor antagonist, atropine (1 μg/ml), added to the cup enhanced evoked release. (B) Currents recorded from a nicotinic receptor detector patch placed adjacent to an ACh release site on a neurite from a tissue-cultured basal forebrain neuron. The neuron was stimulated to give an action potential once per minute, which traveled down the neurite. The ACh released following each action potential triggered a burst of nicotinic channel openings in the detector patch. Muscarine (10 μM) strongly reduced the amount of ACh released. (A after J. D. Dudar and J. C. Szerb, 1969. *J. Physiol.* 203: 741–762; B after T. G. Allen and D. A. Brown, 1996. *J. Physiol.* 492: 453–466.)

The locus coeruleus neurons fire spontaneously both in vivo and in vitro at a steady low rate, which can then be modified by the release of glutamate, GABA, enkephalins, and other transmitters from their afferent inputs.[136,138] Their firing rate can also be inhibited by norepinephrine, through α_2-adrenoceptors; these hyperpolarize the neuron

[138] Williams, J. T. et al. 1984. *Neuroscience* 13: 137–156.

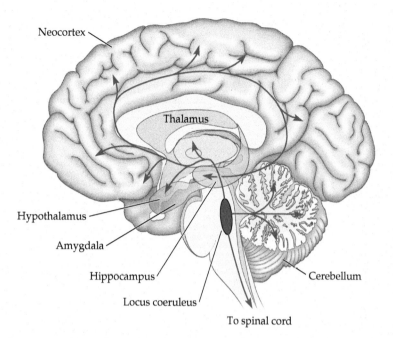

Neocortex

Thalamus

Hypothalamus

Amygdala

Hippocampus

Locus coeruleus

To spinal cord

Cerebellum

FIGURE 14.12 Projections of Norepinephrine-Containing Neurons in the Locus Coeruleus. The locus coeruleus lies in the pons just beneath the floor of the fourth ventricle. Neurons projecting from it innervate widespread regions of the brain and spinal cord.

by opening potassium channels.[139,140] By this means, release of norepinephrine within the locus coeruleus exerts a negative feedback control of the neurons' intrinsic firing rate.[141]

The primary effect of norepinephrine on its target neurons in the hippocampus and cerebral cortex is to inhibit the slow calcium-activated potassium current.[136,142] This action is mediated by β_2-adrenoceptors and involves activation of adenylate cyclase.[143] Its effect is to increase the firing rate of the neuron. Norepinephrine also hyperpolarizes the target neurons by activating α_2-receptors, as it does to the locus coeruleus neurons. The hyperpolarization reduces background activity, while the potassium current inhibition facilitates responses to strong afferent stimulation. These actions enable afferents from the locus coeruleus to augment and sharpen the response of cortical pyramidal cells to the sensory stimulus of interest without increasing noise, as illustrated in Figure 14.13. By such means, the locus coeruleus can increase attention and facilitate learning and memory.[144]

5-HYDROXYTRYPTAMINE (5-HT OR SEROTONIN)
Like the noradrenergic neurons, serotonergic neurons are localized to a few nuclei in the brainstem. These are the **raphe nuclei** that lie directly along the midline from the midbrain to the medulla (Figure 14.14). (The term *raphe* comes from the French for "seam"). In the rat, these nuclei contain only about 20,500 neurons, but their axons innervate wide areas of the brain and extend down the spinal cord.[145] The raphe neurons fire spontaneously at a slow, steady rate of around 1 to 3 Hz, but this rate can be modified by a variety of afferent inputs and is accelerated when an animal is awake or aroused and active.[146] The raphe neurons have 5-HT receptors and are subject to autoinhibition[147] by locally released 5-HT through activation of inwardly rectifying potassium channels.[148,149]

There are a remarkable number and variety of 5-HT receptors.[150,151] One of these, the 5-HT$_3$ receptor, is a ligand-gated cation channel, highly homologous with the nicotinic receptor[152] (so homologous, in fact, that it can actually form a functional chimeric channel with the nicotinic α_4-subunit[153]). These ionotropic 5-HT receptors are widely distributed in the brain both presynaptically and postsynaptically,[154] and also extrasynaptically (see Chapter 18). However, only a few true synaptic currents produced by serotonergic fiber stimulation have been reported, so presumably the receptors respond to diffusely released 5-HT.

All of the other 5-HT receptors are G protein-coupled, differentially activating G_o/G_i, G_q, or G_s proteins (see Chapter 12). These receptors are postsynaptic, presynaptic, and extrasynaptic, and some neurons express more than one type of receptor. Thus, the overall actions of 5-HT on individual neurons and synaptic pathways are complex and variable, and they cannot readily be extrapolated to effects on brain function.[152,153] The overall actions can be more readily deduced from the actions of drugs that mimic 5-HT, block its action on specific receptors, or block its reuptake, or from the effects of individual 5-HT receptor knockouts.[152] For example, projections to the hypothalamus help regulate the sleep–wake cycle[147] and food intake,[155] so that drugs that inhibit 5-HT uptake reduce food intake. These same drugs, which include fluoxetine (Prozac, Sarafem), are used as antidepressants, probably reflecting a general role for 5-HT in controlling affective states.[156] A more focused effect of descending serotonergic fibers is their role in reducing the release of transmitters from nociceptive spinal and trigeminal sensory afferents in the substantia gelatinosa.[157,158]

[139] Aghajanian, G. K., and VanderMaelen, C. P. 1982. *Science* 215: 1394-1396.

[140] Egan, T. M. et al. 1983. *J. Physiol.* 345: 477-488.

[141] Aghajanian, G. K., Cedarbaum, J. M., and Wang, R. Y. 1977. *Brain Res.* 136: 570-577.

[142] Madison, D. V., and Nicoll, R. A. 1986. *J. Physiol.* 372: 221-244.

[143] Madison, D.V., and Nicoll, R. A. 1986. *J. Physiol.* 372: 245-259.

[144] Sara, S. J. 2008. *Nat. Rev. Neurosci.* 10: 211-223.

[145] Jacobs, B. L., and Azmitia, E. C. 1992. *Physiol. Rev.* 72: 165-229.

[146] Vandermaelen, C. P., and Aghajanian, G. K. 1983. *Brain Res.* 289: 109-119.

[147] Piñeyro, G., and Blier, P. 1999. *Pharmacol. Rev.* 51: 533-591.

[148] Wang, R. Y., and Aghajanian, G. K. 1977. *Brain Res.* 132: 186-193.

[149] Penington, N. J., Kelly, J. S., and Fox, A. P. 1993. *J. Physiol.* 469: 387-405.

[150] Barnes, N. M., and Sharp, T. 1999. *Neuropharmacology* 38: 1083-1152.

[151] Filip, M., and Bader, M. 2009. *Pharmacol. Rev.* 61: 761-777.

[152] Barnes, N. M. et al. 2009. *Neuropharmacology* 56: 273-284.

[153] van Hooft, J. A. et al. 1998. *Proc. Natl. Acad. Sci. USA* 95: 11456-11461.

[154] Chameau, P., and van Hooft, J. A. 2006. *Cell Tissue Res.* 326: 573-581.

[155] Garfield, A. S., and Heisler, L. K. 2009. *J. Physiol.* 587: 49-60.

[156] Cowen, P. J. 2008. *Trends Pharmacol. Sci.* 29: 433-436.

[157] Jennings, E. A., Ryan, R. M., and Christie, M. J. 2004. *Pain* 111: 30-37.

[158] Yoshimura, M., and Furue, H. 2006. wJ. *Pharmacol. Sci.* 101: 107-117.

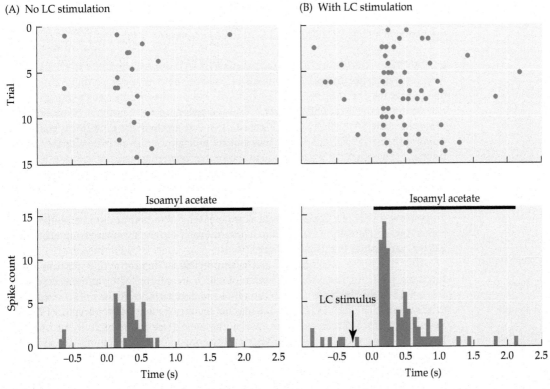

(A) No LC stimulation

(B) With LC stimulation

FIGURE 14.13 Locus Coeruleus Stimulation Sharpens and Enhances Sensory Processing in the Cerebral Cortex. Action potentials were recorded from a single neuron in the piriform cortex of an anesthetized rat for 1 second before and then during a 2-second olfactory stimulus with isoamyl acetate (black bars) applied 14 times (i.e., 14 trials). Each dot in the upper plots represents one action potential. The histograms show the numbers of action potentials recorded, grouped into 50-ms bins. (A) Without locus coeruleus (LC) stimulation. (B) Stimulation of locus coeruleus for 250 ms before the olfactory stimulus. Such stimulation increased the reliability of the response (there are fewer blank horizontal lines in the upper plot) and sharpened it, by increasing the clustering of the action potentials within the first few hundred milliseconds and reducing the jitter in the delay to the first action potential. (After S. J. Sara, 2008. *Nat. Rev. Neurosci.* 10: 211–223; S. Bouret and S. J. Sara, 2008. *Eur. J. Neurosci.* 16: 2371–2382.)

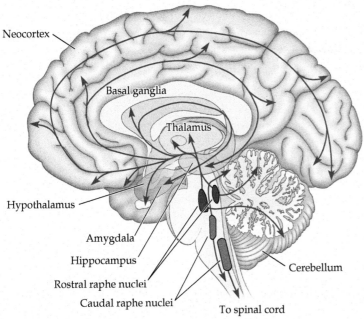

FIGURE 14.14 Neurons Containing 5-Hydroxy-tryptamine (5-HT) Form a Chain of Raphe Nuclei Lying along the Midline of the Brainstem. More caudal nuclei innervate the spinal cord, while more rostral nuclei innervate nearly all regions of the brain.

Thus, the drug sumatriptan, which selectively activates 5-HT$_{1D}$ receptors, can suppress the symptoms of migraine and trigeminal neuralgia. 5-HT also contributes to the expression of aggression in a range of animal species, including crustacea.[159]

DOPAMINE   Dopamine (3-hydroxytyramine) is an intermediary in the synthetic pathway to norepinephrine (see Appendix B). However, some important groups of neurons do not have the enzyme dopamine β-hydroxylase that converts dopamine to norepinephrine, so dopamine is the end product.[160] These **dopaminergic** neurons are concentrated in special nuclei in the brainstem (Figure 14.15). One group in the arcuate nucleus sends axons to the hypothalamus, where they control prolactin secretion from pituitary lactotrophs.[161] The other three groups are in the ventral tegmental area and substantia nigra (the latter so called because the neurons contain neuromelanin and stain black). Axons from these neurons project to the neostriatum in the basal ganglia, limbic structures such as the nucleus accumbens, and the prefrontal cortex. As with other catecholaminergic systems, a very few dopaminergic neurons reach out to many target cells—there are about 7000 neurons in the substantia nigra, but each neuron gives rise to an estimated 250,000 varicosities in the basal ganglia.[162]

Also, like other catecholamine-releasing neurons, dopaminergic neurons show spontaneous firing, the rate and rhythm of which are controlled by afferent inputs.[163] Dopamine release may occur from the soma and dendrites, and many of its effects are extrasynaptic. The released dopamine may act on one or more of five receptors (D1–5). Activating D1 or D5 receptors stimulates adenylate cyclase and phospholipase C, while D2, 3, and 4 receptors inhibit adenylate cyclase, open potassium channels, and inhibit calcium currents (see Chapter 12). Thus, the postsynaptic action of released dopamine varies with different target neurons and can be complex.[164] Nearly all dopaminergic neurons have autoreceptors, on both their terminals and soma–dendrite regions. These are mostly D2 receptors whose activation inhibits neuron firing (if on the soma or dendrites) or inhibits dopamine release (if at the terminals).

The physiological importance of the dopaminergic projection to the basal ganglia became apparent when it was discovered that it was much reduced in individuals with **Parkinson's disease** (a disease affecting motor control; see Chapter 26).[165] In Parkinson's disease there is a selective degeneration of the dopaminergic neurons in the substantia nigra, resulting in the loss of dopaminergic terminals in the striatum. This finding led to one of the most astonishing advances in medical treatment, namely that giving the precursor of

[159] Kravitz, E. A. 2000. *J. Comp. Physiol. A* 186: 221-238.

[160] Carlsson, A. et al. 1958. *Science* 127: 471.

[161] van den Pol, A. N. 2010. *Neuron* 65: 147-149.

[162] Yurek, D. M., and Sladek, J. R., Jr. 1990. *Annu. Rev. Neurosci.* 13: 415-440.

[163] Diana, M., and Tepper, J. M. 2002. In *Handbook of Experimental Pharmacology*, volume 154, part 1. Springer-Verlag, Berlin. pp. 1-62.

[164] Nicola, S. M., Surmeier, D. J., and Malenka, R. C. 2000. *Annu. Rev. Neurosci.* 23: 185-215.

[165] Ehringer, H., and Hornykiewicz, O. 1960. *Klin. Wochenschr.* 38: 1236-1239.

[166] Birkmayer, W., and Hornykiewicz, O. 1962. *Arch. Psychiatr. Nervenkr.* 203: 560-574.

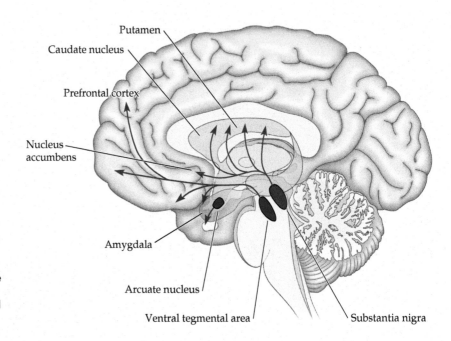

FIGURE 14.15   Neurons Containing Dopamine Are Found in Nuclei in the Hypothalamus and Midbrain. Those in the arcuate nucleus project to the median eminence of the hypothalamus, forming the tuberoinfundibular system. Dopamine neurons in the substantia nigra project to the caudate nucleus, putamen and nucleus accumbens (collectively called the striatum) of the basal ganglia, forming the nigrostriatal pathway. Dopamine neurons in the ventral tegmental area project to the nucleus accumbens, amygdala, and prefrontal cortex, forming the mesolimbic and mesocortical systems.

dopamine, L-dihydroxyphenylalanine (L-DOPA), increased the amount of dopamine in the residual terminals and dramatically reversed the motor deficits.[166,167]

Other dopaminergic projections serve different functions. The projection from the ventral tegmental area to the nucleus accumbens is a reward signaling system, with the neurons increasing their activity in anticipation of or in response to pleasurable events.[107,168] This area is the principal site of action of the addictive drug cocaine, which inhibits the dopamine transporter and increases the amount of dopamine released in the nucleus accumbens.[169] This effect, and the accompanying behavioral response, is abolished in transgenic mice in which the normal dopamine transporter is replaced with one that is insensitive to cocaine.[170] As noted previously, another addictive drug, nicotine, also increases dopamine release in the nucleus accumbens, though by a different mechanism. The projection to the prefrontal cortex is thought to participate in cognitive functions[171] and to control affective states such as schizophrenia;[172] nearly all drugs currently used to treat schizophrenia work by blocking dopamine receptors.

HISTAMINE   Histamine was first identified as a mediator of inflammation. However, when the first antihistamines were introduced (in the 1930s, to treat hay fever, rashes, and insect bites), their main side effect was to make the recipient sleepy. This provided the first clue that histamine might also be important in the brain—a role that has been amply confirmed.[173] There is a dense aggregation of histamine-containing neurons in the tuberomammillary nucleus of the dorsal hypothalamus (Figure 14.16). From there, histaminergic fibers project to wide areas of the brain, including other parts of the hypothalamus, the cerebral cortex, hippocampus, amygdala, and basal ganglia as well as down the spinal cord. Histamine also acts as a transmitter in some invertebrates, for example at arthropod photoreceptor synapses.[174]

There are three subtypes of histamine receptors in the brain, all G protein-coupled: H_1, H_2, and H_3. H_1 receptors (the original antihistamine receptors) are the principal postsynaptic receptors. They activate the G protein G_q to stimulate phospholipase C (see Chapter 12) and depolarize neurons by inhibiting potassium currents (including M-currents[118]) (Figure 14.17A). H_2 receptors are also postsynaptic—their main effect is to inhibit the slow calcium-activated potassium current and increase action potential discharges[175] (Figure 14.17B), which they do by activating adenylate cyclase and increasing cyclic AMP. In contrast, H_3 receptors act as autoinhibitory receptors.[176] They are located on the somata and dendrites of the histaminergic neurons, where they reduce their natural firing rate (Figure 14.17C), and on their terminals, where they reduce transmitter release.

[167] LeWitt, P. A. 2008. *New England J. Med.* 359: 2468-2476.

[168] Schultz, W., Dayan, P., and Montague, R. R. 1997. *Science* 275: 1593-1599.

[169] Kalivas, P. W., and Duffy, P. 1990. *Synapse* 5: 48-58.

[170] Chen, R. et al. 2006. *Proc. Natl. Acad. Sci. USA* 103: 9333-9338.

[171] Seamans, J. K., and Yang, C.R. 2004. *Prog. Neurobiol.* 74: 1-58.

[172] Howes, O. D., and Kapur, S. 2009. *Schizophr. Bull.* 35: 549-562.

[173] Haas, H. L., Sergeeva, O. A., and Selbach, O. 2008. *Physiol. Rev.* 88: 1183-1241.

[174] Stuart, A. E, Borycz, J., and Meinertzhagen, I. A. 2007. *Prog. Neurobiol.* 82: 202-227.

[175] Haas, H. L., and Konnerth, A. 1983. *Nature* 302: 432-434.

[176] Arrang, J. M., Garbarg, M., and Schwartz, J. C. 1983. *Nature* 302: 832-837.

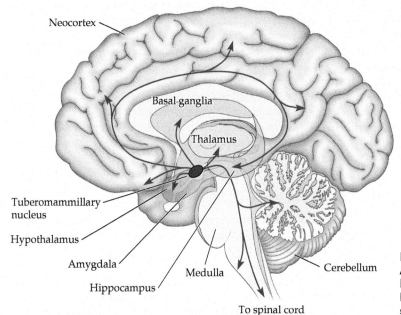

FIGURE 14.16   Histamine-Containing Neurons Are Localized to the Tuberomammillary Nucleus in the Hypothalamus. These neurons have diffuse projections throughout the brain and spinal cord.

(A) H$_1$ action

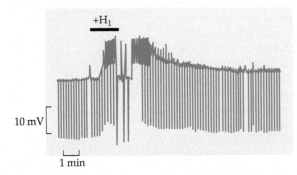

(B) H$_2$ action

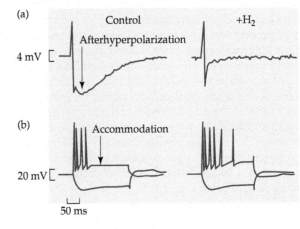

(C) H$_3$ action

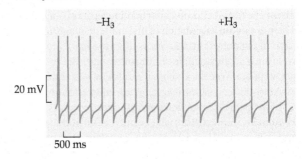

FIGURE 14.17 Effects of Stimulating Three Different Histamine Receptors. (A) Record from a cell in the pontine reticular formation. Downward deflections are transient voltage responses to brief hyperpolarizing constant current injections. Application of histamine (bar) caused depolarization and induced action potential firing (truncated by the recorder). When the cell was repolarized during the response to histamine, the brief current injections produced a larger voltage deflection, showing that the membrane conductance was reduced. This finding was attributed to the reduction of a resting potassium conductance. (B) Stimulating H$_2$ receptors in a human hippocampal pyramidal cell (a) eliminates the long-lasting calcium-dependent afterhyperpolarization following an action potential and (b) reduces accommodation during action potential discharges produced by a 250-ms depolarizing current. (C) Stimulating H$_3$ autoreceptors slows action potential discharges in a tuberomammillary histaminergic neuron. These records show the spontaneous activity of a neuron recorded when H$_3$ receptors were blocked with the selective H$_3$ antagonist thioperamide (–H$_3$) and then when the receptors were unblocked by omitting the thioperamide (+H$_3$). (After H. Haas and P. Panula, 2003. *Nat. Rev. Neurosci.* 4: 121–130.)

[177] Lin, J. S. 2000. *Sleep Med. Rev.* 4: 471–503.

[178] Abe, H. et al. 2004. *Mol. Brain Res.* 124: 178–187.

[179] Kubota, Y. et al. 2002. *J. Neurochem.* 83: 837–845.

[180] Ercan-Sencicek, A. G. et al. 2010. *New England J. Med.* 362: 1901–1908.

[181] Holton, P. 1959. *J. Physiol.* 145: 494–504.

[182] Burnstock, G. 1972. *Pharmacol. Rev.* 24: 509–581.

[183] Abbracchio, M. P. et al. 2009. *Trends Neurosci.* 32: 19–29.

As might be anticipated from the wide distribution of their efferent fibers, tuberomammillary histaminergic neurons affect many brain functions. One notable role is in regulating sleep. Their activity is closely coupled to the sleep–wake cycle (Figure 14.18). They are more active during the awake state and induce cortical arousal through their direct projections to the thalamus and cortex and by activating other ascending arousal systems.[177] Blockade of the histamine H$_1$ receptors on their target neurons explains the somnolent effect of the original antihistamines. A projection to the suprachiasmatic nucleus and to other regions also affects the sleep–wake cycle through an alteration in circadian rhythm.[178]

Histaminergic neurons also control motor behavior. Mice in which histamine levels have been reduced by deleting the synthetic enzyme histidine decarboxylase show exaggerated responses to locomotor stimulants;[179] and a mutation in the gene encoding this enzyme has recently been found in a human family exhibiting Tourette syndrome,[180] a neurological disorder in which the affected person shows uncontrolled jerky spontaneous movements and verbal expostulations.

Adenosine Triphosphate (ATP)

ATP is an essential transmitter and chemical messenger in the PNS. This discovery stems from the pioneering work of Pamela Holton, who first showed that ATP was released from peripheral nerve endings when their axons were stimulated,[181] and by Geoffrey Burnstock, who established its transmitter function in the autonomic nervous system (see Chapter 19) and dubbed ATP-releasing nerves *purinergic*.[182] It is now recognized that ATP also plays a significant role in intercellular communication in the CNS.[183] There are two types of receptors for ATP: P2X receptors, which are ligand-gated cation

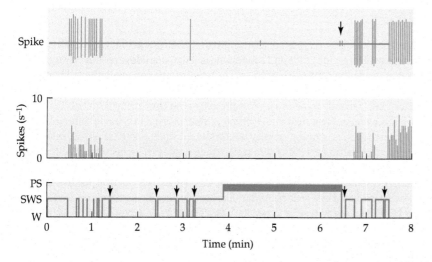

FIGURE 14.18 Histaminergic Neuron Activity Is Related to the Awake State. The top record shows action potential discharges (labeled "Spike") from a single histaminergic neuron in the tuberomammillary nucleus of an unanaesthetized mouse with an extracellular recording electrode. The trace below is a ratemeter output of action potential frequency (Spikes s^{-1}). The bottom diagram shows the awake-sleep state of the mouse, as judged from the electroencephalogram. W = awake; SWS = slow-wave sleep; PS = paradoxical sleep. The neuron fired only when the mouse was awake, and was completely silent when the mouse was asleep. It also stayed silent when the mouse woke up for just very short periods (arrowheads). (Adapted from K. Takahashi et al., 2006. *J. Neurosci.* 26: 10292-10298. © 2006 Society for Neuroscience.)

channels,[184] and G protein-coupled receptors called P2Y receptors.[185] Seven types of P2X receptor subunits and eight different P2Y receptors are known. Many of the P2X receptors and some of the P2Y receptors (most widely, the P2Y1 receptor) are expressed on neurons and glial cells in the brain.

ATP acts as a fast transmitter on P2X receptors at a few synapses in the brain.[186,187] At some synapses, it acts as the sole transmitter,[188] but more often it is co-released with another transmitter.[189] However, the wide distribution of P2X receptors in the CNS (including in presynaptic terminals[186]) suggests that most of them respond to diffusely released ATP, like the nicotinic ACh receptors. Their principal function may be to deliver a charge of calcium, since these receptors have a high conductance for calcium ions.[184] ATP (or more potently, adenosine diphosphate [ADP]) can also excite neurons in the hippocampus by stimulating P2Y1 G protein-coupled receptors, which induce a depolarizing cation current[190] or inhibit the M-current.[191] Chapter 18 discusses the release of ATP through the opening of a special type of transmembrane channel, the pannexin channel.

Neuroglial cells also possess ATP receptors, which may be involved in neuron-to-glial cell signaling.[192] It is envisaged that: (1) ATP released from neurons activates glial cell purinoceptors to increase intracellular calcium ion concentration; (2) the increased intraglial calcium in turn releases ATP and other chemical mediators from the glial cells onto the neurons to alter their activity; and (3) the ATP so released also activates neighboring glial cells to spread the signal.[193] Thus, recent research has shown that glial cells can be depolarized by ATP that is released from specialized release sites along axons,[193] as well as from purinergic nerve terminals; that ATP released following nerve injury activates microglial cells and causes them to release ATP through pannexin channels (see Chapter 10);[194] that ATP-mediated microglial activation contributes to the long-term regulation of pain transmission in the spinal cord;[195] and that in the nucleus tractus solitarius, ATP released from glial cells onto neighboring chemosensitive neurons drives the central respiratory response to produce changes in arterial blood pH and carbon dioxide tension.[196]

Extracellular ATP is rapidly dephosphorylated by ecto-nucleotidases to adenosine, which joins a pool of adenosine extruded from neurons and glial cells by transporters, producing a constant but fluctuating interstitial adenosine concentration of between 25 and 250 nM.[197] Adenosine can activate another family of G protein-coupled receptors on neurons called adenosine receptors. Some of these (A1 and A2$_a$ receptors) are sufficiently sensitive to adenosine to be activated at the normal levels of interstitial adenosine, thus producing a tonic reduction of neuron excitability and transmitter release.[198] This is important in the regulation of sleep.[199] For example, accumulation of adenosine during periods of wakefulness depresses the activity of neurons in the tuberomammillary nucleus, thus precipitating sleepiness. This explains the stimulant action of caffeine, since caffeine blocks adenosine receptors. Thus, mice in which the gene for A2$_a$ is deleted are unusually aggressive and no longer respond to the stimulant effect of caffeine.[200]

[184] Surprenant, A., and North, R. A. 2009. *Annu. Rev. Physiol.* 71: 333-359.

[185] Abbracchio, M. P. et al. 2006. *Pharmacol. Rev.* 58: 281-341.

[186] Edwards, F. A., Gibb, A. J., and Colquhoun, D. 1992. *Nature* 359: 144-147.

[187] Pankratov, Y. et al. 2006. *Pflügers Arch.* 452: 589-597.

[188] Robertson, S. J., and Edwards, F. A. 1998. *J. Physiol.* 508: 691-701.

[189] Jo, Y. H., and Role, L. W. 2002. *J. Neurosci.* 22: 4794-4804.

[190] Bowser, D. N., and Khakh, B. S. 2004. *J. Neurosci.* 24: 8606-8620.

[191] Filippov, A. K. et al. 2006. *J. Neurosci.* 26: 9340-9348.

[192] Fields, R. D., and Burnstock, G. 2006. *Nat. Rev. Neurosci.* 7: 423-436.

[193] Thyssen, A. et al. 2010. *Proc. Natl. Acad. Sci. USA* 107: 15258-15263.

[194] Samuels, S. E. et al. 2010. *J. Gen. Physiol.* 136: 425-442.

[195] Tsuda, M., Tozaki-Saitoh, H., and Inoue, K. 2010. *Brain Res. Rev.* 63: 222-232.

[196] Gourine, A. V. et al. 2010. *Science* 329: 571-575.

[197] Dunwiddie, T. V., and Masino, S. A. 2001. *Annu. Rev. Neurosci.* 24: 31-55.

[198] Haas, H. L., and Selbach, O. 2000. *Naunyn Schmiedebergs Arch. Pharmacol.* 362: 375-381.

[199] Basheer, R. et al. 2004. *Prog. Neurobiol.* 73: 379-396.

[200] Ledent, C. et al. 1997. *Nature* 388: 674-678.

Peptides

There are differences between peptide transmitters (or **neuropeptides**) and small molecule transmitters such as amino acids and monoamines. First, peptides are split off from larger precursor molecules by peptidase enzymes. The precursors are made in the cell bodies and then packaged (with their peptidase enzymes) into large secretory (i.e., dense-core) vesicles (see Figure 15.8). Second, peptides are often present in the same nerve terminals that release small-molecule transmitters such as the amino acids. However, they are in different vesicles that surround the active zone and so may be co-released when electrical activity increases.[25] Third, in the mammalian nervous system at least, the peptides act exclusively as indirect transmitters, mainly through G protein-coupled receptors (see Chapter 12), and tend to straddle the boundary between transmitter and hormone. The best example of true peptidergic transmission is that mediated by a gonadotrophin-like peptide (luteinizing hormone-releasing hormone, or LHRH) in frog sympathetic ganglia[201] (see Figure 19.2B); most peptides seem to have a less clearly identifiable, more complex effect in the mammalian brain.

Peptides are good immunogens, so antibodies have been used extensively to identify the neurons, fiber tracts, and nerve terminals that contain them or their precursor molecules.[202] However, peptides do not readily enter the brain, and relatively few non-peptide chemicals capable of stimulating or blocking their receptors have been discovered, so their specific functions at individual synapses are often difficult to determine. As pointed out in Box 14.2, there are more than 60 neuropeptides in the brain, too many to be discussed individually. Instead, we have selected for illustration five peptides with different functions: two, substance P and the opioid peptides, with a particular (but not exclusive) connection to pain perception; the orexins, which regulate feeding and the sleep–wake cycle; and two closely related peptides, vasopressin and oxytocin (see also Chapter 18), which appear to play an interesting role in how animals (and humans) interact with each other.

Substance P

Substance P is a peptide with 11 amino acids, having the composition Arg-Pro-Lys-Pro-Gln-Gln-Phe-Phe-Gly-Leu-Met. It is a member of the family of tachykinins. There are two other tachykinins in the mammalian CNS, the neurokinins (NKs) A and B, but many more in non-mammalian vertebrates and invertebrates.[203] Substance P is so called because in 1931 von Euler and Gaddum first detected its biological activity in a *powder* (whence P) made from extracts of horse intestine and brain.[204] Substance P and other neurokinins act on a group of G_q-coupled receptors called NK receptors. Substance P preferentially targets NK1 receptors but can also activate NK2 and NK3 receptors at high concentrations.

Substance P is highly concentrated in primary afferent pain-sensing neurons and their unmyelinated axons, and in the central endings of these neurons in the substantia gelatinosa in the dorsal horn of the spinal cord.[205] When primary afferent fibers are stimulated, substance P (along with glutamate) is co-released and then depolarizes the target dorsal horn neurons.[206] Its role in nociceptive (pain) transmission has been examined using NK1 receptor antagonists and mice in which the NK1 receptor has been genetically deleted (NK1 knockouts). It is not involved in the transmission of acutely painful stimuli, such as a tail-pinch or burn, but NK1 knock-out mice showed a reduced response to the prolonged pain produced by injecting a painful inflammatory substance.[207,208] The gradual increase in the firing of dorsal horn neurons during repeated C-fiber stimulation (termed "wind-up") that is associated with sensitization to painful stimuli was also strongly reduced in these animals.[209] Rather disappointingly, however, NK1 antagonist drugs seem not to have any significant effects on inflammatory pain in humans.[210] Substance P is also strongly expressed in some supraspinal regions, such as the substantia nigra.[208] It may be involved in the control of affective states, since mice in which the NK1 receptor gene has been deleted show behavioral changes similar to mice treated with antidepressant drugs.[211]

Opioid Peptides

Opioid peptides are a family of endogenous neuropeptides that interact with opioid receptors (as do exogenous substances such as morphine). They include the pentapeptides

[201] Kuffler, S. W. 1980. *J. Exp. Biol.* 89: 257–286.

[202] Hökfelt, T. et al. 2000. *Neuropharmacology* 39: 1337–1356.

[203] Severini, C. et al. 2002. *Pharmacol. Rev.* 54: 285–322.

[204] von Euler, U. S., and Gaddum, J. H. 1931. *J. Physiol.* 72: 74–87.

[205] Hökfelt, T. et al. 1975. *Science* 190: 889–890.

[206] Otsuka, M., and Yoshioka, K. 1993. *Physiol. Rev.* 73: 229–308.

[207] Cao, Y. Q. et al. 1998. *Nature* 392: 390–394.

[208] De Felipe, C. et al. 1998. *Nature* 392: 394–397.

[209] Suzuki, R., Hunt, S. P., and Dickenson, A. H. 2003. *Neuropharmacology* 45: 1093–1100.

[210] Hill, R. 2000. *Trends Pharmacol. Sci.* 21: 244–246.

[211] Yan, T. C., Hunt, S. P., and Stanford, S. C. 2009. *Neuropharmacology* 57: 627–635.

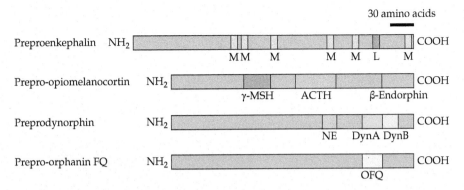

FIGURE 14.19 **Four Precursor Proteins that Generate the Opioid Peptides** and other peptide hormones by peptidase cleavage. M = met-enkephalin; L = leu-enkephalin; γ-MSH = γ-melanocyte-stimulating hormone; ACTH = adrenocorticotropic hormone; NE = α-neoendorphin; DynA and DynB = dynorphins A and B; OFQ = orphanin FQ/nociceptin. (After T. Darland et al., 1998. *Trends Neurosci.* 21: 215–221; C. Mollereau et al., 1996. *Proc. Natl. Acad. Sci.* 93: 8666–8670.)

leu-enkephalin and met-enkephalin (Tyr-Gly-Gly-Phe-Leu and Tyr-Gly-Gly-Phe-Met), which were originally discovered by Hughes, Kosterlitz, and their colleagues (see Box 14.2), plus several larger peptides containing the enkephalin sequences, such as the α-endorphins, β-endorphins, and the dynorphins (dynorphin A and B, neo-dynorphin).[212] They are formed by peptidase cleavage from four large precursor proteins (Figure 14.19) and stimulate one or more of three opioid receptors labelled μ, δ, and κ (sometimes called MOR, DOR, and KOR for mu-, delta- and kappa-opioid receptor). These are G protein-coupled receptors that activate the pertussis-toxin-sensitive G proteins, G_o and G_i. Like other G_o-coupled receptors, they inhibit calcium channels to reduce transmitter release, activate inwardly rectifying potassium channels to hyperpolarize neurons, and inhibit adenylate cyclase (see Chapter 12).

Opioid peptides are closely involved in the control of pain. Thus, they are strongly expressed in the periaqueductal gray matter of the midbrain and in the dorsal horn of the spinal cord.[213,214] At the latter site, enkephalin-containing fibers innervate nociceptive dorsal horn neurons[215] and inhibit them by activating an inwardly rectifying potassium current.[216] Enkephalin released from descending fibers in the brainstem or from spinal interneurons also inhibits the release of substance P from nociceptive afferent fibers.[217] This probably results from the inhibition of the calcium current required for transmitter release from afferent nerve endings, as is indicated by the experiments on sensory neurons depicted in Figure 14.20.[218] Opioid receptor antagonists and genetic deletion of the opioid receptors[219] both induce hyperalgesia (increased sensitivity to pain), demonstrating that the opioid

212 Weber, E., Evans, C. J., and Barchas, J. D. 1983. *Trends Neurosci.* 6: 333–336.

213 Hökfelt, T. et al. 1977. *Proc. Natl. Acad. Sci. USA* 74: 3081–3085.

214 Marvizón, J. C., Chen, W., and Murphy, N. 2009. *J. Comp. Neurol.* 517: 51–68.

215 Ma, W. et al. 1997. *Neuroscience* 77: 793–811.

216 Marker, C. L. et al. 2006. *J. Neurosci.* 26: 12251–12259.

217 Collin, E. et al. 1991. *Neuroscience* 44: 725–731.

218 Mudge, A. W., Leeman, S. E., and Fischbach, G. D. 1979. *Proc. Natl. Acad. Sci. USA* 76: 526–530.

219 Kieffer, B. L., and Gavériaux-Ruff, C. 2002. *Progr. Neurobiol.* 66: 285–306.

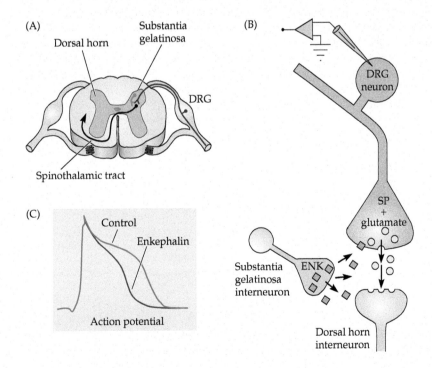

FIGURE 14.20 **Pathway for Transmission of Pain Sensation in the Spinal Cord.** (A,B) Dorsal root ganglion (DRG) cells responding to noxious stimuli release substance P (SP) and glutamate at their synapses with interneurons in the dorsal horn of the spinal cord. Interneurons containing enkephalin (ENK) in the substantia gelatinosa of the dorsal horn block transmission partly by inhibiting transmitter release from terminals of the DRG cells. (C) Intracellular recordings from a DRG cell demonstrate that enkephalin acts by causing a decrease in the duration of the action potential, reflecting reduced calcium current, which would reduce the amount of transmitter released from sensory nerve terminals. (A,B after T. M. Jessell and L. L. Iversen, 1977. *Nature* 268: 549–551; C after A. W. Mudge et al., 1979. *Proc. Natl. Acad. Sci. USA* 76: 526–530.)

peptides play a physiological role in controlling pain. However, these peptides and their receptors are also widely expressed in other parts of the brain not directly concerned with pain, such as the basal ganglia and subcortical limbic areas,[220] suggesting their involvement in other functions.

Another interesting opioid peptide has the dual names orphanin FQ and nociceptin.[221,222] This is because orphanin was identified as the previously unknown ligand for an *orphan* receptor called NOP (formerly called ORL1), hence orphanin,[223] and nociceptin because it *increased* the response to painful stimuli in animals.[224] The "FQ" is added to orphanin because it is identical to dynorphin A (see Figure 14.19) except for two amino acid substitutions: phenylalanine (F) and glutamine (Q). The NOP receptor is homologous with the opioid receptors, couples to their same G proteins, and has the same effects on neurons when stimulated as do opioid receptors.[224] The reason it *increases* pain, rather than reducing it like other opioids, is probably because the NOP receptors are located on different neurons than those with enkephalin or dynorphin receptors. It has been suggested that the NOP neurons normally reduce activity in pain pathways, so that when they are inhibited by nociceptin/orphanin FQ transmission, the pain pathway is enhanced (disinhibited). Nociceptin/orphanin FQ and its receptors are also expressed widely throughout the brain, so this peptide has effects on the brain that are unrelated to pain.[221,222]

Orexins (Hypocretins)

Orexins are hypothalamic peptides that regulate sleep and feeding by promoting awakening and enhancing appetite[225,226] (see Box 14.2 for an account of their discovery). There are two orexins, A and B, which are both generated from the same precursor protein. They act on two G protein-coupled receptors, OX1 and OX2, which mainly activate the G protein G_q and, when stimulated, increase the activity of the target neuron. Orexin-containing neurons are localized to the posterior lateral hypothalamus, but their axons innervate large areas of the brain (Figure 14.21).

The role of orexins in regulating sleep was established by two genetic observations. First, mice in which the DNA sequences encoding the orexins had been deleted showed excessive night-time sleeping.[227] (Mice are nocturnal, so this is equivalent to daytime sleeping in humans.) The second clue came from work on dogs with the sleep disorder **narcolepsy**—a disorder that also quite commonly affects people (about 1 in 2000 in the United States). Individuals with narcolepsy suffer from repeated periods of extreme daytime sleepiness, suddenly falling asleep at the most inconvenient times (sleep attacks); in extreme cases, these episodes are coupled with loss of muscle tone, so that the person collapses (cataplexy). It was found that dogs that have this disorder (Doberman pinschers and Labradors) have specific mutations in the gene encoding the OX2 orexin receptor.[228] Humans who have narcolepsy do not necessarily have this mutation but instead lose orexin-containing

[220] Mansour, A. et al. 1988. *Trends Neurosci.* 11: 308-314.

[221] Darland, T., Heinricher, M. M., and Grandy, D. K. 1998. *Trends Neurosci.* 21: 215-221.

[222] Meis, S. 2003. *Neuroscientist* 9: 158-168.

[223] Reinscheid, R. K. et al. 1995. *Science* 270: 792-794.

[224] Meunier, J. C. et al. 1995. *Nature* 377: 532-535.

[225] Tsujino, N., and Sakurai, T. 2009. *Pharmacol. Rev.* 61: 162-176.

[226] Bonnavion, P., and de Lecea, L. 2010. *Curr. Neurol. Neurosci. Rep.* 10: 174-179.

[227] Chemelli, R. M. et al. 1999. *Cell* 98: 437-451.

[228] Lin, L. et al. 1999. *Cell* 98: 365-376.

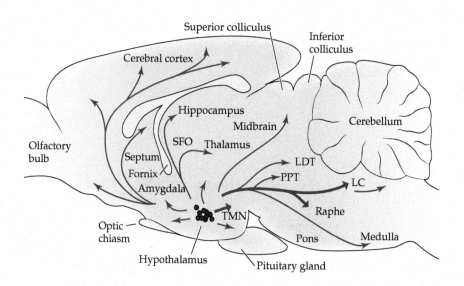

FIGURE 14.21 Orexin-Containing Neurons in the Hypothalamus and Their Axonal Projections. LC = locus coeruleus; LDT = laterodorsal thalamus; PPT = pedunculopontine tegmental area; TMN = tuberomammillary nucleus; SFO = subfornical organ. (After N. Tsujino and T. Sakurai, 2009. *Pharmacol. Rev.* 61: 162-176.)

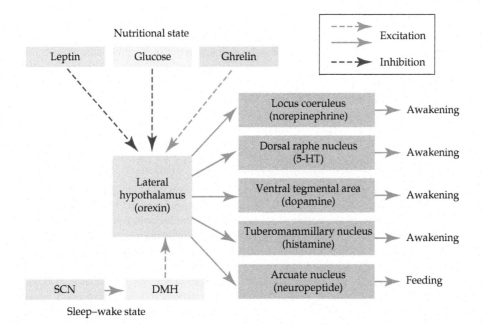

FIGURE 14.22 Integration of Awakening and Feeding Signals by the Orexinergic Neurons in the Lateral Hypothalamus. Orexinergic neurons receive information about the sleep-wake state from the suprachiasmatic nucleus and about the nutritional state from extracellular glucose levels and from the levels of the hormones leptin and ghrelin. They signal awakening and feeding through the various pathways indicated on the right. SCN = suprachiasmatic nucleus; DMH = dorsal medial hypothalamus; dashed lines = afferent signals; solid lines = efferent signals. (After N. Tsujino and T. Sakurai, 2009. *Pharmacol. Rev.* 61: 162–176.)

neurons, so they do not secrete enough orexin.[227] Orexin neurons induce awakening via pathways to the locus coeruleus, dorsal raphe, and tuberomammillary nucleus, activating noradrenergic, serotonergic, and histaminergic neurons, respectively (Figure 14.22). Stimulation of histaminergic neurons could play a role, because the awakening effect of orexin injected into the lateral ventricles of mice is abolished when the histamine H_1-receptor gene is deleted.[229] In turn, the orexinergic neurons receive information about the state of the sleep–wake cycle from the suprachiasmatic nucleus.

Orexinergic neurons also act as sensors of nutritional state and respond to changes in extracellular glucose levels. As shown in Figure 14.23, orexinergic neurons are spontaneously active when the concentration of glucose in the extracellular medium is low (0.2 mM in this experiment). However, increasing the glucose concentration progressively silences the neurons, by activating twin-pore potassium channels (K_{2P} channels; see Chapter 5) and hyperpolarizing the neurons.[230] Orexinergic neurons are also inhibited by the

[229] Huang, Z. L. et al. 2001. *Proc. Natl. Acad. Sci. USA* 98: 9965–9970.

[230] Burdakov, D. et al. 2006. *Neuron* 50: 711–722.

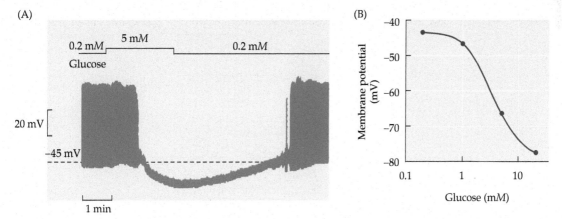

FIGURE 14.23 Extracellular Glucose Concentration Regulates the Firing of Orexin-Containing Neurons. (A) Spontaneous action potentials recorded from an orexin-expressing neuron in a slice of rat hypothalamus in vitro, recorded first in a solution containing 0.2 mM glucose and then on raising the glucose to 5 mM. Glucose hyperpolarizes the neuron and inhibits action potentials. (B) The membrane potential is progressively increased as the glucose concentration is raised from 0.2 mM to 10 mM. (After D. Burdakov et al., 2005. *J. Neurosci.* 25: 2429–2433. © 2005 Society for Neuroscience.)

hormone leptin (secreted by adipocytes, or fat cells, in proportion to the amount of fat they contain) but are activated by another hormone, ghrelin (secreted from the stomach and pancreas as a hunger signal) (see Figure 14.22). Hence, the orexinergic neurons signal low glucose and hunger, which leads to increased food intake, partly by activating neurons that secrete hypothalamic neuropeptide Y (NPY) but mainly by triggering orexin's awakening action. In other words, you have to be awake to eat, and hunger wakes you up. Hence, orexin-containing neurons help coordinate the brain's response to information about the body's nutritional and sleep–wake balance.

Vasopressin and Oxytocin: The Social Brain

Vasopressin and oxytocin are contained in neurons in the supraoptic and paraventricular nuclei of the hypothalamus (see also Chapter 18). They are secreted into the bloodstream from nerve endings in the posterior pituitary gland. Vasopressin promotes water reabsorption from the kidney (it was originally called antidiuretic hormone); oxytocin induces lactation. However, processes of these neurons innervate other parts of the brain (Figure 14.24); thus, these peptides can excite many central neurons.[231]

Both peptides strongly influence the social behavior of animals and humans via direct or indirect connections to the nucleus accumbens, prefrontal cortex, and amygdala. Some of the key observations leading to this conclusion came from experiments on voles.[232] Some voles, such as the prairie vole (*Microtus ochrogaster*), are monogamous: The male forms a strong pair bond with the female, cooperates in rearing the pups, and aggressively repels a strange prairie vole. Other related vole species, such as the meadow vole (*M. pennsylvanicus*) and the montane vole (*M. montanus*), are more promiscuous and do not form tight pair bonds. It was found that this behavioral difference was critically dependent on the expression and distribution of the vasopressin V1A receptor in the male.[233] Thus, intracerebroventricular injection of a V1A receptor antagonist in the normally monogamous male prairie vole increased aggression, disrupted male–female pair bonding, and increased extra-pair bonding,[234] while overexpression of the V1A receptor gene *AVPR1A* dramatically increased pair bonding in the more promiscuous meadow vole.[233] Differences in V1A receptor expression in the two species are related to the presence of a long insert in the noncoding region of the *AVPR1A* gene in the meadow vole.[235] Interestingly, the human gene shows polymorphisms in this region, which have been correlated with the strength of pair bonding in human males.[236]

[231] Raggenbass, M. 2001. *Prog. Neurobiol.* 64: 307-326.

[232] McGraw, L. A., and Young, L. J. 2010. *Trends Neurosci.* 33: 103-109.

[233] Lim, M. M. et al. 2004. *Nature* 429: 754-757.

[234] Winslow, J. T. et al. 1993. *Nature* 365: 545-548.

[235] Young, L. J. et al. 1999. *Nature* 400: 766-768.

[236] Walum, H. et al. 2008. *Proc. Natl. Acad. Sci. USA* 105: 14153-14156.

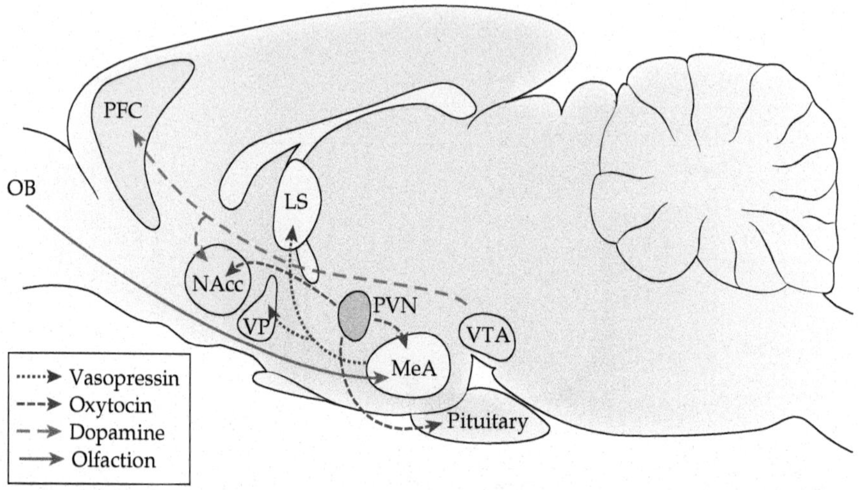

FIGURE 14.24 Proposed Neural Circuits Underlying the Effects of Vasopressin and Oxytocin on Social Interaction. LS = lateral septum; MeA = medial nucleus of the amygdala; NAcc = nucleus accumbens; OB = olfactory bulb; PFC = prefrontal cortex; PVN = paraventricular nucleus; VP = ventral pallidum; VTA = ventral tegmental area. (After L. A. Mc-Graw and L. J. Young, 2010. *Trends Neurosci.* 33: 103-109; L. J. Young et al., 2005. *J. Comp. Neurol.* 493: 51-57.)

Oxytocin has the complementary effect of strengthening pair bonding in female voles. Thus, oxytocin release in the nucleus accumbens is greatly increased after mating, while infusion of oxytocin facilitates pair bonding and blocking oxytocin receptors hinders it.[234] Pair bonding and maternal–pup bonding are also reduced in mice in which the oxytocin receptor or the enzyme CD38 (which facilitates oxytocin release) is disrupted.[237] Facilitation of pair bonding involves a suppression of the normal fear response mediated by the amygdala, which is where the olfactory recognition signal required for social interaction is processed (see Figure 14.24). In humans, this effect translates to an increase in trust and empathy,[238,239] essential prerequisites for interpersonal bonding. Indeed, oxytocin and vasopressin may provide the long-sought chemical basis for at least part of that human emotion termed love.[240,241]

[237] Higashida, H. et al. 2010. *J. Neuroendocrinol.* 22: 373-379.

[238] Baumgartner, T. et al. 2008. *Neuron* 58: 639-650.

[239] Hurlemann, R. et al. 2010. *J. Neurosci.* 30: 4999-5007.

[240] Zeki, S. 2007. *FEBS Lett.* 581: 2575-2579.

[241] Young, L. J. 2009. *Nature* 457: 148.

SUMMARY

- There is a wide variety of chemical transmitters in the CNS. Neurons that use a particular transmitter can be identified by immunohistochemical and other visual methods.

- Many neurons release more than one transmitter, and each transmitter can act on a variety of target receptors. Hence, their postsynaptic effects on individual neurons are often complex.

- The main excitatory transmitter is glutamate. Glutamate acts on two types of ionotropic receptors (AMPA and NMDA receptors) to generate excitatory postsynaptic potentials. It also acts on a metabotropic receptor, mGluR, to produce pre-and postsynaptic modulatory effects.

- GABA and glycine are inhibitory transmitters in the brain and spinal cord. Glycine acts on ionotropic receptors. GABA acts on both ionotropic (GABA$_A$) and metabotropic (GABA$_B$) receptors.

- Cholinergic neurons are concentrated in the basal forebrain. Their axons innervate wide areas of the cerebral cortex and many subcortical regions. They play a role in cortical arousal, attention, and memory. ACh released from these nerves acts on ionotropic nicotinic receptors, which are located mainly on presynaptic nerve endings, and on metabotropic muscarinic receptors.

- The monoamines norepinephrine, 5-HT, dopamine, and histamine are contained in a relatively few neurons clustered in discrete nuclei in the brainstem and midbrain. Axons of noradrenergic, serotonergic, and histaminergic neurons project to wide areas of the forebrain and affect numerous brain functions. Dopaminergic axons project to the basal ganglia and limbic system, and play a specific role in the control of motor function.

- ATP is released as a co-transmitter from many neurons. It acts on ionotropic P2X and metabotropic P2Y receptors on both neurons and neuroglial cells.

- Several different neuropeptides are released from central neurons. Examples described are substance P and the enkephalins, which control pain; orexin, which affects sleep and feeding; and oxytocin and vasopressin, which affect social behavior.

Suggested Reading

General Reviews

Abbracchio, M. P., Burnstock, G., Verkhratsky, A., and Zimmermann, H. 2009. Purinergic signalling in the nervous system: an overview. *Trends Neurosci.* 32: 19–29.

Brown, D. A. 2010. Muscarinic acetylcholine receptors (mAChRs) in the nervous system: some functions and mechanisms. *J. Mol. Neurosci.* 41: 340–346.

Cooper, J. R., Bloom, F. E., and Roth, R. H. 2003. *The Biochemical Basis of Neuropharmacology*, 8th ed. Oxford University Press.

Dani, J. A., and Bertrand, D. 2007. Nicotinic acetylcholine receptors and nicotinic cholinergic mechanisms of the central nervous system. *Annu. Rev. Pharmacol. Toxicol.* 47: 699–729.

Dayan, P., and Huys, Q. J. 2009. Serotonin in affective control. *Annu. Rev. Neurosci.* 32: 95–126.

Haas, H. L., Sergeeva, O. A., and Selbach, O. 2008. Histamine in the nervous system. *Physiol. Rev.* 88: 1183–1241.

Hokfelt, T. 2010. Looking at neurotransmitters in the microscope. *Prog. Neurobiol.* 90: 101–118.

Iversen, S. D., and Iversen, L. L. 2007. Dopamine: 50 years in perspective. *Trends Neurosci.* 30: 188–193.

Krnjevic, K. 2010. When and why amino acids? *J. Physiol.* 588: 33–44.

Livingstone, P. D., and Wonnacott, S. 2009. Nicotinic acetylcholine receptors and the ascending dopamine pathways. *Biochem. Pharmacol.* 78: 744–755.

Lodge, D. 2009. The history of the pharmacology and cloning of ionotropic glutamate receptors and the development of idiosyncratic nomenclature. *Neuropharmacology* 56: 6–21.

McGraw, L. A., and Young, L. J. 2010. The prairie vole: an emerging model organism for understanding the social brain. *Trends Neurosci.* 33: 103–109.

Mesulam, M. 2004. The cholinergic lesion of Alzheimer's disease: pivotal factor or side show? *Learn. Mem.* 11: 43–49.

Sakurai, T. 2007. The neural circuit of orexin (hypocretin): maintaining sleep and wakefulness. *Nat. Rev. Neurosci.* 8: 171–181.

Salio, C., Lossi, L., Ferrini, F., and Merighi, A. 2006. Neuropeptides as synaptic transmitters. *Cell Tissue Res.* 326: 583–598.

Sara, S. J. 2008. The locus coeruleus and noradrenergic modulation of cognition. *Nat. Rev. Neurosci.* 10: 211–223.

Surmeier, D. J. 2009. A lethal convergence of dopamine and calcium. *Neuron* 62: 163–164.

Thiele, A. 2013. Muscarinic signaling in the brain. *Annu. Rev. Neurosci.* 36: 271–294.

Original Papers

Edwards, F. A., Gibb, A. J., and Colquhoun, D. 1992. ATP receptor-mediated synaptic currents in the central nervous system. *Nature* 359: 144–147.

Gourine, A.V., Kasymov, V., Marina, N., Tang, F., Figueiredo, M. F., Lane, S., Teschemacher, A. G., Spyer, K. M., Deisseroth, K., and Kasparov, S. 2010. Astrocytes control breathing through pH-dependent release of ATP. *Science* 329: 571–575.

Kravitz, A. V., Freeze, B. S., Parker, P.R.L., Kay, K., Thwin, M. T., Deisseroth, K., and Kreitzer, A. C. 2010. Regulation of parkinsonian motor behaviours by optogenetic control of basal ganglia circuitry. *Nature* 466: 622–626.

Lin, L., Faraco, J., Li, R., Kadotani, H., Rogers, W., Lin, X., Qiu, X., de Jong, P. J., Nishino, S., and Mignot E. 1999. The sleep disorder canine narcolepsy is caused by a mutation in the hypocretin (orexin) receptor 2 gene. *Cell* 98: 365–376.

Shen, W., Hamilton, S. E., Nathanson, N. M., and, Surmeier, D. J. 2005. Cholinergic suppression of KCNQ channel currents enhances excitability of striatal medium spiny neurons. *J. Neurosci.* 25: 7449–7458.

Stell, B. M., Brickley, S. G., Tang, C. Y., Farrant, M., and Mody, I. 2003. Neuroactive steroids reduce neuronal excitability by selectively enhancing tonic inhibition mediated by α-subunit-containing GABAA receptors. *Proc. Natl. Acad. Sci. USA.* 100: 14439–14444.

Whim, M. D., and Moss, G. W. 2001. A novel technique that measures peptide secretion on a millisecond timescale reveals rapid changes in release. *Neuron* 30: 37–50.

Winslow, J. T., Hastings, N., Carter, C. S., Harbaugh, C. R., and Insel, T. R. 1993. A role for central vasopressin in pair bonding in monogamous prairie voles. *Nature* 365: 545–548.

CHAPTER 15

Transmitter Synthesis, Storage, Transport, and Inactivation

Neurons synthesize and release neuropeptides as well as low-molecular-weight transmitters. Low-molecular-weight transmitters, such as acetylcholine (ACh), γ-aminobutyric acid (GABA), and glutamate, are synthesized in the axon terminal. Several mechanisms ensure that their supply is adequate to meet the demands of release; these include storage in vesicles, rapid changes in the activity of enzymes mediating transmitter synthesis, and long-term changes in the number of enzyme molecules in the terminal. More than one neurotransmitter may be stored in and released from the same nerve terminal. Neuropeptides are synthesized and incorporated into dense-core vesicles in the cell body, then shipped down to release sites in the axon, soma, and dendrites. Axon terminals and varicosities may release transmitters from small clear vesicles at active zones, and peptides or small transmitters from large electron-dense vesicles at the periphery of active zones.

Vesicles and other organelles move by fast axonal transport toward the terminal (anterograde transport) and back to the cell body (retrograde transport). Slow axonal transport moves cytoplasmic proteins and components of the axonal cytoskeleton from the cell body toward the terminal.

The final step in chemical synaptic transmission is removal of the transmitter from the synaptic cleft. Low-molecular-weight transmitters released from synapses are either degraded after release or taken up into glial cells or axon terminals where they are repackaged into vesicles and released again. Neuropeptides and transmitters released outside synaptic terminals diffuse and act distantly. Drugs that interfere with transmitter degradation or uptake can have profound effects on signaling, indicating that such removal processes play an important role in synaptic function.

FIGURE 15.1 Chemical Synaptic Transmission. At chemical synapses, neurotransmitters are synthesized, stored in synaptic vesicles, and released by exocytosis. Transmitters diffuse across the synaptic cleft, activate receptors on the postsynaptic cell, and then are removed by diffusion, uptake, or degradation.

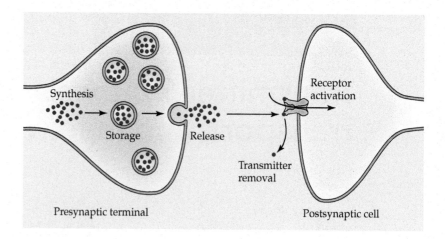

Chapters 11, 12, and 14 have shown that there are many different chemical neurotransmitters. Some are small molecules (less than 1 kilodalton in mass); these include acetylcholine, the amino acids glutamate and GABA, and several monoamines (norepinephrine, dopamine, 5-hydroxytryptamine [5-HT], and histamine). Others (peptides) can be several kilodaltons in size. In this chapter we consider how some of the key transmitters are made (or synthesized); how they are stored in vesicles; how they (or their synthetic enzymes) get to the nerve ending (by axoplasmic flow); and how, after their release by exocytosis, the transmitters are degraded or their postsynaptic action is otherwise terminated (Figure 15.1). Mechanisms of exocytosis were described in Chapter 13; the synthesis and release of gases and lipid transmitters on demand were explained in Chapter 12.

Neurotransmitter Synthesis

Where are transmitter molecules synthesized, and how are transmitter stores maintained and replenished? Are transmitters shipped ready-made to the nerve terminals, or are they assembled there from precursors provided by the cell body? The answers to such questions are different for different transmitters. Low-molecular-weight transmitters are produced within the axon terminal from common cellular metabolites and are stored in small synaptic vesicles (50 nanometers [nm] in diameter). Nitric oxide (NO), carbon monoxide (CO), and the endocannabinoids are also synthesized within terminals. However, since they cannot be packaged in vesicles, they immediately diffuse out of nerve terminals to act on their targets (see Chapter 12). Neuropeptide transmitters, by contrast, are synthesized in the cell body, packaged in large dense-core vesicles (100–200 nm in diameter), and shipped to release sites in the soma, dendrites, and axon terminals.

Principal biochemical pathways for the synthesis and degradation of acetylcholine, GABA, glutamate, catecholamines (dopamine, norepinephrine, and epinephrine), and histamine are shown in Appendix B.

Synthesis of Acetylcholine

Birks and MacIntosh performed one of the first thorough investigations into how transmitters are accumulated in nerve terminals and how transmitter stores are maintained during periods of activity. In their studies of ACh they used terminals of preganglionic axons in the superior cervical ganglion of the cat (Figure 15.2A,B; see also Chapter 19).[1] They cannulated the carotid artery and the jugular vein, perfused the ganglion with solutions containing anticholinesterase, and analyzed the perfusate for ACh. A small amount of ACh was continually released from the ganglion at rest, amounting to 0.1% of the total contents each minute (Figure 15.2C). The fact that the level of ACh in the ganglion remained constant meant that ACh was synthesized continually at rest. Subsequently it was shown that the ongoing rate of synthesis of ACh at rest, determined by

[1] Birks, R. I., and MacIntosh, F. C. 1961. *Can. J. Biochem. Physiol.* 39: 787–827.

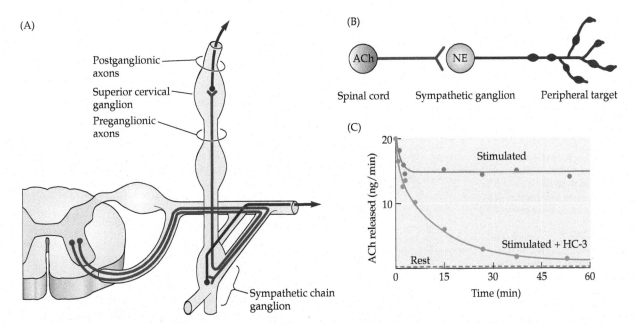

FIGURE 15.2   Measuring the Release of ACh from the terminals of preganglionic axons in the cat superior cervical ganglion. (A) Preganglionic axons reach the superior cervical ganglion from more posterior ganglia in the sympathetic chain. (B) Preganglionic neurons, whose cell bodies lie in the spinal cord, release acetylcholine (ACh) as a transmitter at synapses in sympathetic ganglia. Ganglion cells release norepinephrine (NE) from varicosities along their processes in the periphery. (C) Release of ACh from a cat sympathetic ganglion perfused with oxygenated plasma containing 3×10^{-5} M eserine (physostigmine) to inhibit acetylcholinesterase. In control medium, preganglionic stimulation at 20 stimuli/s causes a sustained, 100-fold increase in the rate of ACh release (solid blue line) compared with release at rest (dashed blue line). Release decreases rapidly during stimulation in the presence of 2×10^{-5} M hemicholinium (HC-3) (solid green line), which blocks choline uptake. (After R. I. Birks and F. C. MacIntosh, 1961. *Can. J. Biochem. Physiol.* 39: 787–827.)

monitoring the incorporation of radioactively labeled choline into ACh, is so high that an amount equal to the entire store of ACh is degraded and resynthesized within the axon terminals every 20 minutes.[2]

Birks and MacIntosh then stimulated the preganglionic nerve with long trains of impulses and found that the quantity of ACh released from the ganglion increased 100-fold, so that an amount corresponding to 10% of the original content was released each minute (see Figure 15.2C). Remarkably, this rate of release was maintained for over an hour with no change in the level of ACh in the ganglion. Thus, during an hour of stimulation an axon terminal can release an amount of ACh equal to many times its original content without having its stores depleted.

The only exogenous ingredient the nerve terminals need to maintain their stores of ACh under such conditions is choline, which is taken up from the surrounding fluid via an active transport process (Figure 15.3). The requirement for extracellular choline was demonstrated both by perfusing the preparation with solutions lacking choline and by blocking choline uptake into the axon terminals with hemicholinium (HC-3). In both cases, the level of ACh in the ganglion and the amount released by stimulation fell rapidly (see Figure 15.2C).

How is ACh synthesis controlled to meet the demands of release? Our understanding of the mechanisms regulating ACh synthesis and storage in cholinergic nerve terminals is surprisingly limited. The enzymatic reactions are summarized in Figure 15.3 and shown in detail in Appendix B. Acetylcholine is synthesized from choline and acetyl coenzyme A (acetyl-CoA, or AcCoA) by the enzyme choline acetyltransferase (ChAT) and is hydrolyzed to choline and acetate by acetylcholinesterase (AChE). Both enzymes are found in the cytosol. Because the reaction catalyzed by ChAT is reversible, one factor controlling the level of ACh is the **law of mass action**. For example, a fall in ACh concentration caused by release would favor net synthesis until equilibrium was reestablished. However, the regulatory mechanisms at work within cholinergic axon terminals are more complex

[2] Potter, L. T. 1970. *J. Physiol.* 206: 145–166.

FIGURE 15.3 Pathways of Acetylcholine Synthesis, Storage, Release, and Degradation.
Acetylcholine (ACh) is synthesized from choline and acetyl coenzyme A (AcCoA) by choline acetyltransferase (ChAT) and is degraded by acetylcholinesterase (AChE). AcCoA is synthesized primarily in mitochondria; choline is supplied by a high-affinity active transport system that can be inhibited by hemicholinium (HC-3). ACh is packaged into vesicles together with ATP for release by exocytosis. Transport of ACh into vesicles is blocked by vesamicol. Vesicular ACh is protected from degradation. After release, ACh is degraded by extracellular AChE to choline and acetate. About half of the choline transported into cholinergic axon terminals comes from the hydrolysis of ACh that has been released. At some synapses, ATP combines with postsynaptic receptors. ATP is hydrolyzed by extracellular ATPases to adenosine and phosphate (P_i); adenosine can combine with presynaptic receptors to modulate release (see Chapter 14).

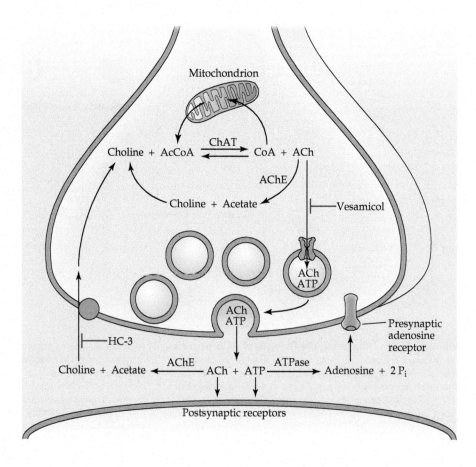

[3] Erickson, J. D. et al. 1994. *J. Biol. Chem.* 269: 21929–21932.

[4] Eiden, L. E. 1998. *J. Neurochem.* 70: 2227–2240.

[5] Prado, M. A. et al. 2002. *Neurochem. Int.* 41: 291–299.

[6] Jope, R. 1979. *Brain Res. Rev.* 1: 313–344.

[7] Parsons, S. M., Prior, C., and Marshall, I. G. 1993. *Int. Rev. Neurobiol.* 35: 279–390.

[8] Axelrod, J. 1971. *Science* 173: 598–606.

than this. For example, under resting conditions the accumulation of ACh is limited by ongoing hydrolysis by intracellular acetylcholinesterase; inhibition of intracellular AChE causes the ACh content to increase.[1,2] Thus, the level to which ACh accumulates represents a steady state between ongoing synthesis and degradation. This is a common feature of the metabolism of low-molecular-weight transmitters. Although it seems wasteful, such constant turnover may be an unavoidable consequence of the mechanisms that ensure an adequate supply of transmitter is always available.

Much of the ACh in nerve terminals is sequestered in vesicles, whereas ACh synthesis and degradation occur in the cytosol. Thus, to have an effect on the rate of synthesis, the release of ACh must reduce the cytoplasmic concentration of ACh, which presumably occurs from the movement of cytoplasmic ACh into newly formed vesicles. Similar interplay between cytoplasmic synthesis and vesicular storage and release is a common feature of the metabolism of low-molecular-weight transmitters. Maintaining the correct balance between ACh synthesis and vesicular uptake is facilitated by the fact that the gene for the vesicular ACh transporter VAChT is contained in the first intron of the gene for the synthetic enzyme ChAT,[3] so that the entire gene forms a cholinergic neuron gene.[4] This process ensures a coordinated expression of the two proteins for synthesis and vesicular uptake through a common gene promoter.[5] In cholinergic nerve terminals in the central nervous system (CNS), the supply of choline and co-substrate acetyl-CoA (made in mitochondria) and the activity of ChAT have also been shown to regulate the rate of ACh synthesis.[6,7]

Synthesis of Dopamine and Norepinephrine

Another mechanism by which the rate of synthesis of substances in cells is controlled is **feedback inhibition**, in which the rate-limiting step in a biosynthetic pathway is inhibited by the final product. A good example comes from studies by von Euler, Axelrod, Udenfriend, and their colleagues on the synthesis, storage, and release of norepinephrine in sympathetic neurons and in secretory cells of the adrenal medulla.[8] Adrenal medullary cells resemble sympathetic neurons in many ways. They share the same embryonic origin, are innervated by cholinergic axons that originate in the CNS, and release a catecholamine in response to stimulation. The term **catecholamine** is used to designate collectively the substances 3,4-dihydroxyphenylalanine (DOPA), dopamine, norepinephrine, and epinephrine—all of which contain a catechol nucleus (i.e., a benzene ring with two adjacent hydroxyl groups) and an amino group (see Appendix B). Mammalian sympathetic neurons release norepinephrine (those in frog release epinephrine); adrenal medullary cells release epinephrine as well as norepinephrine (see also Chapter 19).

Norepinephrine is synthesized from the common cellular metabolite tyrosine in a series of three steps. First, tyrosine is converted to DOPA by the enzyme tyrosine hydroxylase, then DOPA to dopamine by aromatic L-amino acid decarboxylase (AAAD), and finally dopamine to norepinephrine by dopamine β-hydroxylase (Figure 15.4; see also Appendix B). The conversions of tyrosine to DOPA and of DOPA to dopamine occur in the cytoplasm. Dopamine is then transported into synaptic vesicles, where it is converted to norepinephrine by dopamine β-hydroxylase, which is associated with the vesicle membrane. Much of

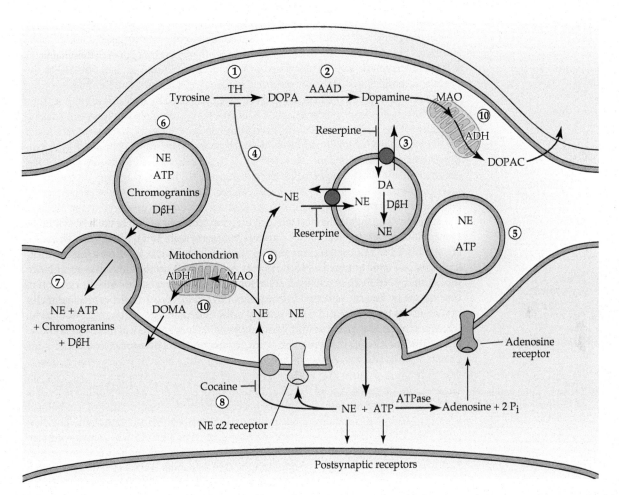

FIGURE 15.4 Pathways of Norepinephrine Synthesis, Storage, Release, and Uptake. (1) Tyrosine is converted to DOPA by tyrosine hydroxylase (TH). (2) DOPA is converted to dopamine (DA) by aromatic L-amino acid decarboxylase (AAAD). (3) Dopamine is transported into vesicles, where it is converted to norepinephrine (NE) by dopamine β-hydroxylase (DβH) (4). Norepinephrine inhibits TH, thus regulating synthesis by feedback inhibition. Transport of dopamine and norepinephrine into vesicles is blocked by reserpine. (5) Vesicles also contain adenosine triphosphate (ATP); (6) large dense-core vesicles contain soluble DβH and chromogranins as well. (7) All soluble components of vesicles are released together. Norepinephrine, ATP, adenosine, and peptides derived from chromogranins can bind to pre- or postsynaptic receptors. Presynaptic receptors for norepinephrine and adenosine are shown. (8) After release, norepinephrine is transported back into the varicosity by an uptake mechanism that is blocked by cocaine. (9) Norepinephrine in the cytoplasm can be repackaged into vesicles for release. (10) Within the varicosity, monoamine oxidase (MAO) and aldehyde dehydrogenase (ADH) in the mitochondria degrade norepinephrine to 3,4-dihydroxymandelic acid (DOMA) and dopamine to 3,4-dihydroxyphenylacetic acid (DOPAC).

the norepinephrine is stored within vesicles; some escapes into the cytoplasm, where it is susceptible to degradation by monoamine oxidase.

Neurons that release dopamine as a transmitter contain tyrosine hydroxylase and AAAD but they lack dopamine β-hydroxylase. Other neurons, as well as adrenal medullary cells, release epinephrine, which is derived from norepinephrine by the action of phenylethanolamine N-methyltransferase.

Typically the first enzyme in a multiple-step pathway is rate-limiting and is inhibited by the final product. In extracts of the adrenal medulla, the activity of tyrosine hydroxylase was found to be two orders of magnitude lower than that of AAAD and dopamine β-hydroxylase, suggesting that tyrosine hydroxylation was the rate-limiting step. Moreover, tyrosine hydroxylase was shown to be inhibited by norepinephrine (and by dopamine and epinephrine as well). Thus, as dopamine, norepinephrine, or epinephrine accumulates, further synthesis is inhibited until a steady state is reached, at which point the rate of synthesis is equal to the rate of degradation and release (see Figure 15.4).

Evidence that feedback inhibition regulates the synthesis of norepinephrine in neurons came from experiments by Weiner and his colleagues on terminals of sympathetic axons innervating the smooth muscles of a duct called the vas deferens.[9] They measured the rate of norepinephrine synthesis in the terminals by bathing the preparation in radioactively labeled precursors and monitoring the accumulation of radioactively labeled norepinephrine. They found that the rate of norepinephrine synthesis was more than threefold greater if the first enzymatic step was bypassed by providing DOPA rather than tyrosine as the precursor, confirming that the conversion of tyrosine to DOPA was rate-limiting.

To test the idea that the rate-limiting step was controlled by feedback inhibition, they varied the concentration of norepinephrine (NE) in the cytoplasm in two ways. First, taking advantage of the fact that sympathetic axon terminals have a specific transport mechanism for NE, they added NE to the bathing fluid, which caused an increase in NE concentration in the terminals and decreased the rate at which NE was synthesized from tyrosine. Conversely, nerve stimulation, which lowers the concentration of NE in the cytoplasm, increased the rate of conversion of tyrosine to NE almost twofold. No such increase was seen, however, if NE was added to the bath during nerve stimulation. Apparently, uptake from the medium was sufficient to maintain the level of NE in the axon terminals and so limit its biosynthesis.

Additional factors affect catecholamine synthesis (Figure 15.5). When axon terminals are stimulated to release norepinephrine, tyrosine hydroxylase acquires a higher affinity for its co-factor tetrahydrobiopterin (see Appendix B) and becomes less sensitive to inhibition by NE.[10] These changes are associated with a reversible phosphorylation of the enzyme by kinases activated by the influx of calcium ions.[11,12] An additional factor that regulates tyrosine hydroxylase activity is the concentration of tetrahydrobiopterin, which is synthesized from guanosine triphosphate.[13] Thus, a variety of mechanisms act to ensure that the rate of synthesis of norepinephrine meets the demands of release.

[9] Weiner, N., and Rabadjija, M. 1968. *J. Pharmacol. Exp. Ther.* 160: 61–71.

[10] Joh, T. H., Park, D. H., and Reis, D. J. 1978. *Proc. Natl. Acad. Sci. USA* 75: 4744–4748.

[11] Zigmond, R. E., Schwarzchild, M. A., and Rittenhouse, A. R. 1989. *Annu. Rev. Neurosci.* 12: 415–461.

[12] Nagatsu, T. 1995. *Essays Biochem.* 30: 15–35.

[13] Nagatsu, T., and Ichinose, H. 1999. *Mol. Neurobiol.* 19: 79–96.

[14] Boadle-Biber, M. C. 1993. *Prog. Biophys. Mol. Biol.* 60: 1–15.

[15] Hamon, M. et al. 1981. *J. Physiol. (Paris)* 77: 269–279.

Synthesis of 5-Hydroxytryptamine (5-HT, Serotonin)

Serotonin is synthesized from tryptophan. The first step, conversion of tryptophan to 5-hydroxytryptophan (5-HTP) by the enzyme tryptophan hydroxylase, is rate-limiting (see Appendix B).[14] 5-HTP is decarboxylated to serotonin (also called 5-HT) by AAAD, the same enzyme that converts DOPA to dopamine. Stimulation of neurons releasing 5-HT causes an increase in the rate of conversion of tryptophan to 5-HT. It has been suggested that this is due to changes in the properties of tryptophan hydroxylase caused by calcium-dependent phosphorylation,[15] similar to the effects of stimulation on tyrosine hydroxylase. Like tyrosine hydroxylase, tryptophan hydroxylase requires the co-factor tetrahydrobiopterin, and serotonin synthesis is thought to be regulated by the availability of this co-factor.

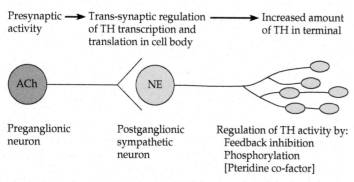

FIGURE 15.5   Regulation of Tyrosine Hydroxylase in sympathetic neurons. The expression of tyrosine hydroxylase (TH) is influenced by the activity of the presynaptic neuron, a process referred to as trans-synaptic regulation. This determines the amount of TH present in the cell and nerve terminal. Within nerve terminals, there is local control of tyrosine hydroxylase activity.

Neurons cannot synthesize tryptophan. Thus, the initial event leading to 5-HT synthesis is the facilitated transport of tryptophan from blood into cerebrospinal fluid (see Chapter 10). Other neutral amino acids (phenylalanine, leucine, and methionine) are transported from the blood into the brain by the same carrier. Thus, an important determinant of the level of 5-HT in serotonergic neurons is the relative amount of tryptophan compared with other neutral amino acids in the diet. As a result, behaviors associated with 5-HT function (see Chapter 14) are particularly sensitive to dietary influences.[16] For example, volunteers fed a low-protein diet for a day and then given a tryptophan-free amino acid mixture showed an increase in aggressive behavior[17] and changes in sleep cycle.[18]

Synthesis of GABA

GABA is synthesized from glutamate by the enzyme glutamic acid decarboxylase (GAD) (Figure 15.6). This reaction was first characterized as part of the so-called GABA shunt—a series of reactions by which α-ketoglutarate can be converted to succinate. The GABA shunt was originally considered to be a brain-specific pathway for glucose metabolism that bypassed part of the Krebs cycle (hence the term "shunt"). The discovery that GABA is the major inhibitory transmitter in the brain, together with the finding that glutamic acid decarboxylase is found only in neurons releasing GABA (see Chapter 14), suggests that the GABA shunt is not of general importance in glucose metabolism.

Kravitz and his colleagues showed that in crustacean inhibitory neurons, physiological levels of GABA inhibit glutamic acid decarboxylase, indicating that feedback inhibition regulates the accumulation of GABA.[19] Several additional regulators of GABA synthesis have been identified in the mammalian brain, including adenosine triphosphate (ATP), inorganic phosphate, and the co-factor pyridoxal phosphate.[20] Two forms of glutamic acid decarboxylase (GAD_{67} and GAD_{65}) are present in brain.[21,22] GAD_{67} has a high affinity for pyridoxal phosphate and so may be constitutively active. GAD_{65} has a lower affinity, and its activity may be rapidly regulated by co-factor availability. Mutant mice lacking GAD_{65} have normal behavior and levels of GABA but are slightly more susceptible to seizures. GAD_{67} knock-out mice show a substantial reduction in brain GABA and die shortly after birth from severe cleft palate.[23]

Synthesis of Glutamate

Glutamate is the major excitatory transmitter in the brain. There is more than one pathway for glutamate synthesis in cells. In neurons, glutamate destined for release as a transmitter is derived primarily from glutamine by a phosphate-activated form of the enzyme

[16] Sandyk, R. 1992. *Int. J. Neurosci.* 67: 127-144.

[17] Moeller, F. G. et al. 1996. *Psychopharmacology (Berl.)* 126: 96-103.

[18] Voderholzer, U. et al. 1998. *Neuropsychopharmacology* 18: 112-124.

[19] Hall, Z. W., Bownds, M. D., and Kravitz, E. A. 1970. *J. Cell Biol.* 46: 290-299.

[20] Martin, D. L. 1987. *Cell. Mol. Neurobiol.* 7: 237-253.

[21] Erlander, M. G. et al. 1991. *Neuron* 7: 91-100.

[22] Soghomonian, J. J., and Martin, D. L. 1998. *Trends Pharmacol. Sci.* 19: 500-505.

[23] Asada, H. et al. 1997. *Proc. Natl. Acad. Sci. USA* 94: 6496-6499.

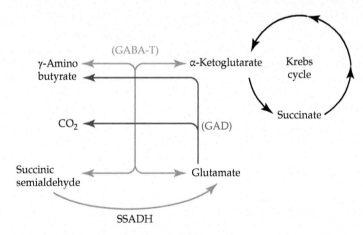

FIGURE 15.6 GABA Synthesis and Metabolism. GABA is synthesized from glutamate by the enzyme glutamic acid decarboxylase (GAD), which requires pyridoxal phosphate as a co-factor. Glutamate is synthesized from α-ketoglutarate by the enzyme GABA α-oxoglutarate transaminase (GABA-T) or from glutamine (see Figure 15.7). GABA is metabolized to succinic acid by GABA-T and succinic semialdehyde dehydrogenase (SSADH). (After R. W. Olsen and G.-D. Li, 2012. In *Basic Neurochemistry: Principles of Molecular, Cellular, and Medical Neurobiology* 8th ed., S. T. Brady et al. [Eds.]. Academic Press, Boston.)

FIGURE 15.7 Pathways for Glutamate Synthesis, Storage, Release, and Uptake in glutamatergic neurons. Glutamate is synthesized from glutamine within mitochondria by a phosphate-dependent form of the enzyme glutaminase. An inorganic phosphate (PO_4) transporter is localized to glutamatergic terminals. After release, some glutamate is taken up into presynaptic terminals; most is taken up by glial cells and converted to glutamine, which is then released and taken up into nerve terminals for conversion to glutamate. EAAT = excitatory amino acid transporter.

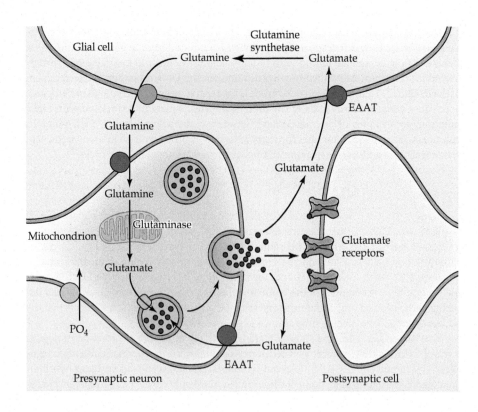

glutaminase[24] (Figure 15.7). Much of the glutamate released by neurons is taken up by glial cells and converted to glutamine. Glutamine, in turn, is released from the glial cells, taken up by neurons, and converted back to glutamate.[25–27]

Short- and Long-Term Regulation of Transmitter Synthesis

The regulatory mechanisms described so far operate rapidly to change the rate of synthesis within nerve terminals. In addition to such short-term effects, there are long-term regulatory mechanisms. A good example comes from the response of the sympathetic nervous system to prolonged exposure of an animal to stress. When the body is stressed, sympathetic neurons are activated. With prolonged activation, the levels of tyrosine hydroxylase and dopamine β-hydroxylase in the cell bodies and terminals of sympathetic neurons increase as much as three- to fourfold.[28,29] The increase is due to the synthesis of new enzyme molecules. Other enzymes of norepinephrine synthesis and degradation, such as AAAD and monoamine oxidase, are not affected.

The increase is triggered by synaptic activation of sympathetic neurons (see Figure 15.5). Such **trans-synaptic regulation** provides a mechanism whereby the synthetic capability of the neurons can be matched to the rate of transmitter release.[30] Experiments on human sympathetic ganglia have demonstrated that electrical stimulation of preganglionic fibers induces a marked increase in the level of the mRNAs for tyrosine hydroxylase and dopamine β-hydroxylase within 20 minutes, suggesting that the regulation of genes involved in norepinephrine synthesis is very rapid and sensitive.[31]

Synthesis of Neuropeptides

Regulation of the stores of peptide transmitters is complicated by the separation between the sites of synthesis and release. Peptides are synthesized on ribosomes, which are found predominantly (but not exclusively[32]) in neuronal cell bodies. This arrangement has two consequences. First, the rate of synthesis of peptides is regulated in the cell body, and the peptides must then be stored in vesicles and transported actively (as we will discuss in the next section). This is a slow process compared with the rapid local control of the synthesis and storage of low-molecular-weight transmitters within the axon terminal. Second, the amount of a

[24] Albrecht, J. et al. 2007. *Front. Biosci.* 12: 332-343.

[25] Palmada, M., and Centelles, J. J. 1998. *Front. Biosci.* 3: 701-718.

[26] Hertz, L. 2004. *Neurochem. Int.* 45: 285-296.

[27] Torres, G. E., and Amara, S. G. 2007. *Curr. Opin. Neurobiol.* 17: 304-312.

[28] Thoenen, H., Mueller, R. A., and Axelrod, J. 1969. *Nature* 221: 1264.

[29] Thoenen, H., Otten, U., and Schwab, M. 1979. In *The Neurosciences: Fourth Study Program.* MIT Press, Cambridge, MA. pp. 911-928.

[30] Comb, M., Hyman, S. E., and Goodman, H. M. 1987. *Trends Neurosci.* 10: 473-478.

[31] Schalling, M. et al. 1989. *Proc. Natl. Acad. Sci. USA* 86: 4302-4305.

[32] Giuditta, A. et al. 2008. *Physiol. Rev.* 88: 515-555.

peptide available for release is limited to the amount on hand in the terminal or extrasynaptic release sites. However, the binding of peptides to their receptors occurs at a much lower concentration (in the range of 10^{-10} to 10^{-8} M) than the binding of low-molecular-weight transmitters, such as ACh, to their receptors (10^{-7} to 10^{-4} M). In addition, the mechanisms by which they are removed from the extracellular space are generally slower. Moreover, neuropeptide receptors, like other metabotropic receptors, act indirectly through intracellular pathways that can provide great amplification (see Chapter 12). As a consequence, only a few molecules of a peptide are needed to influence a target cell, so the demands of release can be met by the supply of molecules transported from the cell body.

Peptides are synthesized as part of larger precursor proteins, which often contain the sequences for more than one biologically active peptide[33] (Figure 15.8). The initial steps

[33] Mains, R. E., and Eipper, B. A. 1999. In *Basic Neurochemistry: Molecular, Cellular, and Medical Aspects*, 6th ed. Lippincott-Raven, Philadelphia. pp. 363–382.

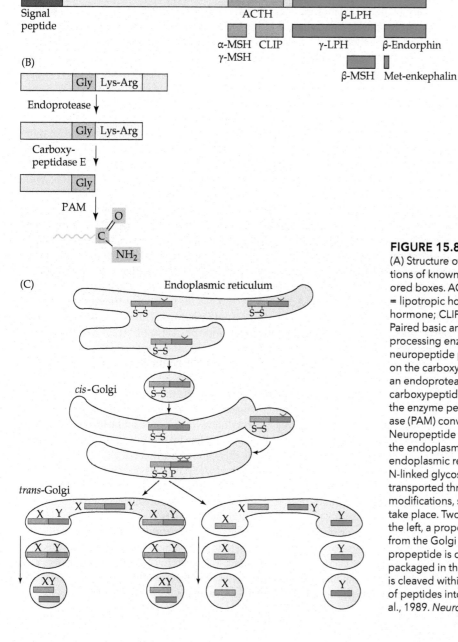

FIGURE 15.8 Synthesis of Neuropeptides.
(A) Structure of bovine pro-opiomelanocortin. The locations of known peptide components are shown by colored boxes. ACTH = adrenocorticotropic hormone; LPH = lipotropic hormone; MSH = melanocyte-stimulating hormone; CLIP = corticotropin-like intermediate peptide. Paired basic amino acid residues—common targets for processing enzymes—are indicated. (B) Processing of neuropeptide precursors usually begins with cleavage on the carboxy-terminal side of the recognition site by an endoprotease. The basic residues are trimmed by carboxypeptidase E. If the peptide ends in glycine (Gly), the enzyme peptidylglycine α-amidating monooxygenase (PAM) converts the carboxy terminus to an amide. (C) Neuropeptide precursors are directed into the lumen of the endoplasmic reticulum by a signal sequence. In the endoplasmic reticulum, disulfide bonds are formed and N-linked glycosylation occurs. The propeptide is then transported through the Golgi apparatus, where further modifications, such as sulfation and phosphorylation, take place. Two packaging schemes are illustrated. On the left, a propeptide is packaged into vesicles budding from the Golgi apparatus; as the vesicle matures, the propeptide is cleaved, resulting in two peptides (X and Y) packaged in the same vesicle. On the right, a propeptide is cleaved within the Golgi apparatus, followed by sorting of peptides into separate vesicles. (After W. S. Sossin et al., 1989. *Neuron* 2: 1407–1417.)

in neuropeptide precursor synthesis are those typical of secreted proteins: synthesis in the endoplasmic reticulum, signal peptide cleavage, processing in the Golgi apparatus, and incorporation into large (100- to 200-nm) dense-core vesicles, sometimes also containing low-molecular-weight transmitters. Later steps are unique to neurons and endocrine cells. They are catalyzed sequentially by: (1) specific endoproteases that cleave the precursor protein into the appropriate peptide molecules; (2) exopeptidases, which remove C-terminal basic residues; and (3) a bifunctional, amidating enzyme that converts the C-terminal peptidyl glycine to the corresponding peptide amide[34,35] (see Figure 15.8B). Proteolytic processing begins in the *trans*-Golgi network and continues within large dense-core vesicles as they are transported to release sites. Some cells synthesize more than one transmitter peptide; these can be differentially sorted into vesicles and targeted to different terminals.[36]

Storage of Transmitters in Vesicles

Low-molecular-weight transmitters, such as ACh and NE, are synthesized and packaged into vesicles in the cytoplasm, including the axon terminal. In electron micrographs synaptic vesicles containing transmitters tend to be small (50 nm in diameter) and appear clear; vesicles containing transmitters (e.g., biogenic amines) and peptides that are released outside synapses (extrasynaptically) are larger (100–200 nm) and have dense cores. The concentration of low-molecular-weight transmitters in vesicles is approximately 0.5 *M*—much greater than that in the surrounding cytoplasm.

The accumulation of transmitters in vesicles is mediated by specific transport proteins. They are members of a large superfamily of solute carrier (SLC) transporters[37] and are described in Chapter 9 (see Figure 9.5 and Table 9.1). An important point to note is that there are fewer types of vesicular transporters than there are neurotransmitters, so some SLCs transport more than one transmitter. Thus, while there are individual vesicular ACh transporters (VAChTs) and three vesicular glutamate transporters (VGLUT1, VGLUT2, and VGLUT3), there is only one vesicular inhibitory amino acid transporter (VIAAT) for both of the two inhibitory transmitters, GABA and glycine, and only one vesicular monoamine transporter (VMAT, with two variants, VMAT1 and 2) for all of the monoamines (i.e., norepinephrine, dopamine, serotonin, and histamine). A vesicular transporter for ATP has recently been identified, the vesicular nucleotide transporter (VNUT, from the SLC17A gene family), which also transports adenosine diphosphate (ADP) and guanosine triphosphate (GTP).[38]

This poor substrate specificity has some interesting consequences. Thus, it means that some vesicles can store and release more than one transmitter. For example, GABA and glycine are both substrates for the inhibitory amino acid transporter, VIAAT. Jonas and his colleagues[39] found that GABA and glycine are both released from the same vesicles in the presynaptic boutons of spinal interneurons. This co-release could be detected because GABA and glycine activate separate postsynaptic receptors, which can be distinguished pharmacologically. The miniature inhibitory postsynaptic currents, which result from transmitter release from a single vesicle, contained components resulting from activation of both of these receptors.

Another consequence is that the wrong transmitter can be taken up by the vesicles and then be released as a "false transmitter" instead of the natural transmitter. This property can be useful. For example, the drug α-methyldihydroxyphenylalanine (α-methyl DOPA), which was once used to reduce blood pressure, is taken up into adrenergic nerve terminals and converted to α-methylnorepinephrine through the normal NE biosynthetic pathway (see Figure 15.4); it is then taken up into the synaptic vesicles on the monoamine transporter (displacing norepinephrine) and can subsequently be released from the adrenergic terminals instead of norepinephrine.[40] Since α-methylnorepinephrine is less effective than norepinephrine in stimulating the postjunctional adrenergic receptors, α-methyl DOPA inhibits noradrenergic transmission and reduces blood pressure. The broad specificity of the monoamine transporters also means that the monoamine transmitters are potentially capable of replacing each other. Thus, when 5-HT levels in the brain are increased, serotonin can be taken up into the synaptic vesicles of dopaminergic neuron terminals in the striatum and subsequently released from these terminals.[41]

[34] Seidah, N. G., and Chretien, M. 1997. *Curr. Opin. Biotechnol.* 8: 602–607.

[35] Steiner, D. F. 1998. *Curr. Opin. Chem. Biol.* 2: 31–39.

[36] Salio, C. et al. 2006. *Cell Tissue Res.* 326: 583–598.

[37] Hediger, M. A. et al. 2004. *Pflügers Arch.* 447: 465–468.

[38] Sawada, K. et al. 2008. *Proc. Natl. Acad. Sci. USA* 105: 5683–5686.

[39] Jonas, P., Bischofberger, J., and Sandkuhler, J. 1998. *Science* 281: 419–424.

[40] Kopin, I. J. 1968. *Annu. Rev. Pharmacol.* 8: 377–394.

[41] Zhou, F. M. et al. 2005. *Neuron* 46: 65–74.

A further point to note is that vesicular uptake mechanisms may not be saturated. This means that the concentration of transmitter in the vesicles (and hence the quantum of transmitter released) is not necessarily constant but may vary in a manner dependent on several factors, including the availability of the transmitter, the proton gradient driving uptake (see Chapter 9), and the intracellular chloride concentration.[42,43] Thus, by patching onto the large presynaptic terminals of the calyx of Held, Takahashi and his colleagues found that the quantal size measured from the miniature postsynaptic currents varied with the amount of glutamate (between 1 and 100 mM) in the patching pipette.[44] The activity of VGLUT is regulated by the concentration of chloride ions in the terminals, which bind to an allosteric site on the transporter protein; this chloride effect is inhibited by some products of metabolism, such as ketone bodies, with a consequent reduction in hippocampal miniature synaptic currents.[45] The reduction in glutamatergic transmission was suggested to explain the antiepileptic effect of a ketogenic diet, which is high in fat and low in protein and carbohydrate.

Co-Storage and Co-Release

Following a suggestion by Sir Henry Dale,[46] neurons are customarily characterized by the transmitter they release—for example, cholinergic neurons (releasing ACh), adrenergic neurons (releasing norepinephrine or epinephrine), glutamatergic (releasing glutamate), and so on. However, it is now clear that many neurons (perhaps the majority) can release more than one transmitter: This effect has been dubbed "co-transmission."[47] In some cases co-transmission occurs because two transmitters are stored in the same vesicle—for example, the co-release of co-stored glycine and GABA[39] described in the previous section. Another example is ATP, which is frequently co-stored with catecholamines or ACh in synaptic vesicles and released as a co-transmitter.[48,49] Alternatively, co-released transmitters are stored in different vesicles but in the same nerve terminal; they may then be differentially released, depending on the frequency and pattern of action potential activity.[50,51] Thus, as described in Chapter 18, effective release of peptides usually requires repetitive action potentials or bursts of action potentials, unlike co-released amino acids or amines (see Chapter 13). A similar distinction has been observed between the pattern of activity required for the release of the same transmitter (5-HT) from clear vesicles at the nerve terminals and dense-core vesicles in the soma of the same neuron.[52]

In the mammalian CNS, the fast transmitters (glutamate or GABA) are often contained in and released from the same nerve terminals as those that store ACh, a monoamine, or a peptide.[53] Thus, the recurrent collaterals of motor axons that excite Renshaw interneurons in the spinal cord, which were originally deduced to be cholinergic,[54] have recently been shown to also release glutamate.[55] Co-release of glutamate and ACh has also been recorded from single axons of cholinergic neurons from the basal forebrain[56] (Figure 15.9). Previous immunocytochemical work had indicated that VGLUT and the ACh-synthesizing enzyme ChAT were sometimes both present in basal forebrain neurons, but their co-release at cortical synapses could not be tested directly using electrophysiological methods because the postsynaptic (muscarinic) action of ACh is slow and temporally dissociated from the afferent nerve impulses (see Chapters 12 and 14). The solution adopted was to generate an autaptic glutamate-transmitting neuronal synapse in single cell culture (see Figure 15.9A,B) and then to use a skeletal muscle myoball containing nicotinic receptors as a fast-responding ACh detector. In this way it could be shown that both transmitters were released simultaneously from the same axon (though not necessarily from the same bouton) (see Figure 15.9C). A similar autaptic approach has been used to show co-release of glutamate with dopamine from single dopaminergic neurons of the ventral midbrain.[57] In such cases, glutamate subserves the basic function of synaptic excitation while the co-released amine (or peptide) provides a more long-lasting modulatory function. Since the latter effect relates most closely to the overall function of the neurons (see Chapter 14), it is useful to preserve their amine- or peptide-based labels, such as cholinergic and so on, as originally suggested by Dale.[46]

Developmental and activity-dependent variations in the proportions of co-released transmitters (e.g., glutamate and GABA) can provide another mechanism of synaptic plasticity.[58]

[42] Erickson, J. D. et al. 2006. *Neurochem. Int.* 48: 643–649.

[43] Edwards, R. H. 2007. *Neuron* 55: 835–858.

[44] Ishikawa, T., Sahara, Y., and Takahashi, T. 2002. *Neuron* 34: 613–621.

[45] Juge, N. et al. 2010. *Neuron* 68: 99–112.

[46] Dale, H. H. 1933. *J. Physiol.* 80: 10–11.

[47] Burnstock, G. 1976. *Neuroscience* 1: 239–248.

[48] Dowdall, M. J., Boyne, A. F., and Whittaker, V. P. 1974. *Biochem. J.* 140: 1–12.

[49] De Potter, W. P., Smith, A. D., and De Schaepdryver, A. F. 1970. *Tissue Cell* 2: 529–546.

[50] Kupfermann, I. 1991. *Physiol. Rev.* 71: 683–732.

[51] Whim, M. D., Church, P. J., and Lloyd, P. E. 1993. *Mol. Neurobiol.* 7: 335–347.

[52] De-Miguel, F. F., and Trueta, C. 2005. *Cell. Mol. Neurobiol.* 25: 297–312.

[53] Seal, R. P., and Edwards, R. H. 2006. *Curr. Opin. Pharmacol.* 6: 114–119.

[54] Eccles, J. C., Fatt, P., and Koketsu, K. 1954. *J. Physiol.* 126: 524–562.

[55] Lamotte d'Incamps, B., and Ascher, P. 2008. *J. Neurosci.* 28: 14121–14131.

[56] Allen, T. G., Abogadie, F. C., and Brown, D. A. 2006. *J. Neurosci.* 26: 1588–1595.

[57] Sulzer, D. et al. 1998. *J. Neurosci.* 18: 4588–4602.

[58] Gutierrez, R., 2015. *J. Chem. Neuroanat.* 13: 9–20.

(A)

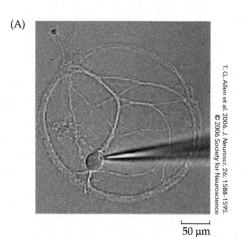

50 μm

(B)

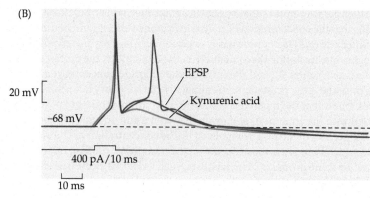

20 mV

–68 mV

EPSP

Kynurenic acid

400 pA/10 ms

10 ms

FIGURE 15.9 Simultaneous Release of Two Neurotransmitters from a Single Neuron. (A) A single cholinergic basal forebrain neuron dissociated from a rat brain was cultured in isolation for 3 weeks. During that time it sent out an axon that branched and went back to innervate the same neuron, forming an autapse. (B) An action potential was initiated by passing current into the neuron soma through a patch electrode. The action potential was conducted along the axon to the autapse, resulting in an excitatory postsynaptic potential (EPSP) and a second action potential in the soma. This EPSP was due to the release of glutamate, since it was reduced by the glutamate receptor antagonist kynurenic acid (1 m*M*). (C) Experimental arrangement. Stimulus was applied through the patch clamp electrode, which also recorded the EPSC produced by release of glutamate from the autapse (see D and E, left columns). A second patch electrode bearing a myoball (a small sphere of muscle membrane containing nicotinic receptors that can detect acetylcholine) was placed close to the axon forming the autapse. Responses of the myoball to ACh released from the autapse are shown in the right-hand columns of (D) and (E). (D,E) Simultaneous recordings of autaptic and myoball currents generated by a single action potential. The autaptic current is blocked by 1 m*M* kynurenic acid (D), showing that it is due to the release of glutamate, whereas the myoball current is blocked by 100 μM of the nicotinic blocker hexamethonium (E), showing that it is due to the release of acetylcholine. (After T. G. Allen et al., 2006. *J. Neurosci.* 26: 1588–1595. © 2006 Society for Neuroscience.)

(C)

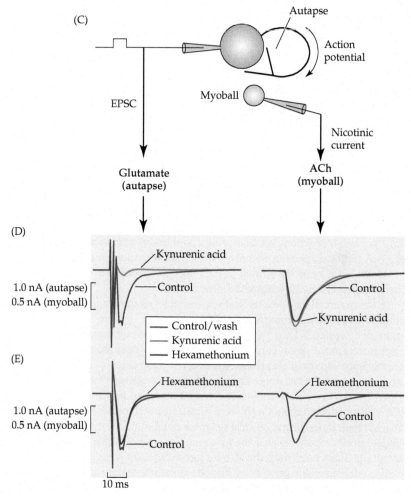

EPSC

Glutamate (autapse)

Autapse

Action potential

Myoball

Nicotinic current

ACh (myoball)

(D)

1.0 nA (autapse)
0.5 nA (myoball)

Kynurenic acid

Control

Control

Kynurenic acid

Control/wash
Kynurenic acid
Hexamethonium

(E)

1.0 nA (autapse)
0.5 nA (myoball)

Hexamethonium

Hexamethonium

Control

Control

10 ms

Axonal Transport

Proteins found in axon terminals must have been shipped there from the cell body, where they are synthesized. The first evidence for movement of material along axons came from experiments by Weiss and his colleagues, who ligated peripheral nerves and described the ballooning out of axons just proximal to the site of constriction, and the subsequent movement of the accumulated material along the axons after the constriction was removed.[59] These effects suggested that normally there is a continuous bulk movement of axoplasm along the axon at the rate of 1 to 2 mm/day, which was given the name **axoplasmic flow**. This idea was buttressed by later experiments using

[59] Weiss, P., and Hiscoe, H. B. 1948. *J. Exp. Zool.* 107: 315–395.

radioactively labeled amino acids[60] and fluorescent proteins[61] to follow the movement of proteins from neuronal cell bodies along peripheral and central axons. Such movement has even been observed in single axons in cell culture (Figure 15.10)[62] and in organelles along living nerve fibers, followed by cinematography.[63]

Rate and Direction of Axonal Transport

Measurement of the time course of accumulation of material proximal to a constriction or in axon terminals demonstrated characteristic differences in the rates of movement within the broad spectrum of components being transported. Structural proteins, such as tubulin and neurofilament proteins, move at the slowest rates (1–2 mm/day), while membrane-enclosed organelles, such as mitochondria and vesicles (including synaptic vesicles packed with transmitter), move much faster (up to 400 mm/day).[64] Such rapid movement could not be accounted for by the bulk flow of cytoplasm, and thus the general term **axonal transport** was adopted.

[60] Droz, B., and Leblond, C. P. 1963. *J. Comp. Neurol.* 121: 325–346.

[61] Dahlstrom, A. B. 2010. *Prog. Neurobiol.* 90: 119–145.

[62] Koehnle, T. J., and Brown, A. 1999. *J. Cell Biol.* 144: 447–458.

[63] Forman, D. S., Padjen, A. L., and Siggins, G. R. 1977. *Brain Res.* 136: 197–213.

[64] Grafstein, B., and Forman, D. S. 1980. *Physiol. Rev.* 60: 1167–1283.

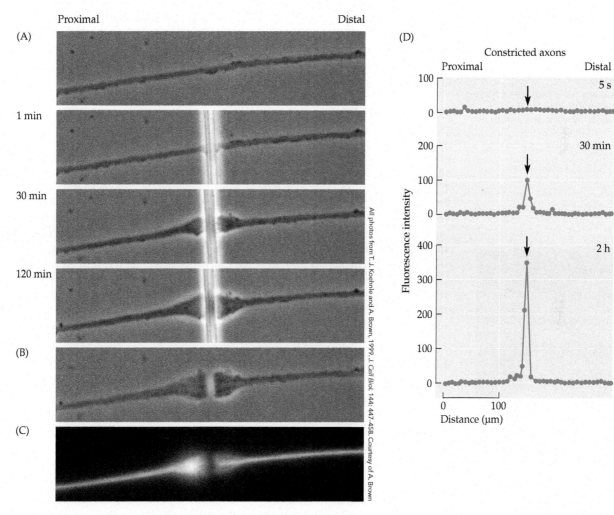

FIGURE 15.10 Slow Axonal Transport is demonstrated by the accumulation of cytoskeletal components at the site of axonal constriction. A single axon from a cultured rat dorsal root ganglion neuron was constricted by pressure from a glass fiber. (A) Phase-contrast images show the axon immediately before constriction and after 1, 30, and 120 minutes. (B) Two hours after constriction, the cell was fixed and the glass fiber removed. (C) Fluorescence micrograph of the axon labeled with anti-neurofilament protein antibodies. (D) Graphs of fluorescence intensity as a function of distance along axons constricted for 5 seconds, 30 minutes, or 2 hours. The time course of accumulation of neurofilament protein at the site of the constriction (arrow) indicated that the average transport rate was approximately 3 mm/day. (D after T. J. Koehnle and A. Brown, 1999. *J. Cell Biol.* 144: 447–458.)

[65] Vallee, R. B., and Bloom, G. S. 1991. *Annu. Rev. Neurosci.* 14: 59-92.

[66] Bartlett, S. E., Reynolds, A. J., and Hendry, I. A. 1998. *Immunol. Cell Biol.* 76: 419-423.

[67] Kuypers, H. G. J. M., and Ugolini, G. 1990. *Trends Neurosci.* 13: 71-75.

[68] Teune, T. M. et al. 1998. *J. Comp. Neurol.* 392: 164-178.

[69] Inoue, S. 1981. *J. Cell Biol.* 89: 346-356.

[70] Allen, R. D., Allen, N. S., and Travis, J. L. 1981. *Cell Motil.* 1: 291-302.

[71] Brady, S. T., Lasek, R. J., and Allen, R. D. 1982. *Science* 218: 1129-1131.

[72] Vale, R. D., and Fletterick, R. J. 1997. *Annu. Rev. Cell Dev. Biol.* 13: 745-777.

[73] Vallee, R. B., and Gee, M. A. 1998. *Trends Cell Biol.* 8: 490-494.

[74] Hirokawa, N. 1998. *Science* 279: 519-552.

[75] Sheetz, M. P. 1999. *Eur. J. Biochem.* 262: 19-25.

[76] Howard, J., Hudspeth, A. J., and Vale, R. D. 1989. *Nature* 342: 154-158.

[77] Svoboda, K. et al. 1993. *Nature* 365: 721-727.

[78] Mandelkow, E., and Hoenger, A. 1999. *Curr. Opin. Cell Biol.* 11: 34-44.

[79] Hirokawa, N., Niwa, S. and Tanaka, Y. 2010. *Neuron* 68: 610-638.

[80] Kodera, N. et al. 2010. *Nature* 468: 72-76.

[81] Baas, P. W., and Brown, A. 1997. *Trends Cell Biol.* 7: 380-384.

[82] Hirokawa, N. et al. 1997. *Trends Cell Biol.* 7: 382-388.

Some proteins and organelles move toward the axon terminal (anterograde transport), and others from the terminal to the cell body (**retrograde transport**).[63,65] Retrograde transport of membrane-enclosed organelles returns material to the cell body for recycling or degradation, and it has been shown to be crucial for the movement of trophic molecules, such as nerve growth factor, from axon terminals back to cell bodies (see Chapter 27).[66]

Neuroanatomists have developed tracers, such as horseradish peroxidase, fluorescently labeled beads, and even viruses, that are carried in anterograde and retrograde directions by axonal transport. Using tracers such as these, it is possible to map synaptic connections, even over long distances, by visualizing individual axons, their terminal arborizations, and their cell bodies.[67,68]

Microtubules and Fast Transport

Although early experiments demonstrated that axonal transport required metabolic energy and relied on intact microtubules, for 30 years little progress was made in understanding its mechanism. Then two technological advances triggered very rapid progress: (1) the development of microscopic techniques that allowed direct visualization of single vesicles within cells,[69,70] and (2) the finding that vesicle movements persisted in cell-free systems, such as extruded squid axoplasm.[71] Studies by Reese, Sheetz, Schnapp, Vale, Block, and their colleagues have demonstrated that transport occurs by the attachment of organelles, such as mitochondria and vesicles, to microtubules. Mechanochemical enzymes, or motors, hydrolyze ATP and use the energy to carry organelles along the microtubule track (Figure 15.11).[72,73]

Microtubules have an inherent polarity; in axons, the plus (i.e., positive, centrifugal) end points toward the distal axon terminal. Anterograde transport is powered by kinesin, which moves organelles toward the plus end, while retrograde transport is powered by cytoplasmic dynein, which moves organelles toward the minus (i.e., negative, centripetal) end (Figure 15.12).[74] Specific receptors on the surface of organelles mediate the attachment of either kinesin or cytoplasmic dynein and thus regulate the direction of organelle movement (Figure 15.13).[75] Remarkably, a single kinesin motor has been shown to pull an organelle along at speeds equivalent to fast axonal transport;[76] each molecule of ATP hydrolyzed produces a step of approximately 8 nm, corresponding to the distance from one αβ tubulin dimer to the next along the microtubule protofilament.[77,78] Differences in the rate of transport of different components arise from differences in the proportion of time they remain on track and in the resistance they encounter trying to penetrate the dense network of cytoskeletal and cross-bridging elements within the axon. In synaptic regions, actin forms the major cytoskeletal protein and myosins are the main molecular motors.[79] Analogous stepping transport by myosin has recently been examined in detail using high-speed atomic force microscopy.[80]

Mechanism of Slow Axonal Transport

Soluble proteins of intermediary metabolism and cytoskeletal elements, such as microtubules and neurofilaments, move from the cell body toward the axon terminal by slow transport.[63] There is considerable debate about whether microtubules and neurofilaments move as intact polymers[81] or if polymerized filaments are stationary and tubulin and neurofilament monomers or oligomers are transported.[82] What is clear is that diffusion cannot account for the axonal transport of cytoskeletal proteins and that an active process is involved.

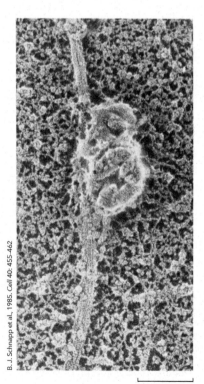

B. J. Schnapp et al., 1985. *Cell* 40: 455-462.

0.1 μm

FIGURE 15.11 Identifying the Organelles and Tracks Mediating Fast Axonal Transport. Electron micrograph of a vesicle attached to a microtubule in extruded squid axoplasm. Before fixation, this organelle was observed by light microscopy moving along a filamentous track at a rate corresponding to fast axonal transport. The electron micrograph shows that the organelle is a synaptic vesicle, and the track is a microtubule. A layer of granular and finely filamentous material coats the glass substrate.

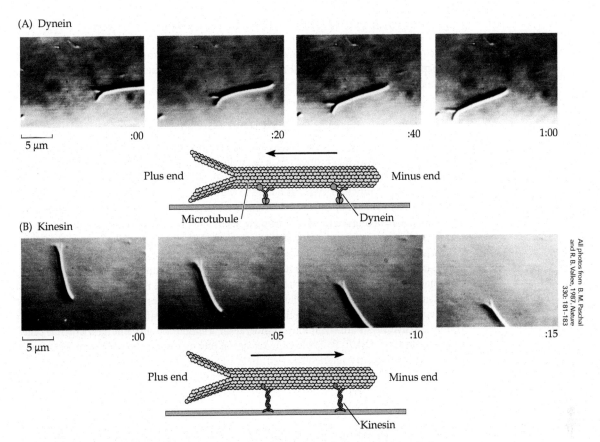

FIGURE 15.12 **The Molecular Motors Dynein and Kinesin Propel Microtubules in Opposite Directions.** (A,B) Sequential images of the movement of microtubule fragments on purified fast-transport motors. Time is indicated in minutes. Purified cytoplasmic dynein (A) or kinesin (B) was adsorbed to a cover slip, and fragments of microtubules were added. When the fragments contacted the surface, they were propelled toward their frayed (distal, or +) end on dynein and toward their compact (proximal, or –) end on kinesin, as illustrated. (After B. M. Paschal and R. B. Vallee, 1987. *Nature* 330: 181–183.)

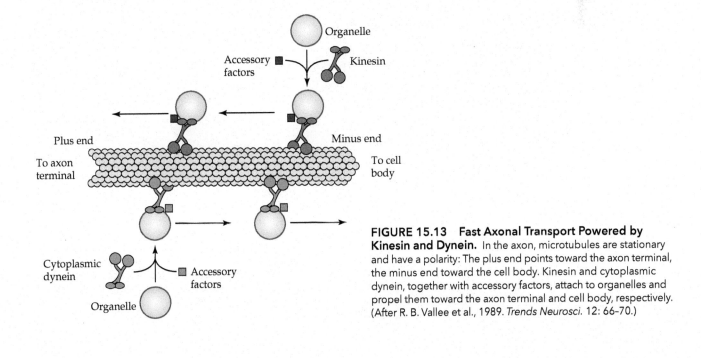

FIGURE 15.13 **Fast Axonal Transport Powered by Kinesin and Dynein.** In the axon, microtubules are stationary and have a polarity: The plus end points toward the axon terminal, the minus end toward the cell body. Kinesin and cytoplasmic dynein, together with accessory factors, attach to organelles and propel them toward the axon terminal and cell body, respectively. (After R. B. Vallee et al., 1989. *Trends Neurosci.* 12: 66–70.)

Removal of Transmitters from the Synaptic Cleft

The final step in chemical synaptic transmission is the removal of transmitter from the synaptic cleft. The mechanisms for transmitter removal include diffusion, degradation, and uptake into glial cells or nerve terminals.

Removal of ACh by Acetylcholinesterase

As described in Chapter 9 the action of ACh is terminated by the enzyme acetylcholinesterase (AChE), which hydrolyzes ACh to choline and acetate. Much of the choline is transported back into the nerve terminal and reused for ACh synthesis. At the vertebrate skeletal neuromuscular junction, AChE is bound to the synaptic basal lamina—that portion of the muscle fiber's sheath of extracellular matrix material that occupies the synaptic cleft and junctional folds (Figure 15.14).[83] There are 2600 catalytic subunits of AChE per square micrometer of synaptic basal lamina[84] (compared with the 10^4 ACh receptors per square micrometer in the postsynaptic membrane).

It might seem inefficient to have acetylcholinesterase situated between the axon terminal and the postsynaptic membrane, forcing molecules of ACh to traverse a minefield of degradative enzymes before having an opportunity to interact with their postsynaptic receptors. However, if the dimensions of the cleft and the rates of ACh diffusion, binding, and hydrolysis are taken into consideration, a simple scheme emerges, which is called the **saturated disk**.[85] Following the release of one quantum, the concentration of ACh increases almost instantaneously (within less than a millisecond) across the width of the cleft to a level high enough (0.5 mM) to saturate both ACh receptors and esterase within a

[83] McMahan, U. J., Sanes, J. R., and Marshall, L. M. 1978. *Nature* 271: 172-174.

[84] Salpeter, M. M. 1987. In *The Vertebrate Neuromuscular Junction.* Alan R. Liss, New York. pp. 1-54.

[85] Bartol, T. M. et al. 1991. *Biophys. J.* 59: 1290-1307.

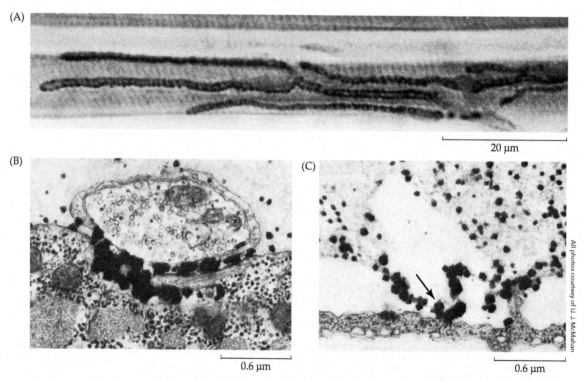

All photos courtesy of U. J. McMahan

FIGURE 15.14 Acetylcholinesterase Is Concentrated in the synaptic basal lamina at the skeletal neuromuscular junction. (A) Light micrograph of a neuromuscular junction in a frog cutaneous pectoris muscle stained by a histochemical procedure for acetylcholinesterase. The dark reaction product lines the synaptic gutters and junctional folds. (B) Electron micrograph of a cross section of an axon terminal from a muscle stained for acetylcholinesterase as in (A). The electron-dense reaction product fills the synaptic cleft and the junctional folds. (C) Electron micrograph of a damaged muscle in which the nerve terminal, Schwann cell, and muscle fiber have degenerated and been phagocytized, leaving only empty basal lamina sheaths (see Chapter 29). The damaged muscle was stained for acetylcholinesterase; reaction product is associated with the synaptic basal lamina (arrow).

disk approximately 0.5 μm in diameter centered on the release site. Binding of ACh to its receptors and to AChE is rapid compared with the rate at which AChE can hydrolyze ACh (it takes AChE 0.1 ms to hydrolyze one molecule of ACh). Therefore, the fraction of ACh molecules released that bind initially to postsynaptic receptors is determined by the ratio of receptors to esterase; thus, approximately 70% of the ACh molecules bind to AChE and approximately 30% to ACh receptors.[86] Binding causes a precipitous fall in ACh concentration. The concentration then remains low because AChE can hydrolyze ACh molecules much faster (10 molecules/ms) than they are released from receptors as the channels close (mean open time, τ, = 1 ms; see Chapter 11). Thus, by 0.1 ms or so after release, the concentration of ACh in the cleft has fallen to levels that make the probability of two ACh molecules being available to bind and open another receptor negligible.

Such an analysis predicts that inhibition of acetylcholinesterase should have a more pronounced effect on the duration of the synaptic potential than on its amplitude, which is the case. Amplitude is increased 1.5-fold to 2-fold, and the duration is increased 3-fold to 5-fold.[87] Thus, the organization of the neuromuscular junction and the density and kinetic properties of ACh receptors and AChE combine to produce a synapse that is capable of very rapid responses and efficient use of ACh.

Acetylcholinesterase seems to have a similar function in cholinergic nerve–nerve synapses, such as those in autonomic ganglia, in that its inhibition prolongs the synaptic current.[88,89] However, much of the AChE at these sites is located on the presynaptic fibers,[90,91] where it probably has the additional function of reducing the ACh overspill during repetitive nerve activity. Cholinesterase inhibitors produce a much more dramatic enhancement and prolongation of the slow synaptic current produced by repetitive afferent stimulation; this results from stimulation of muscarinic ACh receptors outside the immediate area of the synapse[92] (see Chapters 14 and 17).

Removal of ATP by Hydrolysis

The action of ATP, like that of ACh, is rapidly terminated by hydrolysis.[93] Ecto-ATP diphosphohydrolase (ecto-ADPase or ecto-apyrase) hydrolyzes ATP to ADP and ADP to AMP. AMP is converted to adenosine by ecto-5′-nucleotidase. Both enzymes are found on glial cells, and at synaptic sites on neurons. At many synapses, adenosine modulates transmission by combining with receptors on pre- and postsynaptic cells.[94] ATP and adenosine are also mediators of extrasynaptic communication between neurons, glia, and blood vessels (see Chapter 18). The action of adenosine is terminated by uptake and by adenosine deaminase, which degrades adenosine to inosine.

Removal of Transmitters by Uptake

The actions of dopamine, norepinephrine, glutamate, 5-HT, glycine, and GABA are terminated by uptake of the transmitter into presynaptic nerve terminals, postsynaptic cells, or glial cells by specific transport proteins.[95,96] Transmitters transported into nerve terminals can be repackaged and released again. This process was first shown for norepinephrine uptake into sympathetic nerve endings by Julius Axelrod and his colleagues.[97,98] They found that radioactively labeled NE was accumulated in sympathetically innervated tissues, that this was prevented by sympathetic denervation, and that the labeled NE could be released again by sympathetic nerve stimulation.

The properties of these membrane transporters are described in detail in Chapter 9. There are separate membrane transporters for norepinephrine, dopamine, and 5-HT, and for the amino acids glutamate, GABA, and glycine. These are distinct from the vesicular transporters and show less substrate overlap (though there is some overlap between the norepinephrine and dopamine transporters). The transporters for the monoamines are important targets for several drugs used to treat psychiatric disorders, such as depression, and also for some recreational drugs, such as cocaine and the amphetamines[95] (see Chapter 14).

There appear to be no specific uptake mechanisms for peptide transmitters. Their transmitter action is terminated by diffusion, or in some cases by peptidase hydrolysis.[99]

[86] Kuffler, S. W., and Yoshikami, D. 1975. *J. Physiol.* 251: 465–482.

[87] Katz, B., and Miledi, R. 1975. *Proc. R. Soc. Lond. B* 192: 27–38.

[88] MacDermott, A. B. et al. 1980. *J. Gen. Physiol.* 75: 39–60.

[89] Rang, H. P. 1981. *J. Physiol.* 311: 23–55.

[90] Weitsen, H. A., and Weight, F. F. 1977. *Brain Res.* 128: 197–211.

[91] Davis, R., and Koelle, G. B. 1978. *J. Cell Biol.* 78: 785–809.

[92] Brown, D. A., and Selyanko, A. A. 1985. *J. Physiol.* 365: 335–364.

[93] Zimmermann, H. 2006. In *Novartis Foundation Symposium 276: Purinergic Signalling in Neuron-Glial Interactions.* Wiley, Chichester, UK, pp. 113–128.

[94] Dunwiddie, T. V., and Masino, S. A. 2001. *Annu. Rev. Neurosci.* 24: 31–55.

[95] Gether, U. et al. 2006. *Trends Pharmacol. Sci.* 27: 375–383.

[96] Iversen, L. 2006. *Brit. J. Pharmacol.* 147 (Suppl. 1): S82–S88.

[97] Hertting, G. et al. 1961. *Nature* 189: 66.

[98] Hertting, G., and Axelrod, J. 1961. *Nature* 192: 172–173.

[99] Isaac, R. E., Bland, N. D., and Shirras, A. D. 2009. *Gen. Comp. Endocrinol.* 162: 8–17.

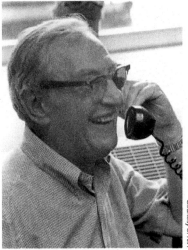

Julius Axelrod, 1970

SUMMARY

- ACh, norepinephrine, epinephrine, dopamine, 5-HT, histamine, ATP, GABA, glycine, and glutamate are low-molecular-weight transmitters. Neuropeptides form a second group of transmitters.

- Many neurons release more than one transmitter, typically a low-molecular-weight transmitter and one or more neuropeptides.

- Low-molecular-weight transmitters are synthesized in the cytoplasm, including that of varicosities and axon terminals, packaged in small vesicles, and stored for release. Feedback mechanisms control the number and activity of enzymes that catalyze transmitter synthesis, therefore maintaining an adequate supply of transmitter.

- Neuropeptides are synthesized in the cell body, processed and packaged in large dense-core vesicles in the Golgi apparatus, and transported to the axon and dendrites.

- Slow axonal transport moves soluble proteins and components of the cytoskeleton from the cell body to the axon terminal at a rate of 1 to 2 mm/day.

- Fast axonal transport moves vesicles and other organelles at speeds of up to 400 mm/day either toward the release sites (anterograde transport) or toward the cell soma (retrograde transport). Fast transport is mediated by molecular motors that move organelles along microtubules.

- The final step in chemical synaptic transmission is the removal of transmitter from the synaptic cleft by diffusion, degradation, or uptake. Prompt transmitter removal is important for normal synaptic function.

Suggested Reading

General Reviews

Axelrod, J. 1971. Noradrenaline: Fate and control of its biosynthesis. *Science* 173: 598–606.

Chen, N. H., Reith, M. E., and Quick, M. W. 2004. Synaptic uptake and beyond: the sodium- and chloride-dependent neurotransmitter transporter family SLC6. *Pflügers Arch.* 447: 519–531.

Cooper, J. R., Bloom, F. E., and Roth, R. H. 2003. *The Biochemical Basis of Pharmacology*, 8th ed. Oxford University Press, New York.

Edwards, R. H. 2007. The neurotransmitter cycle and quantal size. *Neuron* 55: 835–858.

Guedes-Dias, P., and Holzbauer, E. L. F. 2019. Axonal transport: Driving synaptic function. *Science* 366: 199. doi: 10.1126/science.aaw9997.

Hediger, M. A., Romero, M. F., Peng, J. B., Rolfs, A., Takanaga, H., and Bruford, E. A. 2004. The ABCs of solute carriers: physiological, pathological and therapeutic implications of human membrane transport proteins. Introduction. *Pflügers Arch.* 447: 465–468.

Hirokawa, N., Niwa, S., and Tanaka, Y. 2010. Molecular motors in neurons: transport mechanisms and roles in brain function, development, and disease. *Neuron* 68: 610–638.

Hökfelt, T., Broberger, C., Xu, Z. Q., Sergeyev, V., Ubink, R., and Diez, M. 2000. Neuropeptides—an overview. *Neuropharmacology* 39: 1337–1356.

Iversen, L. 2006. Neurotransmitter transporters and their impact on the development of psychopharmacology. *Brit. J. Pharmacol.* 147, Suppl. 1: S82–88.

Prado, M. A., Reis, R. A., Prado, V. F., de Mello, M. C., Gomez, M. V., and de Mello, F. G. 2002. Regulation of acetylcholine synthesis and storage. *Neurochem. Int.* 41: 291–299.

Seal, R. P., and Edwards, R. H. 2006. Functional implications of neurotransmitter co-release: glutamate and GABA share the load. *Curr. Opin. Pharmacol.* 6: 114–119.

Torres, G. E., and Amara, S. G. 2007. Glutamate and monoamine transporters: new visions of form and function. *Curr. Opin. Neurobiol.* 17: 304–312.

Vallee, R. B., and Bloom, G. S. 1991. Mechanisms of fast and slow axonal transport. *Annu. Rev. Neurosci.* 14: 59–92.

Original Papers

Allen, T. G., Abogadie, F. C., and Brown, D. A. 2006. Simultaneous release of glutamate and acetylcholine from single magnocellular "cholinergic" basal forebrain neurons. *J. Neurosci.* 26: 1588–1595.

Birks, R. I., and MacIntosh, F. C. 1961. Acetylcholine metabolism of a sympathetic ganglion. *Can. J. Biochem. Physiol.* 39: 787–827.

Brady, S. T., Lasek, R. J., and Allen, R. D. 1982. Fast axonal transport in extruded axoplasm from squid giant axon. *Science* 218: 1129–1131.

Forman, D. S., Padjen, A. L., and Siggins, G. R. 1977. Axonal transport of organelles visualized by light microscopy: Cinemicrographic and computer analysis. *Brain Res.* 136: 197–213.

(An accompanying movie, *Movement of Organelles in Living Nerve Fibers*, is available at the following website: http://www.alp.mcgill.ca/Pub/Pub_Main_Display.asp?LC_Docs_ID=4911)

Howard, J., Hudspeth, A. J., and Vale, R. D. 1989. Movement of microtubules by single kinesin molecules. *Nature* 342: 154–158.

Jonas, P., Bischofberger, J., and Sandkühler, J. 1998. Corelease of two fast neurotransmitters at a central synapse. *Science* 281: 419–424.

Kodera, N., Yamamoto, D., Ishikawa, R., and Ando, T. 2010. Video imaging of walking myosin V by high-speed atomic force microscopy. *Nature* 468: 72–76.

Kuromi, H., and Kidokoro, Y. 1998. Two distinct pools of synaptic vesicles in single presynaptic boutons in a temperature-sensitive *Drosophila* mutant, *shibire*. *Neuron* 20: 917–925.

McMahan, U. J., Sanes, J. R., and Marshall, L. M. 1978. Cholinesterase is associated with the basal lamina at the neuromuscular junction. *Nature* 271: 172–174.

Schnapp, B. J., Vale, R. D., Sheetz, M. P., and Reese, T. S. 1985. Single microtubules from squid axoplasm support bi-directional movement of organelles. *Cell* 40: 455–462.

CHAPTER 16

Synaptic Plasticity

The efficacy of transmission at a synapse is not fixed, but can vary as a consequence of patterns of ongoing activity. Short trains of presynaptic action potentials can produce either facilitation of transmitter release from the presynaptic terminal that persists for several hundred milliseconds, or depression of release lasting for seconds, or a combination of both. More prolonged trains of presynaptic action potentials produce post-tetanic potentiation (PTP), an increase in transmitter release that can last for several minutes. An intermediate phase of enhancement, classified as augmentation, decays with a time course similar to that of synaptic depression. These changes in synaptic efficacy are closely linked to accumulation of calcium in the presynaptic cytoplasm during activity, and its subsequent extrusion.

At many synapses repetitive activity can produce not only short-term changes, but also alterations in synaptic efficacy that last experimentally for hours or even days. The two phenomena of this type are known as long-term potentiation (LTP) and long-term depression (LTD). LTP is mediated by an increase in calcium concentration in the postsynaptic cell that sets in motion a series of second-messenger systems that recruit additional receptors into the postsynaptic membrane and, in addition, increase receptor sensitivity. LTD appears to be associated with smaller increases in postsynaptic calcium concentration and is accompanied by a reduction in the number and sensitivity of postsynaptic receptors. LTP and LTD appear to involve presynaptic mechanisms as well. Because of their persistence for long periods, LTP and LTD have been postulated to be substrates for various forms of learning and formation of memory.

So far we have discussed excitatory and inhibitory synaptic transmission in terms of a single action potential arriving at the presynaptic nerve terminal, causing depolarization, calcium entry, and transmitter release, followed by a postsynaptic potential change. Under such circumstances, except for statistical variations, the postsynaptic responses at any given synapse are relatively stable. During everyday activity, however, synapses in the nervous system are not usually activated by the arrival of an occasional presynaptic action potential. Instead, constant streams of action potentials invade the terminals—sometimes regularly with clocklike intervals, other times in bursts of varying frequency and duration. Such ongoing activity can have marked effects on the efficacy of synaptic transmission, with changes that occur over a wide range of timescales.

Short-Term Changes in Signaling

Facilitation and Depression of Transmitter Release

When a brief train of stimuli is applied to a presynaptic nerve, the amplitude of the resulting postsynaptic potentials may progressively increase (**synaptic facilitation**), decrease (**synaptic depression**), or undergo a combination of both. This process is illustrated in Figure 16.1A, which shows end plate potentials recorded from a frog neuromuscular junction, produced by a short train of impulses to the motor nerve. The end plate potentials were reduced in amplitude by lowering calcium in the bathing solution so that the initial quantum content of the potentials was low (less than 10). The amplitudes of the potentials (measured from the starting point of each rising phase) increase progressively during the train. Furthermore, the effect outlasts the stimulus train, so that the response to a test stimulus occurring 230 milliseconds (ms) later is still larger than the first response in the sequence. So in this experiment, repetitive stimulation resulted in facilitation.

Transmitter release can also be subject to synaptic depression if the number of quanta released by a train of stimuli is large. A similar experiment on a muscle in higher calcium concentration is shown in Figure 16.1B. Here the quantal release is very large, but the responses have been reduced in amplitude by blocking the postjunctional acetylcholine (ACh) receptors with curare. During repetitive stimulation, the responses become progressively smaller in amplitude. As with facilitation, depression outlasts the stimulus train (not shown) and can persist for several seconds. After a long train of repetitive stimulation, depression can be severe, reducing the amplitude of the synaptic potential to less than 20% of its previous value.

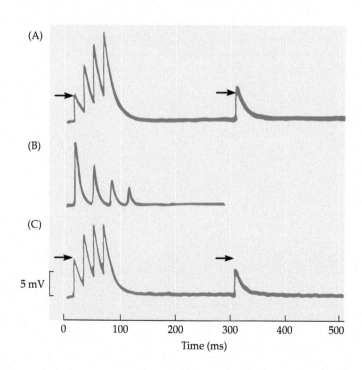

FIGURE 16.1   Facilitation and Depression at the Vertebrate Neuromuscular Junction. (A) When muscle is bathed in a low-calcium solution to reduce the quantum content of the response, the amplitudes of end plate potentials increase progressively during a train of four impulses. The response to a test pulse occurring 230 ms later is still facilitated (arrows indicate initial amplitude). (B) Similar experiment with a curarized preparation in a high-calcium solution. The response amplitudes decrease progressively during the train. (C) Interaction between facilitation and depression in normal calcium. The second response is facilitated, but there is no subsequent increase in response amplitude because of the onset of depression. The test response recorded 230 ms after the end of the stimulus train is still depressed. (A,C after A. Mallart and A. R. Martin, 1968. *J. Physiol.* 196: 593-604; B after A. Lundberg and H. Quilisch, 1953. *Acta Physiol. Scand.* 30: 121-129.)

Figure 16.1C illustrates how facilitation and depression can interact at intermediate levels of release. During the train of impulses, the initial facilitation is overridden by depression. Although the overall amplitude of the response increases because of summation, there is no increase in amplitude of the individual responses after the second response. Later, when the test pulse is given, facilitation has worn off and only depression remains.

Post-Tetanic Potentiation and Augmentation

A relatively long, high-frequency train of stimuli (commonly called a *tetanus* because such a train of stimuli applied to a muscle or to its motor nerve produces a tetanic muscle contraction) usually results in synaptic depression but is followed a few seconds later by an increase in synaptic potential amplitude that can persist for tens of minutes. This is called **post-tetanic potentiation** (PTP). Figure 16.2 shows an example from an experiment on a cell in a ciliary ganglion from a chicken, treated with curare to reduce the amplitude of the excitatory postsynaptic potential (EPSP). In addition, in order to prevent the synaptic potential from triggering an action potential, the cell was hyperpolarized (long downward deflection) before stimulating the presynaptic nerve. The first upward deflection is an electrical coupling potential (see Chapter 11); the second, slower depolarization is the EPSP, produced by release of ACh from the presynaptic terminal. It is the EPSP that is of interest. Initially the EPSP was only about 4 mV in amplitude (because of curarization). The presynaptic nerve was then stimulated at 100 pulses/second for 15 seconds (1500 stimuli), which caused a transient depression of the EPSP (not shown). Fifteen seconds later, however, a single test stimulus produced an EPSP well over 20 mV in amplitude (see Figure 16.2B)—so large, in fact, that it exceeded threshold and produced an action potential! The EPSP amplitudes produced by subsequent test shocks then declined (see Figure 16.2C–E), but the response was still twice the pre-tetanic amplitude 10 minutes after the end of the tetanic stimulation (see Figure 16.2F).

PTP is also associated with an increase in the rate of ongoing spontaneous, or tonic, transmitter release from the nerve terminal. The spontaneous appearance of individual miniature synaptic potentials is accelerated after the tetanus and then declines to resting level over the same time course as the potentiation itself.[1,2]

An intermediate phase of enhancement of transmitter release by repetitive stimulation has been designated **augmentation**.[3] It is produced by stimulus trains of moderate duration, comes on more slowly than facilitation, and decays over a period of several seconds. At the frog neuromuscular junction, augmentation and facilitation together can increase synaptic potential amplitude by a factor of more than five.

[1] Liley, A. W. 1956. *J. Physiol.* 133: 571–587.

[2] Martin, A. R., and Pilar, G. 1964. *J. Physiol.* 175: 16–30.

[3] Magleby, K. L., and Zengel, J. E. 1976. *J. Physiol.* 257: 449–470.

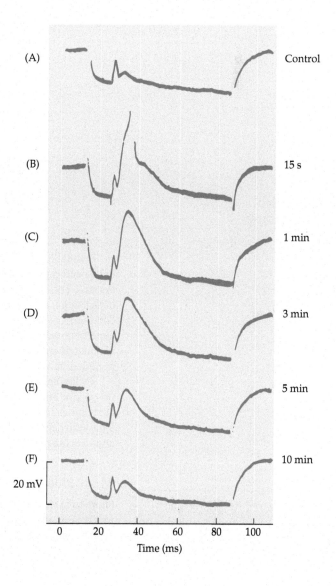

FIGURE 16.2 Post-Tetanic Potentiation (PTP) of the excitatory postsynaptic potential (EPSP) in a chick ciliary ganglion cell, produced by preganglionic nerve stimulation. Potentials were recorded with an intracellular microelectrode. To prevent action potential initiation, the EPSP amplitude was reduced with curare and a hyperpolarizing pulse applied though the recording electrode before each stimulus. (A) The control record shows electrical coupling potential (brief depolarization) followed by a small EPSP. (B) Response recorded 15 seconds after the end of a train of 1500 stimuli applied to the preganglionic nerve. The EPSP amplitude is more than six times greater than control, giving rise to an action potential. Amplitude of coupling potential is unchanged. (C–F) Test stimuli at 1, 3, 5, and 10 minutes after the tetanus produce slow decline of potentiation, with the EPSP in the last record still more than twice the control value. (From A. R. Martin and G. Pilar, 1964. *J. Physiol.* 175: 16–30.)

FIGURE 16.3 Time Courses of Activity-Induced Changes in synaptic transmission. Graphs indicate the amplitude of the synaptic response to a test stimulus—relative to that recorded before a conditioning stimulus train—as a function of time after the end of the train. (A) Facilitation has two components: a larger one decaying with a time constant of about 50 msec and a smaller one with a decay time constant of about 250 msec. (B) Recovery from depression is complete, and augmentation is largely dissipated after 10 seconds. (C) Post-tetanic potentiation (PTP) lasts for more than 10 minutes. (D) Long-term potentiation (LTP) and long-term depression (LTD) can last well beyond 10 hours.

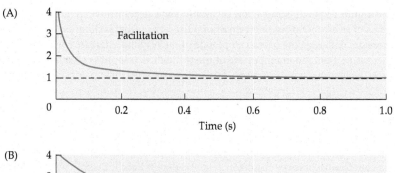

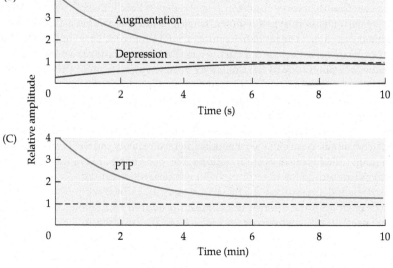

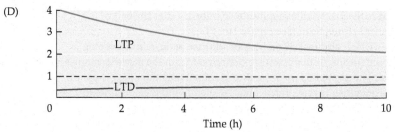

Facilitation, depression, augmentation, and PTP, although first observed at the vertebrate neuromuscular junction, occur throughout the vertebrate and invertebrate nervous systems. Their characteristic time courses are summarized in Figure 16.3A–C. The decay of facilitation is not a simple exponential process, but instead has two components. A small component decays over a relatively long period with a time constant of about 250 ms. Superimposed on that is a much larger and briefer component with a decay time constant of about 50 ms.[4] Decay of augmentation and recovery from depression both occur over periods of several seconds. PTP usually decays with a time constant of several minutes.

Facilitation, depression, augmentation, and PTP are referred to as short-term changes in synaptic efficacy, to distinguish them from two changes that last much longer, found at synapses in the central nervous system (CNS)—long-term potentiation (LTP) and long-term depression (LTD), discussed later in the chapter. As shown in Figure 16.3D, LTP and LTD can persist for hours.

Mechanisms Underlying Short-Term Synaptic Changes

Short-term changes in synaptic efficacy during and following repetitive activity are related to increases or decreases in the number of quanta of transmitter released from the presynaptic terminals and not, for example, to a change in the size of an individual quantum or to a change in the sensitivity of the postsynaptic membrane.[1,5,6] As discussed in Chapter 13,

[4] Mallart, A., and Martin, A. R. 1967. *J. Physiol.* 193: 679–694.

[5] del Castillo, J., and Katz, B. 1954. *J. Physiol.* 124: 574–585.

[6] Kuno, M. 1964. *J. Physiol.* 175: 100–112.

the amount of transmitter released by any one stimulus depends on the size of the readily releasable pool of synaptic vesicles within the terminal and on the fractional release from the pool (i.e., the average probability that any vesicle will be released). The fractional release, in turn, is dependent on the amount of calcium that enters the terminal through voltage-activated calcium channels. Traditionally, facilitation and potentiation have been ascribed to increases in release probability mediated by increases in available calcium, and depression to depletion of the releasable pool of vesicles. Experiments over the past 50 years have revealed a rather more complicated picture.

FACILITATION   Experimental evidence obtained by Katz and Miledi in 1968 suggested that facilitation of transmitter release during a train of action potentials in the presynaptic terminal might be related to a progressively increasing residue of calcium left over from the previous stimuli.[7] The residual amounts, themselves insufficient to trigger release, would add to the next bolus of incoming calcium, thereby increasing the release probability. The decay of facilitation over time would then represent the return of intracellular calcium to its resting level. This idea that calcium accumulation is involved in some way is supported by observations at a variety of synapses that buffering intracellular calcium concentration with calcium chelators attenuates facilitation.[8]

Subsequent studies have indicated that increased cytoplasmic calcium has additional effects that can contribute to facilitation. For example, experiments on glutamatergic synapses in the auditory brainstem of the rat have shown that facilitation is also accompanied by a progressive increase in calcium influx with each impulse during a conditioning train.[9,10] During facilitation, calcium currents through the channels increase, and subsequently return to normal, with a time course similar to that of facilitation of transmitter release. The increase in calcium current is due to an increase in the voltage sensitivity of calcium channel activation. Although increased calcium influx through individual channels is a major contributor to facilitation, direct effect of bulk calcium accumulation still plays a role.[11,12]

DEPRESSION   Depression of synaptic potentials is seen only after a relatively large quantal release, which suggests that one underlying factor is depletion of vesicles from the nerve terminal during the conditioning train.[1,13] However, early experiments on the frog neuromuscular junction indicated that depression is accompanied by a reduction in release probability as well.[14] Similar experiments on cultured rat hippocampal neurons have led to the same conclusion.[15]

Experiments on calyx of Held synapses have shown depression of presynaptic calcium currents by prior conditioning pulses.[16,17] As with facilitation, the amount of depression depends on the amount of calcium entering the cytoplasm during the conditioning period. During repetitive activation at low frequencies, this reduction in calcium current and the consequent reduction in release probability are the major factors underlying depression.

At stimulus frequencies of 100 or more per second and with normal levels of transmitter release, depletion of the available pool contributes as well, accounting for as much as 50% of the reduction in release. At these frequencies, calcium currents are first facilitated and then depressed, and recovery from depression occurs over a period of several tens of seconds. In spite of the early facilitation of calcium current during the train, the corresponding excitatory postsynaptic currents show immediate depression due to depletion. Subsequent recovery occurs in two phases, the first over a period of seconds, reflecting recovery from depletion, and the second with a time course parallel to that of recovery from depression of the presynaptic calcium current.

AUGMENTATION AND PTP   Like facilitation and depression, augmentation and PTP are associated with increased intracellular calcium concentration. Experiments on the neuromuscular junction of the frog showed that if calcium is removed from the bathing solution during application of the conditioning train, then no potentiation occurs.[18] At the crayfish neuromuscular junction, PTP is reduced in magnitude and duration by treatments that interfere with calcium uptake and release by mitochondria, suggesting that calcium influx during the tetanus may be accompanied by rapid mitochondrial calcium loading.[19] In that event, excess mitochondrial calcium might be released slowly, thereby prolonging the elevation of cytoplasmic calcium concentration and maintaining

[7] Katz, B., and Miledi, R. 1968. *J. Physiol.* 195: 481–492.

[8] Zucker, R. S., and Regehr, W. G. 2002. *Annu. Rev. Physiol.* 64: 355–405.

[9] Cuttle, M. F. et al. 1998. *J. Physiol.* 512: 723–729.

[10] Borst, J. G. G., and Sakmann, B. 1998. *J. Physiol.* 513: 149–155.

[11] Neher, E., and Sakaba, T. 2008. *Neuron* 59: 861–872.

[12] Xu, J., He, L., and Wu, L.-G. 2007. *Curr. Opin. Neurobiol.* 17: 352–359.

[13] Mallart, A., and Martin, A. R. 1968. *J. Physiol.* 196: 593–604.

[14] Betz, W. J. 1970. *J. Physiol.* 206: 629–644.

[15] Sullivan, J. M. 2007. *J. Neurophysiol.* 97: 948–950.

[16] Forsythe, I. D. et al. 1998. *Neuron* 20: 797–807.

[17] Xu, J., and Wu, L.-G. 2005. *Neuron* 46: 633–645.

[18] Rosenthal, J. L. 1969. *J. Physiol.* 203: 121–133.

[19] Tang, Y.-G., and Zucker, R. F. 1997. *Neuron* 18: 483–491.

the potentiation. PTP is not dependent on sodium entry, as it can be produced by trains of artificial depolarizing pulses applied to the nerve terminal in the presence of tetrodotoxin (TTX).[20] In that circumstance, the magnitude of the potentiation is increased with increasing extracellular calcium concentration, and in very high calcium (83 mM), PTP can last for more than 2 hours.

In the calyx of Held, high-resolution fluorescent dye techniques have been used to measure calcium transients produced by single presynaptic stimuli. After induction of PTP, presynaptic calcium influx increased by about 15%.[21] At the peak of PTP, average cytoplasmic calcium concentrations increased from a resting value of about 50 nM to over 200 nM. The calcium concentration then declined to its resting level with a time course that paralleled that of the decay of PTP.[22,23]

The increase in presynaptic calcium influx indicates that PTP and augmentation are due, at least in part, to an increase in transmitter release probability. The sustained increase in release may also reflect an increase in the size of the releasable pool. One technique for estimating the releasable pool size is to induce rapid, ongoing transmitter release until the pool is exhausted and then estimate how much has been released. Depletion experiments on synapses between cultured hippocampal neurons indicate that augmentation is due to an increase in release probability, with no apparent increase in the size of the releasable pool of transmitter.[20] However, depletion experiments on the calyx of Held synapses have shown that during PTP the releasable pool increases in size.[24] In one experiment a 6000-shock tetanus produced synaptic currents reaching a maximum of about four times the control amplitude. The potentiation was accompanied by a maximum increase of about 70% in the size of the releasable pool, and an increase in release probability by a factor of about 2.5. PTP decayed in two phases. The first phase, with a time constant of about 1 minute, was due to a return of the release probability toward its resting value; the second phase extended over a period of 10 to 20 minutes and represented the return of the releasable pool to its resting size.

How does increased intracellular calcium act to modulate calcium channel function? Catterall and his colleagues approached this question by looking at the effects of mutations of Ca$_V$2.1 channels on facilitation and depression.[25] The channels were expressed in cultured superior cervical ganglion (SCG) neurons, and the transfected cells formed cholinergic synaptic connections with adjacent SCG cells in the culture. Mutations were made on the channel α_1-subunits at two nearby locations on the C terminus. At one location, an isoleucine and a methionine residue at adjacent positions (IM) were replaced by two alanines (AA). At the other location, a calmodulin-binding domain (CBD) was deleted. At synapses with IM-AA mutations, facilitation was virtually absent. Deletion of the CBD segment, however, removed almost all of the depression. The authors concluded that changes in calcium channel conductance observed during facilitation and depression of transmitter release are mediated by conformational changes in the channel produced by selective binding of calcium-calmodulin to the C-terminal sites.

Although the experiments we have discussed here provide a general picture of factors underlying short-term plasticity, the actual details may vary considerably from one type of synapse to the next. For one thing, most of the experiments in which changes in calcium channel currents were examined were done on calyx of Held synapses, which contain Ca$_V$2.1 channels with P/Q-type currents. Release of transmitter at synapses in the peripheral nervous system and in some parts of the CNS is subserved predominantly by calcium influx through Ca$_V$2.2 channels with N-type currents, which may have quite different properties.[26] Another factor to consider is the progressive effects of increased calcium concentration inside the presynaptic terminal membrane. In the calyx of Held synapse, the increase in intracellular calcium first mediates facilitation of channel currents; then, as the concentration builds up further, facilitation switches to inhibition. With this scenario, the overall effect of calcium influx can be expected to depend markedly on physical factors, one example being the size of the terminal. In very small terminals with a large surface-to-volume ratio, calcium concentration could build up rapidly so that the overriding effect is inhibitory, whereas in very large terminals the build up could be much smaller, yielding only facilitation. Similarly, differences between presynaptic terminals in the cytoplasmic concentration and distribution of calcium chelators could produce marked differences in synaptic behavior.

[20] Stevens, C. F., and Wesseling, J. F. 1999. *Neuron* 22: 139–146.

[21] Habets, R. L., and Borst, J. G. 2006. *J. Neurophysiol.* 96: 2868–2876.

[22] Korogood, N., Lou, X., and Schneggerburger, R. 2005. *J. Neurosci.* 25: 5127–5137.

[23] Habets, R. L., and Borst, J. G. 2005. *J. Physiol.* 564: 173–187.

[24] Habets, R. L., and Borst, J. G. 2007. *J. Physiol.* 581: 467–478.

[25] Mochida, S. et al. 2008. *Neuron* 57: 210–216.

[26] Catteral, W. A., and Few, A. P. 2008. *Neuron* 59: 882–901.

Long-Term Changes in Signaling

In the CNS, repetitive activity can produce changes in synaptic efficacy that last much longer than those seen at peripheral synapses (see Figure 16.3D). These longer lasting changes have been found in a variety of brain locations and are particularly intriguing because their long duration suggests that they may be associated in some way with memory. Two basic changes can be induced: **long-term potentiation (LTP)** and **long-term depression (LTD)**, defined as a persistent increase (LTP) or decrease (LTD) of synaptic efficacy produced by brief repetitive activation.

Long-Term Potentiation

Long-term potentiation (LTP) was first described by Bliss and Lømo in 1973 at glutamatergic synapses in the hippocampal formation.[27,28] This structure, which lies within the temporal lobe of the brain, consists of two regions known as the hippocampus and the dentate gyrus, which in cross section appear as interlocking C-shaped strips of cortex, plus the neighboring subiculum (Figure 16.4). Its orderly arrangement of cells and input pathways enables recording electrodes to be inserted into the brain of the intact animal and placed in close proximity to known cell types, or even intracellularly, to record synaptic potentials. Similarly, stimulating electrodes can be located in specific input pathways. Bliss and Lømo demonstrated that high-frequency stimulation of inputs to cells in the dentate gyrus produced a subsequent increase in the amplitude of excitatory synaptic potentials that lasted for hours or even for days (Figure 16.5). This is now known as **homosynaptic LTP**. A distinctive property of this form of LTP is **input specificity**: Only the activated synapse is potentiated, while other synapses on the same cell are unaffected. Although LTP has been shown to occur in other regions of the brain, including several neocortical areas, and even in autonomic ganglia,[29] it has been studied most extensively in CA1 pyramidal cells in hippocampal slices in vitro.[30]

LTP has captured the attention of neurobiologists because of its possible role in learning and memory. The dorsal hippocampus is critical to spatial learning in rats, as lesioned animals cannot remember the locations of objects previously tracked down in a maze.[31] If information about locations is stored as activity-driven increases in synaptic weights in the

[27] Bliss, T. V. P., and Lømo, T. 1973. *J. Physiol.* 232: 331–356.

[28] Lømo, T. 2003. Philos. *Trans. R. Soc. Lond., B* 358: 617–620.

[29] Alkadhi, K. A., Alzoubi, K. H., and Aleisa, A. M. 2005. *Prog. Neurobiol.* 75: 83–108.

[30] Malenka, R. C., and Nicoll, R. A. 1999. *Science* 258: 1870–1874.

[31] Moser, E., Moser, M., and Andersen, P. 1993. *J. Neurosci.* 13: 3916–3925.

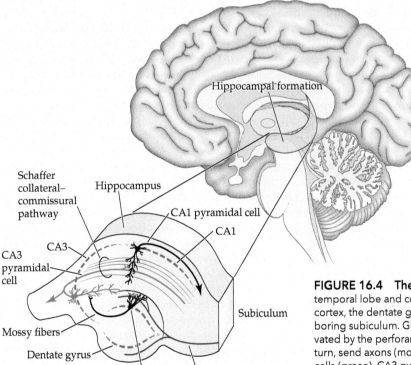

FIGURE 16.4 The Hippocampal Formation lies buried in the temporal lobe and consists of two interlocking C-shaped strips of cortex, the dentate gyrus and hippocampus, together with the neighboring subiculum. Granule cells in the dentate gyrus (black) are innervated by the perforant fiber pathway (red) from the subiculum and, in turn, send axons (mossy fibers) to make synapses on CA3 pyramidal cells (green). CA3 pyramidal cells project axons (Schaffer collaterals) to pyramidal cells in CA1 (black).

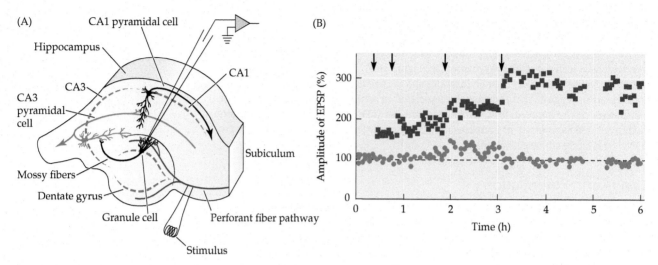

(A)

CA1 pyramidal cell

Hippocampus

CA3

CA3 pyramidal cell

CA1

Mossy fibers

Dentate gyrus

Granule cell

Subiculum

Perforant fiber pathway

Stimulus

(B)

FIGURE 16.5 Long-Term Potentiation (LTP) in the hippocampus of an anesthetized rabbit. (A) Synaptic responses to perforant pathway stimulation were recorded from granule cells in the dentate gyrus. (B) Brief tetanic stimuli (15/s for 10 s) were given at times marked by the arrows. Each tetanus caused an increase in the amplitude of the synaptic response (red squares), eventually lasting for hours. Responses in a control pathway not receiving tetanic stimulation (blue circles) were unchanged. (After T. V. P. Bliss and T. Lømo, 1973. *J. Physiol.* 232: 331-356.)

hippocampus, saturation of hippocampal LTP should impair learning. In one study, LTP was induced to different degrees in different rats; in some rats, saturation was reached, such that synapses could not be further strengthened. In subsequent behavioral tests, spatial learning was profoundly disrupted in rats that received LTP saturation, whereas the rats left with residual synaptic plasticity could still learn.[32]

Associative LTP in Hippocampal Pyramidal Cells

Experiments by T. H. Brown and his colleagues revealed that repetitive activity at one synaptic input to a cell could potentiate synaptic potentials generated by stimulation of another input to the same cell.[33] This is called **associative LTP**. An example is shown in Figure 16.6. Intracellular recordings were made from pyramidal cells in area CA1 of the hippocampus, and two extracellular stimulating electrodes were located in the input pathway (the Schaffer collateral–commissural tract) in such a way as to stimulate subpopulations of axons innervating two different regions on the dendritic arbors of the pyramidal cells (see Figure 16.6A). The stimulus intensities were adjusted so that electrode I evoked a large EPSP in a pyramidal cell, while electrode II evoked a much smaller one. Records of EPSPs produced by electrode II are shown in Figure 16.6B. Brief trains of stimuli (100 Hz for 1 second repeated once again after 5 seconds) applied to electrode I resulted in LTP of the synaptic potentials at that input (not shown), as in the experiments of Bliss and Lømo. The stimuli applied to electrode I had no effect on the smaller EPSP produced by electrode II (see Figure 16.6B, second record). Also, high-frequency stimulation with electrode II did not produce LTP of the smaller response (third record). However, after high-frequency stimulation by I and II together, there was an increase in the size of the EPSPs produced by electrode II (fourth record), lasting for tens of minutes (see Figure 16.6C). This was called associative LTP because the prolonged increased response to input II was produced only when repetitive stimulation of that input was associated with simultaneous stimulation of input I.

Subsequent experiments showed that the magnitude of associative LTP depends on the relative timing of the paired stimulus trains (time-dependent plasticity).[34] In these experiments the potentiating effect was largest when the two trains were coincident, and persisted when the train in the strong pathway followed that in the weak pathway. The potentiation declined as the separation of the trains was increased beyond about 20 ms, and eventually reversed to depression of the weak response with train separations exceeding 200 ms. No associative LTP was observed when stimulating train in the strong pathway *preceded* that in the weak pathway. Instead, paired conditioning trains were followed by depression of the weak response.

The post-tetanic depression seen with train separations exceeding 200 ms, and when strong pathway stimulations came first, possibly occurred simply because no LTP was produced in these circumstances, and its absence unmasked an underlying homosynaptic long-term depression (LTD) produced by the stimulus train in the weak pathway (see Figure 16.12).

[32] Moser, E. I. et al. 1998. *Science* 281: 2038-2042.

[33] Barionuevo, G., and Brown, T. H. 1983. *Proc. Natl. Acad. Sci. USA* 80: 7347-7351.

[34] Levy, W. B., and Steward, O. 1983 *Neuroscience* 8: 791-793.

(A)

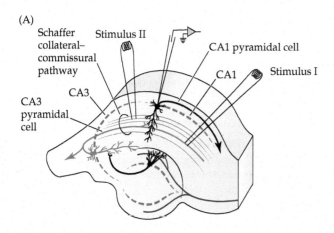

FIGURE 16.6 Associative LTP in a Rat Hippocampal Slice.
(A) Intracellular records were made from CA1 pyramidal cells while stimulating two distinct groups of presynaptic fibers in the Schaffer collateral-commissural pathway (Stimulus I and Stimulus II). The stimuli were adjusted so that responses to stimulation at site I were five times greater than those at site II. (B) Averaged responses to stimulation at site II in control condition, after tetanic stimulation at site I (100/s for 1 s), after a similar tetanus at site II, and after a combined tetanus at sites I and II. Only the combined tetanus produced potentiation; test shock 10 minutes later indicated a twofold increase in response amplitude. (C) Summary of the results in part B showing the time course of the changes in response amplitude. Stimulation at site I had no effect, stimulation at II produced a brief potentiation of the response, and combined stimulation at I and II produced LTP. (After G. Barrionuevo and T. H. Brown, 1983. *Proc. Natl. Acad. Sci. USA* 80: 7347-7351.)

(B)

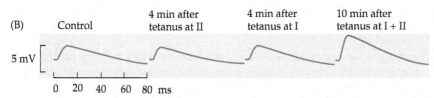

(C)

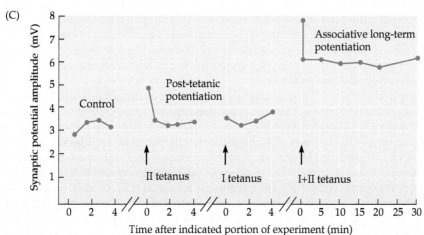

Associative LTP is particularly interesting because it illustrates a possible mechanism for conditioned reflexes, the classic example being conditioning a dog to salivate in response to the sound of a bell.

Like short-term changes in signaling, LTP can be separated into different forms based on their time course of decay.[35] Their induction depends in part on the duration and intensity of the conditioning stimulus. An example is shown in Figure 16.7, which illustrates the response of CA1 pyramidal neurons

[35] Raymond, C. R. 2007. *Trends Neurosci.* 30: 167-175.

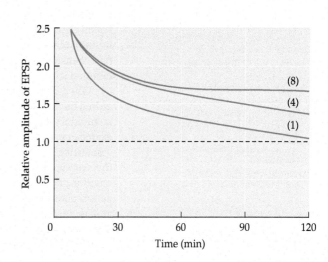

FIGURE 16.7 Three Phases of Decay of LTP in CA1 neurons. A single brief 100-Hz conditioning train applied to the Schaffer collateral pathway (1) increases EPSP amplitude to more than two times normal. The potentiation decays to half its initial value in about 30 minutes. Four conditioning trains (4) produce about the same potentiation, but the decay time is much prolonged. When eight conditioning trains are applied (8), potentiation shows an early decay and then remains at about 1.7 times normal throughout the rest of the recording period. (After C. R. Raymond and S. J. Redman, 2006. *J. Physiol.* 570: 97-111.)

to three different conditioning protocols. A single 100-Hz conditioning train increased the size of the EPSP by about 130%, and the increase decayed back to zero over the next 2 hours. Four conditioning trains produced about the same increase, but the potentiation decayed less rapidly—after 2 hours the EPSPs were still potentiated by 30%. With eight conditioning trains, the decay was still slower, with 80% of the potentiation persisting after 2 hours.

Mechanisms Underlying the Induction and Expression of LTP

Although many synaptic changes associated with LTP have been described in great detail, there is no one single coherent picture of the underlying mechanisms for its induction and expression. For example, some experiments have shown conclusively that in some cells LTP is presynaptic, while in other cells only postsynaptic factors are involved.[36] One or the other may dominate depending on the type of neuron being studied and on the conditions of the experiment. We begin by considering postsynaptic mechanisms for LTP.

An important factor in the postsynaptic expression of LTP is an increase in calcium concentration in the postsynaptic cell. In the CA1 pyramidal cell this increase is accomplished by entry of calcium through N-methyl-D-aspartate (NMDA) glutamate receptors (see Chapter 14). The NMDA receptor forms a cation channel with the unusual characteristic that it is blocked at normal resting potentials. The block is due to occupation of the channel by magnesium ions from the extracellular solution, which are removed when the receptor is depolarized.[37,38] Most glutamate-sensitive cells express both NMDA and non-NMDA ionotropic receptors in their postsynaptic membrane.[39] The non-NMDA receptors are sensitive to α-amino-3-hydroxy-5-methyl-4-isoxazolepropionic acid (AMPA). Both types of receptors are activated by glutamate released from excitatory presynaptic terminals, but in the NMDA receptors calcium entry does not occur until synaptic depolarization by repetitive activation of AMPA receptors is sufficient to remove magnesium block of the cation channels (see Chapter 11).

Involvement of NMDA receptors in LTP is indicated by the fact that NMDA antagonists block the induction of LTP, but do not prevent LTP if they are applied after it has been induced.[40,41] However, entry of calcium through the synaptic channels is not always adequate for the induction of LTP, and the three different phases of LTP illustrated in Figure 16.7 are mediated by different calcium pathways.[42] In dendritic spines and distal dendrites, calcium entry into the cytoplasm through NMDA receptors serves to trigger additional calcium release from the endoplasmic reticulum (ER). Calcium-induced calcium release from the ER depends on activation of ryanodine (Ry) receptors and/or inositol triphosphate (IP_3) receptors (see Chapter 12). Block of Ry receptors selectively inhibits calcium release in synaptic spines and abolishes short-lasting LTP. Block of IP_3 receptors inhibits calcium release along dendrites and abolishes LTP of intermediate duration. Long-lasting LTP that persists beyond the first two phases does not depend on NMDA receptors at all. Instead, it is mediated by calcium entry through L-type voltage-sensitive calcium channels in the cell soma.

The different durations of the increases in synaptic strength induced by the various stimuli imply a difference in the underlying molecular basis of their expression. All persistent changes of synaptic strength ultimately depend on changes in the molecular composition of the synapse. As we will see in Chapter 17, three distinct molecular processes— post-translational, transcriptional, and protein translation processes—contribute to the duration and expression of LTP, and therefore to the different forms of LTP.

When considering the postsynaptic cell as a whole, the dendritic depolarization required to permit calcium entry through NMDA channels can arise from several sources in addition to local synaptic activation of AMPA receptors on single dendritic spines. For example, passive spread of depolarization from other synaptic locations is necessary for associative LTP. The magnitude of the depolarization depends on the distance between the neighboring synapses and the effective space constants of the dendritic branches. In addition, passive depolarization of the cell soma can spread into dendrites, as can somatic action potentials. Finally, dendrites themselves can generate sodium action potentials and, more important, calcium action potentials that provide a source of calcium entry independent of NMDA receptors. These modes of spread of depolarization into dendrites are discussed in Chapter 8.

[36] Lisman, J. E. 2009. *Neuron* 63: 261–264.

[37] Nowak, L. et al. 1984. *Nature* 307: 462–465.

[38] Mayer, M. L., Westbrook, G. L., and Guthrie, P. B. 1984. *Nature* 309: 261–263.

[39] Takumi, Y. et al. 1999. *Ann. NY Acad. Sci.* 868: 474–481.

[40] Collingridge, G. L., Kehl, S. J., and McClennan, H. 1983. *J. Physiol.* 334: 33–46.

[41] Muller, D., Joly, M., and Lynch, G. 1988. *Science* 242: 1694–1697.

[42] Raymond, C. R., and Redman, S. J. 2006. *J. Physiol.* 570: 97–111.

Silent Synapses

One of the major factors in the postsynaptic expression of LTP is the activation of **silent synapses**.[43] In the first few postnatal days, CA1 synapses in rats and mice are virtually devoid of AMPA receptors, so that most do not respond to presynaptic stimulation. As dendritic spines develop, NMDA receptors are expressed first, followed by AMPA receptors, which over the next few weeks appear at roughly half the synapses. Suppose that in a mature synapse some presynaptic excitatory boutons overlie postsynaptic regions on dendritic spines that contain only a few AMPA receptors, or perhaps none at all. Under resting conditions, release of a quantum of glutamate from these boutons will produce little or no response; thus, these synaptic contacts will be silent and only a fraction of the synaptic apparatus will respond to presynaptic excitation (Figure 16.8A). Now suppose that the induction of LTP leads to insertion of AMPA receptors into the postsynaptic membranes of the silent synapses. These will now respond to quanta released from the presynaptic terminal, and the quantum content of the response will increase (Figure 16.8B).

There is now substantial evidence that AMPA receptors in the postsynaptic membrane, which turn over quite rapidly at rest (see Chapter 14), are upregulated during the expression of LTP. The most direct evidence is the demonstration that AMPA receptor subunits are delivered to dendritic spines after repetitive stimulation accompanied by NMDA receptor activation.[44] The AMPA receptor subunit GluA1 (see Chapter 5) was tagged with green fluorescent protein (GFP) and expressed transiently in hippocampal CA1 pyramidal cells. When cell dendrites were examined with laser-scanning and electron microscopy, most of the receptors in the dendrites were found in intracellular compartments, and only about half of the dendritic spines showed fluorescence. After stimulation, tagged receptors were delivered rapidly by exocytosis from intracellular vesicles to extrasynaptic membrane regions on the dendritic shafts.[45] Receptors then diffused to synaptic regions on the dendritic spines, where they were immobilized.[46] Almost all of the spines became fluorescent,

[43] Kerchner, G. A., and Nicoll, R. A. 2008. *Nat. Neurosci.* 9: 813–825.

[44] Shi, S. H. et al. 1999. *Science* 284: 1811–1816.

[45] Makino, H. and Malinow, R. 2009. *Neuron* 64: 381–390.

[46] Borgdorff, A. J., and Choquet, D. 2002. *Nature* 417: 649–653.

(A)

Presynaptic bouton

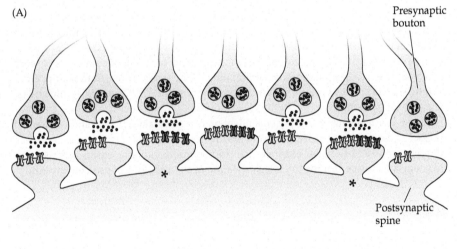

Postsynaptic spine

(B)

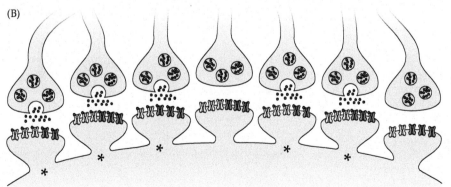

FIGURE 16.8 Proposed Mechanism for Increased Postsynaptic Response during LTP. (A) Release of five quanta of glutamate from presynaptic boutons (indicated by omega figures in the bouton membranes) activates only two postsynaptic spines (asterisks) because many spines contain no AMPA receptors (red receptors) and are "silent." Thus, the quantum content of the response is two, even though five quanta are released. NMDA receptors (yellow receptors) do not respond because depolarization is insufficient to remove the magnesium block. (B) During potentiation, AMPA receptors are inserted into the postsynaptic membranes of the spines and the quantum content of the response is increased to five.

even those that were nearly devoid of label before stimulation. These results indicate that excitatory dendritic spines that are devoid of AMPA receptors receive a full complement of them after repetitive stimulation.

Additional details of the mechanisms for upregulation of AMPA receptor expression and consequent synaptic desilencing have been summarized by Nicoll and his colleagues.[27,43] For example, it has been shown by immunohistochemistry that all Schaffer collateral–commissural synapses contain NMDA receptors but that only a fraction of these contain co-localized AMPA receptors.[47] Correspondingly, electrophysiological experiments reveal many synapses in CA1 pyramidal cells that are activated only by NMDA; these synapses acquire AMPA responses during LTP.[48,49] Still other experiments have demonstrated that after induction of LTP new spines appear on the CA1 pyramidal cell dendrites.[50] Potentiation of the synaptic response by about 80% was accompanied by roughly a 13% increase in measured spine density. A particularly interesting experiment involved the induction of LTP by artificial application of glutamate to individual dendritic spines of CA1 cells.[51] The cells were transfected with GFP so that the spines and spine heads could be visualized readily. Caged glutamate was uncaged in a very small area near a spine by a two-photon laser, in amounts sufficient to produce synaptic currents similar to miniature excitatory postsynaptic currents (EPSCs). Repetitive uncaging (1/s for 1 min) resulted in an increase in spine head volume by about a factor of three. The increase in volume then decayed over a period extending well beyond 1 hour. Presynaptic stimulation of Schaffer collaterals produced the same response. The effect was particularly persistent in small dendritic spines. Enlargement was prevented by NMDA receptor antagonists, and blocked by calmodulin inhibitors.

How does increased cytoplasmic calcium concentration lead to upregulation of AMPA receptor membrane expression? One calcium-dependent biochemical pathway that has been shown to be required for induction of LTP is calcium-calmodulin-dependent protein kinase II (CaMKII).[52] CaMKII is found in high concentrations in the postsynaptic densities of dendritic spines, and intracellular injection of inhibitors of CaMKII prevents the induction of LTP.[53,54] Figure 16.9 shows the sequence of events leading to upregulation and the role that calcium plays. During LTP, the incoming calcium binds to calmodulin to activate CaMKII, which maintains its own activity by autophosphorylation after the calcium concentration has returned to basal levels. CaMKII then has two effects on the AMPA receptors: (1) It phosphorylates receptors present in the membrane, thereby increasing their channel conductance, and (2) it facilitates mobilization of receptors from the cytoplasm into the cell membrane.[55] The synapses return to their previous resting state over time because of constitutive recycling of AMPA receptors into and out of the synaptic membrane.[56]

Long-lasting forms of LTP are dependent on new gene transcription and protein synthesis.[57,58] Several biochemical pathways are involved in linking calcium accumulation in the cell to transcription. For example, activation of modulatory receptors may be linked to adenylate cyclase, leading to phosphorylation of the cAMP response element-binding

[47] Takumi, Y. et al. 1999. *Nat. Neurosci.* 2: 618–624.

[48] Liao, D., Hessler, N. A., and Malinow, R. 1995. *Nature* 375: 400–404.

[49] Isaac, J. T. R., Nicoll, R. A., and Malenka, R. C. 1995. *Neuron* 15: 427–434.

[50] Engert, F., and Bonhoeffer, T. 1999. *Nature* 399: 66–70.

[51] Matsuzaki, M. et al. 2004. *Nature* 429: 761–766.

[52] Schulman, H. 1995. *Curr. Opin. Neurobiol.* 5: 375–381.

[53] Malenka, R. C. et al. 1989. *Nature* 340: 554–557.

[54] Malinow, R., Schulman, H., and Tsien, R. W. 1989. *Science* 245: 862–866.

[55] Malinow, R., and Malenka, R. C. 2002. *Annu. Rev. Neurosci.* 25: 103–126.

[56] Shi, S. et al. 2001. *Cell* 105: 331–343.

[57] Abraham, W. C., and Williams, J. M. 2003. *Neuroscientist* 9: 463–474.

[58] Lynch, M. A. 2004. *Physiol. Rev.* 84: 87–136.

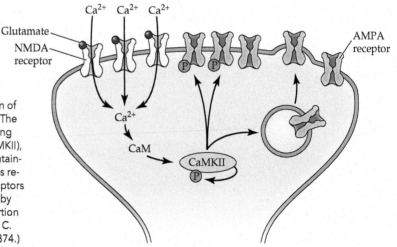

FIGURE 16.9 Role of Calcium in LTP. Activation of NMDA receptors allows calcium entry into the spine. The incoming calcium binds to calmodulin (CaM), activating calcium-calmodulin-dependent protein kinase II (CaMKII), which undergoes autophosphorylation, thereby maintaining its own activity after the calcium concentration has returned to normal. CaMKII phosphorylates AMPA receptors already present in the postsynaptic membrane, thereby increasing their conductance, and facilitates the insertion of new receptors from the cytoplasmic pool. (After R. C. Malenka and R. A. Nicoll, 1999. *Science* 285: 1870–1874.)

protein (CREB). The resulting gene expression involves not only receptor proteins but also other structural and functional proteins, suggesting that an essential long-term consequence of LTP is growth and remodeling of the synapse. The mechanisms whereby new transcripts and proteins are transported from the soma to specific synaptic regions will be discussed in Chapter 17.

Presynaptic LTP

LTP is not only expressed postsynaptically. For example, at mossy fiber synapses on CA3 pyramidal cells, LTP is induced and expressed even when a postsynaptic increase in calcium concentration is completely prevented by blocking both NMDA receptors and voltage-sensitive calcium channels, and loading the postsynaptic cell with high concentrations of a calcium chelator. This observation led to the conclusion that LTP at that synapse was entirely presynaptic.[59] The underlying mechanisms are not at all clear but may involve the recurrent action of glutamate on presynaptic metabotropic glutamate receptors (mGluRs; see Chapter 12), on presynaptic kainate receptors (see Chapter 5), or on presynaptic voltage-activated Ca^{2+} channels.

Several experiments have indicated that presynaptic LTP occurs at CA1 pyramidal cell synapses as well.[60] In these experiments, LTP was associated not with an increase in the amplitude of miniature EPSPs (quantal size), as would be expected from an increase in postsynaptic sensitivity, but rather with an increase in the number of quanta released from the terminal (quantum content). An example is shown in Figure 16.10, where the amplitude distribution of the synaptic potentials is plotted before and after potentiation. In this and other experiments, statistical analysis of the amplitude distributions indicated that the mean quantum content of the potentiated synaptic potential was increased.[61,62]

The results shown in Figure 16.10 could be accounted for in theory by the scheme shown in Figure 16.8, where quantal release is the same before and after conditioning but the observed quantum content is increased because additional postjunctional receptors are made responsive by insertion of AMPA receptors. However, increased release of transmitter during LTP expression has been shown to occur in some instances. For

[59] Nicoll, R. A., and Schmitz, D. 2005. *Nat. Rev. Neurosci.* 6: 863–876.

[60] Voronin, L. L., and Cherubini, E. 2004. *J. Physiol.* 557: 3–12.

[61] Malinow, R., and Tsien, R. W. 1990. *Nature* 346: 177–180.

[62] Beckers, J. M., and Stevens, C. F. 1990. *Nature* 346: 724–729.

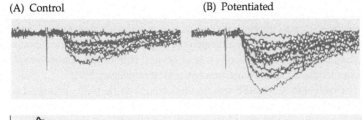

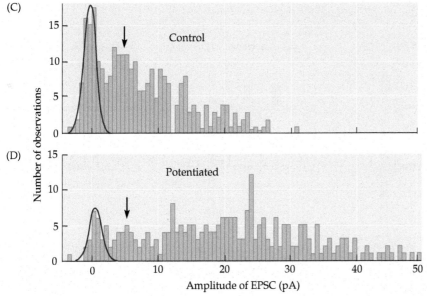

FIGURE 16.10 Change in Quantum Content of synaptic response during LTP. Records from rat hippocampal slice. (A,B) Sixteen superimposed, whole-cell records of synaptic currents in CA1 pyramidal cell before (A) and after (B) conditioning train of stimuli. Note quantal steps in the current amplitudes. After conditioning, the fraction of failures is decreased and there are many more multi-quantal responses. (C,D) Distribution of current amplitudes before (C) and after (D) conditioning. Normal curve is fitted to baseline noise (i.e., failures); arrows indicate mean current produced by a single quantum. After potentiation, the number of failures is reduced and the mean current is increased in amplitude by a factor of almost three, while the single quantum current is unchanged. (After R. Malinow and R. W. Tsien, 1990. *Nature* 346: 177–180.)

[63] Ahmed, M. S., and Siegelbaum, S A. 2009. *Neuron* 63: 372-385.

[64] Bayazitov, I. T., et al. 2007. *J. Neurosci.* 27: 11510-11521.

[65] Castellucci, V. et al. 1970. *Science* 167: 1745-1748.

[66] Lynch, G. S., Dunwiddie, T., and Gribkoff, V. 1977. *Nature* 266: 737-739.

[67] Collingridge, G. L. et al. 2010. *Nat. Rev. Neurosci.* 11: 459-473.

example, FM dye was used to label synaptic vesicles at perforant path synapses on CA1 pyramidal neurons.[63] Dye trapped in the vesicles fluoresces because of its close association with the vesicle lipid membrane, and after vesicle exocytosis the fluorescence is lost as the dye diffuses into the extracellular fluid (see Figure 13.27). Two-photon microscopy was used to observe the loss of fluorescence as vesicles fused during stimulation before and after induction of LTP. The release of vesicles was enhanced significantly during LTP. Interestingly, similar enhancement of release did not occur at synapses formed by Schaffer collaterals on the same cells.

Coexistence of presynaptic and postsynaptic LTP at the same synapse has been demonstrated in CA3 pyramidal cells from transgenic mice in which the fluorescent dye synaptoPHluorin was expressed.[64] Vesicle exocytosis in response to test stimuli was monitored for several hours after induction of LTP, while at the same time postsynaptic potentials (PSPs) were recorded. Tetanization was followed by a large increase in PSP amplitude, accompanied by a smaller, more slowly developing increase in vesicle exocytosis. Thus, LTP can consist of a combination of presynaptic and postsynaptic components.

In summary, LTP in CA1 pyramidal cells has three temporal components. During the conditioning stimulus, calcium influx across the synaptic membrane increases calcium concentration in the cytoplasm and releases additional calcium from the endoplasmic reticulum. Two pathways appear to be involved in such calcium release: one mediated by Ry receptors in dendritic spines, the second by IP$_3$ receptors along the dendrites. These pathways are associated, respectively, with the first and second components of LTP. The increased intracellular calcium then activates CaMKII, as shown in Figure 16.9, leading to increased conductance of existing receptors and insertion of AMPA receptors in the membrane. The third, long-lasting component of LTP appears to depend primarily on calcium entry into the cell soma through voltage-dependent calcium channels and is associated with gene transcription and expression (see Chapter 17). Finally, LTP at CA1 synapses also appears to involve an increase in transmitter release from the presynaptic nerve terminal, possibly lasting throughout the first two phases. Details of the mechanisms associated with the presynaptic changes have yet to be revealed.

Long-Term Depression

One of the earliest demonstrations of long-term synaptic depression (LTD), the inverse of LTP, was in relation to the gill-withdrawal reflex in the sea slug *Aplysia*. Experiments by E. R. Kandel and his colleagues indicated that habituation of the reflex by repeated tactile stimulation of the siphon or mantle was associated with depression of synaptic transmission in an identified gill motor neuron in the abdominal ganglion.[65]

In the vertebrate CNS, LTP was first reported at the Schaffer collateral input to CA1 pyramidal cells[66] and has since been studied in several other regions of the brain.[67]

FIGURE 16.11 Types of Long-Term Depression, classified according to stimulus conditions. Symbols indicate potentiation (+) or depression (-) of the synaptic response after the conditioning stimuli. (A) Homosynaptic LTD is produced by prolonged low-frequency stimulation of the same afferent pathway. (B) Heterosynaptic LTD is produced by tetanic stimulation of a neighboring pathway, which may itself be potentiated after the stimulus train. (C) Associative LTD is produced by low-frequency stimulation of the test pathway together with brief out-of-phase tetani applied to the conditioning pathway. (D) LTD in the cerebellum is produced by coordinated low-frequency stimulation of the climbing-fiber (CF) and parallel-fiber (PF) inputs to Purkinje cells. (After D. J. Linden, 1994. *Neuron* 12: 457-472.)

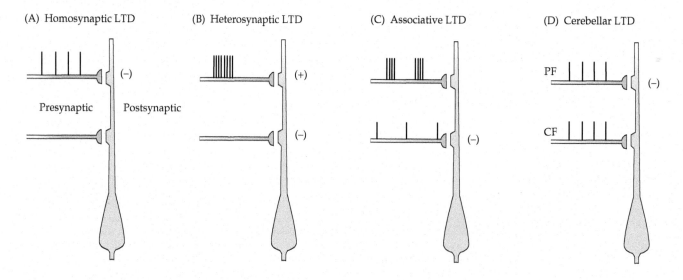

(A) Homosynaptic LTD   (B) Heterosynaptic LTD   (C) Associative LTD   (D) Cerebellar LTD

Presynaptic   Postsynaptic

Homosynaptic LTD is a prolonged depression of synaptic transmission produced by previous repetitive activity in the same pathway (Figure 16.11A). It can be induced by a variety of stimulus protocols, such as prolonged low-frequency stimulation (1–5 stimuli/s for 5–15 min), low-frequency stimulation with paired pulses, or brief high-frequency stimulation (50–100 stimuli/s for 1–5 s). In Schaffer collaterals, homosynaptic LTD is blocked by NMDA receptor antagonists, as well as by pyramidal cell hyperpolarization and postsynaptic injection of calcium chelators.[68,69] However, in other brain locations NMDA antagonists have no effect. Instead, induction of LTD appears to involve metabotropic glutamate receptors (mGluRs).

Figure 16.12 shows an example of homosynaptic LTD in hippocampal CA1 cells. A patch clamp electrode recorded synaptic responses of a single cell, and an extracellular electrode was used to record field potentials produced by synchronous synaptic activity in neighboring cells. Both the single cell and its responding neighbors showed marked depression of the synaptic response after a 10-second tetanic stimulus at 1 stimulus/second (see Figure 16.12A). When the patch clamp (and hence the cell cytoplasm) was loaded with 10 m*M* BAPTA, induction of LTD in the cell was completely eliminated, but post-tetanic depression of the synchronous activity in neighboring cells remained (see Figure 16.12B).

[68] Dudek, S. M., and Bear, M. F. 1992. *Proc. Natl. Acad. Sci. USA* 89: 4363-4367.

[69] Mulkey, R. M., and Malenka, R. C. 1992. *Neuron* 9: 967-975.

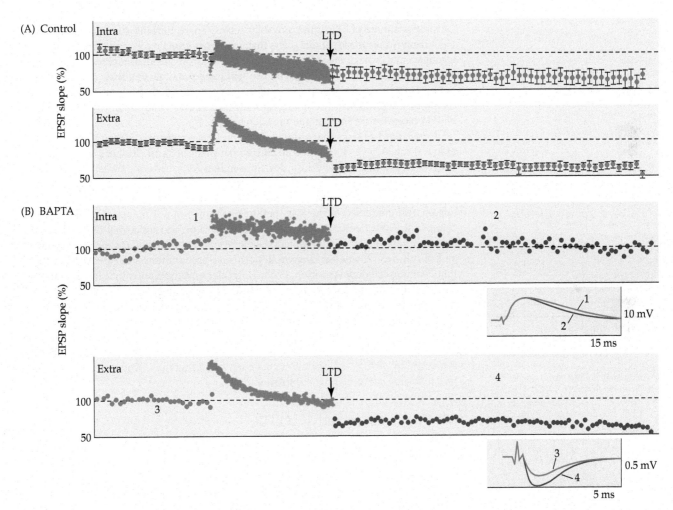

FIGURE 16.12 Homosynaptic LTD in hippocampal CA1 cells. (A) Upper record: Average synaptic responses in five successive trials (mean ± SD), recorded from a single cell with a patch clamp electrode (Intra). Lower record: Simultaneous record of synchronous synaptic activity of a group of cells in the region, recorded by an extracellular microelectrode (Extra). Amplitude of responses is expressed as a percent of the mean control response recorded before repetitive stimulation. Presynaptic stimulation at 1/s for 10 seconds produces initial facilitation and then depression of the synaptic response, followed by LTD. (B) Similar experiment with the patch clamp electrode, and hence the cell cytoplasm, filled with 10 m*M* BAPTA. LTP is completely blocked in the cell but unaffected in neighboring cells. Inserts show intracellular and extracellular synaptic potentials at indicated positions on the traces, before and after repetitive stimulation. (After R. M. Mulkey and R. C. Malenka, 1992. *Neuron* 9: 967-975.)

Heterosynaptic LTD is a prolonged depression of synaptic transmission produced by previous activity in a different afferent pathway to the same cell (Figure 16.11B). This form of LTD was first reported as a correlate of homosynaptic LTP induced in Schaffer collateral input to CA1 pyramidal cells (i.e., induction of LTP in one pathway resulted in depression of transmission at nearby synapses). Later experiments, using chronic recordings from perforant pathway dentate gyrus synapses, showed that the depression could persist for days.[70] The phenomenon is accompanied by a rise in postsynaptic calcium concentration, which in the hippocampus is mediated by NMDA receptor activation.[71] However, it can also be induced by direct postsynaptic depolarization without activation of NMDA receptors. In the dentate gyrus it is blocked by L-type calcium channel blockers.[72]

Associative LTD has been reported to occur with stimulus protocols similar to those used for associative LTP. Combined weak and strong stimulation of two inputs results in depression of the weakly stimulated input (Figure 16.11C). One difference between the protocols for associative LTP and associative LTD is that during induction of LTD the two stimuli are delivered out of phase. As in associative LTP, postsynaptic depolarizing pulses can substitute for the strong synaptic stimulation.[73]

LTD in the Cerebellum

One important site of LTD is the cerebellar cortex. There, Purkinje cells receive excitatory input from two sources: parallel fibers that arise from granule cells and form synapses on secondary and tertiary dendrites; and climbing fibers from the inferior olive nucleus, which make strong synaptic connections on the soma and proximal dendritic tree. Parallel fibers use glutamate as a transmitter, and their synapses contain both mGluR and AMPA receptors. The glutamate receptor in climbing fibers has not been definitely identified. No NMDA receptors are found in the adult cerebellum.[74]

Cerebellar LTD was first studied by Ito and his colleagues.[75] They applied a series of low-frequency (1–4/s) paired stimuli to parallel fiber and climbing fiber pathways (Figure 16.11D) for about 5 minutes. Subsequent responses to parallel fiber stimulation were depressed for several hours. In addition, when application of glutamate to the dendritic field was paired with climbing fiber stimulation, subsequent responses to glutamate were depressed, suggesting that the phenomenon was mediated by postsynaptic changes. Reliable demonstration of cerebellar LTD proved somewhat difficult in vivo, but was established as an unambiguous phenomenon in cerebellar slice preparations[76] and in culture.[77] It was also shown, in both slice preparations and cerebellar cultures, that Purkinje cell depolarization, producing calcium action potentials in the dendrites (see Chapter 7), could substitute for climbing fiber stimulation in inducing LTD.[78,79] However, neither climbing fiber stimulation nor depolarization alone is effective in inducing LTD; co-activation of glutamate receptors, either by parallel fiber stimulation or by direct application of glutamate, is required. In the case of parallel fiber stimulation, LTD is input specific—that is, only the stimulated inputs are depressed. LTD induction is blocked by postsynaptic calcium chelators,[80] and there is a large calcium accumulation following climbing fiber stimulation.[81]

Mechanisms Underlying LTD

Conditions under which LTD can be produced vary considerably, depending on which type is being studied and in what location. One consistent feature is that LTD, like LTP, depends on postsynaptic accumulation of calcium.[68] In the hippocampus, calcium entry appears to be primarily through NMDA receptors, although heterosynaptic LTD can be induced by depolarization alone without receptor activation and is attenuated by L-type calcium channel blockers. This suggests that while local depolarization and calcium accumulation through NMDA receptors produce LTP at the activated input, spread of depolarization to adjacent synaptic regions can produce LTD by calcium entry through voltage-gated calcium channels. In other brain regions free calcium concentration may be elevated by release from intracellular stores by IP_3 after activation of metabotropic glutamate receptors (see Chapter 12). In cerebellar Purkinje cells, where NMDA receptors are absent, calcium entry is through voltage-sensitive calcium channels that generate dendritic action potentials.

[70] Krug, M. et al. 1985. *Brain Res.* 360: 264–272.

[71] Barry, M. F. et al. 1996. *Hippocampus* 6: 3–8.

[72] Christie, B. R., and Abraham, W. C. 1994. *Neurosci. Lett.* 167: 41–45.

[73] Debanne, D., and Thompson, S. M. 1996. *Hippocampus* 6: 9–16.

[74] Levenes, C., Daniel, H., and Crepel, F. 1998. *Prog. Neurobiol.* 55: 79–91.

[75] Ito, M., Sakurai, M., and Tongroach, P. 1982. *J. Physiol.* 324: 113–134.

[76] Sakurai, M. 1987. *J. Physiol.* 394: 463–480.

[77] Hirano, T. 1990. *Neurosci. Lett.* 119: 141–144.

[78] Crepel, F., and Jaillard, D. 1991. *J. Physiol.* 432: 123–141.

[79] Hirano, T. 1990. *Neurosci. Lett.* 119: 145–147.

[80] Sakurai M. 1990. *Proc. Natl. Acad. Sci. USA* 87: 3383–3385.

[81] Ross, W. N., and Werman, R. 1987. *J. Physiol.* 389: 319–336.

Why does calcium accumulation produce LTP in some circumstances and LTD in others? At the moment there is no clear answer to that question except that the difference appears to be related to the increase in concentration. A relatively large increase results in LTP, a smaller increase in LTD. In accordance with this idea is the observation that a stimulus barely able to induce homosynaptic LTP in CA1 cells with normal extracellular calcium concentration produces LTD when extracellular calcium is reduced.[67]

The mechanisms whereby increased cytoplasmic calcium concentration leads to LTD expression appear to be the exact reverse of those responsible for LTP. LTD expression involves a reduction in postsynaptic sensitivity to applied glutamate and a reduction in amplitude of miniature excitatory synaptic potentials.[82,83] Furthermore, during LTD in cultured hippocampal cells, there is a decrease in the number of AMPA receptors clustered in the postsynaptic membrane.[84] These changes are accompanied by dephosphorylation of the GluA1 subunit of the AMPA receptors.[85] As a general rule, during LTP trafficking of AMPA receptors into the membrane, as well as increased receptor sensitivity, is associated with protein kinase (CaMKII) activity, whereas during LTD trafficking of receptors out of the membrane and reduced sensitivity involve activation of protein phosphatase (PP2B). PP2B has a higher affinity than CaMKII for calcium-calmodulin, but its concentration in the cytoplasm is lower. Thus, at low calcium concentrations PP2B is preferentially activated. At higher concentrations, as PP2B becomes saturated, "excess" calcium-calmodulin binds to CaMKII.

Presynaptic LTD

Habituation of the gill withdrawal reflex in *Aplysia* was initially shown to be accompanied by a reduction in the quantum content of the EPSP in the gill motor neuron.[86] This finding bolstered the idea, widely held at the time, that long-term plasticity, like its short-term counterpart, was essentially a presynaptic phenomenon. However, later experiments on LTD in *Aplysia* revealed that postsynaptic mechanisms were involved as well, mimicking those seen in the vertebrate CNS.[87]

In the hippocampus, there is evidence that supports presynaptic involvement in LTD in both CA1 and CA3 neurons.[88,89] One indication of such involvement is provided by the experiments described previously in relation to LTP, in which transmitter release was examined at single synaptic contacts on CA1 pyramidal cell dendrites.[54] As we have already discussed, during LTP the probability of release at any given contact increased markedly. Similarly, after induction of LTD, the probability of release at the dendritic synaptic contacts was reduced by an amount commensurate with the reduction in amplitude of EPSPs recorded from the cell soma.

Long-Term Plasticity at Inhibitory Synapses

Synaptic plasticity has been studied almost exclusively at excitatory synapses, but long-term changes in synaptic transmission following repetitive activation have been observed at inhibitory synapses as well. One mechanism that produces modulation of release at GABAergic synapses, namely depolarization-induced suppression of inhibition (DSI), was discussed in Chapter 12. Depolarization of the postsynaptic cell, say by current injection or by stimulation of excitatory synaptic inputs, causes release into the extracellular space of an endocannabinoid that then binds to a cannabinoid receptor (CB1) on the inhibitory presynaptic terminal. Activation of the presynaptic receptor, in turn, inhibits calcium entry into the terminal during excitation, thereby reducing the release of GABA.

The reduction in GABA release by a short period of postsynaptic depolarization typically persists for less than a minute after the end of the depolarization. However, depression of GABA release lasting for tens of minutes, or more—inhibitory long-term depression, or iLTD—can be produced in CA1 pyramidal cells by repetitive heterosynaptic stimulation.[90] The subsequent depression is blocked in the presence of a CB1 antagonist, indicating that (like the short-term depression) it is mediated by the activation of the cannabinoid receptor. In addition, induction of iLTD is accompanied by protein synthesis in the presynaptic axon, and block of protein synthesis by cycloheximide abolishes iLTD (see Chapter 17). Details of the link between the protein synthesis in the nerve terminal and suppression of GABA release have yet to be determined.

[82] Oliet, S., Malenka, R. C., and Nicoll, R. A. 1996. *Science* 271: 1294–1297.

[83] Murashima, M., and Hirano, T. 1999. *J. Neurosci.* 19: 7326–7333.

[84] Carrol, R. C. et al. 1999. *Nat. Neurosci.* 2: 454–460.

[85] Lee, H.-K. et al. 1998. *Neuron* 21: 1151–1162.

[86] Castellucci, V., and Kandel, E. R. 1974. *Proc. Natl. Acad. Sci. USA* 71: 5004–5008.

[87] Glanzman, D. L. 2009. *Neurobiol. Learn. Mem.* 92: 147–154.

[88] Berretta, N., and Cherubini, E. 1998. *Eur. J. Neurosci.* 10: 2957–2963.

[89] Domenici, M. R., Berretta, N., and Cherubini, E. 1998. *Proc. Natl. Acad. Sci. USA* 95: 8310–8315.

[90] Younts, T. J. et al. 2016. *Neuron* 92: 479–492.

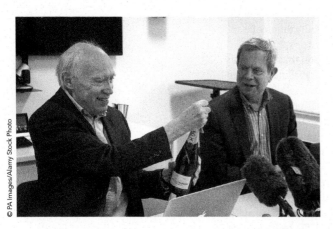

Tim Bliss and Richard Morris, on the news of the Brain Prize, 2016.

[91] Hebb, D. O. 1949. *The Organization of Behavior*. Wiley, New York, NY.

[92] Kessels, H. W., and Malinow, R. 2009. *Neuron* 61: 340-350.

[93] Izquierdo, I., and Medina, J. H. 1995. *Neurobiol. Learn. Mem.* 63: 19-32.

[94] Martinez, J. L., Jr., and Derrick, B. E. 1996. *Annu. Rev. Psychol.* 47: 173-203.

[95] Elgersma, Y., and Silva, A. J. 1999. *Curr. Opin. Neurobiol.* 9: 209-213.

[96] Cain, D. P. 1998. *Neurosci. Biobehav. Rev.* 22: 181-193.

[97] Holscher, C. 1999. *J. Neurosci. Res.* 58: 62-75.

[98] Rogan, M. T., Staubil, U. V., and LeDoux, J. E. 1997. *Nature* 390: 604-607.

[99] McKernan, M. G., and Shinnick-Gallagher, P. 1997. *Nature* 390: 607-611.

[100] Miserendino, M. J. et al. 1990. *Nature* 345: 716-718.

[101] Fanselow, M. S., and Kim, J. J. 1994. *Behav. Neurosci.* 108: 210-212.

Significance of Changes in Synaptic Efficacy

It is a matter of basic belief among those who study nervous system function that learning and memory involve long-term changes in synaptic efficacy, and for this reason the mechanisms underlying LTP and LTD are of particular interest. This interest is strengthened further because both phenomena exhibit a characteristic postulated by Donald Hebb to be required for associative learning,[91] namely that increases in synaptic strength should occur when the presynaptic and postsynaptic elements are coactive. Synapses that exhibit this property are known as Hebbian, and it is sometimes assumed that if the requirement has been satisfied, then learning has occurred. At any rate, numerous correlations have been established between changes in behavior and long-term changes in synaptic efficacy in several regions of the brain.[61,92]

For example, spatial learning in intact animals and LTP in hippocampal slices display several similarities.[93,94,95] Both can be blocked by antagonists of NMDA receptors or metabotropic glutamate receptors and also by inhibitors of calcium-calmodulin protein kinase. However, the nature of the behavioral deficit associated with the block is not always clear. For example, rats under NMDA antagonists have general sensorimotor disturbances that interfere with negotiating a water maze (suggesting that learning ability has been compromised), but they can learn it readily if they first become familiar with the general requirements of the task.[96] Thus, NMDA-receptor-mediated LTP does not seem to be an essential requirement. Similar ambiguities have been encountered with gene deletions—some that eliminate LTP produce a deficit in the spatial learning ability, others do not.[97]

There is growing evidence for the idea that LTP in the amygdala might be a substrate for aversive (or fear) conditioning. Rats trained to associate foot shock with an auditory tone exhibit an exaggerated auditory startle reflex, and cells in the amygdala show an LTP-like increase in their synaptic response to electrical stimulation of the auditory pathway from the medial geniculate nucleus.[98,99] Conversely, induction of LTP at the same synapses by electrical stimulation results in an increase in the response to auditory stimuli.[71] Both effects are blocked by NMDA receptor antagonists.[100,101] In conclusion, while an unequivocal causal relation between LTP and spatial learning tasks has not been established, LTP may play a role in more discrete learning paradigms such as classical conditioning.

SUMMARY

- Short periods of synaptic activation can result in facilitation, depression, or augmentation of transmitter release, or a combination of these effects.

- Facilitation decays gradually over several hundred milliseconds, while synaptic depression and augmentation persist for several seconds.

- Facilitation is related to a persistent increase in cytoplasmic calcium concentration in the presynaptic terminal.

- Longer periods of repetitive stimulation result in post-tetanic potentiation (PTP) of transmitter release, which can last for tens of minutes and, like facilitation, is mediated by an increase in presynaptic terminal calcium concentration.

- In various parts of the CNS, repetitive stimulation can result in long-term potentiation (LTP) or long-term depression (LTD) of synaptic strength.

- LTP in the hippocampal formation is involved in spatial learning and memory.

- The change in synaptic efficacy during LTP or LTD may be homosynaptic, involving only the stimulated input, or heterosynaptic, affecting adjacent synapses on the same dendrite. In addition, heterosynaptic effects may be associative, requiring the coordinate activation of both synapses.

- LTP is produced by an increase in calcium concentration in the postsynaptic cell and involves both the insertion of new receptors into the postsynaptic membrane and an increase in receptor sensitivity.

- Conversely, LTD is mediated by a decrease in the number of postsynaptic receptors and in their sensitivity. It is produced by smaller increases in postsynaptic calcium concentration than those required to produce LTP.

- Both LTP and LTD can also involve changes in transmitter release from the presynaptic terminal.

- Long-term depression can also be produced at inhibitory synapses (iLTD). The depression is mediated by release of an endocannabinoid from the postsynaptic cell by depolarization and its subsequent binding to a presynaptic cannabinoid receptor (CB1).

- Although there are some correlations between LTP and LTD and behavioral tasks involved in learning, no unequivocal causal relation between these long-term synaptic changes and memory formation has been established.

Suggested Reading

General Reviews

Collingridge, G. L., Peineau, S., Howland, J. C., and Wang, Y. T. 2010. Long-term depression in the CNS. *Nature Rev. Neurosci.*11: 459–473.

Lynch, M. A. 2004. Long-term potentiation and memory. *Physiol. Rev.* 84: 87–136.

Massey, P. V., and Bashir, Z. I. 2007. Long-term depression: multiple forms and implications for brain functions. *Trends Neurosci.* 30: 176–184.

Raymond, C. R. 2007. LTP forms 1, 2, and 3: Different mechanisms for the "long" in long-term potentiation. *Trends Neurosci.* 30: 167–175.

Südhof, T., and Malenka, R. C. 2008. Understanding synapses: Past, present, and future. *Neuron* 60: 468–476.

Original Papers

Abraham, W. C., and Williams, J. M. 2003. Properties and mechanisms of LTP maintenance. *Neuroscientist* 9: 463–474.

Barrionuevo, G., and Brown, T. H. 1983. Associative long-term potentiation in hippocampal slices. *Proc. Natl. Acad. Sci. USA* 80: 7347–7351.

Bliss, T. V. P., and Lømo, T. 1973. Long-lasting potentiation of synaptic transmission in the dentate of the anesthetized rabbit following stimulation of the perforant path. *J. Physiol.* 232: 331–356.

del Castillo, J., and Katz, B. 1954. Statistical factors involved in neuromuscular facilitation and depression. *J. Physiol.* 124: 574–585.

Enoki, R., Hu, Y., Hamilton, D., and Fine, A. 2009. Expression of long-term plasticity at individual synapses in hippocampus is graded, bidirectional, and mainly presynaptic: Optical quantal analysis. *Neuron* 62: 242–253.

Ito, M., Sakurai, M., and Tongroach, P. 1982. Climbing fibre induced depression of both mossy fibre responsiveness and glutamate sensitivity of cerebellar Purkinje cells. *J. Physiol.* 324: 113–134.

Kessels, H. W. and Malinow, R. 2009. Synaptic AMPA receptor plasticity and behavior. *Neuron* 61: 340–350.

Mallart, A., and Martin, A. R. 1967. Analysis of facilitation of transmitter release at the neuromuscular junction of the frog. *J. Physiol.* 193: 679–697.

Shi, S. H. et al. 1999. Rapid spine delivery and redistribution of AMPA receptors after synaptic NMDA receptor activation. *Science* 284: 1811–1816.

Weinrich, D. 1970. Ionic mechanisms of post-tetanic potentiation at the neuromuscular junction of the frog. *J. Physiol.* 212: 431–446.

Younts, T. J., et al. 2016. Presynaptic protein synthesis is required for long-term plasticity of GABA release. *Neuron* 92. 479–492

CHAPTER 17

The Molecular and Cellular Biology of Synaptic Plasticity

Chapter 16 has shown that increases in the levels of electrical activity alter the efficacy of synaptic transmission. One fundamental question regarding information storage by synapses is how stable storage can be maintained despite the continuous turnover of molecules at synapses. This chapter describes experiments that, by combining synaptic electrophysiology with molecular and cell biology, have led to understanding the molecular basis underlying long-term plasticity. We discuss two main aspects. The first is how the ongoing patterns of electrical activity change the molecular composition of the synapse. The second is how such molecular changes persist for long periods.

Synaptic plasticity poses challenging cell biology questions, related to the exquisite ability of neurons to control independently the molecular composition and the functional properties of their thousands of synapses and yet coordinate their various parts in a whole, well-integrated response. Long-term synaptic plasticity processes (such as long-term potentiation and long-term depression) are commonly postulated to be the substrates for various forms of learning and memory formation. As we discussed in Chapter 16, there are clear correlative links between synaptic plasticity and learning processes. However, correlation is not causation, and an unequivocal and definitive causal relation between synaptic plasticity and learning and memory has not been established yet, partly due to the lack of established methods to selectively manipulate individual potentiated synapses in vivo. At the end of the chapter we will use what we have learned about the molecular and cellular biology of synaptic plasticity to address causality questions about the necessity and sufficiency of molecular and cellular changes related to synaptic plasticity as a substrate for some forms of memory processes.

[1] Matsuzaki, M. et al. 2004. *Science* 429: 761-766.

[2] Holtmaat, A. and Svoboda K. 2009. *Nat. Rev. Neurosci.* 10: 647-658.

[3] Engert, F., and Bonhoeffer, T. 1999. *Nature* 399: 66-70.

[4] Nagerl, U. V. et al. 2004. *Neuron* 44: 759-767.

[5] Zhou, Q. et al. 2004. *Neuron* 44: 749-757.

[6] Svoboda, K. and Yasuda, R. 2006. *Neuron* 50: 823-839.

[7] Grutzendler, J. et al. 2002. *Nature* 420: 812.

[8] Trachtenberg, J. et al. 2002. *Nature* 420: 788.

[9] Berry, K. P., and Nedivi, E. 2017. *Neuron* 96: 43-55.

[10] Mongillo, G. et al. 2017. *Curr. Op. Neurobiol.* 46: 7-13.

[11] Xu, T. et al. 2009. *Nature* 462: 915.

Structural Plasticity: In Vivo Studies on Spine Dynamics

Chapter 16 has shown that synapses, on electrical stimulation, undergo extensive functional strengthening and weakening of their efficacy. These long-term functional synaptic plasticity changes are paralleled by extensive structural changes (structural plasticity), such as morphological shape remodeling[1] (see Chapter 16) and birth, growth, or disappearance of synapses.[2] Long-term potentiation (LTP) is associated with the growth and formation of dendritic spines,[1,3] whereas long-term depression (LTD) is associated with shrinkage and loss of spines.[4,5] Therefore, measurements of spine volume and dynamics provide an excellent indication of synaptic strength. The advent of two-photon microscopy[6] allowed in vivo longitudinal imaging studies of identified spines from fluorescently labeled neurons in the neocortex of living rodents.[7–9] In the adult brain, dendritic spines are dynamic: They can be transient and volatile[10] or persistent, with lifetimes of several months.[11,12] The spine turnover can be modulated by sensory manipulations.[13]

Transgenic mice in which cortical pyramidal neurons were labeled by the expression of a fluorescent protein were trained to learn a forelimb-reaching motor task. The same apical dendrites of pyramidal neurons were repeatedly imaged before, during, and after motor learning, using transcranial two-photon microscopy (Figure 17.1A).[11] Motor training induced the rapid formation of new dendritic spines in pyramidal neurons of the contralateral motor cortex and a delayed increase in spine elimination, ultimately resulting in total spine density in the trained animals returning to control levels (Figure 17.1B). No change was found in the motor cortex ipsilateral to the trained limb, or in mice that failed to learn.[11] The new spines formed after motor task learning were significantly more stable

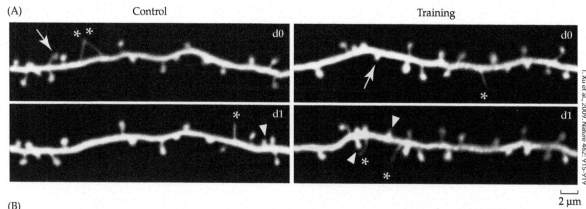

(A) Control · · · Training

d0 / d1

2 μm

T. Xu et al., 2009, *Nature* 462: 915–919

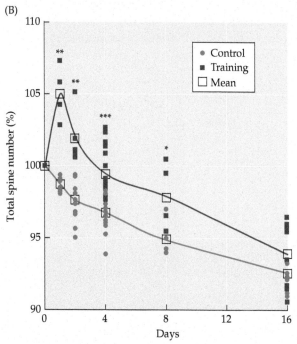

(B)

Control, Training, Mean

FIGURE 17.1 Motor Learning Enhances Spine Dynamics in the Mouse Motor Cortex. (A) Imaging of apical dendrites of pyramidal neurons in the motor cortex during motor learning using transcranial two-photon microscopy. Eliminated spines (arrows), newly formed spines (arrowheads), and filopodia (asterisks) were imaged at 1-day intervals (d0 and d1). (B) Motor training increased transiently the total number of spines in the contralateral motor cortex. (C) Timeline of the repeated imaging of dendritic branches in vivo at day 0 (1st imaging session), day 4 (2nd imaging session) and up to 120 days (3rd imaging session). Spines identified in the first 4 days after training were classified into new and preexisting spines: day 4 (2nd imaging session) vs. day 0 (1st imaging session). (D) New spines were more stable in trained than in control mice. Open black boxes signify the mean. Asterisks = *$P < 0.05$, **$P < 0.01$, ***$P < 0.001$. (After T. Xu et al., 2009. *Nature* 462: 915-919.)

than those formed in control mice that did not undergo the training, and they endured long after training stopped (Figure 17.1C,D).

Learning a novel motor skill task continues to drive spine dynamics and synaptic reorganization, without affecting the stability of synapses formed during the previous learning of the first task, suggesting that different motor behaviors are stored using different sets of synapses.[11] The maintenance of the new spines correlates with the maintenance and the quality of the learned skill.[12] A small fraction of new spines induced by novel experience are preserved throughout the entire life of an animal, possibly representing traces encoding lifelong memories.[12] The prolonged persistence of learning-induced synapses provides a potential cellular mechanism for the consolidation of lasting motor memories.

One prominent feature of in vivo spine dynamics studies is that only a small fraction of the relatively high number of new synapses formed each day are stably maintained over time. A process of selective pruning versus maintaining new synapses would seem necessary for neuronal circuits to store new information without being overloaded and without disrupting previously acquired memories. Sleep might play a role in this process of selective synaptic homeostasis.[14]

Microglial cells are thought to mediate spine elimination, both in the developing[15] and in the adult nervous system,[16] actively engulfing spines tagged for elimination, or nibbling the presynaptic terminal.[17] In the adult mouse hippocampus, synaptic elimination by microglial phagocytosis has been shown to mediate forgetting of a learned **contextual fear conditioning** behavioral task, since depletion of microglial cells or inhibition of microglial phagocytosis greatly prolongs the duration of the memory.[18]

[12] Yang, G. et al. 2009. *Nature* 462: 920–924.

[13] Hofer, S. B. et al. 2009. *Nature* 457: 313–317.

[14] Li, W. et al. 2017. *Nat. Neurosci.* 20: 427–437.

[15] Paolicelli, R. C. et al. 2011. *Science* 333: 1456–1458.

[16] Schafer, D. P. et al. 2012. *Neuron* 74: 691–705.

[17] Weinhard, L. et al. 2018. *Nat. Comm.* 9: 1228.

[18] Wang, C. et al. 2020. *Science* 367: 688–694.

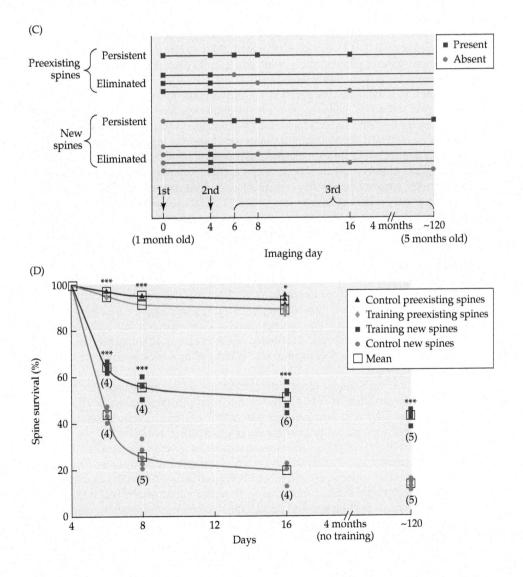

(C)

(D)

Synaptic Protein Turnover and the Transition from Short- to Long-Term Synaptic Plasticity

Enduring changes in the efficacy of synaptic transmission are ultimately determined by changes in the molecular composition of the synapses.[19] The turnover of the synaptic proteome reflects (1) protein traffic into and out of the synapse[20] and (2) rates of synthesis and degradation[21,22]—all processes that are strongly activity-dependent. The exchange rates of synaptic receptors and associated proteins due to activity-dependent traffic into and out of the dendritic spines are rapid (timescale of minutes).[20] The lifetime of synaptic proteins, measured by metabolic labeling, is in the range of hours to days.[21,22] In any event, both the exchange rates and the lifetimes of synaptic proteins are significantly shorter than the typical timescales of long-term plasticity changes.

Short-term forms of synaptic plasticity (see Chapter 16) are sustained by local transient events such as calcium influx and rapid post-translational modifications (e.g., phosphorylation) of existing synaptic proteins, whose lifetimes are in the order of minutes. How can the transition between short-term to long-term synaptic plasticity be supported and consolidated by synaptic proteins with a shorter turnover?

Signaling from Synapses to the Nucleus Activates de Novo Transcription

Activity-dependent de novo RNA transcription is a mechanism to provide synapses with a continuous supply of new proteins to support long-term plasticity.[23,24] Blocking transcription by application of actinomycin D inhibits the maintenance (but not the induction) of a long-lasting form of LTP (late LTP or L-LTP) induced by three trains of strong tetanic stimulation (100Hz, 1 s) in the CA3–CA1 synapse in hippocampal slices (Figure 17.2A), but only if delivered prior to the LTP induction (Figure 17.2B).[23] By contrast, a single train of tetanic stimulation produces a decremental potentiation (early LTP or E-LTP) (see also Figure 16.7) that is insensitive to transcriptional inhibition.

After L-LTP induction, the necessity for transcription of new mRNAs to consolidate the long-term synaptic change requires a bidirectional signaling between stimulated synapses and the nucleus (Figure 17.3A). L-LTP–stimulated synapses communicate to the nucleus via electrical signaling (milliseconds timescale), via regenerative calcium waves (seconds to minutes) or through the physical translocation of signaling proteins (hours). Some of the products of the de novo activity-dependent transcription are relayed back to the activated synapses, where they contribute to the enduring potentiation of those synapses (plasticity-related products) (see Figure 17.3). These mechanisms are not necessarily alternative and, because of their different timing, may generate different waves of activity-dependent transcriptional changes.

A purely electrical signal occurs when glutamatergic excitatory postsynaptic potentials (EPSPs) propagate passively or actively (dendritic spikes) from synapses to the soma, and elicit action potentials at the axon hillock (Figure 17.3B). Action potential firing is the result of the cell-wide integration of all the synaptic inputs to the neuron and is directly linked with de novo transcription in the nucleus that supports L-LTP, via somatic influx of calcium through L-type voltage-gated calcium channels. For instance, action potentials elicited by antidromic stimulation of CA1 neurons, although they do not produce LTP itself, convert a decremental E-LTP, induced by a weak synaptic stimulation, into a prolonged L-LTP[25] (see Figure 17.3B).

Action potentials, under certain circumstances, can backpropagate into the dendrites.[26,27] In experiments recording from connected cortical pyramidal neurons[28] a unitary EPSP was evoked by stimulating a single presynaptic cell, and a single backpropagating action potential was induced by brief current injection into the soma of the postsynaptic cell. When the backpropagating action potential occurred shortly after the EPSP (less than 60 ms), this resulted in LTP (provided this protocol was repeated many times). If the spike occurred in a short window just before the EPSP (< 60 ms), LTD was induced instead.[28] This form of plasticity is called spike timing–dependent plasticity[28,29] and is thought to provide the associative link between postsynaptic and presynaptic activity, required for **Hebbian-type plasticity** (see Chapter 16).

Calcium is the key messenger that links and integrates synaptic activation, action potential firing, and gene transcription in the nucleus. On synaptic activation, calcium enters the

[19] Alvarez-Castelao, B. and Schuman E. M. 2015. *J. Biol. Chem.* 290: 28623–28630.

[20] Choquet, D. and Triller 2013. *Neuron* 80: 691.

[21] Hanus, C., and Schuman, E. M. 2013. *Nat. Rev. Neurosci.* 14: 638–648.

[22] Doerrbaum, A. R. et al. 2018. *eLife* 7: e34202.

[23] Frey, U. et al. 1996. *J. Physiol* 490: 703.

[24] Nguyen, P. V. et al. 1994. *Science* 264: 1104.

[25] Dudek, S. M. and Fields, R. D. 2002. *Proc. Natl. Acad. Sci. USA* 99: 3962–3967.

[26] Stuart, G. J. and Sakmann, B. 1994. *Nature* 367: 69–72.

[27] Magee, J. C., and Johnston, D. 1997. *Science* 275: 209.

[28] Markram, H. et al. 1997. *Science* 275: 213.

[29] Bi, G. Q. and Poo, M. M. 1998. *J. Neurosci.* 18: 10464–10472.

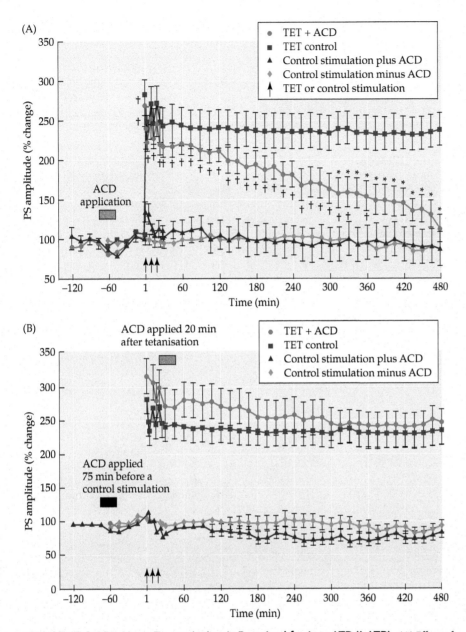

FIGURE 17.2 De Novo Transcription Is Required for Late LTP (L-LTP). (A) Effect of the transcriptional inhibitor actinomycin D (ACD) on L-LTP (population spike [PS] amplitude) in rat hippocampal CA1 slices. Only an E-LTP, and no L-LTP, is observed when ACD is applied before strong tetanic stimulation (TET [100Hz, 1 s, three trains]). (B) ACD applied after induction of LTP does not inhibit L-LTP. Asterisks in (A) indicate statistically significant differences between control LTP and ACD-treated LTP. Crosses in A indicate statistically significant differences between the tetanized input and the non-tetanized control input of the same slices after application of ACD. Error bars indicate +/- standard error of the mean. (After U. Frey et al., 1996. *J. Physiol.* 490: 703-711.)

neuron either via NMDA receptors or via voltage-gated calcium channels. Calcium regulates transcription either by directly entering into the nucleus, or indirectly by activating signaling pathways (see Figure 17.3). Synaptic NMDA receptor–mediated depolarization can also boost calcium entry through dendritic calcium channels and may amplify metabotropic glutamate receptor– (mGluR-) triggered calcium release from the endoplasmic reticulum via ryanodine receptors or inositol triphosphate receptors[30] (see Chapter 16). Regenerative waves of calcium-induced calcium release[31,32] travel from synapses to the nucleus. Both routes of synaptically evoked calcium signaling to the nucleus (soma to nucleus, and synapse to nucleus; see Figure 17.3) ultimately elevate nuclear calcium levels, a signaling end point that activates gene expression programs needed for persistent synaptic adaptations.[33,34]

[30] Berridge M. J. 1998. *Neuron* 21: 13-26.

[31] Nakamura, T. et al. 1999. *Neuron* 24: 727-737.

[32] Ross, W. N. 2012. *Nat. Rev. Neurosci.* 13: 157-168.

[33] Hardingham, G. E. et al. 2002. *Nat. Neurosci.* 5: 405.

[34] Hagenston, A. M., and Bading, H. 2011. *Cold Spring Harb. Perspect. Biol.* 3: a004564.

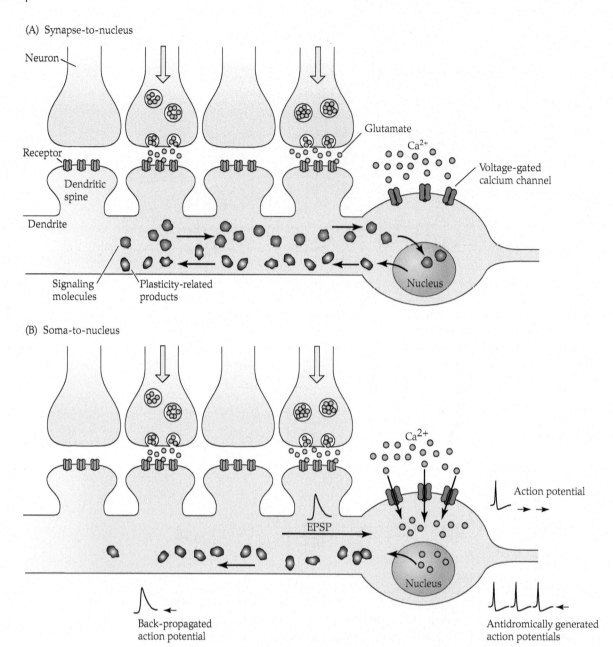

(A) Synapse-to-nucleus

Neuron

Receptor

Dendritic spine

Dendrite

Glutamate

Ca²⁺

Voltage-gated calcium channel

Signaling molecules

Plasticity-related products

Nucleus

(B) Soma-to-nucleus

Ca²⁺

Action potential

EPSP

Nucleus

Back-propagated action potential

Antidromically generated action potentials

FIGURE 17.3 Bidirectional Signals between Stimulated Synapses and Nucleus.
Synaptic activity can signal the nucleus via signaling molecules that translocate to the nucleus to initiate transcription (A) or via electrical signals (EPSP or dendritic spikes) that reach the soma (B). As a result of action potentials produced by synaptic activity, Ca²⁺ enters the soma through voltage-dependent calcium channels, where it directly or indirectly initiates transcription. The products of de novo transcription (plasticity-related products) travel back to the synapses. The soma can signal back to the synapses also by back propagating action potentials (B). (After J. W. Rudy, 2020. *The Neurobiology of Learning and Memory*, 3rd ed. Oxford University Press/Sinauer, Sunderland, MA.)

The route of calcium entry matters: Depending on the location and route of calcium entry into the neuron, distinct signaling pathways are activated, regulating distinct transcriptional and cellular responses.[33,34] For example, synaptic and extrasynaptic NMDA receptors have opposite effects on the transcription activity-dependent gene regulation and neuron survival.[35] Calcium entry through synaptic NMDA receptors induces cyclic AMP response element binding protein (CREB) activity (see next paragraph) and brain-derived neurotrophic factor (BDNF) gene expression. In contrast, calcium entry through extrasynaptic NMDA receptors, triggered by either glutamate exposure or hypoxic or ischemic

[35] Hardingham, A. M., and Bading, H. 2010. *Nat. Rev. Neurosci.* 11: 682–696.

conditions, shuts off CREB activity and activates a pathway that causes mitochondrial dysfunction and cell death.[35.]

A slower signaling from synapses to the nucleus in postsynaptic cells is through the transport of specific proteins.[36-38] Once in the nucleus, proteins activate gene expression, long after initial LTP induction. One protein that undergoes activity-dependent synapse-to-nucleus translocation is ERK (extracellular signal-regulated kinase).[39] The phosphorylated state of pERK is preserved, during transport to the nucleus, by the synaptic protein Jacob, which is phosphorylated (pJacob) by ERK.[37] While the complex pERK–pJacob in the nucleus induces plasticity-related transcription, the activation of extrasynaptic NMDA receptors causes a nonphosphorylated form of Jacob to enter the nucleus and promote neuronal cell death. The phosphorylation state of Jacob allows the nucleus to distinguish between the activation of synaptic or extrasynaptic NMDA receptors.[35]

Early Genomic Targets of Synaptic Activity

The strong stimulation that produces L-LTP promotes the rapid transcription of approximately 300 genes, collectively called immediate early genes (IEGs).[40-42] IEGs are a class of genes whose expression is rapidly (within minutes) and transiently induced by extracellular stimuli, without a requirement for new protein synthesis. Their rapid transcription on synaptic activation is possible because in resting conditions a complex transcriptional machinery is permanently assembled on their promoters and ready to work (Figure 17.4A). The composition of the transcriptional machinery varies for different IEGs and in different cell types.[41,42] A detailed description of the machinery is beyond the scope of this book. The important point is that such a complex machinery is preassembled on the genome and poised for rapid transcriptional response.

DNA sequence motifs within the IEGs promoters, such as the cyclic AMP response element, are constitutively bound by transcriptional activators, for instance CREB (see Figure 17.4A). At rest, this poised state is actively repressed by the association of histone deacetylases and a closed chromatin structure. CREB is a key transcription factor active on electrical activity (reviewed in [43,44]) (Figure 17.4B). Synaptic activity triggers calcium-regulated signaling events that relieve the transcriptional repression of IEGs by inducing CREB phosphorylation, which facilitates the recruitment of histone acetyltransferase CBP (CREB binding protein) to the promoter. The ensuing local histone acetylation (and the detachment and nuclear export of preassembled histone deacetylases) changes the chromatin environment of CREB target genes into an open, relaxed state (see Figure 17.4B), rapidly allowing IEG transcription.

Many IEGs encode DNA binding proteins that function as transcription factors and regulate the expression of a subsequent wave of late-response genes, responsible for the long-term consolidation of plasticity changes (see Figure 17.4A, inset). Other IEGs encode effector proteins that directly regulate the synaptic function, such as the neurotrophin BDNF and Arc (*activity-regulated cytoskeleton-associated protein*)/arg3-1.

Synaptic activity tightly regulates the availability of BDNF at multiple levels: transcription, mRNA transport, translation, secretion, and processing.[45-47] The mammalian BDNF gene has a peculiar organization, with multiple promoters driving the expression of a common exon coding the whole BDNF protein (Figure 17.5A). All BDNF mRNA splicing isoforms encode the same protein, but each isoform shows a distinct subcellular localization and is regulated in a distinct way.[48] This configuration provides extreme regulatory flexibility and precise temporal and spatial control of BDNF activity and localization.

In the cortex, BDNF promoter IV is the most strongly responsive to synaptic activity. At rest, BDNF promoter IV is bound to several transcription factors that recruit repressor complexes (Figure 17.5B). Upon calcium influx, the transcription factors and the chromatin that surrounds BDNF promoter IV are rapidly turned into an active transcriptional state, and the RNA polymerase is recruited for rapid transcription (see Figure 17.5B).

How can we dissect the distinct biological functions of the constitutive versus the activity-dependent pool of BDNF protein? This has been accomplished by generating knock-in mutant transgenic mice, to specifically disrupt the expression of BDNF from promoter IV but not from the other BDNF promoters.[49] Unlike BDNF knock-out mice, which die in the early postnatal days, these knock-in mice live, because they have similar basal levels

[36] Herbst, W. A. and Martin, K. C. 2017. *Curr. Op. Neurobiol.* 45: 78-84.

[37] Panayotis, N. et al. 2015. *Trends Neurosci.* 38: 108-116.

[38] Adams, J. P., and Dudek SM. 2005. *Nat Rev. Neurosci.* 6: 737-743.

[39] Zhai, S. et al. 2013. *Science* 342: 1107-1111.

[40] Flavell, S. W. and Greenberg, M. E. 2008. *Annu. Rev. Neurosci.* 31: 563-590.

[41] Lyons, M. R. and West, A. E. 2011. *Prog. Neurobiol.* 94: 259-295.

[42] Yap, E.-L. and Greenberg, M. E. 2018. *Neuron* 100: 330.

[43] Alberini, C. 2009. *Physiol. Rev.* 89: 121-145.

[44] Silva, A. J. et al. 1998. *Annu. Rev. Neurosci.* 21: 127-148.

[45] Thoenen, H. 1991. *Trends Neurosci.* 14: 165-170.

[46] Park, H. and Poo M. 2013. *Nat. Rev. Neurosci.* 14: 7-23.

[47] Bramham, C. and Messaoudi, E. 2005. *Prog. Neurobiol.* 76: 99-125.

[48] Baj, G. et al. 2011. *Proc. Natl. Acad. Sci. USA* 108: 16813-16818.

[49] Hong, E. J. et al. 2008. *Neuron* 60: 610-624.

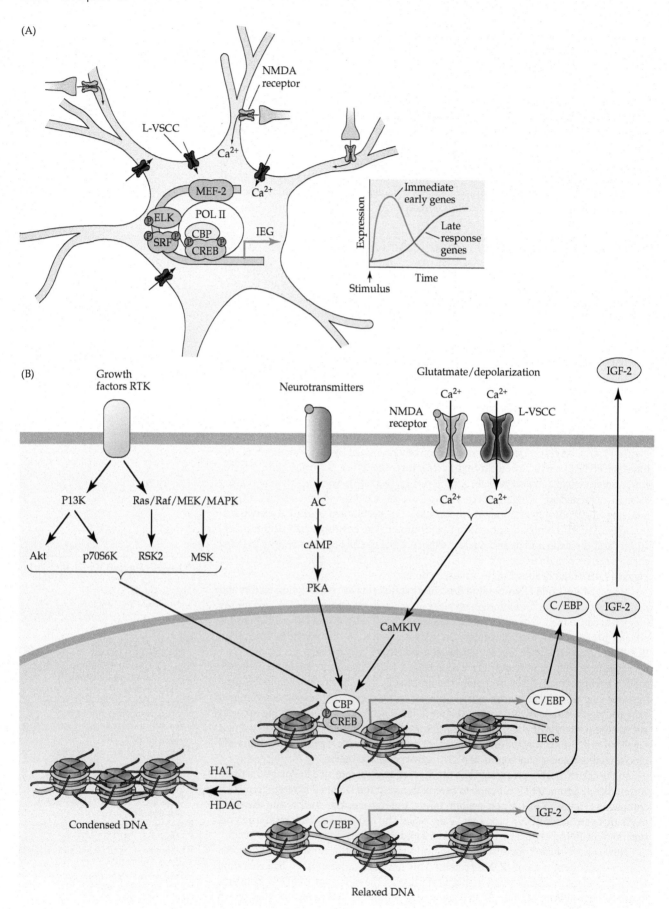

◀ **FIGURE 17.4   Immediate Early Genes Are Poised for Transcription.** (A) Calcium entering via NMDA receptors or via somatic or dendritic L-type voltage-sensitive calcium channels (L-VSCCs) activates preexisting transcription factors, such as CREB and associated proteins, which induce the transcription of immediate early genes (IEGs). Inset: Many IEGs (activated in minutes) encode transcription factors (e.g., FOS and C/EBP) that regulate a subsequent wave of late-response genes (hours) (e.g., *IGF-2*, *Ube3a*). (B) The transcription factor CREB integrates different signaling pathways leading to its phosphorylation at Ser-133 residue, an important step for its activation. CREB phosphorylation can be induced by increase in calcium influx through L-VSCCs or through NMDA receptors. Calcium activates various cytoplasmic signaling pathways, or enters the nucleus directly, where it activates calcium-calmodulin-dependent protein kinase IV (CaMKIV), leading to CREB phosphorylation. The activation of neurotrophin receptor tyrosine kinases (RTK) (for instance by BDNF) and of the downstream signaling pathways (Ras/Raf/MEK/MAPK) also leads to CREB phosphorylation. Another route to CREB phosphorylation is through neurotransmitters binding to their receptors, and regulation of adenylyl cyclase (AC) activity. cAMP recruits protein kinase A (PKA) as another kinase for CREB phosphorylation. At rest, unphosphorylated CREB is already bound to the promoter of target IEGs. Once phosphorylated, CREB recruits, among others, CREB binding protein (CBP), a transcriptional co-activator with histone acetyltransferase (HAT) activity. Acetylation of histones contributes to chromatin relaxation. CREB activation, and the concomitant opening and relaxation of the chromatin, induces the expression of target IEGs (such as C/EBP). C/EBP, in turn, regulates a number of late-response genes, for example, IGF-2. (HDAC: Histone deacetylase) (A after E.-L. Yap and M. E. Greenberg, 2018. *Neuron* 100: 330–348; B after C. M. Alberini and D. Y. Chen. 2012. *Trends Neurosci.* 35: 274–283.)

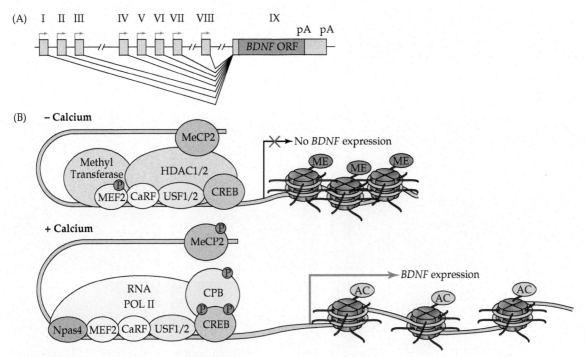

FIGURE 17.5   Organization of the BDNF Gene and Its Multiple Alternative Transcripts. (A) The BDNF gene consists of eight distinct promoters that initiate the transcription of different mRNAs, each of which contains an alternative 5′ exon (blue boxes I to VIII) spliced to a common coding exon (exon IX, *BDNF* Open Reading frame [ORF]), which employs either of two polyadenylation sites (pA). (B) Activation of BDNF exon IV transcription. At rest (top), *BDNF* promoter IV is bound by several transcription factors (CREB, USF, CaRF, MeCP2, and MEF2) that recruit repressor complexes, including histone deacetylases (HDAC1/2) and methyltransferases. The chromatin surrounding the initiation site of *BDNF* transcription synthesis is bound by histones that are methylated (symbol ME in orange circles), and the chromatin is condensed, a state that is correlated with gene repression. Unphosphorylated MeCP2 docks *BDNF* promoter IV to a repressor chromatin locus that further ensures that *BDNF* promoter IV is kept off even though it is poised for transcriptional activation. Synaptic activity-induced calcium influx (bottom) induces phosphorylation of CREB and of MeCP2, releasing the *BDNF* promoter from the repressive locus and changing the epigenetic state of the chromatin surrounding *BDNF* exon IV. This results in the recruitment of the histone acetyltransferase CREB binding protein (CBP), of histone demethylase and in the detachment and nuclear export of the preassembled repressive histone deacetylases (HDAC1/2). The ensuing acetylation of histones (symbol AC in green circles) opens up the chromatin (see also Figure 17.4B), allows the recruitment of the RNA polymerase II and transcription of *BDNF* exon IV ensues (After P. L. Greer and M. E. Greenberg, 2008. *Neuron* 59: 846–860.)

[50] Link, W. et al., 1995. *Proc. Natl. Acad. Sci. USA* 92: 5734–5738.

[51] Lyford, G. L. et al., 1995. *Neuron* 14: 433–445.

[52] Nikolaienko, O. et al. 2017. *Semin. Cell Dev. Biol.* doi: 10.1016/j.semcdb.2017.09.006.

of BDNF, but reduced levels of BDNF promoter IV–dependent mRNA transcripts, following synaptic stimulation. Notably, these mice exhibit a reduction in the strength and number of GABAergic synapses and an impaired inhibitory but not excitatory cortical synaptic transmission. This suggests that the pool of BDNF protein generated from the activity-dependent BDNF transcription regulates synaptic inhibition and therefore cortical excitability.

Arc is a master regulator of synaptic plasticity.[50-52] A rapid, strong, and transient expression of *Arc* mRNA follows electrical stimulation (Figure 17.6A). The newly

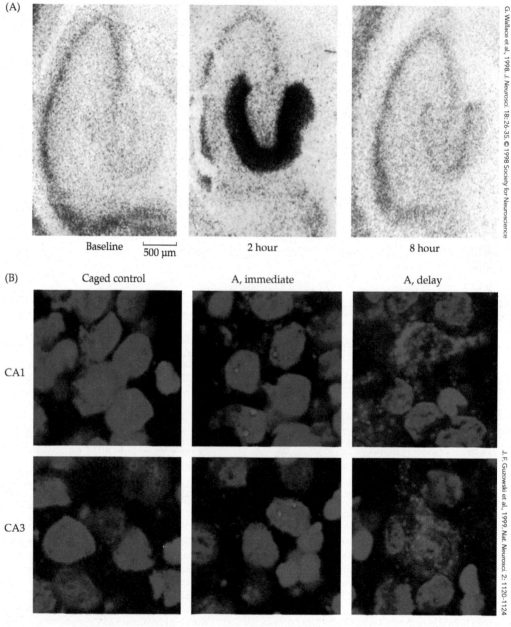

(A)

Baseline   500 µm   2 hour   8 hour

G. Wallace et al., 1998. *J. Neurosci.* 18: 26-35. © 1998 Society for Neuroscience

(B)   Caged control   A, immediate   A, delay

CA1

CA3

J. F. Guzowski et al., 1999. *Nat. Neurosci.* 2: 1120-1124

FIGURE 17.6 Activity-Dependent Transcription of Arc. (A) Kinetics of *Arc* mRNA induction and translocation into granule cell dendrites of rat hippocampus, after a single electroconvulsive seizure. Labeling by a ^{35}S-labeled complementary RNA probe for *Arc* mRNA. Within 1 hour, labeling extended into the dentate molecular layer, indicating transport of *Arc* mRNA up to the distal extent of granule cell dendrites, a distance of up to 300 µm. (B) Subcellular distribution of *Arc* mRNA visualized by fluorescent in situ hybridization in rat CA1 and CA3 hippocampus. Rats were moved from their home cage to environment A for 5 minutes, after which they were either immediately sacrificed (A, immediate) or returned to their home cage for 25 minutes before sacrifice (A, delay). *Arc* RNA appeared first in discrete intranuclear foci (A, immediate) and disappeared from the nucleus, accumulating in the cytoplasm by 30 minutes (A, delay).

transcribed *Arc* mRNA is first detected in the nucleus, and then is translocated to the cytoplasm within 30 minutes (Figure 17.6B). Within 1 hour, *Arc* mRNA is transported to the distal dendrites (see Figure 17.6A). The transcriptional activation of Arc can be used to map neurons that have been activated in response to a given behavioral stimulation, such as the exploration of a new environment (see Figure 17.6B). This activity mapping approach, termed *cellular compartment analysis of temporal activity by fluorescent in situ hybridization (catFISH)*, allows the discrimination of neuronal populations that have been activated by two distinct experiences, by observing the nuclear- and the cytoplasmic-labeled neurons.[53] IEG-based activity mapping has been widely used to identify brain regions that are activated by external stimuli. Characterization of the promoter and enhancer elements responsible for neuronal activity-dependent transcription of IEGs has opened new avenues for live imaging and manipulation of neurons active during learning,[54] as we will see later in the chapter.

Hundreds of activity-regulated IEGs are expressed in the brain, and each cell type expresses a distinct subset of activity-regulated genes.[42,55] Also, the same IEG can trigger distinct transcriptional programs in distinct cells. A good example is provided by the IEG *Npas4*. *Npas4* is a transcription factor that is rapidly induced by neuronal activity in both excitatory and inhibitory neurons. In turn, Npas4 activates distinct late-response genes in inhibitory and excitatory neurons.[56]

Conversely, in any given neuron, different neuronal activity patterns induce the expression of distinct activity-dependent mRNAs,[57] generating transcriptional fingerprints that report on the history of neuronal activity. How distinct types of electrical activity can be decoded by IEGs into distinct modes of genomic regulation is a challenging question under investigation.[58]

Is the activation of CREB by synaptic signals sufficient for expression of genes responsible for L-LTP? This was investigated in cortical slices from transgenic mice, by inducing the expression of a constitutively active form of CREB protein (VP16-CREB).[59] The expression of VP16-CREB in CA1 hippocampal neurons facilitates LTP: L-LTP was established by a single tetanic train, which normally produces only E-LTP. The facilitated L-LTP can also be induced in the presence of transcriptional inhibitors.[59] Indeed, in the transgenic mice the "activity-regulated" mRNA transcripts that support L-LTP are expressed also in basal conditions, because of the constitutively active CREB.

Neuroepigenetics: Stabilizing Activity-Dependent Transcriptional Changes

The expression of IEGs is transient, yet the transcriptional changes induced by synaptic activity, via IEGs, are maintained for periods similar to those of plasticity. Neurons activated during a synaptic plasticity protocol, or during learning, enter a new "transcriptional state," which is maintained and stabilized in the long term. How is this achieved? Changes in chromatin structure are emerging as mechanisms to stabilize the long-term gene expression on synaptic activity.[60,61] These chromatin remodeling changes resemble the epigenetic mechanisms taking place during development and cell fate acquisition, responsible for maintaining cell differentiation (see Chapter 27).

In the context of nondividing postmitotic neurons, **neuroepigenetics** refers to those epigenetic mechanisms, co-opted by neurons, that persistently modify the organization of the chromatin without altering the genome sequence, thus stabilizing the global activity-dependent transcriptional output of the neuron(s).[60,62]

The two canonical epigenetic mechanisms are **post-translational modifications of histone proteins** (acetylation, methylation, and phosphorylation) and dynamic **DNA methylation** (to form 5-methylcytosine). Both of these processes are regulated by synaptic activity-dependent calcium signals.[61]

Mutations in specific components of the activity-dependent transcriptional[42] and epigenetic pathways[63–65] in neurons have been genetically associated with neurodevelopmental and neuropsychiatric disorders in humans. For instance, mutations in human *MeCP2*, a "reader" of methylated DNA, cause the neurodevelopmental disorder Rett syndrome. These observations point to activity-dependent transcription and its epigenetic regulation as key biological mechanisms underlying nervous system functions.

[53] Guzowski, J. F. et al. 1999. *Nat. Neurosci.* 2: 1120–1124.

[54] Kawashima, T. et al. 2013. *Nat. Methods* 10: 889.

[55] Hrvatin, S., et al. 2018. *Nat. Neurosci.* 21: 120–129.

[56] Spiegel, I. et al. 2014. *Cell* 157: 1216–1229.

[57] Tyssowsky, K. M. et al. 2018. *Neuron* 98: 530–546.

[58] Brigidi, G. S. et al. 2019. *Cell* 179: 373–391.

[59] Barco, A. et al. 2002. *Cell* 108: 689–703.

[60] Day, J. J., and Sweatt, J. D. 2011. *Neuron* 70: 813–829.

[61] Campbell, R. R. and Wood, M. A. 2019. *Nat. Rev. Neurosci.* doi: 10.1038/s41583-019-0121-9.

[62] Sweatt, J. D. 2013. *Neuron* 80: 624.

[63] Ebert, D. H. and Greenberg M. E. 2013. *Nature* 493: 327–337.

[64] Nestler, E. J. et al. 2016. *Neuroscientist* 22: 447–463.

[65] Iwase, S. et al. 2017. *J. Neurosci.* 37: 10773–10782.

Early Evidence for Decentralized Protein Synthesis in Neurons

With the nucleus and chromatin being common targets for the thousands of synapses in a neuron, how are the plasticity-related products (PRPs), generated by the activity-dependent transcription, specifically targeted to the activated synapses but not to the rest of the synapses?

One answer to this question is provided by the evidence showing that mRNAs are targeted to dendrites and axons, and that local protein synthesis can occur at postsynaptic and presynaptic sites, where it is modulated by activity.[66-68] Accordingly, the machinery required for protein synthesis, including for polyribosomes, translation factors, endoplasmic reticulum, Golgi secretory outposts, and a selected population of mRNAs, has been found to be present in neuronal processes.

The early observation by Bodian of ribosomes adjacent to synaptic contacts in dendrites of monkey motoneurons [69] was followed by electron microscopic evidence for polyribosomes in distal dendrites of dentate gyrus granule cells[70] (Figure 17.7A). Polyribosomes are found in the dendritic shaft at the base of the spines (Figure 17.7A) and also, more rarely, in the spine neck and head. Evidence for local protein synthesis was first provided by Antonio Giuditta, who demonstrated metabolic labeling of newly synthesized axonal proteins in squid axons separated from the cell bodies.[71] Later, Oswald Steward used autoradiography to show protein synthesis in dendrites of hippocampal neurons that had been mechanically isolated from the cell bodies[72] (Figure 17.7B).

In situ hybridization allowed detection of the first abundant dendritic mRNAs, on a candidate basis: CaMKII (calcium calmodulin kinase)[73] and MAP2 (microtubule-associated protein 2).[74]

The transport of mRNA to most distal dendrites can be stimulated by neuronal activity, as was shown for the mRNAs encoding for the neurotrophin BDNF and its tyrosine kinase receptor TrkB[75,76] (Figure 17.8A) and for *Arc* mRNA[77] (Figure 17.8B). When a topographically localized presynaptic stimulation of the postsynaptic dendritic arbor was performed, newly transcribed *Arc* mRNA was specifically localized in the activated dendritic domain[77] (Figure 17.8B).

mRNA Targeting to Dendrites and Axons

The advent of deep sequencing technologies allowed the systematic and unbiased identification of the collection of dendritic mRNAs (dendritic transcriptome).[78] To enrich for dendritically localized mRNAs, the synaptic neuropil was microdissected from the CA1 region of hippocampal slices, comprising dendrites, axons, glia, and a sparse population of interneurons, but lacking neuronal cell bodies. mRNAs were identified using deep RNA sequencing, and bioinformatic analysis was used to filter out glial, interneuron, endothelial, and mitochondrial mRNAs, yielding around 2550 bona fide dendritic mRNAs.[78] Many of these mRNAs encode proteins known to be present at synapses and dendrites, but it was surprising to find that many dendritic mRNAs encode transcription factors, ribosomal proteins, and mitochondrial proteins. The last might be related to the high energy demand of protein synthesis. A reciprocal cross talk between local translation and synaptic mitochondria has been recently demonstrated.[79]

What about mRNA targeting in axons? The idea of local mRNA translation in axon terminals has a long history[71,80] but was initially well accepted to apply only to developing axons (see Chapter 27), whereas axonal translation in mammalian adult neurons has been a subject of long-standing debate.[81]

Holt and her colleagues used an ingenious experimental approach (axon-TRAP-Ribo Tag) (Figure 17.9) to purify the ribosomes and the associated mRNAs from axonal terminals of developing and of adult mouse retinal ganglion cells innervating the superior colliculus.[82] A tagged ribosomal protein is selectively expressed in retinal ganglion cells, and incorporated into ribosomes, so that when the ribosomes are immunopurified from the superior colliculus, one is sure that they derive from the retinal ganglion cells and not from cells in the optic nerve target region. The tagged ribosomes were immunopurified from the superior colliculus, together with the bound, actively translated mRNAs. Sequencing these mRNAs provided a formal demonstration that axonal terminals of adult (as well as developing) retinal ganglion cells contain a varied and rich repertoire of actively translated mRNAs (axonal translatome)[82] (see Figure 17.9).

[66] Glock, C. et al. 2017. *Curr. Op. Neurobiol.* 45: 169-177.

[67] Van Driesche, S. J. and Martin, K. C. 2018. *Dev. Neurobiol.* 78: 331-339.

[68] Hafner, A. S. et al. 2019. *Science* 364: eaau3644.

[69] Bodian D. 1965. *Proc. Natl. Acad. Sci. USA* 53: 418-425.

[70] Steward, O. and Lewy 1982. *J. Neurosci.* 2: 284-291.

[71] Giuditta, A. et al. 1968. *Proc. Natl. Acad. Sci. USA* 59: 1284-1287.

[72] Torre, E. R. and Steward O. 1992. *J. Neurosci.* 12: 762.

[73] Burgin, K. E. et al. 1990. *J. Neurosci.* 10: 1788-1798.

[74] Garner, C. C. et al. 1988. *Nature* 336: 674-677.

[75] Tongiorgi, E. et al. 1997. *J. Neurosci.* 17: 9492-9505.

[76] Righi, M. et al. 2000. *J. Neurosci.* 20: 3165.

[77] Steward, O. et al. 1998. *Neuron* 21: 741-751.

[78] Cajigas, et al. 2012. *Neuron* 74: 453-466.

[79] Rangaraju, V. et al. 2019. *Cell* 176: 73-84.

[80] Crispino, M. et al. 2013. *Dev. Neurobiol.* 74: 279-291.

[81] Giuditta, A., et al. 2002. *Trends Neurosci.* 25: 400-404.

[82] Shigeoka, T. et al. 2016. *Cell* 166: 181-192.

(A)

(B)

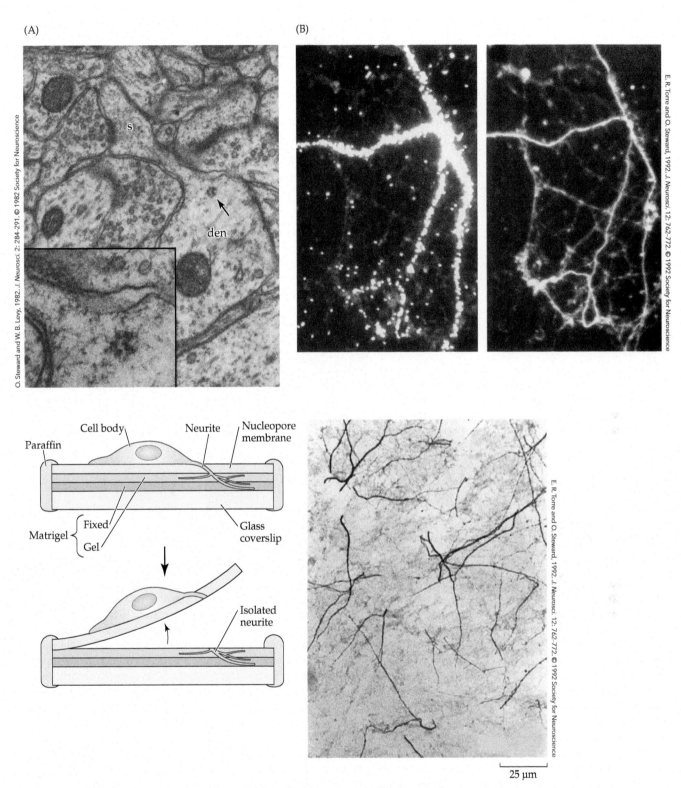

25 µm

FIGURE 17.7   Local Protein Synthesis in Hippocampal Neuron Dendrites. (A, top) Polyribosomes (arrow) in rat hippocampal dentate granule cells viewed by electron microscopy localize at the spine (S) neck-dendritic shaft intersection (den). Inset at lower left: 3× magnified polyribosome cluster, indicated by the arrow in the lower magnification field. (A, bottom left) A sandwich culture system, to isolate dendrites from the soma of rat hippocampal neurons. The porous plating surface permits the passage of neurites but not of cell bodies. A second surface coated with Matrigel (fixed to the coverslip by heating, overlayed with fresh Matrigel) receives the neurites. (A, bottom right) Neurites that remain on the Matrigel surface after peeling off the nucleopore membrane. (B) Isolated neurites from the sandwich cultures were metabolically labeled with ³H-Leu for 30 minutes. Coverslips were stained for MAP2 and exposed for autoradiography. Dark-field and fluorescence observation revealed labeling over isolated neurites (left) that stained positively for the dendritic marker MAP2 (right). (After E. R. Torre and O. Steward, 1992. *J. Neurosci.* 12: 762-772. © 1992 Society for Neuroscience.)

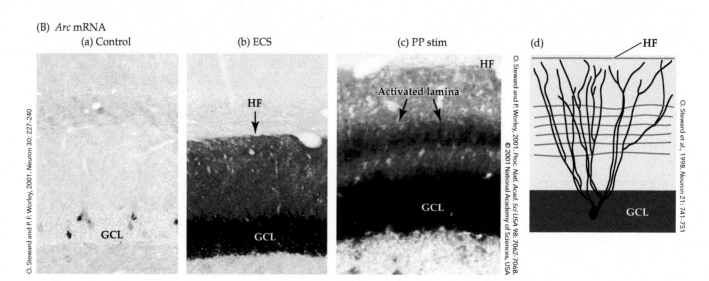

(A) *BDNF* mRNA

Control + Pilocarpine

E. Tongiorgi et al., 2004. *J. Neurosci.* 24: 6842-6852. © 2004 Society for Neuroscience.

FIGURE 17.8 Activity-Dependent Dendritic Transport of mRNA. (A) In situ hybridization for *BDNF* mRNA in the rat hippocampus CA1 region. Left: Control animal Right: Pilocarpine-treated animal (3 hours) with marked enhancement of dendritic signal. (B) In situ hybridization for *Arc* mRNA in dentate gyrus of the rat hippocampus: (a) control; (b) 2 hours after a single electroconvulsive seizure (ECS); arrow points to the hippocampal fissure; (c) after delivering high-frequency trains to the medial perforant path (PP) from the enthorhinal cortex; arrows point to the activated dendritic lamina. (d) Pattern of medial perforant path projections onto dentate granule cell. HF, hippocampal fissure; GCL, granule cell layer.

(B) *Arc* mRNA

(a) Control   (b) ECS   (c) PP stim   (d)

O. Steward and P. F. Worley, 2001. *Neuron* 30: 227-240

O. Steward and P. Worley, 2001. *Proc. Natl. Acad. Sci USA* 98: 7062-7068. © 2001 National Academy of Sciences, USA

O. Steward et al., 1998. *Neuron* 21: 741-751

How are mRNAs targeted to dendrites (and axons)? mRNAs do not travel "naked," but are covered with a host of RNA binding proteins and regulatory RNAs that modulate different aspects of their cellular life (transport, translation, and degradation), forming high-molecular-weight messenger ribonucleoprotein (mRNP) granules.[83] The RNA granules, a reversibly self-assembled boundary-free organelle, are actively transported by motor proteins along the cytoskeleton. Given the small numbers of mRNA copies in dendrites and even more so at individual synapses,[84] it has been proposed that mRNAs do not rest, but continuously patrol the dendrites.[85] Granule-associated mRNAs are transported to their final destination in a translationally repressed state. Synaptic activity releases mRNAs from their translationally repressed state.

Ribosome localization in synaptic compartments is essential for local translation. According to the standard view, the biogenesis of ribosomes occurs in the nucleolus, and ribosomes are transported as assembled organelles. It has therefore been puzzling to observe that mRNAs coding for some (but not all) ribosomal proteins are enriched and translated in both dendrites[78] and axons,[82] and that the axonally synthesized ribosomal proteins incorporate into axonal ribosomes in a nucleolus-independent fashion.[86]

Dendritic and axonal ribosomes might differ from somatic ribosomes in another respect. In mammalian cells, polysomes (clusters of three or four ribosomes engaged with a single mRNA molecule) are commonly thought to represent the translationally active ribosome population. A recent study revealed a surprisingly high number of dendritic and axonal transcripts associated with, and translated by, monosomes (single ribosomes).[87]

[83] Han, T. W. et al. 2012. *Cell* 149: 768-779.

[84] Kosik, K. 2016. *Neuron* 92: 1168.

[85] Doyle, M., and Kleber, M. A. 2011. *EMBO J.* 30: 3540-3552.

[86] Shigeoka, T. et al. 2019. *Cell Rep.* 29: 3605.

[87] Biever, A. et al. 2020. *Science* 367: eaay4991.

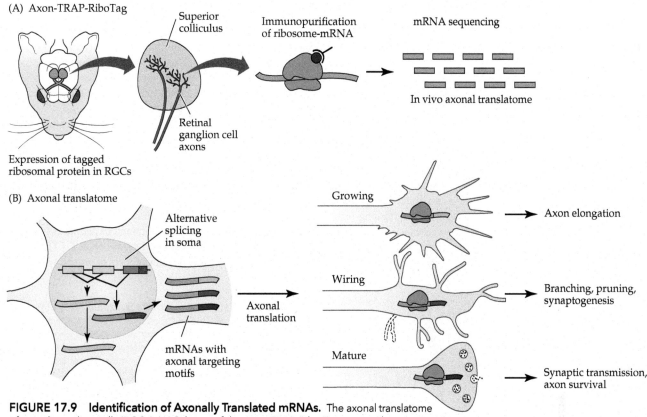

FIGURE 17.9   Identification of Axonally Translated mRNAs. The axonal translatome of retinal ganglion cells (RGCs). (A) Scheme of the Axon-TRAP-Ribo-Tag approach: retina-specific ribosome tagging, immunopurification of tagged ribosomes in axonal terminals from the superior colliculus, and sequencing of the ribosome-associated mRNAs (axonal translatome). (B) The embryonic-to-postnatal axonal translatome comprises genes involved in axon wiring. Adult axons translate mRNAs linked to axon survival and neurotransmission. Axonally translated mRNAs are frequently found to be specific alternative splice variants that carry axon-specific sequence motifs. (After T. Shigeoka et al., 2016. *Cell* 166: 181–192. © 2016 The Authors. Published by Elsevier Inc./CC BY 4.0.)

The mRNA dendritic and axonal localization is regulated by sequences of variable sizes (from tens of nucleotides to several kilobases), usually found in the 3¢ untranslated region (3¢ UTR) of the mRNA. These localization elements, or zip codes, can be a primary RNA sequence (often comprising discontinuous sequence stretches) or a secondary structure formed by the sequence(s). A secondary RNA structure known as a G-quadruplex is present in the 3¢ UTR of many dendritically localized mRNAs, including PSD95 and CaMKIIa, and is necessary and sufficient for their dendritic localization.[88] Zip codes are autonomous and dominant, as they can confer dendritic or axonal localization when inserted onto a reporter mRNA.[89]

The functions of the dendritic pool of mRNA (versus those of the somatic pool) can be investigated by interfering selectively with the mRNA zip code sequences, while leaving the rest of the mRNA (and particularly the coding sequence) unaffected.[90,91] For example, to test the functional role of dendritic translation of CaMKII, the 3¢ UTR of *CamKII* mRNA was mutated by targeted mutagenesis in mice.[90] This caused the *somatic accumulation of the mRNA and the reduction of synaptic CaMKII protein*. In these mice, L-LTP was reduced and behavioral tests for learning and memory showed impairments.

Postsynaptic Protein Synthesis and Synaptic Plasticity

Experiments show that local protein synthesis is required to consolidate CA3–CA1 hippocampal synaptic plasticity.[92,93] Protein synthesis inhibitors were applied either to the cell body or to the apical or basal dendritic fields of CA1 pyramidal cells, each of which receive

[88] Subramanian, M. et al. 2011. *EMBO Rep.* 12: 697–704.

[89] Mayford, M., et al. 1996. *Proc. Natl. Acad. Sci. USA* 93: 13250–13255.

[90] Miller, S. et al. 2002. *Neuron* 36: 507.

[91] An et al. 2008. *Cell* 134: 175–187.

[92] Bradshaw, K. D. et al. 2003. *Eur. J. Neurosci.* 18: 3150–3152.

[93] Vickers, C. A. et al. 2005. *J. Physiol.* 568.3: 803–813.

input from different Schaffer collateral fibers.[92] By stimulating either apical or basal fibers, L-LTP can be produced selectively at synapses of the corresponding region of the dendritic field. When the protein synthesis inhibitor emetine is applied to the entire slice, L-LTP is prevented in both dendritic fields. However, application of emetine just in the apical or basal dendrites blocks L-LTP only in the targeted dendrites, and not in the other dendritic field (Figure 17.10A,B). Local application of emetine to the soma does not affect the production of L-LTP in either region of the dendrites.[92]

A form of L-LTP, lasting at least 5 hours, can be induced and maintained in hippocampal slices where the dendrites of the stratum radiatum are isolated from their cell bodies by microsurgery (Figure 17.10C,D).[93] The magnitude of the potentiation in the isolated dendrites is similar to that recorded from whole neurons. Incubation of the slices with protein synthesis inhibitors blocks the maintenance (but not the induction) of L-LTP in both intact and isolated dendrites (see Figure 17.10D).

Thus, the long-term maintenance of the CA3–CA1 NMDA-dependent L-LTP depends on the *local translation of preexisting mRNAs* and can be maintained in dendrites isolated from their cell bodies. *Protein synthesis is required for the conversion of an E-LTP to late L-LTP.* The induction of E-LTP (and of L-LTP) is, however, independent of protein synthesis.

(A)

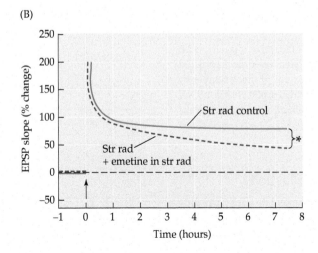

FIGURE 17.10 Local Protein Synthesis and LTP.
(A) Schematic of L-LTP induced by stimulation of two CA1 dendritic domains, in the stratum oriens (basal dendrites of pyramidal neurons) and in the stratum radiatum (apical dendrites). SE: stimulating electrode; RE: recording electrode. (B) When emetine is applied to just the apical or to just the basal dendrites (through the RE), it blocks L-LTP only when the corresponding dendritic field is stimulated, and not the other. Stimulation of apical dendrites (stratum radiatum) is shown. (C) Schematic of L-LTP in CA1 hippocampal slices where the dendrites located in stratum radiatum have been isolated from their cell bodies by a microsurgical cut (D) Late-LTP in both intact (left) and isolated (right) hippocampal slices is blocked by the mRNA translation inhibitor cycloheximide, leaving an E-LTP. Two stimulating electrodes (SE) were used to evoke field EPSPs in two independent pathways. The S1 pathway was used to apply the tetanus stimulation to evoke LTP, while the S2 pathway acted as a control. (A,C after J. W. Rudy, 2020. The *Neurobiology of Learning and Memory*, 3rd ed. Oxford University Press/Sinauer, Sunderland, MA; B after K. D. Bradshaw et al., 2003. *Eur. J. Neurosci.* 18: 3150-3152; D after C. A. Vickers et al., 2005. *J. Physiol.* 568: 803-813.)

(B)

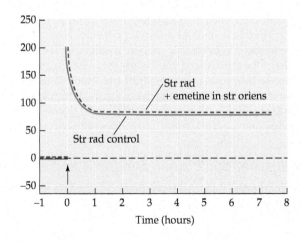

In contrast, the induction of long-term depression (LTD) (see Chapter 16) by activation of metabotropic glutamate receptors (mGluRs) depends on local protein synthesis.[94] Application of mGluR5 agonists to hippocampal slices, or low-frequency stimulation of the presynaptic pathway, reliably induces LTD of evoked excitatory synaptic responses (chemical and electrical LTD, respectively). When hippocampal slices are preincubated with the translation inhibitor anisomycin, the induction of both chemical and electrical LTD is blocked.[94] In contrast, preincubation with the transcription inhibitor actinomycin D has no effect on LTD induction, showing that the translation of mRNAs already present at the synapse is required. In hippocampal slices in which the neuropil has been isolated from the soma, bath application of protein synthesis inhibitors blocks the induction of mGluR-dependent LTD.[94.]

The neurotrophin BDNF evokes, in adult hippocampal slices, an incremental and persistent potentiation of synaptic efficacy (BDNF-LTP), in the absence of synaptic

[94] Huber, K. M. et al. 2000. *Science* 288: 1254–1257.

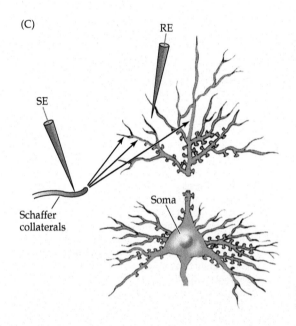

(C)

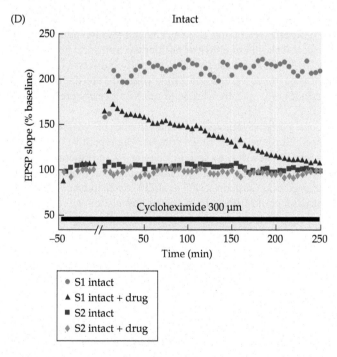

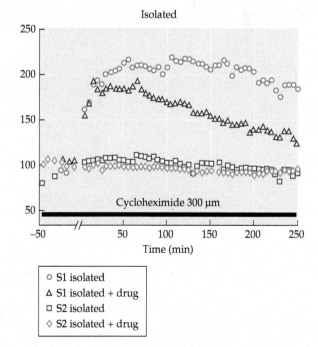

(D)

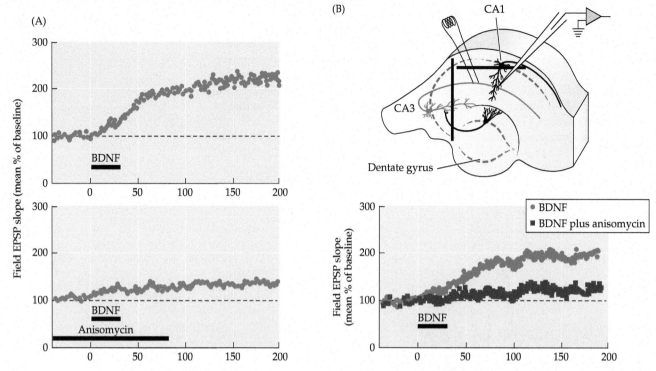

FIGURE 17.11 **Local Protein Synthesis in BDNF-Induced Hippocampal Synaptic Plasticity.** (A) BDNF-induced synaptic potentiation (BDNF-LTP) (top) in adult mouse hippocampal slices is blocked by inhibitors of protein synthesis (bottom). Two representative field EPSPs and their superposition are shown for the indicated time points (arrows labeled 1 and 2). (B) BDNF-LTP at synapses surgically isolated from both the presynaptic and postsynaptic pyramidal cell somata. (Top) Schematic representation showing the placement of the microlesions to isolate CA3 cell bodies from their axons and CA1 cell bodies from their dendrites. Electrophysiological recordings were made in the CA1 dendritic area. DG, dentate gyrus. (Bottom) Blue circles indicate enhancement of synaptic transmission by BDNF. Pretreatment of the slices with anisomycin prevented BDNF-LTP at isolated CA3-CA1 synapses (red squares). Error bars indicate +/- standard error of the mean. (After H. Kang and E. Schuman, 1996. *Science* 273: 1402-1406.)

stimulation of NMDA receptors (Figure 17.11A).[95] BDNF-LTP exhibits an immediate requirement for protein synthesis (see Figure 17.11A) and can also be induced in isolated dendrites, after surgical isolation of either or both presynaptic and postsynaptic somata (Figure 17.11B). BDNF-LTP occludes with electrically induced L-LTP in the CA1 and dentate gyrus hippocampal regions, indicating common mechanisms of expression. Thus, BDNF induces the rapid translation of mRNAs already present in the dendritic spines.

The requirement for local protein synthesis in the maintenance of synaptic plasticity has also been demonstrated at the level of the single synapse,[96] by repetitive two-photon glutamate uncaging in hippocampal slices. As seen in Chapter 16, in response to glutamate uncaging, the volume of the stimulated spine increases, being a fair indicator of local LTP.[1] The spine volume enlargement (structural LTP, or sLTP) can be induced by NMDA receptor stimulation in the absence of Mg ions[1] or by pairing stimulation with postsynaptic spikes (Figure 17.12A).[96] Spine enlargement is restricted to stimulated spines and does not spread to neighboring spines (see Figure 17.12A). The late phase of the sLTP (but not the early phase) is inhibited by pretreatment of hippocampal slices with protein synthesis inhibitors. Persistent sLTP (but not the transient spine enlargement) depends on the activation of BDNF–TrkB signaling, being inhibited by sequestering extracellular BDNF (Figure 17.12B).[96] Application of exogenous BDNF can replace the postsynaptic spikes in the induction of LTP by glutamate uncaging (Figure 17.12C).[96]

In conclusion, not all of the mRNAs necessary to support long-term changes of synaptic plasticity (either LTP or LTD) derive from de novo transcription. Some are present locally,

[95] Kang, H., and Schuman E. 1996. *Science* 273: 1402-1406.

[96] Tanaka, J. I. et al. 2008. *Science* 319: 1683.

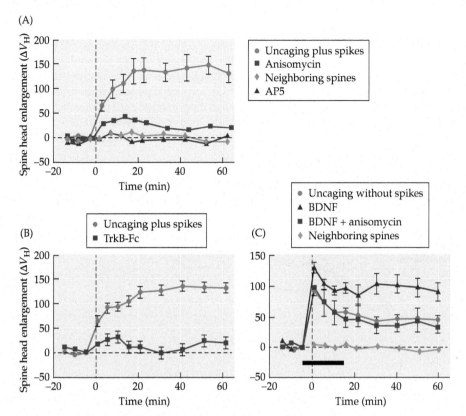

FIGURE 17.12   Single Spine Structural LTP Induced by BDNF Is Protein Synthesis-Dependent. (A) Spine head enlargement (ΔV_H) in CA1 neurons from rat hippocampal slices, induced by repetitive photolysis of caged glutamate with postsynaptic spikes. ΔV_H is specific for the stimulated spine, is NMDA receptor-dependent, and is protein synthesis dependent. (B) Sustained ΔV_H, induced by glutamate uncaging plus post-synaptic spikes, is inhibited by bath application of the BDNF scavenger TrkB-Fc. (C) Exogenous BDNF (black bar) replaces postsynaptic spikes. ΔV_H for spines stimulated by uncaging without spikes in the absence (blue circles) or presence of BDNF, either alone (violet triangles) or with anisomycin (red squares). Green diamonds are neighboring spines. Error bars indicate +/- standard error of the mean. (After J. Tanaka et al., 2008. *Science* 319: 1683–1687.)

albeit in a translationally repressed state, waiting to be activated by a burst of synaptic activity. Thus, new proteins become available at the postsynaptic sites in two waves. The initial wave is the result of early local synthesis; the second wave occurs when the newly transcribed mRNAs reach synapses and become available to be translated on synaptic activation.

Presynaptic Protein Synthesis and Synaptic Plasticity

The studies just discussed show that synthesis of new proteins is required for stabilizing synapses during postsynaptically expressed forms of long-term plasticity. What about local protein synthesis in forms of presynaptic plasticity that involve long-term regulation of neurotransmitter release? Depolarization-induced suppression of inhibition (DSI) and inhibitory long-term depression (iLTD) are, respectively, short-term and long-term modulations of neurotransmitter release at GABAergic synapses, mediated by retrograde endocannabinoid signaling[97] (discussed in Chapters 12 and 16). To investigate presynaptic protein synthesis in iLTD, paired electrophysiological recordings were performed on synaptically connected inhibitory interneurons and CA1 pyramidal cells in rodent hippocampal slices.[98] iLTD was triggered post-synaptically by applying multiple episodes of DSI stimulation (mDSI) (Figure 17.13A).[98] Acute bath application, but not postsynaptic loading, of protein synthesis inhibitors blocks mDSI-iLTD (see Figure 17.13A). Instead, iLTD remains intact when transcription is blocked.[98] The short-term DSI plasticity is not affected by protein synthesis inhibitors (see Figure 17.13A, bottom), showing that protein translation is

[97] Castillo, P. E. et al. 2012. *Cold Spring Harb. Perspect. Biol.* 4:a005728.

[98] Younts, T. J. et al. 2016. *Neuron* 92: 479–492.

essential for long-term, but not short-term, inhibitory plasticity. In addition, translation is required during the induction, but not the maintenance, of iLTD. The presynaptic or post-synaptic locus of protein synthesis in iLTD is directly demonstrated by performing electrophysiological paired recordings between individual hippocampal interneurons and CA1 pyramidal cells (Figure 17.13B). A membrane-impermeable protein synthesis inhibitor (M7GppG) is loaded via patch pipette directly into the presynaptic cell (expressing cannabinoid receptor CB1), resulting in a prolonged inhibition of iLTD (see Figure 17.13B, top). When the same inhibitor is loaded in the postsynaptic pyramidal neuron, iLTD remains intact (see Figure 17.13B, bottom).[98]

In conclusion, in presynaptic terminals of GABAergic inhibitory neurons, protein synthesis is required for long-term but not short-term plasticity. This iLTD involves protein synthesis in the axon but not the soma.[98.]

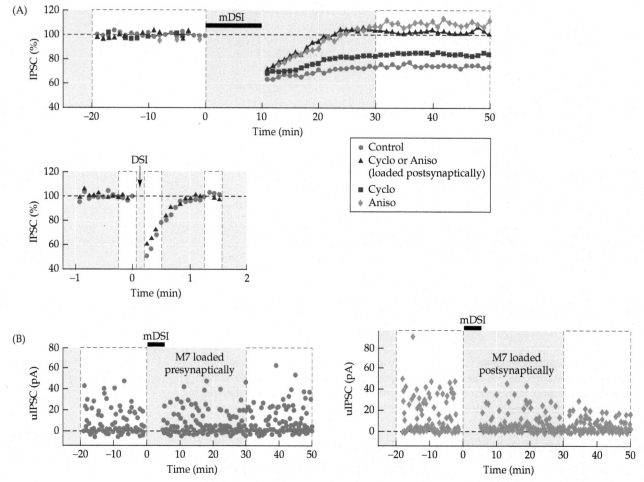

FIGURE 17.13 Presynaptic Protein Synthesis Is Required for Long-Term Plasticity of GABA Release. (A) Top: Whole-cell recordings if inhibitory post synaptic currents (iPSC) from CA1 pyramidal neurons in acute hippocampal slices. Inhibitory LTD (iLTD) is triggered postsynaptically by multiple episodes of depolarization-induced suppression of inhibition (mDSI). iLTD is inhibited by bath application of cycloheximide (Cyclo) or anisomycin (Aniso), but not by postsynaptic loading of the inhibitors via patch pipette. Error bars indicate +/- standard error of the mean. Bottom: Short-term plasticity elicited by a single episode of DSI is not affected by protein synthesis inhibitors. (B) Paired recordings (uIPSC (unitary IPSC)) between hippocampal interneurons and CA1 pyramidal cells. When membrane-impermeable protein synthesis inhibitor M7 is loaded into regular-spiking interneurons, iLTD is abolished (top). iLTD remains intact when M7 is loaded into postsynaptic pyramidal neurons (bottom). M7 is membrane-impermeable protein synthesis inhibitor M7GppG. (After T. J. Younts et al., 2016. *Neuron* 92: 479–492.)

Biochemical Mechanisms of Translational Control in Long-Lasting Synaptic Plasticity

The mRNAs reach the synapses packaged in the mRNP granule, in a translationally repressed state. Synaptic activity relieves the mRNA translational repression by several signaling pathways, which have been mostly characterized for postsynaptic local translation.

Initiation of translation (the assembly of a translationally competent ribosome on the mRNA) is a major target for translational control of synaptic plasticity. Three sensitive points for the regulation of translation initiation by synaptic activity are: (1) phosphorylation of the eukaryotic initiation factor 2α (eIF2α), which controls the formation of the translation initiation complex; (2) mTOR (mammalian target of rapamycin) signaling and phosphorylation of its downstream translation effectors; and (3) phosphorylation of the cytoplasmic polyadenylation element binding protein (CPEB), which controls the polyadenylation of dendritic mRNAs (see [99–101] for general reviews).

A good example of the regulation of translation initiation by synaptic activity is offered by mRNA polyadenylation control. Dormant, translationally repressed mRNAs have a short polyA tail. A long polyA tail, added at the 3¢ end of the mRNA, is required for efficient translation initiation, as we explain shortly. NMDA receptor activation relieves translational repression of a subset of dendritic mRNAs by inducing phosphorylation of CPEB, via CaMKII, thereby regulating the extension of the polyA tail of translationally repressed mRNAs and activating their translation (Figure 17.14A).[102] At rest, polyA tails of mRNAs bound to CPEB are short (Figure 17.14B). In this state, the mRNA is translationally repressed, because the mRNA–ribosome initiation complex cannot form. When synaptic activity induces CPEB phosphorylation, polyA tail elongation occurs (see Figure 17.14B) and the polyA binding protein mediates the formation of the initiation complex at the 5¢ cap of the mRNA (Figure 17.14C).[102] Translation can now start.

Dysregulation of the activity-dependent signaling pathways that engage synaptic protein synthesis has been linked to the pathophysiology of neurological disorders.[99,103] In conclusion, a fine homeostatic regulation of mRNA translation is essential for synaptic plasticity and brain welfare. Exaggerated synaptic translation or sustained translation repression can lead to opposite but equally severe neurological consequences.[99,103] A good example is provided by the Fragile X mental retardation protein (FMRP), whose function is altered by a mutation that results in fragile-X syndrome, the most common form of inherited mental retardation.[104,105] Fragile X syndrome brains show immature long and thin dendritic spines, which are thought to be the cause of mental retardation. Such a phenotype can be reproduced in FMRP knock-out mice.

FMRP is a highly expressed RNA binding protein in the brain. In resting conditions, FMRP is phosphorylated and inhibits translation of several hundred target mRNAs,[104,105] most of which code for synaptic proteins. *Arc* is one of the best-studied mRNA targets of FMRP. The actions of FMRP have been studied in the context of mGluR-dependent LTD whose induction, as we showed earlier, is protein synthesis–dependent.[94,106] Dephosphorylation by mGluR activation disrupts FMRP binding to its mRNA targets and permits their translation (LTD proteins), including the translation of Arc, which induces AMPA receptor internalization (Figure 17.15A). Neurons from FMRP knock-out flies and mice are characterized by excessive constitutive translation of dendritic mRNAs, and by loss of synaptic activity-induced translation.[106] In addition, FMRP knock-out mice show enhanced hippocampal mGluR1-dependent LTD, which becomes independent of protein synthesis (Figure 17.15B). In the absence of FMRP, the baseline translational repression is missing and "LTD proteins" are already available at resting synapses, and are therefore not limiting. This results in enhanced magnitude and translation-independence of mGluR-dependent LTD. Pharmacological reduction of mGluR5 signaling in FMRP knock-out neurons restores both the rate of protein synthesis and the magnitude of LTD to wild-type levels. Thus, FMRP is a translational brake for the synthesis of synaptic proteins at the synapse, and balances the effects of mGluR5 to optimize the levels of synaptic protein synthesis. FMRP appears to affect forms of plasticity that require the activation of local translation for their induction, such as mGluR-dependent LTD, but not the NMDA receptor–dependent L-LTP, which remains normal in FMRP knock-out mice (see Figure 17.15B).[106]

[99] Sossin, W. S. and Costa-Mattioli, M. 2018. *Cold Spring Harb. Perspect. Biol.* doi: 10.1101/cshperspect.a032912.

[100] Costa-Mattioli, M. et al. 2009. *Neuron* 61: 10–26.

[101] Jung, H. et al. 2014. *Cell* 157: 26–40.

[102] Richter 2007. *Trends Biochem. Sci.* 32: 279.

[103] Kapur, M., et al. 2017. *Neuron* 96: 616–637.

[104] Darnell, J. C., and Klann, E. 2013. *Nat. Neurosci.* 16: 1530–1536.

[105] Bassell, G. J., and Warren, S. T. 2008. *Neuron* 60: 201–214.

[106] Sidorov, M. S. et al. 2013. *Mol. Brain* 6: 15.

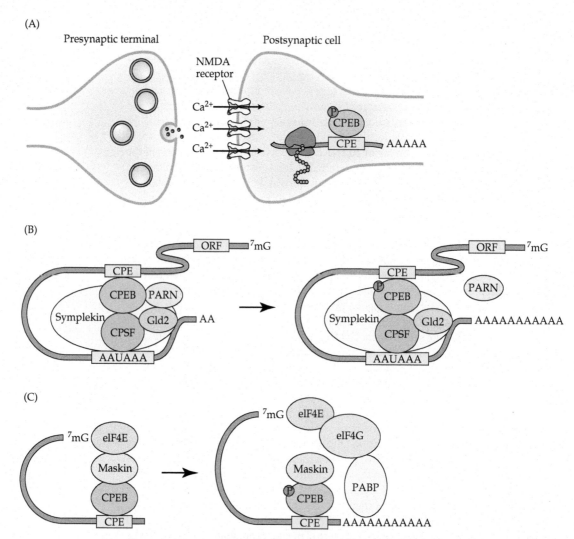

FIGURE 17.14 Translational Control by CPEB at Synapses. (A) Phosphorylation of CPEB, following activation by NMDA receptors (yellow), leads to polyadenylation of translationally repressed mRNAs harboring the CPE sequence. (B) Mechanism of polyadenylation control. mRNAs containing the CPE sequence downstream of the coding region (ORF) assemble into a ribonucleoprotein complex nucleated by CPEB, containing PARN (a deadenylating enzyme) and Gld2 (a polyA polymerase), in addition to CPSF and the scaffold protein symplekin. At rest (left), PARN activity is stronger; the polyA tail remains short. On synaptic activation and CPEB phosphorylation (right), PARN is expelled and Gld2 elongates the polyA tail. (C) mRNA polyadenylation permits the formation of the translation initiation complex between the mRNA cap-binding factors eIF4E and eIF4G. At rest (left), CPEB associates with mRNAs and Maskin, a protein that binds eIF4E, blocking the formation of the translation initiation complex. Following synaptic activation and mRNA polyadenylation (right), the polyA binding protein (PABP) binds the newly elongated polyA tail and recruits eIF4G to the 5′ cap of the mRNA. Translation can now begin. For clarity, other translation factors are omitted. ^{7}mG = 5′ cap of the mRNA. (After J. D. Richter, 2007. *Trends Biochem. Sci.* 32: 279-285. B also based on J. H. Kim and J. D. Richter, 2006. *Mol. Cell* 24: 173-183.)

Degradation of Synaptic Proteins

We saw earlier that synaptic mRNA translation needs to be carefully regulated by homeostatic mechanisms. Synaptic activity can also trigger the local degradation of proteins, by the ubiquitin–proteasome system, as a way of reshaping the synaptic proteome in response to activity.[107,108] Proteasomes are the organelles where proteins that have been tagged for degradation by covalent link of the ubiquitin peptide are proteolytically cleaved. Synaptic activity and NMDA receptor activation induce relocation of proteasomes, which move

[107] Yi, J. J., and Ehlers, M. D. 2005. *Neuron* 47: 629-632.

[108] Bingol, B., and Schuman, E. M. 2005. *Curr. Opin. Neurobiol.* 15: 536-541.

(A)

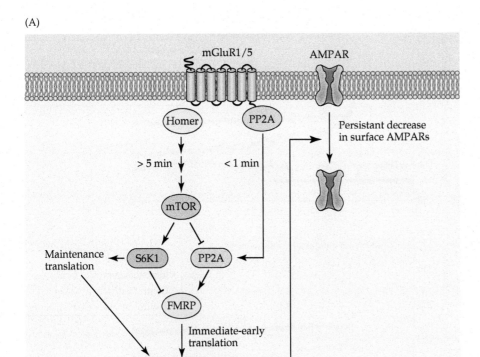

(B)

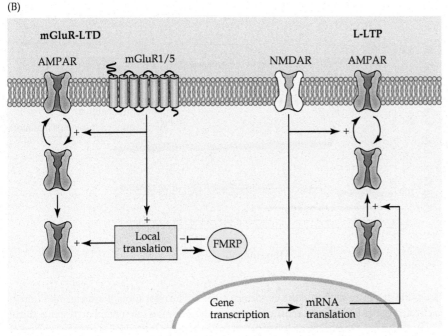

FIGURE 17.15   The Role of FMRP in Translation-Dependent Synaptic Plasticity.
(A) mGluR stimulation rapidly activates protein phosphatase 2A (PP2A), which dephosphory-
lates FMRP, allowing rapid translation of FMRP-bound mRNAs (including *Arc*). As a result, AMPA
receptors (AMPRs) are internalized. mGluRs also induce a slower FMRP re-phosphorylation (by
an mTOR cascade that inhibits PP2A and activates S6K1 kinase), repressing translation of FMRP
targets again. This allows a burst of *Arc* translation. (B) mGluR5 induces LTD by releasing FMRP
translational repression. FMRP and mGluR5 impose opposite regulation on the local mRNA
translation required for mGluR-dependent LTD expression. FMRP regulates local translation of
mRNAs that are already at the synapse and not of mRNAs reaching the synapse after de novo
transcription induced by NMDA receptors (NMDARs) in L-LTP. L-LTP is normal in FMRP knock-
out mice. (A after G. J. Bassell and S. T. Warren, 2008. *Neuron* 60: 201–214; B after M. S. Sidorov
et al., 2013. *Mol. Brain* 6: 15/CC BY 2.0.)

FIGURE 17.16 Coordinated Protein Synthesis and Degradation Are Required for LTP Maintenance.
(A) Top: CA3–CA1 hippocampal L-LTP (field EPSP) is blocked by inhibitors of protein degradation (lactacystin) (cyano filled circles), with respect to the control curve (filled purple triangles). A second independent control pathway was recorded, plus or minus degradation inhibitors (open symbols). Bottom: Protein synthesis inhibitors (anisomycin) block L-LTP (orange filled squares). A second, independent control pathway was recorded, plus or minus translation inhibitors (open symbols). (B) Simultaneous blockade of protein degradation and of protein translation leads to a normal L-LTP (filled green diamonds), identical to control L-LTP (purple triangles). Error bars indicate +/- standard error of the mean. Black bars indicate the application of inhibitors of protein degradation or protein synthesis. (A [top] and B after R. Fonseca et al., 2006. *Neuron* 52: 239-245; A [bottom] after R. Fonseca et al., 2006. *Nat. Neurosci.* 9: 478-480.)

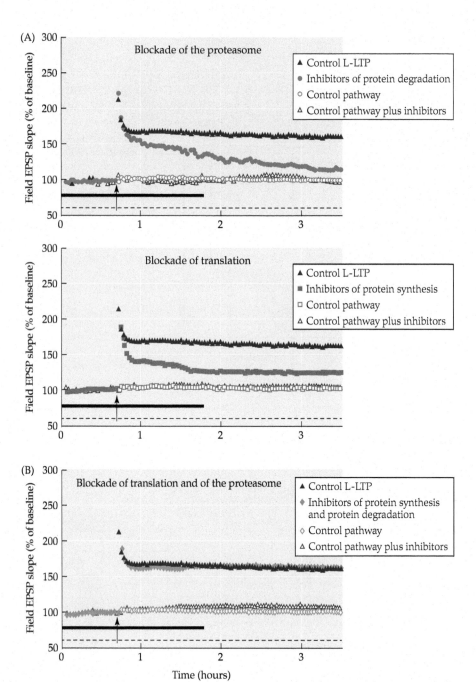

[109] Bingol, B., and Schuman, F. M. 2006. *Nature* 441: 1144- 1148.

[110] Ostroff, L. E. et al. 2002. *Neuron* 35: 535-545.

[111] Fonseca, R. et al. 2006. *Neuron* 52: 239-245.

[112] Greer, P. L., et al. 2010. *Cell* 140: 704-716.

[113] West, A. E., and Greenberg, M. E. 2011. *Cold Spring Harb. Perspect. Biol.* 3: a005744.

from the dendritic shaft into the dendritic spine.[109] The relocation of proteasomes into the activated spines parallels the redistribution of polyribosomes into potentiated spines during LTP.[110] Pharmacological blockade of proteasomes reduces the L-LTP at Schaffer collateral–CA1 synapses, an effect similar to the pharmacological inhibition of translation (Figure 17.16A).[111] Surprisingly, the co-application of proteasome blockers with translational inhibitors largely restores L-LTP (Figure 17.16B). This demonstrates that the maintenance of L-LTP requires a coordinated balance between protein degradation and synthesis, possibly of distinct groups of proteins. Thus, L-LTP might be sustained by the combined action of the synthesis of "positive" proteins and the degradation of "negative" proteins.

Activity-dependent protein degradation therefore represents an additional mechanism for modifying the molecular composition of synapses. A dysregulated degradation of synaptic proteins can lead to neurological conditions. For example, loss of the late-response gene *Ube3a*, an E3 ubiquitin ligase responsible for Arc degradation,[112] causes the neurodevelopmental disorder Angelman syndrome.[113]

MicroRNAs and Synaptic Plasticity

MicroRNAs (miRNAs) are short (22–23 nucleotides) noncoding RNAs that have emerged as important regulators of synaptic plasticity, by regulating local protein synthesis.[114,115] miR-NAs interact with complementary sequences in the 3¢ UTRs of specific mRNA targets, to control their stability and translation.[116] Depending on the degree of complementarity between the miRNA and sequences on target mRNAs, miRNA directs translational repression or mRNA degradation (Figure 17.17A). Neuronal activity influences each step of miRNA biogenesis[114–116] (see Figure 17.17A). The RNA-induced silencing complex (RISC) incorporates the miRNA and presents it to the complementary mRNA. Once this interaction has been made, RISC proteins such as Argonaute cleave or translationally repress the target mRNA (see Figure 17.17A). Since each miRNA interacts with many different target mRNAs, miRNAs represent a sensitive regulation point to control the protein composition of synapses.

Cotransport of neural miRNAs with their target mRNAs in dendrites contributes to the translational repression of mRNAs during their transport. Synaptic activity can release the translation of specific mRNAs from miRNA-mediated repression.[117] Processing of some

[114] Aksoy-Aksel et al. 2014. *Phil. Trans. R. Soc. B* 369: 20130515.

[115] Schratt, G. 2011. *Nat. Rev. Neurosci.* 10: 842–849.

[116] Bartel, D. P. 2009. *Cell* 136: 215–233.

[117] Schratt, G. et al. 2006. *Nature* 439: 283–289.

(A)

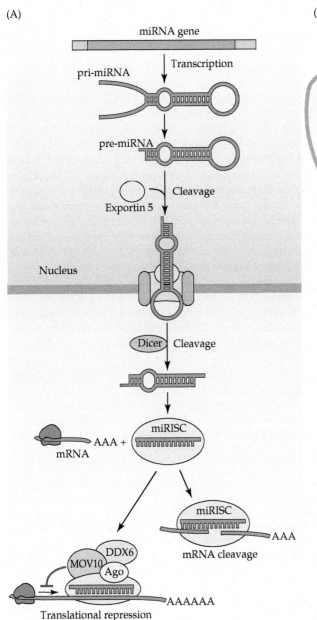

(B)

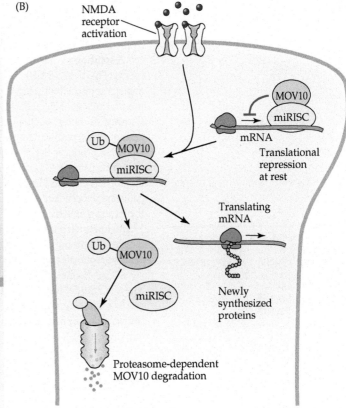

FIGURE 17.17 MicroRNAs and Synaptic Plasticity. (A) Micro-RNA biogenesis. The miRNAs derive from a long primary trancscript (pri-miRNA) that is cleaved to a precursor miRNA (pre-miRNA) in the nucleus. The pre-miRNA is exported to the cytoplasm, where the endoribonuclease Dicer generates the mature miRNA. miRNAs are part of an RNA-induced silencing complex (RISC) containing proteins that engage the miRNAs with their target mRNAs. Depending on the degree of complementarity with the miRNA, the mRNA target can either be degraded or prevented from being translated. (B) NMDA receptor-mediated RISC protein degradation in mammalian neurons. The activity-dependent ubiquitination (Ub) and local degradation of the RISC complex protein MOV10 releases RISC-mediated translational inhibition of target mRNAs, allowing the local translation of several dendritic mRNAs. (A after G. Schratt, 2009. *Nat. Rev. Neurosci.* 10: 842–849; B after S. Banerjee et al., 2009. *Neuron* 64: 871–884.)

pre-miRNAs can also occur locally, in response to single-synapse stimulation, leading to a rapid local increase in the concentration of mature miRNA, associated with a spatially restricted reduction in the translation of a target mRNA.[118]

In *Drosophila*,[119] the protein Armitage, a component of the miRNA–RISC complex, is degraded in regions of the nervous system involved in the induction and establishment of an olfactory memory, concurrently releasing from miRNA suppression the transport and translation of target mRNAs.

Likewise, in mouse hippocampal neurons, the RISC protein MOV10, a homologue of the *Drosophila* protein Armitage, is present at synapses and is rapidly degraded by the proteasome in an NMDA receptor–mediated activity-dependent manner.[120] MOV10 degradation, in response to synaptic activity, allows translation of several miRNA-silenced mRNAs to resume (Figure 17.17B).

Synaptic Tagging and Capture

One important property of L-LTP is *input specificity* (see Chapter 16). When LTP is induced by the stimulation of a group of synapses, it does not occur in other inactive synapses that contact the same neuron. Synapse-specific local translation of mRNAs accounts for some aspects of input specificity, but a question remains: Given that transcription occurs at the soma, what mechanisms ensure that the mRNAs, whose transcription was stimulated by the L-LTP–inducing stimulus, act selectively at the stimulated synapses?

A solution to this problem was suggested by the results of "two-pathways" LTP experiments (Figure 17.18A,B).[121] Two electrodes (S1 and S2) are used to stimulate independent and spatially distinct pathways innervating the same hippocampal CA1 neurons (see Figure 17.18A). As expected, repeated trains of high-frequency stimulation of the S1 pathway ("strong" stimulus) elicit a lasting RNA- and protein-synthesis–dependent L-LTP at the S1 but not the S2 pathway (input specificity) (not shown), whereas a single train to S1 ("weak" stimulus) produces E-LTP (see top left Figure 17.18B, red dots). Surprisingly, when a single train is delivered to S2 either 1–2 hours before (see top right panel in Figure 17.18B) or after (see top left panel in Figure 17.18B) the strong tetanic stimulus to S1, it evokes L-LTP in both pathways. Blockade of protein synthesis (see black bars in Figure 17.18B, lower panels) during the strong stimulation (three trains) inhibits persistent L-LTP in both pathways (see Figure 17.18B lower left panel). However, once the three trains have been delivered to S1, subsequent blockade of protein synthesis during strong stimulus to S2 does not inhibit LTP in S2, that occurs despite protein synthesis inhibition (see Figure 17.18B lower right panel).[121.]

These results can be explained by the synaptic tagging and capture (STC) model.[122] The STC model posits that a strong (L-LTP–inducing) stimulus at S1 synapse(s) generates a dual signal: a local "synaptic tag" and a signal to the nucleus, activating the transcription of new plasticity-related products (PRPs, somatically derived RNAs or proteins). The PRPs are delivered throughout the neuron and are selectively captured, via

[118] Sambandan, S. et al. 2017. *Science* 355: 634–637.

[119] Ashraf et al. 2006. *Cell* 124: 191–205.

[120] Banerjee, S. et al. 2009. *Neuron* 64: 871–884.

[121] Frey, U. and Morris R. G. M. 1997. *Nature* 385: 533–536.

[122] Frey, U. and Morris, R. G. M. 1998. *TINS* 21: 181.

FIGURE 17.18 Synaptic Tag and Capture. (A) "Two-pathways" LTP experiment in a rodent hippocampal slice: two independent pathways–S1 and S2–that project to the same neuronal population in area CA1 are stimulated. (B) Results of the two-pathways LTP experiments. Stimulation with one train (red squares) or with three trains (green diamonds) leads to E-LTP or L-LTP, respectively (top left). Protein synthesis inhibitors (black bars) applied during strong stimulation (three trains) inhibit L-LTP. For a description of the results of the two-pathways LTP experiments (right top and bottom) see text. (C) Top panels: The synaptic tag and capture model. During the induction phase of LTP, strong or weak stimulation of a synapse creates a local synaptic tag. A strong plasticity-inducing stimulation also induces the transcription of plasticity-related products (PRPs) (red dots). The synaptic tag distinguishes the synapses to be potentiated (red hexagon) from other nonstimulated synapses (black hexagon). Bottom panels: Inverse synaptic tagging. Left: LTP-inducing stimuli stimulate de novo transcription of *Arc* mRNA (one of the PRPs) (blue circles). Right: During the late phase of L-LTP, Arc protein, translated in active dendritic regions, is initially delivered into both the potentiated and non-potentiated synapses in the activated domain. Arc protein is then degraded in the active synapses and accumulates in the non-potentiated synapses, being stabilized by the inactive form of CaMKIIβ. (A,B after K. C. Martin and K. S. Kosik, 2002. *Nat. Rev. Neurosci.* 3: 813–820; C after H. Okuno et al., 2018. *Sem. Cell Develop. Biol.* 77: 43–50.)

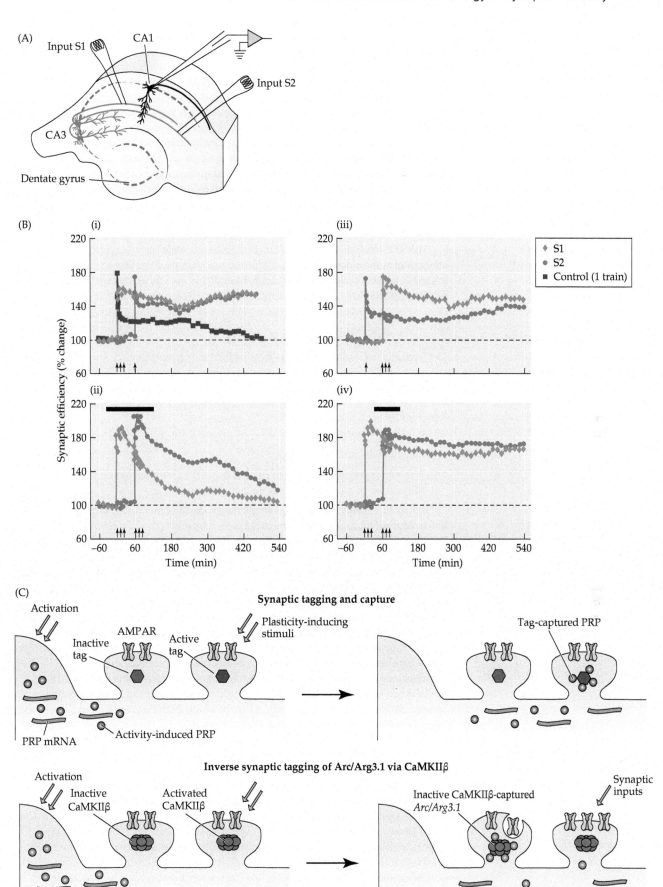

the synaptic tag, by the stimulated S1 synapse(s). This explains input specificity of L-LTP. Also important is that the weak stimulation of another synapse (S2) in the same neuron produces a synaptic tag that can capture the PRPs induced by the strong stimulation of the first S1 synapses. A persistent L-LTP is therefore observed also at S2, which otherwise would express only E-LTP (Figure 17.18C, top panels).

The STC model allows one to make experimentally testable predictions,[123] highlighting the associative and cooperative aspects of LTP: Plasticity factors induced through the strong activation of one input to the neuron might be shared with other weakly stimulated synapses of the same neuron, creating a cooperative association between different synapses, in space and in time. However, cooperation and association are only one side of the coin. The STC model also predicts also that if the availability of plasticity factors becomes limiting, tagged synapses might compete for them. Indeed, competition for plasticity factors between synapses has been demonstrated, under an experimental regime of reduced protein synthesis[124] or when multiple synapses are potentiated.[125]

The STC mechanism provides an example of cell-wide spatial and temporal dendritic integration at the biochemical and molecular level, which occurs on a timescale of hours, instead of the timescale of (tens of) milliseconds typical of the electrical dendritic integration (see Chapter 8).

The Identity of the Synaptic Tag

The "synaptic tag" is an entity defined by the following properties:

1. It is set by weak (E-LTP–inducing) as well as by strong (L-LTP–inducing) stimulations.

2. It is protein synthesis–independent.

3. It is immobile.

4. It has a lifetime of a few hours.

5. It allows the tagged synapses to capture the PRPs generated by the strong stimulation of other synapses of the same neuron.

Rather than being considered a single molecule, the synaptic tag can be considered a self-sustaining molecular process that stays on long enough (a few hours) to capture the incoming PRPs and stabilize the synaptic changes. In this context, signaling pathways that link synaptic activity to local translation meet the requirements for a synaptic tag. Components of this synaptic tagging process, which contribute to the activation of local protein synthesis, include persistently activated, and self-sustaining, kinases, such as PKMζ[126] and CaMKII,[127,128] respectively, and the neurotrophin BDNF and its tyrosine kinase receptor TrkB.[129,130] The latter offer an interesting mechanism as a candidate synaptic tag.

BDNF and TrkB mRNAs are co-expressed in hippocampal and cortical neurons, where they are targeted to dendrites and locally translated, and this had suggested they might form a **local autocrine loop**.[75,76] Experimental evidence for a local autocrine BDNF–TrkB signaling loop activated within a single dendritic spine is presented in Figure 17.19.

We showed in Figure 17.12 that single spine sLTP is blocked by sequestering extracellular BDNF.[96] In the experiment in Figure 17.19, BDNF secretion and TrkB activation are visualized in single spines of rat pyramidal neurons in hippocampal slices, stimulated to undergo sLTP.[130] Glutamate uncaging induces a rapid, NMDA receptor–dependent increase in BDNF–SEP (see Figure 17.19A) and a concomitant TrkB activation in the stimulated spine (see Figure 17.19B) (but not in neighboring spines)[130] Collectively, the data demonstrate a cell-autonomous, activity-dependent postsynaptic local autocrine loop, involving spine-specific BDNF release and TrkB activation in the same spine (see Figure 17.19C).[130] Since BDNF–TrkB signaling is a potent activator of local protein synthesis, this self-perpetuating local autocrine loop may act as a synaptic tag for the capture of incoming PRPs and the selective engagement of the protein-synthetic machinery at the stimulated synapse. We should also consider the possibility that the BDNF acting on this feedforward local synaptic loop is released by astrocytes[131] or by microglia.[132]

[123] Redondo, R. L. and Morris R. 2011. *Nat. Rev. Neurosci.* 12: 17.

[124] Fonseca et al. 2004. *Neuron* 44: 1011.

[125] Sajikumar, S. et al. 2014. *Proc. Natl. Acad. Sci USA* 111: 12217-12221.

[126] Sacktor, T. C. and Hell, J. W. 2017. *Sci. Signal* 10, eaao2327 2017.

[127] Redondo, R. L. et al. 2010. *J. Neurosci.* 30: 4981-4989.

[128] Sanhueza, M. and Lisman J. 2013. *Mol. Brain* 6:10.

[129] Lu, Y. et al. 2011. *J. Neurosci.* 31: 11762-11771.

[130] Harward, S. C. et al. 2016. *Nature* 538: 99.

[131] Vignoli, B. et al. 2016. *Neuron* 92: 873.

[132] Parkhurst et al. 2013. *Cell* 155: 1596.

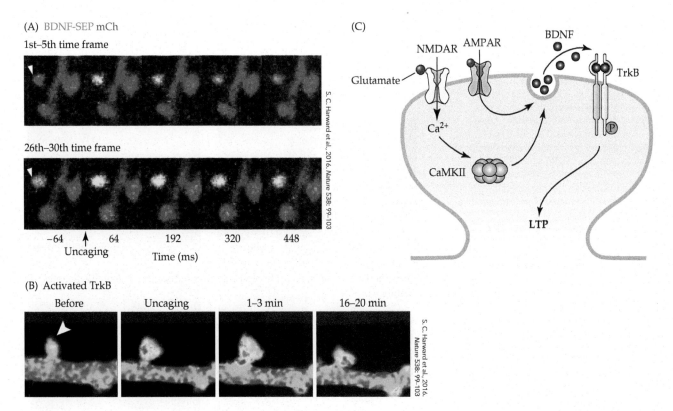

(A) BDNF-SEP mCh

1st–5th time frame

26th–30th time frame

−64   64   192   320   448

Uncaging   Time (ms)

S. C. Harward et al., 2016. *Nature* 538: 99–103

(B) Activated TrkB

Before   Uncaging   1–3 min   16–20 min

S. C. Harward et al., 2016. *Nature* 538: 99–103

(C)

NMDAR AMPAR   BDNF

Glutamate   TrkB

Ca²⁺

CaMKII

LTP

FIGURE 17.19 Local Spine-Specific BDNF–TrkB Autocrine Loop. (A) Two-photon images of glutamate uncaging-evoked changes in BDNF-SEP fluorescence in dendritic spines of CA1 hippocampal rat neurons. Glutamate uncaging induces rapid local release of postsynaptic BDNF in the stimulated spine (white arrowheads), but not in neighboring spines. The secretion of BDNF is visualized by expressing a BDNF molecule fused to a pH-sensitive fluorescent protein (BDNF-SEP), which changes color upon secretion. Each row of images represents the uncaging-triggered BDNF-SEP signal in response to individual uncaging pulses delivered every 448 ms (black arrow). mCh is a member of the red fluorescent protein family, used here as a filler. (B) Glutamate uncaging induces rapid spine-specific activation of BDNF receptor TrkB in the stimulated spine, but not in neighboring spines. The BDNF activation of TrkB receptor was imaged with an activity Förster resonance energy transfer (FRET) sensor. White arrowhead: point of glutamate uncaging. Warmer colors (red, then yellow) indicate higher TrkB activity. (C) Scheme of local spine-specific autocrine BDNF–TrkB signaling. Red circles: glutamate. (From S. C. Harward et al., 2016. *Nature* 538: 99–103.)

Inverse Synaptic Tagging

A complementary mode of tagging synapses was suggested, when it was found that Arc protein selectively accumulates at inactive dendritic spines, in strongly excited neurons[133] (see Figure 17.18C, bottom panels).

Arc is a prototype effector IEG[51] (see Figures 17.6 and 17.8), but its functions are seemingly paradoxical.[134] Activation of NMDA receptors produces a rapid burst of synaptic Arc protein expression, rapidly damped down by an activity- and translation-dependent degradation of its mRNA[135,136] and by Arc protein degradation.[137] Despite being strongly upregulated by stimuli that induce persistent synaptic potentiation, Arc contributes critically to weakening synapses by promoting AMPA receptor endocytosis.[52]

One intriguing finding is Arc accumulation at identified inactive spines in strongly excited neurons.[133] Inactivation of presynaptic release by tetanus toxin, sparsely expressed in a neuronal culture undergoing BDNF-LTP, produces the selective accumulation of Arc protein at postsynaptic sites facing inactive axons (Figure 17.20A). Spines containing high surface AMPA receptors have low Arc levels, and vice versa (Figure 17.20B). Following plasticity-inducing stimulation, which induces spine volume increase, Arc protein accumulates selectively in non-expanded, rather than in expanded, spines.[133]

These findings suggest an *inverse synaptic tagging*, in which Arc targets the non-potentiated synapses within a dendritic domain that has been strongly activated (see Figure 17.18C, bottom panels).[133]

[133] Okuno, H. et al. 2012. *Cell* 149: 886–898.

[134] Steward, O. et al. 2015. *Front. Mol. Neurosci.* 7: 1-15.

[135] Giorgi, C. et al. 2007. *Cell* 130: 179–191.

[136] Farris, S. et al. 2014. *J. Neurosci.* 34: 448–443.

[137] Mabb, A. M. and Ehlers, A. D. 2018. *Sem. Cell Develop. Biol.* 77: 10-16.

FIGURE 17.20 Arc Protein Is Enriched in Inactive Postsynaptic Spines Following de Novo Transcription: Inverse Synaptic Tagging. (A) Top: Scheme of the experiment: Cultured hippocampal neurons, sparsely expressing tetanus toxin light chain fused to GFP (GFP-TeNT), were pre-treated with tetrodotoxin (TTX) for 24 hours, until preexisting Arc was cleared, activated with BDNF for 2 hours, and further incubated for 2 hours before immunostaining for Arc and PSD95 and GFP imaging (for GFP-TeNT expression). TFX, transfection of GFP-TeNT DNA. Arc immunoreactivity is measured in spines facing GFP-TeNT-positive or GFP-TeNT-negative axons (scheme at the bottom of the figure). Bottom left: Large field of the culture. Red: Arc immunostaining. Green: Neurons expressing GFP-TeNT. Blue: PSD95 immunostaining. The region in the yellow box is enlarged on the right. Bottom, right: Arc/Arg3.1-immunoreactivity (IR) signal in the spine facing the GFP-TeNT–expressing axon (synaptically silent) (arrows) was significantly higher than that at adjacent spines that were juxtaposed to GFP-TeNT-negative axon terminals (arrowheads). Such inactive synapse-restricted expression was not observed for the structural postsynaptic protein PSD95. (B) Synaptic Arc content is inversely correlated with surface expression levels of AMPA receptors (GluA1). Left: Spines containing high surface GluA1 signals have low Arc signals (yellow arrows), and vice versa (red arrows). Right: Negative correlation of synaptic Arc and surface GluA1 levels at individual synapses. (After H. Okuno et al., 2012. *Cell* 149: 886–898.)

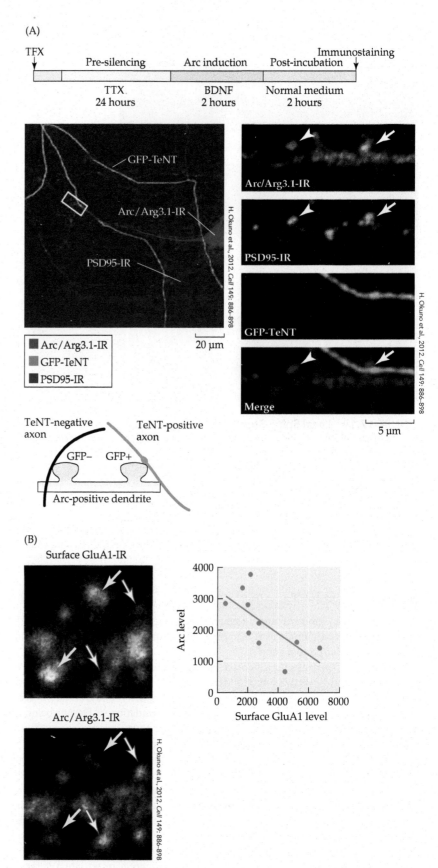

(A)

TFX

Pre-silencing — Arc induction — Post-incubation — Immunostaining

TTX 24 hours | BDNF 2 hours | Normal medium 2 hours

GFP-TeNT

Arc/Arg3.1-IR

PSD95-IR

■ Arc/Arg3.1-IR
■ GFP-TeNT
■ PSD95-IR

20 μm

Arc/Arg3.1-IR

PSD95-IR

GFP-TeNT

Merge

5 μm

H. Okuno et al., 2012. *Cell* 149: 886–898

TeNT-negative axon | TeNT-positive axon

GFP– | GFP+

Arc-positive dendrite

(B)

Surface GluA1-IR

Arc/Arg3.1-IR

Arc level vs Surface GluA1 level

H. Okuno et al., 2012. *Cell* 149: 886–898

The Cellular Basis of Memory

It's clear that memories are manifestations of enduring physical changes in the brain, but the nature of these changes has remained elusive. To describe the memory trace, the German zoologist Richard Semon formulated more than 100 years ago the concept of the **engram** ("the enduring though primarily latent modification in the irritable substance produced by stimulus, I have called an Engram"),[138] whose physical nature and properties were, however, out of reach of the science of his time.

What we have learned about the mechanisms underlying long-term synaptic plasticity offers a conceptual basis for addressing the question of the molecular and cellular properties of memory traces. The goal is to understand the process whereby the network of synapses or neurons that store a given memory is established. Two models are under experimental consideration, the neuronal activation model[139] and the synaptic plasticity and memory model.[140-142] The two models are not necessarily exclusive.[143,144] For example, the formation of neuron ensembles might be implemented by strengthening synaptic connections between neurons of the assembly (see later).

Recently developed techniques allow researchers to genetically tag and manipulate neurons, based on their activity during a learning process. These experimental approaches have begun to establish a causal link between neuronal activity, persistent synaptic changes, and an animal's memory-associated behaviors.

Genetically Tagged Active Neurons

The first step in probing the nature of memory traces (be they neuronal or synaptic ensembles) requires their identification, via the observation of learning-induced changes. The transient expression of IEGs in response to neuronal and synaptic activity provides a route for labeling neurons activated by a learning behavioral task, a procedure known as activity mapping.[53]

A new generation of activity mapping methods exploits IEG promoters that drive the expression of reporter genes, during a defined time window, thereby tagging neurons that have been activated in response to a given learning task.[54]

One intriguing question is whether the same neurons participate in both learning (the acquisition of an ability) and memory (retrieval of the learned response). To address this question, Mayford and his colleagues[145] produced TetTag transgenic mice which express a LacZ reporter gene (encoding β-galactosidase), linked to neural activity, only in a defined time window (Figure 17.21). The transgene expression in those (once active) neurons is

[138] Semon, R. 1904. *Die Mneme als erhaltendes Prinzip im Wechsel des organischen Geschehens*. Wilhelm Engelmann, Leipzig, 1904.

[139] Josselyn, S. A., and Frankland, P. W. *Annu. Rev. Neurosci.* 41: 389–413 2018.

[140] Martin, S. J. et al. 2000. *Annu. Rev. Neurosci.* 23: 649–711.

[141] Neves, G. et al. 2008. *Nat. Rev. Neurosci.* 9: 65–75.

[142] Takeuchi, T. et al. 2013. *Phil Trans. Roy. Soc. B.* 369: 20130288.

[143] Poo, M. M. 2015. *BMC Biol.* doi: 10.1186/s12915-016-0261-6.

[144] Lisman, J. et al. 2018. *Nat. Neurosci.* 21: 309–314.

[145] Reijmers et al. 2007. *Science* 317: 1230.

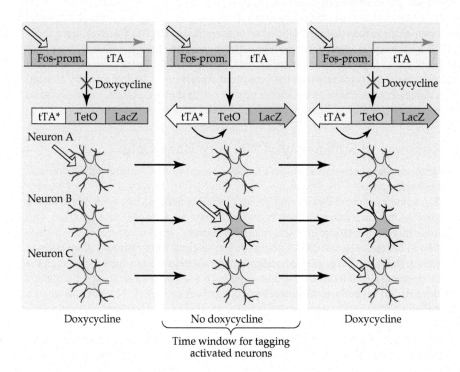

FIGURE 17.21 Genetic Tagging of Active Neurons. Top: In TetTag mice, the promoter of the IEG *c-fos* (Fos-prom.) drives the transcription of tetracycline TransActivator (tTA), a transcription factor that binds to the TetO DNA sequence and activates the transcription of the LacZ reporter (encoding β-galactosidase). tTA is inhibited by doxycycline (DOX). The TetO promoter also drives the transcription of tTA*, a DOX-insensitive version of tTA. Bottom: When the TetTag mice have DOX in drinking water (left panel), neuronal activity (yellow arrow) leads to expression of tTA, but tTA does not trigger LacZ expression (red x) (Neuron A). When mice are switched to a DOX-free diet (middle panel), neuronal activity induces the expression of LacZ (genetic tagging of Neuron B) and of tTA*. The time window is closed by putting mice back on DOX (right panel), and new active neurons (Neuron C) do not express the LacZ reporter. However, neurons that were activated during the "No doxycycline" time window (middle panel) continue to express LacZ (Neuron B). (After L. G. Reijmers et al., 2007. *Science* 317: 1230–1233.)

FIGURE 17.22 Localization of a Stable Neural Correlate of an Associative Memory. Labeling of neurons activated during learning and retrieval of a fear conditioning task. (A) Scheme of the experiment. LacZ expression: red. Expression of an endogenous IEG (ZIF): purple. (B) Example of LacZ and ZIF expression in basolateral amygdala (BLA) neurons. The yellow square in the dark-field picture marks the area shown in the three immunostaining pictures. Yellow arrows mark neurons that express both LacZ and ZIF. Learning and retrieval activate the same set of neurons. CA, central amygdala; LA, lateral amygdala; BLA, basolateral amygdala. (After L. G. Reijmers et al., 2007. *Science* 317: 1230–1233.)

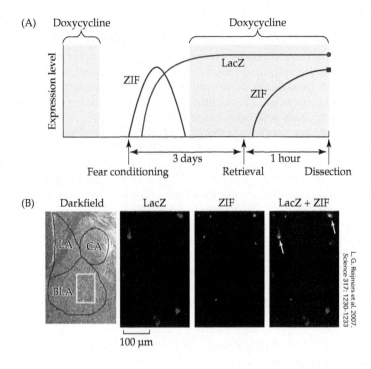

then maintained for a prolonged period, and *no further* labeling of active cells occurs, following closure of the permissive time window (see Figure 17.21). This approach was used to label neurons that were activated while learning a contextual fear conditioning task (Figure 17.22A). Mice were raised in their home cage on a doxycycline (DOX) diet that blocked the expression of the reporter, and no labeling occurred. After DOX was removed from the diet, mice were moved to a new spatial context, where they received a foot shock. This is known to activate neuronal ensembles in the dentate gyrus, cortex, and lateral amygdala. Learning of the fear conditioning task resulted in neurons being tagged by β-galactosidase expression.[145] Mice were then put back in their home cage on a Dox diet. A few days later, mice were moved to the cage where they received the foot shock and tested for fear memory of the task. The neurons activated during this second exposure ("active during test") were identified by immunohistochemistry with antibodies to an endogenous IEG (*Zif268*). Results were that neurons that were labeled during learning of the task ("active during training," β-galactosidase-positive) were reactivated during its recall (i.e., the neurons were double positive for β-galactosidase and Zif268) (Figure 17.22B). The number of reactivated neurons correlated positively with the behavioral expression of the fear memory, indicating a stable neural correlate of associative memory. This shows that learning a task and its subsequent retrieval from memory activate largely the same set of neurons.[145]

Necessity and Sufficiency of Memory Trace Cells

Two strategies have been pursued to get a handle on engram cells, "memory allocation" and "tag-and-manipulate."

Experiments showed that during learning, eligible neurons in a given brain region compete against each other for their recruitment into the memory trace. Neurons with relatively increased intrinsic excitability, during learning, are favored and win this competition to become engram cells, a phenomenon referred to as **memory allocation** of neurons in the trace.[139] For instance, lateral amygdala neurons in which a viral vector is used to increase CREB levels during fear conditioning are more likely to be subsequently activated by fear memory, as measured by IEG activity mapping.[139] These results suggest that relative CREB levels can affect which neurons will be incorporated into a memory trace, by making them more excitable. These "high-CREB" neurons were chosen to test if their post-training ablation disrupts the expression of the established fear memory (Figure 17.23).[146] To ablate specifically these neurons, Sheena Josselyn and her colleagues[146] used

[146] Han et al. 2009. *Science* 323: 1492.

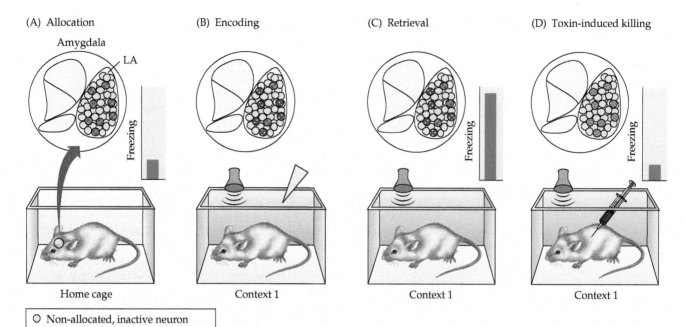

FIGURE 17.23 Selective Erasure of a Fear Memory in Mice. (A) The activity of a subset of lateral amygdala (LA) neurons is experimentally increased, just before training in an auditory fear-conditioning paradigm, by overexpressing CREB. High-CREB allocated neurons (blue) are also engineered to express diphteria toxin receptor. (B) The mouse is then moved to another cage (Context 1) and presented with a tone and a foot shock. Neurons active during the tone and foot-shock pairing are recruited to the trace (shown in red, a subset of the high-CREB [blue] neurons). (C) Fear memory retrieval, associated with above-chance reactivation of engram neurons (red), induces conditioned fear (freezing behavior when the tone is replayed). (D) When diphteria toxin is injected to specifically kill allocated neurons (green), memory retrieval is blocked. Mice show reduced conditioned fear (measured as freezing time during the observation period) when the tone is replayed. (After S. A. Josselyn et al., 2015. *Nat. Rev. Neurosci.* 16: 521-534.)

transgenic mice engineered to express diphtheria toxin receptors selectively in neurons in which high levels of CREB were induced. Since mice do not normally express diphtheria toxin, the toxin was used to selectively kill active high-CREB neurons. The selective deletion of high-CREB neurons, after learning, irreversibly blocked the expression of that fear memory (no freezing response), demonstrating a causal link between the activation of a specific neuronal ensemble in the lateral amygdala and a form of memory (see Figure 17.23).[146] Importantly, mice were capable of learning a new fear conditioning task (showing that overall lateral amygdala function was not compromised), and ablating a similar number of non–CREB-overexpressing cells (nonengram cells) did not disrupt memory. This irreversible loss-of-function experiment demonstrates that the same neurons that are active during fear conditioning are *necessary* for the retrieval of this memory.

In the so called **tag-and-manipulate** strategy, the TetTag method (see Figure 17.21) is used to drive the expression of inhibitory or excitatory optogenetic actuator proteins, during the encoding of a memory, in a time window controlled by a drug (e.g., DOX). The actuator proteins, which persist for several days after closure of the permissive window, are subsequently used for controlling the activity of tagged neurons during memory recall and examining the behavioral effects. This strategy has been used to address the "sufficiency" question: Can a memory response be induced by reactivating the latent trace, in the absence of a sensory external trigger during the memory recall phase?

In groundbreaking experiments, the groups of Mayford[147] and Tonegawa[148] tested if the reactivation of the conditioned neurons is sufficient to retrieve memory. In these gain-of-function experiments, the activated neurons were tagged with IEG promoters driving the

[147] Garner et al. 2012. *Science* 335: 1513.
[148] Liu, X. et al. 2012. *Nature* 484: 381-385.

expression of the excitatory channelrhodopsin-2 (ChR2), which provokes streams of action potentials on blue illumination. The Dox-OFF inducible system was used: In the absence of DOX, dentate gyrus neurons that were active during the formation of a contextual fear conditioning memory start expressing ChR2.[148] In the experiment, animals were first habituated to Context A, with blue-light stimulation while on DOX, and no ChR2 labeling occurred. Mice were then trained by contextual fear conditioning in Context B while off DOX, which allows for tagging of active neurons by the expression of ChR2. Mice were then put again on DOX, so that no new labeling occurred, and their fear response was tested again in Context A, with light stimulation (Figure 17.24A). The results show that illumination of the tagged neurons produces freezing behavior, characteristic of fear conditioning (Figure 17.24B).[148] These gain-of-function experiments show that neurons that participate in learning are *sufficient* for memory retrieval and behavioral output.

Using this approach, a false fear memory was conditioned in the trained animals.[149] Neurons active in a neutral Context A were labeled with ChR2 and later reactivated by light in a different Context B while the animals simultaneously received foot shock. When the animals were returned to the original neutral Context A, they displayed fear response, indicating the recall of a false memory associating the neutral context and the foot shock. A context-specific false memory was therefore "incepted."[149]

The formation of a memory in the absence of experience was demonstrated in an olfactory conditioning paradigm,[150] in which an odor conditioned stimulus is paired with an unconditioned stimulus (e.g., a foot shock) and the resulting association guides future behavior. Frankland and his colleagues replaced the odor with optogenetic stimulation of a specific olfactory glomerulus and the unconditioned stimulus with optogenetic stimulation of distinct inputs into the ventral tegmental area that mediates either aversion or reward.[150] After these intracranial conditioning procedures, presentation of a real odor that

---

[149] Ramirez, S. et al. 2013. *Science* 341: 387–391.

[150] Vetere, G. et al. 2019. *Nat. Neurosci.* 22: 933.

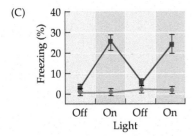

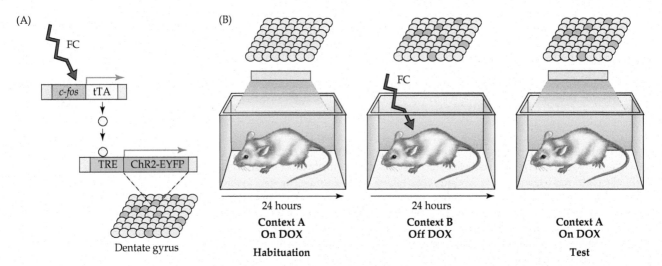

FIGURE 17.24 Optogenetic Reactivation of Genetically Tagged Engram Neurons Is Sufficient to Recall a Contextual Fear Memory. (A) Design of the experiment. Left: Transgenic mice, in which *c-fos* promoter drives the expression of tetracycline TransActivator (tTA), are injected with viruses driving the expression of ChR2–EYFP under the control of the tetracyclin-responsive promoter (TRE) and implanted with an optical fiber reaching the dentate gyrus (DG). DOX removal allows the expression of tTA in neurons that are active in that time window (green circles). EYFP is a green/yellow fluorescent protein. Right: Mice are habituated in context A, with on-off light stimulation while on DOX (habituation), then taken off DOX and fear conditioned in Context B. Mice are put back on DOX, to prevent any subsequent labeling of active DG cells, and tested in context A with on-off epochs of light stimulation (Test). (B) Optical stimulation of genetically tagged engram cells induces post-training freezing. During the habituation sessions, the mice showed no freezing (fear response) during either light-off or light-on epochs (blue line). In contrast, in the Test after fear conditioning, freezing levels during light-on epochs were significantly higher compared with light-off epochs (red line), indicating light-induced fear memory recall. Error bars indicate +/- standard error of the mean. (After X. Liu et al., 2012. *Nature* 484: 381–385.)

corresponded to the targeted olfactory glomerulus (and, importantly, not another odor) induced natural memory recall. The mice either approached or avoided this odor, depending on the valence (positive or negative, respectively) of the unconditioned stimulus pathway that was stimulated during training.[150]

Learning and Memory by Ensembles of Potentiated Synapses

The results just described support the idea that memories are stored in the brain in specific neuronal ensembles.[151,152] In these experiments, neurons are regarded as unitary entities: Neuronal ensembles that are activated by learning, during a time window experimentally controlled, are capable of eliciting memory recall once they are reactivated. What is the nature of the enduring changes that are elicited in these cells by learning?

As noted earlier, in contrast to this neuron-centric view of memory formation, the synaptic plasticity and memory hypothesis asserts that activity-dependent synaptic plasticity is induced at appropriate synapses (synaptic assemblies) during memory formation. These synaptic structural and functional changes are supposed to be both necessary and sufficient for the encoding, and possibly the storage, of a particular memory,[141-143] but this needs to be proven. Indeed, the demonstration of a causal link between a learning-induced change in synaptic efficacy (such as LTP and LTD), at a set of identified synapses, and a correlated memory behavior is still a big challenge (see Chapter 16).[142,143]

Associative fear learning is thought to occur through LTP at cortico-lateral amygdala synapses.[153] An association between a neutral conditioned stimulus (a tone) and an aversive unconditioned stimulus (a foot shock) occurs when corticothalamic projections carrying information about the conditioned stimulus fire coincidently with unconditioned stimulus-associated depolarization of postsynaptic lateral amygdala cells. Optogenetic stimulation of postsynaptic neurons, at the time of tone delivery, results in the formation of an artificial fear memory without the need for a foot shock.[154] Nabavi and his colleagues[155] successfully replaced the tone with optogenetic stimulation of presynaptic auditory cortical inputs to the lateral amygdala, to generate an associative fear conditioned response. The learned optical conditioned stimulus–shock association, then, could be erased by optically-induced LTD in the same presynaptic neural inputs and, afterward, reinstated again, with optically-induced LTP in the same cells.[155] These results support a link between synaptic plasticity and this form of associative memory, but do not provide information on the contribution of individual synapses, or of a specific synaptic assembly, to the memory task.

In order to experimentally identify and manipulate identified synaptic assemblies that have been potentiated in response to a given learning task, new experimental tools are required, to manipulate synapses undergoing plasticity. The mechanism of activity-dependent local translation at synapses, described earlier in this chapter, has been exploited to express reporter or actuator proteins selectively at potentiated synapses, allowing the identification of potentiated synapses in vivo.[156,157] A fluorescent reporter protein, comprising a short stretch of amino acids to target the reporter in the postsynaptic density, is encoded by an RNA that incorporates 5¢ and 3¢ UTR sequences from *Arc* mRNA, which provides activity-dependent translational control. The fluorescent reporter is selectively expressed in NMDA receptor–potentiated spines, with minimal expression in the soma or in other parts of the neuron[156] (Figure 17.25A). This approach was used to drive the expression of ChR2 at potentiated spines in vitro and in vivo.[156] When the spines are stimulated by two-photon glutamate uncaging, the ChR2 protein is locally translated selectively at single potentiated synapses, displaying surface-exposed AMPA receptors[156] (Figure 17.25B,C).

Hayashi-Takagi and his colleagues[157] used this synaptic optogenetic approach to label recently potentiated spines in the primary motor cortex of living mice with a light-sensitive engineered protein, which induces their selective irreversible shrinkage upon blue-light illumination by two-photon microscopy (Figure 17.26A). Motor learning of a hindlimb-related motor skill test induces a remodelling of potentiated spines in a subset of cortical neurons. In vivo photoactivation-induced shrinkage of spines potentiated after learning reveals that the learned motor response is disrupted by the selective photoablation of task-related potentiated spines (Figure 17.26B), but not by identical manipulation of a distinct set of spines potentiated in the same cortical region by a different motor task.[157] This experiment demonstrates that each motor task induces potentiation

[151] Josselyn, S. A. et al. 2015. *Nat. Rev. Neurosci.* 16: 521.

[152] Tonegawa, S. et al. 2015. *Neuron* 87: 918.

[153] Tovote, P. et al. 2015. *Nat. Rev. Neurosci.* 16: 317·

[154] Johansen, J. P. et al. 2010. *Proc. Natl. Acad. Sci. USA* 107:12692-12697.

[155] Nabavi et al. 2014. *Nature* 511: 348.

[156] Gobbo, F. et al. 2017. *Nat. Comm.* 8: 1629.

[157] Hayashi-Takagi, A. et al. 2015. *Nature* 525: 333-338.

(A)

SA-CH

mem
Turq2

SEP-
GluA1

Cherry

Merge

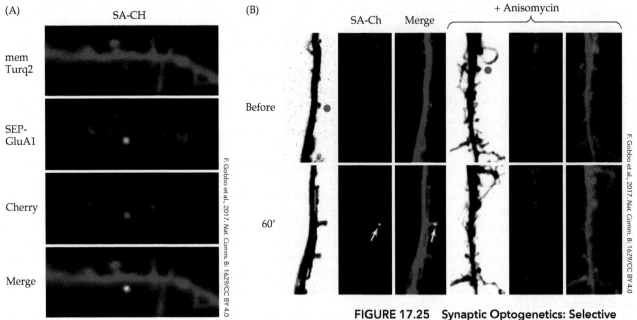

(B)

SA-Ch | Merge | + Anisomycin

Before

60'

F. Gobbo et al., 2017. *Nat. Comm.* 8: 1629/CC BY 4.0

(C)

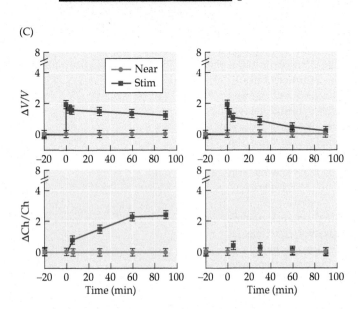

FIGURE 17.25 Synaptic Optogenetics: Selective Expression of Channelrhodopsin-2 (ChR2) at Potentiated Synapses. (A) The vector (SA-Ch) drives the local translation of ChR2-Cherry at potentiated synapses. Imaging of ChR2-Cherry in potentiated spines, after transfection of the SA-Ch vector in cultured hippocampal neurons. ChR2 co-localizes at spines with surface expression of AMPA receptors (SEP-GluA1). SEP-GluA1 is the A1 subunit of the AMPA receptor fused to a pH-sensitive green fluorescent protein (GFP), which becomes fluorescent when exposed to the extracellular environment. memTurq2: neuron filler. Cherry is a member of the red fluorescent protein family. (B) Synapse specificity of ChR2-Cherry (SA-Ch) expression at potentiated synapses. Single dendritic spines of hippocampal neurons expressing SA-Ch were focally stimulated (red dot) by two-photon glutamate uncaging. Sixty minutes after the stimulation the SA-Ch protein is expressed at the stimulated spine (left; see arrowhead), while no SA-Ch expression is seen when protein synthesis is inhibited by anisomycin (right). (C) Time course of SA-Ch expression and spine volume after focal glutamate uncaging. Stimulated spines (red line), but not non-stimulated spines (blue line), showed a volume expansion, paralleled by induction of SA-Ch. The protein synthesis inhibitor anisomycin blocked long term maintenance of spine volume change and accumulation of ChR2-Cherry. (From F. Gobbo et al., 2017. *Nat. Comm.* 8: 1629/CC BY 4.0.)

in a distinct group of synapses. The selective irreversible elimination of this task-related synaptic ensemble leads to the erasure of the corresponding learned motor skill.[158]

These results may shed light on the mechanism for the formation of "engram" assemblies. Accordingly, synaptic strengthening between individual engram cells would be the substrate for memory encoding and storage. By using learning-dependent genetic labeling of neurons, the synaptic properties and connectivity of identified engram cells have been studied. Electrophysiological recordings were performed from hippocampal dentate gyrus engram cells, tagged during a contextual fear conditioning learning task.[158] One day after training, engram cells showed an increase in synaptic strength (measured as an increased AMPA:NMDA receptor ratio) and of dendritic spine density, with respect to neighboring non-engram cells.[158] In another experiment,[159] the synaptic connections between identified engram cells in two different hippocampal regions were investigated. After contextual fear conditioning, an increase in the number and size of spines on CA1 engram cells, receiving

[158] Ryan, T. J. et al. 2015. *Science* 348: 1007–1013.

[159] Choi, J. H. et al. 2018. *Science* 360: 430–435.

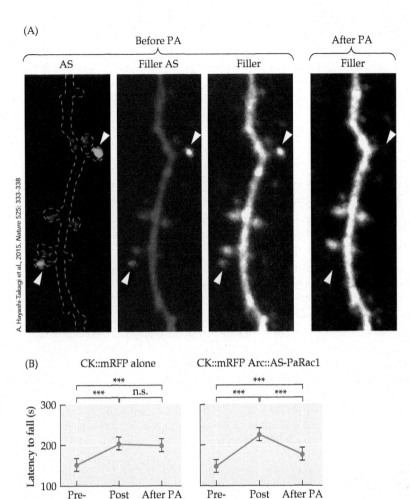

(A)

Before PA | After PA
AS | Filler AS | Filler | Filler

A. Hayashi-Takagi et al., 2015. *Nature* 525: 333-338

(B)

CK::mRFP alone | CK::mRFP Arc::AS-PaRac1

*** | ***
*** | n.s. | *** | ***

300

Latency to fall (s)

200

100

Pre-training | Post training | After PA | Pre-training | Post training | After PA

FIGURE 17.26 Optical Erasure of a Motor Memory by Ablating a Task-Related Synaptic Ensemble (A) Neurons in cultured hippocampal slices were transfected with AS-PaRac1 (AS) and red fluorescent protein (RFP) filler. The AS-PaRac1 vector is transcribed under the control of Arc transcription regulatory sequences. The mRNA harbors the Arc 3′ dendritic targeting element and codes for the PhotoActivated-Rac1 optoprobe (PaRac1), which induces spine shrinkage on blue-light illumination. Selective shrinkage of AS-PaRac1-positive spines by photoactivation (PA). Robust shrinkage (arrowheads) was observed upon photoactivation, while adjacent AS-PaRac1-negative spines were not affected. (B) Erasure of an acquired motor learning by photoactivation of the potentiated spines labeled with AS-PaRac1 in the primary motor cortex. One group of mice was infected with virus driving the expression of the RFP filler (control), while a second group was infected with AS-PaRac1 and the RFP filler. Both groups exhibited significantly better motor performance after training (Post-training), but only the performance of the AS-PaRac1 group was inhibited by photoactivation (After PA). CK::mRFP = CaMKII promoter driving expression of RFP. Arc::AS-PaRac1 = AS-PaRac1 transcribed under the control of Arc transcription regulatory sequences. Error bars indicate +/- standard error of the mean. ***$P < 0.001$ statistical significance. (After A. Hayashi-Takagi et al., 2015. *Nature* 525: 333-338.)

input from CA3 engram cells, was found. This enhanced synaptic connectivity between engram cells was directly correlated with the strength of the memory encoded.[159]

Together, these studies integrate research on synaptic plasticity with the neuron-centred engrams and suggest enhanced structural and functional synaptic connectivity between engram cell as the enduring changes generated by learning.

An attractive corollary to such a hypothesis is that any given neuron may belong to different neuronal assemblies through the potentiation of different subsets of synapses on its dendrites. A particular group membership would be established by activation of one set of potentiated synapses, membership in a different group by activation of another set, and so on. The contribution of memory-specific synaptic ensembles to define specific memory identity out of intermingled memories stored in a shared neuron ensemble is beginning to be investigated.[160,161]

We should also note that shifting the focus, from the neuron-centric view of engram neurons to synaptic assemblies as the unitary elements of the memory traces, naturally brings into play astrocytes[162] and microglia[18] as part of the memory trace.

After the strengthening of synaptic connections between neuronal assemblies, during consolidation, memory traces enter a dormant inactive state. How this dormant, but stable, state is maintained is not known and may involve a long-lasting trace of inhibitory circuits and synapses.[163]

When reactivated, a consolidated trace becomes labile again, a significant parallel with memory studies, as demonstrated by Nader and his colleagues.[164] Retrieving a consolidated memory transiently destabilizes that memory, making it vulnerable and sensitive again to protein synthesis inhibition, eventually leading to reconsolidation of the (new) trace and of the corresponding memory.[165,166] Thus, memories, and the corresponding traces, are

[160] Bilz, F. et al. 2020. *Neuron* 106: 1-14.
[161] Abdou, K. et al. 2018. *Science* 360: 1227-1231.
[162] Santello, M. et al. 2019. *Nat. Neurosci.* 22: 154-166.
[163] Barron, H. C., et al. 2017. *Proc. Natl. Acad. Sci. USA* 114: 6666-6674.
[164] Nader, K. et al. 2000. *Nature* 406: 722-726.
[165] Nader, K. 2015. *Cold Spring Harb. Perspect. Biol.* 7: a021782.
[166] Alberini, C. M., and LeDoux J. E. 2013. *Curr. Biol.* 23: R746.

exquisitely dynamic and the retrieval and reconsolidation process provides a window of opportunity for memory updating or disruption.

Understanding these dynamic and plastic aspects of memory traces might provide insights for weakening maladaptive memories (such as chronic pain and drug addiction) and for enhancing memories to combat cognitive decline.

SUMMARY

- Imaging allows longitudinal visualization of dendritic spines in living mice cortex. Dendritic spines are dynamic.

- Spine turnover is modulated by sensory manipulations or learning. Some learning-induced spines may last months to years.

- The enduring changes in the efficacy of synaptic transmission are determined by dynamic and stable changes in the molecular composition of synapses.

- Activity-dependent RNA transcription is necessary for L-LTP.

- Calcium is the key messenger that links synaptic activation to gene transcription in the nucleus.

- Immediate early genes are the first targets of synapse-to-nucleus signaling. Their rapid activation occurs by preassembling transcription factors at their promoters.

- Many mRNAs are targeted to dendrites and axons in a translationally repressed state, and are translated locally on synaptic activity.

- Biochemical signaling cascades couple neurotransmission to protein synthesis regulatory factors.

- Synaptic tagging and capture ensures translation of newly transcribed mRNAs only at stimulated synapses.

- Neurons activated during a learning task can be genetically tagged by reporter genes transcribed from IEG promoters, during defined time windows.

- The necessity and sufficiency of memory trace cells, forming a neuronal assembly storing certain memories, have been experimentally tested. Specific memories can be erased or recalled in mice by this approach.

- Synaptic ensembles of potentiated synapses can be visualized in vivo, and the selective experimental manipulation of individual potentiated synapses in vivo is becoming possible.

Suggested Reading

General Reviews

Alberini, C. 2009. Transcription factors in long-term memory and synaptic plasticity. *Physiological Rev.* 89: 121–145.

Berry, K. P., and Nedivi, E. 2017. Spine Dynamics: Are They All the Same? *Neuron* 96: 43–55.

Campbell, R. R., and Wood, M. A. 2019. How the epigenome integrates information and reshapes the synapse *Nat. Rev. Neurosci.* https://doi.org/10.1038/s41583-019-0121-9.

Crispino, M. Chun, J. T., Cefaliello, C., Capano, C. P., and Giuditta, A. 2013. Local gene expression in nerve endings. *Dev. Neurobiol.* 74: 279–291.

Gobbo, F., and Cattaneo, A. 2020. Neuronal activity at synapse resolution: reporters and effectors for synaptic neuroscience. *Front. Mol. Neurosci,* in press.

Holtmaat, A. and Svoboda, K. 2009. Experience-dependent structural synaptic plasticity in the mammalian brain. *Nat. Rev. Neurosci.* 10: 647–658.

Josselyn, S. and Tonegawa, S. 2020. Memory engrams: Recalling the past and imagining the future. *Science* 367: eaaw4325.

Jung, H., Gkogkas, C. G., Sonenbert, N., and Holt, C. E. 2014. Remote control of gene function by local translation. *Cell* 157: 26–40.

Kosik, K. S. 2016. Life at low copy number: How dendrites manage with so few mRNAs. *Neuron* 92: 1168–1180.

Lyons, M. R., and West, A. E. 2011.Mechanisms of specificity in neuronal activity-regulated gene transcription. *Prog. Neurobiol.* 94: 259–295.

Poo, M. M., Pignatelli, M., Ryan, T. J., et al. 2015. What is memory? The present state of the engram. *BMC Biology.* doi: 10.1186/s12915-016-0261-6.

Sossin, W. S., and Costa-Mattioli, M. 2018. Translational control in the brain in health and disease. *Cold Spring Harb. Perspect. Biol.* doi: 10.1101/cshperspect.a032912.

Takeuchi, T., Duszkiewicz, A. J., and Morris, R. G. M. 2013. The synaptic plasticity and memory hypothesis: Encoding, storage and persistence. *Phil. Transact. Roy. Soc. B* 369: 20130288.

Yap, E.-L., and Greenberg, M. E. 2018. Activity-regulated transcription: Bridging the gap between neural activity and behavior. *Neuron* 100: 330.

Original Papers

Bradshaw, K. D., Emptage, N. J., and Bliss, T. V. P. 2003. A role for dendritic protein synthesis in hippocampal late LTP. *Eur. J. Neurosci.* 18: 3150–3152.

Cajigas, I. J., Tushev, G., Will, T. J., tom Dieck, S., Fuerst, N., and Schuman, E. M. 2012. The local transcriptome in the synaptic neuropil revealed by deep sequencing and high-resolution imaging. *Neuron* 74: 453–466.

Choi, J.-H., Sim, S.-E., Kim, J.-I., et al. 2018. Interregional synaptic maps among engram cells underlie memory formation. *Science* 360: 430–435.

Frey, U., Frey, S., Schollmeier, F., and Krug, M. 1996. Influence of actinomycin D, a RNA synthesis inhibitor, on long-term potentiation in rat hippocampal neurons in vivo and in vitro. *J. Physiol* 490: 703–711.

Frey, U. and Morris, R. G. M. 1997. Synaptic tagging and long-term potentiation. *Nature* 385: 533–536.

Giuditta, A., Dettbarn, W. D., and Brzin, M. 1968. Protein synthesis in the isolated giant axon of the squid. *Proc. Natl. Acad. Sci. USA* 59: 1284–1287.

Gobbo, F., Marchetti, L., Jacob, A., et al. 2017. Activity-dependent expression of Channelrhodopsin at neuronal synapses. *Nat. Comm.* 8: 1629.

Guzowski, J. F., McNaughton, B. L., Barnes, C. A., and Worley, P. F. 1999. Environment-specific expression of the immediate-early gene Arc in hippocampal neuronal ensembles. *Nat. Neurosci.* 2: 1120–1124. doi: 10.1038/16046.

Hafner, A.-S., Donlin-Asp, P. G., Leitch, B., Herzog, E., and Schuman, E. M. 2019. Local protein synthesis is a ubiquitous feature of neuronal pre- and postsynaptic compartments. *Science* 364: eaau3644.

Han, J.-H., Kushner, S. A., Yiu, A. P., et al. 2009. Selective erasure of a fear memory. *Science* 323: 1492.

Hayashi-Takagi, A., Yagishita, S., Nakamura, M., et al. 2015. Labelling and optical erasure of synaptic memory traces in the motor cortex. *Nature* 525: 333–338.

Huber, K. M., Kayser, M. S., and Bear, M. F. 2000. Role for rapid dendritic protein synthesis in hippocampal mGluR-dependent long-term depression. *Science* 288: 1254–1257.

Kang, H. and Schuman, E. 1996. A requirement for local protein synthesis in neurotrophin-induced hippocampal synaptic plasticity. *Science* 273: 1402–1406.

Liu, X., Ramirez, S., Pang, P. T., et al. 2012. Optogenetic stimulation of a hippocampal engram activates fear memory recall. *Nature* 484: 381–385.

Matsuzaki, M. et al. 2004. Structural basis of long-term potentiation in single dendritic spines. *Science*: 429: 761–766.

Nabavi, S., Fox, R., Proulx, C. D., et al. 2014. Engineering a memory with LTD and LTP. *Nature* 511: 348–352.

Nader, K., Schafe, G. E., and Le Doux J. E. 2000. Fear memories require protein synthesis in the amygdala for reconsolidation after retrieval. *Nature* 406: 722–726.

Okuno, H., Akashi, K., Ishii, Y., et al. 2012. Inverse synaptic tagging of inactive synapses via dynamic interaction of Arc/Arg3.1 with CaMKIIβ. *Cell* 149: 886–898.

Ramirez, S., Liu, X., Lin, P.-A., et al. 2013. Creating a false memory in the hippocampus. *Science* 341: 387–391.

Reijmers, L. G., Perkins, B. L., Matsuo, N., and Mayford, M. 2007. Localization of a stable neural correlate of associative memory. *Science* 317: 1230.

Shigeoka, T. et al. 2016. Dynamic axonal translation in developing and mature visual circuits. *Cell* 166: 181–192.

Steward, O., Wallace, C. S., Lyford, G. L., and Worley, P. F. 1998. Synaptic activation causes the mRNA for the IEG *Arc* to localize selectively near activated postsynaptic sites on dendrites. *Neuron* 21: 741–751.

Tongiorgi, E., Righi, M., and Cattaneo, A. 1997. Activity-dependent dendritic targeting of BDNF and TrkB mRNAs in hippocampal neurons. *J. Neurosci.* 17: 9492–9505.

Vickers, C. A., Dickson, K. S., and Wyllie, D. J. A. 2005. Induction and maintenance of late-phase long-term potentiation in isolated dendrites of rat hippocampal CA1 pyramidal neurons. *J. Physiol.* 568.3: 803–813.

Xu, T. et al. 2009. Rapid formation and selective stabilization of synapses for enduring motor memories. *Nature* 462: 915.

Yang, G., Pan, F., and Gan, W.-B. 2009. Stably maintained dendritic spines are associated with lifelong memories. *Nature* 462: 920–924.

Younts, T. J., Monday, H. R., Dudok, B., et al. 2016. presynaptic protein synthesis is required for long-term plasticity of GABA release. *Neuron* 92: 479–492.

CHAPTER 18

Mechanisms of Extrasynaptic Communication

This chapter deals with the mechanisms and effects of the release of signaling molecules from the soma, dendrites, and axons in the absence of synaptic structures, a form of release called extrasynaptic. Transmitters, peptides, certain proteins, and nucleic acids are released extrasynaptically by exocytosis; gases and other molecules that are released by diffusion are discussed in Chapter 12.

Synaptic and extrasynaptic communication are different and complementary. Synaptic communication is fast and localized; extrasynaptic communication is slow and diffuse. Substances released extrasynaptically sometimes diffuse over a wide range of distances to reach their targets. Their effects last from seconds to days.

Extrasynaptic communication adapts the function of entire circuits to the continuous environmental challenges. One example is the modulation of aggression in lobsters. Aggressive encounters induce a characteristic posture that can be reproduced by injection of serotonin. The tail flipping during aggression makes serotonergic neurons discharge into the neuropil and the blood stream. By acting on central and peripheral neurons and on effector muscles, the levels of serotonin adjust the intensity of aggression. Another example is adaptation to light in the vertebrate retina. Focal illumination evokes exocytosis of dopamine and ATP from amacrine cells. Dopamine increases the visual sensitivity by uncoupling electrical synapses along the retinal pathways; ATP activates glia, which synthesize and release vasodilator and vasoconstrictor molecules. Arterioles respond by increasing blood flow and oxygenation in the illuminated region.

The mechanisms for extrasynaptic exocytosis from the soma and dendrites are known in great detail. Transmitters and peptides are contained in clear and dense-core vesicles, most of which rest at a distance from the plasma membrane. Vesicles may release more than one type of molecule and neurons may release from different extrasynaptic sites. Streams of action potentials or activation of excitatory receptors increase the intracellular calcium concentration and mobilize vesicles to the plasma membrane. Exocytosis lasts milliseconds in small axonal varicosities or hundreds of seconds in large somata and dendrites. The long-lasting exocytosis is maintained by the released molecules. Activation of autoreceptors coupled to phospholipase C produces inositol triphosphate (IP_3). An IP_3-dependent calcium release evokes more exocytosis, closing a positive feedback loop.

A long-distance form of extrasynaptic communication occurs by the flow of signaling molecules in the cerebrospinal fluid (CSF). A few minutes after being released, molecules activate distant regions of the central nervous system (CNS). Yet another form of extrasynaptic communication is through the release of vesicles loaded with cocktails of signaling molecules, including nucleic acids and certain proteins. Extracellular vesicles bind to cell surface receptors and release their contents inside cells.

Meaning of Extrasynaptic Communication for the Nervous System

Earlier chapters have shown that neurons connect to each other, forming stereotyped circuits. Action potentials spread rapidly along the fibers; synapses transfer information in less than a millisecond, and plasticity adapts transmission dynamically to the ongoing changes in electrical activity. Such rapid functioning of neuronal circuits allows a well-trained table-tennis player to detect the trajectory and acceleration of a ball approaching at a speed of 50 to 80 km/h along a few meters. Within 200 to 300 ms, the player's brain coordinates the motion of his entire body to smash the ball precisely in an opposite corner of the table. Two such cycles may occur every second! Let's now add a prelude to our story: Our champion was left by his sweetheart the night before the finals of the tournament, and his mood, lack of attention, and anxiety make him lose the game. In a contrasting example, we may imagine the euphoria of the authors of this book when a chapter is finished! Each such experiences regulates our performance in an opposite direction through the **extrasynaptic release** of signaling molecules that modulate the functioning of entire populations of neurons, glia, and blood vessels.

Neurons may release transmitters at synapses and the same or other molecules extrasynaptically from different regions. Extrasynaptic release may occur onto the heavily packed neuropil, into the CSF, or into the blood stream. In the extracellular space, molecules reach their targets via **volume transmission**[1]—namely, the extracellular diffusion of signaling molecules from their release sites to distant receptors. The effects of extrasynaptic exocytosis start after time lags that depend on the site of release and the arrival of molecules at their targets; how long the effects last depends on the transmitter and its receptor.

Glia are fundamental players in extrasynaptic neurotransmission. They establish reciprocal communication with neurons and may release the same or other signaling molecules to carry their messages. By capturing and releasing signaling molecules, glial cells link the electrical activity of neurons with the physiology of every other cell type in the nervous system.

A remarkable property of extrasynaptic communication is that participating neurons may innervate vast regions of the nervous system. Release from each neuronal segment contributes to modulate entire neuronal circuits. A good example is the modulation of aggression in lobsters studied by Kravitz and his colleagues.[2]

Tuning of Aggression in Lobsters

When two lobsters encounter each other, a sequence of aggressive approaches determines the establishment of social dominance[3] (Figure 18.1). Lobsters display their main weapon, their claws, while flipping their tail and urinating on each other. Gradually, one lobster dominates and the subordinate escapes by walking backward. The onset of aggression has a long latency and once settled continues for tens of minutes, a period far too long to be explained solely by the functioning of hard-wired circuitry but compatible with the duration of hormonal effects.

The aggressive posture in isolated lobsters can be produced by an injection of serotonin solution into the circulation.[4] Conversely, the subordinate posture follows an injection of octopamine, an invertebrate catecholamine chemically similar to dopamine. A key observation to understand such effects came from lobsters in which serotonin had been depleted by treatment with the synthetic drug 5,7-dihydroxytryptamine. Lobsters totally devoid of serotonin are still aggressive; the neuronal circuit that encodes aggression remains fully functional, but it lacks modulation of the strength and duration of its output. Serotonergic neurons are therefore gain-setters, namely they are determinants of the intensity of the aggression response. The serotonin they release acts at different levels, lowering the firing threshold of certain neurons and muscles while increasing the amount of transmitter released by motoneurons[5] and the rate of heartbeat.[6]

The motor program of aggression can be evoked in the isolated nervous system by a bathing application of serotonin. This preparation permitted Kravitz and his colleagues to characterize the contribution of individual neurons and muscles to aggressive behavior. The link between the circuit encoding aggression and the neurons releasing serotonin is through command neurons,[7] a special type of neuron that is necessary and sufficient

[1] Borroto-Escuela, D. O. et al. 2015. *Phil. Trans. R. Soc. B* 370: 20140183.

[2] Kravitz, E. A. 1988. *Science* 241: 1775–1781.

[3] Huber, R. et al. 1997. *Brain Behav. Evol.* 50 (Suppl 1): 60–68.

[4] Livingstone, M. S., Harris-Warrick, R. M., and Kravitz, E. A. 1980. *Science* 208: 76–79.

[5] Glusman, S., and Kravitz, E. A. 1982. *J. Physiol.* 325: 223–241.

[6] Hernández-Falcón, J. et al. 2005. *Cell Mol. Neurobiol.* 25: 329–343.

[7] Edwards, D. H., Heitler, W. J., and Krasne, F. B. 1999. *Trends Neurosci.* 22: 153–61.

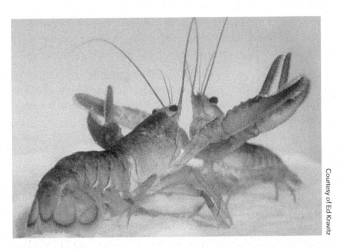

Courtesy of Ed Kravitz

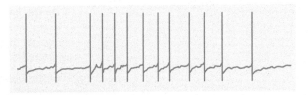

Right 5-HT cell of A-1

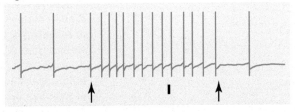

FIGURE 18.1 Aggressive Behavior of Lobsters. (A) When two lobsters meet, they invariably display their large claws. Both lobsters remain claws-up, standing high on the tips of their walking legs and making periodic tail flips. (B) In isolated preparations, the activation (period between arrows) of a neuron that commands the tail flip produces bilateral activation of serotonergic (5-HT) cells in the A1 ganglion. Serotonin that is released acts as a gain-setter for the aggressive behavior. (B after P. M. Ma et al., 1992. *J. Neurophysiol.* 68: 36-54.)

to coordinate a whole motor pattern (see Chapter 20). The activity of particular neurons that command tail flipping markedly increases the firing rate of serotonergic neurons in the first abdominal ganglion (A1 neurons),[8] from a tonic low-frequency firing at 0.5 to 3.0 impulses per second (Hz) to brief bursts of action potentials at 20 Hz.[8] Such a pattern drives the release of serotonin from central branches of the A1 neuron onto the neuropil, where serotonin influences the central activity of the circuitry. In parallel, the peripheral branches of the same A1 neuron discharge into the circulation, where serotonin acts as a hormone to enhance motor effectiveness. An equivalent series of experiments has shown that octopamine modulates as a whole the circuit that produces submissive responses.[2] Moreover, serotonin and octopamine inhibit each other′s effects, acting as physiological antagonists, and either transmitter facilitates the contraction of muscles involved in the corresponding posture.

The work by Kravitz and his colleagues exemplifies a principle of the functioning of the nervous system: Transmitter molecules released extrasynaptically reconfigure the workings of neural circuits in a timescale that ranges from minutes to hours or days. The diverse actions of such molecules adapt temporarily the responses of entire circuits to dynamic challenges.

Early Evidence for Extrasynaptic Release of Transmitters

While the elegant and precise experiments by Bernard Katz and his colleagues demonstrated the way by which neuromuscular transmission occurs within less than a millisecond (see Chapter 14), earlier recordings of electrical events that suggested release of chemicals, made by Elliott, Dixon, and others, had a much longer time course. John Eccles, who had seen similar effects, later commented:

> *I was so impressed by the long latency, 0.1 seconds, and the slow time course, measured in seconds, of the action of a single vagal volley that I continued for many years to regard this time course of an indubitable chemical mediation by ACh as the paradigm for all chemical transmissions.*[9]

Any briefer transmission was believed not to be chemical but electrical. However, Henry Dale made the suggestion that "the fast responses are due to very close apposition of the releasing presynaptic terminals and the slow responses to a remote release"[9]—an explanation that turned out to be correct.

Dale, with his profound understanding of the chemistry of transmission, also guessed about release from different parts of neurons:

[8] Hörner, M. et al. 1997. *J. Exp Biol.* 200: 2017-2033.

[9] Eccles J. 1976. *Notes Rec. R Soc. Lond.* 30: 219-230.

I am still interested, however, in the question why the transmitter and its enzyme systems should be present, not merely at the axon ending, though there apparently in special concentration, but also all along the length of the axon, and apparently in the cell body.[10]

For Dale this observation implied, in addition to the flow of transmitter to axonal terminals, "the fact that the chemical function appeared to be a function not merely of the nerve ending, but of the whole neurone."[10]

Transmitter release outside axonal terminals received unexpected morphological support during the identification of serotonergic and dopaminergic neurons in the brain of rodents. Application of the Falck–Hillarp histological technique to detect biogenic amines from the production of fluorescent derivatives allowed Dalstrom and Fuxe to detect a strong yellowish fluorescence around the cell bodies and projections of neurons in the raphe nucleus (see Figure 14.2). Such fluorescence was prominent in the presence of serotonin uptake blockers. A similar observation made for dopamine, along with the fact that opiate receptors may be distributed far from the release sites of enkephalin and β-endorphin, suggested to Fuxe and his colleagues the concept of volume transmission.[11]

Physiological and pharmacological experiments by Paton and Vizi,[12] Dunn,[13] and others[14,15] suggested that stimulation produced transmitter release from the axons or soma, followed by nonsynaptic effects on the releasing and other neurons.[14,15] Later technical developments permitted elegant ways to detect the extrasynaptic release of transmitter from isolated neurons. By taking advantage of the oxidation properties of the monoamines dopamine, noradrenaline, and serotonin,[16] it is possible to use amperometry to record somatic current spikes on release of quantal packages of transmitter. Other transmitters that are inaccessible to amperometry, such as acetylcholine and ATP,[17–21] can be detected by a patch pipette containing receptors excised from cells that express them natively (nicotinic Ach receptors, see Figure 14.11B) or experimentally (purinergic receptors). Results demonstrated unequivocally the quantal release of transmitter from the soma and other regions of neurons, and inspired the search for the mechanism and functions of extrasynaptic exocytosis. Somatic release of peptides was also added to the story.[22] As John Nicholls later wrote,

It is an irony of science that the first inklings of chemical synaptic transmission were postulated…through studies of the release of adrenaline by the adrenal medulla and of acetylcholine from the vagus nerve to the heart. Both constitute extrasynaptic release.[23]

Mechanisms for Extrasynaptic Exocytosis

This section discusses the mechanism for extrasynaptic exocytosis occurring from different parts of the cell. Emphasis is given to somatic and dendritic release, in which the coupling of stimulation with exocytosis has been analyzed step by step by direct experimentation. The mechanisms for exocytosis have been conserved from invertebrates to vertebrates and resemble those of exocytosis from gland cells,[24] but are remarkably different from the mechanisms for exocytosis at synapses described in Chapter 13.

Extrasynaptic exocytosis can be defined according to the neuronal structure from which it occurs:

- *Somatic and/or dendritic exocytosis*, also called somato-dendritic exocytosis, occurs for long periods of time from the soma or dendrites upon fusion of large numbers of clear (translucid under the electron microscope) or dense-core (with an opaque core under the electron microscope) vesicles.
- *Axonal exocytosis* occurs from varicosities formed along non-myelinated peripheral and central axons. Varicosities may release molecules from clusters of clear or dense-core vesicles without pre- or postsynaptic structures.
- *Perisynaptic exocytosis* occurs in the periphery of presynaptic active zones. Vesicles, usually dense-core vesicles, are not part of the synaptic pool. Perisynaptic exocytosis requires outbursts of electrical activity.
- *Spillover* is a leak of transmitter from the synaptic cleft upon increased presynaptic exocytosis.
- *Release of intracellular vesicles* containing cocktails of signaling molecules. Vesicles flow through the extracellular space and release their contents inside other cells.

[10] Eccles, J. C. et al. (Eds.). 1986. In *Progress in Brain Research*, Vol. 680 Elsevier Science Publishers B.V. (Biomedical Division).

[11] Fuxe, K., et al. 2007. *Brain Res. Rev.* 55: 17-54.

[12] Paton, W. D.,and Vizi, E. S. 1969. *Brit. J. Pharmacol.* 35: 10-28.

[13] Dun, N. J., and Minota, S. 1982. *J. Physiol.* 323: 325-337.

[14] Björklund and Lindvall, 1975. *Brain Res.* 83: 531-537.

[15] Nirenberg et al., 1996. *J. Neurosci.* 16: 436-447.

[16] Jaffe, E. H. et al. 1998. *J. Neurosci.* 18: 3548-3553.

[17] Puopolo, M. et al. 2001. *Neuron* 30: 211-225.

[18] Huang, H. P. et al. 2012. *Front. Mol. Neurosci.* 5: 29.

[19] Bruns, D. et al. 2000. *Neuron* 28: 205-220.

[20] Sun, Y., and Poo, M.-M. 1987. *Proc. Natl. Acad. Sci. USA* 84: 2540-2544.

[21] Gu, Y. et al. 2010. *Neuron Glia Biol.* 6: 53-62.

[22] Huang, L. Y., and Neher, E. 1996. *Neuron* 17: 135-145.

[23] De-Miguel, F. F., and Nicholls, J. G. 2015. *Philos. Trans. R Soc. Lond. B Biol. Sci.* 370: 20140181.

[24] Thorn, P., et al. 2016. *J. Neurochem.* 137: 849-859.

More than one region of a neuron may release extrasynaptically, and neurons may also form synaptic connections.

Peptide Release from Magnocellular Hypothalamic Neurons

Magnocellular hypothalamic neurons are a good example as to how different regions of neurons may release extrasynaptically with relative independence. Morphologically similar magnocellular hypothalamic neurons synthesize, and release independently from the axon or dendrites, either oxytocin or vasopressin, with each peptide producing a remarkable number of physiological effects[25] (see Chapter 14). The somata concentrate in the supraoptic nucleus (SON) and paraventricular nuclei[26] (PVN) of the hypothalamus, where neurons producing either peptide can be identified by specific antibody staining. Long varicose axons may discharge peptide into the blood stream of the neurohypophysis, a type of secretion referred to as neurohumoral. At the other extreme, one or two dendrites emerge from the soma and release the same peptides into the SON or PVN. Electron micrographs show that each compartment of these morphologically simple neurons is heavily populated with dense-core vesicles[27] (Figure 18.2).

Peptide exocytosis in magnocellular neurons has been studied using two main procedures. Morphologically, vesicle fusion can be captured by adding tannic acid (one of the tannins contained in red wine) to the fixative solution during stimulation.[28,29] Tannic acid stabilizes the dense-core vesicles that fuse, allowing one to find dense cores exposed to the extracellular space in electron micrographs (see Figure 18.2B). Alternatively, the amount of peptide released from different regions of the cell can be quantified by radioimmunoassay (Figure 18.3). Such studies have shown that trains of action potentials, but not single impulses, produce exocytosis.[30] The amount of release increases with the frequency of stimulating trains of potentials, peaking at 20 Hz.[30] If trains of impulses alternate with silent periods, such as in dehydration, the peak of exocytosis[31,32] occurs at lower frequency.[32] Serotonergic lobster neurons and other neuron types described later in the chapter display a similar frequency-dependence.

[25] Ludwig, M., and Leng, G. 2006. *Nat. Rev. Neurosci.* 7: 126-136.

[26] Tobin, V., Leng, G., and Ludwig, M. 2012. *Front. Physiol.* 3: 261.

[27] Morris, J. F., and Ludwig, M. 2004. *J. Neuroendocrinol.* 16: 403-408.

[28] Buma, P., and Nieuwenhuys, R. 1987. *Neurosci. Lett.* 74: 151-157.

[29] Pow, D. V., and Morris, J. F. 1989. *Neuroscience* 32: 435-439.

[30] Dreifuss, J. J. et al. 1971. *J. Physiol.* 215: 805-817.

[31] Dutton, A., and Dyball, R. E. 1979. *J. Physiol.* 290: 433-440.

[32] Cazalis, M., Dayanithi, G., and Nordmann, J. J. 1985. *J. Physiol.* 369: 45-60.

(A)

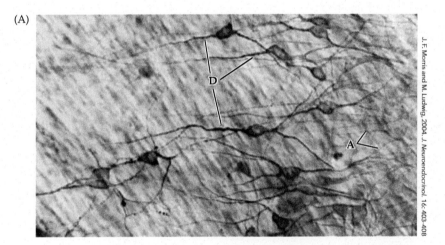

J.F. Morris and M. Ludwig, 2004. *J. Neuroendocrinol.* 16: 403-408

FIGURE 18.2 Dendritic Exocytosis from Magnocellular Neurons.
(A) Morphology of magnocellular neurons of guinea pig stained for vasopressin. Each neuron produces two or three minimally branched dendrites (D). Fine axons (A) project to the right. (B) Electron micrograph showing dense-core vesicle fusion in a dendrite (D) of magnocellular rat neuron. Tannic acid was added to the fixative solution to stabilize the dense-core vesicles that fuse during depolarization with high potassium (arrows).

(B)

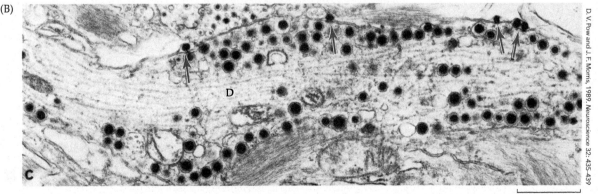

D.V. Pow and J.F. Morris, 1989. *Neuroscience* 32: 435-439

500 nm

[33] Moos, F. et al. 1989. *Exp. Brain Res.* 76: 593–602.

[34] Ludwig, M. et al. 2002. *Nature* 418: 85–89.

[35] de Kock, C. P. et al. 2004. *J. Physiol.* 2004; 561: 53–64.

[36] Ludwig, M., and Stern, J. 2015. *Philos. Trans. R. Soc. Lond. B Biol. Sci.* 370: 20140182.

[37] Huang, H. P. et al. 2007. *Proc. Natl. Acad. Sci. USA* 104: 1401–1406.

[38] McGinty, D. J., and Harper, R. M. 1976. *Brain Res.* 101: 569–575.

[39] Beart, P. M., McDonald, D., and Gundlach, A. L. 1979. *Neurosci. Lett.* 15: 165–170.

[40] Su, M., Li, L., Wang, J., et al. 2019. *Front. Cell Neurosci.* 13: 557.

Regional Regulation of Peptide Release

Magnocellular neurons release differentially from the axon and dendrites. For example, suckling stimulates bursting activity and oxytocin release from axonal terminals in the neurohypophysis,[33] with little or no release from the soma or dendrites. By contrast, during lactation, suckling evokes oxytocin release solely from the dendrites. The oxytocin that has been released from the dendrites activates dendritic receptors, which induce intracellular calcium-induced calcium release without increasing the electrical activity in the soma or nerve terminals.[34] In response, vesicles approach the plasma membrane of the dendrites, increasing the readily releasable pool. Such priming of vesicles (different from the priming of synaptic vesicles described in Chapter 13) increases exocytosis even 90 minutes later, in response to osmotic stimulation, action potentials, activation of peptide receptors, or activation of extrasynaptic NMDA receptors inserted in the dendrites[35] (see Figure 18.3). The large calcium current through NMDA receptors is sufficient to evoke exocytosis in the absence of action potentials. In a second step, the peptide released from dendrites in magnocellular and other neuron types auto-inhibits firing and exocytosis.[36–40] Vasopressin that has been released dendritically first strengthens the ongoing bursts of action potential and facilitates the milk ejection reflex and later auto-inhibits firing and prevents further exocytosis.[36]

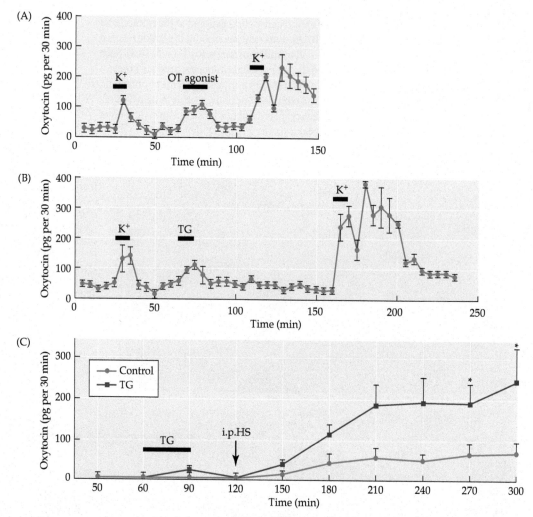

FIGURE 18.3 Dendritic Exocytosis after Priming of the Vesicle Pool. Oxytocin was quantified by radioimmunoassay. (A) After release induced by potassium depolarization, application of the oxytocin (OT) agonist (Thr4, Gly7 oxytocin) evokes further release and primes the vesicle pool. A subsequent potassium depolarization enhances the amount of release. (B) Priming is reproduced by inducing intracellular calcium release by application of thapsigargin (TG) to release calcium from intracellular stores. (C) After vesicle priming by supraoptic nucleus dialysis with thapsigargin, intraperitoneal (i.p.) injection of hypertonic saline (HS) solution evokes larger amounts of oxytocin release from the dendrites. Error bars indicate standard deviation. (After M. Ludwig et al., 2002. *Nature* 418: 85–89.)

Mechanism for Somatic Exocytosis of Serotonin in Leech Retzius Neurons

The mechanisms for somatic and dendritic exocytosis are similar but far different from the mechanism for synaptic exocytosis (see Chapter 13) in three main aspects. First, dense-core vesicles rest at a distance from the plasma membrane. Second, multiple steps mediate excitation and exocytosis, thus making release highly regulated. And third, brief trains of impulses evoke a large-scale exocytosis that starts after a lag and continues for tens to hundreds of seconds. The experimental accessibility of leech Retzius neurons has allowed study of the coupling between stimulation and exocytosis in the soma step by step. Experiments in other neuron types point to a similar general mechanism for somatic exocytosis.[41]

Chapter 20 will describe the structure and function of the leech nervous system. For now it is sufficient to mention that two Retzius neurons in each CNS ganglion have the largest somata and are the major serotonergic producers in the CNS.[42] The morphology of a Retzius neuron filled with fluorescent dye is shown in Figure 18.4. The large (60- to 80-μm diameter) soma of adult neurons is connected to a thick axon. Branches of the primary axon project to the periphery and to the anterior and posterior ganglia. An exuberant arrangement of neurites bearing varicosities emerges from the primary axon to innervate a vast portion of the ipsilateral neuropil. Serotonin is released from dense-core vesicles in the soma, and from clear and dense-core vesicles in the axon.

[41] Trueta, C., and De-Miguel, F. F. 2012. *Front. Physiol.* 3: 319.

[42] Coggeshall, R. E. 1972. *Anat. Rec.* 172: 489–498.

(A)

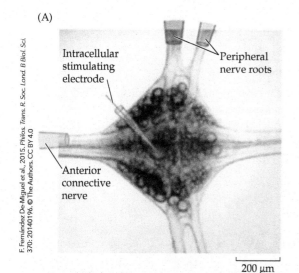

(B)

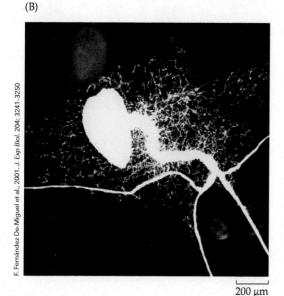

(C) Before Retzius cell stimulation

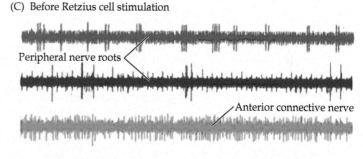

(D) 25 minutes after stimulation

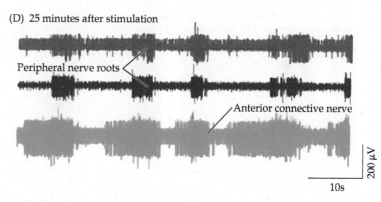

FIGURE 18.4 Serotonin Release from Retzius Neurons Activates the Crawling Circuitry. (A) A CNS ganglion with superimposed representations of extracellular recording electrodes connected to the anterior connective nerve (green) and the peripheral nerve roots (red and blue). An intracellular stimulating electrode (yellow) is inserted in the soma of one Retzius neuron of the pair in the ganglion. (B) Morphology of the Retzius neuron filled with Lucifer yellow fluorescent dye and reconstructed from confocal images. (C) Electrical activity collected from nerve roots before stimulation of the Retzius neuron. The colors refer to the electrodes in (A). Extracellularly recorded action potentials are seen as vertical spikes. The activity from each neuron has a characteristic amplitude in the record. (D) Twenty-five minutes after stimulating a Retzius neuron with 20-Hz trains, the activity in each nerve displays bursts of spikes approximately every 10 seconds, reporting crawling behavior. (C,D from F. Fernández De-Miguel et al., 2015. *Philos. Trans. R. Soc. Lond. B Biol. Sci.* 370: 20140196. © The Authors. CC BY 4.0.)

Timing of Behavioral Responses to Extrasynaptic Exocytosis

Another advantage of the leech is that each CNS ganglion contains the circuitry for behaviors; its activation can be detected from the pattern of activity of motoneurons in the peripheral nerves. An experiment made in an isolated central ganglion illustrates the timing of a response to extrasynaptic release of serotonin.[43] The activity of motoneurons, collected by extracellular suction electrodes connected to peripheral nerves, reports on the activation of behavioral circuits (see also Chapter 20). Figure 18.4 shows that without any stimulation, the activity of different motoneurons (categorized from the amplitude of the individual spikes) is uncorrelated. Stimulation of one Retzius neuron to produce precise trains of 10 impulses at 20 Hz—similar to those that maximize release from these and lobster or magnocellular neurons—reproducibly triggers a long latency and persistent synchronization of the motoneuron activity. The bursts of action potentials approximately every 10 seconds are commands to the muscles that produce crawling[44] (see Chapter 20). Strikingly, the synchronization starts about 10 minutes after the stimulation trains and continues at least for 2 hours.

Activation of the crawling circuit is produced by serotonin released on stimulation of the Retzius neuron, since it fails to appear on stimulation in the presence of the serotonergic antagonist methysergide in the bathing solution or if the frequency of stimulation is reduced to 1 Hz, similar to the baseline firing frequency of serotonergic neurons in leeches, lobsters, and mammals.[45–48]

The long latency and duration of the responses to stimulation of Retzius neurons rely on events occurring between stimulation and the actions of serotonin on targets cells, since crawling can be rapidly elicited by the addition of adequate concentration of serotonin to the bathing fluid.[49] The following sections show the steps in the coupling between stimulation and exocytosis. A convenient way to start is by analyzing the ultrastructure of serotonin release sites.

Ultrastructure of Somatic Release Sites

Autoradiography and electron microscopy experiments by Coggeshall and his colleagues show that the soma of Retzius neurons contains astronomical numbers of dense-core vesicles filled with serotonin.[42,50] Amplified images of neurons stimulated at 1 Hz, which does not evoke exocytosis, show microtubule links between vesicle clusters and the plasma membrane[51] (Figure 18.5A). Such assemblies suggest an active transport of vesicles, which (as

43 De-Miguel, F. F. et al. 2015. *Philos. Trans. R. Soc. Lond. B Biol. Sci.* 370: 20140196.

44 Friesen, W. O., and Kristan, W. B. 2007. *Curr. Opin. Neurobiol.* 17: 704–711.

45 Ma, P. M., Beltz, B. S., and Kravitz, E. A. 1992. *J. Neurophys.* 68: 36–54.

46 García-Pérez, E. et al. 2004. *Biophys. J.* 86: 646–655.

47 Aghajanian, G. K., Foote, W. E., and Sheard, M. H. 1968. *Science* 161: 706–708.

48 Mosko, S. S., and Jacobs, B. L. 1974. *Physiol. Behav.* 13: 589–593.

49 De-Miguel, F. F. et al. 2015. *Philos. Trans. R. Soc. Lond. B Biol. Sci.* 370: 20140196.

50 Rude, S., Coggeshall, E., Van Orden, L. S. III 1969. *J. Cell Biol.* 41: 832–854.

51 De-Miguel, F. F. et al. 2012. *PLOS ONE* 7: e45454.

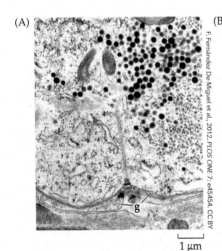

(A)

1 µm

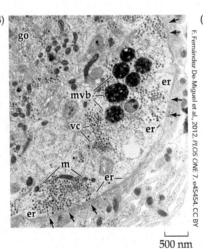

(B)

500 nm

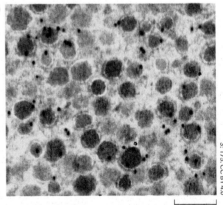

(C)

200 nm

FIGURE 18.5 **Ultrastructure of Somatic Release Sites.**
(A) Pseudocolored electron micrograph of a soma that had been stimulated with 1-Hz trains, which failed to evoke exocytosis. A cluster of vesicles (blue) and surrounding mitochondria (red) are distant from the plasma membrane. Smooth endoplasmic reticulum (green) is scattered between the vesicles and the plasma membrane. Cytoskeleton bundles (yellow) form attachments to the vesicles (not shown) and arrive at the plasma membrane. Mitochondria (red) surround the vesicle clusters. The extracellular side of the cytoskeleton anchoring site receives fingers of the giant glial cell (g) that surrounds the soma. (B) After stimulation with 20-Hz trains, vesicle clusters (vc) are apposed to the plasma membrane (arrows) and flanked by endoplasmic reticulum (er) and mitochondria (m). Multivesicular bodies (mvb) are frequent. Vesicles along the membrane face layers of glia. go = golgi. (C) Vesicle uptake of extracellular horseradish peroxidase from the extracellular medium during fusion provides evidence of exocytosis. The small black spots are colloidal gold particles bound to anti-peroxidase antibody.

we will soon show) takes them to the plasma membrane. Mitochondria are near the vesicle clusters, and endoplasmic reticulum is scattered between the vesicle clusters and the plasma membrane. The plasma membrane does not show any of the active zone material that characterizes presynaptic terminals (see Chapter 13). Another observation is that the soma is surrounded exclusively by layers of glia, without any pre- or postsynaptic structures interacting with Retzius neurons. The distribution of vesicles changes radically in electron micrographs taken after stimulation of neurons with trains at 20 Hz51 (Figure 18.5B). Such frequency is reached physiologically, for example by applying pressure to the skin or by stimulating pressure sensory neurons in the ganglion with microelectrodes.[52] About 50% of the vesicle clusters in those sections appear apposed to the plasma membrane, indicating that electrical stimulation promotes their active transport to the plasma membrane.

The arrival of vesicles at the plasma membrane is followed by their fusion[53] and endocytosis, as shown by an experiment in which the marker horseradish peroxidase added to the extracellular fluid was taken up by vesicles (Figure 18.5C).

Frequency-Dependence of Somatic Exocytosis

It is possible to quantify the amount of exocytosis on stimulation of Retzius neurons by using fluorescent dye FM1-43 in the extracellular medium[54] (Figure 18.6). As mentioned in Chapter 13, the dye penetrates vesicles during fusion and remains after endocytosis. Therefore, the gradual fusion of vesicles in a cluster results in a fluorescent spot just inside the plasma membrane. The number of spots per soma is a measure of exocytosis. As shown in Figure 18.6, the number of fluorescent spots increases with the frequency of stimulation between 5 and 20 Hz. Below 5 Hz a constitutive exocytosis is common in stimulated and non-stimulated neurons. Similar spots are seen in serotonergic raphe neurons of rat using three-photon microscopy to visualize serotonin. Depolarization induces mobilization of the spots to the plasma membrane followed by disappearance, indicating exocytosis.[55]

[52] Velázquez-Ulloa, N. et al. 2003. *J. Neurobiol.* 54: 604–617.

[53] Trueta, C., Kuffler, D. P., and De-Miguel, F. F. 2012. *Front. Physiol.* 3: 175.

[54] Trueta, C., Méndez, B., and De-Miguel, F. F. 2003. *J. Physiol.* 547: 405–416.

[55] Kaushalya, S. K. et al. 2008. *Neurosci. Res.* 86: 3469–3480.

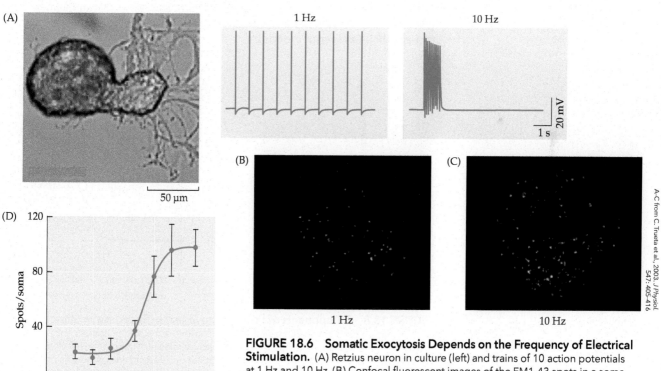

FIGURE 18.6 Somatic Exocytosis Depends on the Frequency of Electrical Stimulation. (A) Retzius neuron in culture (left) and trains of 10 action potentials at 1 Hz and 10 Hz. (B) Confocal fluorescent images of the FM1-43 spots in a soma stimulated with a 1-Hz train. A similar pattern is obtained without stimulation or on stimulation with magnesium substituting for calcium, indicating constitutive exocytosis. (C) The same neuron after being stimulated with a 10-Hz train, showing an increased number of fluorescent spots. (D) Frequency-dependence of exocytosis. Data are mean values plus standard deviation. (D after C. Leon-Pinzon et al., 2014. *Front. Cell Neurosci.* 8: 169. CC BY 3.0.)

A–C from C. Trueta et al., 2003. *J Physiol.* 547: 405–416

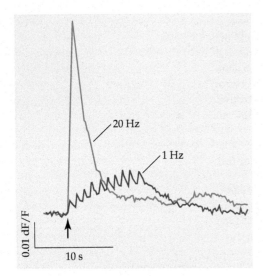

FIGURE 18.7 Frequency-Dependence of Calcium Signaling in Response to Stimulation. Kinetics of intracellular calcium elevations detected by the calcium-sensitive dye Fluo-4 in an isolated Retzius neuron. The traces are responses of the same neuron to trains of 10 impulses delivered at 20 Hz (blue) and 1 Hz (red). The arrow indicates the initiation of stimulation. (After C. Leon-Pinzon et al., 2014. *Front. Cell Neurosci.* 8: 169. CC BY 3.0.)

[56] Bi, G. Q. et al. 1997. *J. Cell Biol.* 138: 999–1008.

[57] Leon-Pinzon, C. et al. 2014. *Front. Cell Neurosci.* 8: 169.

A clue to explain how stimulation frequency is translated into exocytosis came again from electron micrographs. Stimulation of neurons with 20-Hz trains in the presence of magnesium substituting for calcium in the extracellular fluid, to block calcium entry to the neuron, fails to produce mobilization of vesicles, as also happens on stimulation at 1 Hz (see Figure 18.5A). The result is striking for showing that the primary role of calcium entry on stimulation is not to promote exocytosis (as in synapses) but to trigger the active transport of vesicles to the plasma membrane.[56] The way by which this active transport occurs is discussed later, but first is it convenient to discuss how the calcium signal is built up.

Calcium Signaling in Response to Electrical Stimulation

Intracellular calcium elevations in response to stimulation can be detected from the fluorescence of calcium-sensitive dyes.[57] Figure 18.7 shows the remarkably different calcium transients produced by trains delivered at 1 and 20 Hz to the same neuron. On 1-Hz stimulation, the interval between subsequent impulses permits the intracellular calcium concentration in response to each action potential to rise and decrease before the next impulse, thereby producing a slow rising and decaying transient with a shark-teeth shape. In contrast, the transmembrane calcium entry during a rapid 20-Hz train produces a sharp calcium elevation that peaks by 600 ms and decays with a 3-second half-life.

Calcium Channels Activated by Electrical Stimulation

The soma of Retzius neurons[54,57] and of other neurons releasing transmitters is enriched in L-type (Ca_V1) calcium channels. The poor inactivation of L-type channels makes them suitable for calcium permeation during the prolonged stimulation that evokes extrasynaptic exocytosis. Figure 18.8 shows that stimulation in the presence of the L-type calcium blocker nimodipine reduces the fast calcium transient by 90% and abolishes somatic exocytosis.

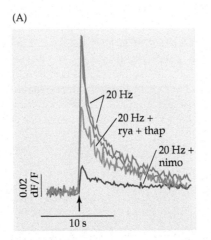

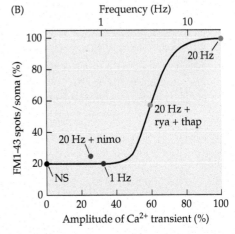

FIGURE 18.8 Components of the Calcium Signal in Response to Stimulation. (A) The calcium transient on 20-Hz stimulation (blue line) is the sum of calcium entry through L-type calcium channels and calcium-induced calcium release. Nimodipine (nimo), which blocks L-type calcium channels, reduces the transient by 90% (red line). A mixture of ryanodine and thapsigargin (rya + thap) that eliminates calcium-induced calcium release reduces the amplitude of the transient by 40% (green line). (B) Number of FM1-43 fluorescent spots as a function of the stimulation frequency (above) and the amplitude of the calcium transient (below). The black curve is the frequency-dependence of exocytosis in Figure 18.6D. Circles are average amplitudes of the calcium transient in each experimental condition. Stimulation at 1 Hz and at 20 Hz in the presence of nimodipine renders constitutive amounts of exocytosis. NS = no stimulation. (After C. Leon-Pinzon et al., 2014. *Front. Cell Neurosci.* 8: 169. CC BY 3.0.)

In adult magnocellular neurons, the calcium entry that evokes dendritic exocytosis occurs principally through N-type (Ca$_V$2.2) calcium channels, since exocytosis can be blocked by w-conotoxin; somato-dendritic release of other peptides such as dynorphin and pituitary adenylate cyclase-activating polypeptide (PACAP)[17,58,59] combines calcium entry through L- and N-type channels. Calcium entry though NMDA receptors also evokes dendritic release of peptides from magnocellular neurons, from dendrites of raphe serotonergic neurons, and from dopamine ganglion neurons of rat, suggesting another conserved mechanism for extrasynaptic exocytosis.[17,35,60]

Amplification of the Fast Calcium Transient

The amplitude of the calcium transient on 20-Hz stimulation of Retzius neurons is much larger than expected from the summation of the calcium that enters through the plasma membrane.[57] Such amplification is produced by the activation of calcium-induced calcium release (see Chapter 12). Figure 18.8 shows that a mixture of ryanodine and thapsigargin, to block calcium-induced calcium release, reduces both the amplitude of the calcium transient and the amount of exocytosis in a similar proportion of about 40%.[57] Figure 18.8B associates the amount of exocytosis with the frequency of stimulation and the amplitude of the calcium transient. The smooth endoplasmic reticulum in the periphery of the soma (see Figure 18.5) is in a key position to release calcium for this amplification.

Dynamics of Somatic Exocytosis

Another striking phenomenon of somatic exocytosis is that each step from stimulation to exocytosis occurs in a logarithmically longer timescale. Figure 18.9 shows that a train of 10 impulses at 20 Hz lasting 0.5 seconds evokes a calcium transient that lasts a few seconds; exocytosis starts tens of seconds later and continues for up to 400 seconds, depending on the number of vesicles in the cluster. Such increasingly longer events are not exclusive to Retzius cells but also exist in other types of neurons.[57]

The latency for the onset of release reflects the transport of vesicles to the plasma membrane. Once exocytosis starts, its kinetics—measured from the development of FM1-43 fluorescent spots (see Figure 18.9)—show that in any given release site, exocytosis continues without any further stimulation. The end of exocytosis produces the plateau of fluorescence.[51] Therefore, each vesicle cluster arriving at the membrane is a functional unit for a large-scale serotonin exocytosis.

One wonders, what is the physiological function of such slow- and large-scale exocytosis? A possible answer comes again from morphology. Figure 18.5 showed that serotonin is released onto thin extracellular spaces surrounded by glia. Such spaces have 100–300 nm in size. With such dimensions, a rapid vesicle fusion may saturate the extracellular transporters and diffusion pathways, causing a serotonin "jam" and a massive inflow of fluid following the osmotic gradient. However, the slow fusion rate of one to

[58] Shibuya, I. et al. 1998. *J. Neuroendocrinol.* 10: 31-42.

[59] Simmons, M. L. et al. 1995. *Neuron* 14: 1265-1272.

[60] de Kock, C. P. J. et al. 2006. *J. Physiol.* 577: 891-905.

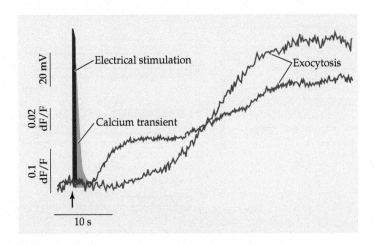

FIGURE 18.9 Time Course of the Main Events of Somatic Exocytosis of Serotonin. The kinetics of the large-scale exocytosis are shown by the fluorescence increases of FM1-43 in two spots from different neurons. The second fluorescence increase in one of the kinetics is produced by release from a second vesicle cluster that arrives at the same release site. (After F. F. De-Miguel et al., 2015. *Philos. Trans. R. Soc. Lond. B Biol. Sci.* 370: 20140196. © The Authors. CC BY 4.0.)

four vesicles per second, quantified from the kinetics of exocytosis and the number of vesicles that fuse, may prevent such adverse effect.[61]

Vesicle Transport to the Plasma Membrane

Two new questions emerge from the previous discussion: How are vesicle clusters transported to the plasma membrane in response to the calcium transient? And how is the large-scale exocytosis maintained long after the end of the calcium transient? We now discuss the structure and function of the transport system, and then will discuss how calcium triggers the transport and how exocytosis is maintained.

Vesicle transport to the plasma membrane uses two complementary transport systems[56] (Figure 18.10). Microtubules and kinesin motors transport the vesicle clusters to the periphery of the cell. In the soma shell, a resting actin cortex forms a barrier for the transport, but as in other neurons and endocrine cells, electrical stimulation and calcium transform the actin cortex into a rail for the vesicle transport,[62–66] which occurs by the coupling to myosin motors. Both transport systems obtain their energy from the cleavage of one ATP molecule[67] per motor step. Any experimental manipulation that alters the structure of the tubulin–kinesin or actin–myosin transport systems reduces the amount of fluorescent spots by 60%. Moreover, the remaining exocytosis occurs with longer delays and from small vesicle clusters (see Figure 18.10).

[61] Noguez, P., Rubí, J. M., and De-Miguel, F. F. 2019. *Front Physiol.* 10: 473.

[62] Tobin, V. A., and Ludwig, M. 2007. *J. Physiol.* 582: 1337-1348.

[63] Wang, Y. F., and Hatton, G. I. 2006. *J. Neurophysiol.* 3933-3947.

[64] Torregrosa-Hetland, C. J., et al. 2011. *J. Cell Sci.* 124: 727-734.

[65] Vitale, M. L., Seward, E. P., and Trifaró, J. M. 1995. *Neuron* 14: 353-363.

[66] Oheim, M., and Stühmer, W. 2000. *Eur. Biophys. J.* 29: 67-89.

[67] Schnitzer, M. J., and Block, S. M. 1997. *Nature* 388: 386-390.

FIGURE 18.10 Vesicle Transport System in Retzius Neurons.
(A) Molecular identification of the rails for the transport system by triple staining with antibodies against tubulin and the vesicle protein synaptophysin, and with phalloidin, which binds to actin filaments. On 1-Hz stimulation (left), vesicles remain internal to the actin cortex. Microtubules enter the actin cortex and arrive at the plasma membrane. On 20-Hz stimulation (right), vesicles appear immersed in the actin cortex (pale blue) and adjacent to the plasma membrane. (B) Kinetics of somatic exocytosis in nine FM1-43 spots from different neurons. (C) Chemicals that affect the tubulin-kinesin (red) or the actin-myosin (green) transport increase the latency of exocytosis, which occurs exclusively from small vesicle clusters, as seen by the small fluorescence amplitude. Each plot contains six traces from different neurons. The compound tested is indicated in each plot. ATA = aurintricarboxylic acid; BDM = 2,3-Butanedione monoxime. (B,C courtesy of Gabriela Torres Platas and Paula Noguez Garrido, in manuscript.)

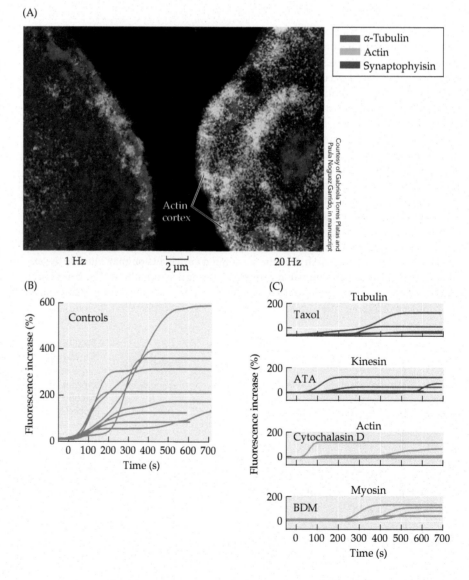

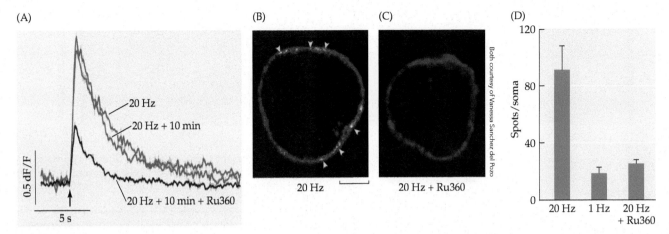

FIGURE 18.11   Calcium Entry to the Mitochondria Is Required for Somatic Exocytosis. (A) Mitochondrial calcium transients measured by fluorescence of the calcium indicator Rhod-2. Incubation of cells for 10 minutes with ruthenium-360 (Ru360), to block calcium entry to the mitochondria, reduces the amplitude of the calcium transient by 60%. The red trace after 10 minutes is a control for the incubation time of Ru360.

(B) Equatorial image of a Retzius neuron stimulated at 20 Hz in the presence of FM1-43. The bright fluorescent spots (arrowheads) indicate exocytosis. (C) Absence of fluorescent spots in a neuron stimulated in the presence of Ru360. (D) Number of FM1-43 spots per soma. The error bars indicate the standard deviation. (A,D courtesy of Vanessa Sanchez del Pozo.)

Calcium-Dependent ATP Synthesis Fuels the Vesicle Transport

Both kinesin and myosin motors cleave one ATP molecule for each step forward.[67,68] For that reason, the absence of massive vesicle transport at rest suggests that ATP synthesis is required for transport to occur. An attractive hypothesis is therefore that the fast calcium transient induces mitochondrial ATP synthesis by interacting with the Krebs cycle.[69]

A series of experiments confirmed this hypothesis. First, intracellular injection of the mitochondrial calcium-sensitive dye Rhod-2 into Retzius neurons showed that electrical stimulation is followed by calcium entry to the mitochondria (Figure 18.11). Second, blockade of calcium entry to the mitochondria by ruthenium-360 reduces the calcium transient by 60% without affecting the cytosolic calcium transient. Third, electrical stimulation of neurons in the presence of ruthenium-360 abolishes the evoked exocytosis, as revealed by the lack of fluorescent FM1-43 spots (see Figure 18.11).

Calculations made by applying thermodynamic theory to the kinetics of exocytosis indicate that dense-core vesicles are transported at 15 to 90 nm/s, depending on the cluster size, along distances ranging from a few hundreds of nanometers to about 6 μM.[51] Surprisingly, the thermodynamic efficiency of the energy expenses is only 6% or less,[61] rather low, given that the fuel motor of many modern cars reaches efficiency levels of about 20%. Data indicate that the low efficiency is due to obstacles imposed by essential structures for exocytosis on the vesicle transport, such as the calcium releaser endoplasmic reticulum and the actin cortex.

A Serotonin- and Calcium-Dependent Feedback Loop Sustains Somatic Exocytosis

By the time vesicles arrive at the plasma membrane, the fast calcium transient has faded out. Exocytosis is then evoked and maintained by calcium that is being released intracellularly, this time in response to the serotonin that has been released either constitutively or on stimulation. Measurements of intracellular calcium[57] in Figure 18.12 show that the fast calcium transient is followed by a persistent calcium elevation tightly localized in the vicinity of the plasma membrane. The kinetics of the persistent calcium elevation and exocytosis develop in parallel (see Figure 18.12B). Voltage clamp recordings show that calcium for the persistent transient does not enter the soma across the plasma membrane. Instead, a third calcium source comes into play. Binding of serotonin that has been released to serotonin type 2 receptors activates phospholipase C, which synthesizes IP_3; activation of IP_3 receptors produces calcium release from smooth endoplasmic reticulum and exocytosis. Preventing binding of serotonin to receptors by the antagonist methysergide eliminates both

[68] Mehta, A. D. et al. 1999. *Nature* 400: 590–593.

[69] Denton, R. M., Mckormack, J. G., and Edgell, N. J. 1990. *Physiol. Rev.* 70: 391–425.

(A)

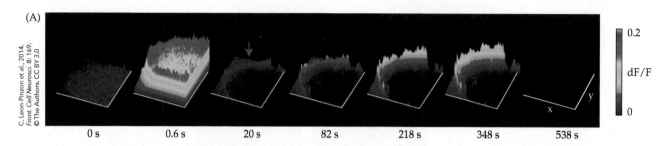

0 s 0.6 s 20 s 82 s 218 s 348 s 538 s

(B)

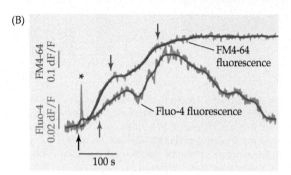

FIGURE 18.12 A Persistent Calcium Increase Sustains Somatic Exocytosis. (A) Sequence of surface plots of Fluo-4 fluorescence reporting the calcium increases on 20-Hz stimulation (t = 0). The frame at 0.6 s shows the peak of the fast calcium transient invading the soma. The following images show the persistent calcium transient in the periphery of the soma. The x and y scale bars = 10 μm; the z-axis is the normalized (dF/F) fluorescence. (B) Kinetics of exocytosis (FM4-64 fluorescence; pink) and calcium (Fluo-4 fluorescence; pale blue) recorded simultaneously on 20-Hz stimulation (black arrow). The smoothed kinetics (red and blue) are superimposed. The fast calcium transient (asterisk) is truncated owing to the image acquisition rate. The kinetics of exocytosis has two increases (red arrows), indicating exocytosis from two subsequent vesicle clusters. The peripheral calcium transient grows following exocytosis (blue arrow). Termination of exocytosis (plateaus in the red trace) is followed by a decrease in the amplitude of the calcium transient. After the second plateau the calcium level returns to baseline. (After C. Leon-Pinzon et al., 2014. *Front. Cell Neurosci.* 8: 169. © The Authors. CC BY 3.0.)

the persistent calcium transient and the large-scale exocytosis (Figure 18.13). A similar effect occurs by preventing the activation of phospholipase C with the compound U-73122. Therefore, the large-scale somatic exocytosis is maintained by a three-step feedback loop:

1. Serotonin that has been released activates autoreceptors
2. Autoreceptors activate intracellular calcium release
3. Calcium evokes serotonin exocytosis

The positive feedback loop fades out when exocytosis ends and calcium returns to base levels. Similar feedback loops maintain somatic and dendritic peptide exocytosis by magnocellular neurons and dorsal root ganglion neurons, pointing to a general mechanism for extrasynaptic large-scale exocytosis.[70]

Proteins Involved in Vesicle Fusion

The way by which vesicles that fuse extrasynaptically interact with the plasma membrane remained mysterious owing to the absence of any distinctive active zone material. However, exocytosis from isolated magnocellular neurons can be abolished by tetanus toxin, which cleaves synaptobrevin 2, a component of the SNARE complex carried by dense-core vesicles. Other conventional members of the SNARE complex are not found in the soma and dendrites of such neurons, suggesting that the extrasynaptic SNARE complex incorporates isoforms of proteins of the fusion complex in presynaptic terminals. This hypothesis is reinforced by findings in dopaminergic neurons, which express isoforms of VAMP2, SNAP-25, and syntaxin 3b unusual at synapses.[71] Moreover, the soma and dendrites of dopaminergic neurons substitute the calcium sensors synaptotagmins 1 and 2 for the higher affinity synaptotagmins 4 and 7—an adequate substitution considering that the fusion of dense-core vesicles is not coupled to calcium channels.[72]

Vesicle Recycling

The recycling of dense-core vesicles is also remarkably different from that in any form of synaptic endocytosis discussed in Chapter 13. Whereas at synapses recycling occurs in the bouton, in somatic exocytosis dense-core vesicles travel back to the Golgi apparatus for recycling (see Chapter 15). Electron micrographs of Retzius neurons that were fixed after

[70] Bao, L. et al. 2003. *Neuron* 37: 121-133.

[71] Witkovsky, P. et al. 2009. *Neuroscience* 164: 488-496.

[72] Mendez, J. A. et al. 2011. *J. Biol. Chem.* 286: 23928-23937.

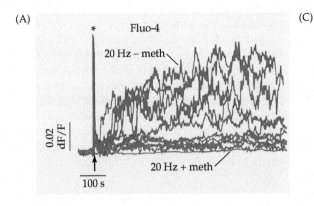

(A)

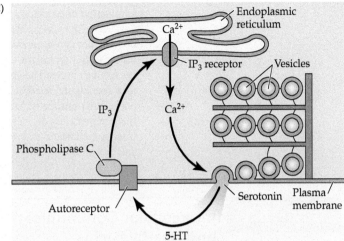

(C)

FIGURE 18.13   A Serotonin- and Calcium-Induced Feedback Loop Maintains Somatic Exocytosis. Kinetics of calcium (Fluo-4 fluorescence) (A) and exocytosis (FM1-43 dye) (B) measured simultaneously under confocal microscope in spots from different neurons. Stimulation of 20 Hz (arrows) was applied in the absence (blue traces) or presence (gray traces) of methysergide (140 µM) to block activation of serotonin (5-HT) autoreceptors. The fast Ca^{2+} transient (asterisk) remains unaffected. (C) Schematic representation of the feedback loop. (After C. Leon-Pinzon et al., 2014. *Front. Cell Neurosci.* 8: 169. © The Authors. CC BY 3.0.)

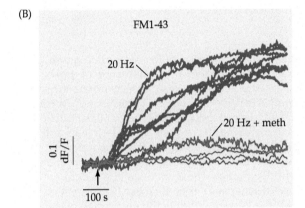

(B)

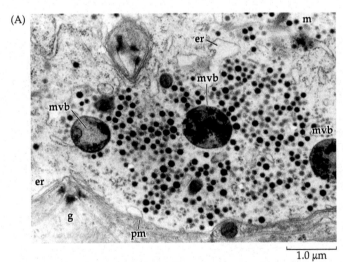

(A)

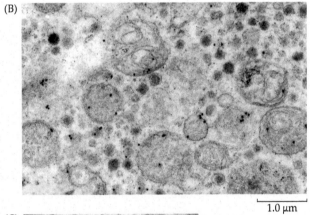

(B)

(C)

FIGURE 18.14   Somatic Dense-Core Vesicle Recycling. (A) Electron micrograph of the soma of a Retzius neuron stimulated at 20 Hz. A dense-core vesicle cluster with multivesicular bodies (mvb) in proximity to the plasma membrane (pm). m = mitochondria; er = smooth endoplasmic reticulum; g = glia. (B) Dense-core vesicles and multivesicular bodies in a neuron stimulated at 20 Hz in the presence of extracellular horseradish peroxidase show small dark gold particles coupled to antiperoxidase antibody. (C) Higher magnification of a multivesicular body with accumulation of gold particles.

stimulation of exocytosis in the ganglion show that dense-core vesicle clusters accumulate adjacent to the plasma membrane (Figure 18.14). Clear vesicles are also formed during endocytosis of dense-core vesicels. After exo- or endocytosis in the presence of extracellular horseradish peroxidase, electrodense gold particles attached to antibodies that recognize horseradish peroxidase appear in electrodense and clear vesicles newly formed by endocytosis (see Figure 18.14B,C), including those inside **multivesicular bodies**. Multivesicular bodies are transported back to regions enriched in Golgi apparatuses to release and recycle their contents. As discussed in Box 18.1, certain other multivesicular bodies fuse with the plasma membrane and release their vesicles to the extracellular space—thus creating an alternative form of extrasynaptic communication.

BOX **18.1** Intercellular Communication Mediated by Endosomes and Microvesicles

Signaling molecules in different tissues may reach distant targets by being transported inside two types of extracellular vesicles: exosomes and endosomes (Figure A).[73] Exosomes are secreted upon fusion of multivesicular bodies with the plasma membrane. Their 40- to 100-nm diameters resemble those of clear and dense-core vesicles. Ectosomes are produced by budding off the plasma membrane. Ectosomes are larger than exosomes, having diameters of 100 to 500 nm. Both types of extracellular vesicles contain cocktails of lipids, proteins, and nucleic acids, the combination of which depends on the cell type and its functional state[74] (see www.microvesicles.org). The mechanisms of release and target recognition of extracellular vesicles are summarized in Figure A.

Regulation of Synapse Formation by Exosome Release in the Neuromuscular Junction

Most research on the role of extracellular vesicles in the nervous system cells is carried out in cultures of neurons and glia. However, direct experimentation in the nervous system has produced exciting results. For example, the neuromuscular synapse of the *Drosophila* fruit fly larva–which is accessible to electrophysiological recordings, genetic and molecular perturbations, and electron microscopy–has allowed the study of how extracellular vesicles regulate the number and size of neuromuscular connections by extracellular vesicle signaling.

The terminals of motoneurons accumulate multivesicular bodies that release exosomes on fusion with extrasynaptic regions of the plasma membrane (Figure B). A type of protein carried by exosomes is Wingless (Wg; the fly orthologue of mouse WNT1), which mediates the expansion synapses during growth of *Drosophila* larvae.[73,75] Wg does not diffuse in aqueous solutions, but is transported by exosomes, forming a dimer with the transmembrane protein Evi (Eveness Interrupted, also known as

Wntless).[76] The expression of Evi coupled to green fluorescent protein (GFP) allows detection of green spots in multivesicular bodies that incorporate Wg-Evi dimers. Electrical stimulation of motoneurons with trains of impulses produces fusion of multivesicular bodies in extrasynaptic regions of the terminals and release of exosomes (see Figure B).[73] The fusion of multivesicular bodies depends on calcium activation of a SNARE complex whose composition is different from that at synapses[77] (see Chapter 13). Once it is released, the Wg-Evi dimer in the membrane of the exosome binds to extrasynaptic receptors in presynaptic boutons and postsynaptic muscle foldings. Reducing the levels of Evi expression reduces the number of neuromuscular synapses in the larva.

Direct experimentation allows one to test several interesting hypotheses on the functional roles of extracellular vesicles. For example, the soma and dendrites of dopaminergic neurons in the substantia nigra concentrate dopamine and its vesicular transporter VMAT2 in clear and dense-core vesicles, but also in multivesicular bodies and tubulovesicular structures derived from smooth endoplasmic reticulum.[78] Such diversity of potential releasing organelles correlates with marked variations in the amplitude and kinetics of amperometric spikes recorded from the soma. Somatic release of dopamine may therefore occur on fusion of clear and dense-core vesicles but also from multivesicular bodies and other membrane structures.

---

[73] Budnik, V., Ruiz-Cañada, C., and Wendler, F. 2016. *Nat. Rev. Neurosci.* 17: 160–172.

[74] Colombo, M., Raposo, G., and Théry, C. 2014. *Annu. Rev. Cell. Dev. Biol.* 30: 255–289.

[75] Packard, M. et al. 2002. *Cell* 111: 319–330.

[76] Korkut, C. et al. 2009. *Cell* 139: 393–404.

[77] Meldolesi, J. 2018. *Curr. Biol.* 28: R435–R444.

[78] Nirenberg, M. J. et al. 1996. *J. Neurosci.* 16: 4135–4145.

(Continued)

BOX 18.1 Intercellular Communication Mediated by Endosomes and Microvesicles (continued)

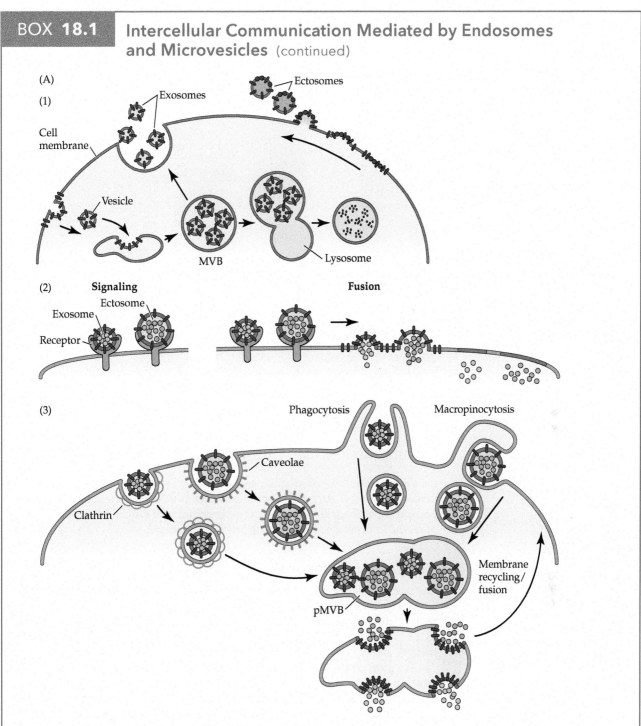

Figure A Communication by Extracellular Vesicles.
Schematic representation of the production and release of exosomes and ectosomes in a cell body. (1) A multivesicular body (MVB) is generated from an endocytic cisterna on accumulation of vesicles. Molecules from the cytosol accumulate at the intracellular surface of the cisterna where 50- to 150-nm-diameter vesicles (yellow) are formed. The newly formed MVB can proceed in two alternative directions (arrows). In one direction, the MVB forms a lysosome, followed by fusion and degradation of its components. In the other direction, the MVB fuses with the plasma membrane (exocytosis) and discharges exosomes to the extracellular fluid. The assembly and release of 100- to 500-nm-diameter ectosomes (horizontal arrows at the top of cell surface) occur at the plasma membrane. (2) Fusion of extracellular vesicles with the plasma membrane (PM) of a target cell. Exosomes and ectosomes bind to surface receptors and fuse with the plasma membrane to discharge their cargoes into the cytosol. The vesicle membranes integrate with the surface of the cell. (3) Uptake is mediated by clathrin and caveolae, or depends on phagocytosis and micropinocytosis. After uptake, vesicles are incorporated into cisternae, then into a pseudo-multivesicular body (pMVB), to end with vesicle fusion and discharge to the cytosol. The membrane of the vesicles is retrieved and reused for release of newly formed vesicles (not shown). (After J. Meldolesi, 2018. *Curr. Biol.* 28: R435–R444.)

(Continued)

Intercellular Communication Mediated by Endosomes and Microvesicles (continued)

(B)

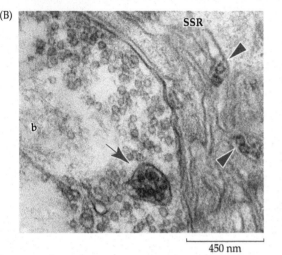
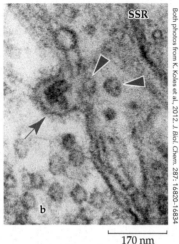

450 nm   170 nm

Figure B **Exosome Release in Neuromuscular Junctions of *Drosophila* Larvae.** (1) Electron micrograph of a synaptic bouton (b) containing a multivesicular body (arrow). The arrowheads point to small vesicles in foldings of the subsynaptic reticulum (SSR) of the muscle cell. (2) A multivesicular body (arrow) fusing with the perisynaptic membrane of a presynaptic bouton (b). The extracellular vesicles in the SSR (arrowheads) might have been released from the bouton.

Coexisting Forms of Extrasynaptic Communication

It has been shown that the retrograde spread of electrical activity to the soma and dendrites produces well-regulated forms of somatic and dendritic exocytosis. Here we discuss how bursts of impulses traveling along axons evoke release from varicosities in non-myelinated axons and from perisynaptic vesicles in presynaptic boutons.

Exocytosis from Axonal Varicosities

The axons of non-myelinated neurons that release acetylcholine, monoamines, ATP, and peptides commonly display varicosities. Autonomic peripheral neurons form varicose contacts on smooth muscle, cardiac muscle, viscera, and ganglion cells[79–81] (see Chapter 19). In the CNS, varicose axons are abundant in the hippocampus, basal ganglia, and amygdala,[82–84] and occur in lower proportion in the cortex.

As a general rule, varicosities along axons appear about every 5 μm and contact their targets in passing (*en passant*; Figure 18.15). Certain varicosities form morphological synapses, but most lack active zones, suggesting that they release extrasynaptically.[84,85] The proportion of synaptic versus nonsynaptic contacts varies from one cell type to another and among different target regions of the nervous system. Moreover, under the electron microscope, varicosities display an abundance of clear and dense-core vesicles (see Figure 18.15). Both vesicle types may coexist, and release of more than one type of molecule is common.[86,87] Figure 18.15 shows responses of smooth muscle to transmitter release from a single varicosity on stimulation of sympathetic nerve.[88] The variations in the rise time and amplitude of the evoked responses are similar to those that occur spontaneously, indicating that the evoked potentials are responses to single quanta.

Perisynaptic Release

In a series of elegant experiments, John Nicholls and his colleagues showed that Retzius neurons maintained in culture, in spite of being adult, survive for weeks and form unidirectional

[79] Luff, S. E. 1996. *Anat. Embryol. (Berl).* 193: 515-531.

[80] Tachibana, S., Takeuchi, M., and Fujiwara, T. 1985. *J. Electron Microsc. (Tokyo)* 34: 136-138.

[81] Baluk. P., and Fujiwara, T. 1984. *Neurosci. Lett.* 51: 265-270.

[82] Hökfelt, T. 1968. *Z. Zellforsch Mikrosk Anat.* 91: 1-74.

[83] Contant, C. et al. 1996. *Neuroscience* 71: 937-947.

[84] Umbriaco, D. et al. 1995. *Hippocampus* 5: 605-620.

[85] Descarries, L. et al. 1996. *J. Comp. Neurol.* 375: 167-186.

[86] Nusbaum, M. P., Blitz, D. M., and Marder, E. 2017. *Nat. Rev. Neurosci.* 18: 389-403.

[87] Hökfelt, T. et al. 2018. *Front. Neural Circuit.* 12: 106.

[88] Cunnane, T. C., and Stjarne. L. 1984. *Neuroscience* 13: 1-20.

Both photos from K. Koles et al., 2012. *J. Biol. Chem.* 287: 16820-16834

chemical synapses with pressure sensory neurons. Retzius neurons are always presynaptic and release quanta of serotonin from clear vesicles (**perisynaptic release**). Release depends on calcium, and the synapse shows facilitation and depression on repeated stimulation. The electron micrograph in Figure 18.16A shows that the synaptic vesicle pool is surrounded by perisynaptic dense-core vesicles that rest distantly from the plasma membrane. Antibody staining shows that such perisynaptic vesicles are also filled with serotonin.[89]

Amperometric recordings from similar terminals formed by the axonal stump of Retzius neurons plated singly allow one to capture oxidation spikes of serotonin quantal release from both synaptic clear and perisynaptic electrodense vesicles. Action potentials produced by a microelectrode in the soma are rapidly followed by small spikes produced by about 4700 serotonin molecules.[90] Subsequent action potentials increase the presence of large spikes produced by about 90,000 molecules (see Chapter 13) released from perisynaptic dense-core vesicles (Figure 18.16B). The latency for exocytosis from dense-core vesicles after an action potential is about 17 ms, and spikes continue to appear after stimulation, as explained by the distance between resting dense-core vesicles and the plasma membrane.

The amount of serotonin released from the synapse in response to a 20-Hz train of 10 impulses that produces early facilitation and late depression is about 60 quanta. Since each quantum contains 4700 molecules, a train releases about 282,000 serotonin molecules. The effect of such dynamic release along the train is quite significant in the small synaptic contact. However, such molecules would fill only three dense-core vesicles! This simple counting suggests that, as it happens in reality, most of the transmitter that is released perisynaptically gets lost before arriving at receptors.

Somatic versus Synaptic Release

We can now calculate the amount of serotonin released by the soma on a 20-Hz train. The plot in Figure 18.6 shows that approximately 80 vesicle clusters arrive at the plasma membrane, after subtracting the constitutive exocytosis. By assuming an average of 500 vesicles per cluster, the amount of serotonin released is $80 \times 500 \times 90,000 = 3.6 \times 10^9$ molecules. That means that 3.6 billion molecules can be released from the soma in response to a single 20-Hz train! The actual number increases because the axon is also a massive serotonin releaser. Such is the magnitude of serotonin extrasynaptic release that activates the crawling circuitry in Figure 18.4.

As it is released, serotonin diffuses among the labyrinth of thin layers of glia (see Figure 18.5) and is also taken up by the glia. It is not surprising, then, that diffusion of serotonin produces the long latency between the onset of exocytosis and the onset of behavior.

Transmitter Spillover

A different form of extrasynaptic communication takes place through the leak of transmitter from the synaptic cleft and its recognition by extrasynaptic receptors. Early experiments made in cerebellar synapses suggested that with increases in presynaptic activity, the transmitter that is being released saturates its uptake and leaks from the synaptic cleft,[91] a phenomenon called **spillover**. In brain slices of hippocampus, which allow controlled stimulation and recording of inhibitory and excitatory synapses,[92] Nicoll and his colleagues have shown that repeated stimulation of GABAergic synapses onto CA1 pyramidal cells with brief 50-Hz trains prolongs postsynaptic inhibition.[92] This occurs because GABA spillover activates extrasynaptic GABA_B metabotropic receptors. Blocking

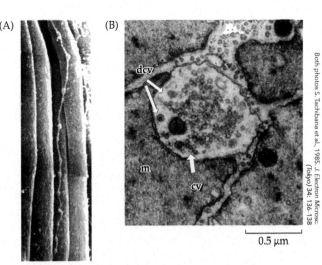
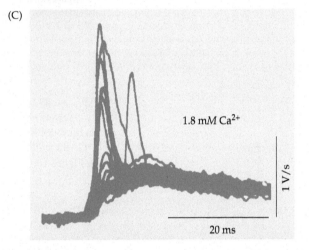

FIGURE 18.15 Exocytosis from Varicosities. (A) Scanning electron micrograph of a varicose axon innervating smooth muscle of the bladder. (B) Transmission electron micrograph of a varicosity with a cluster of clear vesicles (cv; thick arrow) and dense-core vesicles (dcv; thinner arrows). Synaptic structures are absent. m = muscle fiber. (C) Superimposed evoked responses to release from a single varicosity on nerve stimulation. (C after T. C. Cunnane and L. Stjarne, 1984. *Neuroscience* 13: 1–20.)

[89] Kuffler, D. P., Nicholls, J., and Drapeau, P. 1987. *J. Comp. Neurol.* 256: 516–526.

[90] Bruns, D., and Jahn, R. 1995. *Nature* 377: 62–65.

[91] Silver, R. A. et al. 1996. *J. Physiol.* 493: 167–173.

[92] Isaacson, J. S., Solís, J. M., and Nicoll, R. A. 1993. *Neuron* 10: 165–175.

(A)

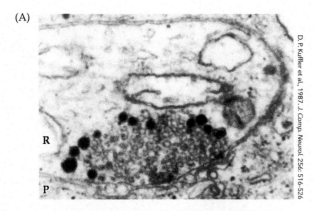

D. P. Kuffler et al., 1987. J. Comp. Neurol. 256: 516–526

(B)

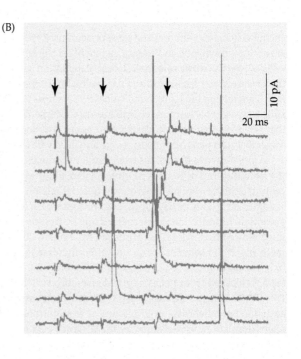

FIGURE 18.16 Synaptic and Perisynaptic Release of Serotonin.
(A) Electron micrograph of a synapse made in culture between a presynaptic Retzius neuron (R) and a postsynaptic pressure sensory neuron (P). The axonal bouton contains clear vesicles, some of which are docked in an active zone. Dense-core vesicles cap the synaptic cluster. (B) Successive amperometric recordings of serotonin release from a terminal in a single Retzius cell. Small spikes follow individual action potentials (arrows); large spikes increase their presence along the train. Recordings were made under low (1 mM) external calcium. (B from D. Bruns and R. Jahn, 1995. *Nature* 377: 62–65.)

GABA$_B$ receptors with CGP 35348 prevents the elongation of the postsynaptic response; conversely, the amplitude and duration of the inhibition are enhanced by the GABA uptake inhibitor SKF 89976A (Figure 18.17).

GABA spillover also inhibits glutamate release from excitatory synapses onto CA1 cells (see Figure 18.17) by activation of presynaptic GABA$_B$ receptors.[92] Inhibition of GABA

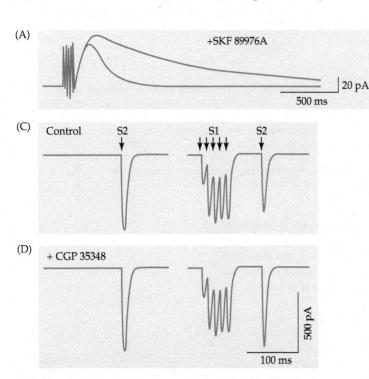

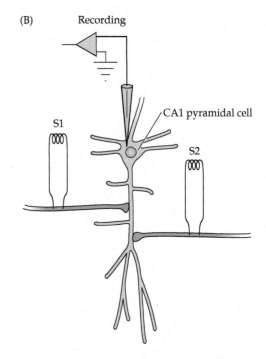

FIGURE 18.17 GABA Spillover in Hippocampal Synapses.
(A) Inhibition of GABA uptake by SKF 89976A increases the amplitude and decay time of postsynaptic currents in response to a brief train of stimulation. (B) Inhibition of glutamate release by GABA spillover. Stimulation electrodes S1 and S2 stimulate excitatory and inhibitory fibers that connect to CA1 pyramidal cells. The recording (Rec) electrode collects the responses from CA1 cells. (C) A test stimulus delivered by electrode S2 produces a large excitatory current. A conditioning train of five pulses at 50 Hz delivered by electrode S1 produces release and spillover of GABA; a second test pulse produces a reduced excitatory current. (D) The inhibition of the excitatory current is prevented by the GABA$_B$ metabotropic receptor blocker CGP 35348. (After J. S. Isaacson et al., 1993. *Neuron* 10: 165–175.)

uptake again enhances the effect of spillover. Altogether, GABA spillover moves the balance toward inhibition over excitation in CA3 cells. Glutamate spillover in cerebellar synapses has also been shown by another series of experiments. Its effects include activation of silent synapses and a normalization of the activity of nearby synapses[93-95] (see Chapter 16).

As discussed in Chapter 10, spillover of transmitters may activate receptors and transporters on surrounding glia.[96,97] Calcium recordings from glia during neuronal stimulation suggest that glia contribute to synaptic communication by forming "tripartite synapses" (pre- and postsynaptic terminals plus glia), an interesting topic under active study and debate.[98] Dopamine, noradrenaline, and ATP are also proposed to spill over. However, spillover requires a demonstration of the synaptic origin of release, and such transmitters are mostly released extrasynaptically.

Modulation of Visual Sensitivity and Blood Flow in the Retina

Earlier in this book we used the retina to exemplify different levels of the workings of the nervous system. Here we use the retina to exemplify how extrasynaptic release integrates adaptation to illumination with increases in blood flow and oxygenation in the illuminated region.

Modulation of retinal function incorporates classic transmitters, gases, cannabinoids, and peptides. However, only two transmitters that are released extrasynaptically are needed for the purpose of this chapter: dopamine and ATP. Dopamine acts as a gain-setter of visual sensitivity by modulating electrical activity at chemical and electrical synapses.[99] ATP activates Müller glial cells and induces synthesis and release of vasodilators and vasoconstrictors.[100]

Dopamine Release in the Retina

Dopamine is released mainly by dopaminergic amacrine (DA) cells, and in smaller amounts by catecholamine-containing amacrine cells. Figure 18.18 schematizes a DA cell

[93] Kerchner, G., and Nicoll, R. 2008. *Nat. Rev. Neurosci.* 9: 813-825.

[94] Coddington, L. T., Nietz, A. K., and Wadiche, J. I. 2014. *Cerebellum* 13: 513-520.

[95] Arnth-Jensen, N., Jabaudon, D., and Scanziani, M. 2002. *Nat. Neurosci.* 5: 325-331.

[96] Reist, N. E., and Smith, S. J. 1992. *Proc. Natl. Acad. Sci. USA* 89: 7625-7629.

[97] Dani, J. W., Chernjavsky, A., Smith, S. J. 1992. *Neuron* 8: 429-440.

[98] Durkee, C. A., and Araque, A. 2019. *Neuroscience* 396: 73-78.

[99] Roy, S., and Field, G. D. 2019. *J. Pharmacol. Sci.* 140: 86-93.

[100] Newman, E. A. 2015. *Philos. Trans. R. Soc. Lond. B Biol. Sci.* 370: 20140195.

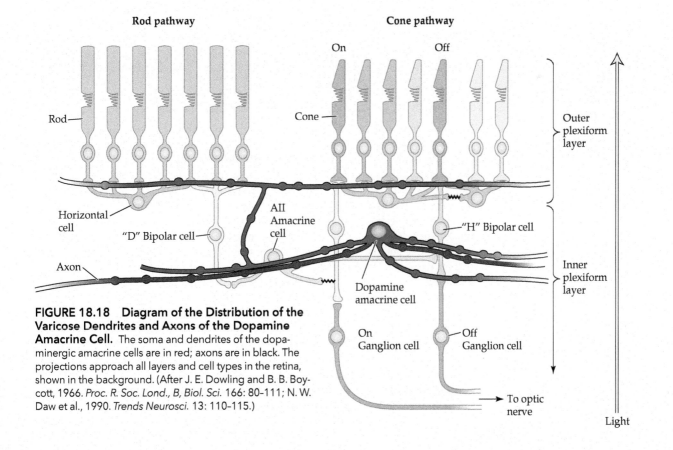

FIGURE 18.18 Diagram of the Distribution of the Varicose Dendrites and Axons of the Dopamine Amacrine Cell. The soma and dendrites of the dopaminergic amacrine cells are in red; axons are in black. The projections approach all layers and cell types in the retina, shown in the background. (After J. E. Dowling and B. B. Boycott, 1966. *Proc. R. Soc. Lond., B, Biol. Sci.* 166: 80-111; N. W. Daw et al., 1990. *Trends Neurosci.* 13: 110-115.)

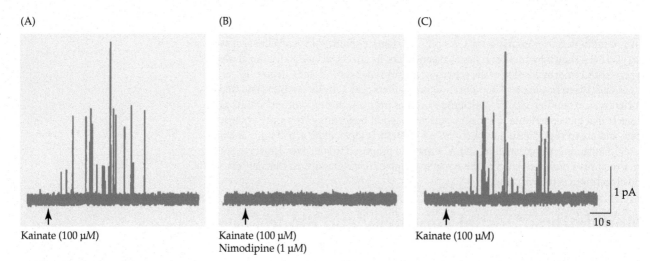

(A) Kainate (100 µM)

(B) Kainate (100 µM) Nimodipine (1 µM)

(C) Kainate (100 µM)

1 pA

10 s

FIGURE 18.19 Bursts of Dopamine Release from Isolated DA Cells. (A) Application of kainate (bar) depolarizes the soma and evokes a burst of exocytosis events that outlast the presence of kainate. Spikes are quanta of dopamine detected by carbon fiber amperometry. (B) Nimodipine abolishes exocytosis in the presence of kainate. (C) Exocytosis recovers on nimodipine (a Ca_V1 calcium channel blocker) washout. (After M. Puopolo et al., 2001. *Neuron* 30: 211-225.)

and its interactions with other cell types. Long, thick, bistratified dendrites bearing spines and varicosities interact with every cell type of the retina.[101] Usually more than one varicose axon per cell emerges from the soma and dendrites and extends over the inner plexiform layer, where connections between ganglion cells and bipolar cells are established.

Somatic Exocytosis of Dopamine

Electrical activity has been recorded from DA cells isolated from transgenic mice that express red fluorescent protein under the control of tyrosine hydroxylase, the enzyme that synthesizes dopamine. Spontaneous action potentials induce release of small numbers of dopamine quanta that can be recorded by amperometry; a large-scale release can be induced by kainate, which mimics excitatory inputs onto DA cells, depolarizing the cell and producing bursts of action potentials. Depolarization and exocytosis are coupled through activation of L-type calcium channels (Ca_V1; Figure 18.19). The extracellular dopamine affects most retinal cell types, some at considerable distance from the release sites.[102]

Modulation of Light Adaptation by Dopamine

In dark-adapted retinae of fish, amphibia, rodents, and primates, most cell types are coupled by gap junctions.[103] A bright light shone onto a small area of photoreceptors produces a visual response and the extrasynaptic exocytosis of dopamine from the DA cells.[101] The physiological effects of dopamine on retinal cell coupling have been explored by injection of intracellular tracers and recordings of electrical responses from individual cells.[104]

Horizontal cells are electrically coupled in the dark-adapted retina.[104-107] A few photons (for example, from a star shining in the dark sky) activate one or a few cones and their transmission line to ganglion cells. Active, electrically coupled horizontal cells in darkness inhibit a large population of surrounding photoreceptors, integrating a large visual field that operates with low resolution (see Chapter 22). Dopamine that is released on illumination acts on D1[105] receptors of horizontal cells; activation of these receptors uncouples horizontal cells through the production of cyclic AMP, activation of protein kinase A, and phosphorylation of connexin-36.[105] In this form of light adaptation, shrinking of the visual field of horizontal cells produces sharper vision in smaller areas (Figure 18.20). Dopamine also uncouples photoreceptors[108,109,110] and the networks established by amacrine II (AII) cells,[111] which connect the rod pathway to the cone pathway. All these effects disconnect the dim-light visual pathway and bias the visual sensitivity for bright light conditions.

It is a sobering thought that knowledge of the circuitry of the brain will probably not on its own explain how the brain works. For example, without knowing the detailed

[101] Hirasawa, H., Contini, M., and Raviola, E. 2015. *Philos. Trans. R. Soc. Lond. B Biol. Sci.* 370: 20140186.

[102] Veruki, M. L., and Wässle, H. 1996. *Eur. J. Neurosci.* 8: 2286-2297.

[103] Bloomfield, S. A., and Volgyi, B. 2009. *Nat. Rev. Neurosci.* 10: 495-506.

[104] Piccolino, M., Neyton, J., and Gerschenfeld, H. M. 1984. *J. Neurosci.* 4: 2477-2488.

[105] Zhang, A. J., Jacoby, R., and Wu, S. M. 2011. *J. Comp. Neurol.* 519: 2125-2134.

[106] Xin, D., Bloomfield, S. A. 1999. *J. Comp. Neurol.* 405: 75-87.

[107] Mangel, S. C., and Dowling, J. E. 1987. *Proc. R. Soc. Lond. B Biol. Sci.* 231: 91-121.

[108] Ribelayga, C., Cao, Y., and Mangel, S. C. 2008. *Neuron* 59: 790e801.

[109] Jackson, C. R. et al. 2009. *J. Neurochem.* 109: 148e157.

[110] Jin, N. G., and Ribelayga, C. P. 2016. *J. Neurosci.* 36: 178e184.

[111] Voigt, T., and Wässle, H. 1987. *J. Neurosci.* 7: 4115-4128.

(A)

(B)

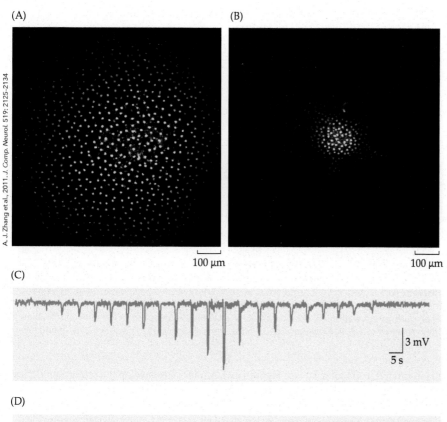

A. J. Zhang et al., 2011. *J. Comp. Neurol.* 519: 2125-2134

100 μm

100 μm

(C)

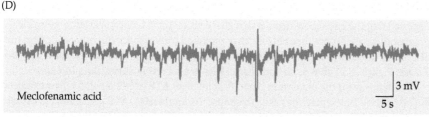

3 mV

5 s

(D)

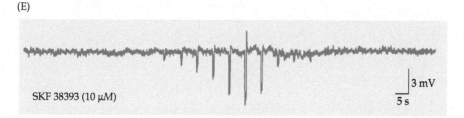

Meclofenamic acid

3 mV

5 s

(E)

3 mV

5 s

SKF 38393 (10 μM)

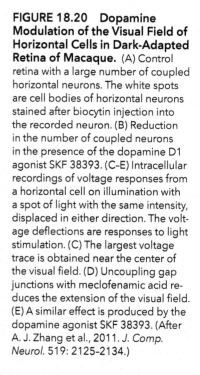

FIGURE 18.20 Dopamine Modulation of the Visual Field of Horizontal Cells in Dark-Adapted Retina of Macaque. (A) Control retina with a large number of coupled horizontal neurons. The white spots are cell bodies of horizontal neurons stained after biocytin injection into the recorded neuron. (B) Reduction in the number of coupled neurons in the presence of the dopamine D1 agonist SKF 38393. (C–E) Intracellular recordings of voltage responses from a horizontal cell on illumination with a spot of light with the same intensity, displaced in either direction. The voltage deflections are responses to light stimulation. (C) The largest voltage trace is obtained near the center of the visual field. (D) Uncoupling gap junctions with meclofenamic acid reduces the extension of the visual field. (E) A similar effect is produced by the dopamine agonist SKF 38393. (After A. J. Zhang et al., 2011. *J. Comp. Neurol.* 519: 2125–2134.)

connections of the cells in the retina, one cannot begin to guess how light is transduced to give rise to action potentials in the optic nerve. The anatomy on its own, and even the properties of the synapses, do not reveal the essential role of extrasynaptically released dopamine in the retina.

ATP and Glia as Mediators of Neurovascular Coupling

The extrasynaptic release of transmitters in response to illumination has another fundamental consequence: It couples the neuronal activity in the active region of the brain with a dramatic increase in blood flow. Such neurovascular coupling, demonstrated early on by Roy and Sherrington,[112] is not only fundamental for the workings of the brain but is also the basis for observing brain activity with magnetic resonance imaging (MRI).

A special type of glial cell in the retina, the Müller cell, is equivalent to astrocytes outside the retina. Müller cells exhibit receptors to multiple transmitters, and respond to their increased levels by releasing the same transmitter or other molecules. Like other types of

[112] Roy, C. S., and Sherrington, C. S. 1890. *J. Physiol.* 11: 85-108, 158-7-158-17.

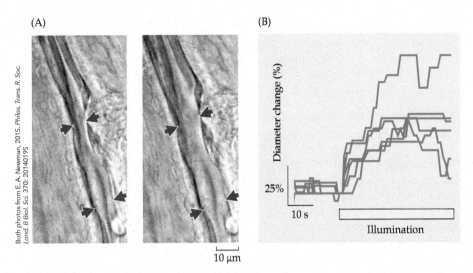

FIGURE 18.21 **Neurovascular Coupling Mediated by Glial Cells.** (A) Stimulation of the retina with flickering light produces dilation of arterioles in an acutely isolated rat retina. The photograph on the left was taken before illumination; the photograph on the right was taken during illumination. (B) Dilation of retinal arterioles in response to flickering illumination of the retina. (From E. A. Newman, 2015. *Philos. Trans. R. Soc. Lond. B Biol. Sci.* 370: 20140195.)

glia discussed in Chapter 10 (see Figure 10.1), Müller cells envelop the retinal capillaries with their end feet.[113] Based on the fact that glial cells register the overall levels of activity of their neighboring neurons, Paulson and Newman[114] put forward an original idea: They suggested that the end feet of depolarized glial cells might act on capillaries to cause localized vasodilation. Several lines of evidence provided by Newman and others confirm the idea. Thus, through glial signaling, active neurons can be supplied with extra oxygen and glucose. Figure 18.21 shows dilation of arterioles in a rat retina during illumination.

The pathway for the increase in blood flow involves ATP.[115] Müller glial cells are targets of ATP released from amacrine cells in response to illumination. ATP stimulates purinergic receptors on Müller cells, leading to the production of IP$_3$ and release of intracellular calcium. This is the beginning of the cascade of intracellular messengers shown in Figure 18.22,

[113] Biesecker, K. R. et al. 2016. *J. Neurosci.* 36: 9435-9445.

[114] Paulson, O. B., and Newman, E. A. 1987. *Science* 237: 896-898.

[115] Newman, E. A. 2013. *J. Cereb. Blood Flow Metab.* 33: 1685-1695.

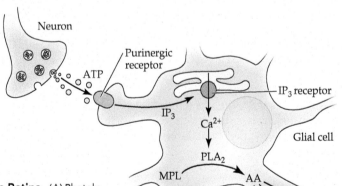

FIGURE 18.22 Neurovascular Coupling in the Retina. (A) Photolysis of caged calcium evokes a calcium increase in the glia followed by dilatation of an arteriole. (B) Metabolic pathway from glia to blood vessel contraction. Exocytosis of ATP from neurons stimulates purinergic receptors (pink) on glial cells, which produce IP$_3$ and intracellular calcium release. Calcium activates phospholipase A2 (PLA$_2$), which converts membrane phospholipids (MPL) to arachidonic acid (AA). Arachidonic acid is metabolized to the vasodilators prostaglandins (PGs) and epoxyeicosatrienoic acids (EETs), and to the vasoconstrictor 20-hydroxy-eicosatetraenoic acid (20-HETE). (A after M. R. Metea and E. A. Newman, 2006. *J. Neurosci.* 26: 2862-2870; B after E. A. Newman, 2013. *J. Cereb. Blood Flow Metab.* 33: 1685-1695.)

which ends with the production of the vasodilators prostaglandin E_2 and epoxyeicosatrienoic acids (EETs), and the vasoconstrictor 20-hydroxy-eicosatetraenoic acid (20-HETE). The immediate result is the dilation of arterioles near the illuminated area. Astrocytes in the brain produce similar effects.[116]

Cerebrospinal Fluid as a Source of Volume Transmission

The cerebrospinal fluid (CSF), with its ever-changing load of signaling molecules, allows long-distance communication between brain regions. The demonstration that the oxytocin diluted in the CSF can evoke contractions in isolated rabbit uterus gave the first insight as to the role of CSF in long-distance communication. Since then, the origin and functions of substances and precursor cells carried by the CSF flow have been a matter of study and debate.[117,118] Three complementary phenomena contribute to such communication. One is the dynamic liberation of transmitters, peptides, microRNAs, growth factors, and proteins into the CSF. The second is the continuous flow of CSF. The third is the bidirectional exchange of molecules across the ependymal cell layer that separates the CNS from the CSF.

The Ependymal Cell Layer

Ependymal cells are the major players in the flow of information between the neuropil and the CNS (see also Box 10.1). The ventricles and central canal of the spinal cord are lined by a layer of ependymal cells, which have a unique combination of properties of glia and epithelial cells. However, their glial characteristics and embryonic origin, the glial markers they express, and their precursor cell capabilities[119-121] dominate their classification as a special type of glia.

The layer of ependymal cells permits bidirectional exchange of fluid and substances between the CSF and CNS.[122] In addition, the synchronous beating of the cilia of ependymal cells, which face the CSF, determines the posterior-to-anterior direction and speed of the CSF flow. By contrast, in the subarachnoid spaces that surround the brain, the CSF flow is driven by the arterio-venous pressure gradient.

In the ventricles, a population of modified ependymal cells and capillaries form the **choroid plexus**, which produces about 80% of the CSF; the rest is contributed by the ependyma and blood vessels.[117] The production of CSF varies along the 24-hour period; more CSF is produced at night, and its renewal three to five times per day makes the episodic fluctuations in the levels of circulating molecules significant for signaling.[118]

A third type of modified ependymal cell are the tanycytes, which substitute the beating cilia for microvilli and send a long projection into the CNS. Tanycytes capture substances from the CSF by endocytosis and it is suggested that after incorporation in multivesicular bodies, such substances are released in the CNS by the tanycytes' projections.[123] The fourth major cell type contributing to the ependymal layer is neurons. Neuronal processes that reach the CSF capture and may release signaling molecules, as discussed next.

Exchange and Flow of Signaling Molecules between the CNS and CSF

The exchange of signaling molecules between the CSF and the CNS occurs in three complementary ways:

1. Diffusion over short distances

2. Diffusion via perivascular spaces aided by pumping driven by the vascular system

3. Selective uptake and release by neuronal structures exposed to the CSF

The complex composition of the CSF includes an abundance of most transmitters[124] and peptides. All are secreted by the choroid plexus, glia, and axon terminals that arrive at the periventricular ependyma.[125] The ciliary beating, essential for appropriate CSF flow, is modulated by transmitters and peptides. On the other hand, the absence of ciliary beating is lethal, resulting in the accumulation of CSF and the development of hydrocephaly.[120]

[116] Attwell, D. et al. 2010. *Nature* 468: 232-243.

[117] Veening, J. G., and Barendregt, H. P. 2010. *Cerebrospinal Fluid Res.* 7: 1.

[118] Skipor, J., and Thiery, J. C. 2008. *Acta Neurobiol. Exp. (Wars)* 68: 414-428.

[119] Johansson, C.B. et al. 1999. *Cell* 96: 25-34.

[120] Ohata, S., and Alvarez-Buylla, A. 2016. *Trends Neurosci.* 39: 543-551.

[121] Moreno-Manzano, V. 2019. *Curr. Opin. Pharmacol.* 50: 82-87.

[122] Milhorat, T. H. 1975. *J. Neurosurg.* 42: 628-645.

[123] Rodríguez, E. M. et al. 2005. *Int. Rev. Cytol.* 247: 89-164.

[124] Fania, C., et al. 2017. *PLOS ONE* 12: e0179280.

[125] Bruni, J. E. 1998. *Microsc. Res. Tech.* 41: 2-13.

(A)

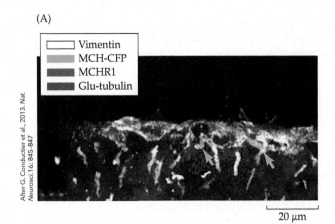

After G. Conductier et al., 2013. *Nat. Neurosci.* 16: 845-847

FIGURE 18.23 Acceleration of Ciliary Beating by MCH (Melanin-concentrating Hormone) Release. (A) Confocal optical section of the ependymal layer. MCH fibers (green arrowheads) and MCH receptor 1 (MCHR1; pink) are in close proximity to ependymal cells immunostained for vimentin marker (white). Tubulin staining (red) shows cilia (arrows). (B) Ciliary beating frequency (CBF) in response to MCH, serotonin (5-HT), and ATP. (C) Ciliary beating frequency on stimulation of MCH cells is reduced by the MCH antagonist H-6408. Error bars are the standard error. (After G. Conductier et al., 2013. *Nat. Neurosci.* 16: 845-847.)

(B)

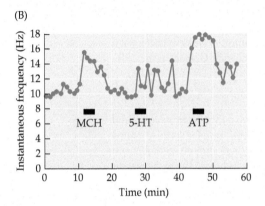

(C)

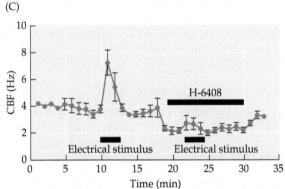

Serotonin accelerates the ciliary beating (Figure 18.23) in brainstem slices of rat by activating serotonin receptors, IP_3 production, and intracellular calcium release[126] (the same pathway described for somatic serotonin release). Another accelerator of ciliary beating is melatonin concentrating hormone (MCH),[127] a peptide that is produced in the hypothalamus and released by terminals arriving at the ependymal cell layer and CSF. Stimulation of MCH cells in brain slices of mouse or perfusion of peptide accelerate ciliary beating (see Figure 18.23). By contrast, application of the MCH antagonist H-6408 reduces the basal beating and suppresses the effect of electrical stimulation of MCH neurons.

Other experiments injecting peptides into the CNS have shown their diffusion over long distances to reach the CSF. For example, β-endorphin appears in the CSF approximately 10 minutes after being injected into the striatum of rats. In other experiments, stimulation of release by electrical microstimulation of the arcuate nucleus increases β-endorphin levels in the CSF after a few minutes.[128,129]

Signaling molecules[130] flowing in the CSF reach distant regions. Vasopressin administered into the lateral ventricle of the cat flows at about 1 cm/min to arrive in about 2 minutes at the ventral surface of the brainstem. A similar flow speed can be measured in the aqueduct of human brains by MRI.[131–133]

Perivascular Pumping

The distribution of CSF contents into the brain is aided by perivascular pumping. The arterial pulsations pump liquid through the perivascular space toward the outer surface of the brain.[134,135] The differences between pumping and passive diffusion are striking. Measurements of the diffusion velocity of exogenous horseradish peroxidase after intraventricular or cisternal injection in the brain show a diffusion velocity below 1 mm/hr. However, the pulsations of cerebral arteries induce horseradish peroxidase to appear along all the microvessels of the neuraxis within 5 minutes.

In other experiments, sexual behavior was evoked by intraventricular but not by intravenous administration of gonadotropin-releasing hormone (GnRH) in the periaqueductal

126 Nguyen, T. et al. 2001. *J. Physiol.* 531: 131-140.

127 Conductier, G., Brau, F., Viola, A., et al. 2013. *Nat. Neurosci.* 16: 845-847.

128 Bach, F. W., and Yaksh, T. L. 1995. *Brain Res.* 690: 167-176.

129 MacMillan, S. J., Mark, M. A., and Duggan, A. W. 1998. *Brain Res.* 794: 127-136.

130 Tricoire, H. et al. 2003. *Reprod. Suppl.* 61: 311-321.

131 Greitz, D. 1993. *Acta Radiol. Suppl.* 386: 1-23.

132 Wagshul, M. E. et al. 2006. *J. Neurosurg.* 104: 810-819.

133 McCormack, E. J., Egnor, M. R., and Wagshul, M. E. 2007. *Magn. Reson. Imaging* 25: 172-182.

134 Rennels, M. L. et al. 1985. *Brain Res.* 326: 47-63.

135 Hadaczek, P. et al. 2006. *Mol. Ther.* 14: 69-78.

gray region. The soma and axon of neurons that produce GnRH are abundant in the median eminence of the brain[136,137] and release GnRH into the CSF. Perivascular pumping sends peptide to the periaqueductal gray region, which has little GnRH innervation[137] but is rich in GnRH receptors.[137,138]

Uptake of Peptides by Neuronal Structures

Some examples of the release of substances to the CSF were mentioned in previous paragraphs. Here we mention two examples of uptake by neuronal structures that are in contact with the CSF. Experiments using autoradiography to detect the fate of radio-iodinated nerve growth factor (NGF) after intraventricular injection[139] show that NGF appears inside cholinergic neurons in the basal forebrain, with a peak occurring 18 hours after the injection. Likewise, neurons in the raphe nucleus selectively capture insulin-like growth factor and leukemia inhibitory factor from the CSF.

[136] Skinner, D. C. et al. 1997. *Endocrinology* 138: 4699-4704.

[137] Caraty, A., and Skinner, D. C. 2008. *Endocrinology* 149: 5227-5234.

[138] Leblanc, P. et al. 1988. *Neuroendocrinology* 48: 482-488.

[139] Ferguson, I. A. et al. 1991. *J. Comp Neurol.* 313: 680-692.

SUMMARY

- Neurons may release transmitters and peptides by exocytosis from the soma, axon, and dendrites in the absence of synaptic structures.

- Extrasynaptic release occurs from clear or dense-core vesicles. More than one type of molecule can be released by the same neuron and from the same vesicle.

- Extrasynaptic release from the axons, soma, and dendrites may occur independently from each other, following specific local mechanisms.

- The soma and dendrites may release large amounts of molecules for long periods of time through a multistep process.

- The large-scale exocytosis from the soma and dendrites is sustained by a positive transmitter- and calcium-dependent feedback loop.

- Extrasynaptic receptors may be far from the release sites.

- In the retina, extrasynaptic communication integrates the function of neuronal circuits, glia and blood vessels.

- The exchange of substances between the CFS and the CNS permits communication between distant structures.

Suggested Reading

Borroto-Escuela, D. O., Agnati, L. F., Bechter, K., Jansson, A., Tarakanov, A. O., and Fuxe, K. 2015. *Phil. Trans. R. Soc. B* 370: 20140183.

Budnik, V., Ruiz-Cañada, C., and Wendler, F. 2016. Extracellular vesicles round off communication in the nervous system. *Nat. Rev. Neurosci.* 17: 160–172. doi: 10.1038/nrn.2015.29.

Coddington, L. T., Nietz, A. K., and Wadiche, J. I. 2014. The contribution of extrasynaptic signaling to cerebellar information processing. *Cerebellum* 13: 513–520.

Descarries, L., and Mechawar, N. 2000. Ultrastructural evidence for diffuse transmission by monoamine and acetylcholine neurons of the central nervous system. *Prog. Brain Res.* 125: 27–47.

Durkee, C. A., and Araque, A. 2019. Diversity and specificity of astrocyte-neuron communication. *Neuroscience* 396: 73–78.

Fuxe, K., Dahlström, A., Höistad, M., Marcellino, D., Jansson, A., Rivera, A., Diaz-Cabiale, Z., Jacobsen, K., Tinner-Staines, B., Hagman, B., Leo, G., Staines, W., Guidolin D., Kehr, J., Genedani, S., Belluardo, N., and Agnati, L. F. 2007. From the Golgi-Cajal mapping to the transmitter-based characterization of the neuronal networks leading to two modes of brain communication: wiring and volume transmission. *Brain Res. Rev.* 55: 17–54.

Huang, H. P., Zhu, F. P., Chen, X. W., Xu, Z. Q., Zhang, C. X., and Zhou, Z. 2012. Physiology of quantal norepinephrine release from somatodendritic sites of neurons in locus coeruleus. *Front. Mol. Neurosci.* 5: 29.

Kravitz, E. A. 1988. Hormonal control of behavior: Amines and the biasing of behavioral output in lobsters. *Science* 241: 1775–1781.

Roy, S., and Field, G. D. 2019. Dopaminergic modulation of retinal processing from starlight to sunlight. *J. Pharmacol. Sci.* 140: 86–93.

Veening, J. G., and Barendregt, H. P. 2010. The regulation of brain states by neuroactive substances distributed via the cerebrospinal fluid; a review. *Cerebrospinal Fluid Res.* 7: 1.

Original Articles

Alpár, A. Zahola, P., Hanics, J., Hevesi, H., Korchynska, S., Benevento, M., Pifl, C., Zachar, G., Perruigini, J., Severi, I., et al. 2018. Hypothalamic CNTF volume transmission shapes cortical noradrenergic excitability upon acute stress *EMBO J.* 37: e100087.

Bao, L., Jin, S.-X., Zhang, C., Wang, L.-H., Xu, Z.-Z., Zhang, F.-X., Wang, L.-C., et al. 2003. Activation of delta opioid receptors induces receptor insertion and neuropeptide secretion. *Neuron* 37: 121–133.

Bering, E. A. 1955. Choroid plexus and arterial pulsation of cerebrospinal fluid: Demonstration of the choroid plexuses as a cerebrospinal fluid pump. *AMA Arch. Neurol. Psychiat.* 73: 165–172.

Contant, C., Umbriaco, D., Garcia, S., Watkins, K. C., and Descarries, L. 1996. Ultrastructural characterization of the acetylcholine innervation in adult rat neostriatum. *Neuroscience* 71: 937–947.

Ferguson, I. A., Schweitzer, J. B., Bartlett, P. F., and Johnson, E. M. 1991. Receptor-mediated retrograde transport in CNS neurons after intraventricular administration of NGF and growth factors. *J. Comp Neurol.* 313: 680–692.

Isaacson, J. S., Solís, J. M., and Nicoll, R. A. 1993. Local and diffuse synaptic actions of GABA in the hippocampus. *Neuron* 10: 165–175.

Kuffler, D. P., Nicholls, J., and Drapeau, P. 1987. *J. Comp. Neurol.* 256: 516–526.

Leon-Pinzon, C., Cercós, M. G., Noguez, P., Trueta, C., De-Miguel, F. F. 2014. Exocytosis of serotonin from the neuronal soma is sustained by a serotonin and calcium-dependent feedback loop. *Front. Cell Neurosci.* 8: 169.

Mendez, J. A., Bourque, M. J., Fasano, C., Kortleven, C., and Trudeau, L. E. 2011. Somatodendritic dopamine release requires synaptotagmin 4 and 7 and the participation of voltage-gated calcium channels. *J. Biol. Chem.* 286: 23928–23937.

Odette, L. L., and Newman, E. A. Model of potassium dynamics in the central nervous system. 1988. *Glia* 1: 198–210.

Paulson, O. B., and Newman, E. A. 1987. Does the release of potassium from astrocyte endfeet regulate cerebral blood flow? *Science* 237: 896–898.

Puopolo, M., Hochstetler, S. E., Gustincich, S., Wightman, R. M., and Raviola, E. 2001. Extrasynaptic release of dopamine in a retinal neuron: activity dependence and transmitter modulation. *Neuron* 30: 211–225.

Sun, Y., and Poo, M.-M. 1987. Evoked release of acetylcholine from the growing embryonic neurons. *Proc. Natl. Acad. Sci. USA* 84: 2540–2544.

Trueta, C., Méndez, B., and De-Miguel, F. F. 2003. Somatic exocytosis of serotonin mediated by L-type calcium channels in cultured leech neurones. *J. Physiol.* 547: 405–416.

PART IV

Integrative Mechanisms

Beyond the mechanisms that individual neurons, glial cells, and synapses use to communicate, of prime interest for neurobiology is the behavior of an animal as a whole. The first of the two chapters in this section, Chapter 19, deals with an essential function of the nervous system: the constant performance of "housekeeping tasks." The cardiovascular, respiratory, and intestinal needs of an animal must be regulated by the autonomic nervous system as the animal flies, swims, runs, feeds, or walks. In this chapter the biophysical, molecular, and chemical mechanisms described previously for neurons come together. Indeed, many key discoveries, such as the identification of transmitters, were first made at sympathetic and parasympathetic synapses. In addition, we will show that the autonomic nervous system is not truly autonomous, and interacts with emotions and hormonal aspects of the functions of the brain.

Similarly, Chapter 20 describes how the complex behavior of relatively simple animals is brought about by the integrated actions of nerve cells. Examples include the way in which ants and bees forage for food and then, in an extraordinary manner, find their way home using receptors that respond to ultraviolet light or to magnetic fields. Crayfish illustrate how the visual system integrates information from the ever-changing environment to decide on a particular behavior. In the leech, the circuits between identified individual sensory neurons, interneurons, and motor neurons have been traced and their biophysical properties analyzed. Such information provides a basis for explaining how complex movements are initiated and carried out by the animal.

CHAPTER 19

Autonomic Nervous System

The autonomic nervous system controls essential functions of the body. Thus, neurons of the autonomic nervous system supply smooth muscles in the eye, lung, gut, blood vessels, bladder, genitalia, and uterus. They regulate glandular secretion, blood pressure, heart rate, cardiac output, and body temperature, as well as food and water intake. In contrast to speedy conduction and muscle contractions required for limb movements, these housekeeping or vegetative functions are slower, last longer, and are not under the direct control of the will.

Four distinct groupings of neurons make up the autonomic nervous system. The **sympathetic division** consists of neurons with myelinated axons that leave the spinal cord through ventral roots from thoracic and lumbar segments. They form synapses on nerve cells in sympathetic ganglia situated alongside and at a distance from the spinal cord, and on chromaffin cells in the adrenal medulla. Sympathetic postganglionic axons are unmyelinated and extend over long distances to target areas. The **parasympathetic division** consists of axons leaving through certain cranial and sacral nerves. They form synapses in ganglia situated in or close to the target organs. Parasympathetic postganglionic axons are, in general, shorter than those of the sympathetic nervous system. A third, highly complex division consists of millions of nerve cells in the intestinal wall, the **enteric nervous system**. The fourth division comprises neurons in the spinal cord, hypothalamus, and brainstem. Within the central nervous system (CNS), boundaries between the autonomic and somatic nervous systems are not sharply defined.[1] Functionally, however, there are good grounds for retaining the parasympathetic denomination of the sacral outflow shown in Figure 19.1.[2]

Synaptic and extrasynaptic transmission coexist in the autonomic nervous system with extraordinary diversity, and make use of nearly all the known transmitters. Principles of transmission and integration that were first revealed at autonomic synapses include the chemical nature of synaptic and extrasynaptic transmission, reuptake of transmitter, autoreceptors on presynaptic terminals, co-release of more than one transmitter at a single terminal, and the role of second messengers (see also Chapter 12). In autonomic ganglia, the transmitters include acetylcholine (ACh) and peptides. Parasympathetic postganglionic nerve terminals release acetylcholine as the primary transmitter, which acts on muscarinic receptors in the target organs, and also release nitric oxide (NO) and peptides. Postganglionic sympathetic neurons release norepinephrine, epinephrine, acetylcholine, purines, or peptides as primary transmitters. Autonomic neurons co-release peptides together with adenosine triphosphate (ATP).

Whereas much is known about the regulation of activity in smooth muscle and gland cells, less information is available about integrative mechanisms in the CNS that regulate autonomic functions. The periodic 24-hour cycle of activity, known as circadian rhythm, influences many autonomic functions. Experiments in which recordings were made from specific neurons in the retina and in the hypothalamus (see also Chapter 22) have revealed cellular mechanisms that generate the rhythm.

The name *autonomic* implies an independent system that runs on its own. In part, this is true. The autonomic nervous system controls blood vessels outside the CNS, the heart, glands, and smooth muscle throughout the gut, bronchi, bladder, and spleen, without our having to make conscious decisions. By a simple act of will one cannot increase the diameter of the pupil or the blood flow through one's little finger. It is possible of course to cheat the system, to some extent, by using tricks; thus, the generation of emotion by deliberately thinking of an exam, a dental appointment, or a film starlet can stimulate the sympathetic nervous system to increase the heart rate.

In practice, the performance of the autonomic nervous system is closely linked to voluntary movements. Exercise results in appropriate diversion of blood to the muscles and in stimulation of sweat glands; the action of standing up from a recumbent position requires circulatory adjustments so as to maintain blood flow to the brain. Ingestion of a meal reroutes blood to the stomach and intestines. By turning activity on or off in a widespread group of target cells, the autonomic nervous system deals with the housekeeping and maintenance work of the body. The brain establishes the priorities, setting in motion digestion, reproduction, micturition, defecation, or focusing in dim light, through mechanisms that are not decided by our conscious will.

Of key concern for human beings are disorders of the autonomic nervous system that lead to conditions such as asthma, constipation, diarrhea, ulcers, hypertension, heart disease, stroke, and retention of urine (or lack thereof). We simply take for granted the regulation of essential bodily functions. For instance, it is remarkable that all the readers of this book have body temperatures of about 37°C and blood pressure values of about 120/80 mm Hg, in spite of their very different metabolic rates (and states of mind while reading).

Recent experiments and classic work on the autonomic nervous system represent such an extensive and varied field that a comprehensive review is impossible in this chapter. Indeed, entire textbooks[3,4] and specialized journals[5–7] are devoted to important functions of the autonomic nervous system. A large amount of information is available about mechanisms that control the enteric nervous system and bladder, diameter of the pupil, and secretion by glands, and that regulate respiration, temperature, body weight, appetite, and reproduction.[8–10]

In this chapter, as in others, the main emphasis is on a few select examples that illustrate cellular, molecular, and integrative mechanisms. We will show that although much is now known about the autonomic nervous system, many questions remain, particularly about integrative mechanisms in the CNS; there the distinction between autonomic and somatic systems has no hard-and-fast boundaries. It is convenient to begin with a brief description of the principal features of the peripheral autonomic nervous system.

Functions under Involuntary Control

Sympathetic and Parasympathetic Nervous Systems

Figure 19.1 shows the principal anatomical features of the autonomic nervous system. Virtually all the organs of the body are supplied by autonomic neurons. Even skeletal muscle fibers, which receive no direct innervation, depend on the autonomic nervous system—their blood supply is regulated according to need. Sympathetic preganglionic neurons are situated in the intermediolateral horn of the spinal cord of segments T1 to L3 (see Appendix C-8). Their myelinated axons pass through ventral roots to form synapses in ganglia situated alongside the vertebral column and peripheral to it (see Figure 19.1A). From these ganglia, unmyelinated axons run to the tissues. By contrast, the parasympathetic outflow is restricted to cranial nerves III, VII, IX, and X and sacral roots S2, S3, and S4 (see Figure 19.1B). The parasympathetic ganglia are located close to or in the tissues themselves. Hence, the parasympathetic myelinated preganglionic axon is long, whereas the unmyelinated postganglionic axon is short.

The actions of the two systems are often, but not always, antagonistic (Table 19.1). For example, excitation of sympathetic neurons leads to dilatation of the pupil, increased heart rate, and decreased gut motility. Parasympathetic excitation produces opposite effects, such as pupillary constriction, slowed heart rate, and increased gut motility. However, glandular secretion can be increased by activation of either system. Both systems can cause smooth muscles to contract or to relax, depending on the transmitter that is released and the types of receptors that are present on the muscle.

[1] Espinosa-Medina, I. et al. 2016. *Science* 354: 893–897.

[2] Jänig, W. et al. 2017. *Auton. Neurosci.* 206: 60–62.

[3] Burnstock, G., ed. 1990-99. *The Autonomic Nervous System.* 8 vols. Harwood Academic, New Jersey.

[4] Robertson, D., ed. 2004. *Primer on the Autonomic Nervous System,* Academic Press, London.

[5] *J. Autonomic Nervous System*

[6] *Autonomic Neuroscience*

[7] *J. Autonomic Pharmacology*

[8] Cooper, J. R., Bloom, F. E., and Roth, R. H. 2002. *The Biochemical Basis of Pharmacology.* Oxford University Press, New York.

[9] Fowler, C. J., Griffiths, D., and de Groat, W. C. 2008. *Nat. Rev. Neurosci.* 25: 7324–7332.

[10] Spyer, K. M., and Gourine, A. V. 2009. *Philos. Trans. R. Soc. Lond., B, Biol. Sci.* 364: 2603–2610.

(A) Sympathetic

(B) Parasympathetic

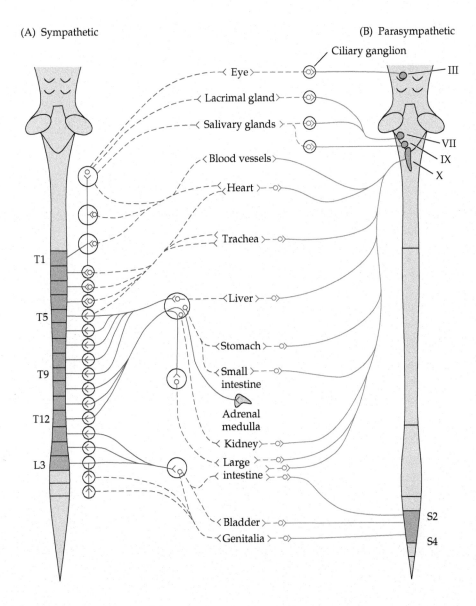

FIGURE 19.1 The Autonomic Nervous System and the target organs that it innervates. Solid lines are myelinated preganglionic axons; dashed lines are unmyelinated postganglionic axons. (A) Principal features of the sympathetic nervous system, including the paravertebral ganglia, peripheral ganglia, and adrenal medulla. Research studying the genetics and development of the sympathetic and parasympathetic neurons suggests that the sacral parasympathetic outflow is formed from sympathetic neurons, not parasympathetic neurons, and so should really be classified as part of the sympathetic nervous system. (B) The parasympathetic nervous system has more restricted output and targets that it innervates in comparison with the sympathetic nervous system.

A major difference between the two autonomic systems is that, while the parasympathetic nervous system functions in a focused manner, the sympathetic nervous system tends to be thrown into action as a whole, with widespread generalized consequences for the body. The sympathetic system is typically activated under conditions of *fright, fight,* and *flight,* as well as during intense exercise. The symptoms are familiar; they include dilated pupils, dry mouth, pounding heart, sweating, and enhanced emotions. The systemic effects of sympathetic neuronal activity are enhanced further by chromaffin cells in the adrenal medulla. These cells are modified ganglionic neurons. They receive cholinergic input from preganglionic axons and secrete epinephrine, norepinephrine, peptides, and ATP as hormones into the bloodstream.[11,12] Epinephrine in the blood reinforces and extends sympathetic activity. It can reach and bind to receptors in smooth muscle of bronchi, far from sympathetic nerve endings; epinephrine also binds to receptors in blood vessels that are insensitive to norepinephrine (see Box 19.1). Unlike norepinephrine, epinephrine produces vasodilatation as well as contraction of blood vessels.

By contrast, the parasympathetic nervous system is more focused in its activity. It is surely a considerable advantage that the pupil can constrict in bright light and that the lens of the eye accommodate for viewing nearby objects selectively, without concomitant and ill-timed arousal of bladder contractions or even more embarrassing parasympathetic effects.

[11] Crivellato, E., Nico, B., and Ribatti, D. 2008. *Anat. Rec. (Hoboken)* 291: 1587–1602.

[12] Fulop, T., Radabaugh, S., and Smith, C. 2005. *J. Neurosci.* 25: 7324–7332.

TABLE 19.1

Characteristic actions of adrenergic sympathetic and cholinergic parasympathetic nervous systems

Organ	Adrenergic sympathetic		Cholinergic parasympathetic
	Action[a]	Receptor[b]	Action
Eye			
Iris			
Radial muscle	Contracts	α_1	—
Circular muscle	—	—	Contracts
Ciliary muscle	(Relaxes)	β	Contracts
Heart			
Sinoatrial node	Accelerates	β_1	Decelerates
Contractility	Increases	β_1	Decreases (atria)
Vascular smooth muscle			
Skin, splanchnic vessels	Contracts	α	—
Skeletal muscle vessels	Relaxes	β_2	—
Nerve endings	Inhibits release	α_2	—
Bronchiolar smooth muscle	Relaxes	β_2	Contracts
Gastrointestinal tract			
Smooth muscle			
Walls	Relaxes	α_1, β_2	Contracts
Sphincters	Contracts	α_1	Relaxes
Secretion	—	—	Increases
Myenteric plexus	Inhibits	α	Activates
Genitourinary smooth muscle			
Bladder wall	Relaxes	β_2	Contracts
Sphincter	Contracts	α_1	Relaxes
Metabolic functions			
Liver	Gluconeogenesis	α/β_2	—
	Glycogenolysis	α/β_2	—

[a]Accounts of the actions of the autonomic nervous system on target organs listed in this table that are not dealt with in this chapter are given in reviews and textbooks of physiology and pharmacology (see references in text).

[b]Not all the adrenergic receptors or effector cells are included; purinergic, peptidergic, and cholinergic mechanisms are dealt with in the text. Whereas epinephrine acts on all the adrenergic receptors, norepinephrine is effective on α_1, α_2, and β_1-receptors but only weakly on β_2. The various types of adrenergic and muscarinic receptors are characterized by the specific agonists and antagonists that bind to them and by their molecular structures.

Transmission in Autonomic Ganglia

Certain mechanisms of transmission in the autonomic nervous system have already been described in earlier chapters (see Chapters 11, 12, 14, and 18). These include synaptic and extrasynaptic release, the co-release of multiple transmitters from nerve endings, modulatory actions of autonomic transmitters, the properties of receptors that use second messengers, and the effects of acetylcholine and epinephrine on cardiac muscle. The way in which such mechanisms interact to influence signaling is well illustrated by experiments made on transmission in autonomic ganglia. These synapses serve to demonstrate integrative processes occurring in the CNS that are even more complex.

Autonomic ganglia constitute topographically divergent relay stations—that is, each preganglionic fiber innervates many ganglionic neurons, and hence can excite many postganglionic fibers. Perhaps unsurprisingly, the degree of topographical amplification, expressed as the number of ganglion cells innervated by each preganglionic fiber, increases with animal size (at least, in mammals)—for example, from 60 cells in the mouse cervical sympathetic ganglion to 420 in that of the rabbit.[13] There is also topographical convergence in that each ganglion cell is innervated by up to 16 preganglionic fibers.[13] Of these, one or two make "strong" connections in which the synaptic potential is suprathreshold and almost invariably generates a postganglionic action potential, whereas the others form weak connections in which the individual synaptic potentials are mostly subthreshold and generate action potentials only when they summate or are otherwise amplified. The normal frequency of natural action potential activity in mammalian sympathetic fibers is between 0.5 and 5 impulses per second (0.5–5 Hz),[13,14] rising to 10–20 Hz under extreme conditions such as asphyxia.

The mechanism of direct, rapid transmission at autonomic ganglia is similar to that at the skeletal neuromuscular junction. Each presynaptic impulse releases acetylcholine, which acts on nicotinic receptors in the postsynaptic cell to open channels and produce

[13] Ivanov, A., and Purves, D. 1989. *J. Comp. Neurol.* 284: 398-404.

[14] McLachlan, E. M., ed. 1995. *Autonomic Ganglia.* Gordon and Breach, London.

[15] Selyanko, A. A. et al. 1979. *J. Auton. Nerv. Syst.* 1: 127-137.

[16] Rang, H. P. 1981. *J. Physiol.* 311: 23-55.

[17] Mathie, A. A. et al. 1991. *J. Physiol.* 439: 717-750.

[18] Gibbins, I. L., and Morris, J. L. *Cell Tissue Res.* 326: 205-220.

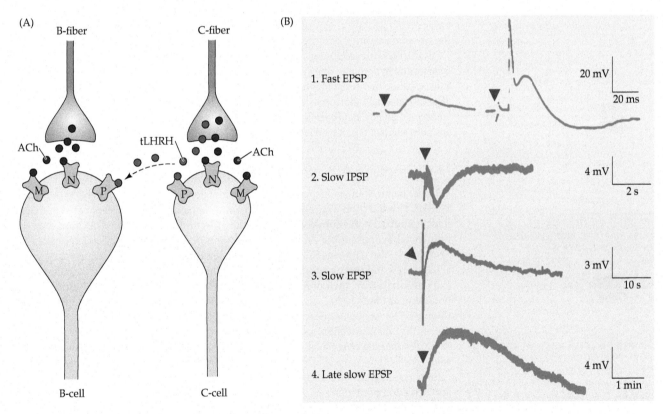

FIGURE 19.2 Four Types of Postsynaptic Potential in Bullfrog Sympathetic Ganglion Cells. (A) Arrangement of sympathetic lumbar ganglion cells in the frog. Large B-cells (50–70 μm diameter) receive a single preganglionic myelinated B fiber descending from the upper spinal cord via the sympathetic chain. These release ACh to act on nicotinic (N) and muscarinic (M) receptors on the B-cell. The smaller (<50 μm) C cells receive pregan-glionic unmyelinated C-fibers from the seventh and eighth spinal roots. Most of these fibers co-release both ACh and the peptide tLHRH (teleost luteinizing hormone releasing hormone). N = nicotinic receptor; M = muscarinic receptor; P = peptide receptor. (B) Microelectrode recordings of: (1) the fast EPSP in a B-cell following a single preganglionic stimulus giving a subthreshold EPSP and (right) a stronger stimulus giving a larger EPSP with a superimposed action potential; (2) a slow inhibitory postsynaptic potential (SIPSP, lasting 2 s) in a C-cell after stimulating the seventh and eighth spinal roots with 13 stimuli at 20 Hz (this results from activation of muscarinic [M] receptors on the C-cell because the nicotinic receptors were blocked with curare); (3) a slow cholinergic EPSP lasting 30 s in a B-cell due to activation of muscarinic receptors following four stimuli at 50 Hz to the sympathetic chain above ganglion; (4) the peptidergic late slow EPSP in a B-cell lasting about 300 s after stimulating the central portions of spinal nerves 7 and 8 (50 stimuli at 10/s). This is due to release of teleost luteinizing hormone releasing hormone (tLHRH) from synaptic boutons on C-cells and subsequent intra-ganglionic diffusion to B-cells (dashed lines in part [A]). Note the differences in time scales for the different responses. (After Y. N. Jan et al., 1979. *Proc. Natl. Acad. Sci. USA* 76: 1501-1505.)

a fast depolarization (see Chapters 11 and 14).[13–18] As at the neuromuscular junction, a single presynaptic action potential is followed by one in the postsynaptic cell (Figure 19.2). The nicotinic receptors, however, differ in their subunit composition from those at the motor end plate, being made up of α- and β-subunits but without γ-, δ-, or ε-subunits (see Chapters 5 and 27).[19–21]

Transmission between the preganglionic axon and the ganglion cell is far more elaborate than would at first appear. Thus, a very different picture emerges with repetitive stimulation of the presynaptic axon. Under these conditions, the ganglion is not simply a throughway, but is a site of complex interactions. With trains of impulses, prolonged depolarizing or hyperpolarizing, long-latency, synaptic potentials arise in the ganglion cell.[22,23] They summate to produce a steady, subthreshold depolarization maintained for seconds, minutes, or even hours. During the depolarization, a single presynaptic action potential can now give rise to multiple impulses in the postsynaptic cell. Both the fast and the slow synaptic potentials are evoked by the release of acetylcholine from the presynaptic nerve terminals. As before, the fast, direct synaptic potential (see Figure 19.2A) results from activation of nicotinic ACh receptors. The slow potential (see Figure 19.2B) is due to activation of muscarinic ACh receptors that are coupled to G proteins (see Chapter 12). Cholinesterase activity at sympathetic synapses is generally lower than that at neuromuscular synapses, and the enzyme is located primarily on the presynaptic cholinergic terminals[24] instead of on the postsynaptic membrane. Hence, anticholinesterase compounds only modestly enhance nicotinic transmission at autonomic synapses.[16] They do, however, strongly facilitate the synaptic activation of muscarinic receptors.[25]

Kuffler and his colleagues found that a second transmitter also contributes to slow depolarizing and hyperpolarizing synaptic potentials in frogs. Certain presynaptic axons release a decapeptide that resembles luteinizing hormone-releasing hormone (LHRH). (LHRH is also known as gonadotropin-releasing hormone [GnRH]; see Figure 19.8.) Hence, in frog autonomic ganglia, neuronal firing and excitability are controlled by both ACh, secreted synaptically, and by LHRH, secreted perisynaptically by presynaptic neurons (see Chapter 12).

M-Currents in Autonomic Ganglia

What is the mechanism responsible for the slow depolarizations produced by ACh and LHRH? This question was resolved by Brown, Adams, and their colleagues, who identified an unusual potassium current carried by **M-channels**—so called because they are influenced by muscarinic ACh receptors[26] (and in frogs, also by LHRH receptors[27]). M-channels, also known as KCNQ or K_V7 channels (see Chapter 5), have a high open probability at rest and make a substantial contribution to the resting potassium conductance. With depolarization, their probability of opening increases. An unusual property of the M potassium channels is that activation of muscarinic receptors causes these channels to *close* (Figure 19.3). As a consequence, the resting influx of sodium ions is no longer balanced by the resting potassium efflux and the cell depolarizes.

After their discovery in autonomic ganglia, M-channels were found in neurons in the spinal cord, hippocampus, and cerebral cortex.[28,29] M-channel closure produced by transmitters results from activation of phospholipase C.[30–32] This in turn leads to hydrolysis and depletion of membrane phosphatidylinositol-4,5-bisphosphate—a molecule that is required for channel opening (see Chapter 12).

What is the physiological importance of M-currents in autonomic ganglia? The principal effect of the M-current is to raise the threshold for firing an action potential. Thus, when a neuron with an M-current is depolarized, it fires only one or two action potentials and then becomes silent. The steps that cause this to happen are:

> Initial depolarization opens M-channels → M-channels generate an outward potassium current → potassium current counteracts inward sodium current in initial phase of action potential → prevents full action potential from developing

[19] Ullian, E. M., McIntosh, J. M., and Sargent, P. B. 1997. *J. Neurosci.* 17: 7210-7219.

[20] Listerud M. et al. 1992. *Science* 254: 1518-1521.

[21] Rust, G. et al. 1994. *Eur. J. Neurosci.* 6: 478-485.

[22] Kuffler, S. W. 1980. *J. Exp. Biol.* 89: 257-286.

[23] Jan, Y. N., Jan, L. Y., and Kuffler, S. W. 1980. *Proc. Natl. Acad. Sci. USA* 77: 5008-5012.

[24] Koelle, G. B. 1962. *J. Pharm. Pharmacol.* 14: 65-90.

[25] Brown, D. A., and Selyanko, A. A. 1985. *J. Physiol.* 365: 365-387.

[26] Brown, D. A., and Adams, P. R. 1980. *Nature* 283: 673-676.

[27] Adams, P. R., and Brown, D. A. 1980. *Brit. J. Pharmacol.* 68: 353-355.

[28] Brown, D. A., and Passmore, G. M. 2009. *Brit. J. Pharmacol.* 156: 1185-1195.

[29] Hansen, H. H. et al. 2008. *J. Physiol.* 586: 1823-1832.

[30] Suh, B. C., and Hille, B. 2008. *Annu. Rev. Biophys.* 37: 175-195.

[31] Delmas, P., and Brown, D. A. 2005. *Nat. Rev. Neurosci.* 6: 850-862.

[32] Hernandez, C. C. et al. 2008. *J. Physiol.* 586: 1811-1121.

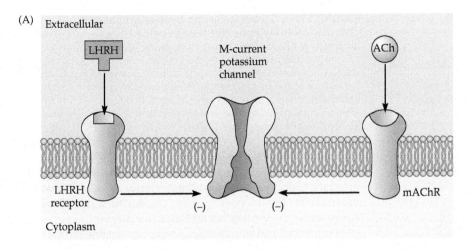

(A)

(B)

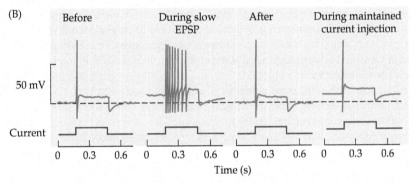

FIGURE 19.3 Inhibition of Potassium Currents in Sympathetic Ganglion Cells modulates responses to presynaptic stimulation. (A) Binding of ACh to muscarinic receptors (mAChRs) and binding of LHRH to its receptor both inhibit M-current potassium channels. (B) The effect of the decrease in the M-current during the slow synaptic potential is to increase the excitability of the ganglion cell. Depolarizing current pulses applied through the microelectrode (lower traces) before and after a slow synaptic potential produce a single action potential. During the slow potential, the same current pulse elicits a burst of action potentials. Depolarizing the ganglion cell (to the same extent as occurs during closure of M-channels) by injecting a maintained current has no such effect on the responsiveness of the cell. (After S. W. Jones and P. Adams, 1987. In *Neuromodulation: The Biochemical Control of Neuronal Excitability*. Oxford University Press, New York.)

When the M-current is suppressed through closure of the K+ channels by the transmitter, this series of steps does not happen and the neuron fires repetitively (see Figure 19.3). In other words, the neuron switches from **phasic-firing** to **tonic-firing** mode when the M-current is suppressed. Some sympathetic neurons (e.g., in prevertebral ganglia) do not have M-currents, and they fire tonically rather than phasically.[33] Cells that do possess M-currents may be induced to fire spontaneous action potentials by strong inhibition of M-current (see, for example, the effect of synaptically released LHRH on frog ganglion cells in Figure 12.7C). Inhibition of M-current also reduces the threshold nicotinic current needed to generate a postsynaptic action potential.[34] This enhances synaptic gain through the ganglion so that some previously subthreshold synaptic potentials become suprathreshold, increasing the overall frequency of postsynaptic action potential generation.

M-channels have a major effect on firing patterns in the autonomic nervous system. In cells with large M-currents, such as those that cause dilatation of the pupil, presynaptic inputs do not fire tonically and the output is roughly one to one.[35] By contrast, cells in lumbar ganglia that cause vasoconstriction receive a continuous bombardment from presynaptic inputs. This inhibits their M-currents through the muscarinic effect of acetylcholine. Accordingly, they fire tonically at varying frequencies, depending on the input, and produce greater or reduced tonic vasoconstriction. These results fit with the special requirement of discontinuous, episodic dilatation of the pupil on demand and maintained control of blood vessel diameter. Tonic and phasic discharges have additional effects; they can determine which types of transmitters are released by the terminals of a ganglion cell onto its targets.

Transmitter Release by Postganglionic Axons

Although acetylcholine is the principal transmitter used by postganglionic parasympathetic axons, they can co-release nitric oxide (NO)[36] and peptides (Figures 19.4 and 19.5). For example, ACh released by parasympathetic axons causes salivary glands to secrete by acting on muscarinic receptors. With high-frequency stimulation, the same axons also liberate a

[33] Wang, H.-S., and McKinnon, D. 1995. *J. Physiol.* 485: 319–325.

[34] Kullmann, P. H., and Horn, J. P. 2006. *J. Neurophysiol.* 96: 3104–3113.

[35] Jänig, W., and McLachlan, E. M. 1992. *Trends Neurosci.* 15: 475–481.

[36] Toda, M., and Okamura, T. 2003. *Pharmacol. Rev.* 55: 271–324.

Parasympathetic axon varicosity

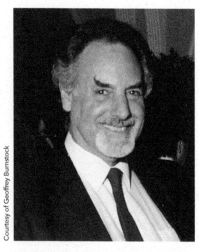

FIGURE 19.4 **Co-transmission by Parasympathetic Postganglionic Neurons** that release both acetylcholine and vasoactive intestinal peptide (VIP). Parasympathetic nerve fibers supplying the salivary gland secrete both transmitters, which are stored in separate vesicles. Stimulation at low frequencies releases acetylcholine but not VIP, while at higher frequencies both transmitters are released, causing vasodilatation and secretion of saliva. (After G. Burnstock. 1983. In *Dale's Principle and Communication Between Neurones.* Neville N. Osborne, ed., pp. 7–35. Pergamon Press: Oxford.)

peptide called vasoactive intestinal peptide (VIP). VIP, originally found in gut and brain, causes vasodilatation, increased intracellular calcium concentration, and increased secretion of saliva that is not blocked by atropine, which is an antagonist for muscarinic receptors.[37]

For sympathetic postganglionic neurons, norepinephrine is the principal transmitter. Sympathetic axons innervating sweat glands and blood vessels in skeletal muscle, however, secrete acetylcholine instead of norepinephrine.[38] Sympathetic nerve fibers also secrete ATP and peptides, which are co-released with the conventional transmitters as described in Chapter 18. The locations of some of the transmitters used in intestinal reflexes are shown in Figures 19.4 and 19.5.

Table 19.1 shows the principal locations of adrenergic receptors in the body and their mechanisms of action. With the advent of molecular biology, it became clear that the amino acid sequences are similar in the α_1- and α_2- as well as the β_1-, β_2-, and β_3-adrenergic receptors, and also in the muscarinic receptors activated by ACh. All of these receptors contain seven transmembrane segments, are coupled to G proteins, and use second messengers (see Chapter 12) (Box 19.1).

Purinergic Transmission

In a remarkable series of experiments, Burnstock and his colleagues demonstrated the existence of a major class of sympathetic transmitters, the purines: ATP and adenosine.[39] Certain sympathetic nerve fibers secrete ATP from their terminals, either as the principal transmitter or together with norepinephrine or acetylcholine. The experiments showing that ATP is a sympathetic transmitter were originally designed for a quite different purpose. Burnstock and Holman[40] recorded intracellularly from smooth muscle fibers of the reproductive system to investigate sympathetic postganglionic transmission, which at the time was thought to be mediated by norepinephrine. Their recordings of spontaneous miniature potentials constituted an important finding, because before this time, quantal release had

[37] Burnstock, G. 2006. *Trends Pharmacol. Sci.* 27: 166–176.

[38] Guidry, G. et al. 2005. *Auton. Neurosci.* 123: 54–61.

[39] Burnstock, G. 1995. *J. Physiol. Pharmacol.* 46: 365–384.

[40] Burnstock, G., and Holman, M. E. 1961. *J. Physiol.* 155: 115–133.

[41] Kasakov, L. et al. 1988. *J. Auton. Nerv. Syst.* 22: 75–82.

Geoff Burnstock

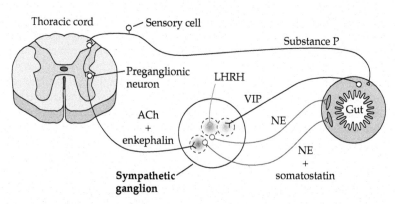

FIGURE 19.5 **Localization of Transmitters** and neuropeptides in neurons of the sympathetic nervous system. All known transmitters are found in the intestine. LHRH = luteinizing hormone-releasing hormone; NE = norepinephrine; VIP = vasoactive intestinal peptide. (After T. Hökfelt et al., 1980. *Nature* 284: 515–521.)

| BOX **19.1** | The Path to Understanding Sympathetic Mechanisms |

The development of concepts about mechanisms of transmission in the autonomic nervous system spanned many years. The original work of Henry Dale in the 1930s and 1940s showed that excitatory and inhibitory transmission in target organs is extremely complicated. One source of confusion arose from the idea that epinephrine might be the transmitter molecule liberated by sympathetic nerves (as originally suggested by Elliott in 1904). It was not until von Euler[42] discovered that norepinephrine, not epinephrine, is the principal transmitter released by sympathetic nerves that the distinction between hormonal and transmitter actions could be accounted for.

Epinephrine released from the adrenal medulla reaches receptors in cells that are not innervated by sympathetic axons—for example, on smooth muscle fibers of bronchioles in the lung. It can also act on receptors that are insensitive to norepinephrine released from sympathetic nerve fibers. A major advance was made by Ahlquist,[43] who devised the scheme for classifying α- and β-adrenergic receptors by comparing specific agonists and antagonists. This classification was essential for explaining the varied excitatory and inhibitory sympathetic actions that occur on blood pressure, smooth muscle, the gut, bronchi, and glands.

The discovery that some sympathetic axons release acetylcholine (ACh) or purines was also essential.

An understanding of the transmitters and receptors used by the autonomic nervous system has allowed new drugs to be developed for treatment of diseases. One example is provided by the control of bronchioles in the lung. Bronchoconstriction occurs in asthma or severe anaphylactic reactions of the immune system. To initiate relaxation of smooth muscle in the bronchi, β_2-receptors are activated by giving epinephrine or a more specific agonist (such as salbutamol, a β_2-agonist used for the treatment of asthma), but not norepinephrine, which has little or no effect on β_2-receptors. Bronchodilatation allows the patient to breathe again. Another example is provided by the beta-blockers that are widely used and highly effective in the treatment of high blood pressure, coronary artery disease, and glaucoma. As their name implies, these drugs act by blocking the actions of norepinephrine and epinephrine on β-receptors in the heart, smooth muscle of blood vessels, kidney, and eye.[44]

---

[42] von Euler, U. S. 1956. *Noradrenaline.* Charles Thomas, Springfield, IL.
[43] Ahlquist, R. P. 1948. *Am. J. Physiol.* 153: 586–600.
[44] Black, J. W., and Prichard, B. N. 1973. *Br. Med. Bull.* 29: 163–167.

---

been observed only at the skeletal neuromuscular junction. Later, however, Burnstock and his colleagues[41] showed that norepinephrine is not the sole transmitter and that the sympathetic neurons co-release a purine (i.e., ATP) and a peptide (neuropeptide Y). The miniature potentials in the smooth muscle are in fact due to ATP, rather than norepinephrine, acting directly on ion channel receptors.

Two main families of purine receptors (known as purinergic, or P, receptors) have been identified, sequenced, and cloned (see Chapters 5 and 14). A family of eight or more P1 receptors is situated in pre- and postsynaptic structures in the periphery and in brain. They are activated preferentially by adenosine and are G protein-coupled. Although ATP is the transmitter liberated from presynaptic endings, enzymes rapidly break it down to adenosine, which is the natural agonist for the P1 receptors. ATP does act directly on a family of P2 receptors[45] in the central and the peripheral nervous systems, where it regulates endocrine secretion and smooth muscle contractility and activates nociceptive C-fibers.[46]

Sensory Inputs to the Autonomic Nervous System

This description of the autonomic nervous system has failed to mention essential components: sensory inputs and reflex regulation. Indeed, in textbooks of physiology and pharmacology, the autonomic nervous system is often treated as though it functioned as a purely motor system for smooth muscle, cardiac muscle, and glands.

One reason for neglect of autonomic regulation is the paucity of our knowledge. Mechanisms of smooth muscle contraction, such as blood vessel constriction and dilatation, the forward propulsion of material through the gut, and bladder emptying seem relatively straightforward compared with, say, playing tennis. And yet the integration that is required is far from simple. On the afferent side, sensory receptors in the eye, lungs, blood vessels, viscera, and other target tissues provide information about the organs concerned[10,47] (see Figure 19.5). These include nociceptive receptors that signal information about painful stimuli.

---

[45] Soto, F., Garcia-Guzman, M., and Stühmer, W. 1997. *J. Membr. Biol.* 160: 91–100.
[46] Giniatullin, R., Nistri, A., and Fabbretti, E. 2008. *Mol. Neurobiol.* 37: 83–90.
[47] Saper, C. B. 2002. *Annu. Rev. Neurosci.* 25: 433–469.

A deceptively simple and well-studied reflex is the response of the circulation to changes in body position. With the human body lying flat, the brain is supplied by blood without differences in pressure between the legs and the head. The assumption of a vertical stance causes a drop in blood pressure above the level of the heart, as blood accumulates in the gut and legs. In the absence of autonomic regulation, loss of consciousness results from standing up, owing to diminished blood flow through the brain.[4] The receptors that signal the need for a change in the pattern of circulation are situated in a large artery in the neck, the carotid artery. The endings are stretch receptors embedded in a swelling of the arterial wall, known as the carotid sinus. Distension of the wall causes increased firing, as shown in Figure 19.6.

The sensory axons run to the brainstem and terminate in a well-defined nucleus (the nucleus of the solitary tract). These neurons project to neurons in the brainstem reticular formation, which in turn project to the autonomic preganglionic neurons. In the horizontal position, a high rate of sensory firing gives rise to inhibition of cardiovascular sympathetic outputs (see Figure 19.6). Blood pressure, heart rate, and cardiac output are depressed, and blood vessels in the skin and gut are dilated, when one is lying down. With assumption of vertical posture, the pressure in the artery falls and the rate of firing of the carotid sinus

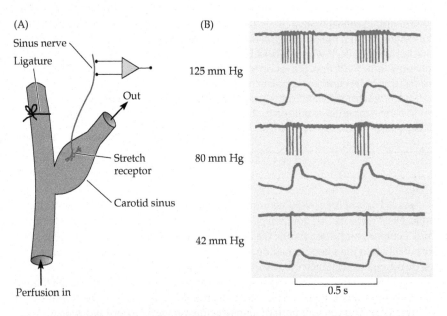

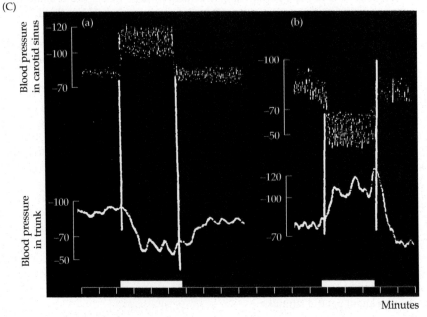

FIGURE 19.6 Firing of Carotid Sinus Stretch Receptors in response to raised blood pressure. (A) Experimental arrangement for recording from sensory nerve fibers in the carotid sinus while it is distended by the circulation or, as in the diagram, artificially perfused. (B) Relationship between blood pressure (lower traces) and the firing of a single afferent fiber from the carotid sinus at different levels of mean arterial pressure (from top down: 125, 80, and 42 mm Hg, measured with a manometer). (C) A classic record made in 1924. The head of this animal was supplied with blood from a different animal so that blood pressure in the head arteries could be controlled separately by the experimenters. (a) Increased pressure in the head caused a fall in systemic blood pressure in the trunk of the animal. (b) Decreased pressure in the head caused an increase in systemic pressure. Such records were made before electrical recordings were possible; experimenters determined blood pressure using a mercury manometer and registered the movements with a fine pointer on a smoked drum. (B After E. Neil, 1954. *Arch. Middlesex Hosp.* 4: 16; C after G. V. Anrep and E. H. Starling, 1925. *Proc. R. Soc. Lond. B.* 97: 463–487.)

axons is reduced dramatically, removing the central inhibition. The resulting release of sympathetic activity causes blood vessels in the skin and gut to constrict, and cardiac output and heart rate to rise. The increase in pressure maintains blood flow through the brain.

The ancient recordings in Figure 19.6C, made by Anrep and Starling using a pointer that scratched the surface of a rotating smoked drum, still provide good illustrations of these effects.[48] It was the same E. H. Starling who, with W. M. Bayliss in 1902, first coined the word *hormone* and proposed the concept of hormonal action while they worked on the control of secretion in the gut.

The description of the reflex presented in Figure 19.6 appears simple. But the central sympathetic and parasympathetic integrative mechanisms for rerouting blood where it is urgently needed remain a black box.[10] This is also the case for other autonomic reflexes for which the sensory and motor limbs are known—for example, enteric, excretory, and respiratory reflexes.[4,49]

The Enteric Nervous System

Local regulatory reflexes in the gut (see Figure 19.5) are extremely complex and are brought about by vast numbers of neurons. The enteric nervous system contains more than 10 million nerve cells arranged in the wall of the intestine as sensory neurons, interneurons, and motor neurons. Every known transmitter is represented there (and many of them were first discovered in the gut). To analyze the intrinsic circuits is difficult because of the profuse local reflexes and numbers of connections.[50,51] Functional analysis has been a major challenge even in simpler systems, such as the viscera of the lobster (mentioned in Chapter 20). When Selverston and his colleagues[52] began to study the stomatogastric ganglion, with its complement of only 30 neurons, it seemed that it could perhaps be worked out completely. Yet although great progress has been made by electrical recordings from identified neurons and although principles of general significance for neurobiology have been discovered, a complete understanding is still not at hand. What appeared at first to be a simple circuit for regulating gut functions turned out to be plastic and modifiable rather than static and hard-wired.

Regulation of Autonomic Functions by the Hypothalamus

Hormones provide an essential aspect of control of the autonomic nervous system. The secretion of hormones by glands (such as the thyroid, ovary, and adrenal cortex) is regulated by releasing factors secreted in the CNS (discussed in the sections that follow). The hormones in turn act back on the CNS to regulate the secretion of releasing factors, creating a feedback loop.

The hypothalamus (Figures 19.7 and 19.8) is a brain area that controls integrative autonomic functions, including body temperature, appetite, water intake, defecation,

[48] Starling, E. H. 1941. *Starling's Principles of Human Physiology.* Churchill, London.

[49] Cameron, O. G. 2009. *Neuroimage* 47: 787-794

[50] Obaid, A. L. et al. 2005. *J. Exp. Biol.* 208: 2891-3001.

[51] Altaf, M. A., and Sood, M. R. 2008. *Dev. Disabil. Res. Rev.* 14: 87-95.

[52] Selverston, A. I., and Ayers, J. 2006. *Biol. Cybern.* 95: 537-554.

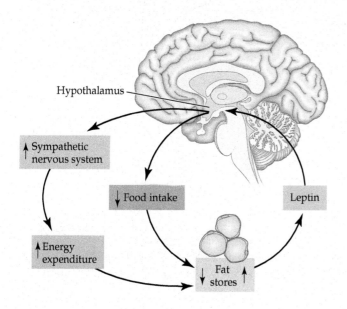

FIGURE 19.7   Mechanism by Which Leptin Regulates Body Weight. Leptin peptide is secreted into the circulation by adipose cells in fat depots. It acts on neurons in the hypothalamus that inhibit the intake of food and increase the expenditure of energy by activating the sympathetic nervous system. As a result, the fat content of the body decreases. (After K. Rahmouni et al., 2004. In D. Robertson (ed.), *Primer on the Autonomic Nervous System.* Academic Press, London.)

FIGURE 19.8 Hypothalamus and Pituitary Gland in the human brain. (A) Sagittal section of brain, with the area shown in (B) outlined. (B) Nuclei of the hypothalamus and adjacent structures. (C) Connections of hypothalamic neurons with the neurohypophysis (posterior pituitary gland) and adenohypophysis (anterior pituitary gland). Axons run directly to the neurohypophysis. There the terminals secrete hormones into the circulation. By contrast, releasing hormones released by neurons in the hypothalamus reach the adenohypophysis in high concentration through a dedicated group of blood vessels called the hypophyseal portal system (red dashed lines). There they activate secretory cells, which liberate hormones into the circulation. DA = dopamine, GnRH = gonadotropin-releasing hormone, TRF = thyroid hormone-releasing factor, OX-VP = oxytocin-vasopressin.

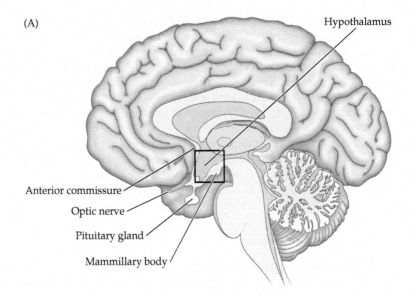

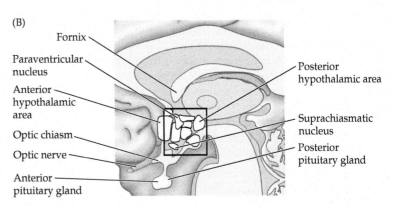

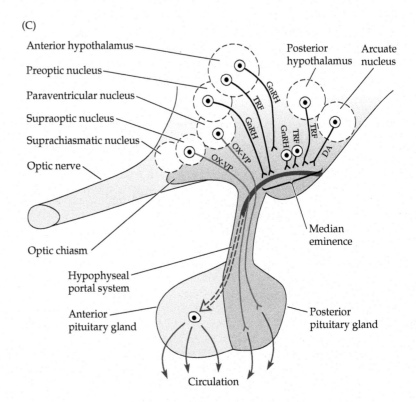

micturition, heart rate, arterial pressure, sexual activity, lactation, and on a slower times-cale, growth.[53] The precision of these homeostatic mechanisms enables us to keep our body temperature at about 37°C, our blood pressure at about 120/80 mm Hg, our heart rate at 70 beats/minute, and our intake and output of water at 1.5 liters/day. In addition, the hypothal-amus makes it possible for food to be propelled inexorably along the alimentary tract with appropriate secretions for digestion and absorption at every level. The hypothalamus is also a brain area in which appetite, emotions, and responses to bodily exercise are regulated. Emotions are coupled to autonomic responses. Even the thought of food leads to secretion of saliva, and the anticipation of exercise gives rise to increased sympathetic activity.

Appetite is regulated by a remarkable series of steps involving cells that store fat.[54,55] When adipocytes are activated by β_3-receptors, they secrete a 167-amino acid protein known as leptin, which acts on cytokine receptors situated in the membranes of neurons in a variety of hypothalamic nuclei. Leptin gene expression is increased by overfeeding and reduced by starvation (see Figure 19.7). Other delicately controlled functions are the ex-traordinarily precise and regular rhythms generated by the hypothalamus. Slow rhythms include those that control endocrine secretion. For example, sexual and reproductive func-tions oscillate with periods of weeks that depend on secretion of peptide hormones by hy-pothalamic cells. These act on the anterior pituitary gland to stimulate secretion of other hormones into the bloodstream.

Hypothalamic Neurons That Release Hormones

A well-studied example of hormonal release is provided by neurons in the hypothalamus that secrete gonadotropin-releasing hormone (GnRH, which is the same as LHRH).[56] A prime action of these neurons is to secrete GnRH into a portal system of blood vessels that flow directly from the hypothalamus to the anterior pituitary gland (see Figure 19.8). Neurally released GnRH thereby acts selectively on a gland that is not directly innervated, enabling the CNS to control hormonal secretion. Thereafter, the releasing hormone is di-luted in the major vessels of the circulation and cannot, for example, influence transmission in autonomic ganglia. In the anterior pituitary gland (adenohypophysis), GnRH stimulates specific cells to secrete gonadotropin—a hormone that is essential for sexual and reproduc-tive rhythms and functions.

This brief, oversimplified account cannot do justice to the beautiful experiments of G. W. Harris, who first demonstrated that the local release of a releasing hormone from the hypothalamus could provide an essential control mechanism.[57] His description of delivery of a chemical message through a system of blood vessels (the hypophyseal portal system; see Figure 19.8C) by highly localized transport was a revolutionary concept.

Distribution and Numbers of GnRH Cells

GnRH cells are dispersed throughout the hypothalamus, with no clearly defined nucleus or aggregate. The previous section dealt only with those GnRH cells close to the anterior pitu-itary gland (in the median eminence) that promote its gonadotropin secretion (see Figure 19.8). The release of the releasing hormone itself is also influenced by hormones, such as those secreted by the ovary that feed back into the brain and by synaptic inputs mediated by a variety of transmitters, including norepinephrine, dopamine, histamine, glutamate, and γ-aminobutyric acid (GABA).[58]

One extraordinary feature of the GnRH cells is their small number: 1300 in rats and 800 in mice.[59] Rats and mice (and human beings) would become extinct without these few, scattered cells in the brain. A second remarkable feature is their development (see Chapter 29). During embryonic days 10 to 15 in rats, the precursor cells first appear in a region known as the olfactory placode. This is the region destined to be the future olfactory mu-cosa. After dividing, the cells migrate along axons of the olfactory nerve and end up in the hypothalamus.[60] The pathways and molecular mechanisms of GnRH cell migration have been studied in embryos, in newborn opossums, and in culture systems.[61] Since all the cells can be reliably marked by specific antibodies to GnRH, they can be counted quanti-tatively at the site of origin and as they migrate. Other types of neurons migrate along the

[53] Eikeles, N., and Esler, M. 2005. *Exp. Physiol.* 90: 673-682.

[54] Rahmouni, K., Haynes, W. G., and Mark, A. L. 2004. In *Primer on the Autonomic Nervous System.* Academic Press, London. pp. 86-89.

[55] Williams, K. W., Scott, M. M., and Elmquist, J. K. 2009. *Am. J. Clin. Nutr.* 89: 9855-9905.

[56] Lee, V. H., Lee, L. T., and Chow, B. K. 2008. *FEBS J.* 275: 5458-5478.

[57] Harris, G. W., and Ruf, K. B. 1970. *J. Physiol.* 208: 243-250.

[58] Bhattarai, J. P. et al. 2011. *Endocrinology* 152: 1551-1561.

[59] Wray, S., Grant, P., and Gainer, H. 1989. *Proc. Natl. Acad. Sci. USA* 86: 8132-8136.

[60] Cariboni, A., Maggi, R., and Parnevalas, J. G. 2007. *Trends Neurosci.* 30: 638-644.

[61] Tarozzo, G. et al. 1998. *Ann. NY Acad. Sci.* 839: 196-200.

[62] Tarozzo, G. et al. 1995. *Proc. R. Soc. Lond., B, Biol. Sci.* 262: 95-101.

[63] Burbach, J. P. et al. 2001. *Physiol. Rev.* 81: 1197-1267.

[64] Amar, A. P., and Weiss, M. H. 2003. *Neurosurg. Clin. N. Am.* 14: 11-23.

[65] Kosterin, P. et al. 2005. *J. Membr. Biol.* 208: 113-124.

[66] Blau, J. et al. 2007. *Cold Spring Harb. Symp. Quant. Biol.* 72: 243-250.

[67] Saper, C. B., and Fuller, P. M. 2007. *Cold Spring Harb. Symp. Quant. Biol.* 72: 543-550.

[68] Colwell, C. S. 2011. *Nat. Rev. Neurosci.* 12: 553-569.

[69] Kononenko, N. I. et al. 2008. *Neurosci. Lett.* 436: 314-316.

[70] Piggins, H. D., and London, A. 2005. *Curr. Biol.* 15: 455-457.

[71] Pandi-Perumal, S. R. et al. 2006. *FEBS J.* 273: 2813-2838.

[72] Ralph, M. R. et al. 1990. *Science* 247: 975-978.

[73] Davidson, A. J., Yamazaki, S., and Menaker, M. 2003. *Novartis Found. Symp.* 253: 110-121.

same axonal pathway as the GnRH cells. Before reaching the hypothalamus, however, they branch off along other axons to reach distinctively different destinations.[62]

Figure 19.8 shows that in addition to the GnRH cells in the hypothalamus, there exist specific populations of neurons that secrete other hormones required for autonomic functions. Metabolism, thyroid function, absorption of salts by the kidney, and growth all depend on releasing hormones that are secreted into the portal system and that act on the anterior pituitary gland.

Specific hypothalamic neurons in the supraoptic and paraventricular nuclei (see Figure 19.8) innervate the posterior pituitary gland directly. As we discussed in detail in Chapter 18, their endings, soma, and dendrites release antidiuretic hormone (ADH, also known as vasopressin) and oxytocin into the blood, extracellular fluid, and cerebrospinal fluid (CSF).[63-65] Hence, the control of water absorption by the kidney and the contractions of the uterus depend directly on the firing of hypothalamic neurons.

Circadian Rhythms

Of particular importance in the life of an animal are the circadian rhythms that control the day–night or sleep-wake cycle. In the absence of all external synchronizing cues, 24-hour rhythmical cycles are maintained by an internal clock for prolonged periods (weeks or months) in invertebrates as well as vertebrates,[66-68] and even in explants or isolated neurons in culture.[69] The internal timing mechanism can be altered (or entrained) by providing regularly spaced light and dark stimuli. Autonomic functions are strongly influenced by biological clocks that act on the pineal gland to regulate the secretion of **melatonin**[70,71] (Box 19.2).

In mammals, a key structure in the hypothalamus for generating the rhythm of the internal clock is the suprachiasmatic nucleus (SCN). An important input to this nucleus is from the eye.[72,73] After destruction of the suprachiasmatic nucleus in rats, light and

BOX 19.2 Melatonin

Melatonin is synthesized in the pineal gland from 5-hydroxytryptamine (serotonin; see page B-3, Appendix B) in a two-step process by the enzymes arylalkylamine-N-acetyltransferase (AA-NAT) and hydroxyindole-O-methyltransferase (HIOMT). It is secreted continuously from the pineal gland but in much larger amounts at night than during the daytime because light reduces the rate at which it is synthesized. The effect of light is conveyed from the retina to the suprachiasmatic nucleus (SCN; see the section on "Circadian Rhythms" in this chapter) and thence to the spinal outflow of the cervical sympathetic nerves and from the postganglionic cervical sympathetic nerve to the pineal gland. The light-induced increased activity in the SCN *reduces* sympathetic discharge activity to the pineal gland—thus, sympatho-pineal activity is greatest in the dark (the opposite of that in the SCN). The noradrenaline released by these hyperactive nighttime sympathetic fibers increases melatonin secretion by increasing the amount of AA-NAT (the rate-liming step in melatonin synthesis), by an effect on transcription.

Melatonin helps synchronize the body's circadian rhythms. It does not directly induce sleep in humans but assists in resetting the sleep-wake cycle when the normal rhythm is disturbed. For this reason it is some-

times taken as a medicine to combat jet lag. More important, it is essential for the maintenance of the annual seasonal reproductive cycles in many mammals and birds. This is because melatonin inhibits the secretion of GnRH, and hence the secretion of the sex hormones follicle-stimulating hormone (FSH) and luteinizing hormone (LH), which are required for female sexual development and reproduction. In temperate climates, the long periods of darkness in winter cause a prolonged secretion of melatonin, which inhibits sexual and reproductive activity. Reproductive activity is therefore restricted to other times of year with shorter nights, when the secretion of melatonin is briefer.

In frogs, melatonin has a completely different function, in controlling skin color. Daylight secretion of melatonin alters the distribution of melanin in frog skin melanocytes in such a way as to lighten the overall skin color; the converse occurs at night. In contrast, melatonin has no effect on skin color in humans.

(A)

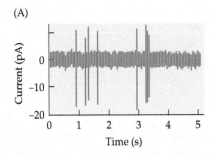

(B)

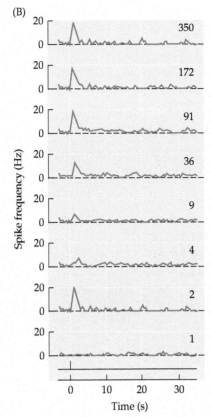

FIGURE 19.9 Recordings from an In Situ Retinal Ganglion Cell in response to illumination by a small spot shone onto the cell soma. (A) Spontaneous firing in darkness. (B) Effect of different-intensity flashes (50-ms duration, 480-nm wavelength, 40-m diameter). The flash monitor is shown in the bottom trace, and the relative intensity is indicated by numbers on the right of each trace. Responses were averaged over several trials. (After M. T. Do et al., 2009. *Nature* 457: 281-287.)

dark entrainment of endogenous rhythms becomes lost. Locomotor activity, drinking, sleep–wake cycles, and rhythms of hormone secretion become disrupted. If fetal hypothalamic tissue containing the SCN is transplanted to a host previously rendered arrhythmic by a complete lesion of the SCN, then rhythmicity is restored with a free running period corresponding to that of the donor genotype.[74] Information about cellular and molecular mechanisms that produce regular night and day cycles has been obtained in both invertebrates and vertebrates.[75,76,77]

Until recently, there was an apparent paradox concerning the way in which light and dark could entrain the day–night cycle. This paradox arose from the properties of neurons in the visual cortex, which do not respond at all to changes in the level of illumination, but rather only to bars, edges, and moving patterns. Even in the retina, recordings from ganglion cells had shown that the best stimulus for them to fire is not the level of illumination but contrast (see Chapters 2, 3, and 22). This problem has been resolved by the discovery of a small number of specialized ganglion cells that are themselves photoreceptors. These photoreceptive ganglion cells contain the pigment melanopsin and respond to diffuse illumination (Figure 19.9). Their axons project to the suprachiasmatic nucleus rather than to the lateral geniculate nucleus. If all the rod and cone receptor responses are abolished, the pupil still constricts in bright light and the day–night rhythm can still be entrained.[78,79,80,81]

In neurons of the suprachiasmatic nucleus, the frequency of spontaneous action potentials increases during the day and decreases at night, as shown in Figure 19.10. By what mechanism is the rhythm produced? This problem has been investigated in slices of rat SCN in culture where GABA has been shown to be a major transmitter.[82] Yarom and his colleagues[83] have shown that certain groups of suprachiasmatic neurons in a slice respond to GABA with depolarization and increased rates of firing during the day (see Figure 19.10A). The same concentration of GABA applied at night causes hyperpolarization and a decrease in firing rate (see Figure 19.10B). Hence, as in developing CNS,[84] GABA can be an excitatory or an inhibitory transmitter[85] (see Chapters 11 and 27). The type of response depends on the level of internal chloride. As described

[74] Kaufman, C. M., and Menaker, M. J. 1993. *J. Neural Transplant. Plast.* 4: 257-265.

[75] Numano, R. et al. 2006. *Proc. Natl. Acad. Sci. USA* 103: 3716-3721.

[76] Siepka, S. M. et al. 2007. *Cold Spring Harb. Symp. Quant. Biol.* 72: 251-259.

[77] Lowrey, P. L., and Takahashi, J. S. 2004. *Annu. Rev. Genomics Hum. Genet.* 5: 407-441.

[78] Berson, D. M., Dunn, F. A., and Takao, M. 2002. *Science* 295: 1070-1073.

[79] Hattar, S. et al. 2002. *Science* 295: 1065-1070.

[80] Güler, A. D. et al. 2008. *Nature* 453: 102-105.

[81] Do, M. T. et al. 2009. *Nature* 457: 281-287.

[82] Choi, H. J. et al. 2008. *J. Neurosci.* 28: 5450-5459.

[83] Wagner, S. et al. 1997. *Nature* 387: 598-603.

[84] Cherubini, E., Gaiarsa, J. L., and Ben-Ari, Y. 1991. *Trends Neurosci.* 14: 515-519.

[85] Albus, H. et al. 2005. *Curr. Biol.* 15: 886-893.

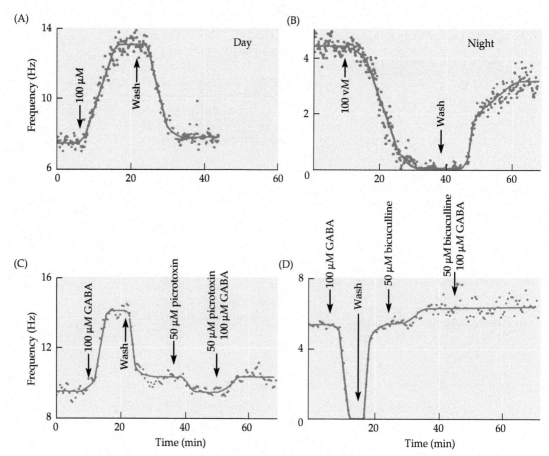

FIGURE 19.10 Circadian Rhythm of a Slice of Rat Suprachiasmatic Nucleus Maintained in Culture. GABA was applied at different times while extracellular recordings were made from neurons. GABA gave rise to increases in action potential frequency in the daytime (A) and to decreases at night (B). (C,D) Recordings show that the effects of GABA were blocked by GABA antagonists picrotoxin (C) and bicuculline (D). The change from excitation to inhibition can be accounted for in terms of changed intracellular chloride concentrations, which were assessed by whole-cell patch recordings (not shown). The conductance change produced by GABA remains unchanged during the day–night cycle. (After S. Wagner et al., 1997. *Nature* 387: 598–603.)

in Chapter 11, when the internal chloride concentration is low, the chloride equilibrium potential (E_{Cl}) is more negative than the resting potential. Opening of channels by GABA allows chloride ions to enter and the membrane to hyperpolarize. With raised internal chloride concentrations, E_{Cl} shifts to a value positive with respect to the resting membrane potential. As a result, GABA causes chloride ions to move out of the cell and gives rise to a depolarization. The change from inhibition to excitation is actively regulated by the activity of NKCC1 and KCC2 chloride transporters[86,87] (see Chapter 9). The mechanisms by which those transporters are differentially regulated during the day–night cycle are not yet known.

Common proteins that are associated with periodicity throughout the animal kingdom have been revealed by genetic techniques. Genes and proteins that control circadian rhythms have been identified and cloned in *Drosophila*[88] (Box 19.3). In many species these proteins, one of which is known as PER (PERIOD), have been observed in pacemaker regions such as the suprachiasmatic nucleus.[75] In flies, deletion of the *per* gene abolishes circadian rhythm. Reintroduction of the *per* gene reestablishes the rhythm.[89] Although no link has been found between regulatory proteins and intracellular chloride concentration, it is gratifying that one can now begin to explain circadian rhythms in terms of genes and ion concentrations in well-defined groups of neurons.

[86] Wagner, S., Sagiv, N., and Yarom, Y. 2001. *J. Physiol.* 537: 853–869.

[87] Belenky, M. A. et al. 2010. *Neuroscience* 165: 1519–1537.

[88] Saez, L., Meyer, P., and Young, M. W. 2007. *Cold Spring Harb. Symp. Quant. Biol.* 72: 69–74.

[89] Zehring, W. A. et al. 1984. *Cell* 39: 369–376.

BOX 19.3 Genetic Clocks

An early clue to the presence of a genetic circadian clock was provided by the experiments of Ronald Konopka and Seymour Benzer (1971) on fruit flies (*Drosophila melanogaster*). Noting that the adult fly normally hatched from the pupa at dawn, irrespective of the amount of light, as though it had an internal 24-hour clock, Konopka and Benzer made a series of random mutations in the male fly's DNA with chemical agents, and observed what happened to the fly's internal clock. They found two mutations, one leading to a shortened hatching cycle of about 19 hours and the other with a lengthened cycle of about 28 hours (Figure A). They also found that these differences carried through into the locomotor activity of the adult flies monitored under constant infrared light. Crossbreeding suggested that both mutations affected the same gene and that the gene controlled the *period* of an internal oscillator.

Further work on *Drosophila* led to the identification of the *per* (*period*) gene and its protein product, PER, and showed both the *per* mRNA and PER protein showed a basic 24-hour cycle, the mRNA preceding the protein by about 6 hours. It was suggested that the 24-hour cycle might be caused by feedback inhibition of *per* transcription by PER protein. To do this, PER has to enter the nucleus and bind to the *per* gene promoter. It does this by combining with another molecular clock protein, TIM (TIMELESS). The PER/TIM complex then inhibits the endogenous transcriptional activation of the *per* and *tim* genes by a nuclear protein complex termed the CYC/CLOCK complex (Figure B). The basic 24-hour cycle is maintained by additional phosphorylation steps and ancillary genes and proteins. An analogous genetic molecular clock involving homologs of *per* and *tim* has been identified in the mouse.

The 2017 Nobel Prize in Physiology or Medicine was awarded to Jeffrey Hall and Michael Rosbash (Brandeis University) and Michael Young (Rockefeller University) for their work unraveling the *Drosophila* molecular clock.

Konopka, R. J., and Benzer, S. 1971. Clock mutants of *Drosophila melanogaster*. *Proc. Natl. Acad. Sci. USA* 68: 2112-2116.

Foster, R., and Kreitzman, L. 2004. *Rhythms of Life*. Profile Books: London.

Young, M. W. 2000. Life's 24-hour clock: molecular control of circadian rhythms in animal cells. *Trends Biochem. Sci.* 25: 601-606.

(A)

Normal

Short period

Long period

Flies emerging per hour

Days

Cyclical Emergence of Normal and Mutated Adult Fruit Flies from Their Pupae. Random genetic mutations of male flies were generated by exposure of their X-chromosomes to ethyl methyl sulfonate. X-mutated males were individually mated with wild-type female flies and their progeny reared in a 12 × 12 hour light/dark cycle. Several hundred pupae from selected matings showing abnormal patterns of adult emergence were then transferred to a rearing box, samples collected at hourly intervals over several days and the numbers of pupae from which adult flies emerged during each hour counted. The graphs show time plots of the numbers of emergent flies per hour (A) from progeny of normal males, (B) from mutated male progeny showing a more rapid emergent cycle (short period), and (C) from mutated male progeny showing a slower emergent cycle (long period). (Adapted from R. J. Konopka and S. Benzer. 1971. *Proc. Natl. Acad. Sci. USA* 68: 2112-2116.)

(B)

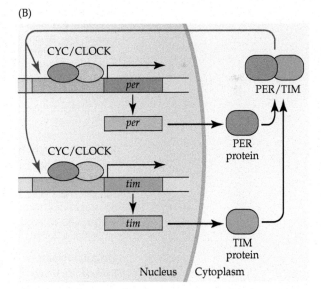

Elements of the Molecular Clock in *Drosophila melanogaster*. Within the nucleus, the CYC/CLOCK protein complex interacts with elements in the promoter region of the per and tim genes to drive their transcription and translation to produce PER and TIM proteins in the cytoplasm. These proteins interact to form the PER/TIM complex. This complex translocates into the nucleus and interacts with the promotor region of the per and tim genes to inhibit the enhancing effect of CYC/CLOCK. Light induces the degradation of TIM to align the clock to the light-dark cycle. (After U. Bhadra et al., 2017. *Sleep Med*. 35: 49-61.)

SUMMARY

- The autonomic nervous system regulates essential functions of all internal organs and is itself regulated by hormonal and sensory feedback.

- Parasympathetic effects are focused, whereas sympathetic effects are widespread and more generalized.

- ACh is the principal transmitter used for transmission in autonomic ganglia at parasympathetic nerve endings and at certain sympathetic nerve endings.

- Norepinephrine is the principal transmitter for most sympathetic endings. Other transmitters include acetylcholine, peptides, and ATP.

- A single molecule—for example, LHRH, which is also known as GnRH—can act as a transmitter at synapses and as a hormone in the brain.

- Analysis of effects mediated by the autonomic nervous system is complex, owing to the variety of receptors and the large numbers of peptide and non-peptide transmitters.

- Epinephrine released as a hormone into the circulation from the adrenal medulla reaches receptors in target cells that are not affected by transmitter released from nerve endings.

- The hypothalamus is the region of the brain that controls the overall activities of the autonomic nervous system and also regulates the secretion of hormones.

- The hypothalamus, in turn, is influenced by higher centers of the CNS and by hormones.

- Cells in the suprachiasmatic nucleus (SCM) in the hypothalamus show an endogenous circadian (24 hour) variation in day-night firing frequency determined by an internal molecular clock. The timing of the clock is set (entrained) by the response of special cells in the retina to ambient light. In turn, the SCN induce a reciprocal (night/day) variation in melatonin synthesis and secretion by the pineal gland. Melatonin secretion helps synchronize the body's circadian and seasonal hormonal activity.

Suggested Reading

General Reviews

Burnstock, G. 2008. The journey to establish purinergic signaling in the gut. *Neurogastroenterol. Motil.* 20 (Suppl 1): 8–19.

Cooper, J. R., Bloom, F. E., and Roth, R. H. 2002. *The Biochemical Basis of Pharmacology.* Oxford University Press, New York.

Delmas, P., and Brown, D. A. 2005. Pathways modulating neural KCNQ/M (K$_v$7) potassium channels. *Nat. Rev. Neurosci.* 6: 850–862.

Foster, R. G., and Kreitzman, L. 2017. *Circadian rhythms: A Very Short Introduction.* Oxford University Press, Oxford, UK.

Fu, Y., Liao, H. W., Do, M. T., and Yau, K. W. 2005. Non-image forming ocular photoreception in vertebrates. *Curr. Opin. Neurobiol.* 15: 415–422.

Robertson, D. 2004. *Primer on the Autonomic Nervous System.* Academic Press, London.

Siepka, S. M., Yoo, S. H., Park, J., Lee, C., and Takahashi, J. S. 2007. Genetics and neurobiology of circadian clocks in mammals. *Cold Spring Harb. Symp. Quant. Biol.* 72: 251–259.

Suh, B. C., and Hille, B. 2008. PIP2 is a necessary cofactor for ion channel function: how and why? *Annu. Rev. Biophys.* 37: 175–195.

Williams, K. W., Scott, M. M., and Elmquist, J. K. 2009. From observation to experimentation: leptin action in the mediobasal hypothalamus. *Am. J. Clin. Nutr.* 89: 9855–9905.

Original Papers

Banks, F. C., Knight, G. E., Calvert, R. C., Thompson, C. S., Morgan, R. J., and Burnstock, G. 2006. The purinergic component of human vas deferens contraction. *Fertil. Steril.* 85: 932–939.

Brown, D. A., and Passmore, G. M. 2009. Neural KCNQ (K$_v$7) channels. *Brit. J. Pharmacol.* 156: 1185–1195.

Güler, A. D., Ecker, J. L., Lall, G. S., Haq, S., Altimus, C. M., Liao, H. W., Barnard, A. R., Cahill, H., Badea, T. C., Zhao, H., Hankins, M. W., Berson, D. M., Lucas, R. J., Yau, K. W., and Hattar, S. 2008. Melanopsin cells are the principal conduits for rod-cone input to non-image forming vision. *Nature* 453: 102–105.

Kuffler, S. W. 1980. Slow synaptic responses in autonomic ganglia and the pursuit of a peptidergic transmitter. *J. Exp. Biol.* 89: 257–286.

Merlin, C. Gegear, R. J., and Reppert, S. M. 2009. Antennal circadian clocks coordinate sun compass orientation in migratory monarch butterflies. *Science* 325: 1700–1704.

Numano, R., Yamazaki, S., Umeda, N., Samura, T., Supino, M., Takahashi, R., Ueda, M., Mori, A., Yamada, K., Sakaki, Y., Inouye, S. T., Menaker, M., and Tei, H. 2006. Constitutive expression of the Period1 gene impairs behavioral and molecular circadian rhythms. *Proc. Natl. Acad. Sci. USA* 103: 3716–3721.

Spyer, K. M., and Gourine, A. V. 2009. Chemosensory Pathways in the Brainstem Controlling Cardio-Respiratory Activity. *Philos. Trans. R. Soc. Lond.* 364: 2603–2610.

Wagner S., Sagiv, N., and Yarom, Y. 2001. GABA-induced current and circadian regulation of chloride in neurones of the rat suprachiasmatic nucleus. *J. Physiol.* 537: 853–869.

CHAPTER 20

Walking, Flying, and Swimming: Cellular Mechanisms of Sensorimotor Behavior in Invertebrates

Throughout this book we present examples of how invertebrate neurons have been used to discover fundamental mechanisms of the workings of the nervous system. Principles of general validity for the generation and conduction of action potentials and for synaptic transmission were derived from the squid giant axon and giant synapse. Experiments on invertebrates have also provided crucial insights into cellular and molecular mechanisms of how nerve cells integrate information to coordinate behavior. Because of their simplified nervous systems and wide diversity, animals such as flies, bees, ants, worms, snails, lobsters, and crayfish offer several advantages for studying how nerve cells integrate information to produce coordinated behavior. First among these advantages is that invertebrate behavior is elaborate and often highly stereotyped, thus more readily analyzed. Second, given the accessibility of many invertebrate nervous systems compared with those of vertebrates, it is often possible to recognize individual nerve cells and study them using electrophysiological and molecular techniques. Third, one or a pair of neurons in invertebrates exerts a function that involves hundreds or thousands of functionally redundant neurons in the central nervous system (CNS) of a mammal.

Invertebrates with less accessible nervous systems, such as ants and bees, have complex behaviors that exemplify an important principle: Measurements of behavior provide insights into integrative mechanisms. Desert ants walk and bees fly over long distances, taking meandering paths while foraging for food. Once it has found a food source, however, the ant or bee orients toward its nest and returns there directly, in a straight line. Somehow, the individual ant or bee calculates the position from which it started, and heads straight for home. This navigation requires the integration of information provided by polarized light from the sun, magnetic fields, and learning. Crustaceans have provided several examples of the organization of neuronal circuits. Crayfish leave their burrows under low light intensities and return when the light levels increase. Different light levels activate particular visual and command neurons. Some of these neurons evoke exiting from the burrow; others evoke returning to the burrow.

If one's goal is to work downward from behavior to the properties and connections of individual neurons, neither the ant nor the bee provides an experimentally favorable preparation, owing to the small size and large number of cells in its CNS. The leech, by contrast, provides a convenient preparation for analyzing how behavior is generated by networks of neurons. Leeches swim, crawl, select suitable victims to feed on, and make love to other leeches of the same species, all directed by a CNS composed of experimentally accessible ganglia. About 400 neurons in each ganglion have been identified by visual inspection and by direct electrical recording. Thus, in individual leech neurons one can measure their biophysical properties, trace their connections, search for the genes they express, and define their roles in behavior.

The sophisticated computations made by the nervous system of ants, bees, crayfish, and leeches make these invertebrates appealing for studying cellular mechanisms of behavior. Invertebrates display a wide variety of stereotyped behaviors, with various levels of complexity, that are comparable to behaviors of vertebrates. Behaviors such as reflexes, locomotion, feeding, reproduction, or aggression and other forms of social behaviors are produced by relatively small numbers of neurons, each having a significant contribution to the overall behavior. In contrast, equivalent behaviors in vertebrates typically require far more neurons.

[1] Bailey, C. H., and Kandel, E. R. 2008. *Prog. Brain Res.* 169: 179-198.

[2] Shimahara, T., and Tauc, L. 1975. *J. Physiol.* 247: 321-341; and Kandel, E. R. 1979. *Behavioral Biology of Aplysia.* W. H. Freeman, San Francisco, CA.

[3] Wiese, K., ed. 2002. *The Crustacean Nervous System.* Berlin, Germany.

[4] Muller, K. J., Nicholls, J. G., and Stent, G. S., (Eds.) 1981. *Neurobiology of the Leech.* Cold Spring Harbor Laboratory, Cold Spring Harbor, NY.

[5] Shain, D. H., ed. 2009. *Annelids in Modern Biology.* Wiley-Blackwell, Hoboken, NJ.

[6] Atwood, H. L., ed. 1982. *Biology of Crustacea.* Academic Press, New York.

[7] Beadle, D. J., Lees, G., and Kater, S. B. 1988. *Cell Culture Approaches to Invertebrate Neuroscience.* Academic Press, London, UK.

[8] Wehner, R., and Muller, M. 2006. *Proc. Natl. Acad. Sci. USA* 103: 12575-12579.

[9] Merkle, T., and Wehner, R. 2008. *J. Exp. Biol.* 211: 3370-3377.

[10] Muller, M., and Wehner, R. 2010. *Curr. Biol.* 20: 1368-1371.

From Behavior to Neurons and Vice Versa

Invertebrates with large neurons permit us to find out which neurons take part in a circuit and how their electrical activity, branching patterns, and connectivity contribute to coordinated behavior. One can follow circuits from sensory inputs to motor outputs and explore the basis of unconscious decision-making processes. One can also follow molecular events occurring cell by cell as the animal modifies behavior as a result of experience. It is also possible to study how circulating transmitters or hormones modulate the circuits and diversify the behavioral responses (see Chapter 18).

The nervous system of each invertebrate species has its own set of advantages and disadvantages for analyzing the neural basis of behavior—indeed, beware the scientist who claims to have the ideal system!

The literature on crustaceans, insects, and particularly the sea slug *Aplysia* (which has been extensively studied by Tauc, Kandel, and their colleagues) is far too extensive to be dealt with in a book of this size.[1] Indeed, entire monographs are available on these systems.[2–7] Accordingly, as in other chapters, here we use selected examples for detailed discussion of circuitry and behavior. For complementary reasons, we have singled out for discussion the nervous systems of ants, bees, crayfish, and leeches. In ants and bees, behavioral analysis is the starting point. This has revealed neuronal mechanisms that provide the animals with information about how their motion is driven by sensory cues such as polarized light and magnetic fields in the outside world. Experiments on crayfish illustrate how decisions can be made at an early stage of visual processing and how commands initiated by single neurons can produce a behavioral response. The leech features more limited behaviors than do the others and has a highly stereotyped CNS with fewer and usually larger neurons. Thus, the leech provides preparations in which one can study in great detail how the properties, connections, and functions of individual identified nerve cells contribute to behavior.

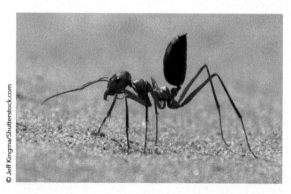

FIGURE 20.1 The Desert Ant *Cataglyphis bicolor.* It is able to return home in a direct path after having searched for food. (After R. Wehner, 1994. *Fortschr. Zool.* 31: 11-53.)

Navigation by Ants and Bees

Essential for understanding the workings of the nervous system is the quantitative analysis of behavior. The extraordinary performance of invertebrate nervous systems can be appreciated by considering complex navigation by ants, which meander over long distances searching for food and then unerringly find their way home.[8–10]

(A)

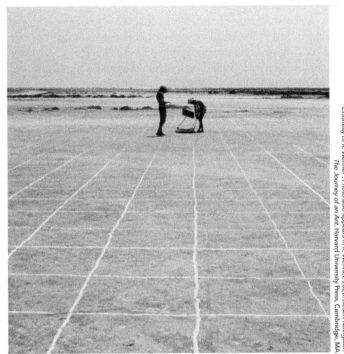

(B)

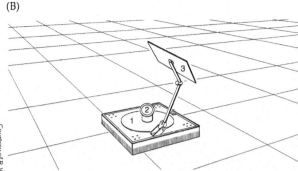

FIGURE 20.2 Measuring the Movements of an Ant on the Desert Floor. (A) A desert ant is tracked as it migrates along the desert floor using a rolling optical laboratory cart to follow the ant and control the portion of sky it can observe. (B) The experimenter moves the cart, keeping the ant centered within the optical setup. The horizontal aperture (1) can be fitted with filters that cut out all light except ultraviolet light or light polarized in just one direction. A small aperture (2) sits atop a circular tube, and the screen (3) is used to prevent the ant from seeing sunlight directly. Since the cart has a frame, the little ant cannot see the skyline or markers on the ground and is also shielded from the wind. The white lines are 1 m apart and are painted on the desert floor to enable the observers to track the ant's progress accurately. (B after R. Wehner, 1994. *Fortschr. Zool.* 39: 103-143.)

The Desert Ant's Pathway Home

Wehner and his colleagues have conducted experiments to analyze how desert ants, *Cataglyphis bicolor* (Figure 20.1) and related species, are able to wander for long distances in search of food and then return toward the nest in a straight line. A particularity of desert ants is that pheromones are useless for this purpose because of their volatility in the high temperatures of the desert. Instead, the ants' behavior reflects inputs from polarized light and magnetic fields, proprioception, an internal clock, and learning. The principle of the experiments conducted by Wehner and his colleagues' is illustrated in Figures 20.2 and 20.3.[11,12] An area of desert in Tunisia around the nest and the food supply of the ants is marked out in squares, as shown in Figure 20.2. A single ant is then followed as it walks to the food source and back. An ant can wander for hundreds of meters (m) in search of food, then return to the nest with an error of about 1 m, less than 1% (in this respect the ant is doing far better than at least one author of this book, who does not have the mathematical skills for making computations of this sort). Figure 20.3 illustrates a tortuous, 19-minute outward path from nest to food. The journey back home, by contrast, takes about 6 minutes; it is direct, unhesitating, and the small error to find the nest is compensated for in the last moments. Experiments show that the ant integrates all the information about the

[11] Wehner, R. 1997. In Lehrer, M. (Ed.), *Orientation and Communication in Arthropods*. Birkhauser, Basel, Switzerland, pp. 145-185.

[12] Collett, M., Collett, T. S., and Wehner, R. 1999. *Curr. Biol.* 9: 1031-1034.

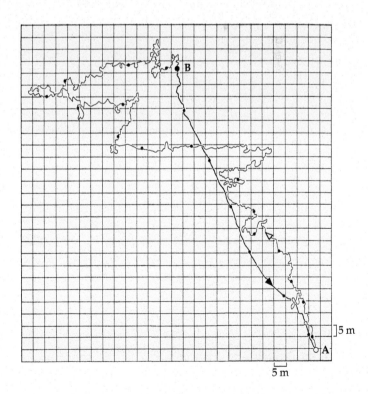

FIGURE 20.3 Pathways Taken by an Ant from its nest (A) to a source of food (B) and back. The distance between sequential dots on the trace represents the distance traveled in 1 minute. The ant follows a tortuous path (> 592 m) until it happens upon the food. Then, it heads straight home (140 m) with amazing accuracy. (After R. Wehner, 1994. *Deutsch. Zool. Ges.* 87: 9-37.)

]5 m

5 m

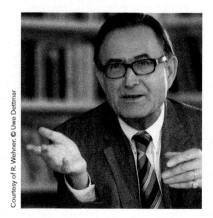

Rüdiger Wehner

[13] Bregy, P., Sommer, S., and Wehner, R. 2008. *J. Exp. Biol.* 211: 1868–1873.
[14] Muller, M., and Wehner, R. 1994. *J. Comp. Physiol.* A 175: 525–530.

movements that lead it to the food, keeping track of both the angles turned (as with a compass) and the distances traveled (as with an odometer).

How does the ant do this? Spatial cues and useful landmarks do not abound in the desert, although objects and odors near the nest do provide information for finding the nest hole at short distances.[13] This finding was shown by experiments in which the ant made the round trip while able to view only a portion of the sky.[14] To eliminate the sun and all other cues, the experimenter walked along with the ant, pushing a cart that kept the ant centered under an aperture to the sky (see Figure 20.2B). Inserted into the aperture were filters that determined the direction, wavelength, and angle of polarization of the light seen by the ant through the aperture to the sky. In the absence of the sun, landmarks, and odors, and with only the polarization of light from the sky to guide it, the ant headed straight for home.

Polarization of electromagnetic radiation such as light refers to the situation in which the electrical vector of an electromagnetic wave is restricted to a single plane of at least two possible planes (and the magnetic vector is accordingly restricted to the orthogonal plane). With appropriate filters, one can separate one polarized light from another (this is how lenses in cinema theaters separate the images arriving to each eye to generate three-dimensional sensation in our brain). Light from the sun becomes polarized as it traverses the atmosphere, as we can appreciate when a properly oriented polarizing filter darkens the sky by blocking light polarized in a different direction. If the sun shines at any angle other than vertical, an asymmetrical pattern of polarization orientations occurs, as shown

(A)

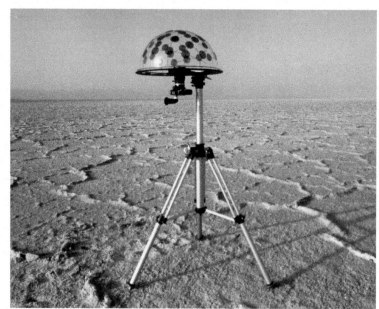

(B)

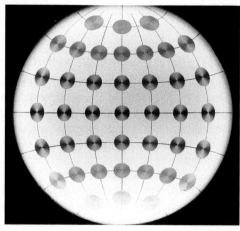

FIGURE 20.4 Patterns of Polarized Light. (A) An array of polarizing filters is mounted in a transparent dome that is oriented parallel to the horizon. (B) Thus, each filter is oriented toward, and reveals the polarization of light from, a different part of the sky. For a person standing at the equator with the sun shining directly overhead, the patterns would be completely symmetrical. (C,D) Different patterns of polarization are produced with the sun at two different positions (indicated by the red dot in each panel); thus, by observing the pattern of polarization, an ant need observe only a small part of the heavens to compute the position of the sun and thereby navigate successfully. (A,B after R. Wehner, 1994. *Deutsch. Zool. Ges.* 87: 9–37; C,D after R. Wehner, 1997. In Lehrer, M. [Ed.], *Orientation and Communication in Arthropods.* Birkhauser, Basel, Switzerland.)

(C)

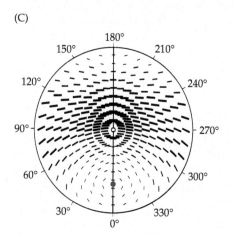

(D)

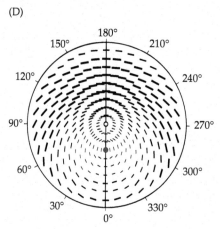

in Figure 20.4. Although human eyes cannot detect polarized light, those of desert ants can (as can the eyes of other arthropods, such as bees, wasps, and crustaceans).[15,16] The pattern of polarized light defines the position of the sun, whether or not it can be seen directly, and thus provides the required navigation compass.

The odometer function for the pathfinding process appears to be generated by summing proprioceptive information associated with the locomotory movements of the ant's legs (so it is a pedometer rather than an odometer!), in which each step is associated with covering a certain distance. This integration of locomotory information was shown by ingenious experiments in which the stride length of individual ants was altered, just as they were about to start their return journey to the nest. Some ants had their legs (and thus their strides) lengthened by gluing on stilts made of boar's hairs; these ants routinely overshot the nest on the homeward journey before initiating the local searching movements that told the experimenters that the ants *thought* they were near home. Conversely, ants whose legs and strides were shortened by amputation of distal leg segments initiated the local searching movements before they reached the vicinity of the nest.[17,18]

Polarized Light Detection by the Ant's Eye

The dome-shaped compound eye of an insect consists of a multifaceted array of radially oriented photo-detecting units called ommatidia. Each ommatidium has its own nerve tract and sees the world from its own perspective.[19] Ants have nine distinct, elongated photoreceptor cells (rhabdomeres) per ommatidium, some whose peak sensitivity is for green light and others whose peak sensitivity is for ultraviolet (UV) light. As with vertebrate photodetection (see Chapter 22), the visual response in ants and other insects starts when light is absorbed by pigment molecules (rhodopsin) closely packed on subcellular organelles in each rhabdomere. In insect rhabdomeres, however, these organelles take the form of closely packed sausages (i.e., microvilli) oriented perpendicular to the long axis of the cell, instead of the stacks of disks in vertebrate rods and cones. This difference enables certain specialized ommatidia to respond preferentially to light that is polarized in a particular orientation. The sensitivity of these ommatidia to polarization arises from the fact that the microvilli are stacked precisely parallel to one another along the entire length of their UV-sensitive rhabdomeres (Figure 20.5). As a result, the rhodopsin molecules in the microvilli are arranged in uniform register with respect to the electrical vector of the incident light.[20]

[15] Muller, K. J. 1973. *J. Physiol.* 232: 573-595.

[16] Wehner, R. 1989. *Trends Neurosci.* 12: 353-359.

[17] Wittlinger, M., Wehner, R., and Wolf, H. 2006. *Science* 312: 1965-1967.

[18] Wittlinger, M., Wehner, R., and Wolf, H. 2007. *J. Exp. Biol.* 210: 198-207.

[19] Zollikofer, C., Wehner, R., and Fukushi, T. 1995. *J. Exp. Biol.* 198: 1637-1646.

[20] Goldsmith, T. H., and Wehner, R. 1977. *J. Gen. Physiol.* 70: 453-490.

(A)

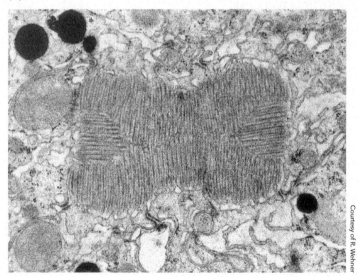

Courtesy of R. Wehner

(B)

FIGURE 20.5 Arrangement of Photoreceptors Responsive to Polarized Light. (A) Electron micrograph of an ommatidium in the dorsal region of the eye of an ant. (B) The microvilli in the ommatidium are arranged in a precisely orthogonal manner, summarized schematically. Heavy lines separate the eight numbered photoreceptors. Photoreceptors 1 and 5 respond preferentially to light polarized at right angles to that preferred by the other photoreceptors. Elsewhere in the eye, the microvilli are not at right angles like this. (B after R. Wehner, 1996. *Nova Acta Leoplodina NF* 72: 159-183.)

FIGURE 20.6 Polarized Light Detectors in the Eye of the Desert Ant. (A) The arrangement of photoreceptors (ommatidia) in a single, compound eye. The receptors for polarized light, used by the ant to navigate, lie in the dorsal rim of the eye, within the area bounded by black dots. (B) Scanning electron micrograph of the eye of the ant. (After R. Wehner, 1994. *Deutsch. Zool. Ges.* 87: 9-37.)

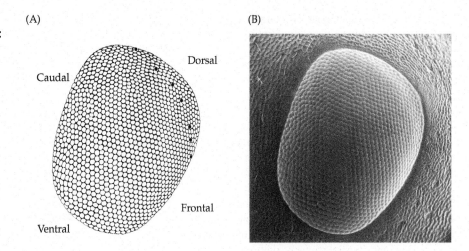

(A)

Dorsal

Caudal

Ventral

Frontal

(B)

In the desert ant, these specialized ommatidia lie within the dorsal rim area of the eye, so they are normally oriented skyward (Figure 20.6). Since rhodopsin absorbs light optimally along the long axis of the molecule, one particular plane of polarized light will be most effective in generating electrical signals in that rhabdomere. Moreover, the orientations of the microvilli in different UV-sensitive rhabdomeres of the dorsal rim ommatidia are aligned precisely at 90° to one another (see Figure 20.5), an arrangement seen only in those photoreceptors concerned with polarized light. This orthogonal arrangement of receptors in one ommatidium is optimal for sensing the angle of polarization, by comparing the outputs of the orthogonally oriented receptors. A single photoreceptor on its own could not differentiate between differences of intensity, wavelength, and polarization. Similar arrangements of polarized light receptors exist in the dorsal rim of bee eyes and in crustacean eyes.

Evidence that polarized light is essential for the ant's navigation has been provided by the following experiments: First, if the eye is covered by a contact lens leaving only the dorsal rim exposed, the ant can still take a direct way home. Second, if the dorsal rim of the eye is blocked, pathfinding becomes disturbed. Third, if the pattern of polarization reaching the ant's eye is shifted by appropriate filters (placed on the cart), the ant's return course becomes deviated by a precise and calculable extent.

Strategies for Finding the Nest

For navigation to be successful, information arriving at the eye must be correlated with a celestial map in which the position of the sun determines the orientations of polarized light. As the ant walks away from the nest, constant reference is made to the complex but regular pattern in the sky by the ommatidia. This provides the nervous system with information about the direction of travel. The compound eye is hemispherical, and this allows for a faithful spatial representation of orientations like those shown in Figure 20.6. A further complication arises because the sun is not stationary. Hence, the ant has to compensate for the shifting pattern of polarization during the day as it travels. That it can do so has been shown in experiments in which an ant is placed at a spot removed from the nest, kept there, and then released at a later time. An ant that has become familiar with the sun's rate of movement for at least one day is able to correct its trajectory in an appropriate manner, as though it had learned the patterns of polarized light at different times of day. In addition to the polarized light compass, the sun itself and external objects situated along the path can be used to aid navigation.[21]

Distinctive features of the terrain and objects are of principal importance in the last part of the return to the nest, which constitutes a tiny hole in the desert. If the homing vector has led to an error, such that the ant has not arrived precisely at its nest, a new strategy is introduced.[14] The ant makes a series of exploratory loops increasingly large but always returning to the starting point. This represents an optimal strategy for reconnoitering without getting lost.

Interestingly, using a computational approach in which the known properties of ant navigation already described are applied, one can produce models or even robots that

[21] Collett, M. et al. 1998. *Nature* 394: 269-272.

FIGURE 20.7 Mobile Robot Known as Sahabot, devised by Wehner and his associates. The robot is equipped with six polarized light sensors arranged in pairs. Each pair forms a polarization-detecting unit, with properties resembling those of the neuron shown in Figure 20.11. Each unit can be tuned to a specific direction of polarization. The robot is able to navigate with this polarized light compass, successfully recreating the behavior of the ant. For example, it can be driven along a tortuous path and then compute the shortest way back to the starting point. (After R. Wehner, 1997. In Lehrer, M. [Ed.], *Orientation and Communication in Arthropods.* Birkhauser, Basel, Switzerland.)

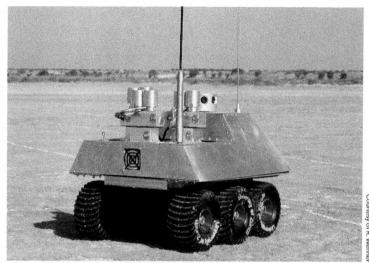

Courtesy of R. Wehner

accurately mimic the navigational behavior of the desert ant using cues provided by polarized light (Figure 20.7). Such models illustrate the possibility of computing trajectories in this way but do not, of course, provide evidence that this is the system the ant uses.

Additional Mechanisms for Navigation by Ants

No seasoned explorer would be comfortable venturing out with just one navigation system—Steve Wozniak, a cofounder of Apple Inc., is reported to drive about with four or more GPS devices—which, in turn, requires procedures for weighing conflicting information. Ants are no exception to this rule. In addition to the coupled polarization compass and pedometer system, the desert ant *Cataglyphis* can also use direct observations of the sun and wind in finding its path through a visually sparse environment, and it weighs these two inputs differently depending on how high the sun is in the sky.[22]

Learning Their Way

The description of the navigation mechanisms we have discussed thus far may make a strong impression that the nervous system of ants integrates information in a purely mechanical manner, like the robot in Figure 20.7. However, ants complement their navigation by learning visual cues and odors that help them find food and compensate for errors in the return path integration. Ants learn certain odors to find their nest and other odors to find food by using different strategies.[23] Learning the odors of the nest requires repetitive training, and the memory of these odors disappears soon after the odors fade. The odors of food, by contrast, have a stronger impact: They can be learned after a single exposure, several odors can be memorized, and the memories persist for life.

Another form of learning appears early in the foraging lives of desert ants. During "learning walks," ants gaze at the nest entrance by turning around continuously.[24] One wonders, how do ants keep their orientation in these turns? Orientation is maintained by detection of the geomagnetic field. Changing the horizontal component of the magnetic field makes the ants change their gaze as predicted by experimental alterations.

Yet another form of learning occurs in ants that work inside nests but are inexperienced outside. Desert ants construct satellite entrances to their nests that can be several meters from the main entrance and from each other. The inside working ants are frequently transported from one entrance to another by an experienced forager (Figure 20.8). If a worker is accidentally dropped en route, it may take the next "taxi" to its destination, if available. If not, however, workers are able to reorient themselves and return home using their memory of the cues along their trajectory, in spite of the fact that they did not use their stride odometer while being carried.[25] This observation shows that the worker have acquired a memory of features of the track from visual

[22] Muller, M., and Wehner, R. 2007. *Naturwissenschaften* 94: 589–594.

[23] Huber, R., and Knaden, M. 2018. *Proc. Natl. Acad. Sci. USA* 115: 10470–10474.

[24] Fleischmann, P. N. et al. 2017. *J. Exp. Biol.* 220: 2426–2435.

[25] Pfeffer, S. E., and Wittlinger, M. 2016. *Science* 353: 1155–1157.

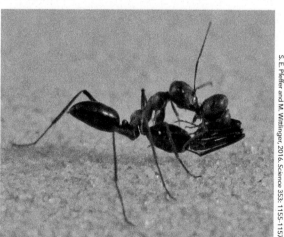

S. E. Pfeffer and M. Wittlinger, 2016. Science 353: 1155-1157

FIGURE 20.8 A Working Ant Being Carried to another nest by a forager.

cues along the pathway. Thus, foraging ants (carriers) use pedometers to measure their travel distance, whereas the workers rely on visual odometry.

The independence and redundancy of the stride odometer and the optic learning paradigms illustrate how these "simple" desert ants have adapted alternative possibilities for navigating in desert conditions. Remarkably, ants inhabiting different visual environments use different sets of strategies for pathfinding.[26,27]

Navigation in Bees

Bees also use a magnetic compass to orient themselves while searching for a target, in addition to visual cues and polarized light.[28,29] Collett and his colleagues demonstrated this phenomenon in experiments in which they trained bees to collect sugar from a small bottle cap on a board.[30] For orientation, a black cylinder was placed in a constant compass direction at a fixed distance from the bottle cap. The cylinder and the sucrose were moved to different places on the board between trials. Periodically, the bottle cap was removed, leaving only the cylinder. The exploration of the board by a trained bee was monitored by video recording. Figure 20.9 shows the trajectory of a bee as it approached and later left the cylinder and the food source. What is clear is that the bee turned so as to face south before landing and again faced south shortly after taking off. In this way, it viewed the visual cue and the attractant (sugar) each time from a constant direction. Observation of the sky alone was not a sufficient explanation for this behavior. Bees faced south in the rain, under a completely overcast sky, or when the sky compass was eliminated. From such observations, one can conclude that somehow the animal can distinguish south from north, east, or west.

The fact that bees are sensitive to magnetic fields was shown by training bees under a tarpaulin, using imposed magnetic fields that shifted the magnetic north. The bees oriented themselves again to the *south*, but this direction was the south of the imposed magnetic field. How changes in imposed magnetic fields produce changes in behavior and pattern recognition is not known. These are sensory mechanisms not known to be represented in our nervous system but present in birds, fish, turtles, and certain invertebrates, some of which have been shown to have magnetoreceptors.

[26] Collett, T. S., and Graham, P. 2004. *Curr. Biol.* 14: R475–R477.

[27] Cheng, K. et al. 2009. *Behav. Processes* 80: 261–268.

[28] Lehrer, M., and Collett, T. S. 1994. *J. Comp. Physiol. A* 175: 171–177.

[29] Dacke, M., and Srinivasan, M. V. 2007. *J. Exp. Biol.* 210: 845–853.

[30] Collett, T. S., and Baron, J. 1994. *Nature* 368: 137–140.

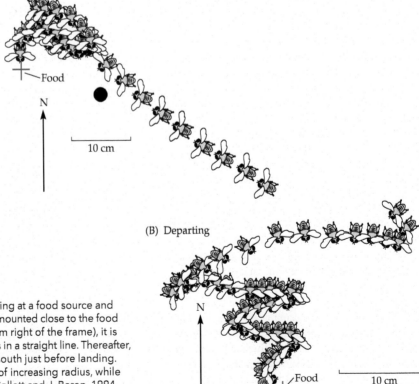

FIGURE 20.9 Trajectory of a Bee landing at a food source and departing from it. A cylinder (black circle) is mounted close to the food source (cross). (A) As the bee arrives (bottom right of the frame), it is oriented toward the cylinder, to which it flies in a straight line. Thereafter, it flies to the food source but turns to face south just before landing. (B) As the bee departs, it flies north in arcs of increasing radius, while facing south (flying backward). (After T. S. Collett and J. Baron, 1994. *Nature* 368: 137–140.)

Without access to proprioceptive information of walking, how do bees judge the distance they have traveled on their flights? By analogy with the proprioceptive leg memory of the ants, one might imagine that bees count wingbeats, but this would lead to errors depending on the speed and direction of the prevailing wind. Instead, it has been shown that bees use a "visually driven odometer" to judge distance. For example, in flying through a tunnel, they maintain their distance between the two walls by balancing the angular velocities of the images impinging on their left and right retinas. In an uncluttered visual environment, they lose their ability to judge distance.[31]

Polarized Light and Twisted Photoreceptors

Ants and bees are evolutionarily related. Thus, it is not surprising that both navigate using receptors for polarized light to provide a compass. The presence of such receptors could, in principle, be a mixed blessing, however. The precise arrays of microvilli allow the heavens to be scanned for the orientatidia of polarized light, as we have seen. But for discriminating shapes and colors, polarization can cause difficulties. For example, as bees fly, they need to identify flowers by their colors. Leaves and petals vary in the way they reflect light in a manner that depends on how waxy the surfaces are; surfaces that are shiny reflect polarized light more than matte surfaces do. Consequently, the angle at which a leaf or petal is illuminated and viewed will affect the amount and the direction of polarized light that is reflected.

The photopigments necessary for color vision in the bee are contained in microvilli (like those of the ant) of specific receptors sensitive to green, blue, or UV light. In the bee eye, as in the ant, the photopigments are arranged in precise, parallel series of rhabdomeres. With variable, uncalibrated contributions by polarized light, the signals regarding color would be ambiguous because the appreciation of color depends not only on wavelength but also on the relative absorption by different classes of color receptors. As Wehner and Bernard[32] put it, "This means that for the bee the hue of a given part of a plant would change, whenever an approaching bee changed its direction of flight and thus, its direction of view—a completely unwanted phenomenon. For example, when zigzagging over a meadow with all its differently inclined surfaces of leaves, the bee would experience pointillistic fireworks of false colors that would make it difficult to impossible to detect the real colors of the flowers." To avoid this problem, the ommatidia of the bee outside the dorsal rim area contain so-called twisted receptors. By light and electron microscopy, it was found that the rhabdomeres were twisted along their long axes. This twist produces a progressive change in the orientation of their microvilli (Figure 20.10), so that they are not in a parallel array throughout the depth of the rhabdomere. Thus, the receptor no longer responds selectively to polarized light. Similar irregularities of the microvilli arrangement are seen in ommatidia outside the dorsal rim in the ant's eye. As in the bee, these ommatidia do not sense the plane of polarized light and can therefore be used for landmark detection.

Neural Mechanisms for Navigation

One satisfactory aspect of the studies on insect navigation we have described thus far is the detailed information now available about the initial sensory mechanisms. At the same time, technical challenges have so far prevented scientists from making the detailed recordings required to fully unravel the integrative steps performed by neurons in the insect ant or bee brain. Neurons in the ant's optic lobe are particularly hard to record because of their small size and because the surrounding sheath is very tough. Thus, Labhart and colleagues studied interneurons in crickets that receive inputs from receptors for polarized light.[33,34] The cricket ommatidia that are sensitive to the plane of polarized light contain rhabdomeres with orthogonally arranged microvilli. These rhabdomeres project to the interneuron, which computes information about the vector of polarization. Figure 20.11 shows electrical recordings from such cells. Their responses are just what would be predicted from behavioral studies with polarized light. Similar neurons have been recorded from the more difficult ant preparation—records were obtained from only six polarization-sensitive neurons in 40 preparations.[35] It is obvious that in spite of the

[31] Srinivasan, M. et al. 1996. *J. Exp. Biol.* 199: 237-244.

[32] Wehner, R., and Bernard, G. D. 1993. *Proc. Natl. Acad. Sci. USA* 90: 4132-4135.

[33] Labhart, T. 1988. *Nature* 331: 435-437.

[34] Labhart, T., Petzold, J., and Helbling, H. 2001. *J. Exp. Biol.* 204: 2423-2430.

[35] Labhart, T. 2000. *Naturwissenschaften* 87: 133-136.

FIGURE 20.10 Twists in Most Bee Photoreceptors Minimize the Influence of Polarized Light.
The inset illustrates the helical twisting of the rhabdomeres in two developing ommatidia (viewed from the side) as one progresses from the tips of the rhabdomeres near the surface of the eye (top) toward the basement membrane (BM). The graph plots the angular position of the transverse axis (TRA; defined in the schematics at right) of various photoreceptors against the depth beneath their tips. Photoreceptors in the dorsal rim of the eye, which are sensitive to polarized light, show no twist (red squares). Elsewhere in the eye, photoreceptors twist either clockwise or counterclockwise (blue circles), as a result of which they do not respond selectively to any particular orientation of polarized light. (After R. Wehner and G. D. Bernard, 1993. *Proc. Natl. Acad. Sci. USA* 90: 4132–4135. © 1993 National Academy of Sciences.)

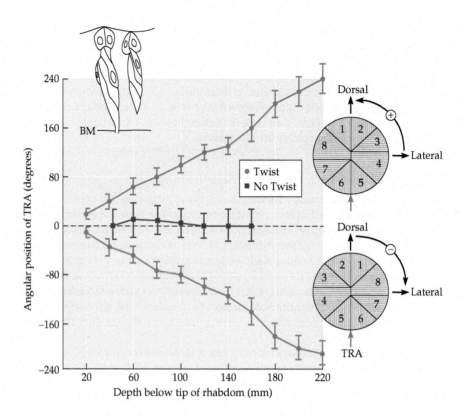

beauty of the experimental paradigms and astute interpretations of the results obtained from experiments made in insects, their nervous systems are not likely to provide significant information about higher levels of behavior. Therefore, to investigate the detailed links between sensory input and motor performance, we must turn to another system.

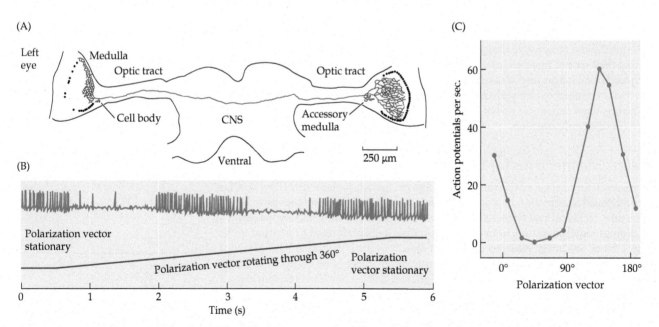

FIGURE 20.11 Electrical Responses of Polarization-Sensitive Interneurons in cricket CNS. The cricket interneurons are large enough to be impaled by microelectrodes. (A) Reconstruction of the interneuron stained by intracellular injection of a histological marker, neurobiotin. This neuron receives its input from the left eye. (B) Responses of a neuron of this type to polarized light as the polarization vector is rotated through 360°. (C) Graphical representation of the response intensity plotted against the angle of the polarization vector. (B,C after T. Labhart, 1988. *Nature* 331: 435–437.)

Deciding between Opposite, Incompatible Behaviors: Neuronal Circuits in the Crayfish

Whatever the behavior of an ant, a bee, or a professor is, it is not randomly produced but a reaction to the quality and magnitude of the animal's external state in combination with its internal state. In this section we show how the nervous system decides its responses to variations in the environmental conditions.

Fishermen know that under dim light at dawn or dusk, lobsters emerge from their burrows to socialize and feed. In darkness or at high light intensities, they return to their burrows. This observation indicates that light triggers opposite attraction and withdrawal locomotor responses. How the nervous system integrates visual information to produce motor responses has been studied in crayfish under controlled laboratory conditions.[36] The stereotyped behaviors of crayfish allow quantitative correlations of their locomotor patterns in response to controlled illumination with the responses of identified visual neurons. Locomotion was quantified in freely moving crayfish by means of infrared optocouplers linked to a computer that detected the animals' movements in either an artificial burrow or an open space. Figure 20.12 shows that a dim light attracted crayfish out of their burrows; once animals wandered into the open space, the onset of a higher-intensity light triggered their withdrawal back to the burrow. Each of these opposing responses comprises a characteristic and mutually incompatible locomotor pattern. During attraction, crayfish walk forward extending their claws; withdrawal consists of walking backward with cycles of tail flipping. These stereotyped and reproducible behaviors can be quantified in terms of the delay (latency) between the onset of light and the exit of the burrow (attraction) or return to the burrow (withdrawal), as a function of the light intensity. The results in Figure 20.12C,D show a clear distinction between the ranges of light that produce attraction and withdrawal. This finding highlights the question of how animals, including humans, categorize the intensity of a stimulus to select one behavior over the other (or others).

[36] De-Miguel, F. F., and Aréchiga, H. 1992. *J. Exp. Biol.* 164: 153–169.

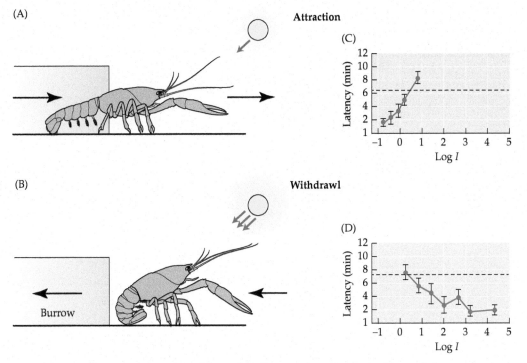

FIGURE 20.12 Attraction and Withdrawal Walking Behaviors Evoked by Light in Crayfish. (A) Low light intensities evoke forward walking attraction with the chelae (claws) extended. (B) When a crayfish is out of its burrow, higher light intensities evoke backward withdrawal locomotion with cyclic tail flipping. (C,D) The latencies of both responses depend on the light intensities. Error bars deptic standard deviation from the data. (After F. Fernández De-Miguel and H. Aréchiga, 1992. *J. Exp. Biol.* 164: 153–169.)

In a second set of experiments, crayfish were maintained on a treadmill that detected the velocity and direction of walking in response to illumination (Figure 20.13). Low light intensities produced the characteristic forward walking of attraction responses; high light intensities evoked backward walking.[37] Direct illumination of the visual fields in the superior part of the eye with low intensities could evoke forward walking; high light intensities applied to visual fields in lower areas of the eye (which receive light preferentially when crayfish are out of their burrows) succeeded in producing backward walking. Moreover, a striking observation was that withdrawal also depended on illumination of photoreceptors in the tail of the crayfish (sensory structures that are uncommon in animals like us). Sectioning the nerve that connects the caudal photoreceptors with the rest of the nervous system made the withdrawal responses slower.

Recordings from individual identified visual neurons in the optic nerve of the crayfish are possible by use of fine extracellular electrodes (see also Chapter 2), unlike in ants or bees. A specific set of 14 "sustaining" neurons reports on the levels of light applied to their visual fields by sustained trains of impulses whose frequencies increase with the light

[37] Wiersma, C. A., and Yamaguchi, T. 1966. *J. Comp. Neurol.* 128: 333–358.

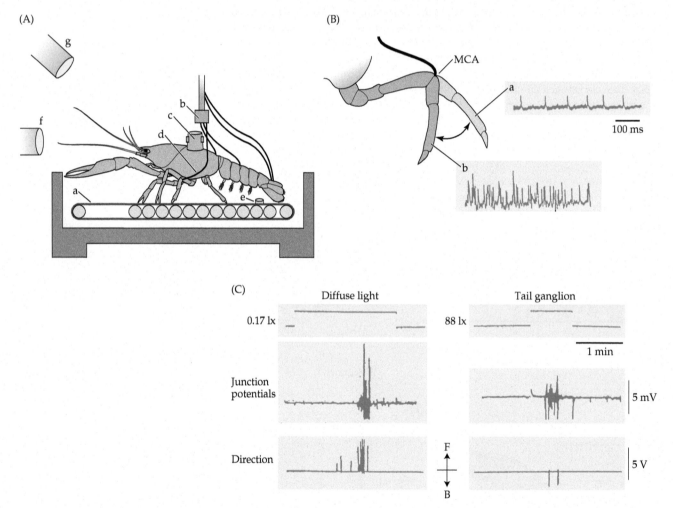

FIGURE 20.13 Locomotor Responses to Illumination in Crayfish Tethered to a Treadmill. (A) The treadmill detected the latency and direction of walking. a is a band roller connected to motion- and direction-detector circuits; b is a connector for electrical recordings of muscle fibers as reporters of motion. c is a tethering cork; d is a recording electrode in the joint for recording muscle activity; e is a light source for illuminating the extraretinal photoreceptor in the sixth ganglion of the tail; f and g are optic fiber lamps for light stimulation. (B) Electrical recordings of muscle activity from the joint of one leg as a reporter of motor responses. Contraction of the joint produced an increase in muscle activity. MCA = the merocarpopodite articulation; a = recording of muscle activity before walking; b = recording during walking. (C) The recordings of muscle activity during walking correlated with the latency and direction of attraction (forward, F) and withdrawal (backward, B) responses. The light pulses and intensities are indicated above the recordings. (After F. Fernández De-Miguel and H. Aréchiga, 1992. *J. Exp. Biol.* 164: 153–169.)

intensity. As seen in Figure 20.14, neurons with visual fields in the central and upper parts of the eye respond to light intensities that attract crayfish. Conversely, a smaller group of four neurons with visual fields in the lower and lateral parts of the eye (O9, O14, O30, and O38) respond to light intensities that induce withdrawal. The increasing response of all sustaining neurons to increasing levels of light raises the question of how withdrawal expresses when the neurons that may evoke attraction are efficiently firing. Recordings from any one sustained neuron during illumination of the visual field of another sustained neuron showed that light intensities that trigger withdrawal inhibit nonselectively the activity of their surrounding neurons. Such observation permits one to hypothesize that the decision-making mechanism occurs in the retina, when activation of the visual input evoking withdrawal inhibits the input that evokes the incompatible attraction response to light. A complementary input reinforces withdrawal when a crayfish wanders out of its burrow and its caudal photoreceptor is activated by the background illumination.

In spite of the fact that the connections between visual neurons and the rest of the locomotor pathway evoking locomotor responses have not been identified, a coherent hypothesis can be proposed about how light intensities evoke attraction or withdrawal. A particular type of neuron discovered by Wiersma in crayfish, the **command neuron**,[38] orchestrates a complete behavior in response to sensory stimulation. Command neurons are widely distributed in animals, where they organize motor responses; in mice, for example, command neurons in the brainstem inhibit locomotor patterns (see also Chapter 26).

In crayfish, stimulation of axons that carry sensory information produces sophisticated patterns of locomotion mediated by command neurons. Stimulation of certain axons produces forward walking such as that in attraction; stimulation of other axons produces backward walking with cyclic tail flipping,[39] such as that seen in withdrawal. The same pattern of backward walking can be evoked by stimulation of the caudal photoreceptor.[40] The way by which command neurons produce rhythmic locomotor patterns in crayfish, lobsters, mollusks, and rodents is by connecting to or being part of circuits that translate the sensory information into alternate bursts of impulses by motoneurons innervating antagonist muscles. Such circuits are called central pattern generators (CPGs). The connections from the visual system to the command neurons and the CPGs producing attraction and withdrawal in crayfish remain elusive. Chapter 26 mentions their activity in the motor systems of mammals. The functioning of the CPGs that control the stomatogastric ganglion of crustacea[41–43] has been described in great detail at the cellular level. The circuit controlling crawling and swimming is described in the next section by using the advantages offered by the nervous system of the leech.

[38] Edwards, D. H., Heitler, W. J., and Krasne, F. B. 1999. *Trends Neurosci.* 22: 153–161.

[39] Bowerman, R. F., and Larimer, J. L. 1976. *Comp. Biochem. Physiol. A Comp. Physiol.* 54: 1–5.

[40] Edwards, D. H., Jr. 1984. *J. Exp. Biol.* 109: 291–306.

[41] Marder, E. et al. 1998. *Ann. NY Acad. Sci.* 860: 226–238.

[42] Wagenaar, D. A. 2015. *J. Exp. Biol.* 218: 3353–3359.

[43] Calabrese, R. L., Norris, B. J., and Wenning, A. 2016. *Curr. Opin. Neurobiol.* 41: 68–77.

FIGURE 20.14 Visual Responses of Crayfish to Light in Relation to Attraction and Withdrawal Behaviors. (A) Visual fields of identified neurons in the eye carrying information about light intensity in crayfish. The clear fields correspond to neurons that responded in the range of light intensities that evoke attraction. The lines indicate the borders of the visual fields in the eye. The shadowed areas are the visual fields for neurons O9, O14, O30, and O38 that responded in the range of light intensities that evoke withdrawal. (B) The firing frequency of visual neurons as a function of the light intensity (*I*) correlates with attraction or withdrawal responses. (After F. Fernández De-Miguel and H. Aréchiga, 1992. *J. Exp. Biol.* 164: 153–169.)

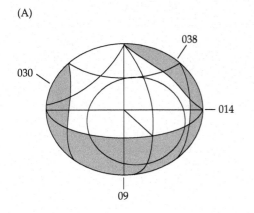

(A)

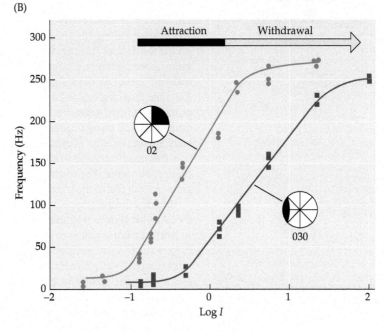

(B)

Analysis at the Level of Individual Neurons: The CNS of the Leech

Since the days of ancient Greece and Rome, physicians have applied leeches to patients suffering from anything from epilepsy, angina, tuberculosis, and meningitis to black eyes and hemorrhoids—an unpleasant treatment that almost certainly did more harm than good to the unfortunate victims. This mania for leeching had one benefit for contemporary biology, however. In the late nineteenth century, the leech nervous system was extensively studied by a roster of distinguished anatomists, including Ramón y Cajal, Sanchez, Gaskell, del Río-Hortega, Odurih, and Retzius.[44] At about the same time, C. O. Whitman, one of the founders of experimental embryology, used another leech species to follow the fates of early embryonic cells[45] (see Chapter 27). Interest in the leech thereafter declined, to be rekindled in 1960 when Stephen Kuffler, David Potter, and John Nicholls applied modern neurophysiological techniques to study leech glial cells (see Chapter 10).[46] This research set the stage for extensive studies of the leech's individual neurons, circuitry, and behavior,[47–49] which in turn led to subsequent studies of leech development[50,51] and regeneration,[52] and of the cell biology or biophysics of its isolated neurons.[53] More recently, various molecular approaches have allowed researchers to create transgenic animals, mutate or knock down the expression of specific genes of interest, and characterize the transcriptional profiles of functionally identified neurons, all within the context of a sequenced genome.[54] Curiously, in recent decades leeches have reentered the realm of medicine, both as a source of novel anticoagulants and, reprising their traditional role in bloodletting, for the minimally invasive postsurgical treatment of venous congestion.[55,56]

With a nervous system containing only about one tenth the number of neurons of the insects and crustacea discussed in the preceding sections, leeches still exhibit stereotyped reflexes such as shortening and local bending in response to mechanical stimuli, along with behaviors involving coordination of the whole body, such as swimming and crawling. Leeches orient by means of sensory cues that allow them to access potential food sources with an efficiency that is the bane of those who swim or trek in leech habitat. Like other animals, leeches modulate their behaviors in response to their physiological state (see Chapter 18) and must choose among mutually incompatible behaviors, such as feeding, mating, swimming, or crawling. Their behaviors are also susceptible to simple forms of learning. Remarkable progress has been made in understanding how these processes are carried out, starting with the properties and connections of individual nerve cells.

Leech Ganglia: Semiautonomous Mini-Brains

The leech body and its nervous system are segmented. That is, various tissues and organs are organized along the anterior–posterior axis into repeating units (segments) that are similar throughout the animal. The leech body contains 32 segments; 21 standard segments make up the midbody, 4 fused segments make up most of the head, and 7 fused segments make up the tail. Each midbody segment is innervated by a morphologically stereotyped ganglion. Even the brainlike ganglia in the head and tail, shown in Figure 20.15, consist primarily of fused segmental ganglia, in which many characteristic features of midbody ganglia are still recognizable.[57] Each ganglion innervates a well-defined territory of the body through bundles of axons that receive and send out continuous multimodal information. Communication between neighboring and distant ganglia in the chain occurs through connective nerves. The coordinated operation of the chain of ganglia is influenced by the brains at each end of the animal.

Perhaps the main appeal of the leech as a neurobiological preparation is the beauty of the living ganglion as it appears under the microscope, with its neurons so recognizable and so familiar from segment to segment, specimen to specimen, and even species to species (Figure 20.16). Each ganglion senses and controls the functioning of its corresponding segment in a relatively independent manner with only about 400 nerve cells,[58] a number that seems quite manageable when compared with the overwhelming numbers of neurons in mammalian nervous systems. As one looks at these limited aggregates of neurons laid out in an orderly pattern, one cannot but marvel at how they, on their own, are responsible for

[44] Payton, W. B. 1981. In K. J. Muller, J. G. Nicholls, and G. S. Stent (Eds.), *Neurobiology of the Leech.* Cold Spring Harbor Laboratory, Cold Spring. Harbor, NY, pp. 27-34.

[45] Maienschein, J. 1978. *J. Hist. Biol.* 11: 129-158.

[46] Kuffler, S. W., and Potter, D. D. 1964. *J. Neurophysiol.* 27: 290-320.

[47] Friesen, W. O., and Kristan, W. B. 2007. *Curr. Opin. Neurobiol.* 17: 704-711.

[48] Nicholls, J. G., and Van Essen, D. 1974. *Sci. Am.* 230: 38-48.

[49] Kristan, W. B., Jr., Calabrese, R. L., and Friesen, W. O. 2005. *Prog. Neurobiol.* 76: 279-327.

[50] Weisblat, D. A., and Kuo, D.-H. 2009. In *Emerging Model Organisms, A Laboratory Manual.* Cold Spring Harbor Laboratory, Cold Spring Harbor, NY, pp. 245-274.

[51] Marin-Burgin, A., Kristan, W. B., Jr., and French, K. A. 2008. *Dev. Neurobiol.* 68: 779-787.

[52] Duan, Y. et al. 2005. *Cell Mol. Neurobiol.* 25: 441-450.

[53] De-La-Rosa Tovar, A., Mishra, P. K., De-Miguel, F. F. 2016. *Front. Cell Neurosci.* 10: 198.

[54] Simakov, O. et al. *Nature* 493: 526-531.

[55] Weinfeld, A. B. et al. 2000. *Ann. Plast. Surg.* 45: 207-212.

[56] Mineo, M., Jolley, T., and Rodriguez, G. 2004. *Urology* 63: 981-983.

[57] Coggeshall, R. E., and Fawcett, D. W. 1964. *J. Neurophysiol.* 27: 229-289.

[58] Macagno, E. R. 1980. *J. Comp. Neurol.* 190: 283-302.

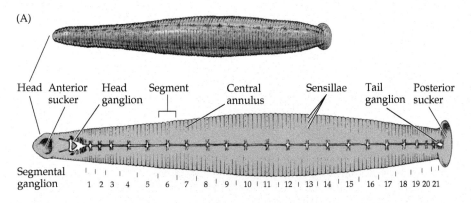

(A)

Head Anterior Head Segment Central Sensillae Tail Posterior
      sucker   ganglion   annulus   ganglion sucker

Segmental
ganglion

1 2 3 4 5 6 7 8 9 10 11 12 13 14 15 16 17 18 19 20 21

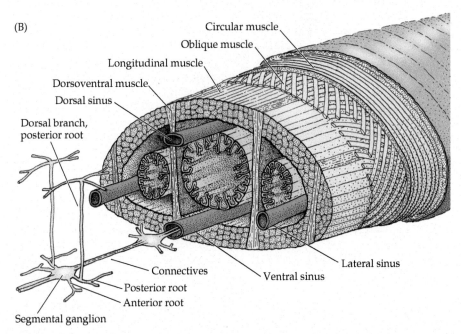

(B)

Circular muscle
Oblique muscle
Longitudinal muscle
Dorsoventral muscle
Dorsal sinus
Dorsal branch,
posterior root

Lateral sinus
Connectives
Ventral sinus
Posterior root
Anterior root
Segmental ganglion

FIGURE 20.15 Central Nervous System of the Leech. (A) The segmented CNS of the leech includes a chain of ganglia that run in the ventral interior of the animal. Over most of the body, five circumferential annuli make up each segment; the central annulus is marked by sensory organs (sensillae) responding to light and touch. (B) The nerve cord lies in the ventral part of the body within a blood sinus. Ganglia, which are linked to each other by bundles of axons (connectives), innervate the body wall by paired roots. The muscles are arranged in three principal layers: circular, oblique, and longitudinal. Dorsoventral muscles flatten the animal. (After J. G. Nicholls and D. Van Essen, 1974. *Sci. Am.* 230: 38–48.)

all the movements, hesitations, avoidance, mating, feeding, and sensations of the animal. In addition to the aesthetic pleasure provided by the preparation, there is the intellectual excitement of trying to solve the circuitry and logic of such a well-organized nervous system. But before one can work out how the animal performs its movements, it is necessary to know about individual cells: their properties, connections, and functions.

Sensory Cells in Leech Ganglia

Unlike the CNS of ants and bees, the CNS of the leech has sensory and motor neurons whose accessibility permits detailed studies of how sensory stimulation produces motor responses. When one strokes, presses, or pinches the skin of a leech, a sequence of movements follows. A segment may shorten abruptly, and the skin may become raised into a series of distinct ridges. Subsequently, the animal bends, writhes, or swims away. Once individual sensory and motor cells have been identified by their shapes, sizes, positions, and electrical properties, one can reliably determine which cells are involved in mediating these reflexes.[59–62]

Figure 20.16 shows three types of sensory cells that have their cell bodies in the ganglion. This is a striking location since in most species the sensory cell bodies are encapsulated in the peripheral nervous system. The neurons labeled T, P, and N in Figure 20.16 owe their names to their selective responses to touch (T), pressure (P), or noxious (N) mechanical stimulation of the skin. One full set of three types of mechanosensory neurons in each side of the ganglion innervates the corresponding side of the skin. Intracellular injection

[59] Nicholls, J. G., and Baylor, D. A. 1968. *J. Neurophysiol.* 31: 740–756.

[60] Stuart, A. E. 1970. *J. Physiol.* 209: 627–646.

[61] Lockery, S. R., and Kristan, W. B., Jr. 1990. *J. Neurosci.* 10: 1816–1829.

[62] Rodriguez, M. J., Perez-Etchegoyen, C. B., and Szczupak, L. 2009. *J. Comp. Physiol. A* 195: 491–500.

(A)

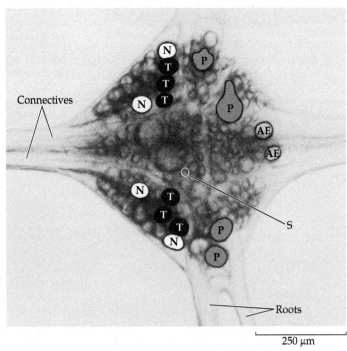

(B)

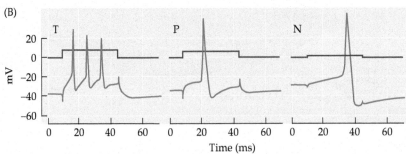

FIGURE 20.16 Leech Segmental Ganglia Contain Individually Identified Neurons. (A) Ventral view of a midbody ganglion. Some individual cell bodies can be clearly recognized by their size and location within the ganglion. For example, the sensory cells responding to touch (T), pressure (P), and noxious (N) mechanical stimulation of the skin are labeled, as are the annulus erector (AE) motoneurons outlined in the posterior part of the ganglion. Identification of other cells in the ganglion is based on more subtle but equally clear-cut physiological or morphological criteria. For example, the S cell, which plays a role in dishabituation and sensitization, is a small and unpaired neuron. (B) Each sensory cell type produces distinctive action potentials. Impulses in T cells are briefer and smaller than those in P or N cells. N cell impulses have a larger afterhyperpolarization than do T or P cells. Current injected into cells through the microelectrode is monitored on the upper traces. (From J. G. Nicholls and D. A. Baylor, 1968. *J. Neurophysiol.* 31: 740–756.)

of current through an intracellular electrode produces action potentials with characteristics that correspond to each neuron type. In that experimental situation, a segment of skin attached to the ganglion by the nerve roots can be stimulated with pulses of calibrated force. As the strength of stimulation applied to the skin is increased, a different type of mechanosensory neuron is recruited. As shown in Figure 20.17A, a light touch of the skin surface produces responses of T cells. The P cells respond only to a marked pressure or deformation of the skin and adapt slowly (Figure 20.17B). The N cells require a stronger mechanical stimulus that may cause damage to the skin, such as a pinch with blunt forceps (Figure 20.17C,D). Similar to the polymodal nociceptors in mammals, one or both N cells also respond selectively to acid, heat, and capsaicin (the burning compound of chili peppers).[63] The modalities

[63] Pastor, J., Soria, B., and Belmonte, C. 1996. *J. Neurophysiol.* 75: 2268–2279.

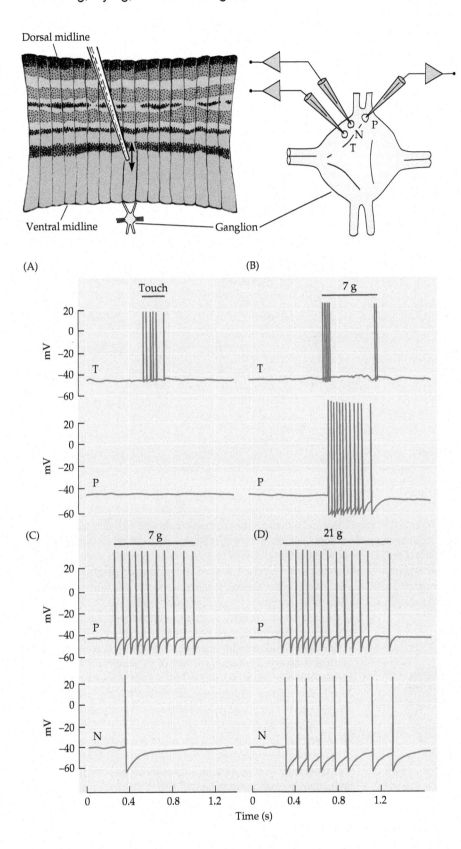

(A)

(B)

(C)

(D)

Time (s)

FIGURE 20.17 Sensory Neurons Respond to Skin Stimulation. A piece of skin and the ganglion that innervates it permit intracellular recordings of T, P, and N sensory cells. Neurons are activated by touching or pressing their receptive fields in the skin. (A) A T cell responds to light touch that is not strong enough to stimulate the P cell. (B) Stronger, maintained pressure evokes a prolonged discharge from the P cell and a rapidly adapting on and off response from the T cell. (C,D) Still stronger pressure is needed to activate the N cell mechanically. g = force in grams. (After J. G. Nicholls and D. A. Baylor, 1968. *J. Neurophysiol.* 31: 740–756; J. G. Nicholls and D. Van Essen, 1974. *Sci. Am.* 230: 38–48.)

and responses of these three mechanosensory neurons resemble those of mechanoreceptors in the human skin (see Chapter 21), which distinguish among touch, pressure, and noxious stimuli. In the leech, however, individual neurons perform the job of many equivalent neurons in a densely innervated region of our own skin, such as the fingertip.

FIGURE 20.18 Receptive Field of a Pressure (P) Sensory Cell. This P cell has an axon that runs out through the root of its own ganglion to supply the skin of the segment in which it is situated. Other axons of smaller diameter pass along the connectives to neighboring ganglia and then through the roots to innervate adjacent (minor) territories. The other P cell in the same side of the ganglion (not shown) innervates a territory closer to the ventral midline but with similar longitudinal extent. There is considerable overlap between the receptive fields of the two cells. Hence, pressure applied to dorsal skin will activate the P cell shown in this figure, pressure applied to ventral skin will activate the other P cell, and pressure applied on lateral skin will activate both P cells. The fact that axons with a small diameter supply the adjacent minor territories has implications for conduction. Conduction of action potentials gets blocked where an axon of small diameter feeds into a larger-diameter axon, as at the points marked by arrows in the diagram at top. (After X. N. Gu, 1991. *J. Physiol.* 441: 755–778.)

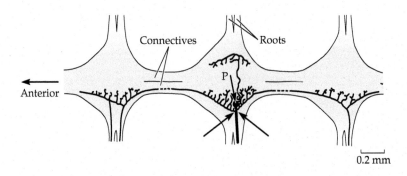

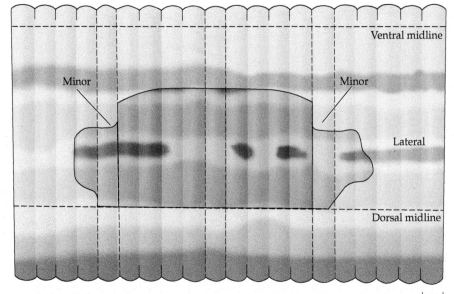

[64] Blackshaw, S. E. 1981. *J. Physiol.* 320: 219–228.

[65] Yau, K. W. 1976. *J. Physiol.* 263: 489–512.

[66] Huang, Y. et al. 1998. *J. Comp. Neurol.* 397: 394–402.

[67] Wang, H., and Macagno, E. R. 1997. *J. Neurosci.* 17: 2408–2419.

[68] Wang, H., and Macagno, E. R. 1998. *J. Neurobiol.* 35: 53–64.

[69] Blackshaw, S. E., and Nicholls, J. G. 1995. *J. Neurobiol.* 27: 267–276.

[70] Blackshaw, S. E., and Thompson, S. W. 1988. *J. Physiol.* 396: 121–137.

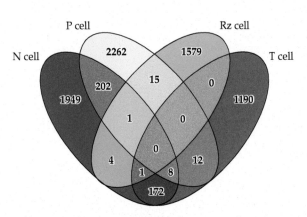

FIGURE 20.19 Venn Diagram showing the number of genes that are differentially expressed among three types of mechanosensory neurons and the neurosecretory Retzius (Rz) neuron, relative to the whole ganglion of the leech. Overlapping regions represent genes that are expressed in two or more cell types. (Courtesy of Elizabeth Heath-Heckman and David Weisblat.)

Figure 20.18 shows that individual sensory neurons innervate well-defined territories, which can be mapped by recording from a cell while applying the mechanical stimuli to different parts of the skin, or by labeling the cell and its projections with a marker, such as horseradish peroxidase.[64] The boundaries of receptive fields can be conveniently identified in relation to landmarks such as segment borders or the coloring of skin, so that one can predict reliably which cells will fire when a particular area is touched, pressed, or pinched. For example, one of the three touch-sensitive T cells innervates dorsal skin, another ventral skin, and the third lateral skin. By contrast, the two P sensory cells divide the skin into roughly equal dorsal and ventral areas. The elaborate and stereotyped branching pattern of a P sensory cell injected with horseradish peroxidase is shown in Figure 20.18. Like P cells, the T and N cells also send axons along the connectives to neighboring ganglia, and then out to innervate minor receptive fields on either side of the major region of innervation.[65] In this system, which has such clear-cut boundaries in the periphery, it has also been possible to determine how the receptive fields become established during development and regeneration.[66–68] Additional sensory cells that respond specifically to light, chemical stimuli, vibration, and stretch of the body wall have been found in the head and in the periphery of the leech.[69,70]

One wonders what molecules determine the physiological differences among the T, P, and N cells shown in Figures 20.16 and 20.17. Starting from painstakingly microdissected pools of approximately 300 neurons of each sensory type (it can now be done with single neurons), it has been possible to construct their distinct **transcriptional profiles**—lists of all the mRNA transcripts expressed by a given cell type, plus their relative abundances (see Chapter 1). It is amazing that, as Figure 20.19 shows, more than 1000 different expressed genes distinguish one cell type from another. Dozens of these genes produce membrane channels of various sorts. It is a fair promise that with an animal such as the leech it is now possible to analyze all the stages of the functioning of the nervous system, from behavior to genes and vice versa.

Motor Cells

The criterion for identifying a motoneuron is that each impulse in the cell is transmitted along its axon and produces monosynaptic responses in the muscle fibers (see also Chapter 26). In the leech, more than 20 pairs of motoneurons in a ganglion supply the various muscles that flatten, lengthen, shorten, or bend the body, while others control the heart (Figure 20.20). Muscles in the leech receive excitatory and inhibitory fibers. Excitation is carried out by acetylcholine. Muscles also receive modulatory peptidergic inputs. Deletion of a single motoneuron can give rise to a specific deficit in behavior.[71] For example, each ganglion contains one annulus erector (AE) motor cell on each side (see Figures 20.16A and 20.20). Impulses in this cell cause the skin of the leech to be raised into ridges, like an accordion. Elimination of one AE motoneuron after injection of a mixture of proteolytic enzymes (pronase) produces a failure in erection in response to appropriate sensory stimuli. This deficit is not permanent, however. Eventually branches of other AE cells sprout and supply the denervated territory.[72]

[71] Bowling, D., Nicholls, J., and Parnas, I. 1978. *J. Physiol.* 282: 169–180.

[72] Blackshaw, S. E., Nicholls, J. G., and Parnas, I. 1982. *J. Physiol.* 326: 261–268.

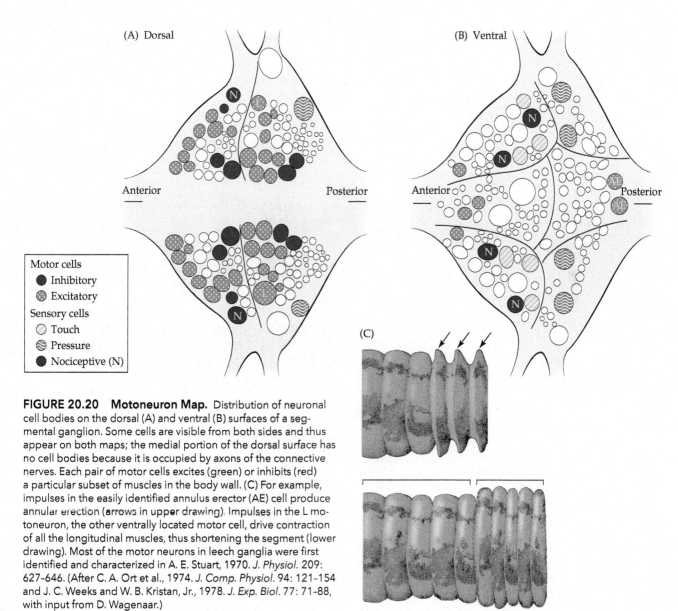

FIGURE 20.20 Motoneuron Map. Distribution of neuronal cell bodies on the dorsal (A) and ventral (B) surfaces of a segmental ganglion. Some cells are visible from both sides and thus appear on both maps; the medial portion of the dorsal surface has no cell bodies because it is occupied by axons of the connective nerves. Each pair of motor cells excites (green) or inhibits (red) a particular subset of muscles in the body wall. (C) For example, impulses in the easily identified annulus erector (AE) cell produce annular erection (arrows in upper drawing). Impulses in the L motoneuron, the other ventrally located motor cell, drive contraction of all the longitudinal muscles, thus shortening the segment (lower drawing). Most of the motor neurons in leech ganglia were first identified and characterized in A. E. Stuart, 1970. *J. Physiol.* 209: 627–646. (After C. A. Ort et al., 1974. *J. Comp. Physiol.* 94: 121–154 and J. C. Weeks and W. B. Kristan, Jr., 1978. *J. Exp. Biol.* 77: 71–88, with input from D. Wagenaar.)

Connections of Sensory and Motor Cells

As shown in Figure 20.20, while the cell bodies of sensory neurons are found mostly on the ventral surface of the ganglion, the cell bodies of most motoneurons are situated closer to the dorsal surface.[60] In the nervous systems of invertebrates, synapses between neurons are usually formed on fine processes (neurites) that accumulate within a central region of the ganglion (the neuropil) but are absent from the cell bodies.[57,73-76]

Examples of the typical ramifications of identified neurons are shown in Figure 20.21. A single sensory cell contacts many postsynaptic targets, and its presynaptic endings are themselves contacted by numerous terminals arising from other neurons that modulate its release of transmitters. Electrical synapses are common, as can be seen by the spread of small markers from an injected neuron into those with which it is electrically coupled (see Figure 20.21C).

The mechanosensory T, P, and N cells make excitatory connections on motoneurons that innervate longitudinal muscles that shorten the leech. For that reason, these are called L motoneurons. Several lines of evidence, including electron microscopy, have shown that the connections are direct (i.e., there are no known intermediary cells; see Figure 20.21C).[77] This fact is important because only if each constituent of a circuit and its properties are known can one pinpoint the sites at which interesting modifications in signaling take place. The mechanism of transmission onto the L motoneuron is different for each type of sensory cell. The N cells act through chemical synapses (with only a hint of electrical coupling), the T cells through rectifying electrical synapses, and the P cells by a combination of both.[77] The same P and N cells also make direct chemical synapses

[73] Muller, K. J., and McMahan, U. J. 1976. *Proc. R. Soc. Lond., B* 194: 481–499.

[74] French, K. A., and Muller, K. J. 1986. *J. Neurosci.* 6: 318–324.

[75] Macagno, E. R., Muller, K. J., and Pltman, R. M. 1987. *J. Physiol.* 387: 649–664.

[76] Baker, M. W. et al. 2003. *J. Neurobiol.* 56: 41–53.

[77] Nicholls, J. G., and Purves, D. 1972. *J. Physiol.* 225: 637–656.

[78] Lewis, J. E., and Kristan, W. B., Jr. 1998. *Nature* 391: 76–79.

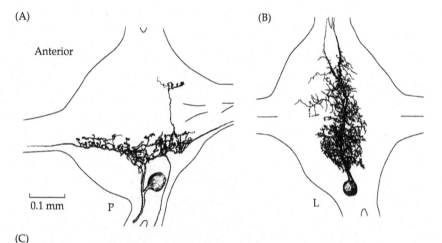

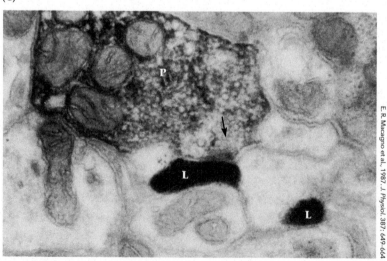

FIGURE 20.21 Structures of Pre- and Postsynaptic Cells labeled by intracellular injection of horseradish peroxidase. (A) The arborization of a pressure (P) cell (shown in Figure 20.18) is profuse, with numerous varicosities. The varicosities represent sites of presynaptic endings that release transmitter. (B) The L motoneuron sends its axons out through contralateral roots. Its processes within the ganglion are smooth and represent postsynaptic sites on which synapses are made. (C) A synapse (arrow) made by a P cell onto an L motoneuron in the neuropil. Both cells were injected with horseradish peroxidase. (A,B after K. J. Muller et al., 1976. *Proc. R. Soc. Lond. B.* 194481-194499.)

E. R. Macagno et al., 1987. *J. Physiol.* 387: 649-664

FIGURE 20.22 Short-Term Changes in Synaptic Plasticity between Sensory and Motor Neurons. (A) Chemical and electrical transmission. A nociceptive (N) or T cell is stimulated twice in succession, and its impulses are recorded (upper trace). Facilitation occurs at the chemical synapse between N and L cells, so the second impulse leads to a larger synaptic potential (facilitation; bottom left). In contrast, at the T–L synapse, no facilitation is seen, which is typical of electrical synapses. (B) Characteristics of transmitter release at different synapses made by a single presynaptic neuron. An N cell is stimulated and responses are recorded in L and annulus erector (AE) cells. Facilitation is greater at the N–AE synapse. (The small, first synaptic potential in the AE cell is marked by an arrow.) (C) When a train of impulses is evoked by stimulating the N cell at a rate of 2 per second (in elevated Ca^{2+}), the synaptic potentials in the AE cell are facilitated to more than double their original size, whereas those in the L cell decrease in amplitude (depression). The x-axis indicates the position number of the synaptic potential in the train. The y-axis gives the height of the synaptic potentials at each position relative to the average size of potentials recorded before the train (set at 100%). (A after J. G. Nicholls and D. Purves, 1972. *J. Physiol.* 225: 637–656; B,C after K. J. Muller and J. G. Nicholls, 1974. *J. Physiol.* 238: 357–369.)

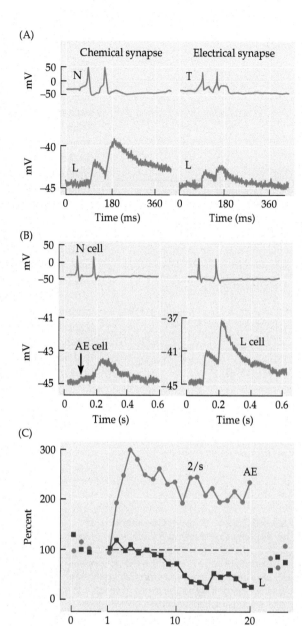

on the AE motoneuron. As illustrated in Figure 20.22, the differing properties of synapses linking specific pairwise combinations of neurons mean that the same cell may be affected differently by otherwise similar presynaptic inputs, and that a given output from one cell can affect two postsynaptic targets differently.

In the leech, as in other animals, the monosynaptic sensory-to-motor connections that produce rapid reflexes are paralleled by indirect connections in which one or more layers of interneurons are interposed between sensory inputs and motor outputs. The polysynaptic routes coordinate more complex directional movements evoked by mechanical stimuli. For example, Kristan and his colleagues have analyzed how a leech bends in response to pressure applied to a segment from different angles. The reflex shown in Figure 20.23 is produced by activation of P and T cells, and the bend directs the segment of the animal away from the stimulus.[48,78] By comparing the frequency of firing of each active P neuron, one can predict the origin of the stimulus.

The information coming from the various P cells is processed by a network of two dozen or so interneurons that select which motoneurons to activate. When a P cell innervating dorsal skin is activated by pressure, it excites excitatory motoneurons that induce contraction of longitudinal muscles near the point of contact and inhibitory neurons on the ventral side. Conversely, when ventral skin is pressed, the ventral muscles contract while those on the dorsal side relax.

FIGURE 20.23 Behavioral Integration by Interneurons in the leech bending reflex. When the skin of a leech is pressed at one point, a reflex bend withdraws that region of the body away from the stimulus. Bending in the appropriate direction occurs by contracting certain muscles and relaxing others. (After J. E. Lewis and W. B. Kristan, 1998. *Nature* 391: 76–79.)

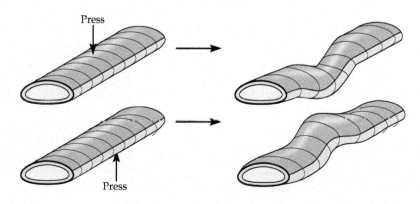

Behavioral Changes in Response to Experience

The sea slug *Aplysia* has been useful for elucidating mechanisms by which transmission can be modified at individual synapses as a result of experience.[1,79–83] In the leech, a complex function of this sort is carried out by the S cell, a single, small and unpaired interneuron in each ganglion (Figure 20.24; see also Figure 20.16A).[84] The S cell receives excitatory inputs from touch and pressure sensory cells and, in turn, excites the L motoneuron, which causes shortening (as already discussed). Each S cell is electrically connected to its homologues in the adjacent ganglia by large, rapidly conducting axons. Injecting different intracellular markers that cannot cross gap junctions into each of two adjacent S cells has shown that their coupling occurs in the midregion of the connective nerve (see Figure 20.24).

The chain of S cells is essential for adaptive types of behavior. Touching a segment of the leech produces a reflex shortening. If the touch is repeated regularly at the same intensity, the shortening becomes progressively weaker—a phenomenon known as **habituation** (Figure 20.25).[85] The sudden arrival of a stronger stimulus that activates P and N cells (as well as T cells) at a different region of the body wall restores the shortening response to touch. This recovery process is known as **dishabituation**. Similarly, if a strong stimulus is applied without previous habituation, **sensitization** occurs; that is, the strength of the response to touch becomes greater than normal. In technically difficult experiments carried out by Muller and his colleagues, the axon of an S cell was cut, or an S cell was killed by injection of the enzyme pronase. Such experimental manipulations did not interfere with shortening or habituation as such, but they disabled dishabituation and sensitization (see Figure 20.25B,C).

[79] Si, K., Lindquist, S., and Kandel, E. 2004. *Cold Spring Harb. Symp. Quant. Biol.* 69: 497-498.

[80] Kandel, E. R. 2001. *Science* 294: 1030-1038.

[81] Glanzman, D. L. 2009. *Neurobiol. Learn. Mem.* 92: 147-154.

[82] Hickie, C., Cohen, L. B., and Balaban, P. M. 1997. *Eur. J. Neurosci.* 9: 627-636.

[83] Walters, E. T., and Cohen, L. B. 1997. *Invert. Neurosci.* 3: 15-25.

[84] Muller, K. J., and Carbonetto, S. 1979. *J. Comp. Neurol.* 185: 485-516.

[85] Sahley, C. L. et al. 1994. *J. Neurosci.* 14: 6715-6721.

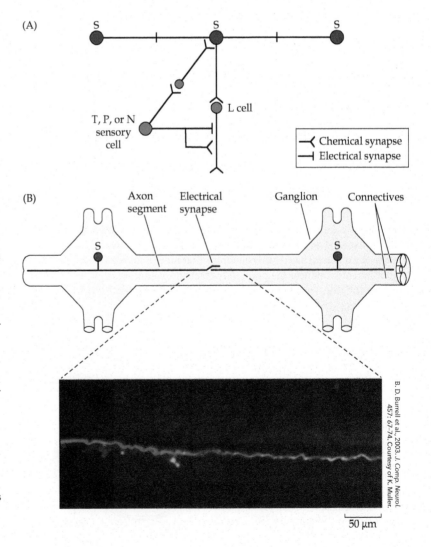

FIGURE 20.24 Known Connections of the Rapidly Conducting S Cells. (A) Electrical and chemical connections of sensory touch (T), pressure (P), and nociceptive (N) cells as well as S cells onto the L motoneuron. Each ganglion contains only one S cell, the axons of which make electrical synapses with its homologues. The S cell chain modulates (but is not required for) rapid shortening in response to sensory stimuli. (B) S cell processes connect to processes emanating from their homologues in neighboring ganglia midway along the interganglionic connective—by electrical synapses. The photomicrograph shows an interganglionic connective from a preparation in which the S cell whose process enters from the left (red) was injected with a mixture of Lucifer yellow (LY; yellow-green) and rhodamine-dextran (RD; red). RD (molecular weight > 10 kDA) cannot cross from cell to cell through electrical junctions, whereas LY (molecular weight ~0.5 kDa) can. Accordingly, the axon of the right-hand S cell became labeled with LY but not with RD. S cell axons regenerate and re-form their connections with very high specificity after injury. The micrograph, which resembles that of a normal animal, was in fact taken from a preparation in which the axon of one S cell had been severed and had re-formed its connections after regeneration. (B after A. Mason and K. J. Muller, 1996. *Eur. J. Neurosci.* 8: 11-20.)

B. D. Burrell et al., 2003. *J. Comp. Neurol.* 457: 67-74. Courtesy of K. Muller.

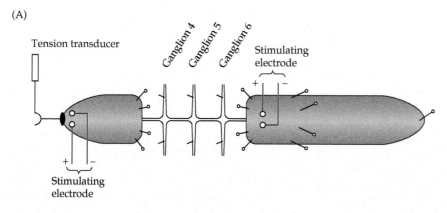

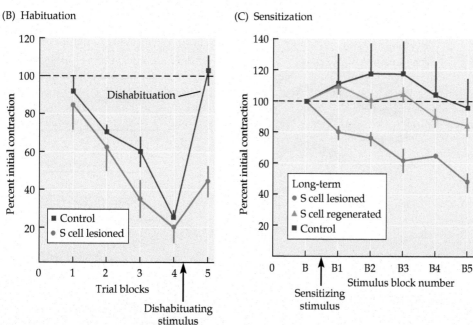

FIGURE 20.25 Habituation, Dishabituation, and Sensitization of leech reflexes, and the role of the S cell. (A) Exposed ganglia are connected to the anterior and posterior parts of the body. Stimuli are applied to anterior or posterior skin by electrodes or by mechanical stimuli that activate touch (T), pressure (P), and/or nociceptive (N) cells. Intracellular recordings are made from S cells, sensory cells, and motoneurons; muscle contractions are measured with a tension transducer. (B,C) Responses to stimuli in control animals (red squares) and animals in which the S cell was lesioned (blue circles), and in some cases regenerated (green triangles). The control animals were subjected to sham operations; the body wall was opened but the S cell was left intact. (B) Responses to weak electrical shocks to posterior skin. In repeated trials, the control animals exhibited habituation; after the

fourth trial, a strong stimulus produced dishabituation. After lesioning an S cell in one segment, only habituation occurred. (C) When a strong sensitizing stimulus was given, the responses of control animals became stronger than normal (sensitization) instead of habituating. After elimination of the S cell, sensitization could no longer be elicited; repeated stimuli produced only habituation. After a severed S cell axon had regenerated, a strong stimulus once again gave rise to sensitization. This experiment demonstrates that a single cell is essential for these complex responses. Error bars indicate the standard error from the mean. (A,C after B. K. Modney et al., 1997. *J. Neurosci.* 17: 6478-6482; B after C. L. Sahley, C. L. et al., 1994. *J. Neurosci.* 14: 6715-6721. © 1994, 1997 Society for Neuroscience.)

A related series of experiments confirmed the importance of the S cell in these processes; in this work, the axon of a single S cell was lesioned and then allowed to regenerate.[86] As expected, breaking the train of transmission along the S cells throughout the length of the animal abolished sensitization. Some weeks later, when the S cell axon had regenerated and re-formed its connections, sensitization could be produced again, as shown in Figure 20.25C.[87] These experiments provide a clear demonstration of the way in which a single cell can play a part in a highly complex response, such as sensitization.

[86] Elliott, E. J., and Muller, K. J. 1983. *J. Neurosci.* 3: 1994-2006.

[87] Modney, B. K., Sahley, C. L., and Muller, K. J. 1997. *J. Neurosci.* 17: 6478-6482.

Circuits Responsible for the Production of Rhythmical Swimming

The locomotor behaviors of ants, bees, crayfish, and leeches already described have common features. First, they are evoked by sensory stimulation. Second, walking, flying, and swimming are rhythmic movements produced by central pattern generators that give rise to alternate cyclic contractions of antagonistic muscles (this also occurs in vertebrates, as we will discuss in Chapter 26). Breathing, chewing, and gastric moments in vertebrates and invertebrates are other examples of rhythmic behaviors.

Mild agitation of the water containing leeches induces them to swim toward the jittering object. Swimming in leeches is a stereotyped forward locomotion generated by repeated serpentine movements of the body (Figure 20.26A). The cycle in each segment consists of the alternate contraction of ventral and dorsal muscles. A wave of such cycles spreads repetitively from head to tail. Again the accessibility of the leech CNS made it intellectually appealing to Stent, Kristan, Friesen, and their colleagues,[88] who searched for the neurons

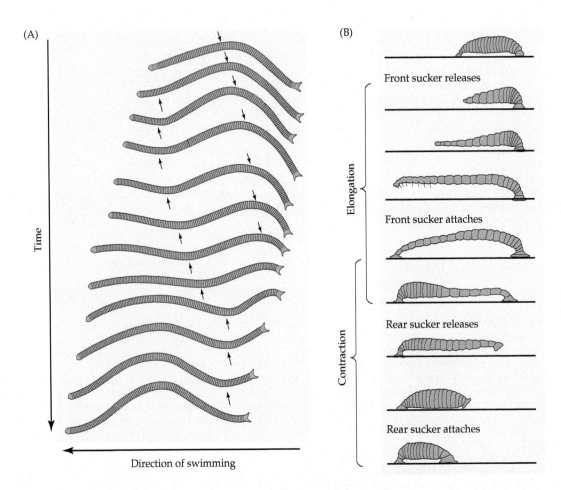

FIGURE 20.26 Locomotory Behaviors of the Leech. (A) In swimming, the leech releases its anterior sucker from the substrate, extends the body forward, and flattens dorsoventrally to generate a blade-shaped profile; then, it releases the posterior sucker and propels itself through the water by passing a wave of rapidly alternating dorsal and ventral flexures from front to back. (B) In vermiform (as opposed to inchworm style) crawling, the animal releases its front sucker and then reaches forward by simultaneously relaxing its longitudinal muscles and contracting its circular muscles to extend the hydrostatic skeleton. After extending, the front sucker attaches and the rear sucker detaches. The animal then shortens by contracting its longitudinal muscles and relaxing its circular muscles, and finally reattaches the rear sucker to complete the cycle. The alternating cycles of extension and contraction also progress from front to back. (A after G. S. Stent et al., 1978. *Science* 200: 1348–1357; B after T. W. Cacciatore et al., 2000. *J. Neurosci.* 20: 1643–1655. © 2000 Society for Neuroscience.)

that initiate, coordinate, and maintain swimming. They were able to record a swim rhythm from chains of ganglia by placing an extracellular suction electrode on a nerve root of one such ganglion, recording the rhythmical output of motoneuron axons in the nerve. Bursts of action potentials occur roughly once per second, a frequency similar to that of the oscillatory waves of the animal as it swims. It is remarkable that a few isolated ganglia or even just one can produce the swimming rhythms; the head and tail ganglia are not essential but send commands that modulate the activity of the whole CNS.[89,90]

A key to the successful analysis of swimming in the leech was the development of a semi-intact preparation. A single midbody ganglion was exposed and immobilized for electrical recordings, attached to the free-moving anterior and posterior ends of the animal by only the intersegmental connectives. Electrical activity from individual neurons could then be recorded with intracellular microelectrodes. The role of each neuron contributing to the circuit could then be tested by stimulating or inhibiting its electrical activity by current injection through the electrode while the two ends of the animal were demonstrably swimming. It was found that peripheral receptors trigger, enhance, depress, or halt swimming. The central pattern generator that produces the oscillations during swimming in the leech requires a small number of identifiable neurons that interact through excitatory and inhibitory synaptic interactions, with some neurons located in adjacent ganglia of the chain. A similar approach was used to characterize the very differently coordinated interneuron circuitry and motor outputs associated with the crawling behavior of the leech (Figure 20.26B).

As in most animals tested (see Chapter 18), biogenic amines modulate the motor activity of leeches.[91-94] Quiescent (sluggish!), non-swimming leeches have lower blood levels of 5-hydroxytryptamine (5-HT or serotonin) than do active leeches. Stimulation of serotoninergic Retzius cells produces massive 5-HT release that increases its concentration in the CNS and blood and promotes swimming in the animal. An analogue of 5-HT (5,7-dihydroxytryptamine, or 5,7-DHT) that selectively destroys the 5-HT neurons in the developing ganglia lowers the levels of 5-HT in embryos. After development, adults that had been depleted of serotonin do not swim spontaneously, but they will do so if immersed in a weak solution of 5-HT.

Why Should One Work on Invertebrate Nervous Systems?

Throughout this book, and from the examples described in this chapter, it is evident that invertebrate nervous systems have been essential for approaching problem after problem relating to the biophysics, cell biology, and development of nerve cells. Particularly striking is the conservation of fundamental mechanisms in species after species through evolution. Often, experiments on an invertebrate have produced the very insight needed for starting the investigation of similar problems in a mammal. For example, a great impetus for the development of the slice technique for mammalian brain came from the work on invertebrate ganglia in which identified neurons could be seen directly in the microscope as they were impaled. Hartline's work on the horseshoe crab eye[95] provided the key stimulus for Kuffler's experiments on the cat retina.[96] At the same time, it would be futile to hope to understand how the visual cortex of a monkey carries out its functions from studies made on an invertebrate. Moreover, technical developments designed for studying such circuits are now commonly used in vertebrates.

What then is the point of studying, say, navigation by ants or bees? First, one can guess that even though we do not see polarized light or sense magnetic fields, the underlying principles for analyzing sensory information and translating it to an effective output will be used again in higher nervous systems, in one way or another. Second, the work on invertebrates illustrates a fundamental attitude toward biology—neurobiology is not restricted to the study of *the* brain (i.e., ours). Rather, there is an inherent fascination in trying to understand how the tiny, finite brain of an invertebrate can do wonderful and sophisticated computations that are essential for its survival. The way in which a leech swims, an ant navigates, a bee dances, a sea slug learns, a cricket sings, or a fly flies are all problems of interest in their own right.[97]

[88] Stent, G. S. et al. 1978. *Science* 200: 1348-1357.

[89] Mullins, O. J., and Friesen, W. O. 2012. *J. Neurophysiol.* 107: 2730-2741.

[90] Puhl, J. G., Masino, M. A., and Mesce, K. A. 2012. *J. Neurosci.* 32: 17646-17657.

[91] Calvino, M. A., and Szczupak, L. 2008. *J. Comp. Physiol. A* 194: 523-531.

[92] Glover, J. C., and Kramer, A. P. 1982. *Science* 216: 317-319.

[93] Willard, A. L. 1981. *J. Neurosci.* 1: 936-944.

[94] Brodfuehrer, P. D. et al. 1995. *J. Neurobiol.* 27: 403-418.

[95] Hartline, H. K. 1940. *Am. J. Physiol.* 130: 690-699.

[96] Kuffler, S. W. 1953. *J. Neurophysiol.* 16: 37-68.

[97] Baca, S. M. et al. 2008. *Neuron* 57: 276-289.

SUMMARY

- The properties of individual neurons and glia are similar between vertebrates and invertebrates. However, invertebrate nervous systems generally have far fewer cells and correspondingly simpler organizations than those of vertebrates.

- Correlated with their comparative simplicity, invertebrate behaviors, though tremendously sophisticated, are often more stereotyped than those of vertebrates and thus more amenable to study. Quantitative measurements of these behaviors shed light on fundamental principles in neurobiology.

- Ants and bees routinely carry out remarkable navigational feats using multiple sensory systems in parallel, including visual cues, the direction of polarization of light, the ability to orient with respect to an external magnetic field, and several forms of learning.

- Studies of crayfish have shown how the visual system categorizes visual responses in deciding between opposite, incompatible behaviors.

- In the leech and some other invertebrate preparations, much or all of the nervous system contains relatively large, identifiable, and experimentally accessible cells. In such preparations it is possible to analyze from the fundamental properties of neurons and connections to behaviors.

- The study of the invertebrate CNS is fascinating in its own right and need not be directed toward understanding mechanisms in the human brain.

Suggested Reading

General Reviews

Bailey, C. H., and Kandel, E. R. 2008. Synaptic remodeling, synaptic growth and the storage of long-term memory in Aplysia. *Prog. Brain Res.* 169: 179–198.

Cheng, K., Narendra, A., Sommer, S., and Wehner, R. 2009. Traveling in clutter: Navigation in the Central Australian desert ant *Melophorus bagoti. Behav. Processes* 80: 261–268.

Collett, M., Chittka, L., and Collett, T. S. 2013. Spatial memory in insect navigation. *Curr. Biol.* 23: R789–R800.

Freas, C. A., and Schultheiss, P. 2018. How to navigate in different environments and situations: Lessons from ants. *Front. Psychol.* 9: 841.

Friesen, W. O., and Kristan, W. B. 2007. Leech locomotion: Swimming, crawling, and decisions. *Curr. Opin. Neurobiol.* 17: 704–711.

Heinze, S. 2017. Unraveling the neural basis of insect navigation. *Curr. Opin. Insect Sci.* 24: 58–67.

Katz, P. S. 2016. Evolution of central pattern generators and rhythmic behaviours. *Phil. Trans. R. Soc. B* 371: 20150057. doi: 10.1098/rstb.2015.0057.

Leonard, J. L., and Edstrom, J. P. 2004. Parallel processing in an identified neural circuit: the Aplysia californica gill-withdrawal response model system. *Biol. Rev. Camb. Philos. Soc.* 79: 1–59.

Marder, E., and Bucher, D. 2007. Understanding circuit dynamics using the stomatogastric nervous system of lobsters and crabs. *Annu. Rev. Physiol.* 69: 291–316.

Srinivasan, M. V. 2010. Honeybees as a model for vision, perception, and cognition. *Annu. Rev. Entomol.* 55: 267–284.

Walters, E. T., and Cohen, L. B. 1997. Function of the LE sensory neurons in *Aplysia. Invert. Neurosci.* 3: 15–25.

Wehner, R., Hoinville, T., Cruse, H., and Cheng, K. 2016. Steering intermediate courses: desert ants combine information from various navigational routines. *J. Comp. Physiol. A Neuroethol. Sens. Neural Behav. Physiol.* 202: 459–472.

Original Papers

Bao, L., Samuels, S., Locovei, S., Macagno, E. R., Muller, K. J., and Dahl, G. 2007. Innexins form two types of channels. *FEBS Lett.* 581: 5703–5708.

De-Miguel, F. F., and Arechiga, H. 1992. Sensory inputs mediating two opposite behavioural responses to light in the crayfish *Procambarus clarkii. J. Exp. Biol.* 164: 153–169.

Gu, X. 1991. Effect of conduction block at axon bifurcations on synaptic transmission to different postsynaptic neurones in the leech. *J. Physiol.* 441: 755–778.

Lewis, J. E., and Kristan, W. B., Jr. 1998. Quantitative analysis of a directed behavior in the medicinal leech: Implications for organizing motor output. *J. Neurosci.* 18: 1571–1582.

Modney, B. K., Sahley, C. L., and Muller, K. J. 1997. Regeneration of a central synapse restores nonassociative learning. *J. Neurosci.* 17: 6478–6482

Srinivasan, M., Zhang, S., Lehrer, M., and Collett, T. 1996. Honeybee navigation en route to the goal: Visual flight control and odometry. *J. Exp. Biol.* 199: 237–244.

Wittlinger, M., Wehner, R., and Wolf, H. 2006. The ant odometer: stepping on stilts and stumps. *Science* 312: 1965–1967.

PART V

Sensation

We know the world through our senses. We reach out and touch nearby objects to feel their shape and texture, and sample the taste of objects in our mouth to see if they are edible. Our eyes and ears respond to visual and auditory signals from afar. In this section we examine the mechanisms by which our brain acquires, analyzes, and acts on this rich variety of sensory information. Chapter 21 provides an overview of the conversion of environmental events into neuronal signals, a process called transduction. It introduces key concepts such as sensitivity, selectivity, receptor potentials, and rate of adaptation and then describes in more detail how chemical stimuli collected by the tongue and nose are converted into electrical signals.

Chapter 22 describes how light produces changes in the membrane potential of photoreceptors in the eye and then outlines how photoreceptor responses are processed in the retina to produce the signals sent by retinal ganglion cells to the center of the brain.

By discussing how sensory receptors transduce mechanical stimuli impinging on the skin, Chapter 23 covers touch sensation, including texture discrimination and pain, another sensory experience that can arise from excitation of skin receptors. The example of tactile whiskers on the muzzle of rodents is used to illustrate how the sensory signals are processed to produce an organized topographic map of whisker location on the somatosensory cortex.

Chapter 24 describes the processing of auditory signals, starting with hair cells in the cochlea and progressing centrally to the auditory cortex. This is followed by a discussion of transduction by hair cells in the vestibular apparatus.

Chapter 25 examines how information from primary sensory cortex is processed in higher-order cortical areas where *meaning* might emerge from stimuli. Finally, Chapter 26 discusses how the nervous system integrates hierarchical information to produce commands that evoke movement. Additional information about this topic in invertebrate nervous systems can be found in Chapter 20.

CHAPTER 21

Sensory Transduction

While the things that surround us are, of course, of real substance and material, we can possess knowledge about the world only after signals connected to or emanating from these things are acquired by our sensory systems. Neuronal sensory receptors are the gateways through which these signals pass. Receptors set the stage for all the analyses of sensory events that are subsequently made within the central nervous system (CNS). They define the limits of sensitivity and determine the range of stimuli that can be detected. Each type of receptor is specialized to respond preferentially to only one type of stimulus energy, called the adequate stimulus. For instance, rods and cones in the eye respond to light (see Chapter 22). The stimulus, whatever its modality, is always converted (transduced) to an electrical signal—the receptor potential. The sensory percept—the experience felt by the individual—is determined by the identity of the activated receptor. Thus, if you press your hand against your eye (do not try this experiment), your eye converts the inappropriate mechanical signal into nerve impulses that, once processed in the brain, are sensed as flashes of light. The strength and duration of a stimulus are coded in the magnitude and duration of the electrical response. Recognition of the location of the signal is determined by the anatomical location of the receptor.

Sensory receptors are exquisitely sensitive to their **adequate stimulus**. For example, a few molecules of a specific odorant, once bound to olfactory receptors in the nose, can be detected. A few quanta of light trapped by receptors in the retina are sufficient to produce a visual sensation. Air pressure waves reach the inner ear, where acoustic hair cells convert mechanical displacements of 10^{-10} meters (0.1 nanometers [nm]) into electrical signals that give rise to detection of a sound.[1] Equally remarkable are electroreceptors in some fish that can detect electrical fields of a few nanovolts per centimeter.[2,3] This signal is similar in magnitude to the field that would be produced if two wires connected to opposite poles of an ordinary flashlight battery could be dipped into the Atlantic Ocean—one wire at Bordeaux, the other at New York!

Sensory receptors have a well-defined range of stimuli to which they respond. For example, our auditory hair cells respond to sounds only within a frequency range of about 20 to 20,000 Hz. The response to light by receptors in our retina is restricted to wavelengths between about 400 and 750 nm; shorter (near-ultraviolet) and longer (near-infrared) wavelengths go undetected. Each system is tuned to the particular needs of the organism—whales and bats can hear much higher frequencies than our 20,000 Hz; radiation wavelengths that we cannot see can be detected by other species—snakes detect infrared, and bees ultraviolet, radiation.

While receptors can convert extraordinarily tiny quantities of energy into neural activity provided that energy matches the adequate stimulus (**sensitivity**), receptors are shielded from energy in a modality that does not match the adequate stimulus (**selectivity**). For instance, the mechanical energy required to excite the optic nerve (the pressure on the eye) is untold times greater than the mechanical energy required to excite fingertip skin receptors. What mechanisms provide sensitivity and selectivity to sensory receptor cells? These vary according to the stimulus and receptor type. In **mechanotransduction** by stretch receptors in muscle, touch receptors in skin, and hair cells of the inner ear, the stimulus acts directly on mechanosensitive ion channels to produce the electrical response. By contrast, **chemotransduction** in olfactory neurons operates through G protein-coupling to an olfactory receptor protein. Taste cells employ both direct and G protein-coupled mechanisms, as do nociceptors that mediate sensations of pain.

Stimulus Coding by Mechanoreceptors

Short and Long Receptors

In general, receptors have two functional regions: At one pole of the cell is the **sensory ending** that is activated by the stimulus, and at the other pole is a synaptic region where the signal is passed on to the next neuron in the sensory pathway. In some receptors, such as retinal rods and inner ear hair cells, the electrical signals generated by the transduction itself, or **receptor potentials**, spread passively from the sensory ending to the synaptic pole of the cell (Figure 21.1A). Such receptors are known as **short receptors**. In some cells, passive spread of the receptor potential can reach a surprisingly distant point. For example, in some crustacean[4] and leech[5] mechanoreceptors, and in photoreceptors in the barnacle eye,[6] the receptor potential spreads passively over a distance of several millimeters. In such cells the membrane resistance, and hence the length constant for spread of passive depolarization, is unusually high.

Whereas receptor potentials are usually depolarizing, certain short receptors respond to their adequate stimulus with a hyperpolarizing potential change. This action occurs, for example, in photoreceptors of the vertebrate retina (see Chapter 22) and in cochlear hair cells that have both hyperpolarizing and depolarizing responses. Whatever the polarity of the receptor potential, short receptors release neurotransmitter tonically from their synaptic regions, with depolarization increasing and hyperpolarization decreasing the rate of release.

In **long receptors** (Figure 21.1B), such as those in skin or muscle, information from single receptors must be sent over a much greater distance to reach the next neuron (e.g., from the big toe to the spinal cord in a giraffe). In order to convey the sensory message over a long distance, long receptors perform a second transformation process in which the depolarizing receptor potential gives rise to action potentials. These impulses then carry the message, with no loss of information, from the point of initiation to the receptor's synaptic terminals.

[1] Bialek, W. 1987. *Annu. Rev. Biophys. Biophys. Chem.* 16: 455–478.

[2] Kalmijn, A. J. 1982. *Science* 218: 916–918.

[3] Heiligenberg, W. 1989. *J. Exp. Biol.* 146: 255–275.

[4] Roberts, A., and Bush, B. M. 1971. *J. Exp. Biol.* 54: 515–524.

[5] Blackshaw, S. E., and Thompson, S. W. 1988. *J. Physiol.* 396: 121–137.

[6] Hudspeth, A. J., Poo, M. M., and Stuart, A. E. 1977. *J. Physiol.* 272: 25–43.

(A) Short receptor

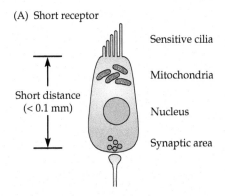

Sensitive cilia

Mitochondria

Nucleus

Synaptic area

Short distance (< 0.1 mm)

FIGURE 21.1 Short and Long Sensory Receptor Cells. (A) Short receptors—such as retinal rods and cones, and mechanosensitive hair cells of the inner ear—are less than 100 μm in length. Thus, receptor potentials generated within the sensory ending spread effectively throughout the cell, altering transmitter release at synaptic areas. (B) Long receptors, such as muscle spindle afferents and cutaneous mechanoreceptors, employ action potentials to conduct their signals to a distant second-order neuron. The amplitude of the receptor potential is encoded in the frequency of action potentials it generates.

(B) Long receptor

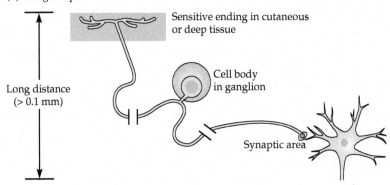

Sensitive ending in cutaneous or deep tissue

Cell body in ganglion

Long distance (> 0.1 mm)

Synaptic area

The number of action potentials per unit of time (frequency) increases in relation to stimulus amplitude. This frequency code is established through the interaction of the maintained receptor current from sensory terminals and the conductance changes associated with the action potential. The increased potassium conductance that occurs on the recovery phase of each action potential drives the membrane potential toward E_K (the potassium equilibrium potential). As this transient increase in potassium conductance fades, the sustained transduction current depolarizes the membrane back to the firing threshold. The stronger the receptor current, the sooner the firing threshold again is reached, and the higher the impulse frequency.

[7] Adrian, E. D., and Zotterman, Y. 1926. *J. Physiol.* 61: 151-171.

[8] Katz, B. 1950. *J. Physiol.* 111: 261-282.

Encoding Stimulus Parameters by Stretch Receptors

The way in which sensory receptors generate electrical signals was studied early on by Adrian and Zotterman,[7] using extracellular recording from sensory nerve fibers arising in vertebrate muscle stretch receptors. Katz was the first to demonstrate the link between sensory stimuli and electrical signals in a mechanoreceptor,[8] when he recorded receptor potentials and showed that stretch caused a depolarization of the sensory ending. When the receptor potential was observed in isolation by blocking the nerve discharge with procaine (a local anesthetic), its amplitude could be seen to increase in a graded fashion with muscle stretch.

Figure 21.2 shows the relationship between receptor potential amplitude and stretch. The function begins with a slope of roughly 0.1 millivolts (mV) (extracellular recording) per millimeter of stretch, but flattens out at higher levels. Thus, the *sensitivity* of the sensory ending—change in millivolts per change in millimeter of stretch—decreases as the stimulus grows. Many sensory receptors take advantage of this nonlinear relationship to provide amplitude coding over a wide range of stimulus intensities. In these receptors the response amplitude increases in proportion to the logarithm of stimulus intensity. This effect is of great utility in receptors, such as hair cells and photoreceptors, that respond to stimuli whose amplitudes vary by several orders of magnitude.

This relationship between stimulus intensity and sensitivity has consequences for the perception of stimuli. In 1846 Weber measured the ability of individuals to discriminate weights held in their two hands and showed that it varied in proportion to the size of the

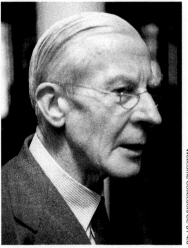

E. D. Adrian

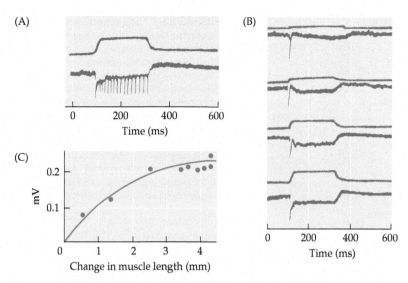

FIGURE 21.2 Receptor Potentials Recorded Extracellularly from a sensory nerve fiber supplying a muscle spindle. The recording electrode is placed as close as possible to the receptor. Downward deflection of the voltage record (lower traces) indicates receptor depolarization. (A) Stretching the muscle (upper trace) produces a receptor potential, on which is superimposed a series of action potentials (lower trace). (B) Four stretches of increasing magnitude applied to the muscle after procaine has been added to the bathing solution. Action potentials (except for the first) are abolished by procaine, but the receptor potentials remain. (C) Plot of receptor potential amplitude against stretch, quanitified as the change in muscle length. (After B. Katz, 1950. *J. Physiol.* 111: 261-282.)

weights. That is, the individuals were just able to detect a 3-gram (g) difference between weights of about 100 g each, whereas weights of 1 kilogram (kg) had to differ by 30 g. In each case, the detectable difference was about 3% of each object's weight. Subsequently, Fechner formalized this relationship, pointing out that it implied a logarithmic relationship between actual stimulus amplitude and perceived stimulus amplitude.[9] The Weber–Fechner relationship is a formulation of the nonlinear connection between stimulus strength and sensation, and its starting point resides in the properties of receptor cells. Although the exact form of the relationship depends on sensory modality, this process applies generally to stimulus perception. The same principal of proportionality pertains to aspects of human behavior that cannot be accounted for merely by receptor cell properties. For example, we are less concerned with a $1.00 increase in the price of a $100.00 item than with the same increase in the price of a $5.00 item.

The Crayfish Stretch Receptor

Stimulus coding was analyzed in detail in crayfish stretch receptors by Eyzaguirre and Kuffler.[10] This preparation is particularly useful because the cell body of the stretch receptor lies in isolation—not in a ganglion, but on its own in the periphery, where it can be seen in live preparations (Figure 21.3A). It is large enough for penetration by intracellular microelectrodes. The cell inserts its dendrites into a nearby muscle strand and sends an axon centrally to a segmental ganglion (Figure 21.3B). In addition, the receptor receives inhibitory innervation from the ganglion. Thus, receptor sensitivity is regulated by the CNS. The muscle fibers into which the receptor inserts receive excitatory and inhibitory innervation.

There are two types of crustacean stretch receptors with distinct structural and physiological characteristics, and their dendrites are embedded in different types of muscle. One responds robustly at the beginning of a stretch, but its response quickly wanes. This decrease in response as the stimulus persists is called **adaptation**. In contrast to such a **rapidly adapting** receptor, the second type of receptor is **slowly adapting**; its response is maintained during prolonged stretch, albeit not as vigorously as at stimulus onset. Typical responses of a slowly adapting and a rapidly adapting stretch receptor are shown in Figure 21.4. In the slowly adapting receptor (see Figure 21.4A), mild stretch of the muscle produces a depolarizing receptor

[9] Boring, E. G. 1942. *Sensation and Perception in the History of Experimental Psychology.* Appleton-Century, New York.

[10] Eyzaguirre, C., and Kuffler, S. W. 1955. *J. Gen. Physiol.* 39: 87-119.

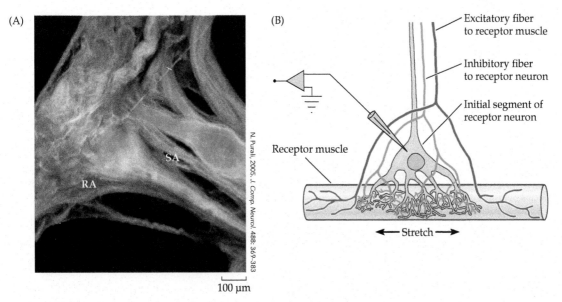

FIGURE 21.3 Crustacean Stretch Receptor. (A) Superimposed picture of tubulin filaments in muscle (gray) and the receptor neurons (red). SA is slowly adapting and RA is rapidly adapting. (B) Relation between stretch receptor neuron and muscle, indicating the method of intracellular recording. The excitatory fiber to the muscle produces contraction; the inhibitory fiber innervates the neuron. Two additional inhibitory fibers are not shown. (B after C. Eyzaguirre and S. W. Kuffler, 1955. *J. Gen. Physiol.* 39: 87–119.)

potential of about 5 mV, lasting for the duration of the stretch. A larger stretch produces a larger potential that depolarizes the cell to above threshold and produces a train of action potentials that propagate centrally along the axon. A similar stretch of the muscle produces only a transient response in the rapidly adapting receptor (see Figure 21.4B).

Muscle Spindles

Stretch receptors in mammalian skeletal muscles show mechanisms of action similar to those in crustaceans. Such stretch receptors were called muscle spindles by early anatomists because of their resemblance to the spindles used by weavers. (Muscle fibers within the spindle are called intrafusal fibers, from the Latin *fusus*, "spindle.") Figure 21.5 illustrates schematically the sensory apparatus of spindles in leg muscles of the cat. The spindle

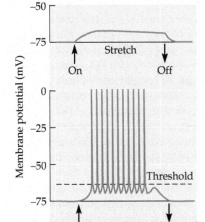

(A) Slowly adapting receptor

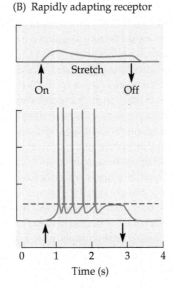

(B) Rapidly adapting receptor

FIGURE 21.4 Responses of Stretch Receptor Neurons to increases in muscle length, recorded intracellularly as indicated in Figure 21.3B. (A) In a slowly adapting receptor, a weak stretch for about 2 seconds produces a subthreshold receptor potential that persists throughout the stretch (upper record). With a stronger stretch, a larger receptor potential sets up a series of action potentials (lower record). (B) In a rapidly adapting receptor, the receptor potential is not maintained (upper record), and during the large stretch, the action potential frequency declines (lower record). (Based on data and simulations in C. Eyzaguirre and S. W. Kuffler, 1955. *J. Gen. Physiol.* 39: 87–119.)

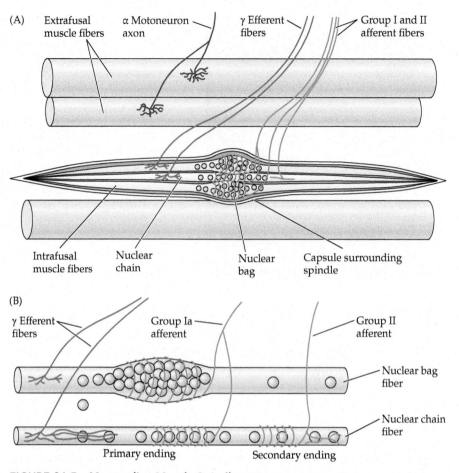

(A)

Extrafusal muscle fibers

α Motoneuron axon

γ Efferent fibers

Group I and II afferent fibers

Intrafusal muscle fibers

Nuclear chain

Nuclear bag

Capsule surrounding spindle

(B)

γ Efferent fibers

Group Ia afferent

Group II afferent

Nuclear bag fiber

Nuclear chain fiber

Primary ending

Secondary ending

FIGURE 21.5 Mammalian Muscle Spindle. (A) Scheme of mammalian muscle spindle innervation. The spindle, composed of small intrafusal fibers, is embedded in the bulk of the muscle, which is made up of large muscle fibers supplied by α motoneurons. Intrafusal fibers are supplied by γ efferent (fusimotor) fibers. Group I and Group II afferent fibers carry sensory signals from the muscle spindle to the spinal cord. (B) Simplified diagram of intrafusal muscle types and their innervation. (B after J. K. S. Jansen and P. B. C. Matthews. 1962. *J. Physiol.* 161: 357–378.)

consists of a capsule containing 8 to 10 intrafusal fibers. In the central, or equatorial, region there is in each fiber a large aggregation of nuclei. Their arrangement provides the basis for the classification of intrafusal fibers as bag or chain fibers, depending on whether the nuclei are grouped together centrally or are arranged linearly.

Two types of sensory neurons innervate each muscle spindle. The larger nerve fibers, Group Ia afferents, have diameters of 12 to 20 micrometers (μm) and conduct impulses at velocities up to 120 meters per second. (For a summary of the fiber classifications referred to here and elsewhere, see Chapter 8.) Their terminals are coiled around the central parts of both bag and chain fibers to form the **primary endings**. The smaller nerve fibers, Group II afferents, are 4 to 12 μm in diameter and conduct more slowly. They contact only chain fibers, where they form **secondary endings**. The muscle spindle also is innervated by motoneurons (**fusimotor fibers**, or γ motoneurons). They cause intrafusal fibers—which contain contractile elements at both ends—to contract and thereby stretch the central nuclear region where the sensory endings are situated, causing them to fire impulses. This interaction provides a mechanism for the efferent control of muscle spindle sensitivity described in Chapter 26.

A surprising new complication in the sensory mechanisms of the muscle spindle has been found by Bewick,[11] who has shown that the primary *sensory* nerve endings in the spindle release the transmitter glutamate. This is unusual, for sensory neurons generally *receive* input, they do not modulate other targets. The function of the transmitter in the spindle is to boost the sensitivity of the stretch receptors themselves.

[11] Bewick, G. S. 2015. *J. Anat.* 227: 194–213.

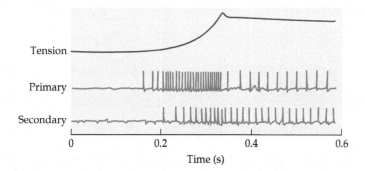

FIGURE 21.6 Specific Muscle Spindle Responses.
Recordings of action potentials from single primary (Group Ia) and secondary (Group II) sensory afferent fibers originating in a cat muscle spindle. The primary fiber greatly increases its discharge rate as tension develops during the stretch; during the maintained phase of the stretch, it quickly adapts to a lower rate. The secondary fiber increases its firing rate more slowly as tension develops and maintains its discharge during the steady stretch. (After J. K. S. Jansen and P. B. C. Matthews, 1962. *J. Physiol.* 161: 357-378.)

Responses to Static and Dynamic Muscle Stretch

When a rapid stretch is applied to a muscle and to the spindles within it, receptor potentials and bursts of impulses arise in Group Ia and II sensory fibers. There is, however, a clear difference in the characteristics of the discharges in the two endings (Figure 21.6). The primary endings, connected to the larger Group Ia axons, are sensitive mainly to the rate of change of stretch. The frequency of discharge is therefore maximal during the dynamic phase, while stretch is increasing, and subsides to a lower steady level while the stretch is maintained. The secondary endings, connected to the smaller Group II fibers, are relatively unaffected by the rate of stretch but are sensitive to the level of static tension.[12] The Group Ia (dynamic) and Group II (static) afferents are analogous to the rapidly adapting and slowly adapting receptors in the crayfish muscle and in other sensory systems.

Mechanisms of Adaptation in Mechanoreceptors

In muscle spindles, the viscoelastic properties of intrafusal fibers allow a gradual decrease in deformation of the sensory terminals.[13] A variety of processes have been shown to contribute to adaptation of crustacean stretch receptors.[12,14-16] In the slowly adapting stretch receptor, trains of impulses lead to an increase in internal sodium concentration and activation of the sodium pump. The net outward transport of positive charges by the pump reduces the amplitude of the receptor potential and hence the discharge frequency. Yet another factor contributing to adaptation is an increase in potassium conductance. For example, during a train of impulses in crayfish stretch receptors, calcium entry through voltage-activated channels causes the opening of calcium-activated potassium channels. The effect of this increase in potassium conductance is to "short out" the receptor potential, reducing its amplitude and the frequency of the sensory impulses. The rapidly adapting crayfish stretch receptor shows prompt adaptation of its firing rate even when a steady depolarizing current is applied experimentally. During imposed stretch, calcium influx through the transduction channels activates nearby calcium-dependent potassium channels to hyperpolarize the cell.[17]

Adaptation in the Pacinian Corpuscle

The Pacinian corpuscle is a rapidly adapting cutaneous mechanoreceptor[18] whose sensory terminal is enclosed in an onion-like capsule made of layers, called lamellae. Pressure applied slowly to the capsule produces no response at all; if pressure is applied quickly and then maintained, only one or two action potentials are generated at stimulus onset. However, the receptors are exquisitely sensitive to vibration up to frequencies of 800 Hz, and they continue to fire as the vibration is maintained. Although Pacinian corpuscles are found generally in subcutaneous tissue, they are particularly common around footpads and claws of mammals, and in the interosseous membranes bridging the bones of the leg and forearm, where they act as sensitive detectors of ground vibration.[19] A similar structure, the Herbst corpuscle, is found in the legs, bills, and cutaneous tissue of birds (and in the tongues of woodpeckers, where they presumably detect vibrations caused by insects). Speculation about the physiological function of Herbst corpuscles includes detection by the duck's bill of aquatic vibrations caused by small prey and, in soaring birds, detection of vibration of flight feathers caused by improper aerodynamic trim.[20] In Chapter 23 we will describe the role of Pacinian corpuscles in the fingertip in sensing texture.

[12] Matthews, P. B. 1981. *J. Physiol.* 320: 1-30.

[13] Fukami, Y., and Hunt, C. C. 1977. *J. Neurophysiol.* 40: 1121-1131.

[14] Nakajima, T., and Takahashi, K. 1966. *J. Physiol.* 187: 105-127.

[15] Nakajima, S., and Onodera, K. 1969. *J. Physiol.* 200: 187-204.

[16] Sokolove, P. G., and Cooke, I. M. 1971. *J. Gen. Physiol.* 57: 125-163.

[17] Erxleben, C. F. 1993. *Neuroreport* 4: 616-618.

[18] Bell, J., Bolanowski, S., and Holmes, M. H. 1994. *Prog. Neurobiol.* 42: 79-128.

[19] Quilliam, T. A., and Armstrong, J. 1963. *Endeavour* 22: 55-60.

[20] McIntyre, A. 1980. *Trends Neurosci.* 3: 202-205.

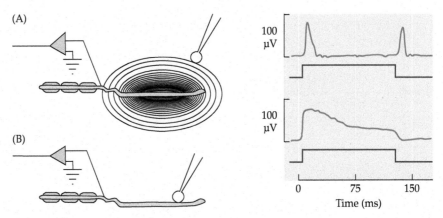

FIGURE 21.7 Adaptation in a Pacinian Corpuscle. (A) A pressure step (lower trace on right) applied to the body of the intact corpuscle produces a rapidly adapting receptor potential (upper trace), as a result of a transient wave of deformation that travels through the capsule to the nerve terminal. A similar response occurs on removal of the pulse. (B) After removal of the capsule layers, pressure applied to the nerve terminal produces a receptor potential that lasts for the duration of the pulse. (After W. R. Loewenstein and M. Mendelson, 1965. *J. Physiol.* 177: 377–397.)

Adaptation in the Pacinian corpuscle was studied in detail by Werner Loewenstein and his colleagues, who showed that it was due, in part, to the dynamic mechanics of the capsule.[21] When a mechanical pulse was applied to an isolated, intact corpuscle, a brief receptor potential appeared at the onset and withdrawal of the pulse (Figure 21.7A). The responses to sustained pressure are transient because compression of the sensory ending is relieved by redistribution of fluid within the capsule. After the capsule was stripped carefully from the nerve ending, the receptor potential decayed only slowly during the pulse (Figure 21.7B). Nonetheless, even when the receptor potential was prolonged, there was still only a brief burst of action potentials in the afferent axon (not shown in the figure); that is, the properties of the axon itself are matched to those of the intact receptor. We can conclude that the neuron and the structure in which it is embedded work together to form a pulse and vibration receptor.

Transduction by Mechanosensory Cells

Mechanosensitive ion channels are found in a wide variety of cell types and organs, including endothelial cells of blood vessels, baroreceptors in the carotid sinus, touch and pressure receptors in the skin, muscle stretch receptors, and mechanosensitive hair cells of the inner ear.[22–24] Two mammalian mechanoreceptor proteins, Piezo 1 and Piezo 2, have been isolated (see Chapter 5). Piezo 1 is found predominantly in tissues exposed to changes in fluid pressure, whereas Piezo 2 is expressed principally in sensory neurons such as dorsal root ganglion cells, and less extensively in lung and bladder. The channels are permeable to cations, as would be expected from their role in producing receptor depolarization, and have conductances on the order of 25 picosiemens (pS).

The structure of mouse Piezo 1 has been deduced from high-resolution (0.4-nm) cryo-electron microscopy (see Chapter 5). High-resolution structure of Piezo 2 has not been revealed, but in sensory neurons the channel is extensively spliced to produce isoforms with distinct functional properties, such as their rate of inactivation, ion permeability, and modulation by intracellular calcium.[25] Altogether, trigeminal ganglion neurons express 17 different splice variants of Piezo 2. Lung and bladder, however, express only a single isoform. Isoforms expressed in neurons subserving nociception and thermoreception differ in relative abundance from those expressed in neurons involved in proprioception and fine touch, suggesting that an important determinant of the functional properties of the receptors is the isoform composition of the Piezo 2 channels.

In crayfish stretch receptors, the current underlying the receptor potential is associated with an increase in permeability to sodium and potassium,[26,27] as well as to divalent cations[28] and to larger organic cations such as tris (tris [hydroxymethyl] amino methane) and arginine. The increase in conductance produced by stretch is unaffected by tetrodotoxin[29]

[21] Loewenstein, W. R., and Mendelson, M. 1965. *J. Physiol.* 177: 377–397.

[22] Ingber, D. E. 2006. *FASEB J.* 20: 811–827.

[23] Garcia-Anoveros, J., and Corey, D. P. 1997. *Annu. Rev. Neurosci.* 20: 567–594.

[24] Szczot, M. et al. 2017. *Cell Reports* 21: 2760–2771.

[25] Chalfie, M. 2009. *Nat. Rev. Mol. Cell. Biol.* 10: 44–52.

[26] Brown, H. M., Ottoson, D., and Rydqvist, B. 1978. *J. Physiol.* 284: 155–179.

[27] Rydqvist, B., and Purali, N. 1993. *J. Physiol.* 469: 193–211.

[28] Edwards, C. et al. 1981. *Neuroscience* 6: 1455–1460.

[29] Nakajima, S., and Onodera, K. 1969. *J. Physiol.* 200: 161–185.

but can be altered by some local anesthetics.[30] Receptor potentials in vertebrate muscle spindles also are due to increased cation permeability.[31]

Mechanosensitive Hair Cells of the Vertebrate Ear

Mechanosensitive **hair cells** of the inner ear are located in two fluid-filled structures that subserve two separate functions, hearing and balance. The cells in the first structure, the **cochlea**, respond to acoustic vibration (sound pressure waves), and those in the second, the **semicircular canals**, respond to head posture and motion. We will discuss in Chapter 24 the structural and functional specializations that support auditory and vestibular signals. For now it will suffice to point out that hair cells in the cochlea are stimulated by movements within the acoustical frequency range—in humans, from 20 to 20,000 Hz. The semicircular canals—the vestibular end organs of the inner ear—are constructed quite differently and respond to the much lower frequencies associated with head movement. Here, mass loading of the saccule and utricle by an overlying **otolithic membrane** makes these epithelial sheets sensitive to linear acceleration. The hair cells in the semicircular canals are stimulated by angular acceleration during head rotation. Both for an acoustic hair cell and a vestibular hair cell, deflection of a bundle of modified microvilli, or stereocilia, that project from the cell's apical surface results directly in the opening of mechanosensitive ion channels.

Structure of Hair Cell Receptors

Hair cells and the surrounding supporting cells form epithelial sheets that separate dissimilar fluid spaces of the inner ear. The basolateral membranes of hair cells are bathed by perilymph, similar in ionic composition to extracellular fluid, with high sodium and low potassium concentration (Figure 21.8). The apical, hair-bearing surface of the hair

[30] Lin, J. H., and Rydqvist, B. 1999. *Acta Physiol. Scand.* 166: 65-74.

[31] Hunt, C. C., Wilkinson, R. S., and Fukami, Y. 1978. *J. Gen. Physiol.* 71: 683-698.

(A)

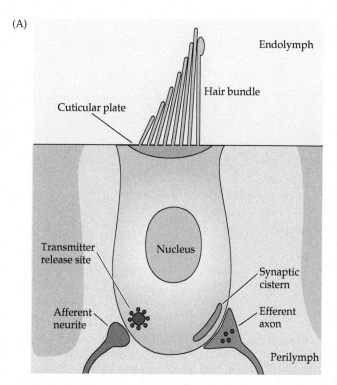

(B)

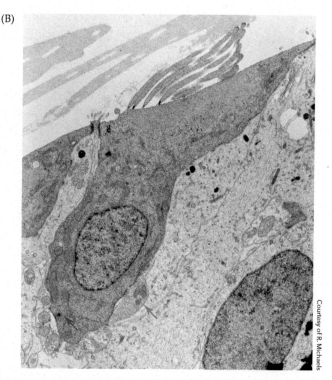

Courtesy of R. Michaels

FIGURE 21.8   The Mechanosensitive Hair Cell. (A) Schematic drawing highlighting the functional specializations of the hair cell. A bundle of specialized microvilli called stereocilia projects from the cuticular plate into the endolymphatic space. In some hair cells, a true cilium, the kinocilium, is found at one side of the hair bundle (not shown). Below the nucleus, hair cells form synapses with afferent and efferent neurons. Synaptic vesicles surround a dense body opposite the ending of an afferent neuron. Efferent neurons projecting from the brainstem form cholinergic synapses. Inside the hair cell, a synaptic cistern lies in close apposition to the plasma membrane underlying the efferent contact. (B) Transmission electron micrograph of a hair cell from chick inner ear. The hair bundle was bent over during fixation. This type of hair cell has an expanded cuticular surface. Afferent contact, on left, is associated with a ribbon (red arrow). A synaptic cistern associated with the efferent contact (blue arrow) is not visible at this magnification.

cell faces endolymph, a solution similar in some ways to cytoplasm, having high potassium and low sodium and calcium concentrations. Hair cells make synaptic contact with afferent fibers on their basolateral surfaces. Many hair cells also receive synaptic input from efferent neurons from the brainstem.

There are anywhere from a few dozen to hundreds of stereocilia (i.e., modified microvilli containing polymerized actin filaments), of graduated length, on different types of hair cells. The longest stereocilia are found on hair cells of the semicircular canals, the shortest in the high-frequency region of the cochlea. Within any one bundle, the stereocilia occur in an organ pipe or staircase array of ascending height. In many hair cells, a single true cilium, the kinocilium (containing a 9 + 2 microtubule array), is found near the middle of the tallest row of stereocilia (see Figure 21.8A). Cochlear hair cells have kinocilia early in development, but these disappear later. During bundle deflection the stereocilia behave like rigid rods and bend at this insertion point.[32] A variety of lateral linkages cause the assembly of stereocilia to move as a unified hair bundle.

Transduction by Hair Bundle Deflection

It has been believed for many years that electrical responses in hair cells are produced by deformation of the hair bundle.[33,34] However, direct experimental confirmation required the development of sensitive techniques for producing and measuring very small movements while recording from hair cells. Auditory and vestibular epithelia from ectothermic (so-called cold-blooded) vertebrates, such as turtles and frogs, have proved particularly advantageous for these experiments. Procedures used for nanostimulation of hair cells in the turtle inner ear are shown in Figure 21.9A. A microelectrode records the hair cell's membrane potential while a glass fiber attached to a piezoelectric manipulator pushes the hair

[32] Flock, A., Flock, B., and Murray, E. 1977. *Acta Otolaryngol.* 83: 85–91.

[33] Flock, A. 1965. *Cold Spring Harb. Symp. Quant. Biol.* 30: 133–145.

[34] Lowenstein, O., and Wersall, J. 1959. *Nature* 184: 1807–1808.

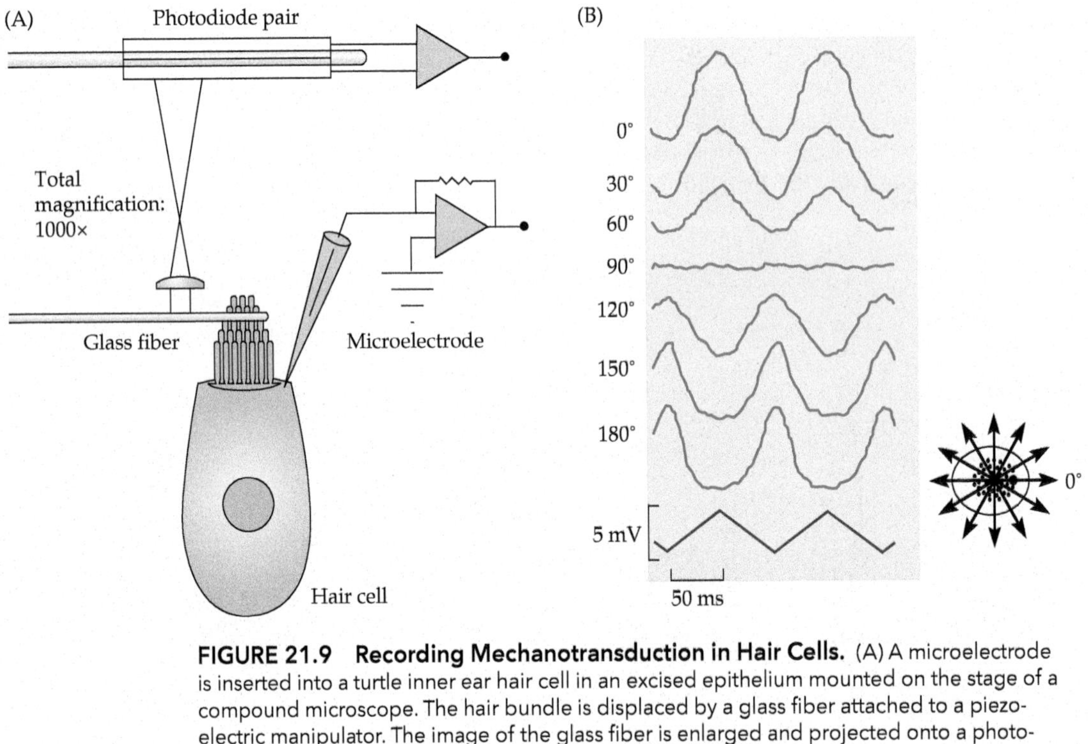

FIGURE 21.9 Recording Mechanotransduction in Hair Cells. (A) A microelectrode is inserted into a turtle inner ear hair cell in an excised epithelium mounted on the stage of a compound microscope. The hair bundle is displaced by a glass fiber attached to a piezoelectric manipulator. The image of the glass fiber is enlarged and projected onto a photodiode pair so that motion causes a differential signal between them. Movements as small as 1 nm can be detected with this method. (B) Receptor potentials recorded from a hair cell in the excised saccule of a frog during bundle deflection at various angles. The kinocilium at the center of the tallest row of hairs lies at 0°. Maximal responses occur for motion toward and away from the kinocilium; no response is seen during motion at right angles to that line. (A after A. C. Crawford and R. Fettiplace, 1985. *J. Physiol.* 364: 359–379; B after S. L. Shotwell et al., 1981. *Ann. NY Acad. Sci.* 374: 1–10.)

bundle. Movements as small as 1 nm can be detected by projecting the image of the glass fiber, or the hair bundle itself, onto a pair of photodiodes. Such a stimulus produces a voltage change of 0.2 mV in the hair cell.[35]

Hudspeth and colleagues carried out a series of elegant experiments that revealed many of the details of transduction in vestibular hair cells of the frog.[36–38] In one series of experiments they demonstrated directly the functional orientation of the hair bundle by varying the direction of stimulation with a piezoelectric manipulator. Deflections toward the kinocilium depolarized the cell, while movement away resulted in hyperpolarization. Bundle deflection perpendicular to that axis caused no change in membrane current.[39] The results of such an experiment are seen in Figure 21.9B, where the magnitude of the voltage change generated in the hair cell varies with the angle of bundle deflection.

Tip Links and Gating Springs

What structural feature of the hair bundle might underlie the directional selectivity of transduction? Pickles and colleagues used the scanning electron microscope to describe a unique class of extracellular linkages connecting the top of one hair with the side of the adjacent taller hair.[40] They observed these **tip links** (Figure 21.10A) only along the axis of mechanical stimulation (i.e., oriented up and down the staircase). The position of the tip links suggested that they might be involved in mechanotransduction, and treatments that break the tip link abolish transduction.[41,42] Indeed, extracellular recordings[43,44] as well as calcium imaging[45,46] indicated that the channels activated by mechanical stimuli are located at the very top of the stereocilia.

Quantitative measures of transduction and the identification of tip links are combined in the **gating spring** hypothesis of mechanotransduction in hair cells. Deflection of the hair bundle in the positive direction (i.e., toward the taller hairs) separates the tips to stretch a gating spring, thus pulling open the transduction channel (Figure 21.10B). When the bundle is pushed away from the tallest hairs, the spring is compressed and the channel closes. Although such a scheme might seem somewhat fanciful, a direct physical connection between bundle mechanics and channel gating is required to explain the great speed at which transduction occurs in hair cells, with time constants of opening of about 40 microseconds (μs).[47–49] Furthermore, the energetics and mechanics of transduction are consistent with this model. For example, it is possible to measure a decrease in bundle stiffness as the transduction channels open, as though this molecular motion relieves some tension on the gating spring.[50] While the mechanism requires a springlike element, the tip link itself is

[35] Crawford, A. C., and Fettiplace, R. 1985. *J. Physiol.* 364: 359–379.

[36] Hudspeth, A. J., and Corey, D. P. 1977. *Proc. Natl. Acad. Sci. USA* 74: 2407–2411.

[37] Hudspeth, A. J., and Jacobs, R. 1979. *Proc. Natl. Acad. Sci. USA* 76: 1506–1509.

[38] Corey, D. P., and Hudspeth, A. J. 1979. *Nature* 281: 675–677.

[39] Shotwell, S. L., Jacobs, R., and Hudspeth, A. J. 1981. *Ann. NY Acad. Sci.* 374: 1–10.

[40] Pickles, J. O., Comis, S. D., and Osborne, M. P. 1984. *Hear. Res.* 15: 103–112.

[41] Crawford, A. C., Evans, M. G., and Fettiplace, R. 1991. *J. Physiol.* 434: 369–398.

[42] Assad, J. A., Shepherd, G. M., and Corey, D. P. 1991. *Neuron* 7: 985–994.

[43] Hudspeth, A. J. 1982. *J. Neurosci.* 2: 1–10.

[44] Jaramillo, F., and Hudspeth, A. J. 1991. *Neuron* 7: 409–420.

[45] Beurg, M. et al. 2009. *Nat. Neurosci.* 12: 553–558.

[46] Lumpkin, E. A., and Hudspeth, A. J. 1995. *Proc. Natl. Acad. Sci. USA* 92: 10297–10301.

[47] Corey, D. P., and Hudspeth, A. J. 1983. *J. Neurosci.* 3: 962–976.

[48] Crawford, A. C., Evans, M. G., and Fettiplace, R. 1989. *J. Physiol.* 419: 405–434.

[49] Basu, A. et al. 2016. *eLife* 5: e16041.

[50] Howard, J., and Hudspeth, A. J. 1988. *Neuron* 1: 189–199.

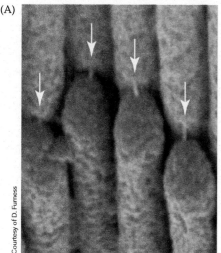

(A)

Courtesy of D. Furness

200 nm

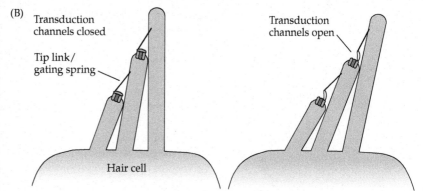

(B)

Transduction channels closed

Tip link/ gating spring

Hair cell

Transduction channels open

FIGURE 21.10 Tip Links on Hair Cell Stereocilia. (A) Scanning electron micrograph of a rat cochlear hair cell showing extracellular fibers that run from the tips of shorter stereocilia to the sides of adjacent taller stereocilia. (B) Tip links are positioned so that deflection of the hair bundle in the excitatory direction extends the tip link and pulls open the transduction channel (right), while the opposite motion relaxes the tip link (left), allowing the channel to close. Current models include a springlike element within the transduction apparatus (but not the tip link itself), with mechanosensitive channels located at the tops of stereocilia.

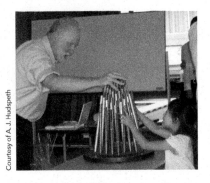

A. J. Hudspeth (left), demonstrating the mechanisms of transduction of the sensory hair bundle.

[51] Kazmierczak, P. et al. 2007. *Nature* 449: 87–91.

[52] Ohmori, H. 1985. *J. Physiol.* 359: 189–217.

[53] Denk, W. et al. 1995. *Neuron* 15: 1311–1321.

[54] Ranade, S. S., Syeda, R. and Patapoutian, A. 2015. *Neuron* 87: 1162–1179.

[55] Fettiplace, R. 2016. *Biophys. J.* 111: 3–9.

[56] Gillespie, P. G. and Muller, U. 2009. *Cell* 139: 33–44.

[57] Hudspeth, A. J., and Gillespie, P. G. 1994. *Neuron* 12: 1–9.

[58] Libby, R. T., and Steel, K. P. 2000. *Essays Biochem.* 35: 159–174.

[59] Gillespie, P. G., Wagner, M. C., and Hudspeth, A. J. 1993. *Neuron* 11: 581–594.

[60] Ricci, A. J., and Fettiplace, R. 1997. *J. Physiol.* 501: 111–124.

[61] Martin, P. Mehta, A. D., and Hudspeth, A. J. 2000. *Proc. Natl. Acad. Sci. USA* 97: 12026–12031.

[62] Kemp, D. T. 1978. *J. Acoust. Soc. Am.* 64: 1386–1391.

[63] Lonsbury-Martin, B. L., and Martin, G. K. 2003. *Curr. Opin. Otolaryngol. Head Neck Surg.* 11: 361–366.

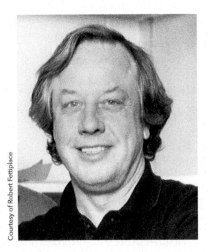

R. Fettiplace

composed of cadherin 23 and protocadherin 15, making it too stiff to serve this function;[51] thus, the molecular identity of the gating spring remains under investigation.

Transduction Channels in Hair Cells

What types of channels are opened in the tips of hair cells? These appear to be nonselective cation channels that have considerable calcium permeability. The single-channel conductance is large, greater than 100 pS.[41,52,53] Strikingly, single-channel conductance increases as one progresses from low- to high-frequency hair cells. From conductance measurements and measurements of total transducer current, it is possible to calculate that each hair cell has only about 100 transduction channels. This corresponds to perhaps as few as two channels per stereocilium!

The very small number of channels in each hair cell makes biochemical and molecular biological investigation especially challenging. Hair cell transduction channels have no intrinsic voltage dependence, nor are they ligand gated in any traditional sense. It may be, therefore, that there are no strong homologies between these and voltage- or ligand-gated ion channels. Four candidate proteins have been identified in hair cells of the cochlea and vestibular apparatus (see Chapter 5).[54] Mutations in one protein (TMC1) result in deafness in mice. However, it has yet to be demonstrated that expression of the protein actually forms a channel. Thus, it may play an auxiliary, rather than a direct, role in transduction.[55]

Adaptation of Hair Cells

Hair cells, whether in the cochlea or semicircular canals, are extraordinarily sensitive, with threshold responses to bundle motion of less than 10^{-9} m.[56] This leads to speculation that an adaptive process exists to maintain sensitivity in the face of a so-called background stimulus. For example, vestibular hair cells in the saccule and utricle must remain sensitive to subtle head movements while continuously being subject to gravitational force acting on the overlying otolithic membrane (see Chapter 24). Indeed, it has been shown by direct measurement that hair cells adapt to a prolonged displacement by establishing a new set point for their operating range, with no loss of sensitivity. This form of set point adaptation is thought to arise from the action of a non-muscle myosin that exerts tension on the transduction channels by pulling against the actin core of the stereocilium.[57] Myosins have been cloned from the inner ear,[58] and specific antibodies have been used to show that myosin 1C is located near the tips of stereocilia in frog hair cells.[59] This myosin-based adaptation depends on calcium influx and is relatively slow. It may be most prominent in vestibular hair cells. The more rapid adaptation seen in auditory hair cells may arise from calcium ions acting directly on the transduction channel, causing it to close.[60]

The tight coupling between mechanical input and transduction channel gating implies that feedback might occur during transduction.[61] Thus, when the hair bundle is deflected, the calcium that enters through the open transduction channels can produce a further change in hair bundle stiffness or position. Similarly, alteration of hair cell membrane potential can move the hair bundle by changing the driving force for calcium entry. These feedback processes can give rise to mechanical resonance (or ringing) in bundle motion. Fettiplace and Crawford explored this phenomenon in auditory hair cells of the turtle using flexible glass fibers to deflect the hair bundle directly.[36] A 75-nm step to the butt end of the glass fiber caused a smaller deflection of the tip attached to the bundle (Figure 21.11). The tip motion was smaller because the bundle was relatively stiff compared with the wispy glass fiber. Furthermore, although the imposed movement was square, the fiber tip showed a small oscillation that was coincident with an oscillatory receptor potential recorded from the hair cell. In other words, the glass fiber pushed the bundle, and the bundle *pushed back*! This oscillatory motion of the hair bundle results from transducer channel gating. The reciprocal interaction between bundle deflection and membrane potential contributes to the production of what are called ear sounds (i.e., otoacoustic emissions) that can be generated in most species, including humans.[62] The ability to elicit otoacoustic emissions from the ear has provided a way for audiologists to assess hair cell function directly, even in infants and comatose patients.[63] In Chapter 24 we will show how

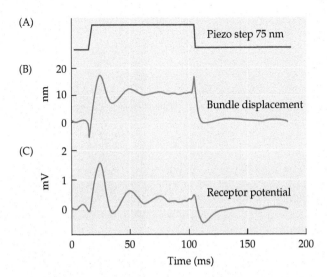

(A) Piezo step 75 nm

(B) Bundle displacement

(C) Receptor potential

Time (ms)

FIGURE 21.11 **Intrinsic Movements of Mechanosensitive Hair Bundles.** (A) A flexible glass fiber attached to a piezoelectric element is stepped and used to deflect the stereociliary bundle of a turtle hair cell (as in Figure 21.9A). (B) Bundle motion reported by a photodiode detector. (C) The oscillating receptor potential obtained with an intracellular microelectrode aligns with the oscillatory movement of a glass fiber attached to the hair bundle. For the voltage record, the ordinate is membrane potential relative to resting potential (-50 mV). The frequency of damped oscillations is 39 Hz. Results suggest that the hair bundle moves the glass fiber. (After A. C. Crawford and R. Fettiplace, 1985. *J. Physiol.* 364: 359-379.)

the active properties of hair cells—their own motion in response to efferent inputs from the brain—act to amplify very weak sounds and attenuate very loud sounds.

Olfaction

Mechanotransduction in the ear attains high sensitivity by tightly coupling the stimulus energy to the hair cell's membrane potential. In contrast, great sensitivity is obtained in olfaction (smell) and vision, and in some forms of taste by chemical amplification—that is, second messenger pathways in which enzymatic cascades produce large numbers of intermediate products, thereby increasing by a thousand-fold the effect of one activated receptor molecule.

Olfaction is poorly developed in humans compared to dogs or pigs or butterflies. But at the same time, considerable effort (and advertising dollars) goes into human olfactory behavior (consider the numbers of soaps, deodorants, and perfumes that are aimed at securing a socially acceptable personal bouquet). In fact, olfactory signals are essential to human survival, stimulating feeding, reproduction, and mother–infant bonding.[64,65] Detection and discrimination of the unique blend of odors linked to those behaviors begins with a large family of molecular receptors in the olfactory receptor neurons.

Olfactory Receptors

Mammals detect odors with a patch of about 100,000 olfactory receptor neurons whose axons project through a thin portion of the frontal skull (the cribriform plate) to the olfactory bulb (Figure 21.12). The long cilia of the olfactory receptors extend into the nasal cavity, where they lie in a layer of mucus, approximately 50 μm thick in humans, that is entirely replaced every 10 min. The mucous layer protects the sensory epithelium, washing out potentially toxic airborne compounds, and all odorants must dissolve through this to reach the sensory cilia. An odorant-binding protein helps concentrate hydrophobic odorants in this aqueous layer.[66] Olfactory receptors are continuously replaced throughout the animal's lifetime. Each receptor lives for several weeks, and new receptors arise from a layer of basal cells in the olfactory epithelium.[67]

The Olfactory Response

Early measurements of olfactory responses were made by Adrian[68] and Ottoson.[69] Since then, evidence has accumulated that odorant molecules interact with receptors in the ciliary membrane to depolarize the olfactory receptors. The resulting action potentials then travel along the receptor axon into the CNS. Patch clamp techniques have been used on isolated olfactory receptors to localize the point of generation of

[64] Stern, K., and McClintock, M. K. 1998. *Nature* 392: 177-179.

[65] Brennan, P. A., and Kendrick, K. M. 2006. *Philos. Trans. R. Soc. Lond., B, Biol. Sci.* 361: 2061-2078.

[66] Pevsner, J. et al. 1988. *Science* 241: 336-339.

[67] Farbman, A. I. 1994. *Semin. Cell Biol.* 5: 3-10.

[68] Adrian, E. D. 1953. *Acta Physiol. Scand.* 29: 5-14.

[69] Ottoson, D. 1956. *Acta Physiol. Scand.* 35: 1-83.

FIGURE 21.12 Olfactory Epithelium. (A) Section through the olfactory epithelium of a mouse. Individual olfactory neurons are labeled with antibodies to a single molecular receptor. (B) Scanning electron micrograph of the olfactory epithelium of a hamster. The olfactory receptor neurons (O) have a long dendrite (D) that extends to the surface, and an axon (Ax) that projects from the epithelium to the olfactory bulb. The long sensory cilia at the tip of the dendrite form a dense mat in this preparation and are not individually resolved.

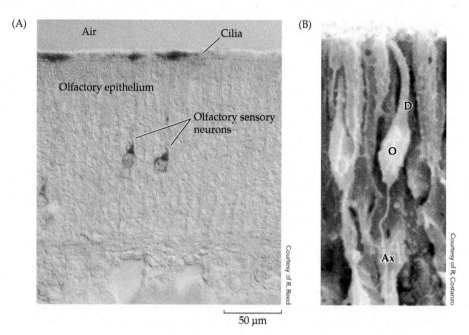

odorant-induced currents and to record their magnitude and time course.[70] An example of such an experiment on a cell isolated from the olfactory mucosa of a salamander is shown in Figure 21.13.[71] The membrane potential of the cell is held at –65 mV, and a solution containing a mixture of odorant molecules (approximately 0.1 mM) in 100 mM KCl is applied from a second pipette by a brief (35 ms) pressure pulse—first to the soma, and then to the distal portion of the dendrite and the cilia. Pipette solution applied to the soma produces a rapid inward current, which is due to the local increase in potassium concentration. The time course of the potassium response provides a measure of the speed of application and subsequent dissipation of the solution by diffusion into the surrounding bath. A second, smaller and slower inward current appears when the odorants reach the apical dendrite.

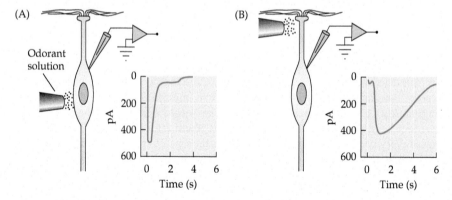

FIGURE 21.13 Responses of Isolated Olfactory Cells from a salamander. A patch clamp electrode is used to record whole-cell current. A solution containing 0.1 mM odorant mixture in 100 mM KCl is applied to the cell by a brief (35 ms) pressure pulse. (A) When solution is applied to the cell body, there is a rapid, transient inward current due to the increased KCl concentration, followed by a smaller, slower current as the odorant reaches the apical end of the dendrite. The time course of the fast inward current is indicative of the time course of application and dissipation of the electrode solution. (B) When the solution is applied to the dendrite, there is only a small, rapid current due to the KCl, but a large current, due to the odorant, lasts for several seconds after the electrode solution has washed away. (After S. Firestein et al., 1990. *J. Physiol.* 430: 135–158.)

[70] Maue, R. A., and Dionne, V. E. 1987. *J. Gen. Physiol.* 90: 95–125.

[71] Firestein, S., Shepherd, G. M., and Werblin, F. S. 1990. *J. Physiol.* 430: 135–158.

Solution applied to the apical dendrite and cilia produces only a small potassium response. However, the odorant itself produces a large inward current that outlasts the time of application by several seconds. The experiment shows that the region of sensitivity to the odorants is the distal dendrite and cilia, and the prolonged time course of the dendritic response is consistent with the idea that the conductance change is produced by a second-messenger system whose activity outlasts the initial odorant binding reaction.

Cyclic Nucleotide-Gated Channels in Olfactory Receptors

The depolarization produced by odorants arises from the opening of nonselective cation channels, permeable to Na+, K+, and Ca2+ (Figure 21.14).[72,73] The channels, which are activated by intracellular cAMP, are closely related to the cation channels opened by cyclic guanosine monophosphate (cGMP) in rod photoreceptors (see Chapter 22).[74] However, although several features of the olfactory transduction cascade are similar to that in photoreceptors, an increase in light intensity leads to a *decrease* in cyclic nucleotide concentration and consequent *hyperpolarization*. During depolarization of the olfactory cells, the influx of calcium opens calcium-activated chloride channels, further contributing to the receptor potential.[75-77] Enhancement of the receptor potential by activation of chloride channels seems like an anomaly, as activation of chloride channels in most cells would be expected to oppose, rather than enhance, membrane depolarization. However, the receptor regions of olfactory cells have an intracellular chloride concentration similar to that of the mucus in which they are bathed. Thus, the chloride equilibrium potential, rather than being close to the resting membrane potential, is near 0 mV, and opening chloride channels results in outward chloride flux (i.e., inward, positive current).[78] Activation of the receptors leads to a relatively rapid response. Using a preparation of isolated olfactory cilia, Breer and colleagues showed that a tenfold increase in cAMP concentration occurred within 50 ms of odorant application.[79] In addition, odor detection is highly sensitive. Activation of only a few ion channels is required to initiate action potentials. This is because of the high input resistance of the receptors, and suggests that only a few odorant molecules may be necessary for olfactory detection.[80]

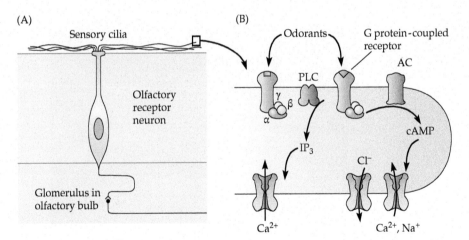

FIGURE 21.14 Transduction in Olfactory Cilia. (A) The molecular receptors for olfactants are found in sensory cilia that project into the mucous layer of the olfactory epithelium. Depolarizing receptor potentials in these long receptors give rise to action potentials that propagate along the olfactory receptor neuron's axon into the CNS. (B) Odorant molecules bind to specific G protein-coupled receptors in the plasma membrane of the olfactory cilia. This frees the α-subunit to activate adenylate cyclase (AC) and raise the concentration of cyclic adenosine monophosphate (cAMP), which causes nonselective cation channels to open, depolarizing the membrane. Calcium-gated chloride current can enhance this effect. Other pathways may involve the activation of phospholipase C (PLC) and the consequent rise in IP3 to act directly on plasma membrane calcium channels.

[72] Nakamura, T., and Gold, G. H. 1987. *Nature* 325: 442-444.

[73] Pifferi, S., Boccaccio, A., and Menini, A. 2006. *FEBS Lett.* 580: 2853-2859.

[74] Dhallan, R. S. et al. 1990. *Nature* 347: 184-187.

[75] Kleene, S. J., and Gesteland, R. C. 1991. *J. Neurosci.* 11: 3624-3629.

[76] Kurahashi, T., and Yau, K. W. 1993. *Nature* 363: 71-74.

[77] Pifferi, S. et al. 2009. *J. Physiol.* 587: 4265-4279.

[78] Kleene, S. J. 2008. *Chem. Senses* 33: 839-859.

[79] Breer, H., Boekhoff, I., and Tareilus, E. 1990. *Nature* 345: 65-68.

[80] Menini, A., Picco, C., and Firestein, S. 1995. *Nature* 373: 435-437.

Coupling the Receptor to Ion Channels

How is odorant binding coupled to the gating of cAMP-dependent cation channels? The mechanism of activation is outlined in Figure 21.14B. The odorant first binds to G protein-coupled receptors (GPCRs). The activated G protein releases its α-subunit, which triggers synthesis of cAMP by adenylate cyclase. The cAMP-activated channels then open, allowing influx of cations, thereby producing membrane depolarization. The prominence of smell in our sensory repertoire is indicated by the fact that more than half of GPCRs, which are the largest superfamily of membrane proteins in the human genome, are classed as odorant receptors.[81]

There is also evidence that some olfactory neurons use G protein activation of phospholipase C and production of inositol triphosphate (IP3) in transduction (see Figure 21.14B).[82] In this case, IP3 may act directly to open calcium channels in the plasma membrane.[83] IP3 appears to be especially important for invertebrate olfaction,[84] less so for vertebrates, as transgenic mice lacking cAMP-gated channels had no residual ability to discriminate odors.[85]

Odorant Specificity

Mammals can discriminate a very large number of odors,[86] and the existence of an enormous number of olfactory receptor proteins provides the substrate for this capability. Only one receptor protein is expressed in each olfactory receptor neuron, but each receptor has a broad range of binding affinities and recognizes a spectrum of odors, rather than being highly selective.[87,88] One approach to understanding this issue has been to examine the anatomical organization of olfactory neurons expressing specific cloned receptor molecules, using in situ hybridization or expression of recombinant proteins. Each particular odorant receptor was found in a restricted area of the olfactory epithelium.[89,90] Different families of receptors genes were expressed in zones extending along the length of the epithelium (Figure 21.15A,B), with any given gene expressed in only a small number of neurons. Olfactory receptor neurons expressing the same molecular receptor project to a single pair of medial and lateral glomeruli in the first central relay station, the olfactory bulb (Figure 21.15C).[91,92]

[81] Antunes, G., and Simoes de Souza, F. M. 2016 *Methods Cell Biol.* 132: 127-145

[82] Boekhoff, I. et al. 1990. *EMBO J.* 9: 2453-2458.

[83] Restrepo, D. et al. 1990. *Science* 249: 1166-1168.

[84] Ache, B. W., and Zhainazarov, A. 1995. *Curr. Opin. Neurobiol.* 5: 461-466.

[85] Brunet, L. J., Gold, G. H., and Ngai, J. 1996. *Neuron* 17: 681-693.

[86] Castro, J. B., Ramanathan, A., and Chennubhotla, C. S. 2013. *PLOS ONE* 8: e73289.

[87] Serizawa, S. et al. 2003. *Science* 302: 2088-2094.

[88] Lewcock, J. W., and Reed, R. R. 2004. *Proc. Natl. Acad. Sci. USA* 101: 1069-1074.

[89] Ressler, K. J., Sullivan, S. L., and Buck, L. B. 1993. *Cell* 73: 597-609.

[90] Vassar, R., Ngai, J., and Axel, R. 1993. *Cell* 74: 309-318.

[91] Mombaerts, P. et al. 1996. *Cell* 87: 675-686.

[92] Bozza, T. et al. 2002. *J. Neurosci.* 22: 3033-3043.

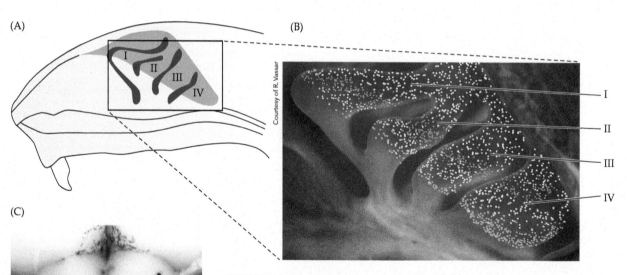

FIGURE 21.15 Expression of Specific Odorant Receptor Genes by Subsets of Olfactory Receptor Neurons. (A) The olfactory epithelium of a rat lies on a series of convolutions of the nasal cavity called turbinates—labeled I to IV. Bands of olfactory receptor neurons label positively for olfactory receptor mRNAs. (B) Probes for different mRNAs label nonoverlapping populations of neurons (depicted as green, yellow, blue, and white dots). (C) Olfactory receptor neurons expressing one receptor gene project to unique glomeruli in each olfactory bulb. (A after R. Vassar et al., 1993. *Cell* 74: 309-318.)

Courtesy of R. Vassar

A. L. Tadenev et al., 2011. *Proc. Natl. Acad. Sci. USA* 108: 10320-10325

This specific innervation pattern is maintained on the way to the bulb by fasciculation of "like" axons. Thus, the receptor proteins determine both odor specificity of the olfactory receptor neurons and convergence of their axons to specific glomeruli. These features of olfactory organization are still more intriguing when one recalls that olfactory receptor neurons turn over every few weeks throughout the lifetime of the organism![93] The mechanisms producing this selective innervation pattern remain largely unknown.

In addition to the main olfactory epithelium, many mammals possess a vomeronasal organ which detects pheromones that stimulate mating and other social behaviors. Vomeronasal receptor neurons (VRNs) project to an accessory olfactory bulb, which in turn projects to the limbic system. VRNs express additional families of molecular receptors. G protein-coupled vomeronasal receptor 1 and 2 (VR1 and VR2)[94–96] superfamilies each include more than 100 genes in mice, some of which specifically bind known pheromones.[97] G protein-coupled formyl peptide receptors mediate immune cell responses to bacteria but also appear to be expressed specifically in VRNs,[98] as are trace-amine-associated receptors.[99] Formyl peptides and trace amines are present in urine and so could contribute to assessment of the gender, social status, or health of individuals.[100] Each vomeronasal neuron may express just one type of molecular receptor, and the pattern of expression differs between male and female rats.[101]

Mechanisms of Taste (Gustation)

Discussions of taste and smell are often combined because both senses are activated by chemical stimuli arriving from the outside world. Indeed, some taste stimuli (tastants) act on GPCRs in ways quite similar to those discussed for olfaction. However, other tastants, principally salts and acids, act directly on membrane conductances, and taste receptor cells differ anatomically from olfactory receptor neurons.

Taste Receptor Cells

Taste receptors are ciliated neuroepithelial cells and are found in taste buds on the tongue surface (Figure 21.16). Like olfactory receptors, taste cells are regenerated throughout life. Unlike olfactory receptors, taste cells do not have axons, but form chemical synapses with afferent neurites within the taste bud. Microvilli project from the apical pole of the taste cell into the open pore of the taste bud, where they come into contact with tastants dissolved in saliva on the tongue's surface. Strikingly, only a subset of cells within the taste bud actually responds to tastants (see Figure 21.16B).[102] A second class of cells fails

[93] Reed, R. R. 2004. *Cell* 116: 329–336.
[94] Dulac, C., and Axel, R. 1995. *Cell* 83: 195–206.
[95] Matsunami, H., and Buck, L. B. 1997. *Cell* 90: 775–784.
[96] Ryba, N. J., and Tirindelli, R. 1997. *Neuron* 19: 371–379.
[97] Boschat, C. et al. 2002. *Nat. Neurosci.* 5: 1261–1262.
[98] Riviere, S. et al. 2009. *Nature* 459: 574–577.
[99] Liberles, S. D., and Buck, L. B. 2006. *Nature* 442: 645–650.
[100] Tirindelli, R. et al. 2009. *Physiol. Rev.* 89: 921–956.
[101] Herrada, G., and Dulac, C. 1997. *Cell* 90: 763–773.
[102] DeFazio, R. A. et al. 2006. *J. Neurosci.* 26: 3971–3980.

(A)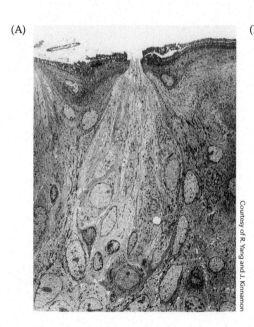

(B)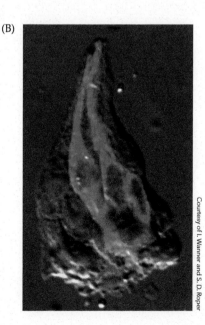

FIGURE 21.16 Taste Receptor Cells Are Found in Taste Buds within the lingual epithelium. (A) A transmission electron micrograph of a taste bud in the tongue of a rat. Individual taste receptor cells have microvilli that project into the taste pore to sample the saliva. (B) An individual taste bud dissected from the tongue of a rat. The taste receptor cells are labeled with an antibody to gustducin, a G protein involved in taste transduction.

to respond to tastants. Instead, there is ultrastructural evidence that they receive chemical synaptic input from the taste cells. Communication between the two cell types may be mediated by ATP[103] and serotonin.[104]

Taste Modalities

Taste stimuli are usually subdivided into five categories: salt, sour, bitter, sweet, and umami, the last being a Japanese word for the taste of monosodium glutamate (MSG), or more generally, amino acid (i.e., meat). Each category has its own transduction mechanism; sweet and umami follow similar molecular pathways but are activated by different molecules (Figure 21.17). The mechanisms fall into two classes, both of which result in depolarization of the taste receptor membrane: (1) direct action of the tastant on ion channels, or (2) coupling of tastant receptors to ion channels through second-messenger pathways involving GPCRs.[105]

There is good agreement that the taste of salt is mediated by direct flux of sodium (or other monovalent cations) through channels in the apical membrane of the taste cell that are open at rest.[106] Sodium is present at higher concentration in salty foods (>100 mM) than in saliva, and it simply diffuses into the cells down its electrochemical gradient, thereby producing depolarization. The candidate channels are similar to epithelial sodium channels (ENaCs) found in frog skin and kidney. They are voltage-insensitive and are blocked by the diuretic compound amiloride. The functional channels consist of three subunits.[107] The α-subunit has been detected in lingual epithelium,[108] and mice in which the ENaC α-subunit was genetically ablated lose their taste for sodium.[109]

Sour taste is produced by the high concentration of protons in acidic foods. Protons may act by entering taste cells through the same amiloride-blockable sodium channels.[110] Alternatively, protons may depolarize the cells by blocking normally open potassium channels.[111] A third mechanism is seen in frog taste cells, which have cation channels that are activated by protons.[112] Recently a protein, otopetrin-1, has been identified as a possible sour taste receptor for strong acids in mice.[113] The protein, originally associated with the vestibular system, has 12 predicted transmembrane domains and, like the frog protein, generates large inward currents in response to extracellular acidification.

In addition to acting at the taste cell's cilia, salts and protons may percolate through the taste pore (a paracellular pathway) to act on the same or other ion channels (including some that are amiloride-insensitive) in the basolateral membranes of the cell.[103] This illustrates what seems to be a general principle of gustation—that is, several parallel transduction pathways can exist for any one class of tastants.

[103] Finger, T. E. et al. 2005. *Science* 310: 1495–1499.

[104] Huang, Y. J. et al. 2005. *J. Neurosci.* 25: 843–847.

[105] Shigemura, N. and Ninomiya, Y. 2016. *Int. Rev. Cell. Mol. Biol.* 23: 71–106.

[106] Roper, S. D. 2015. *Pflügers Arch.* 467: 457–463.

[107] Canessa, C. M. et al. 1994. *Nature* 367: 463–467.

[108] Li, X. J., Blackshaw, S., and Snyder, S. H. 1994. *Proc. Natl. Acad. Sci. USA* 91: 1814–1818.

[109] Chandrashekar, J. et al. 2010. *Nature* 464: 297–301.

[110] Gilbertson, T. A., Roper, S. D., and Kinnamon, S. C. 1993. *Neuron* 10: 931–942.

[111] Kinnamon, S. C., Dionne, V. E., and Beam, K. G. 1988. *Proc. Natl. Acad. Sci. USA* 85: 7023–7027.

[112] Okada, Y., Mitamoto, T., and Sato, T. 1994. *J. Exp. Biol.* 187: 19–32.

[113] Tu, Y-H et al. 2018. *Science* 359: 1047–1050.

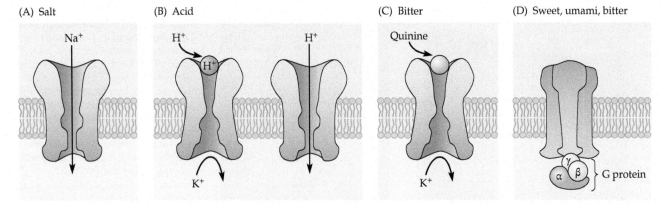

(A) Salt   **(B)** Acid   **(C)** Bitter   **(D)** Sweet, umami, bitter

FIGURE 21.17 Mechanisms of Taste Transduction. Tastant molecules range from protons (acids) to simple salts to complex organic compounds. This wide range of chemical stimuli is transduced by a multiplicity of mechanisms. Salts (A) and acids (B) can permeate ion channels in the sensory ending or block normally open potassium channels. Acid permeation leads to the sour taste. (C) Some bitter compounds also block potassium channels to cause depolarization. (D) Sugars and amino acids (umami) interact with G protein-coupled receptors to initiate second-messenger cascades. Though the sugar and umami receptors are different, they act through similar G-protein mechanisms and are thus shown on the same sketch. All these mechanisms lead eventually to depolarization, voltage-gated calcium influx, and increased release of transmitter onto associated afferent dendrites.

Sweet, umami, and some bitter tastes are mediated by GPCRs, probably acting through phospholipase C and IP3 to release calcium from internal stores (see Chapter 12)[114] and thereby activating calcium-dependent cation channels.[115] In addition, the intracellular messenger cAMP is activated by gustducin, a G protein specific to taste cells.[116] Sensitivity to sweet, bitter, and umami is reduced in gustducin knockout mice.[117]

A growing number of molecular receptors for sweet, bitter, and umami have been identified in recent years. The family of GPCR molecules T1R1, T1R2, and T1R3 may be expressed in sweet receptor cells. A large family of GPCRs, the T2Rs, serve the taste of the widely varying class of bitter compounds.[118,119] Finally, unusual forms of metabotropic glutamate receptors have been implicated in mediating umami taste.[120]

It is important to note that taste, as a percept, results from sensations in addition to those reported by the taste buds. The aromas detected by olfaction, as well as by texture and temperature, which are sensed by other somatosensory neurons, all contribute to the ultimate identification and appreciation of food (ice cream is pleasurable due to all of these features combined). An example in which taste buds are not involved at all is the hot taste of chili peppers. The hot taste arises from activation of temperature-sensitive fibers in the tongue by the compound capsaicin. The capsaicin receptor channel has been cloned and shown to be a heat-sensitive transient receptor potential (TRP) channel (see next section).[121]

Temperature and Pain Sensation

Temperature Transduction

Skin temperature changes are transduced by free nerve endings through the activation of TRP ion channels, which are cation permeable and produce membrane depolarization. The temperature range of channel activation depends on channel type. Four different heat-sensitive TRP channels, TRPV1 to TRPV4, are activated over different temperature ranges above about 25°C (Figure 21.18).[122] A cold-sensitive channel, TRPM8, responds to temperatures below about 25°C.[123] Menthol and eucalyptol also activate this channel, which explains the cooling sensation evoked by these compounds. ANKTM1, a member of the TRP family, responds to noxious cold (<17°C).[124]

[114] Zhang, Y. et al. 2003. *Cell* 112: 293-301.

[115] Zhang, Y. et al. 2007. *J. Neurosci.* 27: 5777-5786.

[116] McLaughlin, S. K., McKinnon, P. J., and Margolskee, R. F. 1992. *Nature* 357: 563-569.

[117] Danilova, V., Damak, S., Margolskee, R. F., and Hellekant, G. 2006. *Chem. Senses* 31: 573-580.

[118] Adler, E. et al. 2000. *Cell* 100: 693-702.

[119] Matsunami, H., Montmayeur, J. P., and Buck, L. B. 2000. *Nature* 404: 601-604.

[120] Chaudhari, N., Landin, A. M., and Roper, S. D. 2000. *Nat. Neurosci.* 3: 113-119.

[121] Caterina, M. J. et al. 1997. *Nature* 389: 816-824.

[122] Lumpkin, E. A., and Caterina, M. J. 2007. *Nature* 445: 858-865.

[123] Reid, G. 2005. *Pflügers Arch.* 451: 250-263.

[124] Kwan, K. Y., and Corey, D. P. 2009. *J. Gen. Physiol.* 133: 251-256.

(A)

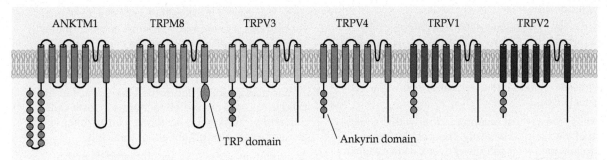

(B)

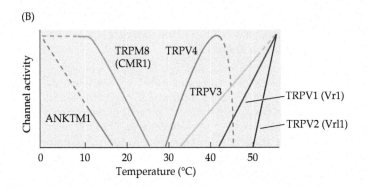

FIGURE 21.18 TRP Channels and Temperature Coding. (A) TRP channels comprise six putative membrane-spanning units and cytoplasmic amino and carboxyl terminals. (B) Heat-sensitive TRPs have different thermal activation ranges. In some cases chemical compounds also activate the receptor, producing a sensation of cooling (menthol on TRPM8) or heating (chili peppers on TRPV1). TRPV1 is also known as vanilloid receptor type 1, VR1, while TRPV2 is also known as VLR1. TRPM8 is also known as the cold and menthol receptor 1 (CMR1). Activation curves are averaged across multiple studies; dashed portions are extrapolated. (After A. Patapoutian et al., 2003. *Nat. Rev. Neurosci.* 4: 529-539.)

Signaling of Pain and Itch

Sensations of pain and itch arise from both direct and indirect actions on ion channels in nociceptive nerve terminals, although there are also distinct pathways for itch (pruritus).[125–127] Painful heat (hotter than about 43°C) causes nonspecific cation channels (TRPV1) to open in C-fiber endings.[128,129] Calcium and sodium ions enter and depolarize the cell, causing action potential generation. Prolonged exposure of these endings to capsaicin eventually causes calcium accumulation and cell death. For this reason capsaicin is used as a long-term analgesic, presumably relieving chronic pain by killing C-fiber afferents.[130,126] Acids also may act to open cation channels directly, and an acid-sensitive ion channel (ASIC) has been cloned from nociceptive neurons.[131,127] Mechanical stimuli leading to skin damage can also produce direct activation of nociceptive endings.

Responses to a wide range of nociceptive substances are mediated by a variety of GP-CRs.[132] These excite the nociceptive endings by acting on TRP channels of the vanilloid (TRPV1–4), melastin (TRPM2 and 8), and ankyrin (TRPA1) families. They enable the nerve terminals to respond to amines, such as histamine and serotonin, peptides, purines and nucleotides, steroids (bile acids), proteases (serine and cysteine), and other noxious substances. These substances are released by epidermal cells as the skin is damaged by mechanical forces (e.g., an abrasion) or by burning.[133]

Histamine and serotonin are prominent stimulants of pain and itch. Histamine acts through Histamine 1 (H1) receptors, and serotonin evokes pain and itching by activating 5-HT2B and 5-HT7 receptors. Separate itch-sensitive cells express non-histaminergic receptors and are sensitive to agents such as mucunain, which are associated with chronic itch.[134] Bradykinin is the prototypic algesic peptide of inflammation, and induces acute pain by activation of B2 receptors. B1 receptors play a more prominent role during persistent pain. Bradykinin and other chemicals in damaged skin also act to increase the excitability of (i.e., sensitize) nociceptive endings activated by other stimuli. For example, in the presence of bradykinin, responses to noxious heat are increased and occur at a lower temperature than normal.[127]

[125] Davidson, S. and Giesler, G. J. 2010. *Trends Neurosci.* 33: 550-558.

[126] Bautista, D. M., Wilson, S. R., and Hoon, M. A. 2014. *Nat. Neurosci.* 178: 175-182.

[127] Basbaum, A. I., Bautista, D. M. et al. 2009. *Cell* 139: 267-284

[128] Bevan, S., and Yeats, J. 1991. *J. Physiol.* 433: 145-161.

[129] Cesare, P., and McNaughton, P. 1996. *Proc. Natl. Acad. Sci. USA* 93: 15435-15439.

[130] Szallasi, A., and Blumberg, P. M. 1996. *Pain* 68: 195-208.

[131] Waldmann, R. et al. 1997. *Nature* 386: 173-177.

[132] Geppetti, P. et al. 2015. *Neuron* 88; 635-639.

[133] Malaviya, R., Morrison, A. R., and Pentland, A. P. 1996. *J. Invest. Dermatol.* 106: 785-789.

[134] Reddy, V. B., Azimi, E., Chu, L., and Lerner, E. A. 2018. *J. Invest. Dermatol.* 138: 461-464.

SUMMARY

- Each type of sensory receptor is exquisitely sensitive to one type of stimulus modality, its adequate stimulus. The receptor is shielded from stimuli of other modalities.

- Short and long receptors differ morphologically and functionally. Short receptors encode stimulus amplitude directly in the amplitude of the receptor potential. Long receptors convert the receptor potential amplitude into a frequency code of action potential firing.

- The response of most receptors varies with the logarithm of the stimulus intensity. This enables receptors to maintain their sensitivity over a wide dynamic range.

- Most sensory receptors adapt during maintained stimuli. Adaptation arises from both mechanical and electrical factors. Rapidly adapting receptors are able to respond to rapidly repetitive stimuli, such as vibration.

- Mechanosensitive hair cells of the inner ear couple movement directly to the gating of ion channels by physical connection. The tip link that connects adjacent stereocilia is stretched by deflection of the hair bundle and so pulls open an ion channel.

- Olfactory neurons employ G protein-coupled membrane receptors that lead to the opening of cAMP-gated cation channels in the plasma membrane.

- Each member of the large family of olfactory receptor proteins is expressed in a small number of olfactory receptors. All neurons expressing a particular receptor protein project to a single glomerulus in the olfactory bulb.

- Amino acids, sugars, and some bitter compounds bind to G protein-coupled receptors in taste cells. Salt and protons (sour) act directly on ion channels to generate receptor potentials in taste cells.

- Temperature sensations are mediated by activation of TRP ion channels in sensory nerve terminals. Channels TRPV1–4 respond to skin temperatures rising above about 25°C, TRPM8 to skin temperatures falling below about 25°C.

- Pain and itch are caused by a range of nociceptive and pruritogenic substances that activate a variety of G protein-coupled receptors in nociceptive and, in some cases, separate itch sensory nerve terminals. These, in turn, activate cationic TRP channels, leading to nerve terminal depolarization and action potential generation.

Suggested Reading

General Reviews

Behrens, M., Briand, L., de March, C. A., Matsunami, H., Yamashita, A., Meyerhof, W., and Weyand, S. 2018. Structure-function relationships of olfactory and taste receptors. *Chem. Senses* 43: 81-87.

Fettiplace, R. 2009. Defining features of the hair cell mechanoelectrical transducer channel. *Pflügers Arch.* 458: 1115–1123.

Gillespie, P. G., and Müller, U. 2009. Mechanotransduction by hair cells: models, molecules, and mechanisms. *Cell* 139: 33–44.

Hudspeth, A. J. 2008. Making an effort to listen: Mechanical amplification in the ear. *Neuron* 59: 530–545.

Kleene, S. J. 2008. The electrochemical basis of odor transduction in vertebrate olfactory cilia. *Chem. Senses* 33: 839–859.

Roper, S. D., and Chaudhari, N. 2009. Processing umami and other tastes in mammalian taste buds. *Ann. NY Acad. Sci.* 1170: 60–65.

Touhara, K., and Vosshall, L. B. 2009. Sensing odorants and pheromones with chemosensory receptors. *Annu. Rev. Physiol.* 71: 307–332.

Vega, J. A., García-Suárez, O., Montaño, J. A., Pardo, B., and Cobo, J. M. 2009. The Meissner and Pacinian sensory corpuscles: revisited new data from the last decade. *Microsc. Res. Tech.* 72: 299–309.

Vollrath, M. A., Kwan, K. Y., and Corey, D. P. 2007. The micromachinery of mechanotransduction in hair cells. *Annu. Rev. Neurosci.* 30: 339–365.

Original Papers

Beurg, M., Fettiplace, R., Nam, J. H., and Ricci, A. J. 2009. Localization of inner hair cell mechanotransducer channels using high-speed calcium imaging. *Nat. Neurosci.* 12: 553–558.

Crawford, A. C., and Fettiplace, R. 1985. The mechanical properties of ciliary bundles of turtle cochlear hair cells. *J. Physiol.* 364: 359–379.

DeFazio, R. A., Dvoryanchikov, G., Maruyama, Y., Kim, J. W., Pereira, E., Roper, S. D., and Chaudhari, N. 2006. Separate populations of receptor cells and presynaptic cells in mouse taste buds. *J. Neurosci.* 26: 3971–3980.

Eyzaguirre, C., and Kuffler, S. W. 1955. Processes of excitation in the dendrites and soma of single isolated sensory nerve cells of the lobster and crayfish. *J. Gen. Physiol.* 39: 87–119.

Howard, J., and Hudspeth, A. J. 1988. Compliance of the hair bundle associated with gating of mechanoelectrical transduction channels in the bullfrog's saccular hair cell. *Neuron* 1: 189–199.

Hudspeth, A. J., and Corey, D. P. 1977. Sensitivity, polarity and conductance change in the response of vertebrate hair cells to controlled mechanical stimuli. *Proc. Natl. Acad. Sci. USA* 74: 2407–2411.

Kazmierczak, P., Sakaguchi, H., Tokita, J., Wilson-Kubalek, E. M., Milligan, R. A., Muller, U., and Kachar, B. 2007. Cadherin 23 and protocadherin 15 interact to form tip-link filaments in sensory hair cells. *Nature* 449: 87–91.

Loewenstein, W. R., and Mendelson, M. 1965. Components of adaptation in a Pacinian corpuscle. *J. Physiol.* 177: 377–397.

Ricci, A. J., Crawford, A. C., and Fettiplace, R. 2003. Tonotopic variation in the conductance of the hair cell mechanotransducer channel. *Neuron* 40: 983–990.

Riviere, S., Challet, L., Fluegge, D., Spehr, M., and Rodriguez, I. 2009. Formyl peptide receptor-like proteins are a novel family of vomeronasal chemosensors. *Nature* 459: 574–577.

Zhang, Y., Hoon, M. A., Chandrashekar, J., Mueller, K. L., Cook, B., Wu, D., Zuker, C. S., and Ryba, N. J. 2003. Coding of sweet, bitter, and umami tastes: different receptor cells sharing similar signaling pathways. *Cell* 112: 293–301.

CHAPTER 22

Transduction and Transmission in the Retina

Our perception of scenes containing objects and background, color, movement, and depth begins with signals evoked by light in the retina. The visual responses to light start at photoreceptors known as rods and cones. Rods are highly sensitive to light and can be activated by a single photon. Color and daylight vision depend on cones, which are less sensitive to light. Our color vision depends on three types of cones, categorized according to the light wavelengths to which they respond. Some cones respond best to short (S) blueish wavelengths, others to medium (M) greenish wavelengths, and yet others to long (L) reddish wavelengths. Certain retinal pathways combine inputs from rods and cones.

Photoreceptors of vertebrates produce unusual signals that give rise to transmission through the retina. In darkness, photoreceptors are depolarized and release glutamate continuously from their synaptic endings. Light absorption by visual pigments leads to a cascade of biochemical reactions. As a result, nucleotide-gated cation channels in the membrane close, causing photoreceptors to hyperpolarize. Light thereby reduces ongoing transmitter release onto postsynaptic horizontal and bipolar cells.

Signals from photoreceptors reach ganglion cells, whose axons form the optic nerve and constitute the sole output from the eye. The intervening cells between photoreceptors and ganglion cells are bipolar, horizontal, and amacrine cells. Like rods and cones, bipolar and horizontal cells produce graded local potentials, not action potentials. As we described in Chapter 2, signaling by individual neurons in the retina and at successive levels of the visual system is best analyzed in terms of receptive fields, which are the building blocks for perception. In the visual system, the receptive field is the area of the retina that, on illumination, enhances or inhibits the activity of a neuron. Signaling in ganglion cells compares the luminance or colors between the small center and the surround in the visual field. Small parvocellular (P) and large magnocellular (M) retinal ganglion cells carry information to deeper visual centers. P cells mediate fine spatial discrimination and some have color sensitivity. Information from the center of the retina, a region called the fovea, is carried by P cells. Larger M cells respond better to moving stimuli and to small changes in luminance contrast. A third type of ganglion cell is the konio (K) cell, which carries information about space and blueish contrasts.

A small number of specialized ganglion cells respond directly to illumination. Such intrinsically photosensitive retinal ganglion cells carry information to visual and nonvisual centers about levels of background illumination and control pupillary constrictions; they also synchronize circadian rhythms.

The performance of nerve cells in the retina is described more fully here than in Chapters 1 and 2, which illustrated the principles of signaling and organization. Here we describe first the principal anatomical features of the visual pathways, to put in perspective the details of retinal organization that follow, and then the stepwise transformation of signals through the retina as light is trapped by visual pigments and generates changes in electrical currents. Chapter 18 dealt with the modulation of retinal function by light.

The Vertebrate Eye

The retina in the eye acts as a self-contained outpost of the brain. It collects information, analyzes it, and hands it on to higher centers through the well-defined optic nerve pathway for further processing. The initial step in visual processing is the formation on each retina of an inverted image of the outside world (Figure 22.1). Essential for clear vision are (1) correct focus of the image by adjustment of the thickness of the lens (accommodation); (2) regulation of light entering the eye by the pupil diameter; (3) convergence of the two eyes to ensure that matching images fall on corresponding points of both retinas; and (4) eye movements that compensate for self-generated or forced movements of the head. Our vision is not uniformly detailed across the visual field but is most acute in the center. We can read small print at the center of gaze, but not in the peripheral field of vision. This loss of acuity arises more from decreased receptor density and changes in connectivity in the peripheral retina than from optical effects.

Anatomical Pathways in the Visual System

The pathways emerging from one eye are illustrated in Figure 22.2, which depicts some of the major landmarks of the visual system in a rat brain. The retinal ganglion cell axons enter the optic nerve; about half cross at the optic chiasm. In each hemisphere of the brain, axons from the equivalent areas of both eyes end in a part of the thalamus called

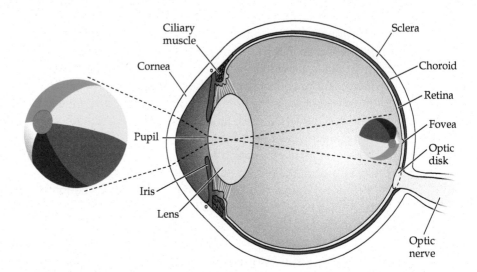

FIGURE 22.1 Structure of the Vertebrate Eye. Cross section through the right eye seen from above and showing the projection of a visual object onto the retina. Activation of ciliary muscle changes the thickness of the lens and the opening of the pupil. The retina is interrupted by the exit of ganglion cell axons at the optic disk to form the optic nerve. Nearby lies the retinal fovea, where visual acuity is best because of the high density of photoreceptors and the thinning of the overlying cellular layers.

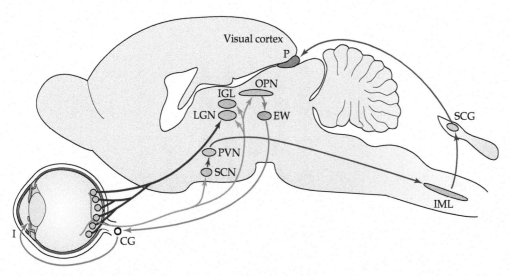

FIGURE 22.2 Central Targets of Retinal Ganglion Cells. The great majority of retinal ganglion cells respond to light transduced by photoreceptors and transmitted via bipolar cells, and send their axons to the lateral geniculate nucleus (LGN) of the thalamus. From there, information flows to visual cortex (see Chapter 2). These classic retinal ganglion cells (thick violet lines) carry information about color, shape, movement—all the details that give us form vision and the ability to analyze the visual world. Another major target is the superior colliculus (not shown), which is involved in response to movement. A small minority of retinal ganglion cells are intrinsically photosensitive due to the expression of the photopigment melanopsin. These intrinsically photosensitive retinal ganglion cells (ipRGCs; thin green lines) project to the LGN and also to the suprachiasmatic nucleus (SCN) (see Chapter 19), and then through the paraventricular nucleus (PVN) to form the retinohypothalamic tract (red lines), which drives circadian rhythms. This circuit involves the intermediolateral nucleus (IML) of the spinal cord, and the superior cervical ganglion (SCG) that ultimately stimulates melatonin release from the pineal gland (P). Other ipRGCs project to the intergeniculate leaflet (IGL), the olivary pretectal nucleus (OPN) and from there to the Edinger-Westphal nucleus (EW) to activate motoneurons in the ciliary ganglion (CG) that control muscles of the iris (I; blue lines). (After D. M. Berson, 2003. *Trends Neurosci.* 26: 314–320.)

the lateral geniculate nucleus (see also Chapter 2). Because of optical reversal by the lens, which projects the left visual field onto the right side of each retina, each cerebral hemisphere sees the visual field on the opposite side. The bundle of ganglion cells that carry information on background illumination projects to nonvisual areas that synchronize circadian rhythms and control the pupillary reflex that modulates the amount of light arriving at the retina.[1]

Layering of Cells in the Retina

Among the reasons the retina is inviting for physiological research is the neat layering and stereotyped morphology of the relatively few nerve cell types—there are only five main classes.[2-5] The arrangement of various cells is illustrated in Figure 22.3. On the deep surface, farthest from the lens and pupil, lie the **photoreceptors**, composed of the **rods**, which are concerned with dim-light color-blind vision, and **cones**, which are used with daylight illumination when we can perceive color. Cones are connected to the **bipolar cells**, which in turn connect to the **ganglion cells**, whose axons are the optic nerve fibers. The connectivity of rods is more complex; their bipolar cells connect to an intervening interneuron, a special type of amacrine cell named the **amacrine type II (AII cell)**, that piggybacks onto the cone circuitry.

Apart from this through-line, there are other cells that make predominantly lateral (i.e., side-to-side) connections. These are the **horizontal cells** and the **amacrine cells** (see Figure 22.3). Only ganglion cells and some amacrine cells generate action potentials. Photoreceptors, horizontal cells, and bipolar cells generate only locally graded signals. Within each of these major classes there are subgroups exhibiting important

[1] Do, M. T. H. 2019. *Neuron* 104: 205-226.

[2] Boycott, B. B., and Dowling, J. E. 1969. *Philos. Trans. R. Soc. Lond. B, Biol. Sci.* 255: 109-184.

[3] Sterling, P., and Demb, J. B. 2003. In *Synaptic Organization of the Brain.* Oxford University Press, New York.

[4] Balasubramanian, V., and Sterling, P. 2009. *J. Physiol.* 587: 2753-2767.

[5] Masland, R. H. 2001. *Nat. Neurosci.* 4: 877-886.

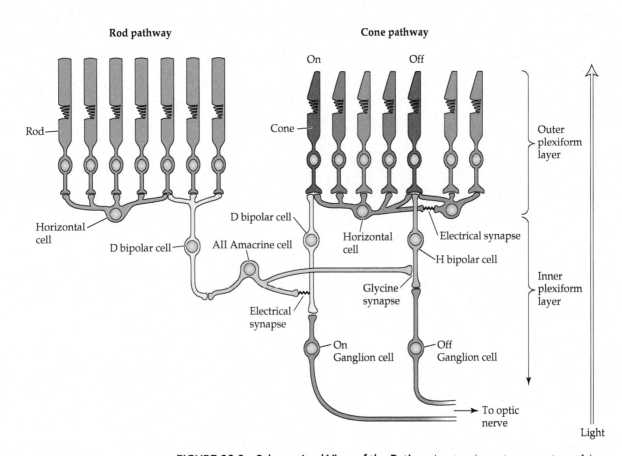

FIGURE 22.3 Schematized View of the Retina showing the main connections of the rod and cone pathways. Light enters the retina from below in this scheme and is absorbed by the rods and cones. Signals are initiated in the outer segments. Rods and cones make synaptic connections onto bipolar cells and horizontal cells in the outer plexiform layer. Horizontal cells connect with each other by electrical synapses and with adjacent rods and cones by GABAergic inhibitory synapses. In the fovea a single cone may connect to a bipolar cell. Bipolar cells make synapses with ganglion cells and amacrine cells (in the figure the AII type) in the inner plexiform layer. Rod bipolar cells on the right make use of the cone pathway via AII amacrine cells. AII cells connect via electrical synapses with the "on" depolarizing (D) bipolar cells of the cone pathway; glycinergic inhibitory synapses connect AII cells with the "off" hyperpolarizing (H) bipolar cells of the cone pathway. Certain peripheral ganglion cells have intrinsic light responses mediated by direct absorption of melanopsin and also receive connections from rods and cones (not shown). The colors of the cones indicate their peak light sensitivity arbitrarily. (After J. E. Dowling and B. B. Boycott, 1966. *Proc. R. Soc. Lond., B, Biol. Sci.* 166: 80–111; N. W. Daw et al., 1990. *Trends Neurosci.* 13: 110–115.)

differences in structure and function. Müller cells and astrocytes constitute the satellite glial cells of the retina. Their contribution to integration of the functioning of the retina was described in Chapter 18.

Phototransduction in Retinal Rods and Cones

Photoreceptors are functional units for light perception. They set the stage for vision and define how the outside world can be perceived; their spectral range varies depending on their type and among species. For example, many invertebrates can detect ultraviolet light. Human photoreceptors normally do not detect ultraviolet light, but they can outperform photoreceptors of some fellow mammals. Cats, lacking appropriate receptors, are color-blind (though we are too at night, when all cats look gray). However, the sensitivity of mammalian rods in darkness is such that a single quantum of light can give rise to an experimentally measurable signal, and only 2 to several quanta are needed for a conscious sensation.[6]

---

[6] Barlow, H. B. 1956. *J. Opt. Soc. Am.* 46: 634–639.

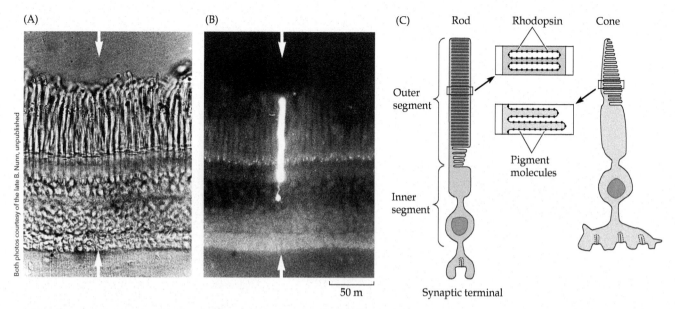

FIGURE 22.4 Photoreceptors in Retina. (A,B) Rod in toad retina injected with a fluorescent dye, Lucifer yellow, as seen in visible light (A) and ultraviolet light (B). Arrows mark identical points on the retina. (C) Diagram of a rod and a cone. The principal features of photoreceptor structure are (1) an outer segment within which light is absorbed by visual pigments; (2) an inner segment containing the nucleus and other "housekeeping" structures; and (3) the synaptic terminal, which releases glutamate onto second-order cells and receives synaptic inputs. In the rod, the pigment rhodopsin (black dots) is embedded in membranes arranged in the form of disks, which are not continuous with the outer membrane of the cell. In the cone, the pigment molecules are on infolded membranes that are continuous with the surface membrane. The outer segment is connected to the inner segment by a narrow stalk. The synaptic endings continually release transmitter in the dark. (C after D. A. Baylor, 1987. *Invest. Ophthalmol. Vis. Sci.* 28: 34–49.)

Three types of cones in humans contribute to color vision. A small number of cones respond to short short (S) blueish wavelengths, a larger number respond to medium (M) greenish wavelengths, and the rest respond to long (L) reddish wavelengths. With less-sensitive cone photoreceptors, about 200 quanta produce a conscious sensation.[7] We can detect subtle tints and differences in contrast or color on a bright day, when the light intensity is several decades greater.

Arrangement and Morphology of Photoreceptors

The rods and cones constitute a densely packed array of photodetectors in the inner layer of retina (i.e., adjacent to the pigment epithelium) that is farthest from the cornea and incoming light. With the exception of one small retinal area, the fovea, light must traverse layers of transparent cells and fibers before reaching the light-absorbing outer segments of receptors (Figure 22.4). In humans, which are diurnal, the pigment epithelium absorbs the light that is not absorbed by the photoreceptors, thereby reducing the scattering of light within the eye and increasing spatial resolution. In cats, which are nocturnal, the absence of the pigment epithelium and properties of the choroid produce a reflection and give light a second chance to be captured by photoreceptors, thereby increasing visual sensitivity at the expense of spatial resolution, which is reduced by the scattering of reflected light.

As shown in Figure 22.5, cones are closely packed in the human fovea, with a density of 160,000/mm^2, whereas rods are excluded from that area.[8] The cones in the fovea are more slender than those in peripheral parts of the retina.[3] Since the fovea contains no rods, it constitutes a blind spot in very dim light, such as at night. That is why we cannot see a star when we try to focus on it directly, but we can see it if we set our focal point right beside it. A different blind spot corresponds to the region of the retina through which the optic nerve fibers leave the eye; at this spot, the optic disk, there are no photoreceptors at all (see Figure 22.5).

[7] Koenig, D., and Hofer, H. 2011. *J. Vis.* 11: 21.

[8] Osterberg, G. 1935. *Acta Ophthalmol. Supp.* 6: 1–103.

(A)

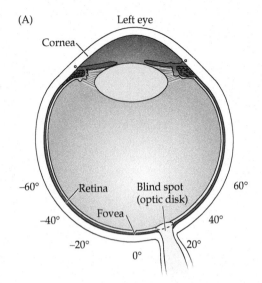

(B)

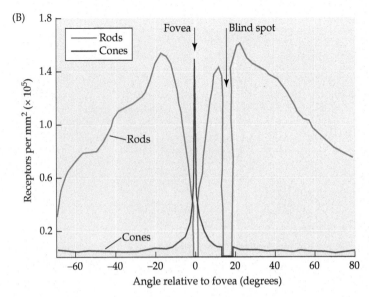

FIGURE 22.5 Distribution of Rods and Cones in the Human Retina. (A) Opposite the cornea, the retina covers an area expressed as a visual angle relative to the position of the fovea. (B) Cones are concentrated in the fovea, where rods are absent. Photoreceptors are absent from the blind spot, where axons of ganglion cells form the optic nerve. (After B. Wandell. 1995. *Foundations of Vision*. Sinauer/Oxford University Press: Sunderland, MA. Data from G. Osterberg, 1935. *Acta Ophthalmol. Supp*. 6: 1–103.)

[9] Helmholtz, H. V. 1962/1924. *Helmholtz's Treatise on Physiological Optics*. Dover: New York.

[10] Liang, J., Williams, D. R., and Miller, D T. 1997. *J. Opt. Soc. Am. A* 14: 2884–2892.

[11] Roorda, A. et al. 2002. *Opt. Express* 10: 405–412.

[12] Hofer, H., Singer, B., and Williams, D. R. 2005. *J. Vis.* 5: 5.

[13] Curcio, C. A. et al. 1991. *J. Comp. Neurol.* 312: 610–624.

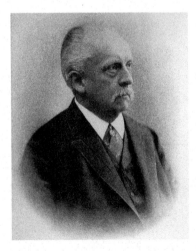

Hermann von Helmholtz (1821–1894) made equally important and original contributions to the study of medicine, hearing, neurophysiology, and thermodynamics. It seems refreshing to read his prose today.

As Helmholtz wrote in 1867,

There is in the retina a remarkable spot which is placed near its center…and which…is called the fovea or pit…[It] is of great importance for vision since it is the spot where the most exact discrimination is made. The cones are here packed most closely together and receive light which has not been impeded by other semi-transparent parts of the retina. We may assume that a single nervous…connection…runs from each of these cones through the trunk of the optic nerve to the brain…and there produces its special impression so that the excitation of each individual cone will produce a distinct and separate effect upon the sense.[9]

Although it was shown later that the connectivity of photoreceptors with the output cells of the retina is much more complex, it is extraordinary that Helmholtz could write this paragraph before the word *synapse* or even the cell doctrine existed.

Mosaics of Color Photoreceptors

The distribution of cones in the living human retina and their contribution to color perception can be studied using **adaptive optics ophthalmoscopy**,[10,11] which allows for identification of individual cones according to their position and wavelength sensitivity. Figure 22.6A shows a cone mosaic formed by the outer segments of individual cones. The wavelength that best excites each cell can be determined by laser focal illumination of individual cones with short, medium, or long wavelengths. The appropriate wavelength bleaches (activates) the pigment in the cone to reflect light differently. After recovery, identified cones can be illuminated alone or in combination with their surrounding cones to analyze perception.

The false colors in Figure 22.6A show that in the fovea, L and M cones outnumber S cones. The proportions of M and L cones vary widely among individuals, from 0.4:1 M:L to 16:1 M:L.[12] S cones contribute only 5% to the population, being scattered around the center of the fovea[13] (not shown). Figure 22.6B shows the distribution of rods and cones in the periphery of the fixed retina, outside the fovea of a macaque. The cones are much larger than the rods, which due to their small size cannot be identified individually using adaptive optics ophthalmoscopy. However, Figure 22.6 shows an immunostaining of S cones in the macaque retina.

(A)

(B)

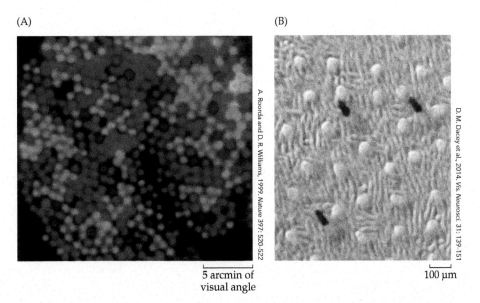

A. Roorda and D. R. Williams, 1999. *Nature* 397: 520-522

D. M. Dacey et al., 2014. *Vis. Neurosci.* 31: 139-151

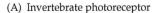

5 arcmin of
visual angle

100 μm

FIGURE 22.6 Distribution of Photoreceptors in the Mammalian Retina. (A) Cone mosaic in the fovea of a living human retina, obtained with adaptive optics ophthalmoscopy. Cones responding to S, M, and L wavelengths are pseudocolored blue, green, and red, respectively. S cones represent a smaller proportion of the mosaic than M and L cones. (B) Peripheral segment of a fixed macaque isolated retina with cones (large spots) and rods (small spots). The size of cones is much larger than in the fovea. Blue cones are immunostained.

Electrical Responses of Vertebrate Photoreceptors to Light

As described earlier, many sensory receptors respond to appropriate stimuli by graded local depolarization that may initiate action potentials. Although the majority of invertebrate photoreceptors behave in this way (Figure 22.7A),[14] the responses of most vertebrate photoreceptors to light are very different. Figure 22.7B exemplifies this difference with the responses of a turtle rod recorded with an intracellular microelectrode.[15] In the dark, the photoreceptor is depolarized by a continuous positive current flowing into the outer segment. Light turns off the ongoing inward current, leaving the always-present outward potassium current to hyperpolarize the cell. The next two sections deal with how light is absorbed by photoreceptors and the mechanisms that underlie the production of electrical signals.

[14] Fuortes, M. G., and Poggio, G. F. 1963. *J. Gen. Physiol.* 46: 435-452.

[15] Baylor, D. A., Fuortes, M. G., and O'Bryan, P. M. 1971. *J. Physiol.* 214: 265-294.

(A) Invertebrate photoreceptor

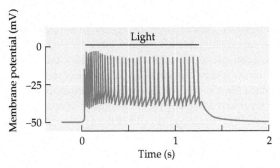

(B) Vertebrate photoreceptor

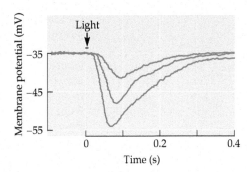

FIGURE 22.7 Responses of Photoreceptors. (A) Photoreceptors of an invertebrate (a horseshoe crab) respond to light with a depolarization that gives rise to impulses. This is the usual type of response elicited from sensory receptors activated by various stimuli, such as touch, pressure, or stretch (see Chapter 21). (B) Photoreceptors of a vertebrate (a turtle) respond with a hyperpolarization that is graded according to the intensity of the flash. (A after M. G. Fuortes and G. F. Poggio, 1963. *J. Gen. Physiol.* 46: 435-452; B after D. A. Baylor et al., 1971. *J. Physiol.* 214: 265-294.)

Visual Pigments

The visual pigments that absorb light are heavily concentrated in membranes of the outer segments of rods and cones. Each rod contains approximately 10^8 pigment molecules. They are aggregated on several hundred discrete disks (approximately 750 in a monkey rod) that do not make contact with the outer membrane (see Figure 22.4C). By contrast, cones have pigment-laden infoldings that are continuous with the plasma membrane. Pigment molecules make up about 80% of the total disk protein. The visual pigment is so closely packed on outer segment membranes that the distance between two visual pigment molecules in a rod is less than 10 nanometers (nm).[16] This dense packing of sensitive molecules in serial layers of membranes traversed by light enhances the probability that a photon will be trapped on its way through the outer segment.

Absorption of Light by Visual Pigments

Rhodopsin is the visual pigment of rods. The high density of rhodopsin and its stability make it an efficient light-trap on photoreceptor disks. Light is absorbed by the retinal moiety (see the next paragraph) of rhodopsin in rods and by related pigments in cones. The events that occur when this happens have been studied by psychophysical, biochemical, and physiological techniques. The absorption characteristics of the visual pigments have been measured quantitatively by spectrophotometry.[17,18] When different wavelengths of light are shone through a solution of rhodopsin, the blue-green light at a wavelength of about 500 nm is absorbed most effectively. The absorption spectrum is similar when small spots of light of different wavelengths are shone onto single rods under the microscope. An elegant correspondence has been demonstrated between the absorption characteristics of rhodopsin and our perception in dim light. Quantitative psychophysical measurements made in humans show that blue-green light at about 500 nm is optimal for perception in the dark. Night vision is color-blind because there is only one type of rod. In daylight, when rods are inactive and cones are active, the visual system uses the different responses of the cones to see color.

Molecular Physiology of Rhodopsin

The relation between the structure and the function of rhodopsin has been studied by electrophysiology, molecular sequencing, and crystallography.[19] Visual pigment molecules consist of two moieties: (1) a protein known as opsin and (2) a covalently bound chromophore (i.e., a chemical group producing color in a compound), 11-*cis* vitamin A aldehyde, known as **retinal.**

Opsin is a member of the large family of seven transmembrane domain proteins that includes metabotropic neurotransmitter receptors, such as adrenergic and muscarinic receptors. Like rhodopsin, molecules in this family exert their effects through second messengers by activating G proteins (see Chapter 12). The primary sequence of opsin consists of 348 amino acid residues with seven hydrophobic regions of 20 to 25 amino acids, comprising seven transmembrane helices.[20] The amino terminus is located in the extracellular space (and within the disk in rods), and the carboxy terminus is in the cytoplasm (Figure 22.8). The carboxy terminus of human rhodopsin binds the α subunit of the G protein. Retinal binds to a lysine residue in the seventh membrane-spanning segment of opsin. Binding to 11-*cis* retinal stabilizes opsin against thermal transitions that may activate the G protein cascade. The stability of rhodopsin in darkness is extraordinarily high. Baylor calculated that spontaneous thermal isomerization of a single rhodopsin molecule should occur once every 3000 years, or 10^{23} times more slowly than photoisomerization.[21] The same chemical link with opsin and the opsin environment determines the absorption of light by retinal, which by itself would be at a peak wavelength of 460 nm. Interactions of retinal with certain opsin amino acids shift the absorbance to the 500-nm peak of rhodopsin, or to the characteristic peaks of the pigments in the different cones.[22]

[16] Dowling, J. E. 1987. *The Retina: An Approachable Part of the Brain.* Harvard University Press, Cambridge, MA.

[17] Brown, P. K., and Wald, G. 1963. *Nature* 200: 37–43.

[18] Marks, W. B., Dobelle, W. H., and Macnichol, E. F., Jr. 1964. *Science* 143: 1181–1183.

[19] Palczewski, K. et al. 2000. *Science* 289: 739–745.

[20] Nathans, J., and Hogness, D. S. 1984. *Proc. Natl. Acad. Sci. USA* 81: 4851–4855.

[21] Baylor, D. A. 1987. *Invest. Ophthalmol. Vis. Sci.* 28: 34–49.

[22] Imamoto, Y., and Shichida, Y. 2014. *Biochim. Biophys. Acta* 1837: 664–673.

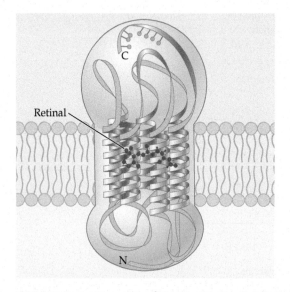

FIGURE 22.8 Structure of Vertebrate Rhodopsin in the Membrane. The helix is partly opened to show the position of retinal (red). C = carboxy terminus; N = amino terminus. (After L. Stryer and H. R. Bourne, 1986. *Annu. Rev. Cell Biol.* 2: 391–419.)

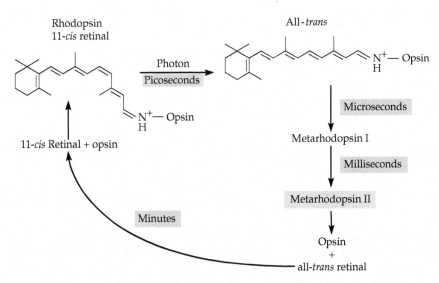

FIGURE 22.9 Bleaching of Rhodopsin by Light. In the dark, 11-*cis* retinal is bound to the protein opsin. Capture of a photon causes isomerization of the 11-*cis* retinal to all-*trans* retinal. The opsin-all-*trans* molecule, in turn, is rapidly converted to metarhodopsin II, which is dissociated to opsin and all-*trans* retinal. The regeneration of rhodopsin depends on interactions between photoreceptors and cells of the retinal pigment epithelium. Metarhodopsin II is the trigger that sets in motion activation of the second messenger system. (After J. E. Dowling, 1987. *The Retina: An Approachable Part of the Brain*. Harvard University Press, Cambridge, MA.)

Once a photon has been absorbed by rhodopsin, retinal undergoes photoisomerization and changes from the 11-*cis* to an all-*trans* configuration. This transition is extremely rapid; it takes place in approximately 10^{-12} seconds. Opsin then undergoes a cascade of transformations through various intermediates.[2] A change in the configuration of the transmembrane helices 6 and 7 changes the configuration of opsin, which interacts with the G protein transducin.[4] One conformation of the protein, metarhodopsin II, is of crucial importance for transduction (discussed in the next section). Figure 22.9 shows the sequence of changes occurring in bleaching and in regeneration of active rhodopsin. Metarhodopsin II appears after about 1 millisecond (ms). Regeneration of rhodopsin is slow, taking many minutes; it entails transfer of retinal between the photoreceptors and the pigment epithelium, where it undergoes transition back to the 11-*cis* configuration, and rebinding to bleached opsin.[23] Cone phototransduction follows a similar chemical cascade with certain differences, such as a less effective amplification and faster signaling and recovery of pigments.[24]

[23] Pepperberg, D. R. et al. 1993. *Mol. Neurobiol.* 7: 61-85.

[24] Shichida, Y. et al. *Biochemistry* 33: 9040-9044.

[25] Baylor, D. A., and Fuortes, M. G. 1970. *J. Physiol.* 207: 77-92.

[26] Luo, D. G., Xue, T., and Yau, K. W. 2008. *Proc. Natl. Acad. Sci. USA* 105: 9855-9862.

[27] Baylor, D. A., Lamb, T. D., and Yau, K. W. 1979. *J. Physiol.* 288: 589-611.

Transduction

How does photoisomerization of rhodopsin give rise to a change in membrane potential? For many years, it was clear that some sort of internal transmitter was required for the generation of electrical signals in rods and cones. One reason is that information about the capture of photons in a rod outer segment must somehow be conveyed from rhodopsin located in the disk, through the cytoplasm to the outer membrane. A second reason is the enormous amplification of the response. Baylor and his colleagues,[25] working on turtle photoreceptors, showed that decreases in membrane conductance and measurable electrical signals were produced when a single photon was absorbed and activated 1 pigment molecule out of about 10^8.

The sequence of events through which activated photopigment molecules change membrane potential has since been elucidated by patch clamp recordings from rod and cone outer segments and by molecular techniques.[26] The scheme for transduction from light to electrical signals is shown in Figure 22.10. In darkness, a continuous *dark* current flows into the outer segment of rods and cones.[27] As a result, they have membrane potentials of approximately –40 mV, which is positive to the potassium equilibrium potential, E_K

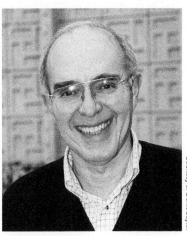

Denis Baylor, 1991

(A)   (B)   Light

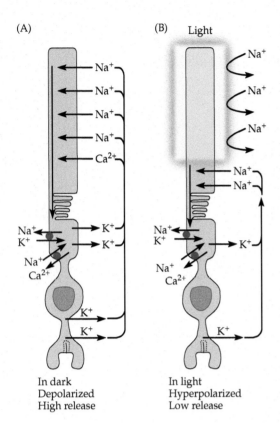

In dark
Depolarized
High release

In light
Hyperpolarized
Low release

FIGURE 22.10   Dark Current in a Rod. (A) In darkness, sodium ions flow through cation channels of the rod outer segment, causing a depolarization; calcium ions also enter through the cation channels. The current loop is completed through the neck of the rod, with the outward movement of potassium through the inner segment membrane. (B) When the outer segment is illuminated, the cation channels close because of a decrease in intracellular cyclic guanosine monophosphate (cGMP), and the rod then becomes hyperpolarized. This hyperpolarization reduces transmitter release. Sodium, potassium, and calcium concentrations of the rod are maintained by pumps and exchangers in the inner segment (red circles); calcium exchangers are also present in the outer segment (see Box 22.1). (After D. A. Baylor, 1987. *Invest. Ophthalmol. Vis. Sci.* 28: 34–49.)

(–80 mV). The inward current in the dark is carried mainly by sodium, moving down its electrochemical gradient through cation channels in the outer segment. Hyperpolarization of the photoreceptor by light is brought about by closure of the channels, allowing the membrane potential to move toward E_K.

In terms of transduction mechanisms, it will be apparent that there are striking similarities between the generation of responses to light by photoreceptors and the responses to odors by olfactory receptors described in Chapter 21.

Properties of the Photoreceptor Channels

The cation channels in the outer segment, under normal physiological conditions, have calcium:sodium:potassium permeability ratios of 12.5:1.0:0.7, and a very low single-channel conductance of around 25 femtosiemens (fS).[28] However, that value depends in part on the activation level[29] and in part on the blocking effect of divalent cations, mainly calcium.[30] Because the sodium concentration is much higher than that of calcium, about 85% of the inward current is carried by sodium. The driving force for potassium movement is of course outward. As calcium ions move through the channels, they are tightly bound to sites within the pore and thus interfere with the passage of other cations. Because of this property, removal of calcium from the solution around the cell allows sodium and potassium to move much more freely through the channel, increasing its conductance to about 25 picosiemens (pS).

Fesenko, Yau, Baylor, Stryer, and their colleagues[28,31,32] have shown that cyclic guanosine monophosphate (cGMP) acts as the internal transmitter from disk to surface membrane and fulfills the requirements of appropriate kinetics and great amplification. As shown in Figure 22.11, a high cytoplasmic concentration of cGMP keeps the cation channels predominantly in an open state. When the cGMP concentration of the fluid facing the inside of the membrane is reduced, channel openings become rare events. Thus, the membrane potential of the photoreceptors is a reflection of the cytoplasmic cGMP concentration—the higher the concentration, the more the cell is depolarized. The cGMP concentration in turn is inversely related to the intensity of ambient light. Increasing light intensity reduces cGMP concentration and reduces the number of open channels. In the absence of cGMP, almost all the channels are closed, the membrane potential becomes hyperpolarized, and the resistance of the outer segment membrane approaches that of a channel-free lipid bilayer.

Molecular Structure of Cyclic GMP-Gated Channels

Complementary DNAs for rod outer segment channels have been isolated and the amino acid sequences determined for channel subunits from human, bovine, mouse, and chicken retinas. There is a pronounced sequence similarity between cDNAs of outer segment channel subunits and the subunits of other cyclic nucleotide-gated channels—for example, those found in the olfactory system.[33] Their membrane regions share structural similarities with other cation-selective channels, particularly in the S4 region and the region of the pore (see Chapter 5). The photoreceptor channels are tetramers made up of at least two different subunit proteins, α and β, with apparent molecular sizes of 63 and 240 kilodaltons (kD), respectively. The intracellular nucleotide-binding site is near the carboxy terminus of the α- and β-subunits.[34]

[28] Fesenko, E. E., Kolesnikov, S. S., and Lyubarsky, A. L. 1985. *Nature* 313: 310–313.

[29] Ruiz, M. L., and Karpen, J. W. 1997. *Nature* 389: 389–392.

[30] Taylor, W. R., and Baylor, D. A. 1995. *J. Physiol.* 483 (Pt 3): 567–582.

[31] Stryer, L., and Bourne, H. R. 1986. *Annu. Rev. Cell Biol.* 2: 391–419.

[32] Yau, K. W., and Nakatani, K. 1985. *Nature* 317: 252–255.

[33] Torre, V. et al. 1995. *J. Neurosci.* 15: 7757–7768.

[34] Kaupp, U. B., and Seifert, R. 2002. *Physiol. Rev.* 82: 769–824.

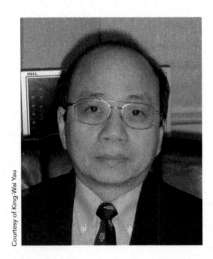

Courtesy of King-Wai Yau

King-Wai Yau

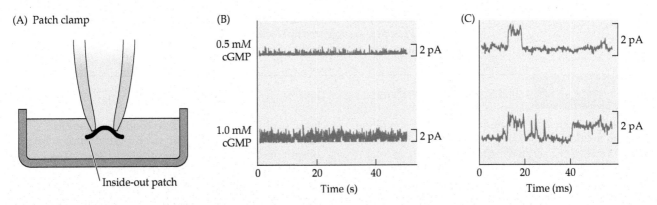

(A) Patch clamp

Inside-out patch

(B)

0.5 mM cGMP ⎤ 2 pA

1.0 mM cGMP ⎤ 2 pA

0   20   40
Time (s)

(C)

⎤ 2 pA

⎤ 2 pA

0   20   40
Time (ms)

FIGURE 22.11 Role of Cyclic GMP in Opening Sodium Channels in rod outer segment membranes (A). (B) Single-channel recordings made from inside-out patches bathed in two concentrations of cGMP. Channel opening causes deflections in the upward direction. The frequency of channel opening is extremely low in control recordings. (C) Addition of cGMP causes single-channel openings, the frequency of which increases with increased concentration. (A after D. A. Baylor, 1987. *Invest. Ophthalmol. Vis. Sci.* 28: 34–49; B,C after A. Zimmerman and D. Baylor. 1986. *Nature* 321: 70–72.)

The cGMP Cascade

The sequence of events leading to reduction in cGMP concentration and consequent closing of the cation channels is shown in Figure 22.12. The decrease in internal cGMP concentration triggered by light is brought about by metarhodopsin II, an intermediary in the bleaching process in which the chromophore separates from the protein (see Figure 22.9). Metarhodopsin II acts on the G protein, **transducin**, which consists of α, β, and γ polypeptide chains.[35,36]

The transient interaction of metarhodopsin II and transducin causes guanosine diphosphate (GDP) bound to the α-subunit to be exchanged for guanosine triphosphate (GTP). This activates the α-subunit, which separates from the β- and γ-subunits, and in turn activates a membrane-bound phosphodiesterase, which is the enzyme that hydrolyzes cGMP. The cGMP concentration falls, fewer sodium channels open, and the rods hyperpolarize. The cascade is terminated by phosphorylation of the carboxy terminus region of the

[35] Stryer, L. 1987. *Sci. Am.* 257: 42–50.
[36] Chen, C. K. 2005. *Rev. Physiol. Biochem. Pharmacol.* 154: 101–121.

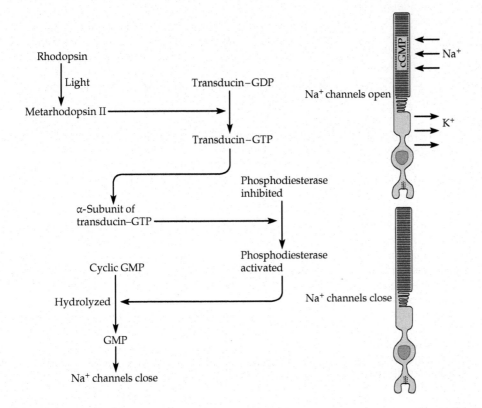

Rhodopsin
↓ Light
Metarhodopsin II ⟶

Transducin–GDP
↓
Transducin–GTP

α-Subunit of transducin–GTP ⟶

Phosphodiesterase inhibited
↓
Phosphodiesterase activated

Cyclic GMP
↓
Hydrolyzed
↓
GMP
↓
Na⁺ channels close

Na⁺ channels open
cGMP ← Na⁺
← K⁺

Na⁺ channels close

FIGURE 22.12 Coupling of Photopigment Activation to G Protein Activation. The G protein transducin binds guanosine triphosphate (GTP) in the presence of metarhodopsin II, leading to activation of phosphodiesterase, which in turn hydrolyzes cyclic GMP. With the reduced concentration of cGMP, sodium channels close. GDP = guanosine diphosphate. (After D. A. Baylor, 1987. *Invest. Ophthalmol. Vis. Sci.* 28: 34–49.)

active metarhodopsin II (Box 22.1). The key role of cGMP in controlling the channels during the response is supported by biochemical experiments. Illumination of photoreceptors can cause a 20% decrease in the internal cGMP concentration.[21]

BOX 22.1   Adaptation of Photoreceptors

The light intensities that humans use for vision range from the detection of single photons to bright sunlight on a tropical beach, a dynamic range of more than 10^{13}. Since pupillary constriction reduces light by only tenfold, adaptation by photoreceptors accounts for most of the wide range of sensitivity[37] and is achieved largely by retinal cones, which are used in daylight and starlight. Although our rods saturate at light levels that we associate with daytime vision, even indoors our cones can adjust to very bright lights, saturating just before light intensities become damaging.

Thus, it is essential to ensure that responses to light can occur at different background levels of illumination. If bright, ambient light were able to close all the nucleotide-gated channels, the receptor would be unable to register any further increase in intensity.

Calcium is one factor of key importance for adaptation of photoreceptors.[38,39] In the dark, the nucleotide-gated channels are open and calcium ions continually flow into the photoreceptor. Calcium is extruded by ion pumps and exchangers in the outer segment (see Figure 22.10).[40] Under conditions of steady illumination, the channels close and calcium entry is reduced. Because calcium is still actively extruded (see Figure 22.10), the intracellular calcium concentration falls. The reduced intracellular calcium concentration opposes closure of the nucleotide-gated channels by several mechanisms.

First, calcium reduces the affinity of channels to cGMP through the calcium-binding protein calmodulin. Lowered calcium concentration therefore increases the affinity of the channels to cGMP, and thereby potentiates channel opening and current flow during illumination. Second, lowered intracellular calcium favors intracellular cGMP accumulation by increasing the activity of guanylate cyclase (i.e., it promotes cGMP synthesis) and inhibiting the activation of phosphodiesterase (i.e., it slows cGMP hydrolysis). Third, lowered intracellular calcium causes phosphorylation of metarhodopsin II and thereby speeds up its inactivation. The rate of termination of the catalytic activity of metarhodopsin II is of importance for transduction, because while it is active, the cascade continues to generate a signal. The phosphorylation of activated rhodopsin is mediated by recoverin,[41] a calcium-binding molecule that is also involved in the inhibition of phosphodiesterase. Dark adaptation, which is the reverse of light adaptation, is principally limited by the regeneration of photopigment, which for full adaptation can take up to 10 minutes for cones and 30 minutes for rods.

Molecular mechanisms for adaptation were analyzed by Baylor and his colleagues,[39] who measured the rate of adaptation of photoreceptor responses in normal and transgenic mice in which 15 amino acids were deleted from the C terminus of rhodopsin, the presumptive site

for phosphorylation of activated rhodopsin (see Figure).[42,43] In a normal rod (see part B of the figure), a flash of light produces an outward current that adapts (i.e., decreases) as expected. Part C of the figure shows the response of a rod in a transgenic mouse to a flash—the response, instead of declining, lasts about 20 times longer than normal. Thus, the 15 amino acids that had been deleted constitute the region of the molecule required for recovery from the effects of a flash of light.

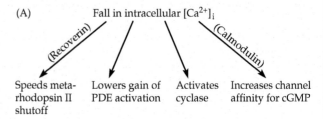

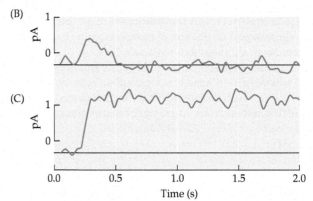

Mechanisms of Adaptation. (A) Diagram showing effects of a fall in the intracellular calcium concentration on mechanisms that influence adaptation of photoreceptors to steady light. (B,C) Responses to flashes of light delivered at time zero were recorded from a rod by suction electrodes. (B) The response elicited by activation of a normal rhodopsin molecule declined as expected. (C) The trace was recorded from a rod in a transgenic mouse in which rhodopsin molecules had been truncated by the deletion of 15 amino acids from the C terminus. The duration of the response was prolonged through failure of the altered rhodopsin molecule to become shut off after the flash. PDE = phosphodiesterase. (A,B after D. A. Baylor, 1996. *Proc. Natl. Acad. Sci. USA* 93: 560–565, B based in part on J. Chen et al., 1995. *Science* 267: 374–377.)

[37] Fain, G. L., Matthews, H. R., and Cornwall, M. C. 1996. *Trends Neurosci.* 19: 502–507.

[38] Baylor, D. 1996. *Proc. Natl. Acad. Sci. USA* 93: 560–565.

[39] Koutalos, Y., and Yau, K. W. 1996. *Trends Neurosci.* 19: 73–81.

[40] Morgans, C. W. et al. 1998. *J. Neurosci.* 18: 2467–2474.

[41] Baylor, D. A., and Burns, M. E. 1998. *Eye (Lond.)* 12 (Pt 3b): 521–525.

[42] Chen, J. et al. 1995. *Science* 267: 374–377.

[43] Fu, Y., and Yau, K. W. 2007. *Pflügers Arch.* 454: 805–819.

Amplification through the cGMP Cascade

Two steps of the cGMP cascade provide the amplification that accounts for the exquisite sensitivity of rods to light. First, a single molecule of active metarhodopsin II catalyzes the serial exchange of transducin-GDP for transducin-GTP. Second, each α-subunit of GTP–transducin activates 12 to 14 molecules of phosphodiesterase in the disk[44] that can hydrolyze a large number of cytoplasmic cGMP molecules. Thereby absorption of one single photon induces many channels to close.

Responses to Single Quanta of Light

The finding that a few quanta of light can give rise to a conscious sensation raises several tantalizing questions. How large is the unitary response; how is it distinguished from ongoing noise; and how is such minimal information transferred faithfully through the retina to higher centers? To measure unitary responses to single quanta, Baylor and his colleagues recorded photoactivated currents of individual rods in retinas from toads.[45] These experiments provide a rare example of the way in which a process as complex as seeing the dimmest possible flashes of light can be correlated with the events that occur in single molecules.[46]

The procedure was to isolate a piece of retina and maintain it in darkness. To measure currents, the outer segment of the rod was sucked into a fine pipette (Figure 22.13). As expected, in darkness a current flowed continuously into the outer segment. As the duration or the intensity of light are increased, the duration and amplitude of the light responses are also increased (Figure 22.14). Flashes of light closed channels in the outer segment, causing a decrease in the dark current. Figure 22.14 shows responses to very dim light flashes, corresponding to one or two quanta of light on the outer segment. The currents are small and quantal in nature. That is, sometimes a dim flash evokes a unitary response, sometimes a doublet, and sometimes nothing at all.

In monkey rods, the current reduction caused by transduction of a single photon is about 0.5 picoamperes (pA). This corresponds to the closure of approximately 300 channels, or about 3% to 5% of the rod channels that are open in the dark, and is the result of the large amplification through the cGMP cascade. Moreover, because of the extreme stability of visual pigments mentioned earlier, random isomerizations and spurious channel closings are rare events. This allows the effects of single-light quanta to stand out against an extremely quiet background. The sensitivity of rods relies on their low noise. In cones, thermal transitions of the visual pigments, spontaneous synthesis of GTP, and membrane channel openings contribute to the background noise and the higher visual threshold. It has been shown that electrical coupling through gap junctions between photoreceptors provides an additional smoothing effect that reduces the background noise and improves the signal-to-noise ratio for responses of rods to single quanta.[47]

[44] Yue, W. W. S. et al. 2019. *Proc. Nat. Acad. Sci. USA* 116: 5144-5153.

[45] Schnapf, J. L., and Baylor, D. A. 1987. *Sci. Am.* 256: 40-47.

[46] Rieke, F., and Baylor, D. A. 1998. *Biophys. J.* 75: 1836-1857.

[47] Bloomfield, S. A., and Volgyi, B. 2009. *Nat. Rev. Neurosci.* 10: 495-506.

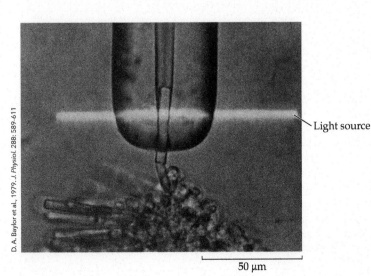

D. A. Baylor et al., 1979. *J. Physiol.* 288: 589-611

Light source

50 µm

FIGURE 22.13 Method for Recording Membrane Currents of a Rod Outer Segment. A suction electrode with a fine tip is used to suck up the outer segment of a rod that protrudes from a piece of toad retina. Slits of light illuminate the receptor with precision. Since the electrode fits tightly around the photoreceptor, current flowing into or out of it is recorded.

(A)

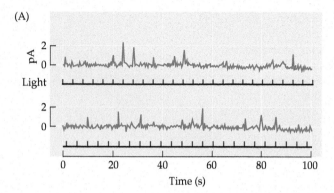

(C)

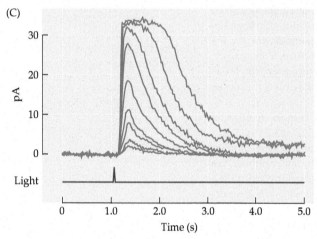

(B)

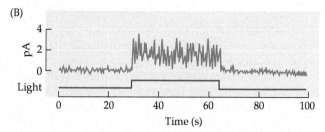

FIGURE 22.14 Recordings Made by Suction Electrode from Monkey Rod Outer Segment. (A) Responses to dim flashes, applied as indicated in the red traces (labeled "Light"), are shown in the two current traces. The currents fluctuate in a quantal manner. Smaller deflections are the currents generated by single photons interacting with visual pigments. Photoisomerizations often failed to occur. (B) Steady, more intense illumination (bottom trace) gives rise to a burst of signals. (C) Responses to flashes of increasing intensity. These currents are the counterpart of voltage traces shown in Figure 22.7B. (After D. A. Baylor et al., 1984. *J. Physiol.* 357: 575-607.)

Cones and Color Vision

Extraordinary insights and experiments by Young and Helmholtz in the nineteenth century defined crucial questions for color vision and at the same time provided clear, unequivocal explanations. Their conclusion that there must be three types of sensory photoreceptors for color in humans has stood the test of time and has been confirmed at the molecular level. To set the stage, we quote again from Helmholtz, who compares the perception of light and sound as well as color and tone. One envies the clarity, force, and timeless beauty of his thinking, especially in view of the confusing, vitalistic concepts that were current at the time:

> *All differences of hue depend upon combinations in different proportions of the three primary colors...red, green and violet...Just as the difference of sensation of light and warmth depends...upon whether the rays of the sun fall upon nerves of sight or nerves of feeling, so it is supposed in Young's hypothesis that the difference of sensation of colors depends simply upon whether one or the other kind of nervous fibers are more strongly affected. When all three kinds are equally excited, the result is the sensation of white light...If we allow two different colored lights to fall at the same time upon a white screen...we see only a single compound, more or less different from the two original ones. We shall better understand the remarkable fact that we are able to refer all the varieties in the composition of external light to mixtures of three colors if we compare the eye with the ear...In the case of sound...we recognize the long waves as low notes, the short as high-pitched, and the ear may receive at once many waves of sound, that is to say many notes. But here these do not melt into compound notes in the same way that colors...melt into compound colors. The eye cannot tell the difference if we substitute orange for red and yellow; but if we hear the notes C and E sounded at the same time, we cannot put D instead of them...if the ear perceived musical tones as the eye colors, every accord might be completely represented by combining only three constant notes, one very low, one very high and one intermediate,*

[48] Dartnall, H. J., Bowmaker, J. K., and Mollon, J. D. 1983. *Proc. R. Soc. Lond. B, Biol. Sci.* 220: 115-130.

[49] Schnapf, J. L. et al. 1988. *Vis. Neurosci.* 1: 255-261.

[50] Nathans, J. 1987. *Annu. Rev. Neurosci.* 10: 163-194.

[51] Nathans, J. 1989. *Sci. Am.* 260: 42-49.

[52] Nathans, J. 1999. *Neuron* 24: 299-312.

[53] Okano, T. et al. 1992. *Proc. Natl. Acad. Sci. USA* 89: 5932-5936.

[54] Jacobs, G. H. 2008. *Vis. Neurosci.* 25: 619-633.

[55] Lamb, T. D. 2009. *Philos. Trans. R. Soc. Lond. B Biol. Sci.* 364: 2911-2924.

[56] Deeb, S. S. 2006. *Curr. Opin. Genet. Dev.* 16: 301-307.

[57] Deeb, S. S., and Kohl, S. 2003. *Dev. Ophthalmol.* 37: 170-187.

[58] Nathans, J. et al. 1986. *Science* 232: 203-210.

simply changing the relative strength of these three primary notes to produce all possible musical effects...But we find a continuous transition of colors into one another through numberless intermediate gradations...the way in which (colors) appear...depends chiefly upon the constitution of our nervous system...It must be confessed that both in man and in quadrupeds we have at present no anatomical basis for this theory of colors.[9]

These farsighted, accurate predictions were validated by quite different sets of observations. First, using spectrophotometry, Wald, Brown, MacNichol, Dartnall, and their colleagues[17,18,48] showed the existence of three types of cones with different pigments in human retina. Second, Baylor and his colleagues recorded currents from monkey and human cones.[49] Three populations of cones were found with distinct but overlapping sensitivities in the short, medium, or long wavelength regions of the spectrum. The wavelengths of light optimal for initiating electrical signals coincided precisely with the absorbance peaks of the visual pigments, which were demonstrated by spectrophotometry as well as by psychophysical measurements of spectral sensitivity (Figure 22.15). Finally, the genes for the three types of cone opsin pigments as well as the gene for rhodopsin were cloned and sequenced by Nathans.[50–52]

What accounts for the ability of different visual pigment molecules to trap specific wavelengths of light preferentially? It turns out that rhodopsin, the rod visual pigment, and all three cone visual pigments contain the same chromophore: 11-*cis* retinal. However, the amino acid sequences of the various opsin proteins differ from one another (Figure 22.16). Differences in just a few amino acids account for the differences in spectral sensitivity. Insights into the evolution of color vision have been gained from comparisons of opsin genes in vertebrates,[22,53] particularly among Old and New World primates.[54] Surprisingly, it has been shown that rhodopsin, the dim-light pigment, was the last to evolve; therefore, night vision appeared after daylight vision.[55] Studies of inherited defects in humans[56,57] provide additional understanding of the molecular basis of color vision.

Color Blindness

Color blindness occurs when one or more types of cones are absent on inheritance. The genes for L and M photopigments are on the X chromosome, while the genes for the S photopigment are on chromosome 7.[58] Nathans has shown that in color-blind people with a genetic defect results in an absence of one of the pigments, more often

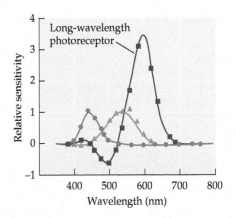

FIGURE 22.15 Comparison of Spectral Sensitivity of Monkey Cones with That Obtained by Human Color Matching. The continuous curves represent color-matching experiments in which the sensitivity at various wavelengths was determined in human participants. The points show results predicted from electrical measurements made by recording currents from single cones, after correcting for absorption in the lens and by pigments on the path to the outer segment. The correspondence between results obtained on single cells and by color matching is extraordinarily good. Note the small sensitivity peak of the long-wavelength photoreceptor (red line) overlapping with the blue sensitivity spectrum. This overlapping allows us to detect violet. (After W. S. Stiles and J. M. Burch, 1959. *Optica Acta* 6: 1–26, plotted by Color and Vision Research Labs, Institute of Ophthalmology, University College London.)

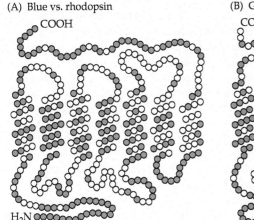

(A) Blue vs. rhodopsin

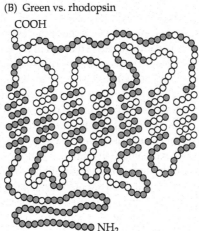

(B) Green vs. rhodopsin

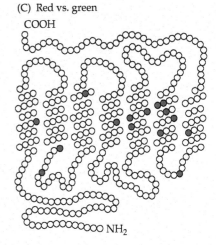

(C) Red vs. green

FIGURE 22.16 Comparisons of Amino Acid Sequences of red, green, and blue pigments with each other and with rhodopsin. Each colored dot represents an amino acid difference. (A,B) Blue and green pigments compared with rhodopsin.

(C) Green and red pigments compared. The sequences of red and green pigments are highly similar. (After J. Nathans et al., 1986. *Science* 11: 193–202, based on P. A. Hargrave et al., 1983. *Biophys. Struct. Mech.* 9: 235–244.)

FIGURE 22.17 **Visible Spectra of Normal Human Vision and Four Types of Color Blindness.** Protanopia is the absence of long-wavelength vision. Deuteranopia is the absence of middle-wavelength vision; the proximity of the absorbance peaks of L and M cones produces similar visual sensitivities in protanopes and deuteranopes. Tritanopia is the rare lack of short-wavelength vision. Below are the spectra of rods and S cone monochromacy. Note that as happens with rods at night, S-cone monochromacy does not produce color perception.

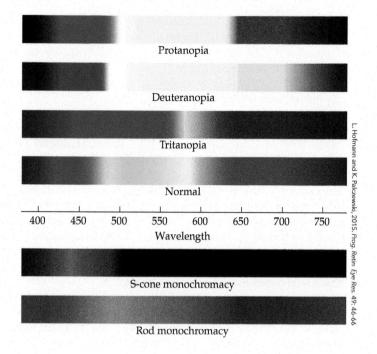

L. Hofmann and K. Palczewski, 2015. *Prog. Retin. Eye Res.* 49: 46-66

L or M. Figure 22.17 compares the visual spectra predicted from the absence of each type of cone. From our present perspective, one can only marvel that explanations at the molecular level so beautifully confirm the brilliant but rigorous speculations of Young and Helmholtz. Their idea that major attributes of color vision and color blindness are to be found within the receptors themselves has now been confirmed by direct physiological measurements[59] and corresponding differences in gene and protein structure.[52]

Integration of Visual Inputs

Receptive Fields of Retinal Neurons

We have seen that responses of individual photoreceptors are color-blind, being produced by one type of visual pigment. Perception of colors results from the combined responses of at least two photoreceptor cells with different color sensitivities. This section shows how inputs from several photoreceptors clustered within small areas of the retina are combined. To understand the mechanisms by which retinal circuits integrate visual responses, it is useful to describe the output of the retina, carried by the ganglion cells.

The **receptive field** is the area of the retina that, on illumination, enhances or inhibits the activity of a neuron. We already mentioned in Chapter 2 that Stephen Kuffler pioneered the experimental analysis of the mammalian visual system by concentrating on the receptive field organization of retinal ganglion cells and the meaning of their signals in the cat. Those experimental conditions made possible the extracellular recording of action potentials from individual ganglion cell axons in the optic nerve. Such recordings revealed two important features of the visual system. The first was that the receptive field of a retinal ganglion cell is organized in a circular, **center-surround** manner. That is, light in the receptive field surround area produces an opposite effect to that in the center (Figure 22.18). The second important feature revealed by ganglion cell recordings was that some retinal ganglion cells are excited by light in their receptive field center—the on-center retinal ganglion cells; in contrast, other ganglion cells are inhibited by light in their receptive field center—the off-center retinal ganglion cells.

Most ganglion cells and other neurons at higher levels in the visual system fire at rest even in the absence of patterned illumination. Appropriate stimuli do not necessarily initiate activity but may modulate the resting discharge; responses of ganglion cells can consist of either an increase or a decrease in action potential frequency. Light produces the most

[59] Rushton, W. A. 1972. Pigments and signals in colour vision. *J. Physiol.* 220: 1P-31P.

(A) On-center field   Off-center field   (B) Diffuse illumination

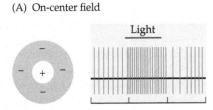 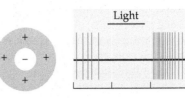

FIGURE 22.18 Receptive Fields of Retinal Ganglion Cells. Retinal ganglion cells have center-surround receptive fields in which light produces opposite effects depending on where it falls. (A) In on-center retinal ganglion cells, a spot of light in the center (indicated by the plus sign) causes increased firing of action potentials (stylized recording on the right, with timing of light indicated by the red bar). The same spot of light falling on the inhibitory surround would reduce activity in these cells. (B) In both on-center and off-center retinal ganglion cells, diffuse light that covers both center and surround produces little or no change in firing. (After S. W. Kuffler, 1953. *J. Neurophysiol.* 16: 37-68.)

vigorous response if it completely fills the center, whereas for most effective inhibition of firing, the light must cover the entire ring-shaped surround but not the center. For both on-center and off-center retinal ganglion cells, the spotlike center and its surround are antagonistic; therefore, if both center and surround are illuminated simultaneously, they tend to cancel each other's contribution, although the center response prevails.

This dichotomy of on and off pathways is now known to be a fundamental property of all vertebrate retinas and establishes an organizing principle for higher visual centers.[60] From these recordings of retinal ganglion cells, it is clear that the eye tells the brain about *patterns* of light and dark. Since photoreceptors can report only light intensity, it must fall to retinal interneurons to provide the analytical steps leading to the more structured retinal output. A small fraction of retinal ganglion cells contain the pigment melanopsin and are intrinsically photosensitive, in addition to being excited by light through the retinal circuitry.[1]

Receptive Fields of Color Perception

The dense packing of cones in the fovea produces hexagonal arrangements with a central cone surrounded by combinations of six others (Figure 22.19), an arrangement ideal for making comparative studies with the visual fields of rods already described in Chapter 2. Under a dim white light background, focal illumination of single M (green) or L (red) cones with a 550-nm wavelength of light (between the peak wavelengths of M and L cones) evokes color perceptions in humans.[61] Flash absorption of a single L cone surrounded by

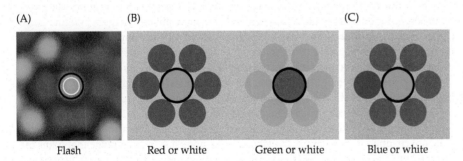

FIGURE 22.19 Percepts on Flash Illumination of Central Cones. (A) Pseudocolored cone arrangement with a central M (green) cone surrounded by L (red) cones. The flash is focused on the central cone. (B) Percepts on a dim white light background. Left: Illumination of a central M cone surrounded by L cones produces predominantly white or red perceptions. Right: Illumination of a central L cone surrounded by M cones produces predominantly white or green perceptions. (C) Blue perceptions can be evoked by illuminating a central M cone on a blue background. In all cases shown here, the majority of perceptions are white. (A from R. Sabesan et al., 2016. *Sci. Adv.* 2: e1600797/CC BY-NC; B,C adapted from B. P. Schmidt et al. 2018. *Sci. Rep.* 8: 8561/CC BY 4.0.)

[60] Schiller, P. H. 2010. *Proc. Natl. Acad. Sci. USA* 107: 17087-17094.

[61] Sabesan, R. et al. 2016. *Science Advances* 2: e1600797.

[62] Schmidt, B. P. et al. 2018. *Sci. Rep.* 8: 8561.

[63] Shekhar, K. et al. 2016. *Cell* 166: 1308-1323.

[64] Kolb, H. 1997. *Eye (Lond.)* 11 (Pt 6): 904-923.

[65] MacNeil, M. A. et al. 1999. *J. Comp. Neurol.* 413: 305-326.

[66] Masland, R. H. 2001. *Curr. Opin. Neurobiol.* 11: 431-436.

[67] Sanes, J. R., and Masland, R. H. 2015 *Ann. Rev. Neurosci.* 38: 221-246.

[68] Wässle, H. et al. 1998. *Vision Res.* 38: 1411-1430.

[69] Mora-Ferrer, C., and Neumeyer, C. 2009. *Vision Res.* 49: 960-969.

[70] Brandstatter, J. H. 2002. *Curr. Eye Res.* 25: 327-331.

[71] Shen, Y., Liu, X. L., and Yang, X. L. 2006. *Mol. Neurobiol.* 34: 163-179.

[72] Herbst, H., and Thier, P. 1996. *Exp. Brain Res.* 111: 345-355.

[73] Zanazzi, G., and Matthews, G. 2009. *Mol. Neurobiol.* 39: 130-148.

[74] tom Dieck, S., and Brandstatter, J. H. 2006. *Cell Tissue Res.* 326: 339-346.

[75] Heidelberger, R., Thoreson, W. B., and Witkovsky, P. 2005. *Prog. Retin. Eye Res.* 24: 682-720.

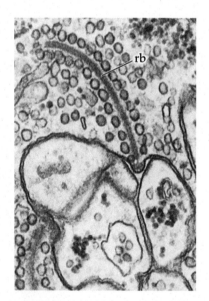

FIGURE 22.20 Ribbon Synapse Made by a Photoreceptor Terminal. Electron micrograph showing clear vesicles aligned on both sides of the ribbon (rb). The synaptic ridge (located between the arrowheads) is wedge-shaped, thus allowing the rod pedicle to contact two postsynaptic processes. Arrowheads point to release sites. (Micrograph from E. Townes-Anderson et al., 1985. *J. Cell Bio.* 100: 175-188.)

M cones evokes white (~60%) or red (~20%) perceptions, the rest being either green or not seen. An opposite arrangement, with an M cone surrounded by L cones, evokes white (~60%) and green (~20%) perceptions, the rest being either red or not seen. Surprisingly, blue perceptions appear when an M cone is illuminated on a blue background.[62] Whereas the stimulation patterns limited to a few cones are enough to produce perception, the on and off sensory fields produced by contrasting monochromatic dim light require additional integration to produce perception, as we showed in Chapter 2.

Synaptic Organization of the Retina

Numerous questions arise about the transmission of signals in the retina. How do rods and cones influence bipolar cells? And how are horizontal and amacrine cells involved in signaling? The analysis of signal processing by these neurons has required a combination of various techniques, including intracellular recording, dye injection, morphological studies, cellular neurochemistry, and identification of transmitters and receptors.

Bipolar, Horizontal, and Amacrine Cells

From the pattern of connections in primate retina, it is clear that the output of the eye is the result of complex integrative processes. For example, the horizontal cells drawn in Figure 22.3 receive synapses from many receptors and in turn feed back onto them. Horizontal cells also end on bipolar cells. Similarly, certain amacrine cells, which receive inputs from bipolar cells, send synapses to bipolar cells as well as to ganglion cells. Horizontal cells and amacrine cells transmit and modify signals traveling through the retina. An additional source of complexity is that each of the major classes of neurons has numerous morphological and pharmacological subtypes. According to physiological, anatomical and transcriptomical criteria, there are 15 major classes of bipolar cells, 2 or more types of horizontal cell, about 40 types of amacrine cells, and about 30 types of ganglion cells.[63–65] It is thought that all morphologically defined retinal cell types have been identified, with distinct functional roles assigned to nearly half of these.[66,67]

Molecular Mechanisms of Synaptic Transmission in the Retina

Virtually all the known neurotransmitters exist in the retina.[68–71] Glutamate is the transmitter liberated by photoreceptors, bipolar cells, and ganglion cells. Horizontal cells secrete γ-aminobutyric acid (GABA). Amacrine cells are diverse; some secrete dopamine (see Chapter 18), others indolamines, acetylcholine, or glycine. Peptides, nitric oxide, and cannabinoids also contribute to retinal signaling.[72]

The continuous, quantal release of glutamate from retinal photoreceptors and bipolar cells is achieved by specialized active zones known as ribbon synapses.[73] Figure 22.20 shows an example of a ribbon synapse, and their functioning is reviewed in Chapter 13. It is enough to mention here that the photoreceptor (and hair auditory cell) terminal contains vesicles that are tethered to a long, flat electron-dense organelle—the ribbon.

The ribbon structure is thought to reflect its specialized function: the ability to sustain high rates of vesicular release modulated by graded changes in presynaptic voltage. In keeping with their functional specialization, ribbons have their own variants of the molecular elements in the canonical fusion complex[74] (see Chapter 13). Ribbons are served by L-type calcium channels with relatively little inactivation and an activation range that spans the resting potential of the cell.[75] Gating of L-type channels supports release from hundreds of vesicles per second from each ribbon.

Receptive Field Organization of Bipolar Cells

The receptive field of a hyperpolarizing (H) bipolar cell is shown in Figure 22.21. A small spot of light shone onto the central part of the field causes a sustained hyperpolarization. Illumination of the annulus, leaving the center dark, causes depolarization. Thus, the central area, driven directly by photoreceptors, is enveloped by

(A) Central illumination

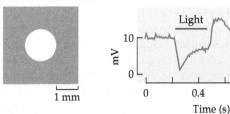

(B) Annular illumination

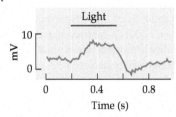

FIGURE 22.21 Receptive Field Organization of a Hyperpolarizing (H) Bipolar Cell. Records made from a bipolar cell in the goldfish retina show a hyperpolarization in response to illumination of the center of the receptive field (A). Annular illumination causes the cell to respond with a depolarization (B). Diffuse light would have little effect on the cell. For a D bipolar cell, illumination of the center would produce depolarization, while illumination of the annulus would produce hyperpolarization. (After A. Kaneko, 1970. *J. Physiol.* 207: 623–633.)

an antagonistic surround. The H bipolar cell in Figure 22.21 is hyperpolarized in the presence of the spot of light. Therefore, it has an off center receptive field. Depolarizing (D) bipolar cells have similarly shaped concentric fields, except that illumination of the center causes depolarization and illumination of the surround causes hyperpolarization. Because it is depolarized when the light goes on, the D bipolar cell has an on-center receptive field. As we mentioned in Chapter 2, the terminology of *on* and *off* responses is used extensively to describe receptive field properties at successive levels of the visual system. An important principle is that a single photoreceptor can contribute to the receptive field centers of both on and off bipolar cells. However, the ribbon synapses are made on the D bipolar cells, whereas cone photoreceptors make separate, conventional-looking synapses at what are called basal junctions on the H bipolar cells, which get their input only from cones.

Responses of Cone Bipolar Cells

Each bipolar cell receives its direct input either from rods or cones. One type of cone bipolar cell, the midget bipolar cell, receives its input from a single cone (see Figure 22.3). As one might expect, midget bipolar cells are found in the through-line at the fovea, where visual acuity is highest. They end on specialized midget ganglion cells. More peripheral cone bipolar cells are supplied by a convergent input from 5 to 20 adjacent cones.

The responses and receptive fields of cone bipolar cells depend on two mechanisms. First, in the dark, the continuous release of glutamate from photoreceptors keeps some bipolar cells depolarized and others hyperpolarized; the effect depends on the postsynaptic glutamate receptors in bipolar cells. Second, light causes photoreceptors to hyperpolarize, thereby reducing glutamate release. Bipolar cells that have excitatory glutamate receptors (H bipolar cells) are depolarized during darkness and become hyperpolarized on illumination when the release of glutamate stops (just as photoreceptors do).[76] Conversely, bipolar cells that have inhibitory glutamate receptors (D bipolar cells) are hyperpolarized during darkness and become depolarized when glutamate release stops on illumination.

H bipolar cells have AMPA or kainate-type cation-selective ionotropic glutamate receptors.[77] In contrast, D bipolar cells have mGluR6 metabotropic glutamate receptors that act through G proteins and second messengers;[78,79] these receptors close a TRP melastatin 1 (TRPM1) cation channel, which opens with light to depolarize the D bipolar cell and reverse the sign of transmission.[80,81] D bipolar cells constitute one of the few retinal cell types in which glutamate has an inhibitory action. Because of the second messenger cascade, signaling in D bipolar cells is slower than in H bipolar cells. Thus, a fundamental property of the visual system—on and off responses to light—originates in the differential response of bipolar cells to glutamate, determined by the glutamate receptors on each cell type.

[76] Kaneko, A., and Hashimoto, H. 1969. *Vision Res.* 9: 37–55.

[77] DeVries, S. H. 2000. *Neuron* 28: 847–856.

[78] Kikkawa, S. et al. 1993. *Biochem. Biophys. Res. Commun.* 195: 374–379.

[79] Masu, M. et al. 1995. *Cell* 80: 757–765.

[80] Nakanishi, S. et al. 1998. *Brain Res Rev.* 26: 230–235.

[81] Koike, C. et al. 2010. *Cell Calcium* 48: 95–101.

Rod Bipolar Cells

Rod bipolar cells are typically supplied by 15 to 45 rods, in accord with the lower spatial sensitivity of night vision. All rod bipolar cells in the vertebrate retina are D type, expressing sign-reversing inhibitory mGluR6 metabotropic glutamate receptors.[82] A change in sign of the signaling may occur at a later post in the circuit. Rather than contacting retinal ganglion cells directly, rod bipolar cells synapse onto AII cells, a subtype among the nearly 40 types of amacrine cells.[83] Each AII cell depolarizes in the light due to the summed input of many rod bipolar cells. AII cells form inhibitory glycinergic synapses onto the axon terminals of cone bipolar cells,[83] by which they influence the activity of retinal ganglion cells.[84] AII cells also form electrical synapses onto the synaptic pedicle of cone bipolar cells, by which the inhibitory response produced by light on photoreceptors is transferred to a different set of ganglion cells (Figure 22.22). It has been suggested that this indirect arrangement results from the later evolutionary arrival of rod photoreceptors to the vertebrate retina, piggybacking onto the preexisting cone circuitry.[85]

Color Vision Combining Rods and Cones

Sharing the retinal pathways generates collaborative possibilities for rods and cones. Jan Purkinje in the nineteenth century wrote in his *Neue Beiträge*:

> *Objectively, the degree of illumination has a great influence on the intensity of color quality. In order to prove this most vividly, take some colors before daybreak, when it begins slowly to get lighter. Initially one sees only black and grey. Particularly the brightest colors, red and green, appear darkest. Yellow cannot be distinguished from a rosy red. Blue became noticeable to me first. Nuances of red, which otherwise burn brightest in daylight, namely carmine, cinnabar and orange, show themselves as darkest for quite a while, in contrast to their average brightness. Green appears more bluish to me, and its yellow tint develops with increasing daylight only.*[86]

The shift to increased sensitivity of the eye to bluish colors experienced under dim light is known as the Purkinje effect. Psychophysical and mathematical analyses indicate that the blue-shifted spectrum of rods accounts for this effect by contributing to the dim-light perception.[87,88]

82 Nomura, A. et al. 1994. *Cell* 77: 361–369.

83 Famiglietti, E. V., Jr., and Kolb, H. 1975. *Brain Res.* 84: 293–300.

84 Wässle, H. 2004. *Nat. Rev. Neurosci.* 5: 747–757.

85 Lamb, T. D. 2009. *Philos. Trans. R. Soc. Lond. B, Biol. Sci.* 364: 2911–2924.

86 J. Purkinje, 1825. Beobachtungen und Versuche zur Physiologie der Sinne. Zweites Bändchem (Observations and Experimentations Investigating the Physiology of Senses). In *Neue Beiträge zur Kenntnis des Sehens in Subjektiver Hinsicht*. Reimer: Berlin.

87 Cao, D. et al. 2008. *Vision Res.* 48: 2586–2592.

88 Barrionuevo, P. A., and Cao, D. 2014. *J. Opt. Soc. Am. A Opt. Image Sci. Vis.* 31: A131–A139.

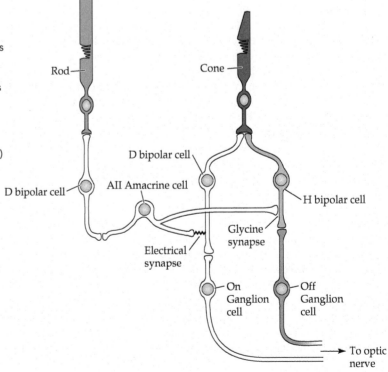

FIGURE 22.22 Pathways from Photoreceptors to Ganglion Cells in the Mammalian Retina. Neurons that depolarize on illumination are white; those that hyperpolarize are shaded. All amacrine cells are depolarized by sign-preserving input from rod D bipolar (RDB) cells. AIIs also make sign-preserving electrical connections onto cone D bipolar (CDB) cells and sign-reversing glycinergic (inhibitory) synapses onto cone H bipolar (CHB) cells. On- and off-center ganglion cells are also shown. (After S. H. DeVries and D. A. Baylor, 1995. *Proc. Natl. Acad. Sci. USA* 92: 10658–10662. © 1995 National Academy of Sciences.)

Horizontal Cells and Surround Inhibition

The responses of D and H bipolar cells to surround illumination are mediated by horizontal cells. Each horizontal cell receives inputs from a large number of photoreceptors. Horizontal cells, like H bipolar cells, respond to illumination of photoreceptors by hyperpolarization (because glutamate release from photoreceptor terminals opens depolarizing ionotropic receptors, and release decreases with illumination). Another feature of horizontal cells is that they are electrically coupled to each other.[89,90] Lucifer yellow dye injected into one horizontal cell spreads readily to others through gap junctions. Thus, one may expect that any one horizontal cell may be influenced by light shone on a large area of retina, because of current flow from its neighbors. However, an interesting feature of the electrical synapses between horizontal cells is that they become uncoupled by dopamine released in response to illumination (see Chapter 18).[91]

Horizontal cells make inhibitory synaptic connections; they release GABA onto photoreceptors and bipolar cells.[92-95] Receptor illumination results in horizontal cell hyperpolarization and a reduction in GABA release. Hence, hyperpolarization of photoreceptors by diffuse light is countered by a reduction in the GABA inhibition coming from horizontal cells. In summary, there is negative feedback onto the photoreceptors through the horizontal cells:

Illumination → photoreceptor hyperpolarization → horizontal cell

hyperpolarization → photoreceptor depolarization

The connections involved in the off-center/on-surround responses of a D bipolar cell (the only ones receiving inputs from cones in humans) are shown schematically in Figure 22.23. For simplicity, the center is represented by a single photoreceptor and the surround by a few

[89] Kaneko, A. 1971. *J. Physiol.* 213: 95-105.

[90] Liu, C. R. et al. 2009. *Neuroscience* 164: 1161-1169.

[91] Tornqvist, K., Yang, X. L., and Dowling, J. E. 1988. *J. Neurosci.* 8: 2279-2288.

[92] Kaneko, A., and Tachibana, M. 1986. *J. Physiol.* 373: 443-461.

[93] Schwartz, E. A. 1987. *Science* 238: 350-355.

[94] Yang, X. L., Gao, F., and Wu, S. M. 1999. *Vis. Neurosci.* 16: 967-979.

[95] Deniz, S. et al. 2011. *J. Neurochem.* 116: 350-362.

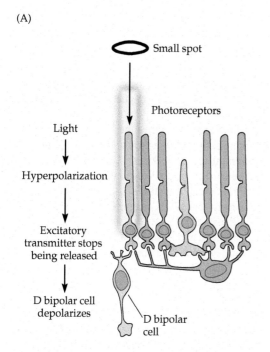 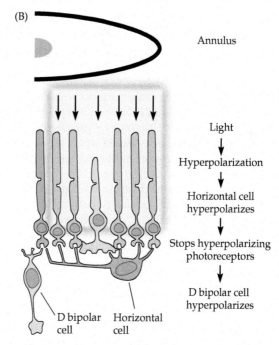

FIGURE 22.23 Connections of Photoreceptors, Bipolar Cells, and Horizontal Cells in the Human Retina. The figure illustrates connections required to elicit responses in D bipolar cells. (A) Light falling on a single rod causes it to become hyperpolarized. As a result, glutamate stops being released and the D bipolar cell becomes depolarized through loss of inhibition. (B) Light falling on the surrounding area in the form of an annulus again prevents glutamate from being released by photoreceptors. As a result, the horizontal cell becomes hyperpolarized; this hyperpolarization prevents the horizontal cell from releasing its inhibitory transmitter, γ-aminobutyric acid (GABA), onto the photoreceptor. The photoreceptor that is connected to the D bipolar cell therefore becomes depolarized (through removal of inhibition). The photoreceptor once again releases glutamate and hyperpolarizes the bipolar cell (not shown). With diffuse light, the depolarizing and hyperpolarizing effects cancel each other out. Thus, horizontal cells play an essential part in the construction of the receptive field properties of bipolar cells.

neighboring receptors connected to a single horizontal cell. The response to illumination of the central photoreceptor is straightforward (see Figure 22.23A). Photoreceptor activation results in hyperpolarization and therefore a reduction in glutamate release. The inhibitory action of glutamate makes the bipolar cell depolarize. The horizontal cell receives a hyperpolarizing input as well, but it is from only one photoreceptor and the effect is small, as is the negative feedback onto the central photoreceptor.

The response to surround illumination involves an extra step (see Figure 22.23B). The horizontal cell, which receives input from several photoreceptors in the surround, is hyperpolarized by illumination. The hyperpolarization reduces GABA release by the horizontal cell. Reduced inhibition of the photoreceptors tends to produce depolarization. The depolarizing feedback effect is minimal on the surround receptors, which are being strongly hyperpolarized by illumination. The central receptor, however, is receiving no illumination; its only input is removal of horizontal cell inhibition. Consequently, the central receptor is depolarized, release of glutamate is increased, and the D bipolar cell is hyperpolarized. Comprehensive reviews and papers describe the morphology and the properties of photoreceptor terminals, bipolar cells, and the feedback synapses of horizontal cells onto bipolar cells.[3,16,96,97]

Significance of Receptive Field Organization of Bipolar Cells

What are the physiological implications of bipolar cell receptive fields? D and H bipolar cells do not simply respond to light. Rather, they begin to analyze information about patterns. Their signals convey information about small spots of light of one color surrounded by light of a different color, about small light surrounded by darkness or about small dark spots surrounded by light. They respond to contrasting patterns of light and dark over a small area of retina. In addition to the broad categories of D and H bipolar cells, approximately 11 types of cone bipolar cells have been distinguished by morphological and immunohistochemical criteria, presumably underlying additional functional specificity.[5,98]

Receptive Fields and Projections of Ganglion Cells

The size of the receptive field of a ganglion cell depends on its location in the retina. Cells situated in the fovea, where visual acuity is highest, have much smaller receptive fields than do cells at the periphery.[99,100]

Consistently, ganglion cells in the monkey retina can be grouped into three main categories, two of which are denoted as **magnocellular** (**M**, large) and **parvocellular** (**P**, small). The M and P terminology is based on the anatomical projections of these neurons to the lateral geniculate nucleus and from there to the cortex. We showed in Chapters 2 and 3 that P ganglion cells project to the four dorsal layers of smaller cells in the lateral geniculate nucleus (the parvocellular division), whereas M ganglion cells project to the larger cells in the two ventral layers (the magnocellular division).

The separate characteristics of neurons in the M and P pathways are maintained at successive levels in the visual system through and beyond the primary visual cortex. In brief, P ganglion cells (also known as midget ganglion cells) have small receptive field centers and high spatial resolution, and most are sensitive to red-green color vision. They provide information about fine detail but require higher contrast stimuli.[98,101] M ganglion cells (also known as parasol ganglion cells because of the shape of their more extensive dendritic arbors, which collect wider inputs) have larger receptive fields than P cells and are more sensitive to small differences in contrast and to movement. A third category of retinal ganglion cells are the **koniocellular** (**K**) cells.[102] K cells carry spatial and contrast information, principally blue on and off contrast responses.[103,104]

Synaptic Inputs to Ganglion Cells Responsible for Receptive Field Organization

The connections of cone D and H bipolar cells with corresponding on- and off-center ganglion cells are very precise. The change in membrane potential of a bipolar cell causes the

[96] Thoreson, W. B. 2007. *Mol. Neurobiol.* 36: 205-223.

[97] Yang, X. F. et al. *Neuroscience* 173: 19-29.

[98] Lee, B. B., Martin, P. R., and Grunert, U. 2010. *Prog. Retin. Eye Res.* 29: 622-639.

[99] Kier, C. K., Buchsbaum, G., and Sterling, P. 1995. *J. Neurosci.* 15: 7673-7683.

[100] Croner, L. J., and Kaplan, E. 1995. *Vision Res.* 35: 7-24.

[101] Kaplan, E., and Shapley, R. M. 1986. *Proc. Natl. Acad. Sci. USA* 83: 2755-2757.

[102] Casagrande, V. A. 1994. *Trends Neurosci.* 17: 305-310.

[103] Szmajda, B. A. et al. 2006. *Proc. Natl. Acad. Sci. USA* 103:19512-19517.

[104] Roy, S. et al. 2009. *Eur. J. Neurosci.* 30: 1517-1526.

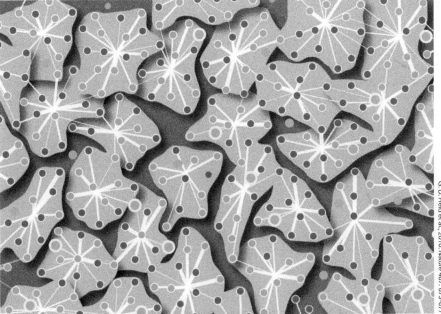

D. M. Dacey et al., 2014. *Vis. Neurosci.* 31: 139-151, based on G. D. Field et al., 2010. *Nature* 467: 673-677

22.24 Distribution of L, M, and S Cones Superimposed on the Receptive Fields of Off Midget Ganglion Cells in the retinal periphery (irregular light gray contours). L cones are red, M cones green, and S cones blue. The mosaic was reconstructed from simultaneous recordings from hundreds of ganglion cells on fine-grain light stimulation to identify each cone input. Cones with input to at least one ganglion cell are highlighted with an annulus. The thickness of the white lines denotes relative strength of the input. The S cone connections (blue circles with a thick yellow outline) are generally weaker.

target ganglion cell to change its membrane potential in the same direction. Consistently, the connections between rods, AII cells, and ganglion cells are so precise that both rods and cones in the same part of the retina supply the same ganglion cell appropriately, but generally by way of different interneurons. Figure 22.24 superimposes the visual fields of the three types of cones on the receptive fields of off midget ganglion cells. Each sensory field has convergence of green and red cones; one or no S cones contribute to the lattice of projections. However, S cones commonly connect to the K ganglion cells.

Amacrine Cell Control of Ganglion Cell Responses

Amacrine cells mediate or contribute to a variety of distinctive types of responses and receptive field properties of retinal ganglion cells.[105,106] Many of these effects are dynamic and depend on the variable range of stimulus intensity, stimulus movement relative to the background scene, or spatial asymmetries in that pattern. For example, together with bipolar cells, amacrine cells show an early stage of processing called **contrast adaptation** or **contrast gain control**.[107]

A retinal ganglion cell's receptive field can also change dynamically in a way that maximizes the cell's sensitivity to spatial features that differ from a surrounding pattern.[108] An example is a cell that can improve its ability to detect an object in a patterned field, such as among tall tree trunks in a forest, as compared with a less regular background. Experiments and modeling have shown that amacrine cells, with their lateral projections, and bipolar cells contribute to the effect, which has been termed **predictive coding**.[108]

Although sensitivity to the direction of movement of stimuli has classically been thought to arise through cortical or tectal connections, there are retinal ganglion cells that detect directional movement of objects against the background. In rabbits it is the starburst amacrine cells that account for sensitivity to direction of movement,[109,110] and starburst amacrine cells with similar properties are found in primates, including humans.[111,112] Small movements of each eye made independently of the other (ocular drift) occur during fixation and are essential for vision. Because ocular drift causes the entire

[105] Baccus, S. A. 2007. *Annu. Rev. Physiol.* 69: 271-290.

[106] Grimes, W. N. et al. *Neuron* 65: 873-885.

[107] Baccus, S. A., and Meister, M. 2002. *Neuron* 36: 909-919.

[108] Hosoya, T., Baccus, S. A., and Meister, M. 2005. *Nature* 436: 71-77.

[109] Fried, S. I., Munch, T. A., and Werblin, F. S. 2002. *Nature* 420: 411-414.

[110] Munch, T. A., and Werblin, F. S. 2006. *J. Neurophysiol.* 96: 471-477.

[111] Rodieck, R. W. 1989. *J. Comp. Neurol.* 285: 18-37.

[112] Rodieck, R. W., and Marshak, D. W. 1992. *J. Comp. Neurol.* 321: 46-64.

visual field to move independently for each eye, it explains the need to detect movement early, at the level of the eye. Therefore, some retinal ganglion cells are wired to respond preferentially to the movement of a small object relative to overall movement of the visual field. Certain amacrine cells provide the processing and connections for sensing such relative motion of objects in a moving field of vision.[113,114] During larger movements called **saccades**, which shift gaze, visual perception is suppressed in part because of central control that is exerted by oculomotor centers, but in addition, some retinal ganglion cell responses are suppressed,[115] apparently by the circuitry that detects global eye movements. Finally, signaling to retinal ganglion cells by a moving stimulus reaches the edge of each ganglion cell's dendritic field before illuminating the cell body; a change in cell sensitivity as a result of the stimulus causes the population of firing ganglion cells to lead the stimulus in what is called motion anticipation.[116]

Coding Information

Throughout the previous discussion, the spike trains from individual neurons have been treated as separate lines from which the brain analyses visual input. Since the firing of ensembles of retinal ganglion cells is crucial for the next levels of analysis into the brain, some studies have compared activity within groups of ganglion cells and identified additional roles of amacrine cells.[117,118] Experiments made in the salamander and mouse retina by Baylor, Meister, Baccus, and their colleagues suggest that the temporal aspects of firing by ganglion cells also can contribute to retinal analysis.[119-122] Thus, when recordings were made simultaneously from ganglion cells with closely adjacent fields, action potentials occurred synchronously for some visual stimuli. For example, a spot of light that straddled the border of two off-center retinal ganglion cells produced synchronous firing. Electrical synapses between amacrine and ganglion cells or between ganglion cells are thought to contribute to coordinated firing, referred to as concerted signaling of ganglion cells.[123,124]

What Information Do Ganglion Cells Convey?

It should be clear that ganglion cell signals tell a different story from that of primary sensory receptors. The sizes, shapes, and dynamic properties of their receptive fields are tuned to detect spatial, temporal, or color contrast, and like bipolar cells from which they derive input, half of the ganglion cells depolarize in response to light. Their synaptic inputs tune them to detect stimuli such as the edge of an image crossing the opposing regions of their receptive field. As we detailed in Chapter 2, higher-order neurons in the visual system construct lines, corners, and all the features that underlie visual object recognition. A very few ganglion cells—those that are intrinsically photosensitive—provide information about the level of ambient illumination.

Intrinsic Responses to Light in Ganglion Cells

Form vision in mammals is served by rods and cones, each with its specific photopigment. Other light-dependent functions, such as pupillary reflexes and entrainment of circadian rhythms, use other sensory receptors and visual pigments. Blind mice that fail to produce rods and cones still exhibit circadian rhythms, and these can be shifted by light exposure at night (entrainment).[125,126] This shift depends on a small population of intrinsically photosensitive retinal ganglion cells (ipRGCs)[127]—about 3% of the total ganglion cells—that express the photoprotein melanopsin and project axons to the suprachiasmatic nucleus (where circadian rhythms are generated)[128] (see Figure 22.2). Melanopsin was first identified in melanocytes of frog skin and is structurally related to rhodopsin. Its 480-nm blue absorption peak is between that of S and M cones.[129] Intrinsically photosensitive retinal ganglion cells depolarize in response to bright light and produce action potentials with a frequency that depends on brightness (Figure 22.25).[130] Accumulating evidence suggests that melanopsin is coupled through a non-transducin G protein to phospholipase C that generates IP_3 and diacylglycerol (DAG), finally to gate cation current through transient receptor potential (TRP)–like channels.[131] This process is similar to the depolarizing phototransduction cascade

[113] Olveczky, B. P., Baccus, S. A., and Meister, M. 2007. *Neuron* 56: 689-700.

[114] Baccus, S. A. et al. 2008. *J. Neurosci.* 28: 6807-6817.

[115] Roska, B., and Werblin, F. 2003. *Nat. Neurosci.* 6: 600-608.

[116] Berry, M. J., 2nd, et al. 1999. *Nature* 398: 334-338.

[117] Shlens, J., Rieke, F., and Chichilnisky, E. 2008. *Curr. Opin. Neurobiol.* 18: 396-402.

[118] Maffei, L., and Galli-Resta, L. 1990. *Proc. Natl. Acad. Sci. USA* 87: 2861-2864.

[119] Meister, M., Lagnado, L., and Baylor, D. A. 1995. *Science* 270: 1207-1210.

[120] Meister, M., and Berry, M. J., 2nd. 1999. *Neuron* 22: 435-450.

[121] Kastner, D. B., and Baccus, S. A. 2013. *Neuron* 79: 541-554.

[122] Jadzinsky, P. D. and Baccus, S. A. 2015. *eLife* 4: e09266.

[123] Brivanlou, I. H., Warland, D. K., and Meister, M. 1998. *Neuron* 20: 527-539.

[124] Schnitzer, M. J., and Meister, M. 2003. *Neuron* 37: 499-511.

[125] Foster, R. G. et al. 1991. *J. Comp. Physiol. A* 169: 39-50.

[126] Freedman, M. S. et al. 1999. *Science* 284: 502-504.

[127] Berson, D. M., Dunn, F. A., and Takao, M. 2002. *Science* 295: 1070-1073.

[128] Hattar, S. et al. 2002. *Science* 295: 1065-1070.

[129] Provencio, I. et al. 1998. *Proc. Natl. Acad. Sci. USA* 95: 340-345.

[130] Berson, D. M., Dunn, F. A., and Takao, M. 2002. *Science* 295: 1070-1073.

[131] Peirson, S. N., Halford, S., and Foster, R. G. 2009. *Philos. Trans. R. Soc. Lond., B, Biol. Sci.* 364: 2849-2865.

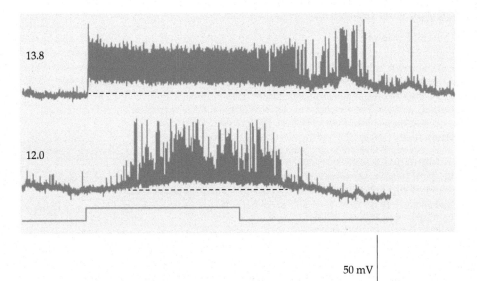

FIGURE 22.25 Phototransduction and Adaptation of an Intrinsically Photosensitive Retinal Ganglion Cell. Electrical activity in response to long light pulses at 500 nm. At low intensity the cell responds with a long latency. Increasing the intensity of illumination accelerates the responses. Activity continues after the light is turned off. Illumination is indicated by the bar below. The numbers on the left are the logarithm of the light intensity. (From D. M. Berson et al., 2002. *Science* 295: 1070-1073.)

known for invertebrates[132,133] (see Figure 22.7A), but differs from the process by which rhodopsin couples to the hyperpolarization of rods and cones.

The intrinsically photoreceptive cells are much more complex than originally expected. They all receive inputs from rods, inhibition from amacrine cells, and excitation from on bipolar cells. Some even have center–surround receptive fields. In addition, each type has a particular response to the speed of motion. Their electrical responses and their projections to the superior colliculus suggest their role as motion and speed visual detectors.[134]

[132] Wang, T., and Montell, C. 2007. *Pflügers Arch.* 454: 821-847.

[133] Berson, D. M. 2007. *Pflügers Arch.* 454: 849-855.

[134] Zhao, X. et al. 2014. *J. Physiol.* 592: 1619-1636.

SUMMARY

- Rod and cone photoreceptors respond to illumination in dim and bright light, respectively.

- Color vision is produced by the combined responses of different types of cones. In humans, S, or blue, cones respond to short wavelengths of light; M, or green, cones respond to medium wavelengths; and L, or red, cones respond to long wavelengths.

- The visual pigments are densely packed on rod and cone membranes.

- Transduction occurs in a series of steps involving a G protein transducing and cyclic GMP.

- In darkness, photoreceptors are depolarized and continuously release glutamate.

- Light causes photoreceptors to hyperpolarize and results in the reduction of glutamate release.

- H bipolar cells are depolarized by glutamate released from photoreceptors in the dark and become hyperpolarized on illumination when the release of glutamate stops.

- D bipolar cells are hyperpolarized by glutamate released from photoreceptors in the dark and become depolarized when glutamate release stops on illumination.

- In the visual system, the receptive field is the area of the retina that, on illumination, enhances or inhibits the activity of a neuron.

- Photoreceptors, horizontal cells, and bipolar cells produce graded local potentials, not action potentials.

- Ganglion cells and amacrine cells generate action potentials.

- Bipolar cells and ganglion cells have concentric receptive fields with on or off centers and antagonistic surrounds.

- Large ganglion cells, known as magnocellular or M cells, have large receptive fields and respond well to movement.

- Smaller ganglion cells, known as parvocellular or P cells, have smaller receptive fields and respond to color and fine detail.

- A small subset of ganglion cells called intrinsically photosensitive retinal ganglion cells (ipRGCs) contain photopigments and responds to illumination even without rods and cones.

Suggested Reading

General Reviews

Brainard, D. H. 2015. Color and the cone mosaic. *Ann. Rev. Vis. Sci.* 1: 519–546.

Chakrabarti, R., and Wichmann, C. 2019. Nanomachinery organizing release at neuronal and ribbon synapses. *Int. J. Mol. Sci.* 20: 2147. Published 2019 Apr 30. doi:10.3390/ijms20092147

Chen, C. K. 2005. The vertebrate phototransduction cascade: amplification and termination mechanisms. *Rev. Physiol. Biochem. Pharmacol.* 154: 101–121.

Dacey, D. M., Crook, J. D., and Packer, O. S. 2014. Distinct synaptic mechanisms create parallel S-ON and S-OFF color opponent pathways in the primate retina. *Vis. Neurosci.* 31: 139–151. doi:10.1017/S0952523813000230

Do, M. T. H. 2019. Melanopsin and the intrinsically photosensitive retinal ganglion cells: Biophysics to behavior. *Neuron* 104: 205–226. doi: 10.1016/j.neuron.2019.07.016

Dowling, J. E. 1987. *The Retina: An Approachable Part of the Brain.* Harvard University Press, Cambridge, MA.

Hofmann, L., and Palczewski, K. 2015. Advances in understanding the molecular basis of the first steps in color vision. *Prog. Retin. Eye Res.* 49: 46–66. Published online 2015 Jul 15. doi: 10.1016/j.preteyeres.2015.07.004.

Imamoto, Y., and Shichida, Y. 2014. Cone visual pigments. *Biochim. Biophys. Acta.* 1837: 664–673. doi:10.1016/j.bbabio.2013.08.009

Sterling, P., and Demb, J. B. 2003. Retina. In G. M. Shepherd (ed.), *Synaptic Organization of the Brain.* Oxford University Press, New York.

Thoreson, W. B., and Dacey, D. M. 2019. Diverse cell types, circuits, and mechanisms for color vision in the vertebrate retina. *Physiol. Rev.* 99: 1527–1573. doi: 10.1152/physrev.00027.2018. PMID: 31140374 PMCID: PMC6689740 (available on 2020-07-01). doi: 10.1152/physrev.00027.2018

Yau, K. W., and Hardie, R. C. 2009. Phototransduction: motifs and variations. *Cell* 139: 246–264.

Zhou, X. E., Melcher, K., and Xu, H. E. Understanding the GPCR biased signaling through G protein and arrestin complex structures. *Curr. Opin. Struct. Biol.* 45: 150–159. doi:10.1016/j.sbi.2017.05.004

Original Papers

Osterberg, G. 1935. Topography of the layer of rods and cones in the human retina. *Acta Ophthalmologica* Supplement 6: 1–103.

Baylor, D. A., Lamb, T. D., and Yau, K. W. 1979. The membrane current of single rod outer segments. *J. Physiol.* 288: 589–611.

Berson, D. M., Dunn, F. A., and Takao, M. 2002. Phototransduction by retinal ganglion cells that set the circadian clock. *Science* 295: 1070–1073.

Boycott, B. B., and Dowling, J. E. 1969. Organization of primate retina: Light microscopy. *Philos. Trans. R. Soc. Lond. B, Biol. Sci.* 255: 109–184.

Chen, J., Makino, C. L., Peachey, N. S., Baylor, D. A., and Simon, M. I. 1995. Mechanisms of rhodopsin inactivation in vivo as revealed by a COOH-terminal truncation mutant. *Science* 267: 374–377.

Croner, L. J., and Kaplan, E. 1995. Receptive fields of P and M ganglion cells across the primate retina. *Vision Res.* 35: 7–24.

Hattar, S., Liao, H. W., Takao, M., Berson, D. M., and Yau, K-W. 2002. Melanopsin-containing retinal ganglion cells: architecture, projections, and intrinsic photosensitivity. *Science* 295: 1065–1070.

Heidelberger, R., Thoreson, W. B., and Witkovsky, P. 2005. Synaptic transmission at retinal ribbon synapses. *Prog. Retin. Eye Res.* 24: 682–720.

Kaneko, A. 1970. Physiological and morphological identification of horizontal, bipolar and amacrine cells in goldfish retina. *J. Physiol.* 207: 623–633.

Kaneko, A., Delavilla, P., Kurahashi, T., and Sasaki, T. 1994. Role of L-glutamate for formation of on-responses and off-responses in the retina. *Biomed. Res.* 15(Suppl. 1): 41–45.

Kuffler, S. W. 1953. Discharge patterns and functional organization of the mammalian retina. *J. Neurophysiol.* 16: 37–68.

Meister, M., Lagnado, L., and Baylor, D. A. 1995. Concerted signaling by retinal ganglion cells. *Science* 270: 1207–1210.

Schnapf, J. L., Kraft, T. W., Nunn, B. J., and Baylor, D. A. 1988. Spectral sensitivity of primate photoreceptors. *Vis. Neurosci.* 1: 255–261.

Trong, P. K., and Rieke, F. 2008. Origin of correlated activity between parasol retinal ganglion cells. *Nat. Neurosci.* 11: 1343–1351.

Zenisek, D., Horst, N. K., Merrifield, C., Sterling, P., and Matthews, G. 2004. Visualizing synaptic ribbons in the living cell. *J. Neurosci.* 24: 9752–9759.

CHAPTER 23

Touch, Pain, and Texture Sensation

The entire body surface is covered with tactile receptors. In this way, the somatosensory system differs from sensory systems whose receptors are clustered within organs, such as the eye, nose, or ear. The sensory system of the skin is essential for identifying shapes and textures; for recognizing, grasping, and manipulating objects; for registering temperature; for directing visual attention; and for avoiding dangerous objects signaled by the pain they evoke. In this chapter we describe the processing that leads from contact of an object with the skin to recognition of the physical properties of that object. The functional organization of the somatosensory system is addressed both in rats and mice, where the whiskers are particularly important, and in primates, where the fingertips are particularly important.

Most somatosensory nerve fibers terminate in tiny accessory structures distributed in different positions within the skin—hair follicles, Meissner's, Merkel's, Pacinian, or Ruffini's corpuscles. But there is another class of fibers that end with no accessory structure—the so-called free nerve endings. Each type of fiber is activated by a specific stimulus and leads to a characteristic sensation. These distinct forms of sensation are called submodalities, and together they make up the modality of somatosensation. The terminations in accessory structures are associated with touch, pressure, stretch, or vibration; free nerve endings are associated with hot, cold, painful, or itchy sensations. The connection between receptor activity and sensation was first posited from studies in anesthetized animals, and has been confirmed by recording from single nerve fibers in the arm of awake humans, who describe the feeling evoked by electrical stimulation of the fiber.

Signals travel to the spinal cord, where they are sorted out into distinct ascending pathways according to the functional category of the receptor. All pathways reach the cerebral cortex after multiple relays. Although stimuli that cause damage lead to activation of the pathway beginning in the free nerve endings, the subjective experience of pain is more complex than the mere perceptual consequence of such activity. Rather, the psychological state of a person, including the expectation of reduced pain (placebo) or of intense pain (nocebo), truly alters the degree of suffering. The modulation resulting from expectations acts through endogenous opioid mechanisms.

At all levels of the ascending somatosensory pathways, neurons are arranged into topographic maps where the spatial relationships of the body are conserved: Adjacent stimulus sites activate adjacent neurons. These maps are grossly distorted because larger territories in the central nervous system (CNS) are dedicated to densely innervated skin areas. The magnified representation of the whiskers in mice and rats is one notable example of map distortion.

The whiskers are represented in layer 4 of cortex by an oversized grid of columns, called barrels. All the neurons in one barrel respond to movement of one whisker on the opposite side of the face. In humans and other primates, the fingertips are densely innervated, providing the tactile input necessary for object manipulation. Cortical map topography can be altered by manipulations during development.

A detailed account of sensory processing, from the skin receptor to the somatosensory cortex, has been established to explain the perception of texture. To identify textures, rats palpate an object with brief touches. The way that the whiskers skip along the surface varies according to the surface's roughness. Whisker motion is converted to spike trains by receptor neurons. Firing rate and temporal patterns of firing in the barrel cortex, together, determine the animal's feeling of texture. In primates there are two channels for sensing texture. The perception of coarse textural features relies on a spatial mechanism—at any given instant, the degree of roughness can be decoded by a "snapshot" of the contrast in firing among slowly adapting neurons with nearby receptive fields. The perception of finely textured surfaces is determined by the excitation of nerve terminations in the Pacinian corpuscles.

From Receptors to Cortex

Receptors in the Skin

Touch receptors are mechanoreceptors: They transduce mechanical energy applied to the skin into the language of the nervous system—that is, sequences of action potentials. The key to this first stage of somatosensation is that each type of touch receptor is sensitive to particular features of mechanical energy and insensitive to all other features. This is because morphological specializations—the structures encapsulating the nerve fiber termination—make that ending respond selectively to one specific type of stimulus. The capsular structures are deformed by mechanical stimuli, and thereby transmit skin deformation to the nerve terminal (Figure 23.1). A single sensory fiber arriving from the spinal cord can branch to innervate from a few to tens of separate capsules in the skin. All capsules innervated by one fiber are of the same type. The encapsulating structure and the nerve terminal within it are called the **receptor complex.**

The **Pacinian corpuscle**, described in detail in Chapter 21, is an intriguing example of how the capsular structure selects the features that reach the nerve termination through the surrounding tissue. The **Merkel's disk** is another structure that filters mechanical energy. This small epithelial cell found under the fingerprint ridges transmits compressive strain to the sensory nerve ending. The responses are sustained during the period of pressure, with firing frequency proportional to the pressure applied to the skin.[1] Another structure, the **Ruffini's corpuscle**, is activated by pressure or compression.[2] Ruffini's corpuscles are located deeper in the skin and have the greatest density at the base of the fingernails, in the tissue overlying joints and ligaments, as well as in the palm.[3] Both the Ruffini complex and the Merkel complex are slowly adapting structures and transmit information about how firmly your hand is grasping an object or how hard your foot is pressing on the floor, the latter of which is essential for balance.

The **Meissner's corpuscle** in the skin of the lips, palm, fingers, and sole of the foot confers on the nerve terminals extraordinary mechanical sensitivity to initial contact and to motion. The receptor complex is a rapidly adapting structure and is strongly activated by low-frequency vibrations, up to 50 Hz.[4] Application of local anesthesia to the superficial skin layers, which affects nerve terminations in Meissner's corpuscles but not in Pacinian corpuscles, diminishes the sense of low-frequency vibration but not high-frequency vibration.[5]

The receptive fields—the area of skin in which stimulation evokes a response—of Meissner and Merkel receptors are small, a few millimeters in diameter, while those of Pacinian and Ruffini receptors are several centimeters in diameter. Most stimuli activate

[1] Iggo, A. and Muir, A. R. 1969. *J. Physiol.* 200: 763-796.

[2] Bolanowski, Jr., S. J. et al. 1988. *J. Acoust. Soc. Am.* 84: 1680-1694.

[3] Pare, M., Smith, A. M., and Rice, F. L. 2002. *J. Comp. Neurol.* 445: 347-359.

[4] LaMotte, R. H., and Mountcastle, V. B. 1975. *J. Neurophysiol.* 38: 539-559.

[5] Mahns, D. A. et al. 2006. *J. Neurophysiol.* 95: 1442-1450.

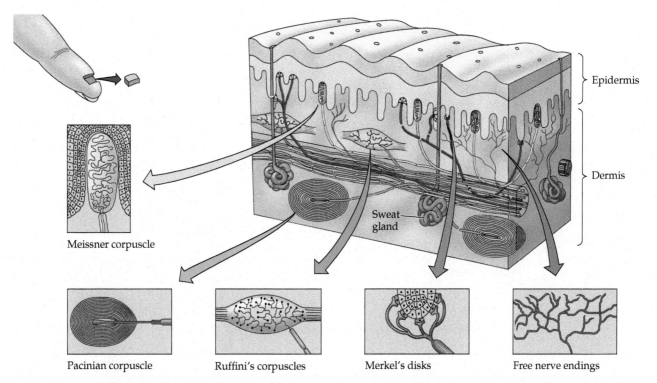

Epidermis

Dermis

Sweat gland

Meissner corpuscle

Pacinian corpuscle

Ruffini's corpuscles

Merkel's disks

Free nerve endings

FIGURE 23.1 Section of Skin Showing the Morphology and Position of Tactile Receptors. This figure refers to glabrous skin (meaning hairless, such as the skin of the palms) in primates. The Meissner's, Pacinian, and Ruffini's corpuscles as well as the Merkel's disk are all specialized structures that filter the mechanical energy that excites the nerve termination. The free nerve endings are—as the name implies—uncovered, which exposes them to substances released by the skin tissues.

several kinds of receptors at once, so that impulses from different classes signal different aspects of the stimulus.[6] For example, if you grasp a vibrating cell phone in your hand, pressure and vibration sensory channels will be activated in parallel.

Hair follicles are innervated by a network of nerve terminals with different morphologies and different positions along the hair shaft and the wall of the follicle. A small hair follicle, like that present in the skin of the body, is illustrated in Figure 23.2A, while a large whisker follicle,[7] like that on the snout of a rat or mouse, is illustrated in Figure 23.2B. The rodent snout whisker is a special hair whose function will be discussed later in the chapter. The nerve endings are excited by any event that leads to torque within the follicle—that is, motion, bending, or pulling of the hair. Because of the dense packing of receptors within follicles, it has been difficult to determine how the selectivity of individual endings varies according to morphology and position. The function of one receptor complex, the Merkel's disk, has been uncovered (Figure 23.3). With a new molecular method that renders the Merkel afferents—and these alone—excitable by blue light, it is possible to identify individual fibers by their response to light pulses and then record their activity in the behaving mouse.[8] The mouse sweeps its whiskers backward and forward to explore the space in front of its snout, a behavior known as *whisking*. The Merkel afferents are excited when the mouse touches a stick with its whiskers, but also when the mouse whisks through the open air; in the latter case, each afferent fiber fires for a particular phase of the whisk cycle. By the overlap of touch signals and self-motion signals, the Merkel afferents carry a message about where in the whisk cycle an object is encountered.

The large difference in Merkel's disk function depending on whether it is situated under the primate fingerprint ridge or in the rodent whisker follicle demonstrates how the nervous system can exploit a given receptor morphology for different roles. Another example is the inner ear hair cell (not to be confused with a skin hair), which has distinct functions according to its location in the vestibular apparatus or the cochlea (see Chapter 24).

All receptors discussed to this point can be grouped together in the category of *low-threshold* inasmuch as they are excited by very light touch. An additional class of

[6] Birder, L. A., and Perl, E. R. 1994. *J. Clin. Neurophysiol.* 11: 534-552.

[7] Rice, F. L., Mance, A., and Munger, B. L. 1986. *J. Comp. Neurol.* 252: 154-174.

[8] Severson, K. S. et al. 2017. *Neuron* 94: 666-676.e669.

(A)

(B)

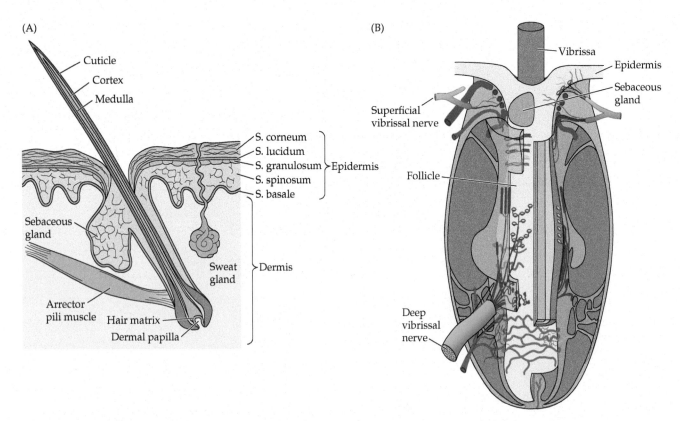

FIGURE 23.2 Hair Follicles. (A) Schematic view of a hair shaft and follicle from the skin of a primate. Nerve terminals are distributed throughout the follicle and wrap around the base of the hair, generating impulses for any hair movement. The muscle contracts to erect the hair in response to cold or arousal. (B) Schematic view of a special hair follicle, that of the large whisker of the snout of a rat or mouse. Nerve terminations enter through the superficial vibrissal nerve and the deep vibrissal nerve to occupy many different locations within the follicle, and their positioning is likely to be closely related to type of hair movement that excites them (vibration, bending, pulling, etc.). As in the case of the unspecialized skin hair in (A), the muscle wrapped around the follicle (not shown) contracts to erect the hair; however, in the case of the whisker, the action is a rhythmic sweeping motion used to collect sensory signals. (B after T. J. Park et al., 2003. *J. Comp. Neurol.* 465: 104–120, courtesy of F. Rice.)

FIGURE 23.3 Function of Merkel's Disks in the Mouse Whisker Follicle. Merkel's disks are shown (right) in magenta. Green structures are nerve terminations, and one afferent fiber is visible extending to the bottom of the image. Merkel afferents were genetically altered to make them fire when exposed to blue light (bottom left, bolt). This allowed the specific class of cells to be identified by microelectrode recording. Then, while the mouse ran on a treadmill, the identified cells fired action potentials when the mouse moved its whiskers backward and forward without contacting any object (purple). The same cells fired when the whiskers touched the vertical pole (green).

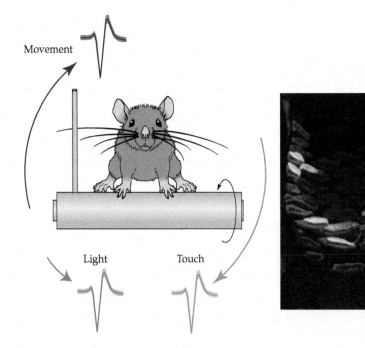

receptor is a **free nerve ending**—one that is not inserted into any specialized capsule or structure (see Figure 23.1). Through a variety of specialized chemical transduction mechanisms, described in Chapter 21, the free nerve endings generate impulses leading to sensations of pain, temperature, itch, or tickle.[6,9,10]

Anatomy of Receptor Neurons

Receptor neurons have three components: (1) a cell body that lies in a dorsal root ganglion situated in the aperture between the vertebrae of the spine, (2) a central branch that joins a dorsal root and projects into the spinal cord, and (3) a peripheral branch that joins other fibers in a peripheral nerve and then terminates as the specialized receptor complex or free nerve ending discussed in the previous section (Figure 23.4). The longest of these peripheral axons, stretching from the cell body to receptor endings in the toe, exceeds 1 meter (m) in length in humans and 3 m in giraffes.

The previous summary applies to the innervation of the skin of the hands, feet, arms, legs, and trunk. For the skin of the face, the cell bodies are in the trigeminal ganglion (instead of the dorsal root ganglion) situated lateral to the brainstem; fibers projecting to the skin travel in the trigeminal nerve—the fifth cranial nerve—and the central processes from these ganglion cells terminate in the trigeminal nuclei of the brainstem.

Because sensory neurons carry signals over long distances, transmission of information to second-order neurons cannot be accomplished by a graded potential like that of the photoreceptor. Instead, action potentials are generated very close to the nerve terminal and travel past the ganglion cell soma and into the spinal cord and brainstem. Thus, sensory neurons are long receptors in the terminology of Chapter 21.

Sensations Evoked by Afferent Signals

An increase in the understanding of touch sensation has come from the method of **microneurography** in humans.[11] A fine metal microelectrode is advanced through the skin of the arm and into the radial, median or ulnar nerves, which contain fibers traveling from the hand to the spinal cord. This setup allows the investigator to record impulses in a conscious individual while applying a stimulus to the skin and to simultaneously monitor the individual's sensations (Figure 23.5). Most fibers have little or no spontaneous activity and fire only when the skin is stimulated. Both the receptive field of a single human nerve fiber as well as the type of stimulus that is most effective in evoking an action potential conform exactly to those previously identified in laboratory animals.[12] A fiber is sensitive to just one submodality—for instance, light pressure, or low-frequency vibration, or high-frequency vibration.[13] A single fiber is sensitive to one or a few distinct skin spots, and receptive field size varies according to receptor submodality.

The advantage of microneurography over animal investigations lies in the fact that people can describe what they feel. From this came the discovery that electrical stimulation

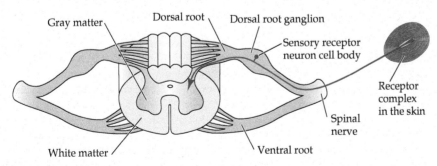

FIGURE 23.4 Morphology of Sensory Receptor Neurons. The cell body lies in a dorsal root ganglion situated in the aperture between the vertebrae of the spine. A central branch joins a dorsal root and projects into the spinal cord; a peripheral branch joins other fibers in a peripheral nerve and then terminates as a specialized cutaneous receptor complex—in this example, a Pacinian corpuscle.

[9] Ikoma, A. et al. 2003. *Arch. Dermatol.* 139: 1475-1478.

[10] Schmelz, M. et al. 2003. *J. Neurophysiol.* 89: 2441-2448.

[11] Vallbo, A. B., and Hagbarth, K. E. 1968. *Electroencephalogr. Clin. Neurophysiol.* 25: 407.

[12] Jarvilehto, T., Hamalainen, H., and Laurinen, P. 1976. *Exp. Brain Res.* 25: 45-61.

[13] Mano, T., Iwase, S., and Toma, S. 2006. *Clin. Neurophysiol.* 117: 2357-2384.

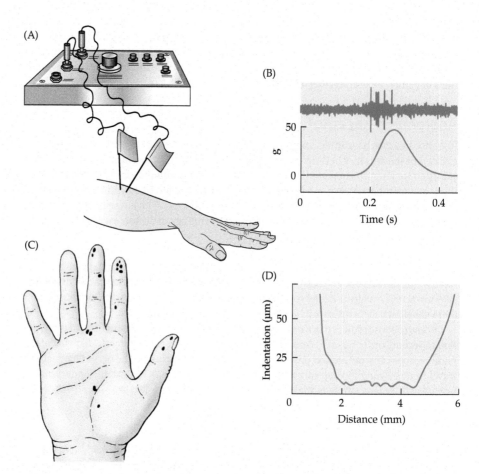

FIGURE 23.5 Microneurography of a Human Nerve. (A) Setup of the experiment. Two microelectrodes penetrate the radial nerve, and the potentials are led by wires to electrical amplifiers. Use of two electrodes allows measurement of conduction velocity. (B) Top: Responses to light pressure of multiple neurons recorded from a peripheral nerve through the same electrode. The units had overlapping receptive fields at the stimulation point. Bottom: Time course of the skin indentation force in grams (g). (C) Receptive fields of rapidly adapting touch receptors (presumably Meissner's corpuscles) in a hand. Fields were mapped by recording discharges from single fibers in the median nerve. Each dot represents the receptive field of one fiber. (D) Indentation (in micrometers) required to produce a response in one unit is plotted against location within the receptive field. The region of maximum sensitivity is about 3 mm in diameter, within which indentations of only a few micrometers are sufficient to produce a response. Points of maximum sensitivity within the region are believed to correspond to the position of individual endings of branches of the same afferent. (A after F. McGlone et al. 2007, *Can. J. Exp. Psychol.* 61: 173–183; B after J. Wessberg et al. 2003. *J. Neurophysiol.* 89: 1567–1575; C,D after R. S. Johanson and A. B. Vallbo, 1983. *Trends Neurosci.* 6: 27–32.)

of a single fiber innervating a mechanoreceptor can evoke an elementary sensation that is experienced as tapping, vibration, or pressure. The sensation feels as if it is occurring at the receptive field location of that fiber. Varying the frequency of impulse generation causes a change in the magnitude of the sensation. For example, increasing the impulse frequency increases the intensity of perceived pressure.

In order for the individual to feel a sensation of pain, impulses are required from many fibers arising from nociceptive free nerve endings, an integrative process known as spatiotemporal summation. Above threshold, the intensity of pain is correlated with the number of action potentials.[14]

Microneurography studies highlight the stimulus specificity of afferent fibers. In addition, they confirm that the activity of a single primary afferent fiber can produce a conscious sensation.[15,16] The threshold of single fibers (e.g., the amplitude of skin indentation required to excite impulses) matches the individuals' threshold for detecting the same

[14] Torebjork, E. 1985. Nociceptor activation and pain. *Philos. Trans. R Soc. Lond. B Biol. Sci.* 308: 227–234.

[15] Johansson, R. S., and Vallbo, A. B. 1979. *J. Physiol.* 297: 405–422.

[16] Ochoa, J., and Torebjork, E. 1983. *J. Physiol.* 342: 633–654.

stimulus.[16] We can deduce that transmission from skin to cerebral cortex is highly reliable, as in vision, and that impulses are delivered from the periphery into a low-noise central processing network: If that network were active in the absence of stimuli, the arrival of additional impulses from one fiber could not be readily detected. Of course, single-fiber activation is not a normal mode of operation—contact with objects produces activity patterns that are complex with respect to time and space. But the signals carried by single fibers constitute the elemental building blocks for meaningful somatic sensations.

With the knowledge of the response properties of afferents from the skin, it is possible to substitute the sense of touch in an amputee. For example, electrical circuits can be embedded in an artificial fingertip to transduce mechanical stimuli into electrical impulses in a way that imitates biological transduction. The artificial fingertip is part of a mechanical hand. Electrical impulses from the synthetic skin are then channeled to the nerve in the upper arm, allowing the individual to feel and manipulate through the substitute hand.[17]

Ascending Pathways

Receptor type, and therefore submodality, is correlated with the diameter of the afferent fiber and its myelination. As we discussed in Chapter 8, diameter and myelination determine conduction velocity. Fibers that carry signals conveying information about gentle (i.e., nonpainful) touch are myelinated and have conduction velocities up to about 60 meters per second (m/s); this class of fiber is called Aβ. Fibers that carry signals about painful stimuli and temperature have conduction velocities from 2 to 10 m/s (Aδ fibers; myelinated) down to 0.2 to 2 m/s (C fibers; unmyelinated). Microneurography shows that activity in Aδ fibers is associated with a rapid stinging or pricking sensation called first pain, whereas activity in C fibers is associated with a burning or aching sensation called second pain. The faster Aδ pain fibers are also responsible for reflexes, which explains how you can jerk your hand away from a scalding pot handle just an instant before you have any sensation of your hand being burned (see Chapter 26 for discussion of such reflexes). Thermoreceptors are innervated by C fibers. Local anesthetic agents block mainly C-fiber activity, suppressing pain and temperature sense while leaving tactile sensibility largely intact.

Chains of neurons with different functional properties follow distinct pathways to the thalamus, and hence to the cerebral cortex. Signals travel to the spinal cord, where they enter one of two ascending pathways, according to the functional category of the receptor. As shown in Appendix C, neuronal activity correlated with sensations such as touch and pressure is carried in dorsal column pathways, while neuronal activity correlated with pain and temperature ascends in the spinothalamic tract. The anatomical separation between fiber types is not absolute, however, as fibers of all types can be found in either pathway.

Within the CNS, somatosensory impulse traffic does not move in only one direction, from nerve terminal to brain; instead, the CNS also sends messages in the reverse direction. Thus, ascending somatosensory pathways are influenced by descending pathways—projections from each level cascade down to preceding levels. Somatosensory cortical areas project densely to the same thalamic, brainstem, and spinal cord sites from which they receive afferent signals. As in the visual system (see Chapters 2 and 3), the precise functions of these feedback connections are not yet known. In general terms, they modulate ascending sensory transmission, facilitating or inhibiting the incoming flow of information. The feedback effects can be highly focused in time and location. For instance, the perception of touch on the skin of the hand is reduced as the arm reaches for an object and then is amplified as the hand palpates its target.[18]

Somatosensory Cortex

The first stage of cortical processing of somatosensory signals occurs in the anterior parietal region—the area targeted by axons from the thalamic ventroposterior nucleus. In primates, input from low-threshold cutaneous receptors—the light pressure and vibration submodalities—reaches a mediolateral strip along the crown of the postcentral gyrus, area 3b in Brodmann's terminology (see Appendix C). A second target of cutaneous inputs is area 1, a strip immediately posterior to area 3b. Input from proprioceptors projects to a mediolateral strip at the anterior border of the somatosensory field (Brodmann's area 3a, just behind motor cortex)

[17] Osborn, L. E. et al. 2018. *Sci. Robot.* 3: eaat3818.

[18] Chapman, C. E., and Beauchamp, E. 2006. *J. Neurophysiol.* 96: 1664-1675.

and a strip at the posterior border (area 2). These areas together are known as **primary somatosensory cortex (S1)** (Figure 23.6), though Kaas[19] argues that only area 3b should be considered primary somatosensory cortex. There is disagreement as to whether the four areas carry out hierarchical processing or parallel processing. One view is that areas 1 and 2 integrate inputs from areas 3a and 3b to generate complex, higher-order response properties; another view is that each of the four areas operates independently on its own thalamic input. The connectivity between the areas and the response properties of neurons in anesthetized monkeys support both positions; the disagreement could be resolved by measuring the activity of neurons and the interactions among these areas in awake, behaving animals.

Lesions to S1 in humans result in a loss of touch sensation on the contralateral side of the body. Although some sensations of touch may eventually be restored, the ability to discriminate shape and texture is disrupted permanently.[20–22] Spatially restricted lesions can be made in animals to provide clearer insights into the sensory functions of specific cytoarchitectonic fields. In monkeys, lesions confined to area 3b produce the severest sensory deficits, spanning multiple tactile functions. Ablation of area 1 results in deficits in texture discrimination, whereas lesions in area 2 impair the ability to discriminate the size and shape of objects.[23,24]

Pain Perception and Its Modulation

The various forebrain regions that play a part in processing nociceptive signals have been identified, but their specific roles have been debated since the early 1900s. Most investigators distinguish between lateral and medial systems. The **lateral system**, whose main components are the lateral regions of the thalamus and S1 and **secondary somatosensory cortex (S2)**, is believed to be involved in processing the sensory discriminative aspects of pain. This system specifies where on the body the sensation arises and, according to the nature of the sensation, what might be the cause. A nociceptive pathway to S1 has been traced, and some of its neurons do respond to noxious stimuli.[25] Also, S1 activation increases in relation to the subjective strength of a painful stimulus, according to functional magnetic resonance imaging (fMRI) studies.[26–28] However, neurosurgical ablation of S1 has effects on the perception of pain that vary widely across individuals.

The **medial system**, whose main components are the medial regions of the thalamus and the insular, anterior cingulate, and prefrontal cortices, is believed to be involved in processing the affective, motivational aspects of pain.[29] Ablation of these regions of cortex profoundly

[19] Kaas, J. H. 1983. *Physiol. Rev.* 63: 206-231.

[20] Weinstein, S. et al. 1958. *J. Comp. Physiol. Psychol.* 51: 269-275.

[21] Schwartzman, R. J., and Semmes, J. 1971. *Exp. Neurol.* 33: 147-158.

[22] Bohlhalter, S., Fretz, C., and Weder, B. 2002. *Brain* 125: 2537-2548.

[23] Randolph, M., and Semmes, J. 1974. *Brain Res.* 70: 55-70.

[24] Semmes, J., Porter, L., and Randolph, M. C. 1974. *Cortex* 10: 55-68.

[25] Kenshalo, D. R. et al. 2000. *J. Neurophysiol.* 84: 719-729

[26] Christmann, C. et al. 2007. *Neuroimage* 34: 1428-1437.

[27] Apkarian, A. V. et al. 2005. *Eur. J. Pain* 9: 463-484.

[28] Davis, K. D. 2000. *Neurol. Res.* 22: 313-317.

[29] Wiech, K., Preissl, H., and Birbaumer, N. 2001. Anaesthesist 50: 2-12.

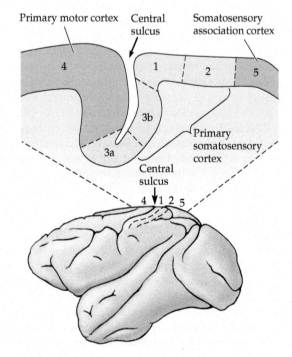

FIGURE 23.6 Organization of Primate Somatosensory Cortex.
The primary somatosensory region is located in the anterior parietal cortex, just behind the central sulcus. The figure depicts the brain of a monkey. The cytoarchitectonic areas (seen in the sagittal section, upper plot) are 3a, 3b, 1, and 2. Area 3b receives dense input from the core of the thalamic ventroposterior nucleus, receiving signals related to light touch. The other somatosensory areas receive less dense thalamic input, arising from shell areas surrounding the ventroposterior nucleus core. Area 1, like area 3b, receives signals related to light touch, while areas 3a and 2 receive signals related to deeper tissues and joints. Areas 4 and 5 are regions that receive dense projections from the adjacent somatosensory cortex and use the information for different functions. Area 4 is part of motor cortex (see Chapter 26), while area 5 integrates somatosensory information with that of other sensory modalities to create a percept of the body in relation to surrounding space.

reduces the subjective unpleasantness of noxious stimuli even as patients are able to sense and discriminate pain on the basis of the conserved lateral system. Moreover, the strength of activation of these areas as observed by fMRI, particularly in the anterior cingulate cortex, is correlated with the judgment of how emotionally distressing the pain sensation is.[26]

Although "pain pathways" from the skin have been identified,[30] it is incorrect to suppose that a specified quantity of nociceptor impulses travels in an uninterrupted stream to the cerebral cortex to produce a proportional quantity of pain. Rather, a given level of nociceptor activation can produce dramatically different subjective experiences under different conditions. A soldier charging into battle may not even notice injuries that would, under other circumstances, produce exceptional pain. In a complementary way, a chronic pain syndrome can exist even without abnormal activity in skin nociceptors.[31] It is the central processing of nociceptor signals, not their mere presence, that gives rise to the sensory and affective experience. Understanding pain thus requires understanding how the stream of impulses arriving from the nociceptors is processed by the rest of the nervous system. And, as pointed out by Melzack,[32] the subjective experience of pain—more than any other experience originating in a sensory organ—is modulated by social, cultural, and personal factors.

The discovery in the 1970s of endogenous opioid receptors in the brain[33–35] implied the existence of brain systems whose normal function must be to modulate the processing of nociceptive signals. The endogenous system acts by the release of peptides (known as **endorphins**) in the spinal cord and in other regions of the CNS, where they inhibit neuronal activity in the pain pathway. The name *endorphin* comes from the fact that these peptides are endogenous and that their chemical structure resembles that of the opiate painkiller morphine. Endorphins act through three major receptors: μ, δ, and κ. The receptor types can be distinguished according to the chemical substance for which they have greatest affinity; for instance, the most effective agonist for the μ-opioid receptors is the opium alkaloid morphine.

Can we control the operation of the endogenous pain modulation system and thereby suppress chronic pain that has outlived its usefulness as an alarm bell? Can we reduce dependence on addictive painkillers? Recent research shows that **placebo** treatment—the suggestion of pain reduction without medication or functional treatment—can effectively reduce even a postoperative pain experience.[36] Effectiveness depends on the degree to which the patient is persuaded that the treatment will work; for instance, placebo treatments that appear from their packaging to be costly are more effective than placebo treatments that appear to be inexpensive.[37] The dependence of placebo treatment on expected efficacy parallels the dependence of an actual painkiller treatment on the expected result—individuals experience more opioid-induced pain suppression when told to expect significant relief.[38] Placebo functions by activating opioid receptors,[39,40] such that placebo-evoked pain suppression is eliminated by blocking μ-opioid receptors.[41] fMRI experiments show that the effectiveness of suggestion in reducing subjective pain is positively correlated with the degree of suppression of activity in anterior cingulate and insular cortices.[38,42,43] Thus, placebo acts directly on the networks that normally generate the unpleasant experience of pain. A fascinating finding is that the expectation of a *negative* outcome can cause an intensification of pain sensations and can cause even a normally innocuous stimulus to be felt as painful.[44] This **nocebo** (from the word *noxious*) effect occurs by driving the endogenous opioidergic system in the opposite direction of the placebo effect.

Just as the patient's expectation of pain reduction can lead to an increased likelihood of that outcome, so can the expectation of a treatment side effect lead to the appearance of that side effect.[45] Individuals were given a placebo cream to combat an itchy rash on the arm, and the placebo cream was packaged to look either like an expensive brand or a cheaper generic product. People were told that the cream could cause increased pain sensitivity as a side effect—an assertion without any pharmaceutical basis. After application of the cream, individuals received a heating probe on the arm and were asked to quantify the pain. Individuals who applied the expensive-looking cream reported twice as much pain—that is, twice as strong a side effect. The increased pain sensitivity was accompanied by increased activation in the anterior cingulate cortex. The fact that expected side effects are actually experienced by patients, and that the strength of the side effect is correlated with the expected strength of real treatment, creates a dilemma for medical professions; patients need to know about the possible occurrence of undesirable effects from any treatment, but knowledge of those undesirable side effects makes them more likely to occur.

[30] Ochoa, J., and Torebjork, E. 1989. *J. Physiol.* 415: 583-599.

[31] Namer, B., and Handwerker, H. O. 2009. *Exp. Brain Res.* 196: 163-172.

[32] Melzack, R. 1973. *The Puzzle of Pain.* Penguin Books: Harmondsworth, UK, pp. 232.

[33] Pert, C. B., and Snyder, S. H. 1973. *Science* 179: 1011-1014.

[34] Terenius, L. 1973. *Acta Pharmacol. Toxicol (Copenh)* 32: 317-320.

[35] Simon, E. J., Hiller, J. M., and Edelman, I. 1973. *Proc. Natl. Acad. Sci. USA* 70: 1947-1949.

[36] Pollo, A. et al. 2001. *Pain* 93: 77-84.

[37] Waber, R. L. 2008. *JAMA* 299: 1016-1017.

[38] Bingel, U. et al. 2011. *Sci. Trans. Med.* 3: 70ra14-70ra14.

[39] Zubieta, J. K. et al. 2005. *J. Neurosci.* 25: 7754-7762.

[40] Zubieta, J. K., and Stohler, C. S. 2009. *Ann. NY Acad. Sci.* 1156: 198-210.

[41] Amanzio, M., and Benedetti, F. 1999. *J. Neurosci.* 19: 484-494.

[42] Wager, T. D. et al. 2004. *Science* 303: 1162-1167.

[43] Petrovic, P. et al. 2005. *Neuron* 46: 957-969.

[44] Benedetti, F. et al. 2006. *J. Neurosci.* 26: 12014-12022.

[45] Tinnermann, A. et al. 2017. *Science* 358: 105-108.

Somatosensory System Organization and Texture Sensation in Rats and Mice

The Whiskers of Mice and Rats

How do impulses from skin receptors eventually lead to the sensation (i.e., registration of the elemental properties) and perception (i.e., recognition of the identity and meaning of the sensation) of the things that we contact? Here we use the sensory pathways originating in the whiskers of mice and rats to illustrate the main principles of the organization and function of touch. We then show how these principles apply to sensation and perception in primates.

Mice and rats are active in dark environments and have poorer vision than primates; their survival depends on their sense of touch. Through the whiskers, the brain builds up percepts of objects: their position, size, shape, and texture.[46] The heart of the tactile system is an array of some 35 long whiskers on each side of the face—thick hairs that the animal flicks forward and backward (there are also shorter, less mobile hairs packed densely around the nose and lips that the animal can use to collect additional information).[47] Contact with an object activates mechanoreceptor terminations located in the whisker follicles, giving rise to neuronal signals (see Figure 23.2B). The first study to use the whiskers as an object of research was carried out by S. Vincent in 1912 for her PhD thesis at the University of Chicago (using rats captured in the city!).[48] She built an elevated labyrinth and found that the total time required to run from the start to the end of the maze and the number of errors (e.g., stepping into dead-end arms) increased dramatically when whiskers were clipped. The whisker-deprived rats were slowed by the need to feel the edge of the platforms with their feet rather than with their whiskers. It is instinctive for rats to step down from an illuminated, raised platform to reach a low, dark space, but they will step down onto an invisible (glass) table only if they can feel it with their whiskers.[49]

Magnification Factor

The behavioral importance of the rodents' whiskers goes hand in hand with the richness of the skin innervation. The whisker pad is the most densely supplied skin area of the body studied so far—about 200 trigeminal ganglion neurons innervate each whisker follicle.[50] In Figure 23.7A, it is evident that the primary somatosensory cortex occupies a greater territory than do the primary sensory fields for vision and audition. And within primary somatosensory cortex, the whisker field is disproportionately large. Although this can be interpreted as a greater magnification of the whiskers' cortical representation with respect to that of other body parts (i.e., in terms of square millimeters of skin projecting to square millimeters of cortical surface), it can also be interpreted as conservation, across body areas, of the relationship between receptor density and cortical territory. In other words, the number of tactile receptors projecting to each square millimeter of cortical surface is constant. According to this relationship, the richly innervated whisker follicles gain a large territory.

Topographic Map of the Whiskers and Columnar Organization

To visualize the organization of the mouse somatosensory cortex, Woolsey and van der Loos[51] separated the cerebral cortex from the underlying structures. Then, they flattened the curved cortex between two slides and sectioned the slab in a tangential plane that yielded a large horizontal expanse of layer 4 in a single section. Once the tissue was stained, distinct clusters of densely packed neurons were visible. The gridlike arrangement of the 35 clusters resembled wine casks, calling out for the name **barrels** (Figure 23.7B). The insight of Woolsey and van der Loos was that the spatial arrangement of the barrels replicated exactly the spatial arrangement of the whiskers on the snout. Every whisker on the snout was given a label (e.g., D3) and could be readily matched with one cortical barrel (again, D3). Within a few years, the prediction of a connection from each whisker to its own cortical barrel was extended from mice to rats and confirmed by many physiological studies.[52-55] Thus, the receptive fields of the neurons in barrel D3 are centered on the so-called principal whisker, D3. Whiskers surrounding the principal whisker may also excite cells to a lesser degree. Neurons in the layers above and below layer 4, which receive their main sensory input from layer 4, also receive a strong input from the principal whisker.[52] So the neuronal

[46] Diamond, M. E. et al. 2008. *Nat. Rev. Neurosci.* 9: 601–612.

[47] Brecht, M., Preilowski, B., and Merzenich, M. M. 1997. *Behav. Brain Res.* 84: 81–97.

[48] Vincent, S. B. 1912. *Behav. Monogr.* 1: 1–82.

[49] Schiffman, H. R. et al. 1970. *Animal Behav.* 18: 290–292.

[50] Welker, E., and Van der Loos, H. 1986. *J. Neurosci.* 6: 3355–3373.

[51] Woolsey, T. A. and Van der Loos, H. 1970. *Brain Res.* 17: 205–242.

[52] Armstrong-James, M., Fox, K., and Das-Gupta, A. 1992. *J. Neurophysiol.* 68: 1345–1358.

[53] Petersen, R. S., and Diamond, M. E. 2000. *J. Neurosci.* 20: 6135–6143.

[54] Simons, D. J. 1978. *J. Neurophysiol.* 41: 798–820.

[55] Welker, C. 1976. *J. Comp. Neurol.* 166: 173–189.

(A)

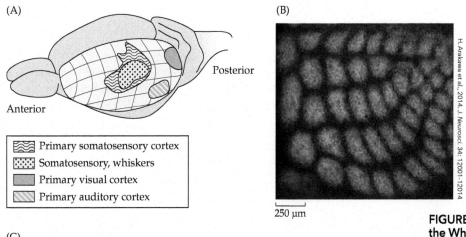

Anterior   Posterior

〰️	Primary somatosensory cortex
⋮⋮	Somatosensory, whiskers
▪	Primary visual cortex
▨	Primary auditory cortex

(B)

H. Arakawa et al., 2014. *J. Neurosci.* 34: 12001–12014

250 μm

(C)

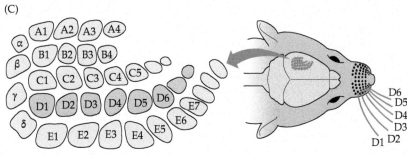

A1 A2 A3 A4
α
B1 B2 B3 B4
β
C1 C2 C3 C4 C5
γ
D1 D2 D3 D4 D5 D6 E7
δ E6
E1 E2 E3 E4 E5

D6 D5 D4 D3 D1 D2

FIGURE 23.7 **Cortical Representation of the Whiskers in Rats and Mice.** (A) Relative positions and sizes of primary sensory cortical fields. (B) Barrels in the mouse somatosensory cortex visible in a tangential section through layer 4. The dark rings are the cell-dense walls of the barrels. (C) Arrangement of the barrels in the left hemisphere of a rat, with each barrel labeled by its corresponding whisker. In the sketch on the right, whiskers D1 through D6, which project to barrels D1 through D6, are shown full-length. The follicles of other whiskers are depicted as dots. (C after M. E. Diamond et al., 2008. *Nat. Rev. Neurosci.* 9: 601–612.)

population extending through all layers forms a cortical column associated with a single whisker, a functional unit anchored by the layer 4 barrel.

Because two whiskers that are adjacent to each other on the animal's face are represented in adjacent cortical barrels, the barrel field constitutes a **topographic map** (Figure 23.7C). Beyond the special case of whiskers, it is common to refer to a brain representation as a map whenever the spatial relationship among sensory receptors is conserved, even if stretched or otherwise distorted, in the central representation of the sense organ. Box 23.1 provides a historical note on the discovery of cortical somatosensory maps.

The map of cortical columns serves to organize the storage of sensory experiences. One demonstration is provided by an experiment in which all whiskers except one—called the trained whisker—were trimmed from the snout of the rats. The animals were then coaxed, in the dark, to perch on one platform, extend the trained whisker across a gap to touch and thus localize a second platform, and jump across the gap to reach a reward (Figure 23.8A). Next, the trained whisker was clipped off and a previously clipped whisker was fixed with glue to a different whisker stub (Figure 23.8B). When the rats were retested, the number of trials necessary to relearn the task was found to increase as a function of the distance between the site of the trained whisker and the new (i.e., attached) whisker (Figure 23.8C). Moreover, the transfer of learning between any two whisker locations was perfectly explained by the spatial distribution of physiological activity within the barrel field map (Figure 23.8D). This experiment suggests the presence of a sensory memory trace governed by the precise topography of the sensory receptors.[56]

Further experiments found that, in humans, tactile learning acquired through a single fingertip is transferred to other fingertips by the same rules as for the whiskers, dictated by the cortical topographic map of the hand.[57] The notion that the map of cortical columns serves to organize the storage of sensory experiences thus seems to generalize from rodents to humans.

Map Development and Plasticity

When a strain of mice is bred to have different numbers of whiskers, the barrel field differs in precise correspondence with the face; thus, extra whiskers (or missing whiskers) are accompanied by extra (or missing) barrels in the matching part of the barrel field.[58,59]

[56] Harris, J. A., Petersen, R. S., and Diamond, M. E. 1999. *Proc. Natl. Acad. Sci. USA* 96: 7587–7591.

[57] Harris, J. A., Harris, I. M., and Diamond, M. E. 2001. *J. Neurosci.* 21: 1056–1061.

[58] van der Loos, H., and Dorfl, J. 1978. *Neurosci. Lett.* 7: 23–30.

[59] van der Loos, H., and Dorfl, J., and Welker, E. 1984. *J. Hered.* 75: 326–336.

BOX 23.1 Variation across Species in Cortical Maps

The expanded representations of particularly sensitive body areas and their locations within distorted maps were described by Adrian beginning in the 1920s in work that opened the modern epoch in the study of somatosensory cortex. The experiments were accomplished by stimulating skin sites while picking up potentials, summated across millions of neurons, through electrodes (tiny spheres of copper) placed on the cortical surface. The line of research was continued by Clinton Woolsey through the 1950s, until microelectrode methods took over. Comparing the cortical skin representation across numerous species, these pioneers found fascinating species-specific maps. Recently, a particularly remarkable cortical map has been discovered: the representation of the pink fleshy appendages, called rays, ringing the snout of the star-nosed mole. These densely innervated tactile probes, which the animal uses to find worms, have an enormous topographically organized cortical representation.

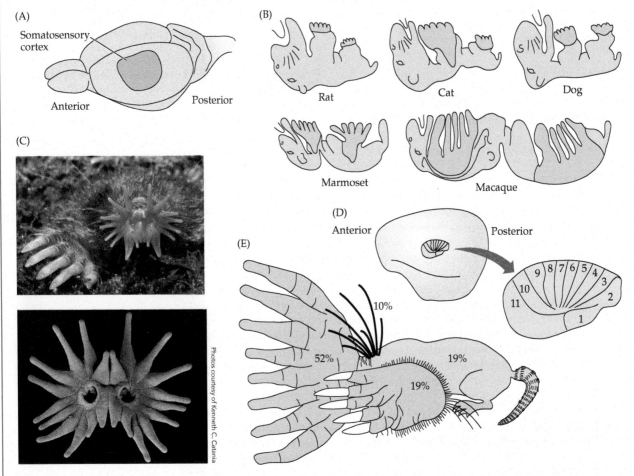

Photos courtesy of Kenneth C. Catania

Cortical Somatosensory Maps. The skin areas that are most important to natural behavior, and are most richly innervated, are associated with expanded cortical representations. (A) View from above of the rodent brain. The location of somatosensory cortex on the cerebral hemisphere, shown here in blue shading, is typical of the general mammalian plan. (B) With the same orientation as in (A), the cortical maps for five species are illustrated. Forelimb and hindlimb are shaded, from which it can be noted that these regions are expanded in the primates—the marmoset and macaque. The maps are not shown in scale to each other. (C) A star-nosed mole. Top: Note the forelimb shaped for digging and the prominent finger-like "rays" around the snout. Bottom: Photomicrograph of the snout, showing the 11 rays per side (22 total) distributed about the central holes—the nostrils. (D) Again, a star-nosed mole. Left: View from the side of the left hemisphere with the snout representation shown in blue. Right: Closer view of the snout representation, in which each ray possesses a separate area. Adjacent rays have adjacent cortical territories. (E) Schematic depiction of the mole's body representation in somatosensory cortex. Percentages indicate the proportion of primary somatosensory cortex responding to the given body part. (B after C. N. Woolsey, 1952. In *The Biology of Mental Health and Disease: The Twenty-seventh Annual Conference of the Milbank Memorial Fund*, H. D. Kruse (Ed.), pp. 193–206. Paul B. Hoeber, Inc., New York; D,E after K. C. Catania and J. H. Kass, 1996. *Bio. Science Rep.* 46: 578–586.)

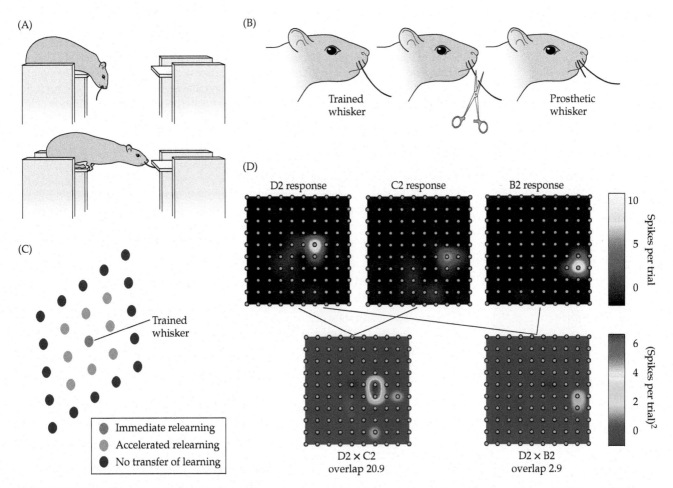

FIGURE 23.8   Role of the Cortical Whisker Map in Sensory Learning. (A) In the gap-crossing task, the rat learned to identify, in the dark, the location of a reward platform by making contact using a single intact whisker, referred to as the trained whisker. In this drawing, the rat first leans into the gap (top sketch) and then extends forward to reach the target (bottom sketch). (B) The trained whisker (left) was clipped off (middle), and a different whisker was fixed to a whisker stump some specific distance from the stump of the trained whisker (prosthetic whisker, right). (C) Schematic depiction of the whisker grid. The speed at which the rat relearned the gap-crossing task depended on the distance from the site of the trained whisker to the site of attachment of the new whisker, indicating that learning was localized. (D) The top three plots show the number of action potentials (spikes per trial) evoked by separate, brief movements of three different whiskers: D2, C2, and B2. The responses were measured across a 10 × 10 grid of microelectrodes placed in the barrel cortex; electrode positions are designated by gray dots. The bottom two plots indicate the degree of overlap in the cortical representation between whisker pairs (D2 × C2, and D2 × B2). This is calculated by multiplying the separate responses of the two whiskers at each electrode; thus, the response scale is (spikes squared per trial) squared. Cortical overlap is higher for the closer whisker pair (D2 × C2) than for the more widely separated whisker pair (D2 × B2). The key result is that the exact quantity of cortical overlap between the representations of any two whiskers perfectly accounts for the degree of learning transfer between those two whisker sites. (After. J. A. Harris et al. 1999. *Proc. Natl. Acad. Sci. USA* 96: 7587-7591. © 1999 National Academy of Sciences, USA.)

Destruction at birth of a whisker follicle will cancel that whisker's module from all maps in the ascending sensory pathway.[60] But once the anatomical connection between one whisker and its corresponding cortical barrel is established a few days after birth, that barrel remains fixed throughout life (see Chapter 28).

The topographic map at the level of cortex is not generated ad hoc from a disordered input—rather, all along the pathway, the neighboring relations are received in an orderly manner from the preceding level. Each barrel receives input from a discrete **barreloid** in the ventroposterior medial nucleus of the thalamus; each thalamic barreloid receives input from a **barrelette** in the brainstem trigeminal nucleus; and each barrelette receives input from a whisker. During development the modular clustering appears in a day-by-day sequence from periphery to cortex.[61]

Although the principal input to a given barrel is its topographically matched whisker, neurons do respond to stimulation of neighboring whiskers, particularly in the column of

[60] Jeanmonod, D., Rice, F. L., and Van Der Loos, H. 1977. *Neurosci. Lett.* 6: 151-156.

[61] Andres, F. L., and Van der Loos, H. 1985. *Anat. Embryol. (Berl.)* 172: 11-20.

neurons above and below the layer 4 barrel. These inputs form the **surround receptive field**. Throughout life, the weighting of the inputs from principal and surround whiskers remains plastic, shifting according to the animal's sensory experience. For example, if some whiskers are trimmed short and others left intact, cortical neurons become more responsive to the whiskers that the animal uses and less responsive to the clipped ones. This form of map plasticity has been attributed mainly to the activity-dependent modification of intracortical synaptic connections.[62–64] The function served by such plasticity may be to allow the remaining sensory input to be processed by a greater number of cortical neurons, thus increasing its impact on behavior.

Plastic reorganization of the cortical somatosensory map is also at work in regions beyond the whisker representation. During the first few weeks after birth, rat pups spend well over half the time in suckling behavior. In the nursing mother rat, the cortical territory representing the ventral skin where her pups suckle increases manyfold, only to retract when the pups are weaned.[65] The significance of this experiment is that map plasticity accompanies the variations in sensory experience that are part of the normal cycle of life.

Texture Sensation through the Whiskers: Peripheral Mechanisms

The maplike organization of somatosensory cortex is essential for detecting the location of a stimulus. We can think of somatotopic organization as the *infrastructure* necessary to maintain spatial information as signals ascend to cerebral cortex. However, there is much more to a stimulus than its location. The *quality* of touch sensation is related to which type of receptor has been activated and the details of the activity in the corresponding neurons. This section and the next provide examples of how touch sensations arise from neuronal activity. Of the many different sensations that originate in the skin, we have selected texture because it allows for interesting comparisons between the rat whisker and the primate fingertip sensory systems; some mechanisms are unique to each, and some mechanisms are common to both.

Texture is defined by local surface material and microgeometry. The perception of texture is important for animal behavior, for example in the selection of nesting materials. Rats sweep their whiskers forward and backward at a frequency of 8 to 12 Hz (mice at 20 Hz), describing large, elegant arcs. As noted earlier, the sweeping action is called whisking and an individual cycle is called a whisk. Whisking is an example of generative sensing—that is, actively moving the receptors to create sensory signals.[66] When the animals set out to identify the texture of an object, they approach it and then palpate its surface with brief, light whisks (Figure 23.9A). To find out how well rats can identify textures, investigators have trained them in the dark to take one action upon contact with one texture and a different action upon contact with a second texture (e.g., turn to the left or right reward location according to the presented stimulus). The rats' performance is remarkably fast and accurate. On an easy task, for instance when one texture is pebbly and the other perfectly smooth, the rats can extract texture identity from just one to six touches per whisker;[67] this translates to a total time between initial contact and texture identification as short as 100 to 600 milliseconds (ms). If the task is made more difficult by using textures that are more alike, rats require more training and more contact time per trial. But after many practice sessions, they are able to make discriminations that are difficult even for humans using a fingertip—for example, selecting between a smooth surface and one with grooves that are 30 micrometers (μm) deep and spaced at 90 μm.[68]

The capacity to discriminate between textures begins with the signal transmitted by the whiskers. On any given whisk, many whiskers touch the surface, but they do so in a seemingly disorderly manner, passing in front of and behind their neighbors. This observation suggests that the sensory system does *not* use the specific spatial arrangement of the whiskers in the sensing of textures. Indeed, if only a few whiskers are left intact (the others clipped), rats can still discriminate textures. So each whisker, by itself, appears to transmit a highly informative message. When moving in air, whisker motion is continuous and fluid. But along a surface, the whisker's trajectory is characterized by an irregular skipping motion made up of intermixed high and low velocities.[69] The underlying process is known as **stick and slip**: The whisker tip tends to get fixed in place (i.e., sticks) and bends until the force applied by the

[62] Diamond, M. E., Armstrong-James, M., and Ebner, F. F. 1993. *Proc. Natl. Acad. Sci. USA* 90: 2082-2086.

[63] Diamond, M. E., Huang, W., and Ebner, F. F. 1994. *Science* 265: 1885-1888.

[64] Celikel, T., Szostak, V. A., and Feldman, D. E. 2004. *Nat. Neurosci.* 7: 534-541.

[65] Xerri, C., Stern, J. M., and Merzenich, M. M. 1994. *J. Neurosci.* 14: 1710-1721.

[66] Diamond, M. E., and Arabzadeh, E. 2013. *Prog. Neurobiol.* 103: 28-40.

[67] von Heimendahl, M. et al. 2007. *PLOS Biol.* 5: e305.

[68] Carvell, G. E., and Simons, D. J. 1990. *J. Neurosci.* 10: 2638-2648.

[69] Arabzadeh, E., Zorzin, E., and Diamond, M. E. 2005. *PLOS Biol.* 3: e17.

(A)

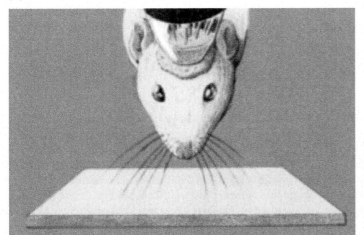

(B)

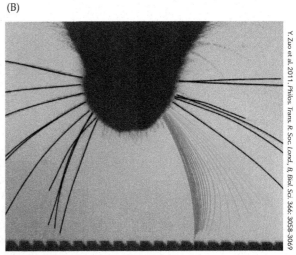

Y. Zuo et al. 2011. *Philos. Trans. R. Soc. Lond. B, Biol. Sci.* 366: 3058-3069

FIGURE 23.9 Texture Discrimination Behavior. (A) This sketch depicts the rat as it leans across a gap to touch a textured plate with its whiskers. The cable on the head of the animal carries neuronal signals to the computer. (B) One frame from a high-speed (1000 frames/second) video. The orientation of the snout of the rat and the texture are similar to that in (A). This texture contains notchlike grooves. One whisker was tracked through a sequence of frames; the traces, from violet to light blue, show the whisker position over 1-ms timesteps. The whisker tip was blocked in a groove and then sprung free as the rat whisked in the posterior direction. Irregular, fast events like this one provide information to the sensory receptors about texture. (A drawn by Marco Gigante.)

follicle muscle overcomes the resistance caused by friction; at this instant, the whisker springs loose (i.e., slips), only to get stuck again.[70] The movement of whiskers on a surface containing grooves resembles their movement along irregular, coarse textures. For instance, Figure 23.9B shows the trajectory of a single whisker as it is released from the groove of a plate. Discrimination can occur because each texture is associated with a distinct trajectory of sticks and slips, and the coarser the texture or the greater the spatial frequency of grooves, the greater is the probability of such slips and the greater their velocity when they occur.

Among sensory receptor neurons, spiking probability increases with progressively higher whisker-bending speed and acceleration.[71] Since whisking along coarse textures leads to higher-velocity slips than does whisking along smooth textures,[69,70] rough texture is translated to a greater rate of neuronal firing,[67,72] which forms a key component of the animals' judgment of roughness.

Texture Sensation through the Whiskers: Cortical Mechanisms

The barrel cortex is critical for texture discrimination. After rats are trained to use their whiskers to discriminate between sandpapers with different grain sizes, the capacity is lost after a lesion of barrel cortex.[73] To substitute the lost capacity, the rats begin to use their forepaw to touch and identify textures.

In a direct test of the proposal that neuronal firing rate distinguishes between different texture sensations, activity was measured in cortical barrels while rats identified a contacted texture as rough or smooth, indicating their choice on each trial by moving to a water reward spout on either the left or right.[67] Success rate was over 80%. On the set of trials when a rat correctly identified the stimulus, the average firing rate of neurons in barrel cortex was higher on each touch for rough trials than for smooth trials. On error trials, the firing-rate code was reversed (i.e., lower for rough than for smooth), meaning that the rat makes its decision (right or wrong) based on the magnitude of whisker-evoked activity in barrel cortex. The temporal pattern of spikes also contributes to the discrimination of texture.[69,74,75]

Rats can make a choice after a single contact, but they frequently make multiple touches before committing to a choice. Does the information contained within somatosensory cortex explain this behavior? To answer this question, investigators measured the quantity of texture information in barrel cortex touch by touch. The texture message did not grow progressively;

[70] Wolfe, J. et al. 2008. *PLOS Biol.* 6: e215.

[71] Shoykhet, M., Doherty, D., and Simons, D. J. 2000. *Somatosens. Mot. Res.* 17: 171-180.

[72] Lottem, E., and Azouz, R. 2009. *J. Neurosci.* 29: 11686-11697.

[73] Guic-Robles, E., Jenkins, W. M., and Bravo, H. 1992. Behav. *Brain Res.* 48: 145-152.

[74] Arabzadeh, E., Panzeri, W., and Diamond, M. E. 2006. *J. Neurosci.* 26: 9216-9226.

[75] Zuo, Y. et al. 2015. *Curr. Biol.* 25: 357-363.

instead, barrel cortex relays texture information to a downstream integrator that accumulates the information until the total quantity of evidence for one texture reaches a boundary.[76,77]

Somatosensory System Organization and Texture Sensation in Primates

Magnification Factor

The whiskers are the critical touch organ in rats and mice; in humans and other primates, the fingertips are the equivalent. Each fingertip is innervated by axons from 250 to 300 sensory neurons (about the same number as the rodent whisker). Because individual axons branch out and terminate in multiple receptor structures, the density of mechanoreceptor terminals reaches the remarkably high value of over 1000 per square centimeter (cm^2). The large number of receptors is responsible for the fine tactual acuity of the fingertips, which enables Braille experts to read at speeds in excess of 100 words a minute or Venetian glass blowers to assess the smoothness of their vases.

The rich fingertip innervation density is, like the whisker innervation of rodents, connected with an expanded cortical representation in which the representation of a 1-cm^2 area of skin on the fingertip occupies a somatosensory cortical area 100 times greater than the representation of a 1-cm^2 area of skin on the shoulder. In humans, innervation density and cortical magnification are high for the lips as well—crucial in the sensory aspects of eating, speaking, and kissing.

Topographic Map of the Skin and Columnar Organization

The magnification of certain areas of skin gives rise to the famous distorted cortical maps. In humans, such maps were discovered in the 1930s in patients undergoing brain operations. As the surgeon electrically stimulated a restricted cortical locus, the patient reported a sensation referred to a particular position on the body; touching that place on the skin led to an evoked potential at the same cortical site.[78] The original scheme, the **homunculus**, was correct concerning the relative locations of the major parts of the body in the coronal plane. Later, details such as the fine organization of the face and the medial-to-lateral sequence of fingers were corrected by using fMRI.[79,80] Like the cortical representation of the whiskers in the mouse and rat, the homunculus is a topographic map because neighboring sites on the skin are represented at neighboring sites in the cortex. Processing of painful stimuli also exhibits a topographic organization within the ascending sensory pathways.[81]

In the 1950s, the use of microelectrodes to record the responses of neuronal clusters to well-controlled stimuli in anesthetized animals led to two crucial advances beyond the basic cortical body map. First, columnar organization was discovered and described for the first time by Lorente de Nó anatomically and then by Mountcastle and his colleagues by use of electrical recordings from primate somatosensory cortex (see also Chapter 3).[82] When the electrode penetrated the cortex at an angle normal to the surface, all neurons responded to the same receptor class and shared overlapping receptive fields on the skin—resembling, conceptually, the columns of V1, primary visual cortex (see Chapter 3). (Barrels in mouse and rat somatosensory cortex are thus a special case of columnar organization.) Second, map topography was worked out in much greater detail. Areas 3b and 1 (Figure 23.10) each contain a map arranged in an elongated mediolateral strip along the postcentral gyrus (also see Appendix C); the two maps are arranged as mirror images reflected about the cytoarchitectonic border.[83] Because a three-dimensional surface (the body) is projected onto a two-dimensional surface (the cortex), map discontinuities are inevitable.

Texture Sensation through the Fingertip: Peripheral Mechanisms

One important way in which fingertip touch differs from whisker touch is that we (primates) manipulate objects with our hands, whereas rodents do *not* manipulate objects with their whiskers. The fingertips provide tactile feedback necessary for the motor control of the hand, such

[76] Zuo, Y., and Diamond, M. E. 2019. *Curr. Biol.* 29: 1415-1424.e5.

[77] Zuo, Y., and Diamond, M. E. 2019. *Curr. Biol.* 29: 1425-1435.e5.

[78] Jasper, H. and Penfield, W., 1954. *Epilepsy and the Functional Anatomy of the Human Brain.* 2nd ed. Little, Brown and Co., Boston.

[79] DaSilva, A. F. et al. 2002. *J. Neurosci.* 22: 8183-8192.

[80] Powell, T. P., and Mountcastle, V. B. 1959. *Bull. Johns Hopkins Hosp.* 105: 133-162.

[81] van Westen, D. et al. 2004. *BMC Neurosci.* 5: 28.

[82] Powell, T. P., and Mountcastle, V. B. 1959. *Bull. Johns Hopkins Hosp.* 105: 133-162.

[83] Merzenich, M. M. et al. 1978. *J. Comp. Neurol.* 181: 41-73.

FIGURE 23.10 Topographic Organization of Somatosensory Cortex in the Owl Monkey. (A) Location of architectonic fields 3a, 3b, 1, and 2. Anterior to the left, posterior to the right. (B) Representations of body surface in areas 3b and 1 of somatosensory cortex. Areas 3a and 2 are largely activated by receptors in deep body tissues, whereas areas 3b and 1 each contain separate representations of cutaneous receptors. The 3b and 1 representations are parallel and are largely mirror images in somatotopic organization. D1–D5, locations of glabrous digit surfaces of hand and foot; digits point in opposite directions in the two representations so that digit tips are rostral in area 3b and caudal in area 1. Vib = mystacial vibrissae; U. Lip = upper lip region; L. Lip = lower lip region; P. Leg = region of posterior portion of leg; A. Leg = region of anterior portion of leg; d = dorsal; v = ventral. Dark regions of cortex indicate representations of the dorsal hairy surfaces of hand and foot. (After J. H. Kaas, 1983. *Physiol. Rev.* 63: 206–231.)

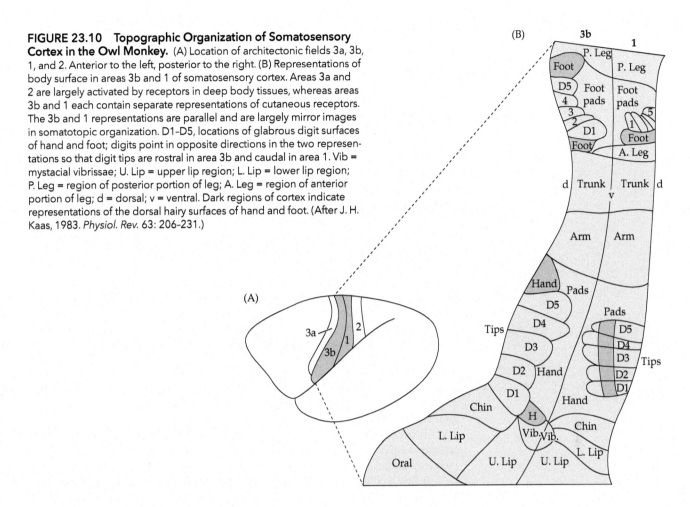

as peeling a banana, holding a pencil, or buttoning a button. While we handle objects, texture is sensed quickly and provides essential information both for identifying the object and for generating the appropriate motor plan. For instance, texture is a crucial part of the sensation that tells us how tightly we must grasp an object to keep it from slipping through our hands.

The mechanisms for sensing texture through the primate fingertip differ in several ways from those of the whiskers.[84] Receptors in the 35 whisker follicles form a discontinuous grid of 35 exquisitely sensitive points, whereas touch receptors in the fingertips are distributed in a continuous, overlapping sheet. The spatial relationships among the whiskers shift from one contact to the next, whereas the layout of fingertip touch receptors is constant over time. Several lines of evidence suggest that the perception of coarse textural features (such as the raised dots of Braille), through the fingertip, does rely on a spatial mechanism—at any given instant, the degree of roughness can be decoded by a "snapshot" (a spatial profile in a short time window) of the contrast in firing among slowly adapting neurons with nearby receptive fields. In contrast, the perceived roughness of finely textured surfaces is determined by the efficacy with which finger motion along the surface excites the rapidly adapting Pacinian receptors. We can view this latter process as a vibration mechanism, and it seems not to depend on comparing the distribution of excitation across separate receptors (as does the spatial mechanism). The reader will have noted that, of the two channels, the vibration mechanism has much in common with how whiskers extract surface properties. This formulation, with its distinct morphological and functional channels for smooth and rough, has been named the **duplex theory** of texture perception. Evidence for the duplex theory is given in the following sections.

COARSE TEXTURES The spatial distribution of receptors allows the primate sensory system to gather signals that turn out to be particularly important for sensing coarse textures. Textures of this sort—for which the center-to-center distance between raised elements is

[84] Diamond, M. E. 2010. *Curr. Opin. Neurobiol.* 20: 319–327.

larger than about 200 μm—can be discriminated simply by pressing the finger against the surface (again, Braille reading is a good example).[57] The fact that finger movement is not necessary points to slowly adapting receptors, presumably of the Merkel type, as the crucial peripheral termination. These receptors do not require motion across the receptive field but rather show an increased firing rate in proportion to the pressure; their spatial resolution of 0.5 to 1 millimeter (mm) matches the limits of human tactile acuity.[2] More direct evidence for slowly adapting coding of coarse textures comes from physiological and psychophysical experiments using stimuli formed by raised dots that vary in height, diameter, and center-to-center spacing.[85,86] Humans rated the roughness of the stimuli, and their estimates were compared with the responses of monkey slowly adapting neurons for the same set of stimuli. The stimuli judged as roughest were the ones that evoked the greatest contrast in firing rate of nearby slowly adapting receptors. Why might *contrast* in firing among adjacent receptors be correlated with roughness? As illustrated in Figure 23.11, if the surface is rough or grainy, adjacent receptors absorb different forces. In contrast, if the surface is smooth, or if there is little space between adjacent grains, force is distributed equally across adjacent receptors.

The division of labor between rapidly and slowly adapting receptors in sensing rough texture is not absolute. There is evidence that rapidly adapting receptors of the Meissner type also contribute to the perception of coarse textures, but the mechanisms are not yet clear. In response to vibration, such receptors fire in phase with each displacement for frequencies up to about 50 Hz.[12,87–89] Some individuals may use vibrations of this kind to identify texture as they move the fingertip along a surface.[90,91]

FINE TEXTURES Slowly adapting receptors only contribute if the separation between pebbles, dots, or ridges is more than about 200 μm; if spacing is less than 200 μm, each slowly adapting receptor averages over the different bumps within its receptive field, and the mechanism of firing contrast no longer works. Therefore, to sense the quality of a fine-grained texture, a finger must move along its surface. The mechanism depends on the temporal firing patterns in rapidly adapting receptors (presumed Meissner receptors) and the firing rate of Pacinian receptors. This conclusion was derived from many different types of experiments.

The first kind of experiment studied the effect of high-frequency adaptation on fine texture sensation. Pacinian receptors (see Chapter 21) register vibrations in the frequency range of 50 to 400 Hz with peak sensitivity for vibrations in the range of about 250 to 300 Hz.[2] If sinusoidal vibrations centered on the Pacinian frequency band are continuously applied to a fingertip, high-frequency vibration sensitivity is lost, and individuals then show a degraded ability to discriminate between fine textures but not between coarse textures. Adaptation of the Meissner rapidly adapting receptor with prolonged vibrations of 10 Hz has a small effect on the sensing of the finest-grain textures.

[85] Connor, C. E. et al. 1990. *J. Neurosci.* 10: 3823-3836.

[86] Connor, C. E., and Johnson, K. O. 1992. *J. Neurosci.* 12: 3414-3426.

[87] Freeman, A. W., and Johnson, K. O. 1982. *J. Physiol.* 323: 21-41.

[88] Coleman, G. T. et al. 2001. *J. Neurophysiol.* 85: 1793-1804.

[89] Lundstrom, R. J. 1986. *Scand. J. Work Environ. Health* 12: 413-416.

[90] Gamzu, E., and Ahissar, E. 2001. *J. Neurosci.* 21: 7416-7427.

[91] Cascio, C. J., and Sathian, K. 2001. *J. Neurosci.* 21: 5289-5296.

(A) 1.5 mm (B) 3.0 mm (C) 4.5 mm

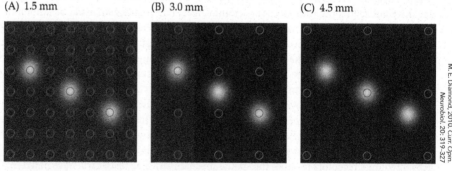

FIGURE 23.11 Scheme for Detection of Coarse Features: Peripheral Mechanisms. Red circles represent regular, raised features on the surface of an object (e.g., grains, dots, pegs). Center-to-center spacing of features is in 1.5 mm in (A), 3.0 mm in (B), and 4.5 mm in (C). In each panel, the receptive fields of three slowly adapting primary afferent neurons are represented by the three light-colored spots. In (A), all three neurons are excited by surface features, so contact evokes little contrast in the firing rate among the three. In (B), two neurons are excited and one is not, causing a contrast in firing rate. In (C), there is also contrast in firing rate, but only one of the three neurons is excited. Due to the contrast in firing rates, (B) would feel roughest.

(A)

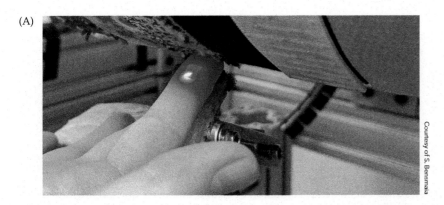

Courtesy of S. Bensmaia

(B)

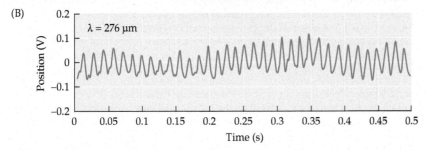

FIGURE 23.12 Skin Vibrations Evoked by Motion across a Fine Texture.
(A) A rotating drum stimulator scans a large set of textures across the finger, fixed to a finger
holder to prevent movement and ensure comfort during the vibration measurements. The
beam of a laser Doppler vibrometer (LDV) is focused on the skin near contact with surface. The
LDV measures skin deflections along the axis of its beam, which is approximately perpendicular to the skin's surface. The LDV exploits the Doppler effect to measure the velocity of the skin
at that location and along that axis. (B) Transducer reading associated with movement along
a surface with a spatial period of 276 μm. Both the frequency and amplitude of the vibrations
varied with spatial period of the probed surface. Surfaces that produced vibrations with a large
amount of power in the frequency range of Pacinian receptors were perceived as roughest.
(B after M. Hollins and S. Bensmaïa, 2007. *Can. J. Exp. Psychol.* 61: 184–195, a portion of Figure
4, pg 189. © 2007 by the Canadian Psychological Association Inc. Permission from the Canadian Psychological Association Inc.)

To collect more evidence, one experiment used an optical device to measure skin
vibrations near the contact point between fingertip and the surface (Figure 23.12). On
each trial, individuals were asked to compare the roughness of two surfaces. A higher
degree of perceived roughness was associated with an increasing intensity of skin vibration *within the range of maximum Pacinian sensitivity*; vibrations at frequencies below or
above the Pacinian peak sensitivity led to lower judgments of roughness.[92] Remarkably,
when individuals were presented the same texture twice, as if they were two separate
stimuli, they judged the texture as rougher on the presentation that evoked stronger vibrations in the Pacinian range.[93]

As a final test, artificial vibrations were added. When the plate surface was made to
vibrate in the preferred Pacinian frequency range while the individual was palpating it, the
texture felt rougher, even when individuals were not aware of the vibration itself.[94]

As with most theories that aim to simplify neurobiology, the duplex theory cannot
fully account for all observations. Textures whose spatial frequencies are partway between coarse and fine are encoded neither by slowly adapting Merkel receptors nor on
rapidly adapting Pacinian receptors; sensing textures of this sort depends largely on contributions of Meissner receptors.[95,96]

Texture Sensation through the Fingertip: Cortical Mechanisms

The evidence described in the previous section concerns the coding of texture by the
peripheral nervous system. In the somatosensory cortex, the distinction between rapidly

[92] Bensmaia, S., and Hollins, M. 2005.
Percept Psychophys. 67: 842–854.

[93] Hollins, M., and Bensmaia, S. J. 2007.
Can J. Exp Psychol. 61: 184–195.

[94] Hollins, M., Fox, A., and Bishop, C.
2000. *Perception* 29: 1455–1465.

[95] Mackevicius, E. L. et al., 2012.
J. Neurosci. 32: 15309–15317.

[96] Weber, A. I. et al. 2013. *Proc. Natl.
Acad. Sci. USA* 110: 17107–17112.

(A) 1.5 mm (B) 3.0 mm (C) 4.5 mm

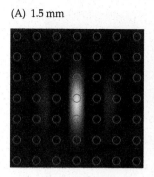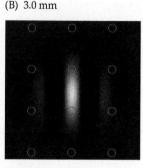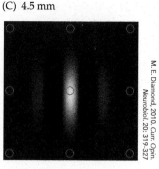

M. E. Diamond, 2010. *Curr. Opin. Neurobiol.* 20: 319-327

FIGURE 23.13 Scheme for Detection of Coarse Features: Cortical Mechanisms.
As in Figure 23.11, red circles represent regular, raised features on the surface of an object (e.g., grains, dots, pegs). Center-to-center spacing of features is 1.5 mm in (A), 3.0 mm in (B), and 4.5 mm in (C). The object surfaces are depicted in relation to the receptive field of a single, slowly adapting cortical neuron. Cortical neurons receive inputs from many peripheral receptors and have complex receptive fields, in this case an elongated excitatory central region (light area) flanked by alternating inhibitory (dark) and excitatory (light) subfields. The texture in (A) evokes a weak response in this neuron because the dots fall on both excitatory and inhibitory regions of the receptive field. The pattern in (B) produces strong excitation of the neuron because two of the dots fall on the central excitatory region and none on the flanking inhibitory subfield. The pattern in (C) excites the neuron to a lesser extent because only one dot falls on the excitatory portion. Thus, this cortical neuron would respond most strongly to a texture with a 3-mm spacing, which would be perceived as rough.

adapting and slowly adapting neurons is less sharp. In area 3b, the somatosensory cortical area with the strongest thalamic input, the responses of neurons are determined by three components within the receptive field: (1) a single, central region of a few millimeters diameter that, when the sensory field is touched, produces excitation at short latency; (2) surrounding regions that, when touched, produce inhibition at nearly the same short latency as the central excitatory field; and (3) a region that overlaps both the short-latency excitatory and inhibitory regions and that, when touched, gives rise to inhibition but at a longer latency.[97] Clearly, whenever object contact activates all three components, for example as the fingertip moves along a surface, the neuronal responses are hard to predict by simply summing the three receptive field components. Nevertheless, neurons have been found whose properties could support the representation of texture. Neurons whose receptive field properties would be expected to cause them to fire at higher rates for contact with coarser textures (Figure 23.13) have been identified; their output could give rise to the percept of roughness.[97–99]

Signals from Pacinian neurons also reach the somatosensory cortex, and some neurons are tuned to give the greatest response to skin vibrations aligned with the peak of Pacinian sensitivity.[4,88,100–107] Thus, vibrations like those illustrated in Figure 23.12B, which occur from movement across a fine surface, can be expected to excite cortical neurons.

It is certain that, in primates, the cerebral cortex does have a role in texture perception, and as in rats, lesions in S1 lead to severe impairments in roughness discrimination. In particular, ablation of Brodmann area 1 has a specific effect on texture discrimination.[23,24] Yet the evidence both from cortical neurons that encode coarse pressure patterns and those that encode high-frequency vibrations has been obtained from monkeys receiving the stimuli passively—cortical activity has not yet been measured while monkeys identify surface roughness. Experiments involving explicit texture judgment will allow correlation of trial-to-trial neuronal output with percept, which is a necessary step to confirm all hypotheses about the neuronal representation of texture.

[97] DiCarlo, J. J., and Johnson, K. O. 2000. *J. Neurosci.* 20: 495-510.

[98] DiCarlo, J. J., Johnson, K. O., and Hsiao, S. S. 1998. *J. Neurosci.* 18: 2626-2645.

[99] DiCarlo, J. J., and Johnson, K. O. 2002. Behav. *Brain Res.* 135: 167-178.

[100] Hyvarinen, J. et al. 1968. *Science* 162: 1130-1132.

[101] Ferrington, D. G., and Rowe, M. 1980. *J. Neurophysiol.* 43: 310-331.

[102] Hyvarinen, J., Poranen, A., and Jokinen, Y. 1980. *J. Neurophysiol.* 43: 870-882.

[103] Burton, H., and Sinclair, R. J. 1991. *Brain Res.* 538: 127-135.

[104] Gardner, E. P. et al. 1992. *J. Neurophysiol.* 67: 37-63.

[105] Sinclair, R. J., and Burton, H. 1993. *J. Neurophysiol.* 70: 331-350.

[106] Lebedev, M. A., and Nelson, R. J. 1996. *Exp. Brain Res.* 111: 313-325.

[107] Zhang, H. Q. et al. 2001. *J. Neurophysiol.* 85: 1805-1822.

SUMMARY

- Low-threshold mechanoreceptors, excited by light contact, form one class of skin receptor. There are several types, each defined by the specialized structure surrounding the nerve termination. The morphology of the structure makes the membrane sensitive to particular properties of mechanical stimuli.

- Another class of skin receptor is the free nerve ending, a terminal that is activated by strong (noxious) mechanical, thermal, or chemical stimuli.

- The method of microneurography—recording and stimulating single nerve fibers in the arm of an awake

- person—elucidates the connection between individual sensory receptor neurons and elemental sensations.

- Different submodalities of skin sensation (e.g., light touch, painful touch, temperature) are relayed by separate anatomical routes to the contralateral thalamic nuclei.

- Primary somatosensory cortex (S1) is the main target of the somatosensory thalamic nuclei. Cortical neurons are excited by skin stimulation, and lesions cause profound tactile deficits (touch, shape, texture, etc.).

- The sense of pain and its emotional effect are influenced by social, cultural, and personal factors. These factors interact with the processing of painful stimuli by modulating the release of endorphins. By a placebo effect, the expectations of an individual can augment the release of endorphins.

- The whisker follicle, the key receptor organ in rodent tactile sensation, contains a rich assortment of receptor types whose functions are beginning to be sorted out.

- The organization of the rodent whisker sensory system introduces several fundamental principles shared with the primate touch system.

- Individual whisker follicles lead, through a chain of synaptic relays, to individual cortical columns called barrels.

- Barrels are arranged as a topographic map of the corresponding whiskers; the whisker map occupies a large territory of cerebral cortex.

- Rats can distinguish between different textures through whisker contact. Contact with a surface causes an irregular whisker trajectory of stops and starts. The pattern of motion and the corresponding temporal firing patter is distinctive for each texture.

- In primates, the fingertips are crucial to many behaviors. They are densely innervated and are associated with a greatly expanded cortical representation.

- The skin is represented by a mosaic of columns in somatosensory cortex. The columns are arranged to produce a distorted map of the skin (more columns for the fingertips and lips). The layout of cortical maps and the properties of single neurons within cortical maps are shaped by sensory experience.

- In primates, there are two channels for sensing texture. The perception of coarse textures is based on the difference in firing rate between adjacent slowly adapting receptors. The perception of fine surfaces is based on motion-evoked vibrations in the skin, transduced by rapidly adapting Pacinian receptors.

Suggested Reading

General Reviews

Apkarian, A. V., Bushnell, M. C., Treede, R. D., and Zubieta, J. K. 2005. Human brain mechanisms of pain perception and regulation in health and disease. *Eur. J. Pain* 9: 463–484.

Bolanowski, S. J., Jr., Gescheider, G. A., Verrillo, R. T., and Checkosky, C. M. 1988. Four channels mediate the mechanical aspects of touch. *J. Acoust. Soc. Am.* 84: 1680–1694.

Diamond, M. E. 2019. Perceptual uncertainty. *PLOS Biol. 17*, e3000430.

Diamond, M. E., Petersen, R. S., and Harris, J. A. 1999. Learning through maps: functional significance of topographic organization in primary sensory cortex. *J. Neurobiol.* 41: 64–68.

Fassihi, A., Zuo, Y., and Diamond, M. E. 2020. Making sense of sensory evidence in the rat whisker system. *Curr. Opin. Neurobiol.* 60: 76–83.

Hollins M., and Bensmaia, S. J. 2007. The coding of roughness. *Can. J. Exp. Psychol.* 61: 184–195.

Johansson, R. S., and Flanagan, J. R. 2009. Coding and use of tactile signals from the fingertips in object manipulation tasks. *Nature Rev. Neurosci.* 10: 345.

Mano T., Iwase S., and Toma, S. 2006. Microneurography as a tool in clinical neurophysiology to investigate peripheral neural traffic in humans. *Clin. Neurophysiol.* 117: 2357–2384.

Melzack, R. 1973. *The Puzzle of Pain.* Harmondsworth: Penguin Books.

Torebjork, E. 1985. Nociceptor activation and pain. *Philos. Trans. R. Soc. Lond., B, Biol. Sci.* 308: 227–234.

Original Papers

Arabzadeh E., Zorzin E., and Diamond, M. E. 2005. Neuronal encoding of texture in the whisker sensory pathway. *PLOS Biol.* 3: e17.

Albert T., Pantev C., Wienbruch C., Rockstroh B., and Taub, E. 1995. Increased cortical representation of the fingers of the left hand in string players. *Science* 270: 305–307.

Pollo, A., Amanzio M., Arslanian A., Casadio C., Maggi G., and Benedetti, F. 2001. Response expectancies in placebo analgesia and their clinical relevance. *Pain* 93: 77–84.

Van Boven, R. W., Hamilton, R. H., Kauffman T., Keenan, J. P., and Pascual-Leone, A. 2000. Tactile spatial resolution in blind Braille readers. *Neurology* 54: 2230–2236.

van der Loos H., and Dorfl, J. 1978. Does the skin tell the somatosensory cortex how to construct a map of the periphery? *Neurosci. Lett.* 7: 23–30.

von Heimendahl, M., Itskov, P. M., Arabzadeh E., and Diamond, M. E. 2007. Neuronal activity in rat barrel cortex underlying texture discrimination. *PLOS Biol.* 5: e305.

Wager, T. D., Rilling, J. K., Smith, E. E., Sokolik A., Casey, K. L., Davidson, R. J., Kosslyn, S. M., Rose, R. M., and Cohen, J. D. 2004. Placebo-induced changes in fMRI in the anticipation and experience of pain. *Science* 303: 1162–1167.

CHAPTER 24

Auditory and Vestibular Sensation

The frequency components of a sound are extracted by the acoustic sensory organ, the cochlea. Other features that ultimately lead to a sound's interpretation as a meaningful signal, such as the location of the sound's source, are extracted later in the auditory pathway. The sensory receptors, the hair cells of the cochlea, are frequency-selective according to their position along the mechanically tuned basilar membrane. This sensory epithelium is tonotopically arranged, distributing sound frequencies along its length. In the mammalian cochlea, each sensory fiber of the eighth cranial nerve innervates a single inner hair cell and so responds best to the same acoustic frequency that activates that hair cell. Efferent feedback from the central nervous system reduces or increases (depending on the situation) hair cell sensitivity and frequency selectivity in the inner ears of reptiles, birds, and mammals (though modern taxonomy classifies birds in Reptilia, this chapter refers to them separately from reptiles such as turtles) . Hair cells of certain vertebrates are electrically tuned to provide acoustic frequency selectivity.

Afferent fibers from the cochlea form synapses in brainstem nuclei. Second-order neurons project to the superior olivary complex or into pathways that ascend through the inferior colliculus to the medial geniculate nucleus of the thalamus. Neurons in primary auditory cortex receive input from both ears and respond to features of sound that are more complex than those encoded in the periphery. The localization of a sound arises from neural computations involving comparisons between inputs to the two ears. Accordingly, the central auditory pathway includes a complex set of synaptic relays and feedback connections at which binaural comparisons are made or other aspects of timing and frequency composition are determined.

Position and motion of the head are transduced by the vestibular apparatus, which consists of three semicircular canals together with the utricle and saccule. Within each of these structures, hair cells (quite similar in morphology to those of the cochlea) are activated by fluid flow induced by rotation or displacement of the head. Vestibular signals travel to the brain in sensory fibers of the eighth nerve but do not normally reach consciousness; they mediate automatic behaviors that maintain body posture and stability. An important mechanism for maintaining stability of gaze is the vestibulo-ocular reflex (VOR). This reflex is mediated by a three-neuron arc that includes sensory neurons, interneurons, and motoneurons.

Mechanosensitive hair cells of the inner ear are receptive to a wide range of stimuli. Hair cells in the ear encode stimulus intensities that vary over six orders of magnitude. Hair cells cover an equally impressive kinetic range, from vestibular coding of head movements that occur at 0.05 Hz to acoustic coding of sounds at more than 100 kHz (in whales and bats). And yet at the molecular level, all vertebrate hair cells operate in essentially the same way—a deflection of the stereocilia causes a receptor potential and subsequent activation of postsynaptic neurons by release of glutamate. The specific range of stimulus frequencies and intensities to which hair cells respond is determined in large part by the accessory structures in which they are embedded. In this chapter we explore the structural adaptations that confer stimulus specificity onto hair cell signaling and follow that signaling through higher levels of processing. We focus mainly on the inner ear of mammals, but important principles also have been learned by studying other vertebrates, particularly at the level of cellular physiology.

As seen in Figure 24.1, the labyrinth of the inner ear includes several elaborately shaped fluid-filled ducts. The tightly wound spiral of the cochlea (from the Greek *kochlias*, "snail") lies ventral to three orthogonally oriented loops of the semicircular canals, part of the vestibular system. In addition, two relatively flat (macular) epithelia, the saccule and the utricle, lie within the central vestibular chamber; these, too, generate signals about head position. A comparison of the labyrinth in reptiles, birds, and mammals illustrates an interesting correlation of structure and function. This point is made in drawings (see Figure 24.1B,C) from von Bekesy,[1] whose studies of inner ear function in the early twentieth century established the basis of cochlear frequency selectivity. As seen in Figure 24.1, the disposition of the semicircular canals is similar in reptiles, birds, and mammals, implying that the function (detecting rotation of the head in space) is similar among vertebrates (these structures exist only in vertebrates). In contrast, the spiraled cochlea of the mammal replaced the shorter auditory end organs of birds and reptiles. This evolutionary progression in auditory structure can be correlated with

[1] von Bekesy, G. 1960. *Experiments in Hearing*. McGraw-Hill, New York.

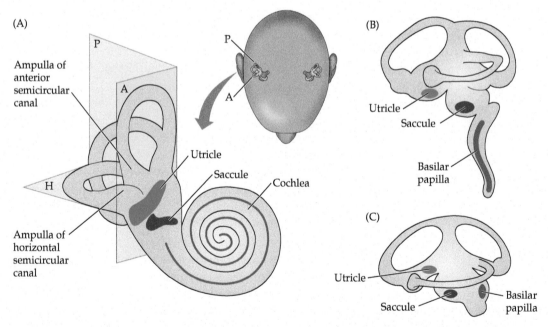

FIGURE 24.1 Sensory Structures of the Inner Ear. The inner ears of (A) mammals (human), (B) birds (chicken), and (C) reptiles (turtle) have in common the orthogonal arrangement of semicircular canals and two macular epithelia, the utricle and saccule. These structures have a similar form across species. In contrast, the auditory sense organ (called the cochlea in mammals and the basilar papilla in other species) increases progressively in length, from 1 mm in turtles, to 5 mm in chickens, to 30 mm in some mammals. The length increase serves as the substrate for expansion into higher-frequency hearing, from 1 to 5 to 20 kHz, respectively. A, the plane containing the anterior semicircular canal; P, the plane containing the posterior semicircular canal; H, the plane containing the horizontal semicircular canal. (B,C after G. von Bekesy, 1960. *Experiments in Hearing*. McGraw-Hill: New York.)

the frequency range of hearing, up to 1 kHz in turtles, 5 kHz in chickens, and 30 kHz in rats. The longer, coiled cochlea of mammals provides a mechanism to expand the high-frequency range of hearing. We will see that several cellular specializations also contribute to the ability to hear higher frequencies. We begin by examining the structure and function of the sensory organs.

The Auditory System

In terrestrial vertebrates, sound waves enter the outer ear, strike the **tympanic membrane** (eardrum), and via mechanical coupling through the **ossicles** of the middle ear, are converted to fluid waves in the cochlea (Figure 24.2A). The fluid waves, in turn, cause vibration of the **basilar membrane**, on which sit sensory **hair cells** in the **organ of Corti**. This process has been summarized poetically by Aldous Huxley:

> Pongileoni's blowing and the scraping of the anonymous fiddlers had shaken the air in the great hall, had set the glass of the windows looking on to it vibrating; and this in turn had shaken the air in Lord Edward's apartment on the further side. The shaking air rattled Lord Edward's membrana tympani; the interlocked malleus, incus and stirrup bones were set in motion so as to agitate the membrane of the oval window and raise an infinitesimal storm of fluid in the labyrinth. The hairy endings of the auditory nerve shuddered like weeds in a rough sea; a vast number of obscure miracles were performed in the brain, and Lord Edward ecstatically whispered "Bach"![2]

The Cochlea

The cochlear duct is divided into three compartments: The **scala media** contains a high-potassium solution, the endolymph. It is separated from the overlying **scala vestibuli** by Reissner's membrane and from the fluid space of the **scala tympani** by intercellular tight junctions between the apical ends of the hair cells and their surrounding supporting cells (see Figure 24.2B). The scala tympani and scala vestibuli contain perilymph, similar in composition to cerebrospinal fluid; the ionic composition of endolymph in the scala media is like that of cytoplasm, with high potassium, low sodium, and calcium ions held to micromolar concentration.[3] The unusual composition of this extracellular fluid is established by ion transport in the **stria vascularis**, a secretory epithelium that lines the lateral wall of the scala media.

There are two distinct groups of hair cells in the mammalian cochlea: **inner hair cells** and **outer hair cells**. Inner hair cells, of which there are about 3500 in each human cochlea, are innervated by dendrites of the auditory nerve and are the primary sensory hair cells of the cochlea. Outer hair cells number about 11,000 in each human cochlea and lie in three or four rows; they modulate the sensitivity and tuning of inner hair cells.

The inner and outer hair cells reside in the organ of Corti on the basilar membrane (Figure 24.2B,C). Bundles of sensory hairs project up from the cell body into an overlying acellular gelatinous sheet, the **tectorial membrane**. Inner and outer hair cells differ by position (inner hair cells are closer to the central axis of the cochlear coil) and innervation pattern. Inner hair cells receive more than 90% of the afferent contacts to the cochlea,[4,5,6] whereas outer hair cells are the postsynaptic targets of the efferent nerve supply (see Figure 24.2C).[7] This differential innervation pattern raises questions concerning the functional roles of these two cell types that will be discussed later in this chapter. The tectorial membrane overlies the hair bundles of both inner and outer hair cells, and differential motion of the tectorial and basilar membranes causes lateral shear to gate the mechanotransduction channels (as detailed in Chapter 21).

Frequency Selectivity: Mechanical Tuning

Interpretation of auditory signals depends on the encoding of their frequency composition. In the mammalian cochlea, transformation of sound frequency into a neuronal representation depends in part on the mechanical properties of the basilar membrane. Its width and

[2] A. Huxley, 1922. *Point Counter Point.* Chatto and Windus Ltd., London.

[3] Wangemann, P. 2006. *J. Physiol.* 576: 11–21.

[4] Brown, M. C. 1987. *J. Comp. Neurol.* 260: 591–604.

[5] Kiang, N. Y. et al. 1982. *Science* 217: 175–177.

[6] Spoendlin, H. 1969. *Acta Otolaryngol.* 67: 239–254.

[7] Warr, W. B. 1975. *J. Comp. Neurol.* 161: 159–181.

(A)

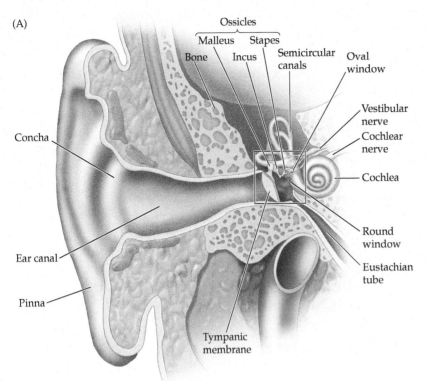

Ossicles
Malleus   Stapes
Bone   Incus   Semicircular
canals
Oval
window

Concha

Vestibular
nerve

Cochlear
nerve

Cochlea

Round
window

Ear canal

Eustachian
tube

Pinna

Tympanic
membrane

FIGURE 24.2   Structure of the Cochlea.
(A) The external, middle, and inner ear, showing the eardrum and its bony connections to
the oval window. (B) The cochlea, showing the
scala media bounded by Reissner's membrane
(which contains endolymph, a high-potassium
solution) and the structural relations among
the basilar membrane and tectorial membrane.
(C) Hair cells form synapses with the terminals
of auditory nerve fibers that have their cell
bodies in the spiral ganglion. Approximately
95% of afferent fibers are postsynaptic to inner
hair cells. As many as 20 afferent fibers are in
contact with a single inner hair cell. Outer hair
cells have few afferent contacts and instead are
the postsynaptic targets of cholinergic efferent
neurons that project from the olivary complex
in the brainstem. Colors depict 4 different types
of synaptic relationship with hair cells.

(B)

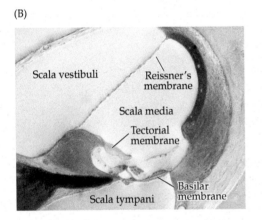

Scala vestibuli

Reissner's
membrane

Scala media

Tectorial
membrane

Basilar
membrane

Scala tympani

(C)

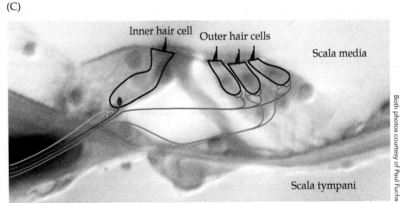

Inner hair cell   Outer hair cells

Scala media

Scala tympani

Both photos courtesy of Paul Fuchs

thickness vary systematically along the length of the cochlea (Figure 24.3). At the base of the
cochlea, near the oval window, the membrane is narrow and rigid, while at the cochlear apex
it is wide and flexible. The consequences of this progressive variation in structure were examined by von Bekesy,[1] who cut a hole in the bony labyrinth that encloses the cochlea and then
used stroboscopic illumination of reflective particles scattered on the basilar membrane to
visualize the pattern of vibration. He observed that high-frequency sounds cause maximal vibration of the thicker, stiffer basal end of the membrane and that low-frequency sounds cause
maximal vibration of the more flexible apical membrane. The basilar membrane works this
way because its resonance frequency—the frequency at which the mechanical energy of an
input vibration is converted to a vibration of the membrane—varies along its length.

As a consequence of the mechanical tuning of the basilar membrane, hair cells at the cochlear base (nearest the stapes footplate) are set in motion preferentially by high-frequency
sound, whereas hair cells progressively farther along the cochlear coil (nearer the apex) are
set in motion by progressively lower-frequency sound (see Figure 24.3A). The resulting
tonotopic map is reflected in the cochlear afferent neurons that innervate single cochlear
hair cells. The frequency selectivity of cochlear afferents is measured by recording action
potentials during presentation of pure tones of various frequencies and intensities. The resulting **tuning curve** of a typical afferent is V-shaped, with "best frequency" defined as the

(A)

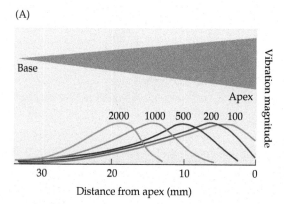

(B)

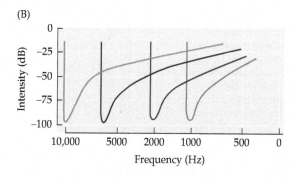

FIGURE 24.3 Cochlear Tuning. (A) The location of maximal displacement of the basilar membrane in the cochlea by sound waves depends on frequency. The curves represent relative displacement at the indicated frequencies (100–2000 Hz). At low frequencies, maximal displacement is near the wider (more flexible) apex; at higher frequencies, maximal displacement is near the narrower (stiffer) base. (B) Shapes of tuning curves of four individual eighth cranial nerve fibers innervating different locations on the cochlea. The sound intensity, in decibels (dB), needed to produce discharges in a fiber is plotted against the frequency of the auditory stimulus. The best frequencies for the fibers (i.e., the frequencies requiring the least stimulus intensity) are 1000, 2000, 5000, and 10,000 Hz. (A after G. von Bekesy, 1960. *Experiments in Hearing*. McGraw-Hill: New York; B after Y. Katsuki, 1961, in W. A. Rosenblith [Ed.], *Sensory Communication*. MIT Press, Cambridge, MA.)

pure tone to which the fiber fires at lowest amplitude (see Figure 24.3B). The characteristic frequency of each sensory fiber is determined by the position along the cochlear duct of the hair cell with which it synapses.

Electromotility of Mammalian Cochlear Hair Cells

The frequency-dependent vibration of cochlear membranes described by von Bekesy provided an elegant basis for cochlear tuning. However, further work showed that vibrations evoked by a pure tone were more broadly distributed than the V-shaped tuning curve of afferents would suggest; thus, the physical properties of those membranes were not, by themselves, adequate to explain the sharp tuning of individual cochlear afferent neurons. Furthermore, it was demonstrated that sharp tuning could be degraded without manipulating the cochlear mechanics,[8,9] for instance by nerve damage, suggesting that some process beyond resonant frequency localization must participate as well.[10] The sharpness of tuning lies in the fact that the outer hair cells of the cochlea (but not the inner hair cells) actively contribute to cochlear vibration through a process called **electromotility**. Outer hair cells shorten in response to depolarization and lengthen during hyperpolarization of their membranes, as though they were tiny muscles (Figure 24.4A).[11,12] The maximal length change that can be induced by electrical stimulation of an outer hair cell is about 4%. For a cell 50 μm long, this corresponds to a maximal length change of 2 μm and is easily observable by light microscopy. The length of a cell is maintained while the potential is held constant. However, such movements are *not* generated by actin–myosin, since agents targeted against actin-based motility and agents that inhibit microtubule assembly and disassembly do not affect Electromotility. Instead, movements result from direct effects of voltage on a charged motor protein, prestin, which is expressed at high levels in the basolateral membrane (Figure 24.4B).[13,14] It is thought that the voltage-dependent conformational changes undergone by prestin are somehow coupled to the cytoskeleton. Electromotility of outer hair cells adds to the vibration amplitude of the cochlear partition (basilar membrane and organ of Corti) during stimulation by sound, and thus increases the deflection of the stereocilia of the inner hair cells.[9,15] In this way, outer hair cells enhance cochlear tuning by adding mechanical energy to movement of the basilar membrane (Figure 24.5). Hearing threshold is dramatically raised if outer hair cell function is disrupted. Given this role as cochlear amplifiers, the efferent innervation pattern of the cochlea that puzzled neurobiologists for decades now makes sense: The central nervous system can regulate cochlear sensitivity by adjusting the *gain* of the amplifier by means of outer hair cell motility.

[8] Ashmore, J. 2008. *Physiol. Rev.* 88: 173–210.

[9] Dallos, P. 2008. *Curr. Opin. Neurobiol.* 18: 370–376.

[10] Gold, T. Hearing. II. 1948. *Proc. R. Soc. Lond. B Biol. Sci.* 135: 492–498.

[11] Brownell, W. E. et al. 1985. *Science* 227: 194–196.

[12] Ashmore, J. F. 1987. *J. Physiol.* 388: 323–347.

[13] Zheng, J. et al. 2000. *Nature* 405: 149–155.

[14] Dallos, P. et al. 2008. *Neuron* 58: 333–339.

[15] Zha, D. et al. 2012. *PLOS ONE* 7: e32757.

FIGURE 24.4 Electromotility of Outer Hair Cells. (A) Whole-cell patch pipettes are used to clamp the membrane potential of outer hair cells isolated from the mammalian cochlea. Depolarization causes the cells to shorten; hyperpolarization makes them longer. Such length changes can be as large as 30 nm/mV. (B) Stretching of the lateral membrane of the outer hair cell generates longitudinal forces. Membrane potential (V_m) drives the prestin motor at the same frequency as that detected by the hair cell, thus amplifying tectorial membrane motion. (B after J. Ashmore, 2008. *Physiol. Rev.* 88: 173–210.)

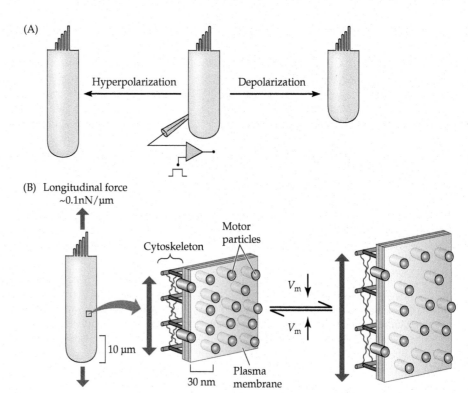

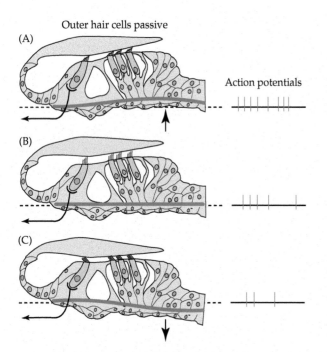

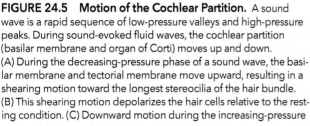

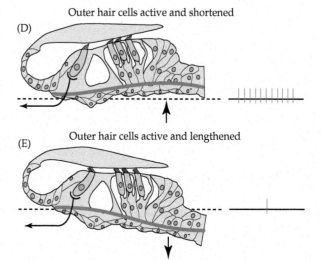

FIGURE 24.5 Motion of the Cochlear Partition. A sound wave is a rapid sequence of low-pressure valleys and high-pressure peaks. During sound-evoked fluid waves, the cochlear partition (basilar membrane and organ of Corti) moves up and down. (A) During the decreasing-pressure phase of a sound wave, the basilar membrane and tectorial membrane move upward, resulting in a shearing motion toward the longest stereocilia of the hair bundle. (B) This shearing motion depolarizes the hair cells relative to the resting condition. (C) Downward motion during the increasing-pressure phase of a sound produces the opposite displacement of the hair bundles, and hair cells are hyperpolarized relative to rest. (D) Active contraction of outer hair cells (set of three cells on the right) during depolarization amplifies the downward motion of the basilar membrane. (E) Active elongation of outer hair cells during hyperpolarization amplifies the upward motion of the basilar membrane. Outer hair cell electromotility modulates the spiking activity of afferent fibers leading from the inner hair cells. The extent of motion is greatly exaggerated here for the purpose of illustration.

Efferent Inhibition of the Cochlea

In mammals, neurons of the superior olivary complex in the brainstem project to ipsilateral and contralateral cochleae (Figure 24.6A).[16] Activation of this pathway causes the release of acetylcholine at efferent synapses onto outer hair cells and suppresses the response of cochlear afferent fibers to sound.[17,18] An example of the reduction in sensitivity of cochlear afferents by efferent inhibition is shown in Figure 24.6B.[19] Of interest is that suppression is maximal near the best frequency for the afferent, reinforcing the role of outer hair cells in cochlear frequency selectivity.

Efferent fibers respond to sound and innervate restricted portions of the cochlea; as a result, feedback inhibition is frequency-specific.[20,21] The effect is to reduce the cochlear response at the relevant frequency, which allows the cochlea to detect differences in intensity of loud sounds that would otherwise saturate the response. In other words, inhibition increases the dynamic range of transduction at that frequency. Efferent feedback also plays a role in protecting the cochlea from loud sound damage.[22] Indeed, when the strength of efferent feedback in mice is modified by genetic engineering, enhanced feedback inhibition is found to protect the mouse from the acoustic injury normally caused by loud sound.[23]

All vertebrate hair cell organs are subject to efferent regulation, and intracellular recordings were first achieved in experimentally tractable preparations, such as the fish lateral line.[24] Studies in the turtle ear showed that activation of the efferent pathway caused large hyperpolarizing inhibitory postsynaptic potentials (IPSPs) in hair cells[25] that would be expected to suppress the hair cell's response to sound. In fact, the inhibition of acoustic sensitivity was even more remarkable, as shown by the intracellular recordings in Figure 24.7A. The hair cell was stimulated with pure tones at three frequencies: one that corresponded to the best or characteristic frequency, one at a higher frequency, and one at a lower frequency. The

[16] Rasmussen, G. 1946. *J. Comp. Neurol.* 84: 141–219.

[17] Galambos, R. 1956. *J. Neurophysiol.* 19: 424–437.

[18] Jasser, A., and Guth, P. S. 1973. *J. Neurochem.* 20: 45–53.

[19] Winslow, R. L., and Sachs, M. B. 1987. *J. Neurophysiol.* 57: 1002–1021.

[20] Wiederhold, M. L., and Kiang, N. Y. 1970. *J. Acoust. Soc. Am.* 48: 950–965.

[21] Liberman, M. C. 1988. *J. Neurophysiol.* 60: 1779–1798.

[22] Rajan, R. 1995. *J. Neurophysiol.* 74: 598–615.

[23] Taranda, J. et al. 2009. *PLOS Biol.* 7: e18.

[24] Flock, A., and Russell, I. 1976. *J. Physiol.* 257: 45–62.

[25] Art, J. J., Fettiplace, R., and Fuchs, P. A. 1984. *J. Physiol.* 356: 525–550.

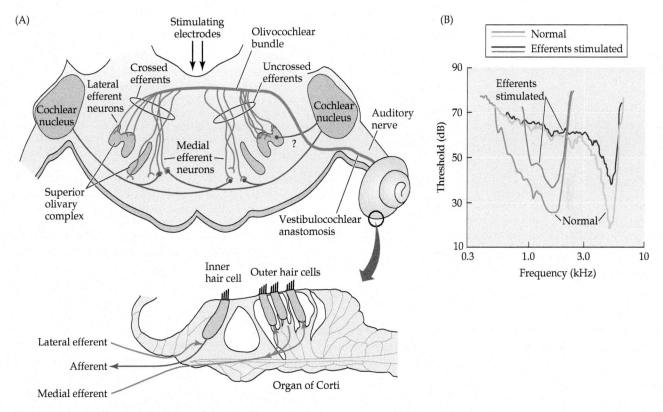

FIGURE 24.6 Efferent Inhibition of the Cochlea.
(A) Efferent neurons reside near the superior olivary complex. Medial efferents give rise to axons that synapse on outer hair cells. The axons of lateral efferents synapse onto type I afferent dendrites beneath inner hair cells. (B) Tuning curves of single cochlear afferent fibers and the effect of inhibition. During inhibition (electrical shocks delivered to efferent axons in the floor of the fourth ventricle), the afferent fiber becomes less sensitive (requiring louder sound to elicit a threshold response). This inhibitory effect is maximal at the center frequency in sharply tuned fibers, so that frequency selectivity is reduced. (A after M. C. Liberman, 1990. *Hear. Res.* 49: 209–224; B after J. J. Guinan and M. L. Gifford, 1988. *Hear. Res.* 37: 29–45.)

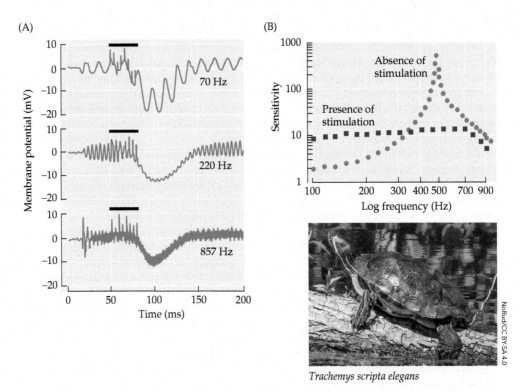

Trachemys scripta elegans

FIGURE 24.7 Effect of Efferent Stimulation on cochlear inner hair cell responses to acoustic stimuli. (A) Middle record: The oscillatory response of a cell to an acoustic stimulus of 220 Hz (its resonant frequency) is inhibited immediately after a brief train of efferent stimuli (indicated by the bar), and the cell is hyperpolarized. Top record: The response to an acoustic stimulus at 70 Hz. The stimulus intensity was adjusted so that the oscillatory response was similar in magnitude to that at 220 Hz. Efferent stimulation produces a hyperpolarization, but an increase, rather than a decrease, in the oscillatory response. Bottom record: The oscillatory response to an 857-Hz stimulus (again adjusted to produce a response similar to that at the resonant frequency) is unchanged by efferent stimulation. (B) Sensitivity of another cell (in millivolts per unit of sound pressure) as a function of frequency in the absence (blue circles) and presence (red squares) of efferent stimulation. Efferent inhibition reduces the response at the resonant frequency and increases the sensitivity at lower frequencies, thereby degrading tuning. (After J. J. Art et al.,1985. *J. Physiol.* 360: 397–421.)

intensities of the tones were adjusted so that each evoked an oscillating receptor potential of the same amplitude. A short train of shocks to the efferent axons hyperpolarized the cell and severely attenuated its response to a tone at 220 Hz (the characteristic frequency). At lower and higher frequencies of acoustic stimulation, activation of the efferents still resulted in hyperpolarization, but the voltage oscillations at high frequencies were unchanged, while those at low frequencies were actually enhanced in amplitude. This differential effect of inhibition results in broadening of the hair cell's frequency response (Figure 24.7B), qualitatively similar to the *detuning* of cochlear afferents in mammals (see Figure 24.6B). The basis for frequency tuning in the turtle ear is described in the next section.

The ion mechanism of cholinergic inhibition was established in chicken hair cells.[26,27] The nicotinic acetylcholine receptors (nAChRs) are ligand-gated cation channels through which sodium and calcium enter the cell, and this leads to the activation of calcium-dependent potassium channels. This two-channel mechanism produces a biphasic change in membrane potential, dominated by the much larger and longer-lasting hyperpolarization. A similar cholinergic inhibitory mechanism is found in mammalian hair cells.[28,29,30] The hair cell's response to acetylcholine is antagonized by α-bungarotoxin, and there is good evidence that two unusual members of the nicotinic receptor family of genes, encoding the α_9- and α_{10}-subunits, form the hair cell nAChR.[31,32]

This synaptic inhibition can explain how efferent synapses on outer hair cells suppress cochlear sensitivity, measured as the response of inner hair cells and their associated

[26] Fuchs, P. A., and Murrow, B. W. 1992. *J. Neurosci.* 12: 800–809.

[27] Martin, A. R., and Fuchs, P. A. 1992. *Proc. R. Soc. Lond., B, Biol. Sci.* 250: 71–76.

[28] Blanchet, C. et al. 1996. *J. Neurosci.* 16: 2574–2584.

[29] Evans, M. G. 1996. *J. Physiol.* 491: 563–578.

[30] Housley, G. D., and Ashmore, J. F. 1991. *Proc. R. Soc. Lond., B, Biol. Sci.* 244: 161–167.

[31] Elgoyhen, A. B. et al. 1994. *Cell* 79: 705–715.

[32] Elgoyhen, A. B. et al. 2001. *Proc. Natl. Acad. Sci. USA* 98: 3501–3506.

afferent neurons. Since outer hair cell electromotility is driven by rapidly alternating acoustic stimuli, the prolonged inhibitory hyperpolarization interrupts that motility. As a result, inhibition reduces the active mechanical contribution of outer hair cells to vibration of the basilar membrane,[33] and so reduces excitation of inner hair cells. In this way the sensitivity and tuning of cochlear afferent neurons are reduced.[20]

It is interesting that electromotility is found only in outer hair cells of the mammalian cochlea. Both prestin (the hair cell motor protein) and the α_{10}-subunit (a component of the hair cell nAChR) have undergone purifying selection during evolution of the vertebrate ear, resulting in isoforms unique to the mammalian cochlea.[34] Nonetheless, efferent inhibition in the turtle produces a similar loss of tuning,[35] implying that some other voltage-dependent process enhances frequency selectivity in non-mammalian hair cells.

Frequency Selectivity in Non-mammalian Vertebrates: Electrical Tuning of Hair Cells

We have seen that the expanded frequency range of mammalian hearing is based on cellular and structural specializations that confer sharp and sensitive mechanical tuning to an extended cochlear duct. And yet, within their range of hearing, non-mammalian vertebrates achieve good acoustic frequency selectivity despite having much shorter basilar membranes that are not mechanically tuned like those of mammals.[36] The studies of Crawford and Fettiplace in the turtle that showed that the mechanosensitive hair cells are frequency-selective through a mechanism of *intrinsic* electrical tuning.[37] Intracellular recordings from a hair cell in the turtle's basilar papilla (the auditory sensory epithelium) are shown in Figure 24.8. When a brief acoustic stimulus (a click) was presented, the hair cell's membrane potential underwent a damped oscillation, or ringing, that occurred at a frequency of about 350 Hz (see Figure 24.8A). This frequency is the same as that of pure tones to which the hair cell was most sensitive, as shown by the frequency sweep experiment in Figure 24.8C. Here, a constant intensity tone was presented to the external ear, and its frequency was gradually

[33] Russell, I. J., and Murugasu, E. 1997. *J. Acoust. Soc. Am.* 102: 1734–1738.

[34] Franchini, L. F., and Elgoyhen, A. B. 2006. *Mol. Phylogenet. Evol.* 41: 622–635.

[35] Art, J. J., and Fettiplace, R. 1984. *J. Physiol.* 356: 507–523.

[36] Manley, G. A. 2000. *Proc. Natl. Acad. Sci. USA* 97: 11736–11743.

[37] Crawford, A. C., and Fettiplace, R. 1981. *J. Physiol.* 312: 377–412.

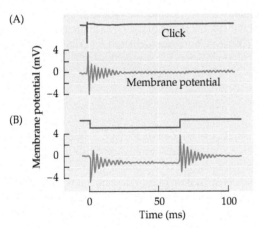

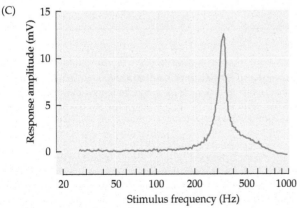

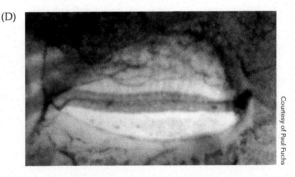

FIGURE 24.8 Hair Cell Tuning in the Turtle Cochlea.
(A) The effect of an acoustic click (indicated by the top trace) on the membrane potential of a hair cell (bottom trace, relative to the resting membrane potential of -50 mV), recorded with an intracellular microelectrode. The click produces a damped oscillation in membrane potential at about 350 Hz, with an initial peak-to-peak amplitude of about 8 mV. (B) A hyperpolarizing current pulse (top trace) applied to the same cell produces similar oscillations at both the onset and termination of the pulse, indicating that the frequency of oscillation is an intrinsic electrical property of the hair cell. (C) When a hair cell with oscillatory responses, such as those seen in (A) and (B), is stimulated with pure tones ranging from 25 to 1000 Hz, the peak-to-peak amplitude of the receptor potential has a sharp maximum at about 350 Hz. (D) Excised turtle inner ear stained with methylene blue. The clear ellipse is the basilar membrane along which the sensory hair cells (horizontal blue band) are tonotopically arrayed from low to high frequencies, left to right. (A–C after R. Fettiplace, 1987. *Trends Neurosci.* 10: 421–425.)

swept from 25 to 1000 Hz. The voltage response in the hair cell peaked near 350 Hz. The voltage ringing produced by an acoustic transient and the tuning curve produced by frequency sweeps are equivalent demonstrations of the hair cell's frequency selectivity.

Figure 24.8B shows the important result uncovered when a microelectrode was used to inject a rectangular current pulse (an electrical transient) into the cell. Voltage ringing was produced with a frequency and rate of decay that were identical to those caused by an acoustic transient. The conclusion from these experiments is that the hair cell's frequency selectivity depends on the electrical properties of the cell membrane. Electrical and acoustic tuning frequencies of hair cells are equivalent and vary systematically along the length of the turtle's basilar papilla, producing a tonotopic array of tuned detectors.

Hair Cell Potassium Channels and Electrical Tuning

What properties of the cell membrane provide this electrical tuning, and how do these properties vary to determine different tuning frequencies? Recordings from hair cells in the frog's saccule (a vestibular receptor) revealed that interactions between voltage-gated calcium channels and **calcium-sensitive** (or Ca²⁺-gated), **voltage-gated potassium** (**BK**) channels can produce voltage ringing.[38,39] Studies of hair cells isolated from the turtle ear[40,41] demonstrated that the characteristic frequency of each cell is determined in a remarkably elegant and straightforward way—namely, by the density and kinetic properties of the BK potassium channels in each cell (Figure 24.9).

In hair cells tuned to lower frequencies, the total potassium conductance is smaller and slower to activate, and thus gives rise to relatively slow voltage oscillations. In higher-frequency cells, the potassium conductance is larger and more rapidly activating. These distinctions extend to the single-channel level (Figure 24.10), where slow BK currents are produced by channels with longer mean open times. Channels with shorter mean open times carry faster currents. Single-channel conductance is the same, so that high- and low-frequency cells also must express different numbers of channels.

The BK channels in hair cells of frogs,[42] turtles,[43] and chickens[44,45] are encoded by a gene whose mRNA is subject to alternative splicing of its composite exons. Some differentially spliced isoforms of the channel are kinetically distinct.[46] Additional variability may be provided by an accessory β-subunit that combines with the channel and slows its gating kinetics.[47] Although BK channels also are expressed in the mammalian cochlea, there is little alternative splicing,[48] and no evidence for electrical resonance in inner or outer hair cells. Nonetheless,

[38] Hudspeth, A. J., and Lewis, R. S. 1988. *J. Physiol.* 400: 237-274.

[39] Lewis, R. S., and Hudspeth, A. J. 1983. *Nature* 304: 538-541.

[40] Art, J. J., and Fettiplace, R. 1987. *J. Physiol.* 385: 207-242.

[41] Art, J. J., Wu, Y. C., and Fettiplace, R. 1995. *J. Gen. Physiol.* 105: 49-72.

[42] Rosenblatt, K. P. et al. 1997. *Neuron* 19: 1061-1075.

[43] Jones, E. M., Laus, C., and Fettiplace, R. 1998. *Proc. R. Soc. Lond., B, Biol. Sci.* 265: 685-692.

[44] Jiang, G. J. et al. 1997. *Proc. R. Soc. Lond., B, Biol. Sci.* 264: 731-737.

[45] Navaratnam, D. S. et al. 1997. *Neuron* 19: 1077-1085.

[46] Jones, E. M., Gray-Keller, M., and Fettiplace, R. 1999. *J. Physiol.* 518: 653-665.

[47] Ramanathan, K. et al. 1999. *Science* 283: 215-217.

[48] Langer, P., Grunder, S., and Rusch, A. 2003. *J. Comp. Neurol.* 455: 198-209.

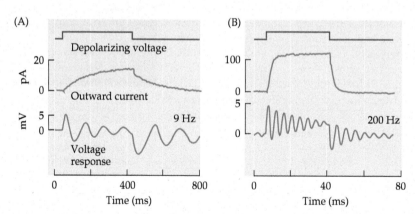

FIGURE 24.9 Tuning Frequency and Potassium Conductance in isolated turtle hair cells measured by whole-cell patch clamp recording. (A) The middle record shows outward current, carried mainly by potassium, produced by a depolarizing voltage command (duration indicated in the top record). Current rises slowly to a maximum of 15 pA. A small current step of the same duration produces oscillatory voltage responses at the beginning and end of the pulse (bottom record) with a resonant frequency of 9 Hz. (B) In another cell, a depolarizing pulse produces a much larger, rapidly rising outward current (middle record; note the changes in current and timescales), indicating a greater density of potassium channels with faster kinetics. The oscillatory response to a small current pulse reveals a concomitant increase in tuning frequency to 200 Hz (bottom record). (After R. Fettiplace, 1987. *Trends Neurosci.* 10: 421-425.)

(A) Low-frequency hair cell   (B) High-frequency hair cell

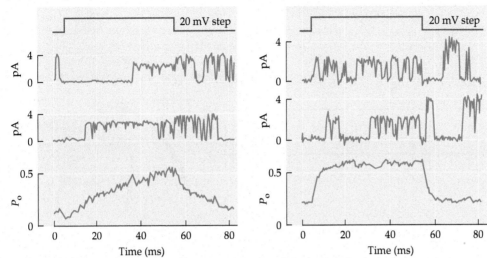

FIGURE 24.10   Single Ca²⁺- and Voltage-Gated Potassium (BK) Channel Currents in turtle auditory hair cells. (A) Cell-attached patch recording from a low-frequency hair cell. The channel opening is upward. The bottom record is the average compiled from large numbers of records, as seen in the middle two traces. Activation and deactivation occur over the course of about 40 ms. (B) Cell-attached patch recording from a high-frequency hair cell. The average record shows activation and deactivation rates that are more rapid for the single BK channel from this cell than the cell in (A). (After J. J. Art and R. Fettiplace, 1987. *J. Physiol.* 385: 207–242.)

as in birds,[49] BK channels appear in rodent cochlear hair cells near the onset of hearing[50] and are more numerous in higher-frequency hair cells.[51,52] The expression of mRNA significantly precedes that of functional channels, and developmental and tonotopic expression patterns appear to be regulated at the level of membrane localization of protein.[53,54]

Synaptic Transmission from Hair Cells to Afferent Fibers

Hair cells are neuroepithelial cells, with the apical pole specialized for mechanotransduction and the basal pole specialized for the release of neurotransmitter. Depolarizing and hyperpolarizing receptor potentials alter the open probability of voltage-gated calcium channels in the hair cell's basolateral membrane. Calcium entry in turn alters the rate of release of neurotransmitter (glutamate) onto the terminal of a postsynaptic afferent neuron. Hair cells, like retinal photoreceptors and bipolar cells, employ so-called **ribbon synapses** for tonic transmitter release[55] (Figure 24.11; see also Chapters 13 and 22). Even in the absence of a stimulus, the membrane potential of the hair cell is above the threshold for gating of voltage-activated calcium channels; consequently, release of glutamate is ongoing and excites the afferent fibers, giving rise to spontaneous action potentials. At frequencies below about 5 kHz, the sinusoidal receptor potential in cochlear hair cells alternately increases and decreases the rate of transmitter release, producing phase-locking in the postsynaptic firing pattern. At frequencies greater than 5 kHz, the hair cell's membrane time constant prevents rapid changes in membrane potential and the resulting afferent activity simply increases above the spontaneous rate for the duration of the tone, without cycle-by-cycle phase-locking (not shown in Figure 24.11).

A type I afferent neuron in the mammalian cochlea has a single dendrite that is postsynaptic to a single ribbon synapse in a single inner hair cell.[56] Afferent action potential activity often exceeds 100 Hz, requiring that the ribbon synapse have an impressive capacity to marshal and release vesicles.[57,58,59] Given that each inner hair cell ribbon tethers only 100 to 200 vesicles,[60] it is still mysterious how the vesicles can be replenished at the required rate.[61,62] A further surprise is that spontaneous transmitter release from ribbon synapses appears to be multivesicular; that is, it can be composed of several vesicles released simultaneously.[63] As we showed in Chapter 13, ribbon synapse function may involve proteins differing from those serving release at other chemical synapses.[64,65]

[49] Li, Y. et al. 2009. *BMC Dev. Biol.* 9: 67.

[50] Kros, C. J. 2007. *Hear. Res.* 227: 3–10.

[51] Engel, J. et al. 2006. *Neuroscience* 143: 837–849.

[52] Wersinger, E. et al. 2010. *PLOS ONE* 5: e13836.

[53] Kim, J. M. et al. 2010. *J. Comp. Neurol.* 518: 2554–2569.

[54] Sokolowski, B. et al. 2009. *Biochem. Biophys. Res. Commun.* 387: 671–675.

[55] Matthews G., and Fuchs, P. 2010. *Nat. Rev. Neurosci.* 11: 812–822.

[56] Liberman, M. C. 1982. *Science* 216: 1239–1241.

[57] Frank, T. et al. 2009. *Proc. Natl. Acad. Sci. USA* 106: 4483–4488.

[58] Griesinger, C. B., Richards, C. D., and Ashmore, J. F. 2005. *Nature* 435: 212–215.

[59] Rutherford, M. A., and Roberts, W. M. 2006. *Proc. Natl. Acad. Sci. USA* 103: 2898–2903.

[60] Sobkowicz, H. M. et al. 1982. *J. Neurosci.* 2: 942–957.

[61] Griesinger, C. B., Richards, C. D., and Ashmore, J. F. 2005. *Nature* 435: 212–215.

[62] Chakrabarti, R., Michanski, S., and Wichmann, C. 2018. *EMBO Rep.*: e44937.

[63] Glowatzki, E., and Fuchs, P. A. 2002. *Nat. Neurosci.* 5: 147–154.

[64] Safieddine, S., and Wenthold, R. J. 1999. *Eur. J. Neurosci.* 11: 803–812.

[65] Roux, I. et al. 2006. *Cell* 127: 277–289.

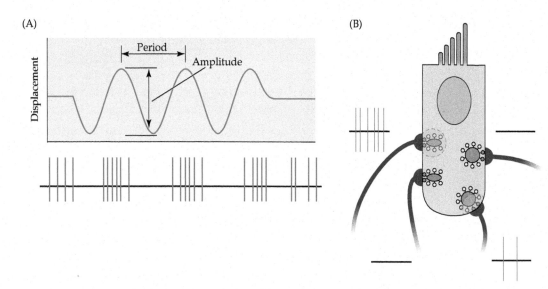

(A)

(B)

FIGURE 24.11 Hair Cell to Afferent Signaling. (A) Type I spiral ganglion neurons are postsynaptic to single ribbon synapses of a single inner hair cell. The ribbon synapse has an electron-dense core to which are tethered about 100 to 200 synaptic vesicles. Sinusoidal stimulation of the hair cell gives rise to phase-locked activity in afferent neurons. (B) Individual afferent fibers contacting a single inner hair cell can have different firing rates, both spontaneous and evoked.

Stimulus Coding by Primary Afferent Neurons

Signaling in the auditory pathway continues with the neurons that receive transmitter released from hair cells. Fibers that carry signals from the cochlea to the brain are part of the vestibulocochlear nerve, also known as the eighth cranial nerve. Their cell body is in the spiral ganglion, and they send their central axons to the cochlear nucleus of the brainstem. Many decades of single-fiber recordings have cataloged the acoustic responses of these primary afferents.[66] Each spiral ganglion neuron responds selectively to the frequency of sound that is optimal for the inner hair cell from which it receives synaptic input. Each inner hair cell is the sole presynaptic partner of a group of type I afferent neurons, numbering from 10 to 30, depending on location in the cochlea (see Figure 24.11). Both acoustic threshold and spontaneous firing rate vary among this pool of afferents,[56] helping extend the dynamic range of the cochlea. Presumably, individual ribbon synapses of an inner hair cell can have different release properties.[67,68] The selective innervation of inner hair cells on the mechanically tuned basilar membrane produces an array of 10,000 or so afferent neurons that serve as **frequency-labeled lines**—the first stage of the tonotopically organized auditory pathway. In addition to this *pitch-is-place* mechanism, phase-locked firing of afferent action potentials to acoustic sinusoids can be used to encode frequency up to about 3 kHz in the guinea pig[69] and up to 10 kHz in the barn owl.[70]

The Brainstem and Thalamus

The main auditory pathways are illustrated schematically in Figure 24.12. Auditory fibers of the eighth nerve travel centrally and send branches to both the dorsal and ventral cochlear nuclei.[71] Second-order axons ascend in the contralateral lateral lemniscus to innervate cells in the inferior colliculus (the nucleus of the lateral lemniscus is a synaptic way station for some of these fibers). Neurons in the ventral cochlear nucleus also provide collateral branches to both the ipsilateral and contralateral superior olivary nuclei. Third-order cells in the olivary nuclei, in turn, send ascending fibers to the inferior colliculus. The ascending pathway then synapses in the medial geniculate nucleus of the thalamus, from which the next neuron projects to the auditory region on the transverse surface of the temporal lobe of the cerebral cortex.

Each level in the auditory pathway is tonotopically mapped. However, individual cells progressively higher in the auditory system have more complex response properties than the

[66] Young, E. D., and Sachs, M. B. 1979. *J. Acoust. Soc. Am.* 66: 1381–1403.

[67] Meyer, A. C. et al. 2009. *Nat. Neurosci.* 12: 444–453.

[68] Grant, L., Yi, E., and Glowatzki, E. 2010. *J. Neurosci.* 30: 4210–4220.

[69] Palmer, A. R., and Russell, I. J. 1986. *Hear. Res.* 24: 1–15.

[70] Koppl, C. 1997. *J. Neurosci.* 17: 3312–3321.

[71] Fekete, D. M. et al. 1984. *J. Comp. Neurol.* 229: 432–450.

FIGURE 24.12 Auditory Pathways. Central auditory pathways are shown schematically on transverse sections of the medulla, midbrain, and thalamus, as well as on a coronal section of the cerebral cortex. Auditory nerve fibers end in the dorsal and ventral cochlear nuclei. Second-order fibers ascend to the contralateral inferior colliculus; those from the ventral cochlear nucleus also supply collaterals bilaterally to the superior olivary nuclei. Further bilateral interaction occurs at the level of the inferior colliculus. Neurons of the inferior colliculus project to the medial geniculate nucleus of the thalamus, which in turn projects to the auditory cortex. (After R. M. Berne and M. N. Levy [Eds.], 1988. *Physiology*, 2nd ed. Mosby: St. Louis, MO.)

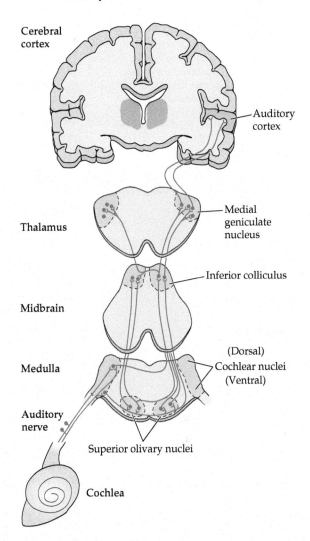

simple V-shaped tuning curves of cochlear afferent neurons (see Figure 24.6B). For example, some cells in the inferior colliculus[72] and auditory cortex[73] are only excited near threshold at their characteristic frequency, and louder tones are inhibitory. With a fresh appreciation that sensory systems promote survival by extracting behaviorally relevant information about important (potentially rewarding or potentially dangerous) events in the surrounding world, neuroscientists have applied so-called naturalistic stimuli—stimulus sets that contain innately meaningful features, for instance acoustic calls—as a way to study auditory cortex.[74]

Sound Localization

The sensitivity and frequency selectivity of the auditory system are key to the animal's ability to locate a sound in space. The selective advantages of acute sound localization are obvious; signals emitted as sound waves can reveal a distant predator or prey in the absence of visual or other cues. However, in contrast to the visual or somatosensory systems, where substantial spatial information derives from the receptor sheet itself, the auditory neuroepithelium contains no direct mechanism to code location. Instead, sound location is computed deeper in the central auditory system on the basis of comparing the timing and intensity of sound arriving at the two ears. The comparison depends on convergence of binaural inputs achieved by extensive, complex crossing over at nearly every level.

The **dorsal cochlear nucleus** subserves largely monaural frequency analysis[75] and provides a direct, tonotopically organized projection onto the contralateral primary auditory cortex, or A1, after relays in the inferior colliculus and medial geniculate nucleus of the thalamus. In contrast, second-order neurons in the **ventral cochlear nucleus** project both ipsilaterally and contralaterally to the superior olivary complex in the brainstem. Most neurons in the **medial superior olive** are excited by stimulation of either ear[76] (and so are designated EE neurons) but respond best when a tone is presented to the two ears with a characteristic delay, first at one ear, then the other. The velocity of sound in air is 340 m/s, so the maximal time difference imparted by the human head (about 18 cm in diameter) is 0.5 ms for a sound arriving along the axis of the two ears; successively more frontal locations impart smaller time differences. Sound arrival time is highly informative at the onset of an acoustic stream and provides less information in the middle of the stream. A second mechanism that conveys location is the phase difference in the sound pressure wave at the two ears.[77,78]

Cells in the **lateral superior olive** receive excitation from the ipsilateral ventral cochlear nucleus (Figure 24.13). Cells in the contralateral ventral cochlear nucleus project across the midline to form synapses in the **medial nucleus of the trapezoid body** (**MNTB**). The cells of the MNTB *inhibit* neurons in the lateral superior olive.[79] Thus, neurons in the lateral superior olive are excited by ipsilateral but inhibited by contralateral sound and so are designated EI neurons. Such an interaction would be useful for detecting differences in the intensity of sound at the two ears. As much as a tenfold difference in intensity is found at high frequencies, for which the head serves as a sound shadow.[80]

Labels in figure: Cerebral cortex; Auditory cortex; Thalamus; Medial geniculate nucleus; Inferior colliculus; Midbrain; Medulla; (Dorsal) Cochlear nuclei (Ventral); Auditory nerve; Superior olivary nuclei; Cochlea

72 Ramachandran, R., Davis, K. A., and May, B. J. 1999. *J. Neurophysiol.* 82: 152-163.

73 Sadagopan, S., and Wang, X. 2008. *J. Neurosci.* 28: 3415-3426.

74 David, S. V. et al. 2009. *J. Neurosci.* 29: 3374-3386.

75 Malmierca, M. S. 2003. *Int. Rev. Neurobiol.* 56: 147-211.

76 Cant, N. B., and Casseday, J. H. 1986. *J. Comp. Neurol.* 247: 457-476.

77 Buell, T. N., Trahiotis, C., and Bernstein, L. R. 1991. *J. Acoust. Soc. Am.* 90: 3077-3085.

78 Kuwada, S. et al. 2006. *J. Neurophysiol.* 95: 1309-1322.

79 Moore, M. J., and Caspary, D. M. 1983. *J. Neurosci.* 3: 237-242.

80 Brungart, D. S., Durlach, N. I., and Rabinowitz, W. M. 1999. *J. Acoust. Soc. Am.* 106: 1956-1968.

FIGURE 24.13 Binaural Connections in the Olivary Complex. Neurons in the ventral cochlear nucleus project to the ipsilateral lateral superior olive (LSO) as well as to the contralateral medial nucleus of the trapezoid body (MNTB) and the contralateral medial superior olive (MSO). Thus, MSO neurons are excited by both ears, and LSO neurons are excited ipsilaterally but are inhibited contralaterally by way of the intervening inhibitory interneuron in the MNTB.

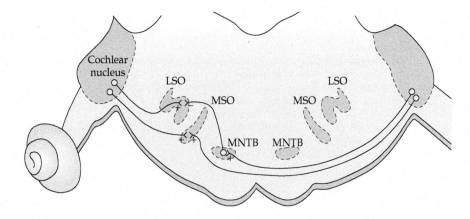

[81] Blauert, J. 1982. *Scand. Audiol. Suppl.* 15: 7-26.

[82] Buell, T. N., and Hafter, E. R. 1988. *J. Acoust. Soc. Am.* 84: 2063-2066.

[83] May, B. J., and Huang, A. Y. 1996. *J. Acoust. Soc. Am.* 100: 1059-1069.

[84] Rice, J. J. et al. 1992. *Hear. Res.* 58: 132-152.

[85] Winer, J. A., and Lee, C. C. 2007. *Hear. Res.* 229: 3-13.

[86] Merzenich, M. M., Knight, P. L., and Roth, G. L. 1975. *J. Neurophysiol.* 38: 231-249.

[87] Reale, R. A., and Imig, T. J. 1980. *J. Comp. Neurol.* 192: 265-291.

[88] Schreiner, C. E., and Winer, J. A. 2007. *Neuron* 56: 356-365.

[89] Hackett, T. A., Preuss, T. M., and Kaas, J. H. 2001. *J. Comp. Neurol.* 441: 197-222.

[90] Romanski, L. M., and Averbeck, B. B. 2009. *Annu. Rev. Neurosci.* 32: 315-346.

[91] Lee, C. C., and Winer, J. A. 2005. *Cereb. Cortex* 15: 1804-1814.

[92] Middlebrooks, J. C., Dykes, R. W., and Merzenich, M. M. 1980. *Brain Res.* 181: 31-48.

[93] Clarey, J. C., Barone, P., and Imig, T. J. 1994. *J. Neurophysiol.* 72: 2383-2405.

[94] Heil, P., Rajan, R., and Irvine, D. R. 1994. *Hear. Res.* 76: 188-202.

[95] Sutter, M. L., and Schreiner, C. E. 1995. *J. Neurophysiol.* 73: 190-204.

Psychophysical studies have shown that localization is accomplished by differences between the two ears in time of arrival or intensity of the incoming sound.[81,82] Thus, if clicks are presented through earphones with different delays, the sound seems to come from the side at which the click arrives first. Humans can detect interaural time differences of as little as 5 μs—remarkable resolution considering that action potentials are approximately 1 ms in duration, which once again emphasizes the importance of precise timing for auditory function. If the clicks are presented simultaneously but are of different intensities, the sound seems to come from the side with the louder click. Both phase and intensity differences vary as a function of frequency. For the human head, phase differences between the two ears are more significant below 2 kHz, whereas intensity differences become more prominent at higher frequencies.

The ability to localize the vertical position of a sound depends strongly on its frequency composition.[83] The external ear and head are not in mirror symmetry above and below. As a consequence, frequency components are differentially reflected depending on whether a sound rises or falls toward the listener.[84]

The Auditory Cortex

Auditory input processed through both dorsal and ventral cochlear nuclei ascends to the auditory cortex. The **primary auditory cortex (A1)** is located on the superior bank of the temporal lobe, corresponding to Brodmann's areas 41 and 42 (see Appendix C) (Figure 24.14). In cats, A1 is on the lateral surface of the brain; many combined anatomical–physiological studies have been performed in this species.[85] Microelectrode recordings in anesthetized animals have shown that A1 has a columnar organization, with cells along a vertical track all giving the strongest response to the same frequency.[86,87] The auditory receptor organ is essentially a one-dimensional map of frequency, so auditory cortex is laid out in isofrequency slablike formation, along which other acoustic dimensions can be mapped.[88]

The auditory cortex in monkeys contains multiple cochleotopic maps, with parallel projections from the medial geniculate nucleus to all these areas.[89] The most posterior of the three areas can be defined as A1 on the basis of its dense thalamic input, robust and short-latency response to pure tones, and well-developed layer 4 replete with granule cells.[90] Surrounding this central "core" is a "belt" and "parabelt" of auditory areas that interconnect with A1 but also with subdivisions of the medial geniculate nucleus. Thus, pathways exist for both serial (from core to belt) and parallel (multiple channels from thalamus to cortex) processing.[91]

By analogy with other sensory cortices, one would expect the tonotopic map of A1 to be subdivided into different functional zones. What acoustic features will be mapped onto cortex? Neurons within an isofrequency slab are clustered according to whether inputs from the two ears summate or suppress.[92] This clustering is thought to reflect binaural computations of sound location carried out in olivary nuclei, although there is no contiguous cortical map of auditory space.[88] And while evidence also exists for systematic variations in intensity and bandwidth coding in A1,[93,94,95] their functional significance remains obscure.

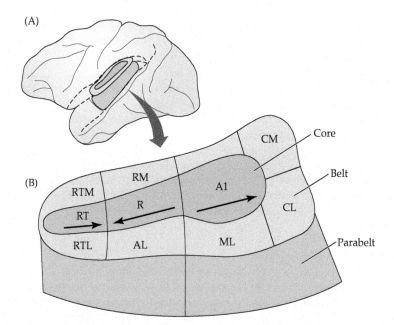

FIGURE 24.14 Organization of Auditory Cortex in Primates. (A) Auditory cortex is found on the superior surface of the temporal lobe and consists of a central core region, surrounded by "belt" and "parabelt" regions that are thought to correspond to higher-level association areas. (B) The core region of primate auditory cortex contains three complete tonotopic maps (low- to high-frequency gradient indicated by arrows). The most caudal map is considered primary auditory cortex (A1). Surrounding the core is the belt region, divided into zones, some of which are tonotopically mapped but less distinctly than A1. Parabelt is still higher order auditory association cortex. A1 = primary or core auditory area; R = rostral core auditory area; RM = rostromedial; RT = rostral temporal core auditory area; RTM = RT medial; RTL = RT lateral; AL = anterolateral belt auditory cortex; ML = middle-lateral belt auditory cortex; CM = caudal-medial belt auditory cortex; CL = caudal-lateral belt auditory cortex. (After L. M. Romanski and B. B. Averbeck, 2009. *Annu. Rev. Neurosci.* 32: 315–346, based on T. A. Hackett et al., 1998. *J. Comp. Neurol.* 394: 475–495.)

Environmental sounds, including vocalizations, consist of constant frequency elements, frequency-modulated elements, and noise bursts.[96] Due to the complexity of such sounds, recognition of acoustic objects must depend on analysis not just of frequency composition but also of how that composition changes in time and the relative timing between different acoustic elements. There is growing appreciation that many cortical neurons are particularly sensitive to the time-varying components of species-specific vocalizations or calls.[97] More than 30 years ago, Suga and colleagues established this principle in studies of echolocating bats,[98] and more recently it has been examined in other species.[99,100] Human vocalizations (i.e., speech sounds) are determined largely by the resonant frequencies of the vocal tract, called **formants**. Vowels are identified by the relative frequencies of the first two formants. Consonants depend more heavily on rapid temporal transitions.[97]

Understanding cortical representation of these complex acoustic objects requires more comprehensive analytical methods, such as reverse correlation. In this approach the response of a single cortical neuron is used to examine the features of a broadband, randomly modulated stimulus leading up to that response. A neuron's selectivity for some combination of spectrotemporal features (called the spectrotemporal response function, or STRF) is defined by its preferred rate (i.e., modulation in time) and scale (i.e., breadth of frequency selectivity). Using these parameters, a hypothetical neuron selective for a vowel sound would have a high scale (narrow spectral bandwidth) and low rate (little temporal modulation). A neuron encoding consonants would have a low scale (broad bandwidth) and high rate (rapid transients).[101]

The processing of auditory signals is complex and not yet understood.[102,103] Behaviorally important sounds must be extracted from a rich and variable acoustic environment.[104] Not only the frequency content but also the sequence in time of incoming sounds must be analyzed in some way[105] (playing a tape recording of human speech backward produces gibberish). In humans, the basic elements of speech, called **phonemes**, are common to all languages and are the sounds first babbled by babies, before particular sounds are selected to be combined into words.[106] These basic sounds are composed of the formants and temporal transitions previously described. One evident challenge for auditory perception is to identify a particular temporal pattern of frequency changes as an acoustic object, even as the absolute frequencies vary with different speakers (male versus female voices, for example). By analogy with the visual system, which contains cells that respond to slits, corners, edges, and other geometrical forms (see Chapter 3), we might expect to find higher-order cells in the human auditory cortex that respond to particular formants or, perhaps, phonemes. Other mammals can provide insights, and the excellent auditory learning capacities of ferrets make them a good target. Ferrets can

[96] Kanwal, J. S., and Rauschecker, J. P. 2007. *Front. Biosci.* 12: 4621–4640.

[97] Young, E. D. 2008. *Philos. Trans. R. Soc. Lond., B, Biol. Sci.* 363: 923–945.

[98] Tsuzuki, K., and Suga, N. 1988. *J. Neurophysiol.* 60: 1908–1923.

[99] Wang, X., and Kadia, S. C. 2001. *J. Neurophysiol.* 86: 2616–2620.

[100] Schnupp, J. W. et al. 2006. *J. Neurosci.* 26: 4785–4795.

[101] Mesgarani, N. et al. 2008. *J. Acoust. Soc. Am.* 123: 899–909.

[102] Nelken, I., and Bar-Yosef, O. 2008. *Front. Neurosci.* 2: 107–113.

[103] Sachs, M. B. 1984. *Annu. Rev. Physiol.* 46: 261–273.

[104] Nelken, I., Rotman, Y., and Bar Yosef, O. 1999. *Nature* 397: 154–157.

[105] Griffiths, T. D. et al. 1998. *Nat. Neurosci.* 1: 422–427.

[106] De Boysson-Bardies, B. et al. 1989. *J. Child Lang.* 16: 1–17.

be trained to generalize vowel identity across variations in fundamental frequency, sound level, and location, while neurons in auditory cortex represent sound identity robustly across acoustic variations.[107] However, in contrast to the other senses, auditory information is extensively processed at subcortical levels, as suggested by its more complex subcortical circuitry. For example, neurons of the inferior colliculus signal interaural time disparities equivalent to those of behavioral threshold.[108]

There is an emerging realization that primary auditory cortex may encode relatively complex auditory features, or even complete auditory percepts,[109] rather than performing the hierarchical assembly of features as in other primary sensory cortices. This organizational plan may reflect the greater challenge of encoding stimuli whose *meaning* depends more on temporal sequence than on spatial features, as for vision and touch. It remains to be seen whether auditory cortex analyzes component features of acoustic stimuli, or more complex assemblies of features that might be regarded as auditory objects.[102]

The Vestibular System

The inner ear contains, in addition to the cochlea, the machinery for detecting the position and movement of the head. Three semicircular canals, one horizontal and two vertical, detect angular motion of the head (rotation), while the macular epithelia, the saccule and utricle (see Figure 24.1), signal linear acceleration. The arrangement of three orthogonally disposed vestibular canals is conserved throughout all vertebrates (with the exception of jawless fishes, such as the lamprey with only two canals and a single otolithic macula).[110] Even invertebrate cephalopod mollusks (e.g., squid, octopuses) have vestibular-like organs, called statocysts.[111] Remarkably, the sensory receptor giving rise to the sense of equilibrium and motion is none other than the hair cell, with morphology and physiology closely resembling those in the auditory hair cell of the cochlea. Of course, specializations to be described later render the vestibular hair cell sensitive to a different set of physical events as compared with the pressure waves of sound.

Vestibular information is essential to the maintenance of posture, efficient locomotion, and stability of gaze. Sometimes referred to as "the silent sense," normal, healthy vestibular function remains largely subconscious. But when something goes wrong, one is acutely aware of vestibular sense. Motion sickness is a temporary but common experience of inappropriate vestibular input, while more serious, longer-lasting deficits can significantly degrade the quality of life. The vestibulo-ocular reflex (VOR) enables one's gaze to remain fixed on a target as the head moves. When this reflex does not work correctly, activities such as driving a car become impossible, since gaze fixation is required to read signs, avoid obstacles, and so on while the car, and hence the head, is in motion.[112]

Vestibular Hair Cells and Neurons

As in the cochlea, the central chamber of the vestibular labyrinth is filled with potassium-rich endolymph. The stereociliary bundles of sensory hair cells project into this space. Consequently, potassium ions enter through open transducer channels to depolarize the hair cell. In contrast to the cochlea, the vestibular labyrinth has only a small negative endolymphatic potential.[113] Hair cell receptor potentials are additionally shaped by a variety of voltage-gated potassium channels whose distributions vary by cell type.[114] As in the cochlea, resting tension within the hair bundle keeps a small fraction of transducer channels open at rest—that is, in the absence of explicit stimulation. Thus, head movements that deflect vestibular hair bundles toward the tallest stereocilia depolarize by opening additional transducer channels, while oppositely oriented deflections hyperpolarize by closing those transducer channels that are open at rest.

Responses of vestibular hair cells to head movements are determined by their location and orientation within the vestibular apparatus. Neither a high-resolution micrograph of a vestibular hair cell nor an intracellular electrical recording would identify a particular cell as being one from the cristae of the semicircular canals or from the maculae of the utricle and saccule.[115] Rather, hair cell structure and function vary topographically in each end organ.[116] The hair cells are of two types (Figure 24.15). Type I vestibular hair cells are

[107] Town, S. M., Wood, K. C., and Bizley, J. K. 2018. *Nat. Comm.* 9: 4786.

[108] Shackleton, T. M. et al. 2003. *J. Neurosci.* 23: 716-724.

[109] Nelken, I. 2004. *Curr. Opin. Neurobiol.* 14: 474-480.

[110] Lowenstein, O., Osborne, M. P., and Thornhill, R. A. 1968. *Proc. R. Soc. Lond., B, Biol. Sci.* 170: 113-134.

[111] Williamson, R., and Chrachri, A. 2007. *Philos. Trans. R. Soc. Lond., B, Biol. Sci.* 362: 473-481.

[112] Land, M. F. 2009. *Vis. Neurosci.* 26: 51-62.

[113] Marcus, D. C. et al. 2002. *Am. J. Physiol. Cell Physiol.* 282: C403-407.

[114] Brichta, A. M. et al. 2002. *J. Neurophysiol.* 88: 3259-3278.

[115] Eatock, R. A. et al. 1998. *Otolaryngol. Head Neck Surg.* 119: 172-181.

[116] Holt, J. C. et al. 2007. *J. Neurophysiol.* 98: 1083-1101.

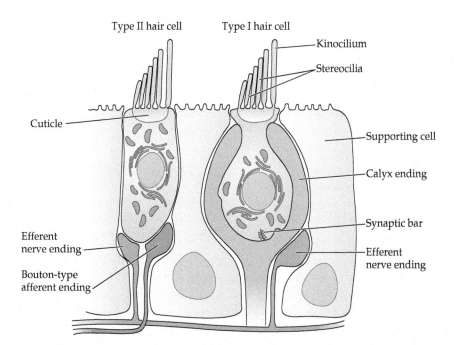

Type II hair cell   Type I hair cell

Kinocilium

Stereocilia

Cuticle

Supporting cell

Calyx ending

Synaptic bar

Efferent
nerve ending

Efferent
nerve ending

Bouton-type
afferent ending

FIGURE 24.15 Vestibular Hair Cells and Neurons. Two types of hair cell are found in all vestibular epithelia. Type I (right) is amphora-shaped and entirely engulfed by the highly specialized calyx afferent ending. Type II (left) is columnar and contacted by bouton-type afferent endings. Vestibular afferent neurons also can be classified by morphology. Calyx-only afferents have the largest-diameter axons and tend to be found near the center of each sensory epithelium. Bouton-only afferents have smaller-diameter axons and tend to be found in the periphery of the epithelium. Dimorphic afferents make both calyx and bouton endings and are scattered throughout the epithelium. Efferent neurons also innervate vestibular epithelia and make contacts directly onto type II hair cells, and onto the calyx ending surrounding type I hair cells. Efferent activation can result in either excitation or inhibition of vestibular afferent activity.

amphora-shaped and enclosed by a specialized afferent nerve terminal, the calyx. The hair cells release glutamate onto the calyx from ribbon-type synapses. Type II hair cells are columnar in shape, have ribbon synapses in apposition to boutonlike endings of afferent neurons, and once again, employ glutamate as a neurotransmitter.

Afferent fibers contact multiple hair cells and are distinguished by the types of synaptic endings they make: calyx-only, bouton-only, and dimorphic (i.e., calyx and bouton).[117] In addition, electrical recordings from vestibular afferents show that they can be divided into regular and irregular subtypes on the basis of their firing patterns.[118] Irregularly firing afferents have larger-diameter axons with calyx or dimorphic endings, and their responses to head movement are more transient, or phasic.[119] Vestibular afferent fibers use an unusual form of sensory coding: They have high spontaneous firing rates, so that head movements are encoded by firing rates that either increase or decrease with respect to the spontaneous rate.

Cholinergic efferent innervation is directed to the calyces on type I hair cells and directly onto type II hair cells (see Figure 24.15). Depending on the species and end organ under study, efferent feedback can be inhibitory, excitatory, or both.[120]

The Adequate Stimulus for the Saccule and Utricle

The vestibular macular epithelia, the saccule and utricle, are commonly referred to as **otolithic organs** because each is overlaid by a mass of calcium carbonate crystals encased in a gelatinous matrix (Figure 24.16). These otoliths (or ear stones) reside in the endolymphatic space in contact with hair cell stereocilia. Head motion results in stereociliary deflection because the inertial load of the otoliths delays the cilia motion relative to that of the head. Because the utricle lies approximately in the horizontal plane when the head is upright, it signals horizontal motion: Change of head angle from horizontal deflects the utricle cilia as the base of the cilia move before the tips. The saccule hangs nearly vertically in the upright head, so it responds maximally to vertical motion, by the same principle. In each instance the effective stimulus is linear acceleration. Constant linear velocity is not a stimulus (during constant-velocity vehicular travel, the vestibular system does not report motion). Hair cell orientations vary systematically within each macular epithelium (see Figure 24.16). In the utricle, the tall edge of each hair bundle (and the position of the kinocilium) points toward a central line of reversal. In the saccule hair, bundles point away. Thus, analysis of linear acceleration must involve integration of both negative and positive changes in afferent activity from each end organ as well the combination of inputs from both the saccule and utricle from both sides of the head.

[117] Goldberg, J. M. 2000. *Exp. Brain Res.* 130: 277–297.

[118] Eatock, R. A., Xue, J., and Kalluri, R. 2008. *J. Exp. Biol.* 211: 1764–1774.

[119] Baird, R. A. et al. 1988. *J. Neurophysiol.* 60: 182–203.

[120] Highstein, S. M. 1991. *Neurosci. Res.* 12: 13–30.

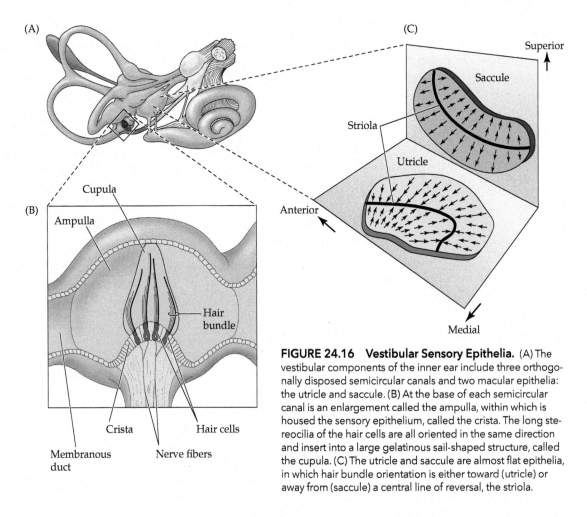

(A)

(B)

Cupula

Ampulla

Hair
bundle

Crista   Hair cells

Membranous   Nerve fibers
duct

(C)

Superior

Saccule

Striola

Utricle

Anterior

Medial

FIGURE 24.16   Vestibular Sensory Epithelia. (A) The vestibular components of the inner ear include three orthogonally disposed semicircular canals and two macular epithelia: the utricle and saccule. (B) At the base of each semicircular canal is an enlargement called the ampulla, within which is housed the sensory epithelium, called the crista. The long stereocilia of the hair cells are all oriented in the same direction and insert into a large gelatinous sail-shaped structure, called the cupula. (C) The utricle and saccule are almost flat epithelia, in which hair bundle orientation is either toward (utricle) or away from (saccule) a central line of reversal, the striola.

The Adequate Stimulus for the Semicircular Canals

The crista ampullaris (shortened to *crista*), which is the sensory epithelium within the enlarged ampulla of each semicircular canal, is composed of hair cells and supporting cells. As the head rotates, inertial drag causes movement of fluid within the semicircular canal and thus displacement of the cupular membrane that stretches across the ampulla (Figure 24.17). The elongated stereociliary bundles of the hair cells project up into the acellular cupula and so are deflected by this motion. If head rotation is constant, the fluid eventually catches up and cupular deflection ceases. Thus, the fluid mechanics of semicircular canals impart a particular sensibility; their hair cells and afferent neurons signal only the change in rotational velocity or angular acceleration (although this principal mechanism is supplemented by cellular and synaptic processes).[121] The orientation of hair bundles is unidirectional within each crista, with the result that fluid motion toward the central vestibular chamber is excitatory for the horizontal canals and inhibitory (i.e., reducing spontaneous firing) for the vertical canals.

The three semicircular canals occupy three orthogonal planes (see Figures 24.1 and 24.17), making their receptors sensitive to three directions of acceleration. In a complex twisting motion, for instance on an amusement park ride, multiple canals are stimulated all at once. The horizontal canal (which actually is tilted upward at about 30°) is positioned in the most external location and is the shortest of the three canals. Turning your head left and right around a vertical axis (e.g., watching a tennis match between two baseline players) evokes fluid movement and thus hair cell activation through this canal. The superior semicircular canal is positioned in the most anterior location; it is vertically oriented, aligned with the sagittal plane. Nodding your head vigorously to agree with a professor's brilliant conclusion—thereby rotating the head through an axis running between the ears—evokes fluid movement and thus hair cell activation through this canal. The posterior semicircular

[121] Highstein, S. M. et al. 2005. *J. Neurophysiol.* 93: 2359-2370.

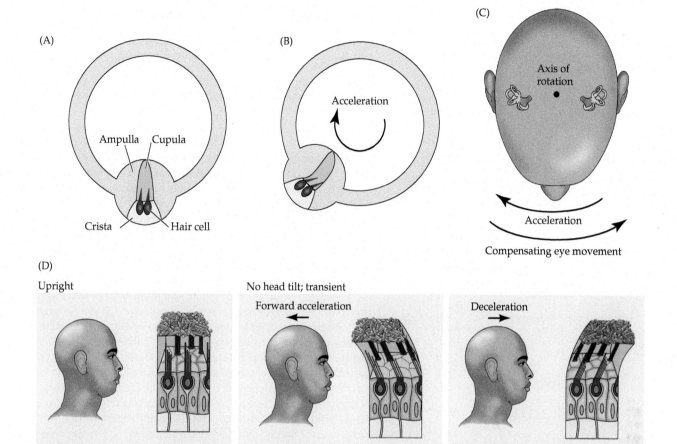

FIGURE 24.17   Stimulation of Vestibular Epithelia.
(A–C) Fluid motion within each semicircular canal deflects the cupula and the inserted stereocilia, causing receptor potentials in the hair cells. Horizontal canals in the two ears provide opposite signals for rotation on the horizontal plane. The right anterior and left posterior canals as well as the left anterior-right posterior canals provide opposing signals about those planes of rotation, approximately 45° from head vertical (also see Figure 24.1). (D) The hair bundles of macular hair cells project into an overlying gelatinous mass containing calcium carbonate crystals (i.e., the otoliths, or ear stones). The otolith provides an inertial load, so that linear acceleration of the head results in differential motion of the epithelium and the overlying otolith, and thus causes receptor potentials in hair cells of each macula. The utricle lies approximately in the horizontal plane of the upright head and the saccule approximately vertically to it, making each relatively sensitive to motion in those planes. The arrows show the direction of utricular hair bundle deflection for horizontal acceleration and deceleration. However, all head motion produces components of motion that affect both maculae. Furthermore, the oppositely oriented hair bundles in each macula give still greater differentiation to the peripheral signal.

canal is also vertically aligned, but is aligned with the coronal plane, oriented at about 90° in relation to the superior canal. The motion that evokes fluid movement and thus hair cell activation through this canal can be envisioned as trying to make your ear touch your shoulder (without raising the shoulder).

The Vestibulo-Ocular Reflex

The vestibulo-ocular reflex (VOR) depends on a simple (three-neuron) circuit by which head motion elicits equal and opposite motion of the eyeballs so that the fovea (the focusing point of the retina; see Chapter 22) can remain fixated on an object of interest in visual space.[122] We will describe one particular example, horizontal head rotation, but in fact all directions of movement activating both cristae and macular epithelia participate in foveation by this mechanism.[123] A rotation of the upright head to the left is compensated by an equal rightward rotation of the eyes (Figure 24.18). Leftward head rotation is excitatory to the left semicircular canal and suppresses activity in the right canal. Left-side canal afferents excite second-order neurons in the vestibular nucleus of the brainstem, which excite motor neurons in the oculo-motor nucleus that in turn activate the medial rectus muscle of the left eye, causing it to rotate

[122] Lorente de Nó, R. 1933. *Arch. Neurol. Psychiatry* 30: 245–291.

[123] Cohen, B., Maruta, J., and Raphan, T. 2001. *Ann. NY Acad. Sci.* 942: 241–258.

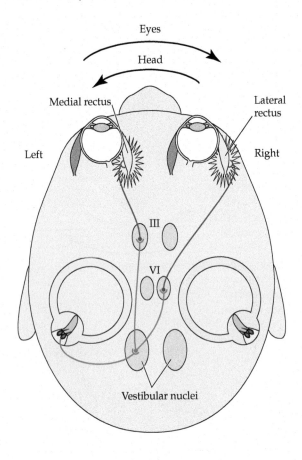

Eyes

Head

Medial rectus

Lateral rectus

Left

Right

III

VI

Vestibular nuclei

FIGURE 24.18 The Vestibulo-Ocular Reflex. Leftward rotation of the head causes excitation of the left horizontal canal and suppression of its contralateral twin. Increased afferent activity causes excitation of principal cells of the vestibular nucleus in the brainstem, which in turn excites motor neurons of the ipsilateral medial rectus and contralateral lateral rectus, causing rightward rotation of the eyes. The net effect is to maintain gaze on a point in space, even as the head is deflected. III and VI are cranial nerves.

rightward. Second-order vestibular neurons also excite motor neurons (in the abducens nucleus) to the lateral rectus muscle of the right eye, causing it to rotate rightward an equal amount. Thus, leftward head rotation is accompanied by coordinate, conjugate, and opposing motions that keep the two eyes fixated on the original visual target. Reduced activity in the right horizontal semicircular canal produces complementary reduction of activity and relaxation of opposing muscles: the left lateral rectus and the right medial rectus.

Under normal conditions the VOR gain (i.e., the ratio of head to eye movement) is 1, and it can operate near normally even with input from only one ear. Obviously, complete loss of the VOR can severely limit normal life activities. Somewhat less devastating is a condition called superior semicircular canal dehiscence, a thinning or complete loss of bone in the floor of the cranial vault at the top of the arch of the posterior (superior) semicircular canal.[124] Such a bony defect allows for transmission of mechanical energy from the cranial fluids to those of the superior semicircular canal, thereby exciting reflex eye movements in the plane of the canal. One disturbing consequence is that loud sounds or impacts absorbed through the head can give rise to eye movements and vertigo. For example, the action and sound of water from a shower result in the shower stall appearing to move! Fortunately, the defect can be repaired surgically.

Higher-Order Vestibular Function

As the "silent sense," vestibular function is largely subconscious, driving or modulating motor activity but not usually giving rise to conscious sensation. This state can change, however, with vertigo and nausea arising from unusual vestibular input (motion sickness) or dysfunction. Happily, in most circumstances one can adapt to that altered condition, gaining sea legs, as it were.

Adaptation of the VOR has been studied extensively. The VOR is highly plastic, and adapts readily to altered sensory input, as wearers of bifocal glasses can attest. In fact, experimental manipulation of the VOR often involves magnifying or reducing lenses that alter the eye's focal length and thus the rate at which the visual scene shifts during eye movement. Subsequently, the VOR gain adapts with experience so that the appropriate compensation is made. This plasticity results from cerebellar modulation of the reflex.[125,126] Purkinje cells in the vestibular portion of the cerebellar cortex (flocculus and nodulus) project directly to inhibit principal neurons of the vestibular nuclei. Changes in synaptic efficacy may take place in the cerebellar Purkinje cells or in their target neurons in the vestibular nuclei.[127,128] As predicted, cerebellar lesions prevent VOR adaptation.[129]

How does vestibular sensation reach consciousness? The answer is confounded by the complication that vestibular sensation usually includes visual, proprioceptive, and tactile stimulation.[130] There is little evidence for a specific primary vestibular region of the cerebral cortex (differently from touch, vision, etc.). Rather, vestibular information reaches many cortical association areas, combining with visual, somatosensory, and motor signals.[131,132] This fact by no means diminishes the importance of the sense of head posture and motion. In addition to being essential for locomotion and visual analysis, vestibular input plays a role in autonomic reflexes, helping maintain blood pressure and respiration with postural changes.[133]

[124] Minor, L. B. 2005. *Laryngoscope* 115: 1717-1727.

[125] Ito, M. 1972. *Brain Res.* 40: 81-84.

[126] Lisberger, S. G. 2009. *Neuroscience* 162: 763-776.

[127] Cullen, K. E. et al. 2009. *J. Vestib. Res.* 19: 171-182.

[128] Blazquez, P. M., Hirata, Y., and Highstein, S. M. 2004. *Cerebellum* 3: 188-192.

[129] Luebke, A. E., and Robinson, D. A. 1994. *Exp. Brain Res.* 98: 379-390.

[130] Angelaki, D. E., and Cullen, K. E. 2008. *Annu. Rev. Neurosci.* 31: 125-150.

[131] Angelaki, D. E., Klier, E. M., and Snyder, L. H. 2009. *Neuron* 64: 448-461.

[132] Ventre-Dominey, J. 2014. *Front. Integ. Neurosci.* 8: 53-53.

[133] Yates, B. J., and Miller, A. D. 1994. *J. Neurophysiol.* 71: 2087-2092.

Sensory Receptor Properties across Modalities

Comparing the properties of hair cells with the properties of photoreceptors (see Chapter 22) gives us insight into some general principles of sensory transduction. The timescale to which a given class of receptors is sensitive is perfectly matched to the timescale of the physical events that they transduce. The visual world around us changes across spans of tens or hundreds of milliseconds; events that we need to process visually—such as a change in facial expression or the movement of a predator—do not occur instantaneously, and little benefit would be gained (at a high cost) in selecting for photoreceptor transduction mechanisms in the millisecond timescale. Accordingly, transduction is slow. Contrast visual events with acoustic events, where relevant information is carried at a timescale of milliseconds. The sound difference between different consonants is distinct across tens of milliseconds.[134] As we have seen earlier in this chapter, the time difference between the two ears, which localizes a sound source, is a fraction of a millisecond. Accordingly, extraordinarily fast auditory hair cell transduction mechanisms have been selected for. Furthermore, consider the hair cells of the vestibular apparatus. Although they are remarkably similar in morphology to the auditory hair cells, the vestibular receptors detect slow variations—those that occur as body and head position shift. Thus, very different forms of receptors (visual vs. auditory) and very similar forms of receptors (auditory vs. vestibular) are all tuned to the physical events in the real world.

Finally, perhaps more for amusement than for neurobiological knowledge, reflect on the way these receptors work. Imagine an auditorium populated by 1,000 top engineers, none of whom has studied this book. If they were tasked with designing a sound-measuring sensor and a position-measuring sensor, not one would think of an instrument that resembles a hair cell, and not one would think of adapting the same instrument for both types of sensing. The nervous system, from its receptors to its high-level cortical circuits, is filled with mechanisms that surprise and thrill us.

[134] Perez, C. A. et al. 2012. *Cereb. Cortex* 23: 670–683.

SUMMARY

- Sound waves are converted into electrical signals by hair cells on the basilar membrane of the cochlea. These signals are passed on to the central nervous system through synapses on terminals of auditory nerve fibers.

- The basilar membrane is tuned mechanically so that it resonates to high frequencies at the basal end and to low frequencies at the apical end.

- Inner hair cells and outer hair cells are positioned on the basilar membrane. The outer hair cell cilia are in contact with the tectorial membrane. For both types of hair cell, membrane voltage is modulated by bending of the hair cell cilia.

- The mechanical response of the cochlear membrane is amplified by voltage-driven motility of outer hair cells, and they serve to lower the hearing threshold.

- Outer hair cells of the cochlea are subject to efferent inhibition by cholinergic brainstem neurons. Efferent inhibition reduces the sensitivity and broadens the frequency response of cochlear afferent fibers.

- In lower vertebrates, frequency selectivity is imparted to hair cells by electrical tuning. Voltage-gated calcium channels and calcium-activated potassium channels interact to enhance the voltage response at the characteristic frequency of each hair cell.

- The central auditory pathway, including cortex, is tonotopically mapped. Response properties of cells in auditory cortex are complex, showing binaural interactions and dependence on temporal combinations of tones. Binaural comparisons of sound intensity and timing are used to compute the locations of sounds in space. These computations are made with synaptic connections in nuclei of the superior olive.

- Stimulus specificity for vestibular hair cells is conferred by the mechanics of their surrounding tissues. Semicircular canals detect angular motion, while the macular epithelia, the saccule and utricle, detect linear acceleration.

- Through the vestibulo-ocular reflex, the vestibular system allows the eyes to maintain their gaze on an object even as the head turns.

Suggested Reading

General Reviews

Ashmore, J. 2008. Cochlear outer hair cell motility. *Physiol. Rev.* 88: 173–210.

Dallos, P. 2008. Cochlear amplification, outer hair cells and prestin. *Curr. Opin. Neurobiol.* 18: 370–376.

Eatock, R. A., Xue, J., and Kalluri, R. 2008. Ion channels in mammalian vestibular afferents may set regularity of firing. *J. Exp. Biol.* 211 (Pt. 11): 1764–1774.

Goldberg, J. M. 2000. Afferent diversity and the organization of central vestibular pathways. *Exp. Brain. Res.* 130: 277–297.

Nelken, I. 2008. Processing of complex sounds in the auditory system. *Curr. Opin. Neurobiol.* 18: 413–417.

Robles, L., and Ruggero, M. A. Mechanics of the mammalian cochlea. *Physiol. Rev.* 81: 1305–1352.

Schreiner, C., and Winer, J. 2007. Auditory cortex mapmaking: principles, projections and plasticity. *Neuron* 56: 356–364.

Young, E. 2008. Neural representation of spectral and temporal information in speech. *Philos. Trans. R. Soc. Lond., B, Biol. Sci.* 363: 923–945.

Original Papers

Crawford, A. C., and Fettiplace, R. 1981. An electrical tuning mechanism in turtle cochlear hair cells. *J. Physiol.* 312: 377–412.

Grant, L., Yi, E., and Glowatzki, E. 2010. Two modes of release shape the postsynaptic response at the inner hair cell ribbon synapse. *J. Neurosci.* 30: 4210–4220.

Highstein, S. M., Rabbitt, R. D., Holstein, G. R., and Boyle, R. D. 2005. Determinants of spatial and temporal coding by semicircular canal afferents. *J. Neurophysiol.* 93: 2359–2370.

Holt, J. C., Chatlani, S., Lysakowski, A., and Goldberg, J. M. 2007. Quantal and nonquantal transmission in calyx-bearing fibers of the turtle posterior crista. *J. Neurophysiol.* 98: 1083–1101.

Hudspeth, A. J., and Lewis, R. S. 1988. Kinetic analysis of voltage- and ion-dependent conductances in saccular hair cells of the bull-frog, *Rana catesbeiana*. *J. Physiol.* 400: 237–274.

Liberman, M. C., Gao, J., He, D. Z., Wu, X., Jia, S., and Zuo, J. 2002. Prestin is required for electromotility of the outer hair cell and for the cochlear amplifier. *Nature.* 419: 300–304.

Nelken, I., Rotman, Y., and Bar Yosef, O. 1999. Responses of auditory cortex neurons to structural features of natural sounds. *Nature* 397: 154–157.

Palmer, A. R., and Russell, I. J. 1986. Phase-locking in the cochlear nerve of the guinea-pig and its relation to the receptor potential of inner hair-cells. *Hear. Res.* 24: 1–15.

Ramanathan, K., Michael, T. H., Jiang, G. J., Hiel, H., and Fuchs, P. A. 1999. A molecular mechanism for electrical tuning of cochlear hair cells. *Science* 283: 215–217.

Winslow, R. L., and Sachs, M. B. 1987. Effect of electrical stimulation of the crossed olivocochlear bundle on auditory nerve response to tones in noise. *J. Neurophysiol.* 57: 1002–1021.

Zheng, J., Shen, W., He, D. Z., Long, K. B., Madison, L. D., and Dallos, P. 2000. Prestin is the motor protein of cochlear outer hair cells. *Nature* 405: 149–155.

CHAPTER 25

Constructing Perception

All the data that can be collected from the outside world are present within the sensory receptors, but neuronal activity does not lead to conscious experience until it can be further elaborated in the cerebral cortex. There, incoming streams of sensory signals are transformed from representations of basic elements into more complex combinations of features; current experiences become meaningful when compared, within cortex, with recent and distant memories as well as with expectations. Knowledge gained from the external world is also used to prepare appropriate motor outputs. How all of this occurs is the subject of this chapter. The cerebral cortex is one of the most densely studied parts of the nervous system and so our aim here is neither to survey every line of research nor to supply conclusions in an encyclopedic manner. Instead, we consider in detail two forms of processing that illustrate fundamental principles: The first is the use of memory to compare two similar stimuli; the second is recognition of an object in the visual field.

Storing a sensation in working memory, recalling, comparing, deciding—such is a chain of operations that we execute thousands of times each day. A monkey can be trained to compare two tactile vibrations, referred to as base and comparison, separated in time by a delay of 1 or more seconds. The base and comparison vibrations are characterized by their frequencies. The monkey must produce different motor responses according to whether the base or the comparison frequency is higher. Neurons in the primary somatosensory cortex (S1) encode vibration frequency by their firing rate, with higher vibration frequency leading to higher firing rate. When a recording electrode is centered in a cortical column made up of rapidly adapting neurons, electrical microstimulation through the *same recording* electrode can substitute for skin deflections in the behavioral task. Thus, sensations can be inserted artificially into the cerebral cortex.

During the comparison task, the activity of neurons in secondary somatosensory cortex (S2) and in frontal cortex differs from that in S1 in several important ways. Cortical neurons beyond S1 can have either ascending or descending firing rates as vibration frequency increases. Whereas the activity of S1 neurons does not persist after presentation of the base stimulus, activity of S2 neurons continues for a brief period, and stimulus-related firing of neurons in frontal cortex continues throughout the entire delay interval. Another important difference is that during the comparison stimulus, S1 neurons encode only the ongoing stimulus, whereas neurons in S2 and in frontal cortex encode the *difference* between the comparison frequency and the base frequency. This comparison is transformed into the subsequent response through premotor cortex and motor cortex. In rats, an analogous sequence of operations has been uncovered, suggesting that common mechanisms underlie working memory across species.[1]

In primates, recognition of objects within a visual scene is mediated by a processing stream in the cerebral cortex running in an anterior direction from the occipital lobe to the inferior temporal lobe (also known as the inferotemporal cortex). Disruption of tissue along this pathway leads to a deficit in object recognition known as agnosia. If the lesion involves a specific region on the ventral surface of the temporal lobe, patients can selectively lose the ability to recognize faces. Measurements of human brain activity, using functional magnetic resonance imaging (fMRI), and of single-neuron activity in monkeys both indicate that neurons at progressively more anterior stages of processing are excited by progressively more complex images until neurons are excited explicitly by objects rather than elemental forms. In both monkeys and humans, a region has been found that seems to be dedicated to the detection and recognition of faces.

We can recognize a familiar object under a variety of viewing angles and lighting conditions. Physiological correlates of such invariance have been found in the form of neurons that are excited according to the identity of an object, independently of the details of how the object is viewed. Progressive increases—both in the complexity of the images that activate neurons as well as in the invariance of neuronal response to viewing conditions—suggest a hierarchical transformation along the posterior–anterior axis.

The posterior–anterior transformation is accompanied by a flow of signals in the opposite direction. Those inputs (known as top–down) serve to direct attention to an expected stimulus location or to salient object features, to activate the recall of images, and to learn associations between visual images that tend to occur in sequence. Objects are frequently recognized by combining information from multiple sensory modalities. The creation of multisensory representations related to real-world objects occurs in association cortex, where unimodal sensory pathways converge.

What Is the Function of Cortical Processing?

Sensory pathways leading from receptors that carry information about touch, taste, hearing, and vision travel across synapses to the thalamus and from there to the cerebral cortex. Signals carrying information about odors travel to the cortex without passing through the thalamus. What operations are carried out on sensory signals once they reach the cortex? Clearly, the answer depends on the sensory modality, and even on the type of stimulus within a modality. For example, although speech and music both enter the nervous system through the acoustic hair cells, they are processed in cortex in very different ways.[2] But one general answer holds up for any sensory input: Intracortical processing serves to integrate and distribute elemental sensory signals in such a way that those signals can gain meaning by linkage with stored knowledge and can be acted on through motor behavior.

This proposal for constructing perception was put forward in a convincing manner by Whitfield.[3] Through analysis of the behavioral effects of lesions in the auditory system, he noted that animals can carry out surprisingly fine sensory discrimination tasks even after ablation of sensory cortex and its connected regions, provided that the task does not require the transformation of "sensory data" into "objects." He therefore postulated that the information present in subcortical centers related to the elemental physical characteristics of a stimulus (tone, wavelength, vibration frequency) can be accessed even by an animal with sensory cortex ablated. However, a deficit appears when the animal is required to endow simple sensations with the quality of belonging to objects. On page 146 of his seminal article, Whitfield concludes that it is the cortex that transforms physical characteristics into the percept of real things that are "out there" in the world. Once intracortical processing converts elemental

[1] Esmaeili, V., and Diamond, M. E. 2019. *Cell Rep.* 27: 3167-3181.e5

[2] Peretz, I. 2006. *Cognition* 100: 1-32.

[3] Whitfield, I. C. 1979. *Brain Behav. Evol.* 16: 129-154.

sensory attributes into percepts of known objects, he continues, the animal appears to be able to use the result of one problem to generalize—that is, to solve a closely related problem. This capacity emerges because, in the late stages of cortical processing, information is organized as objects and concepts, rather than as a set of physical features.

We begin this chapter with a discussion of how tactile stimuli are encoded, stored in memory, and acted on in the course of a behavioral task. The sensory input employed in these experiments is comparatively simple, allowing us to gain a complete picture of its representation at multiple levels of cortex. We then proceed to the visual system and present evidence about how intracortical processing transforms sensory data about images into percepts of objects and movement in the real world. The visual experiments deal with more complex stimuli, so it is difficult to gain a complete quantification of their neuronal representation. Yet the research is compelling because it offers the possibility to connect brain function to perceptual experiences—such as recognizing a face—that are critical to our lives.

Tactile Working Memory Task and Its Representation in Primary Somatosensory Cortex

Behavioral Task

Experiments by Ranulfo Romo and colleagues have provided insights into how stimuli are encoded by neuronal activity and how such activity leads to assessment of the stimuli. In their studies, monkeys are trained to discriminate the difference in frequency between two mechanical vibrations applied sequentially to one fingertip (Figure 25.1A).[4] The first vibration frequency, f_1, and the second vibration frequency, f_2, vary across trials. The first and second stimuli are referred to as the base and comparison, respectively. At the end of the comparison stimulus, the monkey uses its free hand to press a response button, expressing one of two judgments: $f_1 > f_2$ or $f_2 > f_1$. The delay between the base and comparison is 1 second (s) in most experiments, but monkeys can perform the task even with a 10-s delay. The greater the difference between f_1 and f_2, the better the monkey's performance (Figure 25.1B,C). Overall accuracy is similar to that of humans performing the same task.

Neuronal Representation of Vibration Sensations in Primary Somatosensory Cortex

How do neurons encode a sequence of brief, pulsatile indentations applied to the skin? The indentations activate rapidly adapting Meissner's corpuscles which are extraordinarily sensitive to quick indentations (see Chapter 23), and signals are relayed through the spinal cord, brain stem, and thalamus to the primary somatosensory cortex, also known as S1.

Figure 25.2 shows the response of individual S1 neurons to a stimulus train.[5] Action potentials were recorded with an array of microelectrodes inserted into the cortical area receiving input from the stimulated fingertip. More than 50% of neurons exhibited frequency-dependent modulation in firing rate: As vibration frequency increased, firing rate increased (see Figure 25.2A). A large proportion of neurons fired in phase with each indentation; for instance, a vibration of 10 Hz led to a response with intervals of about 100 ms between spikes (see Figure 25.2B). Both kinds of signals—the total number of spikes in the train and the periodicity within the train—carry information about vibration frequency. It may seem intuitive that cortical areas central to S1 use the phase-locked signal, but two observations lead to the surprising conclusion that vibration frequency is extracted from the firing rate instead.

The first observation comes from the comparison between S1 neuronal activity on single trials and the choice made by the monkey on that same trial. The likelihood of the monkey making a correct discrimination on a given trial was unrelated to whether the spike trains were more periodic or less periodic than average on that trial. In contrast, in a small number of single neurons the firing rate fluctuated together with the decision made by the monkey.[5] Since firing rate seems to contribute to the monkey's judgment, it is the better candidate for acting as the critical code.

The second observation comes from altering the stimulus. Having practiced the discrimination task for months using periodic stimuli, the monkeys were then presented with non-periodic stimuli in which indentations were separated by random time intervals

[4] Romo, R. et al. 1997. *Cereb. Cortex* 7: 317-326.

[5] Hernandez, A. et al. 1997. *J. Neurosci.* 17: 6391-6400.

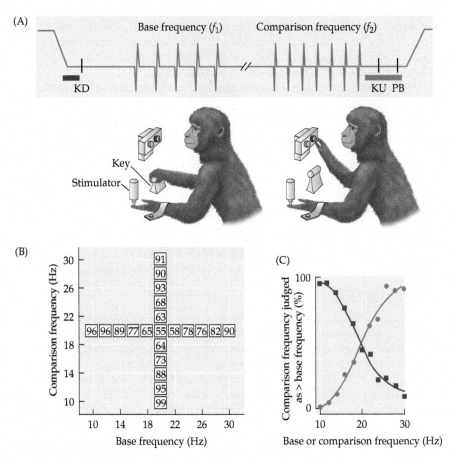

FIGURE 25.1 Vibration Discrimination Task and Performance. (A) The upper plot shows the probe position (y-axis) across time in one trial. The lower drawings show the monkey receiving the stimulus (left) and responding at the conclusion of the trial (right). The experimental sequence is as follows. First, the mechanical stimulator is lowered, indenting one fingertip of the restrained hand. The monkey uses its free hand to press a key down (KD; red bar). Then the monkey receives the first vibration from the stimulator, which oscillates vertically at the base stimulus frequency (f_1). After a delay, the monkey receives the second vibration at the comparison frequency (f_2). The monkey lets the key up (KU) and presses the medial or lateral (blue and red, respectively) response button (PB) to indicate whether f_2 was lower or higher than f_1 (blue bar). (B) Results from a typical session. The horizontal row of boxes indicates the percentage of correct responses at various base frequencies that precede a comparison frequency of 20 Hz. The vertical row indicates the percentage of correct responses at varying comparison frequencies after a base frequency of 20 Hz. Note that the larger differences between f_1 and f_2 led to better performance. The complete experiment included all possible combinations of the base and comparison frequencies (not shown). (C) Results of another typical session presented as curves that illustrate the percent of trials in which the monkey judged the comparison stimulus frequency, f_2, as higher than the base stimulus frequency, f_1. For the red points (squares), f_2 was 20 Hz, and the x-axis gives varying values of f_1. The blue dots show the reverse: f_1 was 20 Hz and the x-axis gives varying values of f_2. Measurement of performance in this manner is known as the psychometric curve; steep curves like these indicate proficient performance of the task and provide a direct way of comparing the animal's performance to neuronal responses. (A-C after A. Hernandez et al., 2002. *Neuron* 33: 959-972. Monkeys after R. Romo & E. Salinas. 2003. *Nat. Rev. Neurosci.* 4: 203-218.)

[6] LaMotte, R. H., and Mountcastle, V. B. 1975. *J. Neurophysiol.* 38: 539-559.

[7] Powell, T. P., and Mountcastle, V. B. 1959. *Bull. Johns Hopkins Hosp.* 105: 133-162.

[8] Salinas, E. et al. 2000. *J. Neurosci.* 20: 5503-5515.

[9] Hernandez, A. et al. 2000. *Proc. Natl. Acad. Sci. USA* 97: 6191-6196.

(see Figure 25.2C). Phase-locked neurons now fired with irregular spike trains mirroring the sequence of skin indentations. If the brain required periodic spike trains to discriminate frequency, performance would degenerate dramatically. Yet the performance was equally strong for periodic and non-periodic stimuli. The choices of the monkey were predictable from the overall firing rate, not the periodicity, of S1 neurons (see Figure 25.2D).[6]

Temporal jitter in a train of skin deflections certainly affects the central processing of stimuli.[7-9] But under the conditions presented here, it is safe to conclude that the percept of vibration frequency is constructed from the firing rate, not the periodicity, of S1 neurons.

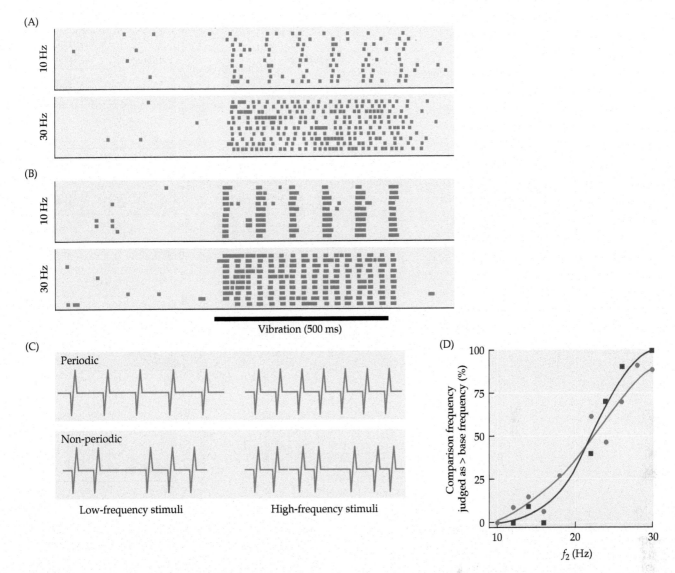

Vibration (500 ms)

FIGURE 25.2 Neuronal Coding of Vibration Frequency in S1. (A) Responses to ten trials with stimulus at 10 Hz (upper plot) and 30 Hz (lower plot). Spike times are blue squares. The black bar indicates the 500-ms period in which the stimulus was presented. This neuron had a low degree of firing periodicity but encoded vibration frequency by firing rate. (B) Responses of a neuron that encoded vibration frequency by periodicity but not by firing rate (since at low-vibration frequency each deflection evoked more spikes). (C) Low-frequency (left) and high-frequency (right) stimuli in a periodic (upper) and non-periodic (lower) stimulus train. (D) The red squares and line are the psychometric curve for

one session derived from the trials in which the base stimulus was 20 Hz (see Figure 25.1C for derivation of such curves). The blue dots and line are a so-called neurometric curve and represent the most accurate performance that an observer of neuronal activity could achieve. The neuron analyzed here encoded vibration frequency by firing rate. For non-periodic stimuli, performance of the monkey and the performance available in S1 neuronal activity were similar, but only for neurons that encoded vibration frequency by firing rate. Neurons that were phase-locked could not encode non-periodic stimuli. (After E. Salinas et al., 2000. *J. Neurosci.* 20: 5503–5515. © 2000 Society for Neuroscience.)

Replacement of Vibrations by Artificial Stimuli

The investigators then tested the effect of stimulating the S1 cells directly, thereby bypassing the pathway from skin to cortex.[10] An artificial stimulus consisted of current injections[11] delivered at the same frequency as the mechanical stimulus for which it substituted (Figure 25.3). Stimulation sites in the S1 cortex were selected with receptive fields on the fingertip at the location of the mechanical stimulating probe. Remarkably, the monkeys were able to discriminate between the frequencies of the tactile base stimulus and the electrical comparison stimulus with the same accuracy as that obtained with two tactile stimuli (see Figure 25.3A,B). The accuracy was also maintained when the base stimulus was electrical (see Figure 25.3C), indicating that the monkeys could form

[10] Lak, A. et al. 2010. Proc. *Natl. Acad. Sci. USA* 17: 7981–7986.

[11] Lak, A., Arabzadeh, E., and Diamond, M. E. 2008. *Cereb. Cortex* 18: 1085–1093.

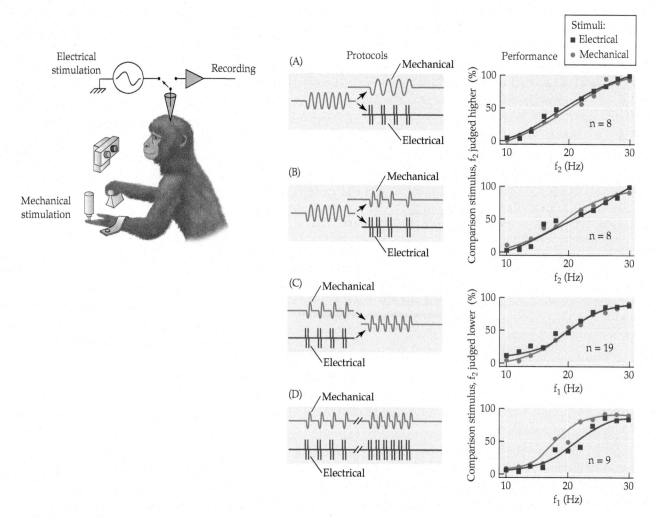

FIGURE 25.3 Replacement of Vibrations by Artificial Stimuli. After training with mechanical stimuli, skin stimuli were replaced by trains of electrical-current bursts (red) injected into S1 at the same frequencies as natural stimuli. In half of the trials, the monkeys compared two mechanical vibrations delivered to the skin. In the other half, one or both of the stimuli were replaced by electrical stimulation in the cortex. The diagrams on the left show four of the protocols used. The curves on the right show the monkeys' performance as psychometric functions (constructed in the manner explained in Figure 25.1C) in the corresponding session with only skin stimuli (blue dots and curve) or electrical stimuli (red squares and curve). (A) All stimuli were periodic. The comparison stimulus could be either mechanical or electrical. (B) The base stimulus was periodic and the comparison stimulus was non-periodic. The comparison stimulus could be either mechanical or electrical. (C) All stimuli were periodic. The base stimulus could be either mechanical or electrical. (D) All stimuli were periodic. In electrical stimulation trials, both base and comparison stimuli were artificial. Tactile stimuli were either sinusoids or trains of short mechanical pulses. (After R. Romo and E. Salinas, 2003. *Nat. Rev. Neurosci.* 4: 203–218, based on R. Romo et al., 1998. *Nature* 392: 387–390; R. Romo et al., 2000. *Neuron* 26: 273–278.)

the working memory of the base stimulus from an artificial input. Even with artificial inputs used as *both* the base and comparison stimuli, monkeys could achieve discrimination levels close to those measured when mechanical stimuli were delivered to the fingertips (see Figure 25.3D).

The use of direct cortical stimuli allowed a further insight into the role of firing periodicity. When the electrical stimulation was non-periodic, the performance remained good and confirmed that firing rate, not temporal pattern, was the feature used by the brain to compute vibration frequency. The monkeys responded to electrical stimulation when the stimulus site was in cortical columns formed by rapidly adapting neurons (see Chapter 23); stimulation of columns formed by slowly adapting neurons produced no behavioral response.

To summarize, the full cognitive operation may be triggered by the signal emanating from a limited number of neurons in one cortical column. The demonstration of artificial sensation has been important for the field of brain–machine interfaces,[12] where one long-term goal is to simulate sensations in the brains of patients with nonfunctional sensory pathways.

[12] Godde, B., Diamond, M., and Braun, C. 2010. *Neurosci. Lett.* 480: 143–147.

Transformation from Sensation to Action

Activity in S1 across Successive Stages of the Task

In the set of experiments described in the previous section, the investigators devised a way of characterizing the relationship between the stimuli and neuronal firing during presentation of the base stimulus, the comparison stimulus, and the delay between the two. Under the assumption that neuronal firing rate has a linear relationship to stimulus frequency, the firing rate (r) within any phase of the task can be described by:

$$r = b + a_1f_1 + a_2f_2$$

where b is the background firing rate (unrelated to any stimulus), f_1 is the base stimulus frequency, and f_2 is the comparison stimulus frequency. For a given neuron, a_1 and a_2 are coefficients that describe how the neuronal discharge rate throughout a trial depends on the stimulus frequencies. The values of a_1 and a_2 can change over the course of the trial. To understand their meaning, an example is useful. Consider first the firing of a neuron in the base period. Suppose that across a set of trials with a variety of stimulus frequencies the neuron's firing rate increases by two spikes per second for each 1-Hz increase in f_1. Then a_1 = 2 for that phase of the task. During this period, the comparison stimulus (with frequency f_2) can have no effect on the firing rate because the stimulus has not yet been presented, so a_2 = 0 (unless, of course, the monkey is reading the computer that runs the experiment and predicts the upcoming stimulus). Consider now the firing of the same neuron during the comparison period. If stimulation during the comparison period itself increases the firing rate by 3 Hz for every 1-Hz increase in f_2, then a_2 = 3. If the base stimulus has no residual effect on the firing rate, then a_1 = 0. However, in a working memory task such as this, the brain must carry a trace of recent events. Therefore, we expect that in some regions of the cortex, neuronal firing during the comparison stimulus must be affected by the value of the past stimulus, f_1. In that case, a_1 will have a non-zero value.

Figure 25.4 illustrates how the neurons in one cortical region can be characterized by their values of a_1 and a_2. Figure 25.4A presents the events of one trial: the base stimulus defined by frequency f_1, the delay, and the comparison stimulus defined by frequency f_2. Figure 25.4B indicates the first cortical region examined, the fingertip representation of S1. Figure

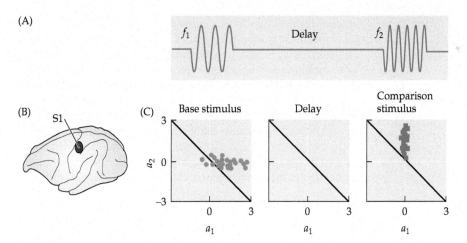

FIGURE 25.4 Neuronal Activity in S1 Cortex Characterized by Firing-Rate Coefficients a_1 and a_2. (A) Time course of the behavior during one trial. (B) Location of recordings sites in S1 cortex. (C) Within the f_1 interval, the delay interval, and the f_2 interval, firing rate can be expressed as $(a_1f_1) + (a_2f_2) + b$. Each point gives the values of a_1 or a_2 for one neuron. Green dots correspond to neurons with significant a_1 coefficients (regardless of a_2); blue squares indicate neurons with significant a_2 coefficients only. During f_1, most values of a_1 are positive and values of a_2 are zero. During the delay, both a_1 and a_2 are zero. During f_2, most values of a_2 are positive and values of a_1 are zero. Points are not plotted if both a_1 and a_2 are zero (as is the case in the middle graph). (After R. Romo and E. Salinas, 2003. *Nat. Rev. Neurosci.* 4: 203–218.)

25.4C shows the activity of one set of S1 neurons during different stages of the task. In all plots, the x-axis gives the value of a_1, and the y-axis gives the value of a_2. During presentation of the base stimulus (left graph of Figure 25.4C), most neurons had a positive value of a_1 because they encoded f_1 by increasing their firing rate as frequency was increased. The values of a_2 were zero, since sensory neurons cannot vary their firing rate according to a future stimulus. During the delay (middle graph), a_1 values returned to zero, indicating that the base stimulus had no residual effect on neuronal discharge. During presentation of the comparison stimulus (right graph), the neurons had a positive value of a_2, while a_1 remained zero.

Activity in Regions beyond S1

The frequency comparison task requires more than the coding of stimulus features in S1 cortex. In the following sections we examine the behavior of cortical regions that operate on tactile signals beyond S1. Figure 25.5 shows the projection of S1 to secondary somatosensory cortex (S2), and then to the inferior convexity of the prefrontal cortex (PFC), a region known to have a role in the memory of sensory stimuli.[13] The medial premotor cortex (MPC) receives input from PFC and also from S2; it is believed to be involved with motor planning. MPC projects to primary motor cortex (M1), which is involved in execution of motor commands (see Chapter 26).

During the base stimulus, neurons in S2 (Figure 25.6A, left graph) showed more complex responses than those in S1 (shown in Figure 25.4C). While responsive S1 neurons only showed an increase in firing rate as stimulus frequency increased, many neurons in S2 showed a *decrease*, reflected as a negative value of a_1. The opposing dependence on frequency—some firing rates rising and others falling as vibration frequency increased—reflects a fundamental transformation of the signal received from S1.

During the base stimulus, a mix of neurons with positive and negative values of a_1 was found in all the frontal lobe areas except M1 (Figure 25.6B–D, left graphs). Latencies were longer in S2 than in S1 and progressively longer in PFC and MPC (not shown). Although S1 is often referred to as "sensory cortex" (and V1 and A1 are referred to as the "sensory cortex" for vision and hearing, respectively), the encoding of tactile vibrations in many regions beyond S1 suggests that sensory cortex extends well beyond the first-order processing region. In M1, very few neurons responded to the first vibration (see Figure 25.6D, left graph), so this region can be considered *not* to participate in sensory processing during this behavior.

During the delay following the base stimulus, many neurons in S2, prefrontal cortex, and medial premotor cortex maintained activity related to the preceding vibration (see Figure 25.6A–C, middle graphs). During presentation of the comparison stimulus, the monkey must decide whether f_2 is greater or less than f_1, and then prepare to press the appropriate response button. Thus, changes in firing rate during the comparison period that are related to the frequency difference, $f_2 - f_1$, are of particular importance. Neurons encoding frequency differences can be identified by the relationship between a_1 and a_2. Referring back to the earlier equation, we see that the case of $a_2 = -a_1$ is particularly significant. Substituting $-a_1$ for a_2 into the equation presented earlier gives the relationship:

$$r = b + a_1 f_1 + a_2 f_2 = b + a_1 f_1 - a_1 f_2$$

$$\text{or } r = b + a_1 (f_1 - f_2)$$

In other words, when points lie close to the line $a_2 = -a_1$, it means that the neuron is responding as a function of $f_1 - f_2$; such neurons appear to *compare* f_1 and f_2. No neurons with such responses were seen in S1 (see Figure 25.4), but they were clearly present in all subsequent cortical areas (see Figure 25.6, right graphs). The dependence on $f_2 - f_1$ is particularly evident during the last 300 ms of the comparison period (red triangles), when the parameters a_1 and a_2 fall closely along the line $a_2 = -a_1$.

[13] Romo, R. et al. 2000. *Neuron* 26: 273-278.

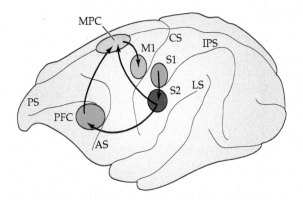

FIGURE 25.5 Cortical Regions Involved in the Vibration Comparison Task. The drawing shows the location of each cortical region. Arrows indicate the expected flow of tactile information. AS = arcuate sulcus; CS = central sulcus; IPS = intraparietal sulcus; LS = lateral sulcus; M1 = primary motor cortex; MPC = medial premotor cortex; PFC = prefrontal cortex; PS = principal sulcus; S1 = primary somatosensory cortex; S2 = secondary somatosensory cortex.

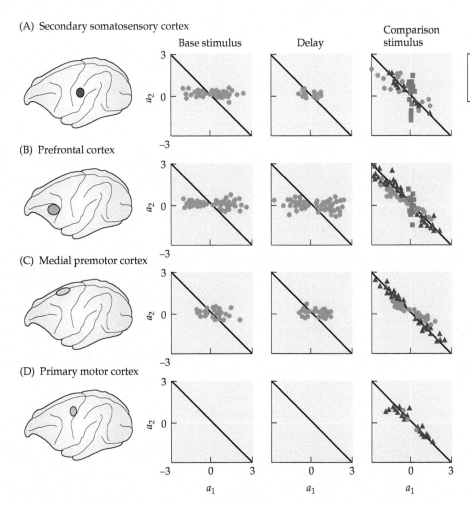

(A) Secondary somatosensory cortex

(B) Prefrontal cortex

(C) Medial premotor cortex

(D) Primary motor cortex

- Significant a_1
- Significant a_2 only
- Last 300 ms of stimulus

FIGURE 25.6 Neuronal Activity beyond S1 Characterized by Firing-Rate Coefficients a_1 and a_2. As in Figure 25.4, green dots indicate neurons with significant a_1 coefficients (regardless of a_2); blue squares indicate neurons with significant a_2 coefficients only. The left set of graphs refers to the base stimulus, the middle set to the delay, and the right set to the comparison stimulus. Red triangles indicate coefficients computed during the last 300 ms of the comparison stimulus. (A) Responses recorded from secondary somatosensory cortex. (B) Responses recorded from prefrontal cortex. (C) Responses recorded from medial premotor cortex. (D) Responses recorded from primary motor cortex. All areas except M1 show stimulus coding during the base stimulus, but (unlike in S1) a_1 can have negative as well as positive values. Neurons continue to represent the base stimulus during the delay, also unlike in S1. During the comparison stimulus, many neurons have firing characterized by the property $a_2 = -a_1$. This is especially so during the final part of the second stimulus, as illustrated by the red triangles. (After R. Romo and E. Salinas, 2003. *Nat. Rev. Neurosci.* 4: 203–218; C also based on A. Hernandez et al., 2002. *Neuron* 33: 959–972.)

Since the comparison task is composed of distinct phases, the time course of signals is particularly pertinent. Figure 25.7 plots the proportion of neurons in different cortical regions that had significant (positive or negative) values of a_1 (green lines) and a_2 (red lines) over time. The proportion of neurons whose firing was described by $a_2 = -a_1$ is illustrated by the blue lines. S1 firing rates were characterized by a_1 during the base stimulus and by a_2 during the comparison stimulus. S2 firing rates were characterized by a_1 during the base stimulus and showed a memory of f_1 during the first 500 ms of the delay period. During the comparison stimulus, many S2 neurons were characterized by a_2 alone, but others were described by $a_2 = -a_1$; the latter neurons encode the difference between the base and comparison stimulus frequencies.

In comparison with S2 neurons, PFC neurons showed a more pronounced memory for the base stimulus and a more prominent representation of the stimulus difference during the comparison period. MPC neurons were characterized by a weaker representation of the

FIGURE 25.7 Time Course of Response Parameters throughout the Trial Period.
Magnitudes of a_1 (green) and a_2 (red) vary from one cortical location to the next. Blue traces indicate neurons whose activity directly represents the comparison between f_1 and f_2 for all different values of the two stimuli (that is, either firing more for $f_2 > f_1$, or for $f_2 < f_1$). Responses are expressed as a percentage of the total number of responding neurons. (After R. Romo et al., 2004. *Neuron* 41: 165–173, based on data from A. Hernandez et al., 2000. *Proc. Natl. Acad. Sci. USA* 97: 6191–6196. © 2000 National Academy of Sciences; A. Hernandez et al., 2002. *Neuron* 33: 959–972; R. Romo et al., 2002. *Nat. Neurosci.* 5: 1217–1225; R. Romo et al., 2003. *Neuron* 38: 649–657.)

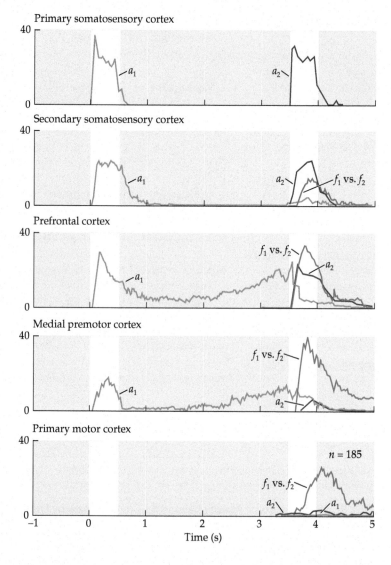

[14] Fassihi, A. et al. 2017. *Curr. Biol.* 27: 1585–1596.

[15] Fassihi, A. et al. 2014. *Proc. Natl. Acad. Sci. USA* 111: 2331–2336.

[16] Stoney, S. D., Jr., Thompson, W. D., and Asanuma, H 1968. *J. Neurophysiol.* 31: 659–669.

current stimulus but by a very strong representation of the stimulus difference. Neurons in M1 showed no stimulus representation or working memory; their activity was related only to the outcome of the stimulus difference, f_2 versus f_1. As would be expected, the responses began later in the comparison period and extended into the interval when the monkeys actually pressed the response button. When rats do the same tactile working memory task (comparing two vibrations received through the whiskers), similar forms of processing have been identified in the cortex, but each region carries out multiple operations.[1,14,15]

Neurons Associated with Decision Making

Monkeys (and humans, when tested with the same stimulus set) sometimes make errors in detecting differences in the frequency of vibration, especially when the difference is small. What is the incorrect message within neuronal activity that leads to errors? Insights can be gained by comparing the activity of an individual neuron on correct versus incorrect trials and, more specifically, by determining to what extent any differences in activity could predict an error. This is referred to as the **choice probability index** for the neuron. A high value means that on trials when the neuron's activity deviates from its average activity in correct trials, there is a high probability of the monkey making an error.[16] An intuitive way of thinking of choice probability index is that if a neuron's index is very high, then when that neuron "makes a mistake," so to speak, the whole brain (and thus the monkey) is likely to make a mistake. Neurons in S1 were found to have a low choice probability index. Typically, they encoded the stimuli accurately, whether the final action turned out to be right or wrong, although the trial-to-trial variability in firing rate of a small number of S1 neurons did predict errors. Neurons in the frontal cortex showed a much higher choice probability index. In MPC, for instance, the choice probability index grew during the delay period and peaked during the comparison period. So errors usually do not depend on a faulty representation of the stimulus in the ascending pathway through S1. Most errors seem to arise through a declining persistence of the representation of f_1 and, consequently, a faulty comparison between f_1 and f_2. Again, similar results have been found in rats.[1]

Earlier we noted that a set of neurons showed firing late in the comparison period that could be characterized by the relation $a_1 = -a_2$. If the activity of these neurons is so closely related to the monkey's task (because their firing rate explicitly encodes the difference between f_2 and f_1), you might expect that they contribute disproportionately to the final decision. In support of this hypothesis, it was found that the monkeys were most likely to make errors on those trials when the neurons whose message is "$a_2 = -a_1$" did not accurately encode the frequency difference: Errors of these neurons were predictive of errors by the monkey.

The transformation of the message carried by neurons from sensory cortex to frontal cortex has been found in other forms of behavior. Monkeys were trained in an easier task, namely, to report on the presence or absence of a mechanical vibration applied to the fingertip. This is known as a **detection task**. Stimulus amplitude varied from trial to trial. On trials with amplitude near the detection threshold (in which monkeys detected the vibration with about 50% likelihood), the firing of neurons in S1 did not predict whether the monkey would detect the stimulus. The firing of neurons in frontal cortex varied in close connection to how the monkey ended up judging the stimulus; frontal cortex neurons seemed to reflect the monkey's subjective feeling. This finding suggests that the neuronal correlates of subjective sensory experience build up from S1 to the frontal lobe.[17]

Analogous findings in rats point again to a general mechanism for decision making in mammals. Neuronal activity in barrel cortex (see Chapter 23), as well as in a frontal cortex target of barrel cortex, was recorded while rats compared the intensity of two vibrations separated by an interstimulus delay, an experimental design adapted to rodents from the studies of monkeys.[18] Durations of both stimulus 1 and stimulus 2 could vary from 100 to 600 ms. Rats overestimated the longer-duration stimulus; thus, the perceived intensity of a vibration grew over the course of hundreds of milliseconds even while the sensory input remained, on average, stationary. The time dependence of the percept allowed the investigators to ask to what extent neurons encoded the ongoing stimulus stream versus the animal's percept. Barrel cortex firing was correlated with the amplitude of the vibration, whereas frontal cortex firing was correlated with the percept: The final frontal cortex population state varied, as did the rat's behavior, according to both stimulus speed and stimulus duration. Just as in monkeys, the transformation of sensory data into the percept appears to involve the integration and storage of sensory cortex signals by frontal cortex. Laboratory rats are docile and intelligent, acting in this and in many other experiments as the perfect species for identifying the most fundamental principles of mammalian sensory processing.

In the experiments described thus far, we have examined the neuronal processing that transforms tactile sensation into a decision. In the next section our goal is once again to characterize intracortical transformations, but now in the visual system. We will examine areas in which cortical neurons represent the features of objects and areas in which cortical neurons represent the object's identity, such as a face.

Visual Object Perception in Primates

Object Perception and the Ventral Visual Pathway

If you are asked to describe what you see, the description will inevitably portray a world made up of meaningful things—for instance, "I see a badly dressed professor at the front of the lecture hall with an illustration of the brain projected behind him," or "I see a piece of chalk that he is hurling at an inattentive student" (preferably not you). It is unlikely that you will describe the scene by the parameters of luminance, contrast, spatial frequency, wavelength, and so on. Yet the objects and people in the scene could not be perceived unless encoded by the early stages of the visual system as elementary features. If pressed to do so, you could perhaps catalog the complete set of elementary features making up the scene, but

[17] Fagg, A. H. et al. 2007. *J. Neurosci.* 27: 11842-11846.

[18] Constantinidis, C., Franowicz, M. N., and Goldman-Rakic, P. S. 2001. *Nat. Neurosci.* 4: 311-316.

it would be laborious and slow. And if the lighting conditions changed, the catalog (luminance, contrast, etc.) would have to be altered.

Describing the same scene according to your knowledge of the world is easy and fast. It does not change if the lighting or the angle of viewing is changed. Whereas the visual world is formed of basic physical features, our subjective experience relates to a world formed of people and things that have significance due to our accumulated knowledge. In this portion of the chapter we present evidence about the processing along the occipito-temporal axis that leads from perception of features to perception of objects.

Chapters 2, 3, and 22 described visual processing from the retina to the posterior pole of the occipital lobe, where the primary visual cortex (V1) is situated. The processing of visual images by the brain is not finished at that point. In humans and other primates, information from V1 radiates outward, in the ventral-anterior direction to the temporal lobe and in the dorsal-anterior direction to the parietal lobe.[19] In this chapter we focus mostly on the **ventral pathway**, the processing stream that underlies how we perceive, identify, and remember objects that we see; we also describe one key function of the **dorsal pathway**, motion perception.

V1 is the point of departure for a series of visual processing steps that take place in the secondary visual cortex (V2), then in V4, and from there in the ventrolateral surface of the temporal lobe where a posterior-to-anterior stream continues in a large area known as inferotemporal cortex (IT). IT consists of several subregions; commonly the posterior part is called TEO and the anterior part TE; TE can be further subdivided into posterior and anterior regions, TEp and TEa, respectively (Figure 25.8). As we will see, neurons in this intracortical stream, at locations progressively farther anterior from V1, are selectively activated by increasingly complex visual images. Since the 1980s onward, much effort has been dedicated to understanding neuronal processing in the ventral visual pathway, and we will present some crucial findings.

Deficits in Object Perception

The difference between seeing elementary forms and perceiving objects was first proposed by Hermann Munk in 1881.[20] Munk was the first scientist to perform precise ablations and careful behavioral observations in laboratory conditions, which led to his sharp insights. His subjects were dogs that received either a lesion restricted to the posterior pole of the occipital lobe or a lesion elsewhere, including regions farther anterior and lateral that are homologous with the primate IT. Dogs with bilateral occipital lobe ablation showed complete blindness, bumping into tables and walls. Those with more anterior lesions, sparing the occipital pole, showed what Munk called "psychic blindness"—they did not collide with furniture, yet they did not recognize by vision previously familiar objects.[20] Psychic blindness was interpreted at the time as a loss of visual memory, or loss of visual images stored in the occipital lobe.

The psychic blindness described by Munk has much in common with the **visual agnosia** syndromes occurring in human patients (in Greek, *agnosia* means "loss of knowledge"). A noted case is patient DF, a young woman who suffered brain damage in 1988 as a result of anoxia from carbon monoxide poisoning.[21] DF had no problem grasping objects placed in front of her or moving through the world without bumping into things, because her dorsal visual pathway was intact. She was unable, however, to indicate the size, shape, and orientation of an object, either verbally or manually: She could perform actions related to objects, but she had no explicit knowledge about the objects' identity. Brain scans revealed that her agnosia was the result of damage to the ventral processing stream.

The most remarkable form of human visual agnosia, **prosopagnosia**, is the selective loss of the ability to recognize people's faces. Although people with prosopagnosia are aware that faces are faces—that is, they know the category of the visual image—they fail to identify faces reliably or to achieve a sense of familiarity from seeing faces of

[19] Parker, A. J., and Newsome, W. T. 1998. *Annu. Rev. Neurosci.* 21: 227-277.

[20] Fellman, D. J., and Van Essen, D. C. 1991. *Cereb. Cortex* 1: 1-47.

[21] Munk, H. 1881. *Ueber die Functionen der Grosshirnrinde; gesammelte Mittheilungen aus den Jahren 1877-80.* Hirschwald, Berlin.

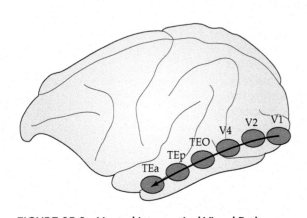

FIGURE 25.8   Ventral Intracortical Visual Pathways. Visual processing areas of the macaque brain. The arrow indicates the posterior-to-anterior flow of information. V1 = primary visual cortex; V2 = secondary visual cortex; V4 = fourth visual cortical area; TEa = anterior part of inferotemporal cortex; TEp = posterior part of inferotemporal cortex; TEO = posterior part of inferotemporal cortex. Parts of the inferotemporal cortex extend to the ventral surface of the temporal lobe, not seen here. Ovals indicate the relative positions, but not the boundaries, of the cortical regions. Analogous processing streams exist in the human brain.

family members, famous persons, and other individuals they previously knew well. They may identify individuals by salient details such as clothing and hairstyle or by nonvisual features such as voice. Although people with prosopagnosia have difficulty forming memories of new faces, they can learn other new objects.

The question has been raised as to whether a deficit in face recognition is truly specific for faces or might be general to other sorts of images that are scanned by the fovea in the same way. The bulk of evidence indicates that a lesion restricted to a specific location in the temporal lobe can produce an agnosia that is genuinely selective to faces.[22] Later we will see that the area whose destruction causes prosopagnosia can be defined as a "face area" by means other than the effects of lesion.

Images That Activate Neurons in the Ventral Stream

Discovery of Responses to Complex Stimuli in Monkeys

In landmark studies, neurons were found in the IT of macaque monkeys that responded selectively to images of behaviorally significant objects, such as hands,[23,24] and additional explorations of IT revealed a set of neurons that responded selectively to faces.[25,26] Thus, there exists a class of temporal lobe neurons that are excited by images of *objects*, not elemental forms such as bars or spots of light (see Chapters 2 and 3).

In humans and monkeys, face identity ("who is it?") and face expression ("what is the state of mind and intention of this individual?") are forms of perception essential to social interaction and survival. Even newborn infants preferentially look at facelike arrangements of features as compared with jumbles of face features or non-biological stimuli, suggesting that our interest in faces is to some extent built into our brain circuitry.[27]

The Special Case of Faces

In the early studies in which face-responsive neurons were found, territories dedicated to this category of stimulus were not detected; only about 30% of neurons were face-responsive.[23,26,28,29] So can we conclude that an area whose principal function is to process such images actually exists? The issue was solved first by identifying with functional magnetic resonance imaging (fMRI) (Box 25.1) a region in the anterior temporal lobe of monkeys in which fMRI signals were elevated selectively by viewing of faces. Once the coordinates were registered, microelectrodes were directed to the same region, where it was found that 97% of neurons responded preferentially to faces (both monkey and human faces) compared with other objects (Figure 25.9).[30] Thus, when correctly targeted, a truly face-selective region can be identified. An elegant experiment established a causal relationship between the activity of face-selective neurons and face perception. The investigators excited small clusters of IT neurons by means of electrical microstimulation while the monkey performed the task of judging whether noisy visual images belonged to "face" or "non-face" categories. Microstimulation of face-selective sites (but not other sites) increased the likelihood of the monkey reporting the presence of a face. The magnitude of the effect depended on the degree of face selectivity of the stimulation site, the size of the stimulated cluster of face-selective neurons, and the exact timing of microstimulation with respect to stimulus onset.[31]

In humans, the physiological evidence for the involvement of the occipito-temporal pathway in object recognition depends largely on brain imaging rather than on electrical recordings. In fMRI experiments, a set of regions in the ventral pathway from occipital to temporal cortex was found to be activated more strongly when individuals viewed real objects as compared with scrambled objects, textures, stationary dot patterns, coherently moving dots, or gratings.[32] When individuals viewed images of objects (faces and cars) broken into blocks, with block size varied from trial to trial (smaller blocks meant greater scrambling), regions that were progressively farther from the occipital pole in the posterior-to-anterior dimension showed less activation as the degree of scrambling increased. These results suggest the existence of a hierarchical axis along which the neuronal properties shift in sensitivity from local object features (which can be conserved even after scrambling) to a more global and holistic representation (the type of representation that is destroyed by scrambling).[33]

[22] Milner, A. D. et al. 1991. *Brain* 114: 405–428

[23] Wada, Y., and Yamamoto, T. 2001. *J. Neurol. Neurosurg. Psychiatry* 71: 254–257.

[24] Desimone, R. et al. 1984. *J. Neurosci.* 4: 2051–2062.

[25] Gross, C. G., Rocha-Miranda, C. E., and Bender, D. B. 1972. *J. Neurophysiol.* 35: 96–111.

[26] Rolls, E. T. 1984. *Hum. Neurobiol.* 3: 209–222.

[27] Perrett, D. I. et al. 1984. *Hum. Neurobiol.* 3: 197–208.

[28] Johnson, M. H. 2005. *Nat. Rev. Neurosci.* 6: 766–774.

[29] Perrett, D. I., Rolls, E. T., and Caan, W. 1982. *Exp. Brain Res.* 47: 329–342.

[30] Baylis, G. C., Rolls, E. T., and Leonard, C. M. 1987. *J. Neurosci.* 7: 330–342.

[31] Tsao, D. Y. et al. 2006. *Science* 311: 670–674.

[32] Afraz, S., Kiani, R., and Esteky, H. 2006. *Nature* 442: 692–695.

[33] Grill-Spector, K. et al. 1998. *Hum. Brain Mapp.* 6: 316–328.

BOX **25.1** Functional Magnetic Resonance Imaging

fMRI has changed neuroscience by allowing investigators to visualize the activation of the brain in healthy people during cognitive tasks. The signal on which the image is based is related to changes in blood volume, oxygen consumption, and blood flow during brain activity. The method relies primarily on measurement of the **blood oxygen level-dependent (BOLD)** signal. As neurons do not have internal reserves for glucose and oxygen, an increase in activity requires more glucose and oxygen to be delivered rapidly through the blood stream. Through a process called the **hemodynamic response**, blood flows to the active neurons and astrocytes at a greater rate than to inactive neurons (see Chapter 10). This extra supply of blood results in a surplus of oxygen-bound hemoglobin in the veins of the active area. The ratio between oxygen-bound and oxygen-free hemoglobin is the BOLD signal obtained by the fMRI machine.

The physical principle for detecting the BOLD signal depends on magnetism: Oxygenated and deoxygenated hemoglobin react differently to the magnetic field that is applied inside the fMRI apparatus. The differential reaction to the magnetic field makes it possible to detect the heightened supply of oxygenated blood present in active brain tissue.

The change in blood flow induced by neuronal activity is not instantaneous; indeed, there is a lag of approximately 1 to 5 seconds. The delay between electrical activity and BOLD signal is known as the **hemodynamic lag**, and it limits the temporal precision with which fMRI can detect neuronal responses to stimuli. The spatial resolution is about 1 mm.

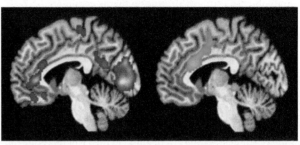

Courtesy of G. Silani

Brain Activity as Revealed by Averaging fMRI Scans across a Group of 20 People. The scans are a view of the midline structures of the right side of the brain in a sagittal plane. To produce the activation shown on the left, participants received pleasant visuo-tactile stimulation; they looked at pictures of agreeable things such as silk and roses while touching the same objects. To produce the activation shown on the right, participants received unpleasant visuo-tactile stimulation; they looked at pictures of disagreeable things such as worms and slugs while touching objects with tactile properties similar to the pictured objects. Areas in which the BOLD signal was significantly higher than that under a control condition (experience of neutral emotions) are denoted in color. Note that the two types of stimulation activated different brain regions, providing some insight into the areas involved with feeling pleasure and disgust.

Presentation of different categories of images activates neurons in different locations.[34] The most category-specific regions are found at the anterior extreme of the ventral pathway in an area known as the **parahippocampal place area** (PPA—where neurons are activated by observation of places, buildings, landscapes) and in the fusiform face area (FFA—activated, as the name implies, by observation of faces).[35,36] This is presumably the center in humans that is homologous with the face-selective region found in monkeys.[30]

A fascinating fMRI experiment suggested that activation in face-selective areas in humans is related to the act of perceiving a face, not just to the processing of images with a facelike form or contour. Individuals viewed "Rubin's vase," a well-known vase–face illusion, for periods of 9 seconds and indicated whether they perceived the vase or else two faces. In those intervals when people perceived faces, there was a larger signal in the face-selective regions of the ventral stream as compared with intervals when they perceived a vase (Figure 25.10). All the while, the physical stimulus remained constant, so the variation in cortical activation could only be correlated with what the individuals perceived.[37]

Perceiving the presence of a face and recognizing the identity of the particular face are related but not equivalent operations. There is evidence that the fusiform face area contributes to both operations. In this region, the magnitude of the fMRI signal is correlated on a trial-by-trial basis with successful identification of the face's owner.[38]

Perceptual Invariance and Neuronal Response Invariance

Although we see a familiar object many times and recognize it each time, its image as it falls on the retina is never exactly the same. If the activity of object-responsive neurons in the temporal lobe truly underlies our identification of objects, one would expect their

[34] Lerner, Y. et al. 2001. *Cereb. Cortex* 11: 287-297.

[35] Grill-Spector, K., and Malach, R. 2004. *Annu. Rev. Neurosci.* 27: 649-677.

[36] Kanwisher, N., and Yovel, G. 2006. *Philos. Trans. R. Soc. Lond., B, Biol. Sci.* 361: 2109-2128.

[37] Downing, P. E. et al. 2006. *Cereb. Cortex* 16: 1453-1461.

[38] Hasson, U. et al. 2001. *J. Cogn. Neurosci.* 13: 744-753.

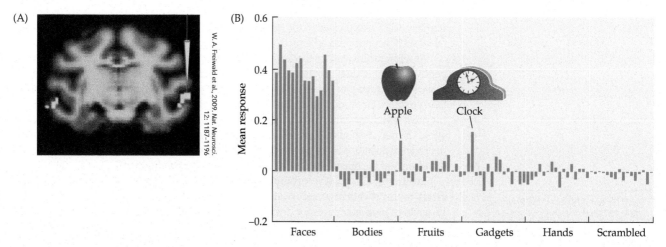

(A)

(B)

W. A. Freiwald et al., 2009. *Nat. Neurosci.* 12: 1187–1196.

FIGURE 25.9 Face-Selective Neurons in Temporal Lobe. (A) Presentation of face images produced a large response in selected areas of the temporal lobe of macaque monkeys. High levels of activity detected in fMRI experiments are colored yellow-red. Electrodes were directed to such areas, as indicated schematically on the right side. (B) Once the electrodes reached the target area, neuronal responses were measured. Six categories of stimulus were presented (pictures of faces, bodies, fruits, gadgets, hands, and scrambled patterns), with 16 individual images per category. The bars give the mean strength of response of all 286 cells tested to all 96 stimuli, and it is clear that most neurons in the selected brain region produced a strong response to face images and much weaker responses to all other categories. The responses to some non-face stimuli, such as the apple and the clock, might have occurred because they contained some facelike features. Mean response (*y*-axis) was calculated as a proportion of each neuron's strongest response to any stimulus. (B after D. Tsao, 2006. *Science* 311: 670–674.)

responses to be to some degree tolerant to changes in viewing conditions that affect object appearance but not identity. Can we confirm such invariance in the human temporal lobe using brain-imaging methods? Each voxel (1 unit of brain volume scanned) in an fMRI experiment reports the strength of activation of many thousands of neurons, giving a spatial resolution far too poor to investigate individual IT neurons (see Chapter 18).

As a way around the spatial constraints, investigators have used an **adaptation procedure** to look for response invariance. The idea is that if the excitation of a neuronal population is related specifically to the viewing of a particular object, then repetition of that image at a high rate will excite the neurons progressively less until their response reaches some low, steady-state level; at that point, the neurons have *adapted*. Next, a new image is presented. If it portrays the same object but is made up of altered elemental features (e.g., size, contrast, or color), then that object will be processed by these same, adapted neurons and the overall

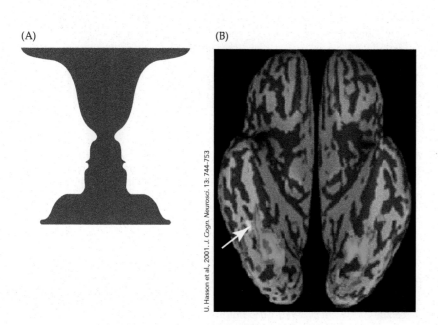

(A)

(B)

U. Hasson et al., 2001. *J. Cogn. Neurosci.* 13: 744–753.

FIGURE 25.10 Brain Activation Directly Correlated with Face Perception. (A) Face-vase illusion. Individuals alternately perceive two faces gazing inward at each other, or else one ornate vase in the middle. It is impossible to perceive the faces and the vase simultaneously. (B) The brain viewed from below. Regions of the ventral surface of the temporal lobe where the signal was stronger when people perceived the vase are in blue; regions where the signal was stronger when people perceived the faces are in yellow-orange. The yellow-orange hotspot, indicated by the arrow, is the fusiform face area. (A after E. Rubin, 1915. *Synsoplevede Figurer: Studier i psykologisk Analyse. Første Del* [*Visually experienced figures: Studies in psychological analysis. Part one*]. Copenhagen and Christiania: Gyldendalske Boghandel, Nordisk Forlag.)

response will be suppressed. If the new image portrays a different object, it will activate a different set of neurons; these, being in the non-adapted state, will give a large response.

As a test for invariance to viewing conditions, the image of one object was shown repetitively to individual people. fMRI signals in a temporal lobe region known as **posterior fusiform** (homologous with the IT in monkeys) continued to adapt even when size, visual field position, direction of illumination, or viewing angle varied from one single image to the next. If viewing conditions remained constant but object identity varied from one image to the next, responses of neurons in this region did not adapt. These results suggest that neuronal populations in the posterior fusiform region fired according to their selectivity for the *identity* of the object, independently of the viewing conditions.[39]

Electrophysiological recordings in monkeys have the single-neuron resolution necessary to investigate response invariance more directly (Figure 25.11). Certain classes of IT neurons in monkeys respond with a similar strength when an image is placed before

[39] Grill-Spector, K. et al. 1999. *Neuron* 24: 187–203.

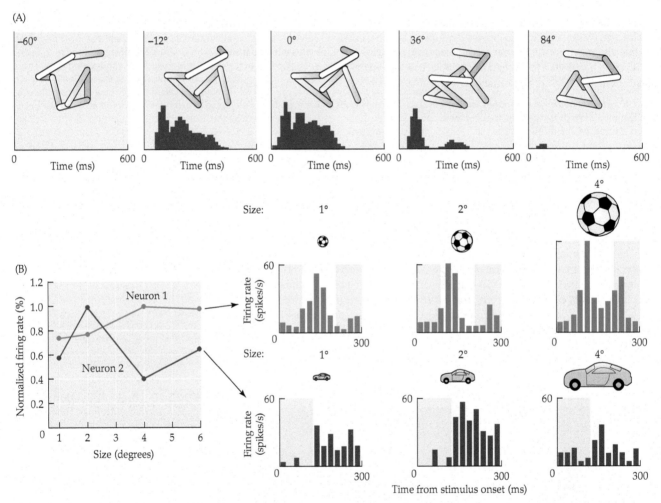

FIGURE 25.11 Responses of Macaque Monkey IT Neurons to Changes in Viewing Angle and Stimulus Size.
(A) Each form resembles a wire paper clip bent into an arbitrary three-dimensional shape. During training, the monkey learned to identify specific wire shapes, with each shape seen from one specific viewing angle. During testing, wire forms were projected onto the screen at the angle familiar to the monkey but also at angles never seen before. The histograms show the activity of one neuron, in firing rate across time, summed over several trials, when a familiar target was presented at different angles (angles of rotation in the horizontal or vertical plane are indicated on each panel). Stimulus onset is at 0 ms. The neuron's response was strong when the form was presented at the familiar viewing angle (central panel; 0°) and at angles ranging from -12° to +36°. For larger rotations, the neuron no longer fired, its response resembling that of unfamiliar objects. Thus, we could say the neuron *recognized* the form unless it was rotated so much as to be unfamiliar. (B) Responses of two IT neurons, one designated in blue and one in red, to presentation of images of a soccer ball and a car. The sizes of the images were changed randomly across presentations, from 1° to 6° of visual field. The graph on the left shows that the neurons fired for the stimulus at levels of 40% to 100% of maximum firing rate even when image size differed. The plots on the right show the two objects at differing sizes. Below each image, the neuronal firing rate, averaged across trials, is plotted for the 300-ms interval immediately after stimulus presentation. (A after N. K. Logothetis et al., 1995. *Curr. Biol.* 5: 552–563; B after D. Zoccolan et al., 2007. *J. Neurosci.* 27: 12292–12307. © 2007 Society for Neuroscience.)

the eyes independently of size, contrast, angle of lighting, blurring, spatial frequency, and position in the visual field.[40] Some of these neurons are excited by a particular face, even when viewed at different angles. Invariance results from exposure to the same object across changing views.[41,42] Theoretical accounts for the generation of invariance have been proposed,[43,44] but collecting adequate experimental data and interpreting the data are difficult. Neuroscientists are currently trying to understand the physiological processes underlying invariance by combining experimental observations with models called artificial neural networks, which are inspired by physics and computer science.[45–47]

Computer programs have now been developed with an impressive ability to classify images rapidly and with a high degree of accuracy.[48] It is not known to what extent the algorithms executed by the artificial neural networks share mechanisms with the processes carried out in the brain.[49]

Dorsal Intracortical Visual Pathways and Motion Detection

While visual perception has been discussed until now in relation to the ventral pathway processing involved in the recognition of objects, another essential function of vision is the analysis of motion. Motion is analyzed by the dorsal, magnocellular–parietal visual pathway (Figure 25.12A; see also Chapter 3). Magnocellular pathway neurons are sensitive to moving stimuli, and this trait is maintained through V1 and V2. From there, the dorsal

[40] Ito, M. et al. 1995. *J. Neurophysiol.* 73: 218-226.

[41] Logothetis, N. K. et al. 1994. *Curr. Biol.* 4: 401-414.

[42] Li, N., and DiCarlo, J. J. 2008. *Science* 321: 1502-1507.

[43] DiCarlo, J. J., and Cox, D. D. 2007. *Trends Cogn. Sci.* 11: 333-341.

[44] Booth, M. C., and Rolls, E. T. 1998. *Cereb. Cortex* 8: 510-523.

[45] Yamins, D. L. and DiCarlo, J. J. 2016. *Nat. Neurosci.* 19: 356-365.

[46] DiCarlo, J. J., Zoccolan D., and Rust, N. C. 2012. *Neuron* 73: 415-434.

[47] Sharpee, T. O. 2016. *Front. Synaptic Neurosci.* 8: 26.

[48] Krizhevsky, A., Sutskever, I., and Hinton, G. E. 2012. In *Advances in Neural Information Processing Systems 25*. Pereira, F. et al. (Eds.). Curran Associates, Inc., pp. 1097-1105.

[49] Baldassi, C. et al. 2016. *Proc. Natl. Acad. Sci. USA* 113: E7655-E7662.

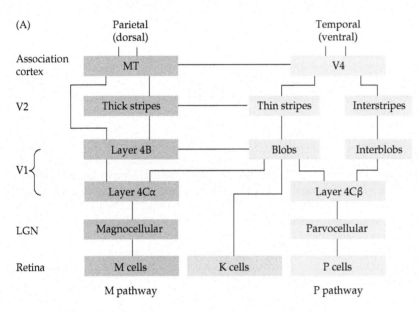

(A)

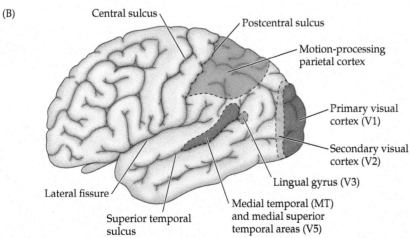

(B)

FIGURE 25.12 Schematic Organization of M, P, and K Channels to Visual Cortex. (A) Functionally distinct layers of the lateral geniculate nucleus (LGN) project to different layers in V1. K cells project to blobs. The M and P cells of 4C may interact preferentially with blob and interblob. Blobs project preferentially to thin stripes in V2. Thin stripes project to V4. Thick stripes in V2 receive input from layer 4B in V1 and project to association area MT (V5). M channels appear to project to dorsal (parietal) visual cortex, where movement is analyzed. P channels project preferentially to area V4, where color vision is processed. Additional details on the architecture of visual cortex are given in Chapter 3. (B) Areas of cortex involved in the dorsal stream of visual processing, as portrayed on a human brain. (A after W. H. Merigan and J. H. R. Maunsell, 1993. *Annu. Rev. Neurosci.* 16: 369-402.)

stream is directed toward the parietal lobe. A key region in the dorsal pathway is the medial temporal (MT) cortex, also known as visual area 5 (V5). Area MT is located in the posterior bank of the dorsal part of the superior temporal sulcus (Figure 25.12B). Selective, bilateral lesion of area MT in humans leads to loss of motion perception (akinetopsia), with other visual functions left intact. One patient described what she saw when pouring a cup of tea: "the fluid appeared to be frozen, like a glacier." She filled the cup over the brim because she could not see the level of liquid rising.[50]

In a comprehensive and elegant series of experiments, Newsome and his colleagues analyzed how the activity of neurons in area MT allows a monkey to assess the direction of movement. In many respects, the results are consistent with those described earlier in the chapter for perception of vibration frequency. The procedure is to teach monkeys to respond to the direction in which a visual stimulus is moving, while cortical recordings are made with a microelectrode. Area MT is retinotopically mapped.[51] Neurons selective for the speed and direction of a moving stimulus are clustered together in columns with a similar preferred direction.[52–55] Such neurons respond poorly or not at all to motion in the opposite, or null, direction. When small regions of MT are chemically lesioned with a neurotoxin, a monkey's ability to detect a moving pattern of dots in a corresponding region of the visual field is impaired.[56]

Area MT is involved in visual tracking. This was shown by experiments in which a monkey was trained to track a moving target with its eyes.[57] The normal pattern of eye movements is seen in the upper record in Figure 25.13, in which the moving target (trajectory begins at time 0) was acquired by a rapid saccade (the downward deflection occurring 200 ms later) and then retained on the fovea by an accurate tracking or smooth pursuit process. After a small injection of neurotoxin (ibotenic acid) into the foveal region of MT cortex, the monkey's ability to track the moving target was markedly impaired. In particular, after the initial saccade, the subsequent tracking velocity was much slower than the target velocity. The deficit is visible in the traces in the lower record in Figure 25.13. That underestimation also applies to the initial saccade made by the lesioned animal. It positioned its eyes as though the estimated velocity were lower than the actual velocity. Somehow, the lesion perturbed the ability of area MT to compute an accurate estimate of target velocity.

How is motion computed in area MT? As stated earlier, cells are clustered into columns of similar preferred direction across the retinotopic map. Thus, the movement of a target across the retina ought to activate those columns aligned with the direction of movement. But moving visual targets will not activate only one such column; they are more likely to exhibit complex patterns of motion that activate many sets of directionally tuned neurons to varying degrees. Thus, it will require some form of neural computation to derive a movement vector.

Newsome and his colleagues studied the neural arithmetic performed by multiple direction columns, using electrical microstimulation to alter eye movements in trained monkeys.[58] The columnar organization means that the cells affected by microstimulation had similar functional properties. The microelectrode that recorded the preferred direction of a column of cells was then used to pass amounts of current to activate that same column during a target-tracking

[50] Zihl, J., Von Cramon, D., and Mai, N. 1983. *Brain* 106: 313-340.

[51] Maunsell, J. H., and Newsome, W. T. 1987. *Annu. Rev. Neurosci.* 10: 363-401.

[52] Zeki, S. M. 1974. *J. Physiol.* 236: 549-573.

[53] Maunsell, J. H. R., and Van Essen, D. C. 1983. *J. Neurophysiol.* 49: 1127-1147.

[54] Albright, T. D. 1984. *J. Neurophysiol.* 52: 1106-1130.

[55] Malonek, D., Tootell, R. B. H., and Grinvald, A. 1994. *Proc. R. Soc. Lond. B, Biol. Sci.* 258: 109-119.

[56] Newsome, W. T., and Pare, E. B. 1988. *J. Neurosci.* 8: 2201-2211.

[57] Dursteler, R. M., Wurtz, R. H., and Newsome, W. T. 1987. *J. Neurophysiol.* 57: 1262-1287.

[58] Groh, J. M., Born, R. T., and Newsome, W. T. 1997. *J. Neurosci.* 17: 4312-4330.

FIGURE 25.13 Involvement of Area MT in Tracking Visual Motion. A monkey was trained to track a moving target (stimulus path shown by red line), and its eye position relative to the target is shown in the upper record. After an initial saccade to center the target on the fovea (the rapid downward eye deflection), the eye closely followed the target path. After injection of a neurotoxin in area MT (lower record), the initial saccade was too large and overshot the target, and subsequent tracking was slower than required, as though the computation of target speed were faulty. (After M. R. Dursteler et al., 1987. *J. Neurophysiol.* 57: 1262-1287.)

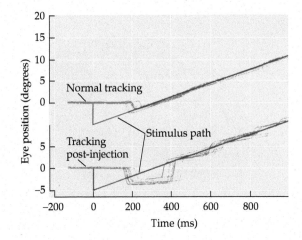

eye movement. The tracking eye movement was compared with and without electrical stimulation to ask how components of the visual motion map sum. Eye position tracked target position closely in the control condition (Figure 25.14A). When electrical stimulation activated an MT column whose directional preference was different from that of the moving target, the resulting eye movement tracked somewhere between the actual direction of the target and the preferred direction of the stimulated cells. The stimulation "pulled" the monkey's eye movement toward the direction associated with the stimulated cells (Figure 25.14B).

The conclusion is that the vectorial average of the activated direction columns ultimately sets the eye movement direction. An appealing feature of these experiments is that the monkey's behavior (eye movements) is a direct measure of the analysis made by higher centers in the cortex. Similar vector averaging will be described for motor cortex in Chapter 26.[59]

Additional insights into the function of area MT came from experiments in which the monkey viewed sequential pairs of random dot stimuli moving in one of four possible directions (Figure 25.15A).[60] The first stimulus was called the sample; it was analogous to what we referred to as the base stimulus in the fingertip vibration experiments. It was followed after a brief delay by a second stimulus referred to as the test, analogous to the comparison stimulus in the fingertip vibration experiment. At the end of each trial, the monkey pressed one of two buttons to indicate whether the direction of motion of the test stimulus was the same as or different from that of the sample. A microelectrode for recording and stimulating was placed in an MT column containing neurons tuned to a specific direction (Figure 25.15B). On trials with no electrical stimulation of area MT, the monkey performed nearly perfectly because the difference in direction between the sample and the nonmatching test stimuli was large (at least 90°). On some trials, microstimulation was applied in area MT during presentation of the sample stimulus; this biased the monkey to choose, as the match, a test stimulus whose motion matched the preferred direction of the stimulated column rather than the direction of the sample stimulus (Figure 25.15C). This experiment indicates that the neuronal activity inserted into the brain through the electrode can be stored and used for future comparison, much like what was shown in the vibration working memory task described earlier in the chapter.

[59] Robinson, D. A., and Fuchs, A. F. 1969. *J. Neurophysiol.* 32: 637–648.

[60] Cohen, R., and Newsome, W. T. 2004. *Curr. Opin. Neurobiol.* 14: 1–9.

(A) No microstimulation of column

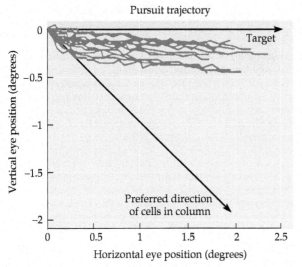

(B) With microstimulation of column

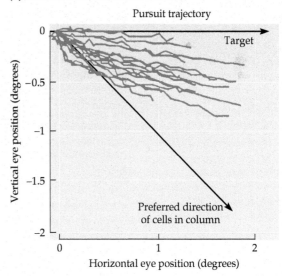

FIGURE 25.14 The Direction of Eye Movements Can Be Altered by Electrical Stimulation in Area MT. (A) Eye movements were recorded in response to a moving visual target. Earlier, an electrode had been inserted into area MT, and the preferred direction of cells in that location was noted. This preferred direction differed from that of the moving target. (B) When this location in area MT was stimulated electrically, the resulting eye movements were biased in the preferred direction of cells in the stimulated region. These results suggest that visual motion is computed as the vector sum of several preferred directions in area MT. (After J. M. Groh et al., 1997. *J. Neurosci.* 17: 4312–4330. © 1997 Society for Neuroscience.)

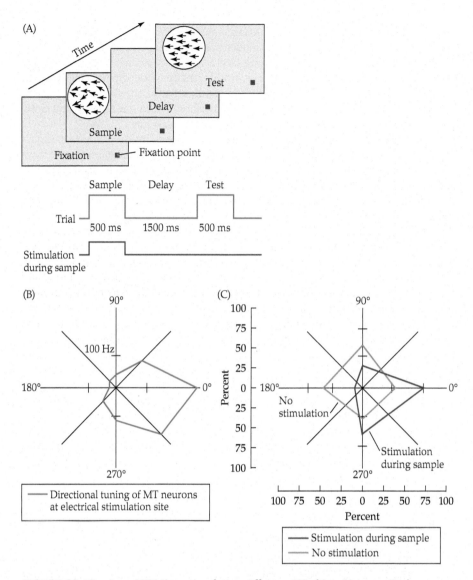

FIGURE 25.15 Area MT Microstimulation Affects a Working Memory Task.
(A) Schematic illustration of the task. After monkeys fixated on the small red square, they were presented with a random dot stimulus for 500 ms (sample). The stimulus consisted of dots moving in a direction determined by a probability distribution whose mean was in one of the four cardinal directions (up, down, left, right). Following a 1500-ms delay period with no image, the test stimulus was presented for 500 ms. The test stimulus consisted of dots moving coherently in either the same direction as in the sample, or in the opposite direction. The monkeys indicated whether the test stimulus matched the direction of the sample by pressing a button. For each sample direction, half of the test stimuli were in the same direction as the sample and half were in the opposite direction. On half of the trials, microstimulation was applied during the sample period. (B) Direction tuning of a sample MT multi-unit site at which electrical stimulation was applied. Firing rate (action potentials/s) is plotted in relation to moving dot direction. The preferred direction of the cells at this site was for motion to the right or down and to the right. (C) Behavioral data from one experiment. The plot shows the percentage of trials on which the monkey reported that the test matched the direction of the sample for each of the four possible sample directions. In the no stimulation condition (green line), the monkey reported a match roughly 50% of the time for all four directions, leading to an average of about 90% correct, as the test actually matched the sample exactly half the time. When microstimulation was applied (red line) to the same site whose tuning is depicted in (B), the monkey reported a match for nearly every trial in which the test stimulus was rightward and for most trials when the test stimulus was downward. By contrast, the monkey almost never reported a match when the test was leftward. This outcome indicates that microstimulation during presentation of the sample biased the monkey's perception of the motion toward the preferred direction of the stimulated cells. (After M. R. Cohen and W. T. Newsome, 2004. *Curr. Opin. Neurobiol.* 14: 169–177, based on J. W. Bisley et al., 2001. *J. Neurophysiol.* 85: 187–196.)

Transformation from Elements to Percepts

Merging of Features

We now return to the discussion of the ventral stream, in which investigators work to understand how neurons in the IT cortex build up responses to complex shapes.[61,62] One set of studies has focused on the selectivity of many of these neurons for two-dimensional boundary shape. The experiments examined posterior processing stages in IT (areas TEO and posterior TEp; see Figure 25.8). For each neuron studied, the monkey was presented in rapid succession with about 1000 stimuli in which shape characteristics varied in small steps to provide a rich and quantifiable dataset. From the responses to the full stimulus set, neurons were fitted with tuning curves. The main result was that combinations of elementary forms, such as oriented curves and contour fragments, formed the tuning curves of these neurons.

In further experiments, three-dimensional shapes were used. Since this entailed an even larger set of potential stimuli, the investigators developed a clever technique whereby new generations of stimuli evolved continuously according to neuronal responsiveness to the stimuli in the previous generation.[61,62] The new generation contained combinations of features that previously were found to excite the neuron. The method allowed the experimenters to quickly converge on the optimal stimulus shape for every neuron. The main result was that the way the IT neurons encoded both two- and three-dimensional images was consistent with a buildup of complex properties based on the integration of simpler properties.

Speed of Processing

The operations necessary to extract meaning from an image—feature selection, recombination, comparison with memory—invoke the idea of an arduous and time-consuming process, yet visual analysis can be effortless and fast. When presented with images that are flashed for as little as 20 to 80 ms, people can make complex judgments about the content of the scene before them. They can reliably determine whether or not the scene contains an animal (motor response: "go") or does not ("no-go"). In a different task, they can determine the presence or absence of food. How much time does the brain need to extract this information? Reaction measures, such as "go" versus "no-go," are imprecise because they include the time required for response execution. A better approach is to look for the first sign in the brain's electrical activity that distinguishes between go versus no-go trials. A scalp potential related to response inhibition on no-go trials becomes evident roughly 150 ms after stimulus onset.[63] Considering that responses begin in V1 at 30 to 100 ms after stimulus onset,[64] we can conclude that the intracortical processing that leads to extraction of high-level image content can be accomplished in some tens of milliseconds.

Fast neuronal processing has been seen in the monkey ventral stream, consistent with human reaction times. For instance, in the face-selective area of anterior temporal lobe, responses distinguish the presence of a face versus another category of image as soon as 130 ms after stimulus onset. The same population of responding neurons identifies the current face from among all faces in the stimulus library 60 ms later.[31]

Normally, inspection of a visual scene is more extended in time, so the claim cannot be made that analysis always involves just one fast pass through the cortex. The timing measures reveal the capacity for incoming signals to rapidly access stored knowledge (for instance, the go/no-go task requires comparison of the new image to the storehouse of what animals look like) and show that any given stage of processing can operate rapidly.

Forms of Coding

We have referred to neuronal coding in a simplified manner, implying that a neuron fires or does not fire for any given stimulus. Closer inspection of neuronal firing shows that this simplification is not accurate. What are the detailed firing patterns of individual neurons, and how do neurons work together to represent the visual world? Are objects represented by activity in a relatively small number of neurons that are each selective for the shape or identity of a specific object (i.e., a sparse code), or are they represented by a pattern of activity across a large number of less selective neurons (i.e., a population code)?

[61] Brincat, S. L., and Connor, C. E. 2004. *Nat. Neurosci.* 7: 880-886.

[62] Yamane, Y. et al. 2008. *Nat. Neurosci.* 11: 1352-1360.

[63] Thorpe, S. J., Fize, D., and Marlot, C. 1996. *Nature* 381: 520-522.

[64] Schmolesky, M. T. et al. 1998. *J. Neurophysiol.* 79: 3272-3278.

The problem is intriguing and challenging. Intuition would suggest that at posterior levels, close to V1, information is encoded by the activity of a very large set of neurons. Since, at anterior levels, neurons are selective to composite features, the coding of an image would be expected to become sparser—a smaller proportion of neurons would be active, with each neuron's activity specifying the presence of some complex visual property. But what happens when the current stimulus matches the preferred stimulus of an entire population?

The experiment described earlier in which the fusiform face area of monkeys was explored provides the beginning of an answer.[31] The region of interest in the anterior temporal lobe was first identified using fMRI responses to face images. Electrodes were advanced to the responding region. Individual neurons were found to respond with different magnitudes to a wide variety of faces so that the exact identity of the presented face was encoded by a population of neurons. By the relative magnitude of response in the population of 94 neurons, it was possible for the experimenter to "decode" which of 96 possible faces was presented on a given trial with an accuracy of 74%.[31]

The distribution of response magnitudes across the population is not the only coding mechanism. One study found that neurons in the monkey IT carried information about the category of stimulus according to *when* they fire.[65] Many cells responded to human and non-primate animal faces with comparable magnitudes but responded significantly more quickly to human faces than to non-primate animal faces. Differences in onset latency may be used to increase the coding capacity as well as to enhance or suppress information about particular object groups by time-dependent modulation.

Top-Down Inputs

Our description of functional processing in the ventral pathway portrayed a cascade of signals from V1 toward the anterior temporal lobe, a so-called downstream flow; this direction of flow is also called feedforward. But information also travels in the anterior–posterior direction—that is, from the frontal cortex and the hippocampus to the temporal lobe and from the temporal lobe back to the occipital lobe. Thus, neurons at every processing center receive feedback from neurons in downstream centers. Understanding of the roles of these **top-down inputs** (to introduce yet more jargon) is still incomplete, but recent work has pointed to several functions.

Imagining or recalling a visual stimulus that is not currently being viewed can produce activation in V1, as revealed by fMRI.[66,67] Since disruption of V1 activity by transcranial magnetic stimulation disrupts visual recall, this activity must constitute one component of the recall of visual memories.[68] Given that the activation cannot originate in the retina, investigators argue that responsibility for re-evoking V1 activity must lie with top–down inputs.

Modulation of cortical processing by attention also is believed to be a top–down function. Directing individuals' attention to different locations in the visual field enhances fMRI signals in cortical areas that are retinotopically aligned with the attended location and inhibits signals in cortical areas that are aligned with the unattended location.[69-71] Attention to objects and faces enhances activation, measured by fMRI, in object- and face-selective regions, respectively.[72-74]

People, as well as monkeys, can readily learn that the presence of one specific image predicts the appearance of a second specific image a short time later (e.g., a plate, then food). Top–down inputs seem to be critical to the formation of associations between image pairs. In an experiment performed in monkeys, recordings were made simultaneously from neurons in two IT areas—area TE, and a region in perirhinal cortex just anterior to TE—while the animals learned associations between pairs of shapes.[75-77] Even in naïve animals, neurons normally fired for specific stimuli, which allowed the experimenters to select two images, image A, "preferred" by the perirhinal neuron, and image B, "preferred" by the TE neuron. The non-preferred stimuli evoked little response before training. Then, the animals began to learn the association: Image A was used as a cue for the appearance of image B. As the monkeys learned that A predicted B, TE neurons began to respond to image A, the cue. The key finding is the relative timing of spikes. When image A appeared, perirhinal neurons responded *before* TE neurons. When image B appeared soon thereafter, perirhinal neurons responded *after* the TE neurons. Thus, TE neurons received signals about their initially preferred stimulus, B, through a posterior-to-anterior flow of visual sensory

[65] Kiani, R., Esteky, H., and Tanaka, K. 2004. *J. Neurophysiol.* 94: 1587-1596.

[66] Ress, D., Backus, B. T., and Heeger, D. J. 2000. *Nat. Neurosci.* 3: 940-945.

[67] Kastner, S. et al. 1999. *Neuron* 22: 751-761.

[68] Kosslyn, S. M. et al. 1999. *Science* 284: 167-170.

[69] Brefczynski, J. A., and DeYoe, E. A. 1999. *Nat. Neurosci.* 2: 370-374.

[70] Macaluso, E., Frith, C. D., and Driver, J. 2000. *Science* 289: 1206-1208.

[71] Tootell, R. B., and Hadjikhani, N. 2000. *Nat. Neurosci.* 3: 206-208.

[72] Avidan, G. et al. 2003. *Neuroimage* 19: 308-318.

[73] O'Craven, K. M., Downing, P. E., and Kanwisher, N. 1999. *Nature* 401: 584-587.

[74] Wojciulik, E., Kanwisher, N., and Driver, J. 1998. *J. Neurophysiol.* 79: 1574-1578.

[75] Naya, Y., Sakai, K., and Miyashita, Y. 1996. *Proc. Natl. Acad. Sci. USA* 93: 2664-2669.

[76] Tomita, H. et al. 1999. *Nature* 401: 699-703.

[77] Naya, Y., Yoshida, M., and Miyashita, Y. 2001. *Science* 291: 661-664.

information, while they received signals that cued the future appearance of stimulus A by an anterior-to-posterior flow of information. Additional experiments identified the frontal cortex as the source of the top–down information flow during cued recall.

Combining Sensory Modalities

Accessing Knowledge by Vision and Touch

Outside the controlled laboratory environment, our experience of the world (or the experience of a monkey or rat) depends on integrating signals from multiple senses. In daily life, once we are familiar with the combined sensory properties of an object, we can recognize that object (a banana, let's say) independently of the modality by which we receive the sensory signal—by sight, texture, shape, or taste. The fact that our knowledge can be accessed and triggered through multiple sensory systems leads to the prediction that some regions of the brain must receive convergent input from several unimodal sensory pathways and, by virtue of that convergence, generate multisensory representations of the world.

The experiment in Figure 25.16 explores the involvement of the cerebral cortex in recognizing an object through multiple sensory modalities.[78] Rats were trained to judge the orientation of a circular object 10 cm in diameter and composed of raised parallel bars alternately colored white and black (see Figure 25.16A). Object orientation was reset by a rotating motor on each trial. When presented with an orientation from 90° (vertical) to 45°, the rat could get a juice reward by licking the left spout; when presented with an orientation from 0° (horizontal) to 45°, the rat could get a juice reward at the right spout (see Figure 25.16B). On each trial, a set of computer-controlled transparent panels and light-emitting diodes allowed the rat to explore the oriented bars through the visual modality alone, using its whiskers in the tactile modality alone, or using both the visual and tactile modalities together. Angles varied in small steps between 0° and 90°. The psychometric performance curves in Figure 25.16C show the proportion of trials in which the rats judged the orientation as vertical when they

[78] Nikbakht, N. et al. 2018. *Neuron* 97: 626-639. e8.

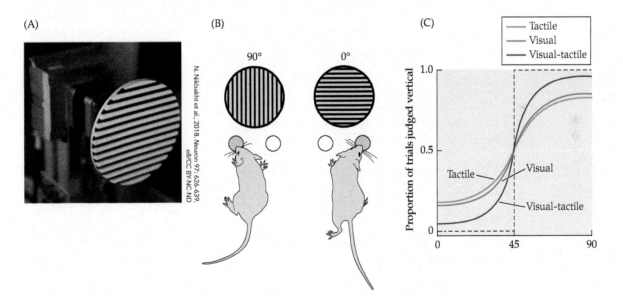

FIGURE 25.16 Visual-Tactile Orientation Categorization Task. (A) Front-side view of the object examined by the rat. Behind the black and white circular object is the rotating motor that sets the grating orientation. (B) Rats were trained to categorize orientations from 90° to 45° in one category and from 0° to 45° in another category. They indicated the category by licking at the left or right juice spouts, and only correct choices were rewarded with juice. Two sample trials, with 90° and 0° angles, are shown. (C) Psychometric curves plot the average performance of rats, across many thousands of trials, in judging the object's orientation as vertical using the three modality conditions: the visual modality alone, the tactile modality alone, or the visual and tactile modalities together. The gray dotted dashed line shows the psychometric curve that would correspond to perfect performance of the task. (B,C after N. Nikbakht et al., 2018. *Neuron* 97: 626-639. e8/CC BY-NC-ND.)

encountered the object using the three different modalities. If the rats could avoid errors even for angles near the boundary of 45°, the psychometric curves would look like the gray dashed line, but animals and humans never generate such an "ideal observer" step function; instead, curves usually take the sigmoid (S-shaped) forms seen in the figure. Note that the visual and tactile modalities alone supported similar levels of performance, whereas the two modalities together provided much better orientation judgment.

Convergence of Sensory Pathways in Association Cortex

Where in the brain do the two distinct sensory channels of vision and touch "work together"? The most likely cortical region would be one receiving input from visual and somatosensory areas. The posterior parietal cortex (PPC) is situated between the somatosensory cortex, which receives tactile input, and the visual cortex (Figure 25.17A) and is a target of projections from both. Responses of two neurons in PPC from tactile, visual, and visual-tactile trials are shown in Figure 25.17B. For the neuron in the left panel, firing rate varied smoothly in relation to the angle of the stimulus. For the neuron in the right panel, firing rate differed sharply according to whether the stimulus was in the horizontal (0–45°) or vertical (45–90°) category; firing did not vary in relation to angles within a category. Both of the examined neurons in PPC, whether they encoded object angle by a graded code (left panel) or object category by a steplike code (right panel), did so independently of the sensory channel(s) through which the rat encountered the object. Indeed, each of the hundreds of studied neurons showed this same property: they were all equally excited by the two sensory channels. The cortical circuit that could produce modality-independent responses is shown in a highly schematic fashion in Figure 25.17C, where purely visual and purely tactile neurons converge on a population that combines the two modalities.

For rodents, vision and touch have likely evolved together to explore the shape, form, and spatial properties of the environment. A rodent might need to maneuver through oriented bars (think of a storm drain along the street), whether those bars are seen or felt. In general, the brain's capacity to call up knowledge about things independently of sensory input channel requires a stage of processing in which the same information is encoded by diverse sensory channels. Regions of cortex that, like PPC, receive projections from early sensory processing areas are referred to as **association cortex**. The functions of association cortical regions

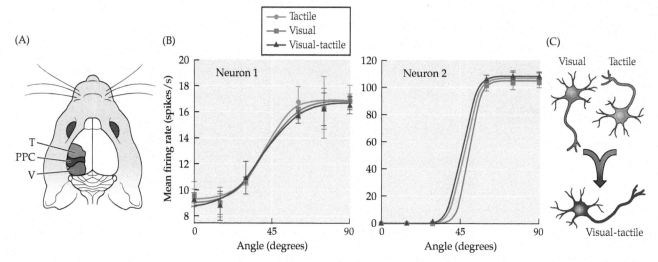

FIGURE 25.17 Encoding of Stimulus Orientation and Stimulus Category in PPC.
(A) The posterior parietal cortex (PPC; red) is located between the visual cortex (V; blue) and somatosensory cortex (T; green), which receives tactile information. The same organization is found in the right hemisphere (not shown). (B) Firing rates computed during stimulus exploration for two PPC neurons in tactile (T), visual (V), and visual-tactile (VT) trials. Error bars are the standard error of the mean (SEM). (C) Proposed scheme for how two unimodal sensory representations may converge to produce a supramodal object representation, like that in PPC. (After N. Nikbakht et al., 2018. *Neuron* 97: 626–639. e8/CC BY-NC-ND.)

can be inferred both from the deficit that emerges when such regions are damaged and from neuronal properties monitored during behavior. A principal function of association cortex is to create representations of the real world using sensory messages as the building blocks. When you feel for your chiming cell phone in your cluttered laptop bag, your percept is that of the external objects, not of your own fingertips—though it is, of course, in the fingertip skin receptors that the tactile information originates. Thus, two sensory modalities, the acoustic tone and the tactile shape, call up the same body of knowledge—the phone.

The rat visual-tactile orientation experiment highlights two properties that underlie the construction of perception through intracortical processing. First, the neuronal responses in PPC are identical across the three sensory modality conditions. Thus, PPC holds the same object representation independently of the input channel. Second, neuronal responses are not "hard-wired," but instead are generated according to behavioral needs. While PPC could receive orientation-tuned signals from earlier stages of visual cortical processing (see Chapters 2 and 3), the reward rule boundary of 45° was set arbitrarily, and its neuronal correlate must also be generated to meet ongoing behavioral demands.

SUMMARY

- All information available about the external world is present in sensory receptors, but sensory signals are perceived as meaningful real-world objects only after elaboration of these signals within the cerebral cortex.

- The sensing, perception, and judgment of a vibration applied to the fingertip has proven to be a useful inquiry. Monkeys can be trained to compare the frequencies of two sequential vibrations, the base stimulus and the comparison stimulus.

- Either the base or comparison stimulus, or both, can be replaced by a train of electrical pulses delivered to somatosensory cortex. The monkeys sense the artificial stimuli as being natural.

- Neurons in S1 encode the base stimulus and the comparison stimulus separately, showing no memory trace or comparison mechanism. Neurons in S2 and in the frontal cortex carry a memory trace for the base stimulus.

- During the comparison stimulus, neurons in the frontal cortex show an explicit computation of the relation between the two stimuli.

- In the premotor cortex, the result of the comparison is transformed into the preparation of the motor act. Primary motor cortex (M1) neurons show no sensory activity but execute the decision transmitted to them.

- Object recognition in the visual modality depends on processing in the ventral pathway, which courses in an anterior direction from the occipital lobe to the inferior temporal lobe (IT).

- Lesions in the ventral pathway can produce highly specific losses in the ability to identify objects.

- In monkeys and humans there are regions dedicated to the processing of faces. Activity in such areas is necessary and sufficient to produce the percept of a face.

- An object may activate a neuron in the inferior temporal lobe (IT) even when viewing conditions change, a property known as invariance.

- The dorsal intracortical pathway proceeds from the occipital lobe to the parietal lobe. Along this pathway, area MT encodes the direction of motion of objects in the visual scene.

- Although it is computationally complex and involves multiple stages, processing of visual images can occur remarkably rapidly.

- Top-down inputs course in the anterior-to-posterior direction and are involved with attention, learning, and recall of earlier images that is cued without the image itself.

- Inputs from multiple primary sensory cortical regions converge in association cortical regions, such as posterior parietal cortex (PPC) in rats. In association cortex, the neuronal representations of encountered objects can be evoked by input from multiple sensory modalities, singly or in combination.

Suggested Reading

General Reviews

DiCarlo. J. J., and Cox, D. D. 2007. Untangling invariant object recognition. *Trends Cogn. Sci.* 11: 333–341.

Grill-Spector, K., and Malach, R. 2004. The human visual cortex. *Annu. Rev. Neurosci.* 27: 649–677.

Kording, K. P., and Wolpert, D. M. 2006. Bayesian decision theory in sensorimotor control. *Trends Cogn. Sci.* 10: 319–326.

Krubitzer, L. 1995. The organization of neocortex in mammals: are species differences really so different? *Trends Neurosci.* 18: 408–417.

Landy, M. S., Banks, M. S., and Knill, D. C. 2011. Ideal-observer models of cue integration. In *Sensory Cue Integration*, Trommershauser, J., Kording, K., and Landy, M. S. (Eds.) Oxford University Press, pp. 5–29.

Parker, A. J., and Newsome, W. T. 1998. Sense and the single neuron: probing the physiology of perception. *Annu. Rev. Neurosci.* 21: 227–277.

Romo, R., and Salinas, E. 2001. Touch and go: Decision-making mechanisms in somatosensation. *Annu. Rev. Neurosci.* 24: 107–137.

Original Papers

Brody, C. D., Hernandez, A., Zainos, A., and Romo, R. 2003. Timing and neural encoding of somatosensory parametric working memory in macaque prefrontal cortex. *Cereb. Cortex* 13: 1196–1207.

Cavada, C., and Goldman-Rakic, P. S. 1989. Posterior parietal cortex in rhesus monkey: II. Evidence for segregated corticocortical networks linking sensory and limbic areas with the frontal lobe. *J. Comp. Neurol.* 287: 422–445.

Ernst, M. O., and Banks, M. S. 2002. Humans integrate visual and haptic information in a statistically optimal fashion. *Nature* 415: 429–433.

Jacobs, R. A. 1999. Optimal integration of texture and motion cues to depth. *Vision Res.* 39: 3621–3629.

Kolb, B., and Walkey, J. 1987. Behavioral and anatomical studies of the posterior parietal cortex in the rat. *Behav. Brain Res.* 23: 127–145.

Lak, A., Arabzadeh, E., Harris, J., and Diamond, M. 2010. Correlated physiological and perceptual effects of noise in a tactile stimulus. *Proc. Natl. Acad. Sci. USA* 17: 7981–7986.

Olcese, U., Iurilli, G., and Medini, P. 2013. Cellular and synaptic architecture of multisensory integration in the mouse neocortex. *Neuron* 79: 579–593.

Romo, R., Hernandez, A., Zainos, A., Brody, C. D., and Lemus, L. 2000. Sensing without touching: Psychophysical performance based on cortical microstimulation. *Neuron* 26: 273–278.

Tsao, D. Y., Freiwald, W. A., Tootell, R. B., and Livingstone, M. S. 2006. A cortical region consisting entirely of face-selective cells. *Science* 311: 670–674.

CHAPTER 26

Initiation and Control of Coordinated Muscular Movements

As with organization in the visual system, the organization of motor control is hierarchical. Smaller, simpler elements are integrated into more complex circuits at higher levels of the nervous system. The motor cells in the spinal cord, which produce all of the body's movements, are controlled by sensory input, feedback loops, and descending motor commands. A simple automatic type of movement is the stretch reflex, such as the knee jerk, in which only two types of neurons are directly involved: a sensory neuron that fires impulses when the muscle is stretched (by the tap of a hammer) and a motor cell that supplies muscles that make the leg move forward. Even at this level, multiple connections of intermediary neurons are necessary for more coordinated contractions of flexors and extensors on both sides of the body. More complex behaviors can be generated by central pattern generators in the central nervous system (CNS). Thus, respiratory movements, which are unfailing, regular, and automatic, arise by use of a motor program that depends on rhythmical activity of command neurons in the brainstem. At the same time, the rate and depth of respiration are modulated by sensory inputs, as well as by voluntary and involuntary commands from higher centers, including the cortex. Walking and running are mediated by programmed neuronal interactions in the spinal cord and in higher centers. These ensure that limbs move appropriately, with the correct phase relations.

Voluntary movements, such as bringing a cup of tea to one's mouth, involve the recruitment of collateral components of motor control, namely anticipation and planning. The trajectory must be designed, synergistic muscles contracted appropriately, and movements rapidly initiated in parts of the body to compensate for shifts in balance and the effect of gravity. When the head and eyes are moved, say to scan the horizon, corollary commands have to be made to allow the image of the world in the mind's eye to remain stationary. For smooth and goal-directed actions to be accomplished, for the head to stay upright and the body to fight against gravity, complex feedback loops are required. They comprise interactions of structures such as the cerebellum, basal ganglia, vestibular apparatus, thalamus, and cortex, as well as stretch reflexes. Sensorimotor integration is carried out in the motor cortex, premotor cortex, and parietal association cortex. Certain individual cortical neurons code for movement of the arm in a particular direction and are arranged in columns like those in the visual cortex.

Cerebellar deficits cause a loss of coordination and balance. Diseases that affect the basal ganglia give rise to spontaneous, disruptive motor outputs and a reduction of voluntary movement. Many aspects of motor control still remain obscure, owing to the complexity of the circuitry and the synaptic mechanisms. It is still not known how the decision is made to pick up a cup of tea or how the cup is moved to one's mouth without spilling a drop, whether the cup is full or half-empty.

For a leech or a fish to swim, for an owl or a cat to catch a mouse, for a bear or a child to ride a bicycle, a blackbird to trill, or a pianist to play a Beethoven sonata, muscles of the body must be brought into play in rapid succession, in a coordinated manner. The intricate mechanisms required for executing even a simple movement, let alone riding a bicycle, pose a major challenge to neurobiologists. How you point your finger is far harder to analyze than how you perceive a moving object. The reason is that in a sensory system such as vision, the stimulus is well defined and one can follow signals from their inception as they spread from photoreceptors to second-, third-, of fourth-order synapses and through the cortex. There, neurons encode in their impulses abstract information about the stimulus, such as a face in the visual field (see Chapter 25). The progression is from simple to ever more complex. By contrast, one cannot in the motor system simply follow signals downward from the top (the cortex) to find out how a voluntary movement of the body is carried out, let alone initiated. The ultimate events in the motor system can be readily studied in terms of muscles, motor nerve cells (motoneurons), and simple reflexes (Figure 26.1). But the descending influences that play upon them arise from a multitude of diverse centers above the level of the spinal cord that also interact with one another. Central mechanisms that underlie our ability to appose our thumb to the digits of the same hand in rapid succession require motor programs and coordinated activity of many separate descending and ascending systems. Our future ability to understand such events depends on knowledge of how the component parts of the motor system, spinal cord, brainstem, vestibular apparatus, cerebral cortex, cerebellum, and basal ganglia work together to plan and execute movements.

As in sensory systems, principles of organization have emerged to simplify the task. Already mentioned is the hierarchical arrangement of motor activation. Increasingly complex motor tasks are organized in successively higher centers. A second principle is that many motor tasks rely for their execution on continual adjustment by feedback. Both negative

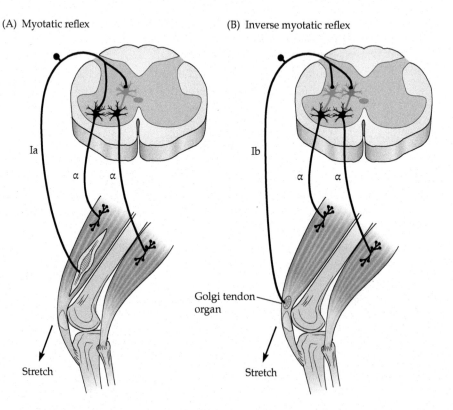

(A) Myotatic reflex

(B) Inverse myotatic reflex

FIGURE 26.1 Organization of Synaptic Connections for Spinal Reflexes. The spinal cord is shown in transverse section, with inhibitory interneurons in blue. (A) In the myotatic, or stretch, reflex, stretch of the muscle spindle generates impulses that travel along Group Ia afferent fibers to the spinal cord and produce monosynaptic excitation of α motoneurons to that same muscle. Impulses also excite interneurons that, in turn, inhibit motoneurons supplying the antagonist muscles. (B) Stretch or contraction of the muscle pulls on the tendon and generates impulses in the Golgi tendon organ's Ib afferent fibers. The Ib fibers inhibit motoneurons that supply the same muscle and excite the antagonists. This is known as the *inverse myotatic reflex*.

and positive feedback loops through the basal ganglia, vestibular apparatus, and cerebellum are essential for the timing and coordination of cortical motor programs. An extra complication in programming motor tasks is that every movement of limbs, trunk, or head occurs in the gravitational field. Hence, the execution of a voluntary movement (for example, raising one leg) must take into account the influence of gravity.

We begin this chapter with spinal reflexes and the control of muscles, and then describe how groups of neurons in the spinal cord and brainstem produce rhythmic, coordinated movements of respiration and locomotion. Next we discuss descending influences from the motor cortex, vestibular apparatus, cerebellum, and basal ganglia.

Adrian, whose name has cropped up in earlier chapters, long ago posed problems regarding motor systems, in sentences that could not be improved on: (1) "The chief function of the central nervous system is to send messages to the muscles which will make the body move effectively as a whole, and for this to take place the contraction of each muscle must be capable of delicate adjustment."[1] and (2) "We may learn a skilled movement by employing certain muscles and therefore certain groups of nerve cells in the motor area of the brain, but when we have learnt it we can carry out the movement with an entirely different set of muscles and nerve cells—we can write our name with a pencil held between the toes when we have learnt to do it with the fingers. We can draw a triangle small or large when we have learned its shape."[2]

The Motor Unit

Sherrington called the spinal motoneuron the **final common path** because all the neural influences that have to do with movement or posture converge on it. The principal motor nerve cells of the spinal cord are called α motoneurons. Smaller γ motoneurons regulate the sensitivity of stretch receptors in muscle, as we will discuss later. (Note: The terms α and γ arose from an early classification of conduction velocity; see Chapter 8.) A single α motoneuron innervates a group of muscle fibers, and together the motoneuron and its target fibers form a functional element known as the **motor unit**. The number of muscle fibers in a motor unit ranges from a few—for example, in muscles used to extend or flex the fingers—to several thousand, in the large weight-bearing muscles of the limbs.

When a motoneuron fires action potentials, all the muscle fibers to which it is connected contract at once. The smoothness of movements is brought about by varying the number and timing of motor units brought into play.[1] Contractions of single motor units are not apparent as small twitches when the whole muscle contracts because the individual activations are asynchronous and are smoothed out by the elastic properties of the muscles. For example, the 25,000 muscle fibers in the cat soleus are supplied by 100 α motoneurons. A contraction of the whole muscle can therefore be graded in 100 steps by **recruitment** of motor units.

Skeletal muscle fibers are not homogeneous: Some are faster in their contractions than others. For example, muscles that contract the fingers, enabling us to play the piano, contract and relax much faster than those that enable us to stand, and their contractile mechanisms fatigue more rapidly. The slowly contracting, fatigue-resistant fibers (*red* muscles) depend on oxidative metabolism for energy production, whereas the fast, rapidly contracting fibers (*white* muscles) depend on glycolysis.

Sensory Information Influencing Muscle Contraction

In order for motor programs to execute voluntary and involuntary movements faithfully, the nervous system must receive sensory information from the muscles themselves. Information about the length and tension of a muscle arises from stretch receptors in structures known as **muscle spindles**. As we described in Chapter 21, muscle spindles lie in the body of the muscle, in parallel with the major contractile fibers. Their **primary endings** send information about tension in the spindle to the spinal cord through the most rapidly conducting nerve fibers in the body, the Group Ia afferent fibers. Impulses arising from primary endings convey information about both the amount of stretch on the central region of the spindle and the rate at which the stretch is increasing. The muscle fibers within the spindle are innervated by slowly-conducting efferent fibers known as γ motoneurons.

[1] Adrian, E. D. 1932. *The Mechanism of Nervous Action*. University of Pennsylvania Press, Philadelphia, PA.

[2] Adrian, E. D. 1946. *The Physical Background of Perception*. Clarendon, Oxford, UK.

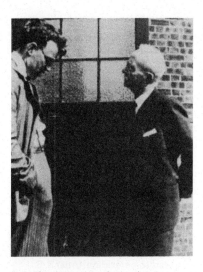

C. S. Sherrington (right) and J. C. Eccles in the 1950s

Muscle tension is also sensed by stretch receptors known as **Golgi tendon organs** in the tendons at either end of the muscle. They send information to the spinal cord through the afferent nerve fibers known as Group Ib, which conduct more slowly than the Ia fibers from spindles (see Box 8.2 for classification of nerve fibers according to conduction velocity and function).

Excitation and Inhibition of Motoneurons

The recruitment and fine control of motoneurons to produce coordinated movements require that influences from many different sources play upon them in the appropriate sequence and with appropriate balance. It is therefore not surprising that a motoneuron is controlled by thousands of synaptic inputs[3] (see Figure 1.13). These inputs convey instructions from higher centers and from sensory receptors in the periphery. The effect on the motoneuron can be excitatory (tending to produce action potentials and contractions) or inhibitory (tending to prevent or reduce contractions). If the excitatory inputs win, muscle fibers contract.

Much is now known about synaptic transmission onto the motoneuron.[4,5] One important excitatory input is from the primary stretch receptors in muscle spindles (Figure 26.2). By painstakingly recording from all the motoneurons supplying a particular muscle (its **motor pool**), Mendell and Henneman[6] showed that each sensory nerve fiber in a muscle spindle sends an excitatory input to as many as 300 motoneurons—virtually all those supplying that muscle.[7]

The arborization pattern of an individual stretch receptor nerve fiber can be seen directly by using intracellular injection of a marker such as the enzyme horseradish peroxidase. The labeled afferent axon branches extensively along the rostrocaudal axis of the spinal cord, where the branches contact members of the motor pool. Close examination of stained individual afferent fibers allows their contacts with individual motoneurons to be mapped (see Figure 26.2). The way in which afferent fibers connect to motoneurons is highly precise: One single sensory fiber makes two to five contacts on the dendritic tree.[8] All the contacts onto a given motoneuron tend to occur within the same general region of the dendritic tree.[9] It is remarkable that a single branch provides these contacts, while other branches of the same axon pass by to supply other motoneurons. Mechanisms that describe how nerve fibers grow and form synaptic connections will be described in Chapter 27.

An impulse in a single sensory nerve fiber arising from a muscle spindle gives rise to only a very small (~200 microvolts [μV]) monosynaptic excitatory potential in a motoneuron. This depolarization is too small on its own to cross the threshold and initiate an action potential. Moreover, not every presynaptic sensory nerve ending releases

[3] Brannstrom, T. 1993. *J. Comp. Neurol.* 330: 439–454.

[4] Eccles, J. C. 1981. *Appl. Neurophysiol.* 44: 5–15.

[5] Hultborn, H. 2006. *Prog. Neurobiol.* 78: 215–242.

[6] Mendell, L. M., and Henneman, E. 1971. *J. Neurophysiol.* 34: 171–187.

[7] Lucas, S. M., and Binder, M. D. 1984. *J. Neurophysiol.* 51: 50–63.

[8] Brown, A. G., and Fyffe, R. E. W. 1981. *J. Physiol.* 313: 121–140.

[9] Burke, R. E., and Glenn, L. L. 1996. *J. Comp. Neurol.* 372: 465–485.

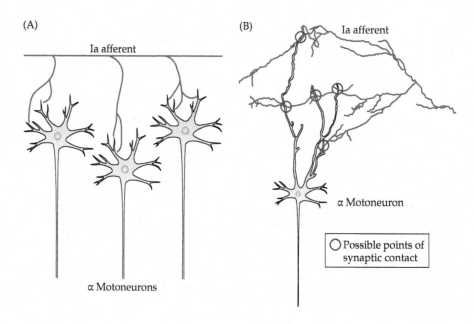

FIGURE 26.2 Contacts between Stretch Receptor Afferents and Spinal Motoneurons. (A) A single muscle spindle (Ia) afferent fiber sends branches to several motoneurons. (B) A more detailed view shows the afferent fiber passing over multiple dendritic branches, indicating possible points of synaptic contact (red circles). Innervation patterns of this kind can be seen experimentally by labeling afferent fibers and motoneurons with histological markers such as horseradish peroxidase. (After R. E. Burke and L. L. Glenn, 1996. *J. Comp. Neurol.* 372: 465–485.)

(A)

Ia afferent

α Motoneurons

(B)

Ia afferent

α Motoneuron

○ Possible points of synaptic contact

transmitter with every impulse—some intermittently fail to release any transmitter. This was first shown by Kuno,[10] who dissected small sensory nerve bundles in dorsal roots and recorded the potentials produced by stimulation of single sensory fibers that terminated in muscle spindles.[11] On its own, a single synaptic potential on the order of 200 μV can be expected to have little influence on the firing pattern of a motoneuron. However, small potentials can sum during brief bursts of activity to produce a buildup of depolarization in a process called temporal summation (Figure 26.3A). In addition, a strong stretch of a muscle such as the soleus can activate all of its 50 Ia stretch receptors, resulting in spatial summation of all the inputs contacting different regions in the motoneuron's dendritic tree (Figure 26.3B). Integration of a multitude of excitatory and inhibitory synaptic inputs determines whether or not the threshold will be reached.

The Size Principle and Graded Contractions

How are motor units recruited to produce smoothly graded movements? As already described, the force of contraction can be increased by bringing in more and more motoneurons, and by increasing their rate of firing. However, further refinement is provided by an unforeseen mechanism: The motoneurons are recruited successively according to their size, small cells first. A motoneuron with a small cell body innervates relatively few muscle fibers, so its activation causes only a modest increase in muscle tension. A large motoneuron contacts many muscle fibers, and an impulse from such a motoneuron gives rise to a large increase in muscle tension. When a contraction begins, small motor units fire, and they produce small increments in tension. As the strength of the contraction is increased, through an act of will or through a reflex, larger units are recruited, each contributing progressively more tension.[12] Finely graded control is thereby achieved, enabling small or large movements to be produced efficiently. The orderly recruitment of motoneurons is referred to as the **size principle**.

In the soleus muscle of the cat, the firing of a small motoneuron may give rise to an increase in tension of about 5 grams (g), whereas a larger motor unit may contribute more than 100 g, and the maximum contraction brought about by all the motor units firing may reach over 3.5 kilograms (kg). Plainly, a small motor unit would be relatively ineffective if brought in when the contraction was near its maximum, and a large unit firing in the lower range would perturb fine movements. The fact that the motor units are recruited in order of increasing size (strength) means that each additional unit adds a relatively fixed fraction (about 5%) to the existing tension.

[10] Kuno, M. 1971. *Physiol. Rev.* 51: 647–678.

[11] Kirkwood, P. A., and Sears, T. A. 1982. *J. Physiol.* 322: 287–314.

[12] Henneman, E., Somjen, G., and Carpenter, D. O. 1965. *J. Neurophysiol.* 28: 560–580.

(A) Temporal summation

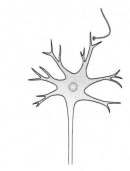

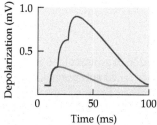

(B) Spatial summation

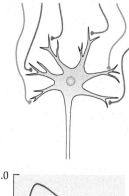

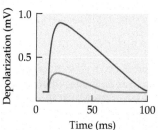

FIGURE 26.3 Temporal and Spatial Summation.
(A) A single action potential in a single Ia afferent produces a synaptic potential in a motoneuron that is only a fraction of a millivolt (mV; bottom blue trace). When the presynaptic fiber fires three action potentials in rapid succession, the synaptic potentials (top red traces) ride on the falling phase of the previous one, so they build up to a larger depolarization—temporal summation. (B) A muscle such as the soleus in a cat may have as many as 100 muscle spindles, and an equivalent number of Ia afferent fibers. These all diverge to contact the majority of motoneurons in the motor pool. Thus, 100 Ia afferents converge onto each motoneuron. A strong stretch of the muscle can activate all the Ia afferents (only a few are shown in the diagram); the individual excitatory postsynaptic potentials add to depolarize the motoneuron by spatial summation.

FIGURE 26.4 The Size Principle. Current flow into a motor nerve cell produces a change in membrane potential that is proportional to the input resistance (r_{input}). Input resistance is inversely proportional to the radius of the cell, so equivalent synaptic currents (i_{syn}) produce greater depolarization ($\Delta V_{syn} = i_{syn}r_{input}$) of smaller motoneurons. The small motoneuron on the left and the large one on the right both receive the same input from Ia afferent fibers. The synaptic current, which is the same in both cells (50 pA), produces a larger depolarization in the smaller motoneuron.

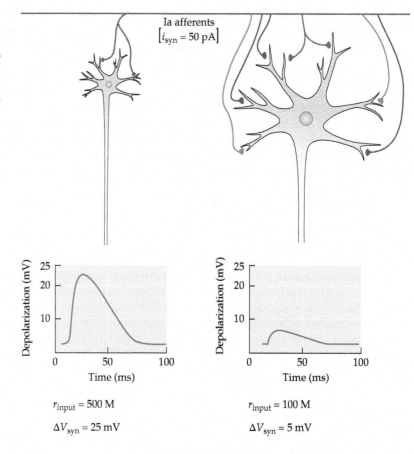

Ia afferents
$[i_{syn} = 50\ \text{pA}]$

$r_{input} = 500\ \text{M}$

$\Delta V_{syn} = 25\ \text{mV}$

$r_{input} = 100\ \text{M}$

$\Delta V_{syn} = 5\ \text{mV}$

The principle that motor unit recruitment adds a fixed fraction, rather than an absolute force increment, to existing muscle tension is also reflected in the sensory aspects of motor activity. We judge weights by the muscular force needed to support them, and we can easily distinguish the difference between 2 and 3 g, but not between 2002 and 2003 g. Again, it is the *relative* change that is important, as enunciated in the Weber–Fechner relationship (see Chapter 21). Indeed, much of our perception of the world is determined in the same way and we act accordingly. You would not mind paying $2003 for an item normally costing $2002, but would be outraged at paying $3 for a $2 item.

How do the cellular and electrical properties of motoneurons explain the size principle? The explanation depends on the electrical properties and sizes of motoneurons. Suppose that all the motoneurons innervating a muscle receive the same synaptic input. The depolarization (voltage) produced by the synaptic current in each motoneuron will depend on its input resistance, which is a function of cell size (Figure 26.4). As we showed in Chapter 8, the input resistance of a nerve cell varies inversely with its radius, just as a thin fuse wire has a greater resistance than a thick one. Thus, any given synaptic current will produce a larger voltage change in small motoneurons, making them more likely to reach threshold than large motoneurons. As the strength of sensory input increases, larger and larger motoneurons will be brought to threshold.

Spinal Reflexes

Reciprocal Innervation

Limb movements are produced by the coordinated contraction of groups of muscles that work together, referred to as **agonists**. Opposing muscles are called **antagonists**. **Extensor muscles** open or extend the joints; **flexor muscles** close or flex the joints and pull the limbs toward the body. When a stretch reflex (see Figure 26.1) is activated by muscle stretch—for example, by a tap on the patellar tendon to produce a knee jerk—the sensory endings in the muscle that extends the leg are deformed and initiate impulses. These impulses are synchronous since they arise from a quick stretch. As already mentioned, a burst of synchronous sensory impulses travels to the spinal cord to excite motoneurons that project back to the muscle that has been stretched. The result is a reflex contraction in the form of a twitch (the leg kicks forward). Normal muscular contractions, however, are produced by *asynchronous* activation of stretch receptor afferent fibers.

It is clear that a complication arises for the performance of natural movements: As one muscle shortens, say the extensor muscle that straightens the knee, it stretches the antagonistic muscles that bend the knee. This bending in turn induces another stretch reflex in the extensor muscle. In principle one would expect such feedback loops to produce tremor. Yet when the knee is straightened or bent, the reflexes normally do not oscillate.

How are oscillations prevented? One mechanism is the inhibitory connection shown in Figure 26.1. A tap to the patellar tendon below the knee, which stretches the extensor muscle, is accompanied by simultaneous inhibition of the α motoneurons that innervate antagonistic flexor muscles. This occurs because the sensory fibers activate spinal interneurons that inhibit the antagonist α motoneurons. The principle of one group of muscles being excited while its antagonists are inhibited was first described by Sherrington, who called it **reciprocal innervation**.[13] In addition, a major function of higher centers such as the basal ganglia (discussed later in the chapter) is to prevent tremor and spasticity from occurring and to guarantee smooth movements.

We have emphasized an artificially produced reflex in this analysis, the knee jerk, because of its simplicity. But naturally induced reflexes produced by stretch receptors play a part in all voluntary and involuntary movements of the body. Without the continuous input from receptors in muscle, the excitability of motoneurons is reduced and they respond poorly or not at all to commands from higher centers.

The stretch-sensitive fibers in muscle spindles known as Group II afferents reinforce the reflex by indirect connections through interneurons in the spinal cord.[14,15] Interneurons that are activated by Group Ib sensory fibers from Golgi tendon organs inhibit the stretch reflex. The axons of Golgi tendon organs[16] activate inhibitory interneurons in the spinal cord (see Figure 26.1B). The Golgi tendon organ endings are *in series* with contracting skeletal muscles. They are sensitive to muscle contraction, which is the principal stimulus that gives rise to their impulses. Contraction of one or two muscle fibers can cause a brisk discharge. Axons from tendon organs activate interneurons that, in turn, *inhibit* α motoneurons supplying their muscle of origin; thus, their action is the opposite of that of spindle afferents.[17–19]

In summary, the stretch reflex has several underlying mechanisms. First, impulses in afferent fibers from the spindles activate motoneurons that supply their own muscles, causing contraction. At the same time, the afferent impulses are transmitted through interneurons to inhibit antagonist muscles. Finally, the muscle contraction itself activates Golgi tendon organ Group Ib afferent fibers that inhibit motoneurons so as to limit ongoing activity.

Flexor Reflexes

Complex combinations of muscular activity, involving multiple joints and sometimes more than one limb, are produced by painful stimuli. The simplest is called the **flexor reflex**, which is activated, for example, when one steps on a sharp object, bangs one's shin against a bench, or touches a hot stove. The response depends on the location and intensity of the offending stimulus, but it has two consistent features: (1) Movement of the affected limb is always primarily flexion and is directed away from the offending stimulus; and (2) if necessary, weight is transferred to the contralateral limb. The input for the reflex arises from responses of nociceptive and tactile receptors in skin.[20] The movement is determined by interplay of networks of excitatory and inhibitory spinal interneurons acting on flexor and extensor motoneurons, respectively, on the side of the stimulus and (if weight transfer is needed) by simultaneous extensor excitation and flexor inhibition on the contralateral side (Figure 26.5). This synaptic activity is organized within the spinal cord at the segmental level, and is supplemented by inputs from higher centers that serve to maintain balance and mediate the appropriate continuation or cessation of movement.

[13] Sherrington, C. S. 1906. *The Integrative Action of the Nervous System*, 1961 ed. Yale University Press, New Haven, CT.

[14] Marchand-Pauvert, V. et al. 2005. *J. Physiol.* 566: 257–271.

[15] Bannatyne, B.A. et al. 2009. *J. Physiol.* 587: 379–399.

[16] Crago, P. E., Houk, J. C., and Rymer, W. Z. 1982. *J. Neurophysiol.* 47: 1069–1083.

[17] Matthews, P. B. C. 1972. *Mammalian Muscle Receptors and Their Central Action*. Edward Arnold, London, UK.

[18] Edin, B. B., and Vallbo, A. B. 1990. *J. Neurophysiol.* 63: 1307–1313.

[19] Windhorst, U. 2007. *Brain. Res. Bull.* 73: 155–202.

[20] Sherrington, C. S. 1910. *J. Physiol.* 40: 28–121.

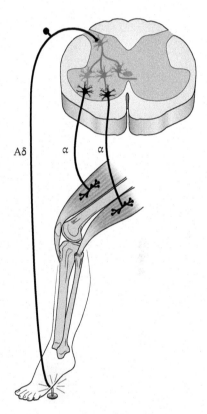

FIGURE 26.5 The Flexor Reflex is a limb-withdrawal reflex, produced in this example by stepping on a tack. Excitation of Aδ pain fibers results in elevation of the thigh (synaptic connections not shown) and flexing of the knee joint by polysynaptic excitation of flexor motoneurons and inhibition of extensors (blue interneuron is inhibitory). Also not shown are contralateral connections that subserve extension of the opposite leg for support.

Motor Control of Muscle Spindles

The sensory responses of muscle spindles are complicated by the fact that the intrafusal muscle fibers themselves are subject to excitation. Excitation is by a dedicated group of motor nerve fibers known as fusimotor, or γ efferent, fibers (Figure 26.6). As the ends of an intrafusal muscle fiber contract, the central region, in which the sensory nerve terminals are imbedded, is stretched, thereby initiating impulses in the sensory nerve fibers. Note that the

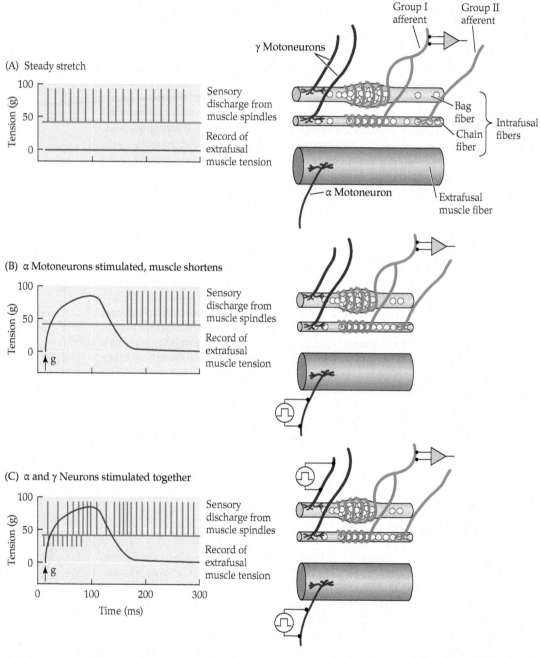

FIGURE 26.6 Efferent Regulation of Muscle Spindles. Records of extrafusal muscle tension (red) and sensory discharge from muscle spindles (blue). (A) Stimulation of γ efferent fibers causes the intrafusal fibers to contract. This contraction stretches the sensory endings of the spindle afferents, causing them to fire. (B) Stimulation of α fibers supplying the main mass of extrafusal muscle fiber causes it to contract. This contraction reduces the stretch on the intrafusal fibers and causes the spindle afferents to stop firing. (C) When α and γ efferent fibers are stimulated together, stimulated tension on the muscle spindles remains unchanged and the sensory discharge continues during contraction of the muscle. (After C. C. Hunt and S. W. Kuffler, 1951. *J. Physiol.* 113: 283–297.)

intrafusal muscle fibers, unlike the main mass of extrafusal muscle fibers, bear no load even if the muscle is lifting many kilograms. This enables them to contract reliably in a graded manner when they are stimulated by their own γ motoneurons. In principle, the spinal cord could command an intrafusal muscle fiber to shorten its length by 50% and be sure to obtain the desired result. By contrast, a motor command to extrafusal muscle fibers via α motoneurons could not guarantee shortening to a precise length. The extent of shortening by extrafusal fibers depends not only on the command but also on the load that has to be lifted.

The role of fusimotor fibers was established in a series of technically difficult experiments on anesthetized cats by Kuffler, Hunt, and Quilliam.[21] They recorded the electrical activity of an individual dorsal root sensory fiber coming from a muscle spindle while at the same time stimulating a single fusimotor γ fiber in the ventral root that supplied the same spindle. Fusimotor stimulation produced an increase in sensory activity, but no increase in tension of the muscle as a whole. Trains of impulses in γ fusimotor neurons either accelerated the sensory discharge produced by stretching the muscle or initiated a sensory discharge in the relaxed muscle.

What is the function of the γ motor system and what is achieved by the efferent regulation of muscle spindle discharges? When the entire muscle is stretched, the intrafusal fibers are stretched as well, producing impulses in the afferent fibers (see Figure 26.6A). Conversely, when extrafusal skeletal muscle fibers contract following α motoneuron stimulation, the intrafusal fibers go slack; the central region of the spindles is no longer stretched, and the sensory discharge stops (see Figure 26.6B). As a result, information about muscle length is not sent to the CNS. If this were all that occurred in response to a motor command, there would be no sensory feedback from the muscle to ensure that the command had been properly executed. Accordingly, motor commands activate both γ and α motoneurons,[22,23] causing the intrafusal muscle fibers to contract in concert with the muscle as a whole (see Figure 26.6C).

The motor innervation of muscle spindles can be thought of as a "gain control" system that continually adjusts the sensitivity of the spindle over all lengths of the muscle. However, the exact functional role of the spindles in programmed movements is not known, because of a lack of knowledge about how the firing of γ motoneurons is regulated by descending influences from higher centers. An example of *co-activation* of α and γ motoneurons is shown in Figure 26.7.[24] The recordings show discharges in spindle afferents of inspiratory muscles during respiration. Figure 26.7A shows that sensory discharges in a spindle from an inspiratory muscle are in fact highest during *inspiration*, when the muscle is contracted and short, not during expiration when it is stretched. This apparent contradiction is explained by the fact that α and γ motoneurons are activated together, so that intrafusal contraction more than compensates for extrafusal shortening. When the γ motoneurons are selectively blocked by a local anesthetic (see Figure 26.7B), the sensory fibers fire only during expiration, while inspiratory muscles are being stretched.

[21] Kuffler, S. W., Hunt, C. C., and Quilliam, J. P. 1951. *J. Neurophysiol.* 14: 29-51.

[22] Sears, T. A. 1964 *J. Physiol.* 174: 295-315.

[23] Allen, T. J., Ansems, G. E., and Proske, U. 2008. *Exp. Physiol.* 93: 391-398.

[24] Critchlow, V., and von Euler, C. 1963. *J. Physiol.* 168: 820-847.

(A) Normal

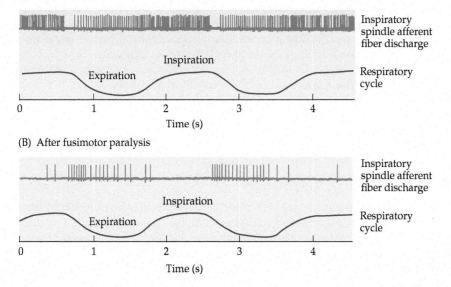

(B) After fusimotor paralysis

FIGURE 26.7 Co-Activation of α and γ Respiratory Motoneurons. (A) Extracellular recording of action potentials arising from a spindle in an inspiratory muscle during the respiratory cycle (lower trace, red). It is at first surprising that the sensory discharge from the inspiratory muscle spindle is highest during inspiration, while the muscles are shortening rather than being stretched. This is due to simultaneous activation of γ fusimotor fibers to the spindle. (B) After the fusimotor fibers are blocked selectively by procaine, the spindles behave passively. The sensory discharge frequency increases during expiration, when the main mass of the muscle is stretched; as expected, sensory firing stops during inspiratory movements when the main mass of the muscle is shortened. (After V. Critchlow and C. von Euler, 1963. *J. Physiol.* 168: 820-847.)

Evidence for co-activation of α and γ motoneurons has also been obtained from experiments on finger movements, where spindle afferents increase their firing even during voluntary isometric contractions, when the joint does not move.[18] An additional complication of spindle mechanisms is that more than one type of γ efferent system has been identified: Certain γ motoneurons increase dynamic responses of spindle afferents (i.e., their responses to the *rate* of stretch); other γ motoneurons increase their static responses (i.e., responses to the *degree* of stretch).[25] Clearly, the motor innervation of spindles prevents the afferent volley of action potentials from being simple indicators of muscle length. That spindle discharges do in fact provide information about the position of limbs and fingers in space is possible only because the CNS continually monitors and modulates the outgoing fusimotor activity.[26]

A major function of extrafusal and intrafusal co-activation is to deal automatically with external perturbations. Suppose a specific rate and extent of shortening of a muscle are programmed. During execution of the program, the α and γ fibers are activated so that the extra- and intrafusal muscles contract in concert, so that as the movement progresses the intrafusal sensory discharge is unchanged from that at rest. Now suppose that contraction of the extrafusal fibers is interrupted by an encounter with an external load. The continuing intrafusal contraction is not interrupted, and "runs ahead" of the bulk of muscle contraction, with the result that the spindle discharge is increased. The increased afferent activity automatically increases the α motoneuron discharge, thereby compensating for the increased external load. The extrafusal fibers then are able to "catch up" with the programmed intrafusal contraction. When the "catching up" has been accomplished, the compensatory intrafusal drive is removed and the contraction is back on its intended track.

It is interesting to note that in theory a γ motor servo mechanism could be effective with no central command at all to the α motoneurons. Contraction of the spindles would simply drive the α motoneurons and produce muscle contraction. This is not the case, however. If γ fibers were to *start* our movements, they could not occur rapidly enough to, say, play Chopin on the piano: The time taken to excite muscles would be far slower than direct activation by α motoneurons. It is also of interest that certain skeletal muscles contain no spindles and are controlled solely by α motoneurons—for example, the extraocular muscles that move the eye.[27] Feedback is visual, and the load on the muscles is constant and irrelevant (apart from minor effects of gravity[28]).

Generation of Coordinated Movements

For several patterned motor acts, sensory feedback is not required to keep them going. For example, during birdsong, movements of the muscles follow each other in a rapid, orderly sequence without sufficient time for a feedback loop to be completed.[29] The next instructions are sent out from the CNS before it can analyze the preceding sound. After the CNS of a leech or a cockroach has been dissected out of the body and deprived of all sensory inputs, it continues to generate impulses in patterns that would normally result in swimming or walking (see Chapter 20). The presence of autonomous **central pattern generators** does not mean that feedback from the periphery is ignored entirely during behavior of the intact animal.[30] For example, if the dorsum of the foot of a walking cat touches a small twig during the swing phase, the foot will be lifted elegantly over the twig. The role of sensory feedback is to modulate ongoing motor programs in accord with the organism's needs and in response to unpredicted challenges imposed by the external world.

We will use two examples—respiration and walking—to illustrate how central pattern generators in the mammalian CNS produce coordinated movements.

Neural Control of Respiration

Ceaseless rhythmical contractions of respiratory muscles ensure that oxygen and carbon dioxide can be exchanged between the blood and the lungs until the moment that one dies. Full-term and premature babies can breathe as soon as they are born; programmed respiratory movements of the rib cage are already made in the embryo (obviously without intake of oxygen). The respiratory rhythm is relentless and unfailing: You can commit suicide by

[25] Durbaba, R., et al. 2003. *J. Physiol.* 550: 263–278.

[26] Smith, J. L. et al. 2009. *J. Appl. Physiol.* 106: 950–958.

[27] Daniel, P. 1946. *J. Anat.* 80: 189–193.

[28] Pierrot-Deseilligny, C. 2009. *Ann. NY Acad. Sci.* 1164: 155–165.

[29] Konishi, M. 2004. *Ann. NY Acad. Sci.* 1016: 463–475.

[30] Briggman, K. L., and Kristan, W. B. 2008. *Annu. Rev. Neurosci.* 31: 271–294.

(A) Movements of rib cage in respiration

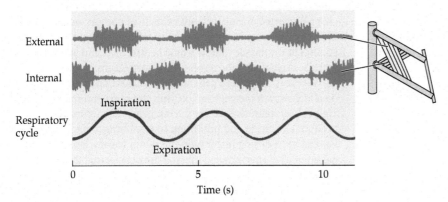

Expiration   Inspiration

(B) Electromyographs of external (inspiratory) and internal (expiratory) intercostal muscles

External

Internal

Respiratory cycle

Inspiration

Expiration

Time (s)

FIGURE 26.8 Movements of Rib Cage and Respiratory Muscles during expiration and inspiration. (A) Actions of the internal intercostal muscles (depressing the ribs during expiration) and external intercostal muscles (raising the ribs during inspiration). As the diaphragm contracts, it expands the lungs. (B) Activity of respiratory muscles in the cat, recorded with needle electrodes. Discharges of the external and internal intercostal muscles are out of phase.

not eating, but you cannot decide not to breathe any more. Nevertheless, this automatic behavior is modulated by sensory feedback and, within limits, can be controlled by the will.

The diaphragm and two antagonistic sets of muscles are responsible for drawing air into the lungs and expelling it. During inspiration, the diaphragm contracts and the rib cage is raised by the external intercostal muscles (Figure 26.8) As a result, the volume of the chest is increased, the lungs expand, and air enters. Expiration is achieved by relaxation of the diaphragm and contraction of the internal intercostal muscles. Other muscles of the thorax and abdomen also contribute to a variable extent, depending on the posture of the animal and the rate and depth of respiration.[31] An example of the respiratory rhythm in muscles of an anesthetized cat is shown in Figure 26.8B. Activity of each muscle is registered by strain gauges and by recording its electrical activity with wire electrodes embedded in the body of the muscle, a technique called electromyography (EMG). Figure 26.8B shows that inspiratory and expiratory muscle contractions are accompanied by bursts of potentials, indicating motor unit discharges; it is apparent that the two sets of muscles contract out of phase.

As in limb muscles, the stretch reflex contributes to movement by maintaining the excitability of motoneurons. When the internal and external intercostal muscles are stretched alternately by commands from the CNS, their Ia afferent fibers fire at high frequencies. Those impulses contribute excitatory synaptic potentials to the homonymous motor neurons (i.e., motor neurons supplying the same muscle) and, through interneurons, contribute inhibition to the motor neurons of antagonist muscles. Figure 26.9 shows the effect on muscle fiber discharge activity as an inspiratory muscle (the levator costae) is stretched by pulling on its tendon. With each inspiration of the animal, the electromyogram shows a burst of spikes.

FIGURE 26.9 Stretch Reflex of an Inspiratory Muscle. During each inspiration the electromyogram (EMG) from a small muscle, the levator costae, shows bursts of action potentials, and the muscle contracts. Stretching the muscle by pulling on its tendon increases the number of impulses in each burst by increasing the reflex drive on the motor unit, without affecting the respiratory rate. (From G. G. Hilaire et al., 1983. *J. Physiol.* 342: 527-548.)

[31] Da Silva, K. M. C. et al. 1977. *J. Physiol.* 266: 499-521.

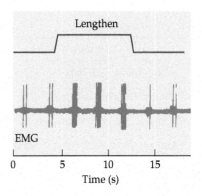

Lengthen

EMG

Time (s)

(A)

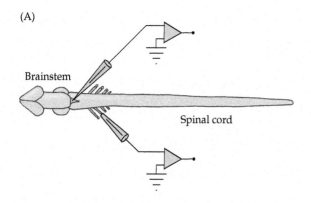

Brainstem

Spinal cord

(B)

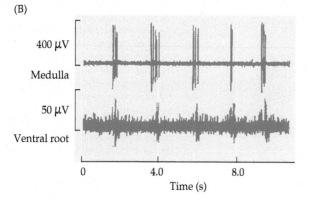

400 μV

Medulla

50 μV

Ventral root

0   4.0   8.0

Time (s)

FIGURE 26.10   Respiratory Rhythm Recorded from Brainstem Neurons in a Neonatal Opossum. (A) Recordings were made from neurons in the brainstem of an isolated CNS. (B) Two brainstem cells discharged regularly with an interburst interval of about 2 seconds (s). The upper trace is from a single neuron in the medulla. Simultaneous recording from a ventral root that supplies the diaphragm (lower trace) shows the corresponding discharge of respiratory motoneurons. (Courtesy of D. J. Zou and J. G. Nicholls, unpublished.)

The activity is enhanced when the muscle is lengthened, but the basic rhythm is hardly altered.

As shown earlier in Figure 26.7, the afferent discharge from muscle spindles is maintained at a high frequency even when the muscles are actively contracting, owing to activity of the fusimotor γ efferent fibers.[24] Fusimotor activity presets muscle spindles for the length change expected during that half cycle. If an unexpected obstruction in the airway were to prevent the expected movement, the sensory endings in the muscle spindle would be stretched, and would fire and increase excitation to the respiratory motoneurons.

Where is the pattern generator for respiration situated and how does it generate the rhythm? Within the pons and medulla there are pools of neurons that fire during inspiration or expiration and produce excitation and inhibition of respiratory motor neurons.[32] For example, during inspiration the motoneurons supplying external intercostal (inspiratory) muscles are depolarized by a barrage of excitatory synaptic potentials arising from neurons in higher centers of the medulla or pons, causing bursts of action potentials. The inspiratory phase is terminated by a burst of inhibitory potentials to the inspiratory neurons from intermingled expiratory neurons.[33]

An example of individual rhythmically active brainstem neurons, recorded from the isolated CNS of a neonatal opossum, is shown in Figure 26.10.[34] The upper trace in Figure 26.10B is an extracellular record from a single neuron in the medulla, showing short bursts of impulses with a period of about 2 seconds. In the lower trace, recordings from a thoracic ventral root show corresponding rhythmic discharges of motoneurons supplying inspiratory muscles, occurring at the same frequency and with a slight delay.

In principle, the rhythmical activation of inspiratory and expiratory motoneurons could be achieved in two ways: (1) Neurons in the brainstem might have inherently rhythmical properties, like heart muscle cells. (2) The rhythm might originate from the activity of excitatory and inhibitory synapses between a network of brainstem neurons; inspiratory command neurons would turn off expiratory neurons, which in time would break free and inhibit the inspiratory neurons, and so on. Endogenously bursting pacemaker neurons have been found in neonatal rats in a region of the ventral medulla called the pre-Bötzinger complex.[32] Experiments made by St. John suggest that those pacemaker neurons may function in relation to gasping rather than to normal respiration.[35]

A major technical problem, as of now, is how to record from the entire population of neurons in an area of the CNS. With electrodes, one can measure either the activity of a small proportion of the population or the average activity of the whole population, which blurs fine details. An alternative is to survey simultaneously the activity of large populations of brainstem neurons, one by one, during inspiration and expiration by optical methods[36] (see also Chapters 1 and 3). Figure 26.11 shows an example of firing by respiratory neurons obtained by calcium imaging. Results such as these have shown that inspiratory and expiratory neurons are intermingled rather than in completely separate pools. Several lines of evidence further suggest that rhythmicity might arise from properties of the network rather than being driven solely by pacemaker cells. As yet, the excitatory and inhibitory connections of the respiratory command neurons in the brainstem have not been traced.

Of importance for the rhythmicity of breathing is the level of carbon dioxide in the arterial blood. Under conditions of reduced CO_2, the rate and depth of respiration are reduced;

[32] Feldman, J. L., Mitchell, G. S., and Nattie, E. E. 2003. *Annu. Rev. Neurosci.* 26: 249–266.

[33] Davies, J. G., Kirkwood, P. A., and Sears, T. A. 1985. *J. Physiol.* 368: 63–87.

[34] Nicholls, J. G. et al.1990. *J. Exp. Biol.* 152: 1–15.

[35] St. John, W. M. 2009. *Philos. Trans. R. Soc. Lond.* B 364: 2625–2633.

[36] Muller, K. J. et al. 2009. *Philos. Trans. R. Soc. Lond.* B 364: 2485–2491.

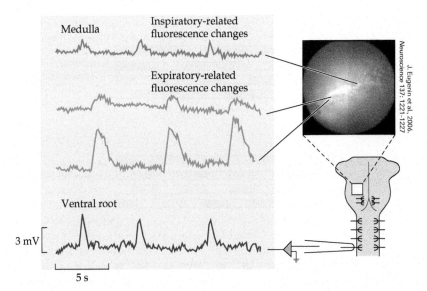

J. Eugenin et al., 2006.
Neuroscience 137: 1221-1227

FIGURE 26.11 Fluorescence Changes in Rostral Medulla (top three traces) and integrated ventral root burst activity to the diaphragm (bottom trace) in an isolated brainstem-spinal cord preparation (stained with calcium-sensitive dye) of a 20-day-old embryonic mouse. On the right are a photograph and drawing of such a preparation with an electrode attached to a cervical ventral root. The approximate region of view is indicated by the white square. Inspiratory-related (top trace, blue) and expiratory-related (second and third traces, green) fluorescence changes are recorded optically from neurons in the rostral medulla. Lines point to cells in the medulla for their respective optical recordings. (From J. Eugenin et al., 2006. *Neuroscience* 137: 1221-1227.)

conversely, respiration is increased by raised levels of CO_2. This effect depends on inputs from chemoreceptors in the carotid arteries and aorta and from neurons and glial cells in the medulla that are sensitive to CO_2 levels.[37,38] The firing patterns of individual medullary neurons that control expiratory and inspiratory motoneurons have been shown to be influenced critically by CO_2. Changes in the steady level of CO_2 are translated into pronounced changes in the frequencies of firing of the interneurons and, therefore, of the respiratory motoneurons.[39] By genetic manipulations, Champagnat,[40] Brunet,[41] and their colleagues have shown that a particular gene known as *Phox2b* is responsible during development for the generation of neurons that respond to increased levels of CO_2. Deletion of the gene in mice gives rise to animals that no longer breathe faster and deeper in a high-CO_2 environment.

We know from everyday experience that modulation of breathing depends on voluntary commands as well as sensory input. You can inhale more deeply when you smell the odor of Kentucky Fried Chicken, maintain expiration for prolonged periods as you sing "Celeste Aida," or hold your breath in an offensive toilet. While the central pattern generator guarantees an unfailing rhythm, it is not fully autonomous. At present, although we know that glutamate and GABA play important roles,[42] we do not yet know whether the respiratory rhythm arises from inherent rhythmicity of brainstem neurons, network properties, or combinations of both.

Neural Control of Locomotion

A striking feature of locomotion is that in vertebrates there is a consistent, highly stereotyped pattern of limb movements. In the walking cat shown in Figure 26.12, the left hindlimb is lifted off the ground first, then the left forelimb, the right hindlimb, and the right forelimb. This sequence provides stabilization by the forelimbs, while the hindlimbs propel the animal: The tendency to turn produced by the hindlimb is counteracted by the forelimbs, thereby preventing rotation and enabling movement to proceed straight forward. Such a sequence is common in vertebrates, including crocodiles, rats, cats, and elephants (but not fish). Even in invertebrates with six legs, such as cockroaches, a similar sequential pattern is observed. During locomotion each leg executes an elementary stepping movement that consists of two phases:[43] (1) a swing phase, during which the leg, having been extended to the rear, is flexed, raised off the ground, swung forward, and extended again to contact the ground, and (2) a stance phase, during which the leg is in contact with the ground, moving backward in relation to the direction taken by the body.

The gait of a cat undergoes striking changes as its speed increases, as shown in Figures 26.12 and 26.13. While the cat is walking, a single leg is raised off the ground at any one time. As the speed increases to a trot, two legs are raised off the ground at once–one foreleg and one hindleg on opposite sides of the animal. Still faster, at a gallop, the two forelegs

[37] Spyer, K. M., and Gourine, A. V. 2009. *Philos. Trans. R. Soc. Lond. B* 364: 2603-2610.

[38] Huckstepp, R. T. et al. 2010. *J. Physiol.* 588: 3901-3920.

[39] Eugenin, J., and Nicholls, J. G. 1997. *J. Physiol.* 501: 425-437.

[40] Champagnat, J. et al. 2009. *Philos. Trans. R. Soc. Lond. B* 364: 2469-2476.

[41] Dubreuil, V. et al. 2009. *Philos. Trans. R. Soc. Lond. B* 364: 2477-2483.

[42] Cifra, A. et al. 2009. *Philos. Trans. R. Soc. Lond. B* 364: 2493-2500.

[43] Pearson, K. 1976. *Sci. Am.* 235: 72-86.

FIGURE 26.12 The Stepping Pattern of a Cat during three different gaits of locomotion: walk, trot, and gallop. The white bars show the time that a foot is off the ground (the swing phase, during which flexor motoneurons are active); the blue bars show the time a foot is on the ground (the stance phase, during which extensor motoneurons are active). During walking, the legs are moved in sequence, first on one side, then on the other. During a trot, a different pattern of interlimb coordination is used: Diagonally opposite legs are raised together. In a gallop, the hindlegs and then the forelegs leave the ground. LF = left foreleg, LH = left hindleg, RF = right foreleg, RH = right hindleg. (After K. Pearson, 1976. *Sci. Am.* 235: 72–86.)

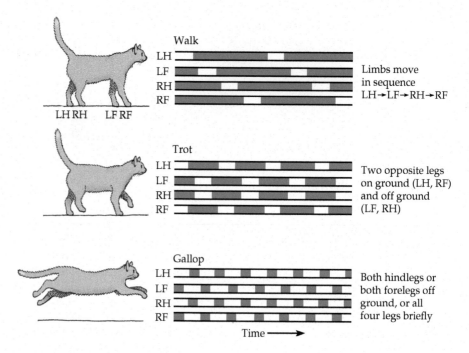

[44] Dasen, J. S., and Jessell, T. M. 2009. *Curr. Top. Dev. Biol.* 88: 169–200.

and then the two hindlegs alternate in leaving the ground. The increase in speed is accomplished by shortening the time that each leg stays on the ground—the stance phase. Thus, as the cat moves faster, each leg is extended for a briefer period before being bent, raised, and moved forward. At all speeds from a slow walk to a gallop, the time spent off the ground by each leg as it swings forward is little altered. There is substantial evidence that intrinsic motor programs are genetically predetermined and appear spontaneously during development, independent of experience.[44]

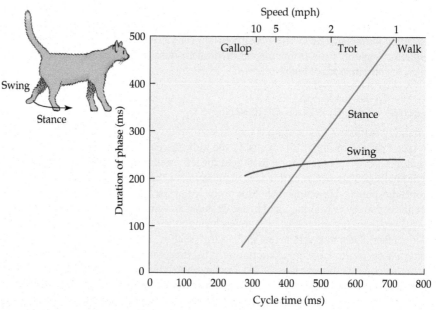

FIGURE 26.13 Constancy of Swing Phase during Locomotion. As the animal moves more and more rapidly (abscissa), the time spent by each foot on the ground (stance phase) becomes progressively shorter (ordinate). The time that each foot spends in the air (swing phase) is almost the same in a walk and a gallop. (After K. Pearson, 1976. *Sci. Am.* 235: 72–86.)

As early as 1911, Graham Brown[45] showed that the elementary circuits required for walking movements in cats appeared to possess semiautomatic properties (see also Guertin[46]). The raising and placing of two hindfeet in alternation could be achieved in a cat after its thoracic spinal cord had been transected.

Experiments made by Shik and Orlovsky[47] and by Nistri,[48] Grillner,[49] and their colleagues have provided evidence for the role of central mechanisms in producing coordinated walking movements. In the experiments of Shik and his colleagues, the upper brainstem of a cat was transected. Such animals can still stand but do not walk or run spontaneously. As shown in Figure 26.14, a cat with such a transection was held with its feet touching a moving treadmill. When a continuous electrical stimulation at 30 to 60 impulses per second was applied through electrodes placed in the cuneiform nucleus (the mesencephalic locomotor region), the cat walked. Displacement of the stimulating electrodes by as little as 0.3 mm abolished the walking response. The stance and swing of the forelegs and the electromyograms recorded during walking appeared normal. Stronger stimulation of the mesencephalic locomotor region by larger currents at the same frequency caused the propulsive forces of the leg muscles to be increased. But while the strength of electrical stimulation could influence the force of the walking movements, the frequency of stepping was not altered, provided that the speed of the treadmill remained constant. Rhythmic discharges of motoneurons that are appropriate for swimming or walking in the intact animal can also be elicited in isolated spinal cord segments of the turtle[50] and in slices of rat spinal cord.[51] Although such spinal cord preparations in vitro have interneurons with properties necessary for producing locomotor patterns,[52] the switching from walk to trot to gallop is not understood.

Sensory Feedback and Central Pattern Generator Programs

Clear parallels emerge in the automaticity of breathing and of walking. For both types of movements, a central program orders the contractions of appropriate groups of muscles in a predestined sequence. For respiratory neurons in the brainstem, the drive depends on the CO_2 in their environment. The drive for the alternation of leg movements during walking or running depends on a descending stimulus supplied by glutaminergic, noradrenergic, dopaminergic, and serotonergic neurons in the mesencephalic locomotor region.[53]

[45] Brown, T. G. 1911. *Proc. R. Soc. Lond. B* 84: 308-319.

[46] Guertin, P. A. 2009. *Brain Res. Rev.* 62: 45-56.

[47] Shik, M. L., and Orlovsky, G. N. 1976. *Physiol. Rev.* 56: 465-501.

[48] Taccola, G., and Nistri, A. 2006. *Crit. Rev. Neurobiol.* 18: 25-36.

[49] Kozlov, A. et al. 2009. *Proc. Natl. Acad. Sci. USA* 106: 20027-20032.

[50] Guertin, P. A., and Hounsgaard, J. 1998. *Neurosci. Lett.* 245: 5-8.

[51] Ballerini, L. et al. 1999. *J. Physiol.* 517: 459-475.

[52] Dougherty, K. J., and Kiehn, O. 2010. *Ann. NY Acad. Sci.* 1198: 85-93.

[53] Pearson, K. G. 2008. *Brain Res. Rev.* 57: 222-227.

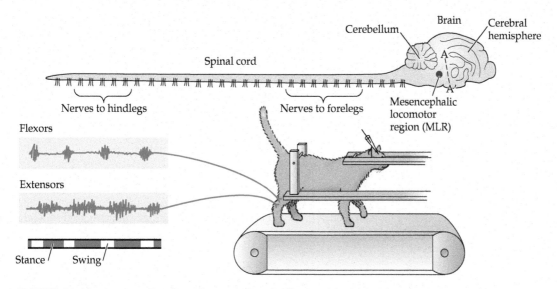

FIGURE 26.14 Locomotion by a Cat on a Treadmill after section of the brainstem (dashed line A-A' in upper figure). Such an animal does not walk spontaneously. Electrical stimulation of the mesencephalic locomotor region (MLR) causes the animal to walk on the treadmill. Electromyographs associated with locomotor activity are recorded by electrodes in limb muscles. The speed of walking or galloping depends on the rate of the treadmill (not shown); increasing the strength or the rate of stimulation increases the strength of limb movements (as though the animal were walking uphill) but not their speed. (After K. Pearson, 1976. *Sci. Am.* 235: 72-86.)

Although sensory input from sensory receptors in the periphery is not required for movement to take place, it does play a major role in regulation. Sensory feedback modulates the frequency and extent of the rhythms to be consistent with the moment-to-moment requirements of the animal. Thus, the rate and depth of respiration depend on the level of blood pH and CO_2, which is sensed by receptors in the brainstem and in aortic and carotid bodies; stretch receptors in the lungs also modulate the rhythm.[54] Similarly, muscle and joint receptors play a key role in modulating the speed of locomotion. For example, the experiment in Figure 26.14 shows the change in gait of a cat from walk to gallop as the speed of the treadmill, upon which the animal is placed, is increased. When the speed of the treadmill is accelerated during constant electrical stimulation of the mesencephalic locomotor region, the locomotion of the cat changes from walking to trotting and then to galloping. Sensory feedback plainly controls the rate of stepping at greater treadmill speeds.[53] As the stance phase shortens, the leg moving to the rear on the treadmill becomes extended more rapidly. It therefore takes less time to reach the point at which afferent signals initiate the swing phase in which the leg is lifted and swung forward. As expected, cutting dorsal roots abolishes the response to different treadmill speeds, but not the walking evoked by electrical stimulation. Afferent feedback has also been shown to control human gait.[55]

Organization of Descending Motor Control

Up to this point we have described how movements made by muscles are initiated and controlled, and illustrated the principles underlying the generation of ongoing rhythmic motor activity. In the following sections we describe descending pathways from cortex, red nucleus, basal ganglia, and vestibular apparatus that converge on motor units to produce programmed movements, as well as their interconnections with each other and with the cerebellum.

Terminology

Knowledge of anatomy is a prerequisite for understanding the physiology of the nervous system. In particular, it is necessary to be able to recognize the names of structures and have some idea of their locations if one is to discuss function. For readers not familiar with the nervous system, terms such as *medial vestibulospinal tract* may seem bewildering, but in fact, anatomists have maintained some rigor in naming fiber tracts so that understanding the name is relatively straightforward. A pathway is named first according to its origin (the *vestibular* nucleus in the brainstem) and then its termination (*spinal* cord). If two or more pathways from the same source run in the spinal cord, their individual locations are specified as *medial* or *lateral*, *ventral* or *dorsal*. Figure 26.15 illustrates the directional terms relative to the main axis of the CNS.

Supraspinal Control of Motoneurons

The major descending pathways to motoneurons are shown in Figure 26.16 (see also Appendix C). These pathways can be classified into two groups, lateral and medial, according to their anatomy and physiological functions.[56]

[54] Mörschel, M., and Dutschmann, M. 2009. *Philos. Trans. R. Soc. Lond. B* 364: 2517-2526.

[55] Nielsen, J. B., and Sinkjaer, T. 2002. *J. Electromyogr. Kinesiol.* 12: 213-217.

[56] Lemon, R. N. 2008. *Annu. Rev. Neurosci.* 31: 195-218.

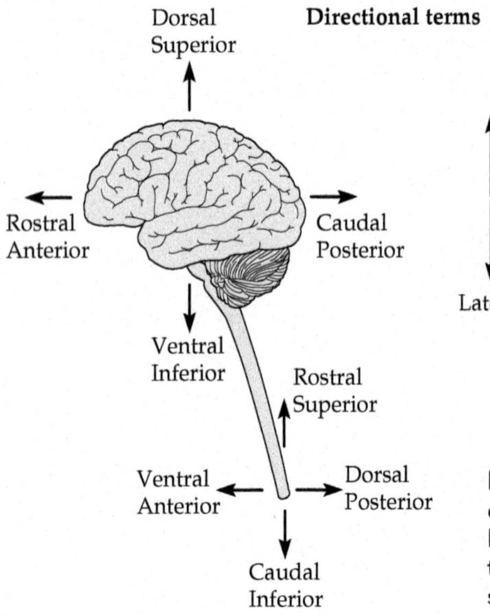

FIGURE 26.15 Directional Terms in the Central Nervous System. Rostral and caudal are toward the nose and tail, respectively. Superior and inferior in a standing human are up and down. Ventral and anterior are toward the front, dorsal and posterior toward the back. Because of the curvature of the neural axis, the top of the brain is both superior and dorsal, and the underside is both inferior and ventral.

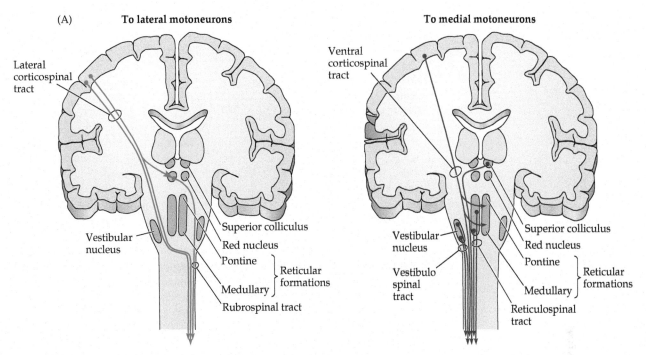

FIGURE 26.16 Major Motor Pathways in the Vertebrate Central Nervous System. Pathways supplying lateral motoneurons (left side, blue) and medial moto-neurons (right side, red) are shown schematically on coronal sections of the cerebral hemispheres, continuing to a longitudinal section of the brainstem and spinal cord. (A) Cells in the primary motor area of the cerebral cortex send axons to the contralat-eral spinal cord to form the lateral corticospinal tract, with collateral connections to the red nucleus. Axons from cells in the red nucleus cross the midline and descend in the rubrospinal tract. The lateral tracts supply monosynaptic and polysynaptic innervation largely to lateral motoneurons (which supply distal musculature; see [B]). Other cortical fibers descend without crossing to form the ventral corticospinal tract, supplying collat-erals to brainstem nuclei. The postural muscles of the body are supplied predominant-ly by the motor regions of the brainstem through the reticulospinal tract, originating in the pontine and medullary reticular formations. The vestibulospinal tract originates in the vestibular nucleus, and the tectospinal tract originates in the superior colliculus. (B) Organization of motoneurons supplying the upper extremities, shown in a trans-verse section of the spinal cord in the cervical region. Muscles of the shoulder and arm are represented most medially, those of the hand most laterally. Extensor motoneurons are located near the margin of the gray matter; flexor motoneurons are more central. (B after E. C. Crosby et al.,1962. *Correlative Anatomy of the Nervous System*. Macmillan: New York, based in part on drawing designed by C. U. Ariëns Kappers.)

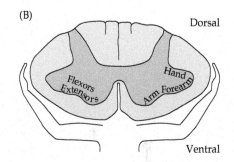

Lateral Motor Pathways

Laterally situated pathways in the spinal cord are primarily concerned with phasic movements and fine manipulations, such as grasping a cup or playing the piano. The **lateral corticospinal tract** (also known as the **pyramidal tract**) originates in the motor and premotor areas of the cerebral cortex, in front of the central sulcus (Brodmann's areas 4 and 6; see Appendix C), as well as from a small strip of the postcentral somatosensory region (known as area 3) of the cerebral cortex (Figure 26.17). Axons originating from pyramidal nerve cells in those regions pass downward through the internal capsule and cerebral peduncles to the medul-lary pyramids, after which most cross the midline (decussate) and continue their descent laterally in the spinal cord. They terminate predominantly on motoneurons and interneu-rons in the lateral gray matter. An important feature is that many of the axons descending from the cortex have terminal branches that end directly on the motoneurons controlling muscles that move the digits.[57,58] In humans and other primates, interruption of the lateral corticospinal tract results primarily in a loss of the ability to move the fingers independent-ly and a deficit in the ability to perform fine, precise tactile movements.[59]

[57] Cheney, D. P., and Fetz, E. E. 1980. *J. Neurophysiol.* 44: 773-791.

[58] Rouiller, E. M. et al. 1996. *Eur. J. Neurosci.* 8: 1055-1059.

[59] Lawrence, D. G., and Kuypers, H. G. J. M. 1968. *Brain* 91: 1-14.

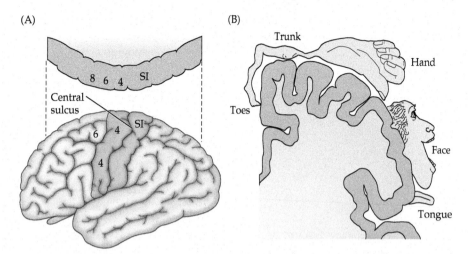

(A)

8 6 4 SI

Central
sulcus

6 4 SI

4

(B)

Trunk

Hand

Toes

Face

Tongue

FIGURE 26.17 Motor Representation on the Cerebral Cortex. (A) Lateral view of the surface of the cerebral cortex. Motor movements result from activation of cells in area 4 of the cerebral cortex (including the cells of origin of the corticospinal tract), which is the primary motor area (M1). The motor system also includes area 6 (premotor area), extending onto the medial surface of the hemispheres. The green strip is the primary somatosensory cortex (SI; see Chapter 23). (B) Sketch of a coronal section through the cerebral hemisphere anterior to the central sulcus. The musculature of the human body is represented in an orderly but distorted fashion, with the leg and foot on the medial surface of the hemisphere and the head most lateral. The very large area devoted to the hand is indicative of the number of neurons involved in manipulations by the digits. (B after W. Penfield and T. Rasmussen, 1950. *The Cerebral Cortex of Man: A Clinical Study of Localization of Function.* Macmillan: New York)

The **rubrospinal tract** originates in the red nucleus (see Figure 26.16) and crosses the midline before descending in the spinal cord to end on interneurons and occasional motoneurons associated with the lateral motor system. Cells in the red nucleus receive excitatory inputs from the motor cortex and from the cerebellum. Although the functional role of the rubrospinal tract is unclear, it is thought to duplicate many of the functions of the corticospinal tract and to constitute a parallel pathway from the cortex.[60] In primates, lesions of the rubrospinal tract have little obvious effect, but interruption of both the rubrospinal and corticospinal tracts severely impairs coordinated positioning of the hands and feet.[61]

Medial Motor Pathways

Medially situated descending tracts provide input to extensor motoneurons that are concerned mainly with sustained activities, such as standing and the adjustment of posture. The medial pathways include the **ventral corticospinal tract**, the lateral and medial **vestibulospinal tracts**, the **pontine** and medullary **reticulospinal tracts**, and the **tectospinal tract**. Except for a small component from the uncrossed ventral corticospinal tract, the descending axons originate primarily in the brainstem (see Figure 26.16). The cells of origin of the lateral vestibulospinal tract lie (as the name indicates) in the lateral vestibular nucleus. Each lateral vestibular nucleus receives input from the ipsilateral vestibular apparatus, in particular from the utricles of the labyrinth (see Chapter 24). The tract descends uncrossed in the spinal cord to provide input to the medial motoneurons supplying postural muscles, with monosynaptic excitatory inputs to extensor muscles and disynaptic inhibitory inputs to flexors. The tract is involved in the maintenance of posture and the regulation of extensor (i.e., antigravity) tone. The pontine reticulospinal tract descends ipsilaterally and ends on segmental interneurons that, in turn, provide bilateral excitation to medial extensor motoneurons. The medullary reticulospinal tract descends bilaterally to provide inhibitory inputs to motoneurons supplying the proximal parts of limbs.

Two other medial brainstem pathways end in the cervical and upper thoracic levels and are concerned with upper body and limb posture, and most particularly with the position

[60] Zelenin, P. V. et al. 2010. *J. Neurosci.* 30: 14533–14542.

[61] Kennedy, P. R. 1990. *Trends Neurosci.* 13: 474–479.

of the head. The medial vestibulospinal tract arises from cells in the medial vestibular nucleus that, in turn, receive inputs both from the semicircular canals in the inner ear (see Chapter 24) and from stretch receptors in neck muscles.[62] The tract descends ipsilaterally to midthoracic levels and is concerned with postural adjustments of the neck and upper limbs during angular acceleration. The tectospinal tract originates in the superior colliculus (tectum) and decussates before descending to upper cervical levels. This pathway mediates orientation of the head and eyes to visual and auditory targets.

Motor Cortex and the Execution of Voluntary Movement

Figures 26.17 and 26.18 show the origin of the corticospinal tracts in primary (M1) and secondary motor areas of the cortex. Motor control is also provided by the somatosensory cortex on the postcentral gyrus.[63,64] Motor cells in the precentral gyrus are arranged in orderly manner according to the location of the musculature they control (see Figure 26.17B). This *somatotopic* representation is highly distorted, with disproportionate representation of the face and hands compared with the trunk. This distortion reflects the relative density of motor innervation devoted to the musculature in each region and, as a consequence, the complexity and subtlety of motor performance.

Motor maps were first demonstrated in 1870 by Fritsch and Hitzig, who produced movements of the body by stimulating the cerebral cortex of animals.[65] The somatotopic representation in humans was later mapped on the brains of patients during neurosurgery by Penfield and his colleagues.[66] Localized stimulation of the cortical surface with brief electrical shocks produced movements of a restricted region of the body, for example a finger, with the location of the contracting muscle depending on the position of the stimulating electrode. Noninvasive recording techniques such as functional magnetic resonance imaging (fMRI) have provided similar maps of the motor cortex.[67,68]

The secondary, or association, motor cortex consists of the premotor cortex (Brodmann's area 6), which lies anterior and somewhat lateral to M1, and the supplemental motor area, also anterior to M1 (see Figure 26.18). Both of these areas, like M1, are somatotopically organized and receive input from sensory association cortex (posterior parietal areas 5 and 7).[69] Premotor cortex is strongly influenced by the cerebellum, and the supplementary motor area is connected with the basal ganglia (see the section "The Cerebellum and Basal Ganglia"). Movements elicited by electrical stimulation in premotor and supplementary motor cortex are complex—for example, a reaching and grasp action—and are often bilateral. Motor-related activity is observed in both of these areas of human brains using fMRI (Figure 26.19). Both areas project somatotopically to the primary motor cortex.

[62] Kaspar, J., Schor, R. H., and Wilson, V. J. 1988. *J. Neurophysiol.* 60: 1765–1768.

[63] Rizzolatti, G, and Wolpert, D. M. 2005. *Curr. Opin. Neurobiol.* 15: 624–625.

[64] Fogassi, L., and Luppino, G. 2005. *Curr. Opin. Neurobiol.* 15: 626–631.

[65] Fritsch, G., and Hitzig, E. 1870. *Arch. Anat. Physiol. Wiss. Med.* 37: 300–332.

[66] Penfield, W., and Rasmussen, T. 1950. *The Cerebral Cortex of Man. A Clinical Study of Localization of Function.* Macmillan, New York, NY.

[67] Porro, C. A. et al. 1996. *J. Neurosci.* 16: 7688–7698.

[68] Rijntjes, M. et al. 1999. *J. Neurosci.* 19: 8043–8048.

[69] Preuss, T. M., Stepniewska, I., and Kaas, J. H. 1996. *J. Comp. Neurol.* 371: 649–676.

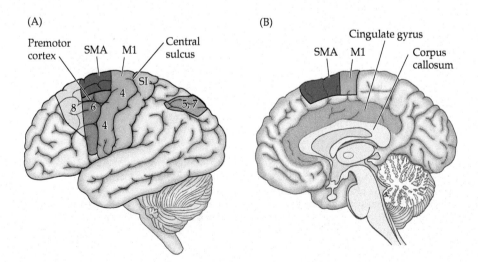

(A)

Premotor cortex SMA M1 Central sulcus

SI

8 6 4

4

5, 7

(B)

Cingulate gyrus

SMA M1 Corpus callosum

FIGURE 26.18 The Association Motor Cortices. (A) The primary and association motor cortices lie anterior to the central sulcus in Brodmann's areas 4 (primary motor cortex, M1) and 6 (premotor cortex and supplemental motor area [SMA]). Frontal eye fields are found in area 8. Primary somatic cortex, SI (areas 3, 1, and 2), and especially association somatosensory cortex (areas 5 and 7), generate commands used in motor planning. (B) Medial surface of the cerebral hemisphere. The cingulate motor area lies between the cingulate gyrus proper and the medial extension of the primary motor and supplementary motor areas.

Tongue   Fingers   Forearm   Eyes

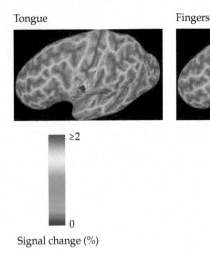

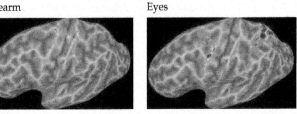

J. D. Meier et al., 2008. *J. Neurophysiol.* 100: 1800–1812

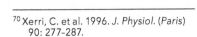

≥2

0

Signal change (%)

FIGURE 26.19 Images of Human Primary Motor Cortex made by fMRI, while the individual moved tongue, fingers, forearm, and eyes. Pseudocolor denotes intensity of signal, with red being the highest. The pattern of activation of cortex resembles that obtained by electrical stimulation.

[70] Xerri, C. et al. 1996. *J. Physiol. (Paris)* 90: 277–287.

[71] Vandermeeren, Y. et al. 2003. *Rev. Neurol. (Paris)* 159: 259–275.

[72] Young, N. A., Vuong, J., and Teskey, G. C. 2012. *J. Neurophysiol.* 108: 1309–1317.

[73] Evarts, E. V. 1965. *J. Neurophysiol.* 28: 216–228.

[74] Evarts, E. V. 1966. *J. Neurophysiol.* 29: 1011–1027.

[75] Krüger, J. et al. 2010. *Front. Neuroeng.* 3: 6.

Somatotopic maps in the sensorimotor cortex are not immutable. In the sensory cortex, repetitive stimulation of fingertips during training sessions leads to enlargement of the corresponding cortical representation of fingertip areas, and expansion of finger areas is seen in the string fingers of violinists and in Braille readers (see Chapter 23). In contrast, paw areas of rats raised in sensory impoverished conditions are reduced.[70]

Similar changes with experience are seen in somatotopic representation in the motor cortex. For example, representations have been shown to change following motor learning.[71] In more recent experiments, development of forelimb motor maps and the effect of experience on development have been studied in neonatal rats.[72] Rats were raised either in small cages (deprived) or in large cages with running wheels, balls, and other toys (enriched). Motor responses to intracortical microstimulation were first seen at postnatal day 35. By postnatal day 45, forelimb motor maps were significantly larger in enriched rats than in the deprived group. In addition, rats between 35 and 44 days of age were trained to reach to a high shelf for food pellets placed in shallow wells. After reach training, the proportion of the motor map devoted to the distal portion of the forelimb (digits and wrist) was 80% on the contralateral (trained) side, compared with 63% on the ipsilateral side.

Cellular Activity and Movement

How is the activity of neurons in motor cortex related to the initiation and performance of a movement? Do individual neurons in M1 cause contraction of a single muscle, direct the strength of contraction of specific muscle groups, control the magnitude of displacement around a joint, or move parts of the body in a particular direction? These questions were first asked by Evarts,[73,74] who recorded the activity of cells in the motor cortex during the performance of trained wrist movements by awake monkeys (Figure 26.20).

In this and other experiments described in the following sections, electrodes were implanted chronically into the motor cortex of monkeys, often for many weeks or even years, to record neuronal activity during trained limb movements.[75] The relations between nerve discharge patterns and various parameters of movement were then examined. For example, by loading the wrist to oppose either flexion or extension, Evarts was able to determine how neural activity was related to force and direction of movement. Some cortical cells fired impulses in association with extension of the wrist, others in association with flexion. In each case the discharge frequency was related to the force required to execute the movement. This behavior of the cortical cells was not unlike the behavior of the spinal motoneurons to

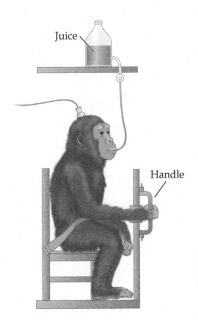

Juice

Handle

FIGURE 26.20 Experimental Arrangement for Recording Cellular Activity related to wrist movement. A monkey, previously trained to move a handle to a designated position, is seated in the chair with its forearm placed in a cuff. The monkey deflects a handle to the left or right between stops, by flexion or extension of the wrist. A system of weights or a torque motor (not shown) is used to load the handle to oppose either flexion or extension. For visually guided movements, the handle position is indicated on a display screen. When the monkey places the handle in the designated position, it receives a reward of fruit juice. Single-unit activity is recorded with a microelectrode positioned in an appropriate area of the brain, by means of a microdrive fixed to the skull.

which they projected. Subsequent experiments showed that this particular kind of behavior is characteristic of corticospinal cells that end directly on spinal motoneurons. Other classes of cells exhibit more complex behavior, depending on other variables, for example the presence of a static load or starting position of the limb.

Higher Control of Movement

One important aspect of the control of voluntary movement is the role of sensory feedback, for example from the visual system or through joint proprioception, or muscle spindles. Movements might be continually reprogrammed as they progress, with ongoing adjustments to compensate for observed deviations from the desired path. Alternatively, a planned movement might be preprogrammed with little or no reliance on feedback control. One argument for this view is that delays in sensory feedback do not permit an adequate degree of control over many observed movements.

Observation made on conscious individuals have indicated that feedback is important but not essential. Marsden and his colleagues found that a man who had been deafferented by a severe peripheral neuropathy affecting dorsal roots could make accurate voluntary movements.[76] He was able to move his fingers, hand, and forearm, and he could outline figures in the air with his eyes closed. However, he was unable to do more complex everyday tasks such as writing, buttoning up his shirt, or holding a cup in one hand. In addition, he could not maintain muscle contractions for more than 1 or 2 seconds without reliance on visual feedback.

A type of motor performance for which feedback is essential is fixating and tracking objects with the eyes during head movements. Eye movements are limited, so the eyes can remain fixed on an object only if the head movement is small. When the head moves or rotates, the eyes first retain their fixation point by moving in the opposite direction, thus keeping the overall visual image stable. They then flick back rapidly and receive a new image on the retina. The sequence repeats until the movement is terminated. These abrupt return deflections are known as **saccades**. The remarkable feature of this process is that sensory information from the eyes themselves and information from the vestibular apparatus are combined to ensure that the image of the visual world remains fixed during the movement. When the visual system receives the new image from the retina at the end of a saccade, it also receives precise information from the vestibular system about the new head position. The two inputs are combined to ensure that each new image is perceived as being at the same location in space as the previous one.[77-79]

Suppose, instead of moving your head, you merely glance at an object that is away from your center of vision. Again your overall visual image remains fixed in space. As there is no head movement, the vestibular system is not involved. Instead, the visual system receives precise information from the motor system about commands sent to the extraocular muscles, and hence about the extent of the eye movement. By contrast, if you move your eye by pushing it very gently with your finger, there is no compensating information from the motor system and movement of the image on the retina is perceived as movement in space.

Cortical Cell Activity Related to Direction of Arm Movements

Irrespective of the role of feedback, movements themselves involve activation of neurons whose activities correlate with a wide variety of movement parameters, such as hand position, joint motion, or specific muscle activation. One such class of cells was found by Georgopoulos and his colleagues while studying cortical cell discharge relating to reaching movements.[80-82] Using multiple electrodes to record the activity of a large number of single units in the arm area of the motor cortex of monkeys during visually guided movements, these researchers found a class of cortical neurons that were directionally selective. These neurons discharged in association with reaching movements in a particular direction but were relatively silent when the direction of movement was changed. Thus, executing the programmed movement involved the recruitment of a specific group of directionally selective neurons to direct the hand to the target location. Preferred directions were not absolute; the discharges fell off as the angle of reach was altered. Furthermore, the preferred

[76] Rothwell, J. C. et al. 1982. *Brain* 105: 515-542.

[77] Wurtz, R. H., 2008. *Vis. Res.* 48: 2070-2089.

[78] Land, M. F. 2009. *Vis. Neurosci.* 26: 561-562.

[79] Watson, T. L., and Krekelberg, B. 2009. *Curr. Biol.* 19: 1040-1043.

[80] Georgopoulos, A. P., Schwartz, A. B., and Kettner, R. E. 1986. *Science* 243: 1416-1419.

[81] Georgopoulos, A. P. et al. 2007. *Proc. Natl. Acad. Sci. USA* 104: 11068-11072.

[82] Merchant, H., Naselaris, T., and Georgopoulos, A. P. 2008. *J. Neurosci.* 28: 9164-9172.

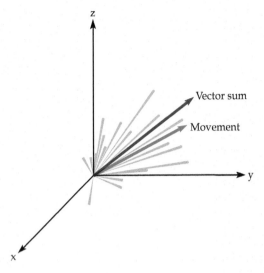

A. P. Georgopoulos et al., 2007. *Proc. Natl. Acad. Sci. USA*
104: 11068–1072. © 2007 National Academy of Sciences

FIGURE 26.21 Encoding Movement in the Motor Cortex. The preferred direction of cortical neurons, shown in three dimensions. The blue arrow indicates the magnitude of the activity recorded from an ensemble of neurons in the motor cortex during a trained movement in the indicated direction. Gray lines represent the activity of single neurons in the ensemble during movement in their individual preferred directions. Each preferred direction is specified by the relative size of the scalar components of the activity vector, projected onto the x-y, x-z, and y-z planes. The direction of the vector sum for the population of individual neurons (red arrow) is similar to that produced by the movement. (After A. P. Georgopoulos et al., 1986. *Science* 243: 1416-1419.)

direction varied with the initial limb position. In one series of experiments, of 2385 recording sites that were analyzed, 985 (41.3%) were directionally tuned.

Figure 26.21 illustrates the activity of a group of neurons in a small area of motor cortex during an arm movement (blue arrow). The angle of the blue arrow indicates the direction of the arm movement in three-dimensional space, and its length indicates the relative intensity of the group discharge. Also shown is the activity of several individual neurons within the group during movements in each of their preferred directions (gray lines). The arrows are scalar projections of the preferred direction vectors onto the x–y, x–z, and y–z planes. The red arrow is the vector sum of all the individual discharges. The direction of the vector sum is close to the direction of the arm movement. This result suggests that the trajectory of the movement is determined by the combined activity of an ensemble of directionally tuned neurons within the group.

Clusters of cells with similar preferred directions are organized in an orderly fashion on the cortex in columns perpendicular to the cortical surface. Figure 26.22A shows the distribution on the anterior bank of the central sulcus of more than 2000 directionally selective columns. The columns are color-coded according to the octant in space occupied by their preferred directions, such as

$$x > 0, y > 0, z > 0 \qquad x > 0, y > 0, z < 0 \qquad x > 0, y < 0, z > 0 \qquad x > 0, y < 0, z < 0$$

and so on. Like colors appear in organized clusters over the surface. More detailed analysis indicates that the columns are centered by minicolumns, each about 30 μm in diameter,

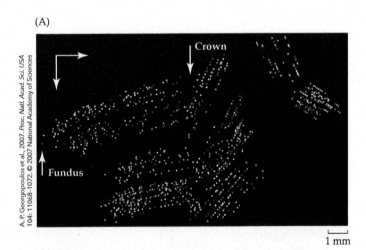

FIGURE 26.22 Mapping of Directionally Selective Columns of Neurons in Motor Cortex. (A) Distribution on the anterior bank of the central sulcus of preferred directions of more than 2000 directionally selective columns of neurons. The columns are color-coded according to which of the eight possible octants in space is occupied by their preferred directions (e.g., x, y, z, positive; x, y, positive, z negative, etc.). Like colors appear in organized clusters over the surface. A = Anterior; L = Lateral. (B) Columns in the clusters are centered by minicolumns, about 30 μm in diameter, with closely similar preferred directions and arranged in a lattice with an average separation of 240 μm. The preferred direction of cells becomes progressively dissimilar as distance (D) from the center of the column increases (not shown). (After A. P. Georgopoulos et al., 2007. *Proc. Natl. Acad. Sci. USA* 104: 11068-11072. © 2007 National Academy of Sciences.)

with closely similar preferred directions and arranged in a lattice with an average separation of 240 μm (Figure 26.22B). The preferred direction of cells becomes progressively dissimilar as distance from the center of the column increases.

Conscious Movements

Many years ago Benjamin Libet and his colleagues performed experiments on people to examine the role of conscious intent in the initiation of voluntary movement.[83] They used electroencephalography to record *readiness potentials* that preceded voluntary movements. Individuals were asked to make a spontaneous movement, such as lifting a finger, and afterward to report the time at which they decided to make the movement. To indicate the decision time, the individuals watched a display screen on which a spot revolved around a clock face, and recalled the spot position at the time the decision was made. The decision time was compared with the time of occurrence of the readiness potential associated with the movement. Surprisingly, the onset of cerebral activity consistently preceded the reported time of intention by several hundred milliseconds. In other words, the neural processing required for planning and executing the movement began without conscious input. The timing indicates that the conscious decision to move did not initiate the neuronal activity responsible for the movement. It also suggests that the reverse may be true: Some component of the neuronal activity may result in conscious awareness of the decision to move. These observations have been confirmed repeatedly, most recently by recording neuronal activity with fMRI.[84]

Sensory-Motor Interaction

As one considers higher aspects of motor function, the boundary between sensory and motor systems becomes blurred. For example, the activity of certain cells in prefrontal cortex of monkeys and humans, known as **mirror neurons**, is related to both the execution and the visual observation of movements. Thus, Rizzolatti and his colleagues have shown that the same neuron fires when a monkey performs an action, such as grasping a stick, as when it observes another monkey doing the same thing.[85] Such mirror neurons may play a part in learning how to perform specific movements by copying the actions of others.

The Cerebellum and Basal Ganglia

The Cerebellum

The principal anatomical features of the cerebellum are shown in Figure 26.23 and Appendix C. The cerebellum participates in motor control through extensive interconnections with the motor cortex and the vestibular system, which is concerned with balance.[86,87] The lucid summary of cerebellar motor function given by Adrian more than 70 years ago still seems elegant, clear, and accurate:

> The cerebellum has the...immediate and quite unconscious task of keeping the body balanced whatever the limbs are doing and of insuring that the limbs do whatever is required of them. Its actions show what complex things can be done by the mechanism of the nervous system in carrying out the decisions of the mind. If I decide to raise my arm, a message is dispatched from the motor area of one cerebral hemisphere to the spinal cord and a duplicate of that message goes to the cerebellum. There, as a result of interactions with other sensory impulses, supplementary orders are sent out to the spinal cord so that the right muscles come in at the exact moment when they are needed, both to raise my arm and keep my body from falling over. The cerebellum has access to all the information from the muscle spindles and pressure organs and so can put in the staff work needed to prevent traffic jams and bad coordination. If it is injured the timing breaks down, muscles come in too early or too late and with the wrong force. The staff work needs to be elaborate, particularly when the body has to be balanced on two legs and uses its arms for all manner of movement, but it is done by the machinery of the nervous system after the mind has given its orders. The cerebellum has nothing to do with formulating the general

[83] Libet, B. et al. 1983. *Brain* 106: 623-642.

[84] Bode, S. et al. 2011. *PLOS ONE* 6: e21612.

[85] Cattaneo, L., and Rizzolatti, G. 2009. *Arch. Neurol.* 66: 557-560.

[86] Glickstein, M., Strata, P., and Voogd, J. 2009. *Neuroscience* 162: 549-559.

[87] Glickstein, M., Sultan, F., and Voogd, J. 2011. *Cortex* 47: 59-80.

FIGURE 26.23 Position and Primary Architecture of the Cerebellum. (A) Location of the cerebellum in relation to the midbrain and brainstem, and its major anatomical features. (B) Somatotopic representation of the body in the anterior and posterior lobes. Roman numerals indicate cerebellar regions.

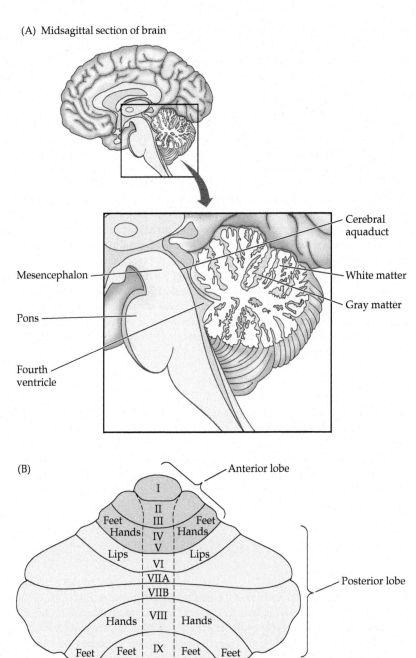

(A) Midsagittal section of brain

Cerebral aquaduct
White matter
Gray matter
Mesencephalon
Pons
Fourth ventricle

(B)

Anterior lobe
I
II
III
Feet
Hands
IV
V
Lips
VI
VIIA
VIIB
Hands
VIII
Hands
Feet
Feet
IX
Feet
Feet
Feet
Hands
Lips
Posterior lobe
X
Flocculonodular lobe

plan of the campaign. Its removal would not affect what we feel or think, apart from the fact that we should be aware that our limbs were not under full control and so should have to plan our activities accordingly.[2]

However, as we discuss later in this chapter, recent experiments have shown that cerebellar function is not limited strictly to motor activity and can be involved in "formulating the general plan of the campaign."

One feature of the cerebellum is that the projections are arranged in a highly ordered manner. Thus, spinal inputs form multiple somatotopic representations on the cerebellar cortex, and these overlie motor representations in the same regions (see Figure 26.23B). Posture and stance are influenced mainly by the output from cells situated in the midline of the cerebellum, whereas fine movements depend on those situated more laterally.

Connections of the Cerebellum

The cerebellum receives proprioceptive, vestibular, and other sensory inputs from the entire body, as well as a massive projection from motor and association cortex. These multiple connections allow actual or intended movements to be compared during their execution with plans provided by the cortex.[88,89] Figure 26.24 shows the afferent and efferent pathways to and from the cerebellum.

The lateral hemispheres receive inputs from a wide area of cerebral cortex (via relay nuclei in the pons) and from the red nucleus (via the inferior olive). The flocculonodular lobe receives inputs from the vestibular nucleus.[90] The medial zone of the cerebellar cortex receives proprioceptive and cutaneous input from all levels of the spinal cord. For this reason, Sherrington referred to the cerebellum as "the head ganglion of the proprioceptive system."[91]

Output from the cerebellar cortex is solely through the axons of **Purkinje cells**, all of which are inhibitory. The Purkinje cell axons project onto cells of the deep cerebellar nuclei and onto vestibular nuclei, again in an orderly fashion. Those from the flocculus and nodulus (vestibulocerebellum) project directly to the vestibular nuclei. The remainder project to the deep nuclei in a regular progression from medial to lateral across the cerebellum. Purkinje cells situated in the midline of the cerebellar cortex project to the fastigial nucleus, which projects to the vestibular nucleus and the reticular formation to influence the vestibulospinal and reticulospinal tracts—that is, the medial motor system concerned with stance and balance. Purkinje cells situated more laterally project to the interposed nucleus, and the most lateral project to the dentate nucleus.[92] Those nuclei send their outputs to the motor cortex via the ventrolateral nucleus of the thalamus. They exert their primary influence on the lateral motor system and thereby influence the musculature of the body concerned with fine movements. The interposed nucleus also projects to the red nucleus. Somatotopic order is maintained in each cerebellar cortical region and carried on through each nuclear projection.

[88] Thach, W. T., Goodkin, H. G., and Keating, J. G. 1992. *Annu. Rev. Neurosci.* 15: 403-442.

[89] Llinás, R., Leznik, E., and Makarenko, V. I. 2002. *Ann. NY Acad. Sci.* 978: 258-272.

[90] Tan, J., Epema, A. H., and Voogd, J. 1995. *J. Comp. Neurol.* 356: 51-71.

[91] Sherrington, C. S. 1933. *The Brain and Its Mechanism.* Cambridge University Press, London, UK.

[92] Habas, C. 2010. *Cerebellum* 9: 22-28.

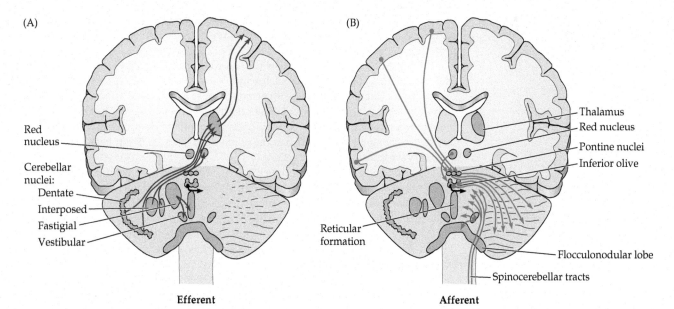

(A)   Efferent

(B)   Afferent

Red nucleus

Cerebellar nuclei:
Dentate
Interposed
Fastigial
Vestibular

Thalamus
Red nucleus
Pontine nuclei
Inferior olive

Reticular formation

Flocculonodular lobe

Spinocerebellar tracts

FIGURE 26.24. Efferent and Afferent Pathways of the Cerebellum shown in relation to the underlying nuclei, cerebral hemispheres, brainstem, and spinal cord. (A) Outputs from the cerebellum (left side, red) are through the dentate, interposed, and fastigial nuclei. Fibers from the dentate nucleus supply the contralateral motor cortex through the ventrolateral nuclei and parts of the ventroposterolateral nuclei of the thalamus. The interposed nuclei project to the contralateral red nucleus. The fastigial nucleus projects to the vestibular nucleus and the pontine and medullary reticular formations, contributing to the medial motor system. (B) Inputs (right side, blue) to the lateral hemispheres of the cerebellum are from wide areas of the cerebral cortex, through the pontine nuclei. Afferent input from the red nucleus is relayed through the inferior olive. More medially, the cerebellum receives extensive input from the spinocerebellar tracts. The flocculonodular lobe is supplied by the vestibular nucleus.

FIGURE 26.25 Pathways between the Cerebellum and Regions of the Cerebral Cortex. Each region of the neocortex has its own pathway to and from the cerebellum. (After V. Benagiano et al., 2018. *J. Comp. Neurol.* 526: 769-789.)

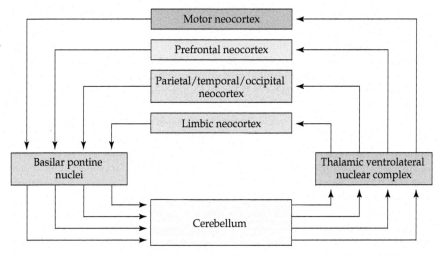

FIGURE 26.25 Pathways between the Cerebellum and Regions of the Cerebral Cortex. Each region of the neocortex has its own pathway to and from the cerebellum. (After V. Benagiano et al., 2018. *J. Comp. Neurol.* 526: 769-789.)

Recent experiments have shown that cerebrocerebellar connections are more extensive than the simple input and output pathways shown in Figure 26.24.[93] Segregated pathways descend to the pontine nuclei not only from motor areas of the neocortex, but also from prefrontal, associative, sensory, and limbic areas (Figure 26.25). In addition, the circuits to these areas are completed by ascending fibers from the ventrolateral thalamus. These feedback connections enable the cerebellum to be involved in a wide variety of non-motor tasks, including sensory perception, cognition, learning, memory, and language. (For specific references see Benagiano.[93])

Synaptic Organization of the Cerebellar Cortex

In few, if any, regions of the CNS have the functional connections of the incoming axons and the output been traced as fully as in the cerebellum.[94] In intact preparations and in slices, a variety of techniques, including anatomical and molecular studies as well as optical and electrical recordings, have been used to reveal the pattern of connections and their physiological mechanisms.

The cytoarchitecture of the cerebellum was revealed by Ramón y Cajal[95] and studied later in detail by light and electron microscopy. The cerebellar cortex is composed of three cellular layers (Figure 26.26). The innermost layer is packed with 10^{10} to 10^{11} **granule cells**—approximating the sum of all other cells in the nervous system! They send axons to the outermost (molecular) layer to form a system of **parallel fibers**, each extending several millimeters along the folium. Also in the granule cell layer are **Golgi cells**, which make inhibitory synapses onto granule cells.

The second cortical layer is occupied by Purkinje cells, whose axons, as already mentioned, constitute the sole output from the cerebellum. The Purkinje cell dendrites extend into the outer molecular layer of the cortex, with their planar arborizations oriented at right angles to the streams of parallel fibers. The parallel fibers make excitatory synaptic contacts onto spiny processes of the distal dendrites of the Purkinje cells. Figure 26.26 shows the way in which the Purkinje cells are stacked in a row along a folium, with the parallel fibers extending through them, rather like the wires laid on telephone poles. It is estimated that each Purkinje cell receives inputs from more than 200,000 parallel fibers!

Each parallel fiber engages a beamlike set of Purkinje cells, extending along the folium and projecting in an orderly manner to the underlying cerebellar nuclei. The significance of this arrangement is that such a beam of Purkinje cells can span all the inputs from muscle spindles and joints in a limb (for example, the shoulder, elbow, and wrist joints of the arm), and thereby has the ability to provide integrated sensory information for regulating complex movements. The second cortical layer also contains **stellate** and **basket cells**, which provide inhibitory inputs to Purkinje cells from remote parallel fibers. The arrangement resembles the lateral inhibition seen in sensory systems.

[93] Benagiano, V. et al. 2018. *J. Comp. Neurol.* 526: 769-789.

[94] Ito, M. 1984. *The Cerebellum and Neural Control.* Raven, New York, NY.

[95] Ramón y Cajal, S. 1995. *Histology of the Nervous System.* 2 vols. Oxford University Press, New York, NY.

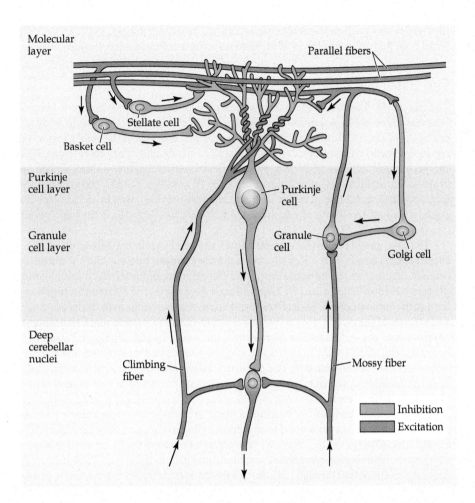

Molecular layer

Parallel fibers

Stellate cell

Basket cell

Purkinje cell layer

Granule cell layer

Purkinje cell

Granule cell

Golgi cell

Deep cerebellar nuclei

Climbing fiber

Mossy fiber

Inhibition

Excitation

FIGURE 26.26 Synaptic Organization of the Cerebellum. The axons of deep nuclear neurons form the output paths of the cerebellum. Mossy fiber inputs excite granule cells, whose axons ascend to the molecular layer to form a parallel fiber network. Parallel fibers form excitatory synapses on Purkinje cells, stellate cells, basket cells, and dendrites of Golgi cells. Climbing fibers form excitatory synapses on Purkinje cells. Both climbing fibers and mossy fibers make excitatory connections with cells in the deep cerebellar nuclei. Red indicates excitation, blue inhibition. Arrows indicate the direction of flow of electrical activity. (After S. Ramón y Cajal. Translated from the French by Neely and Larry Swanson, 1995. *Histology of the Nervous System of Man and Vertebrates.* Vol. 2. Oxford University Press, New York.)

Information flowing into the cerebellum from cortico-pontine relays and sensory systems is carried by **mossy fibers** that make excitatory synapses with granule cells, Golgi cells, and deep nuclear neurons.[96] Mossy fiber excitation of parallel fibers (the axons of granule cells) causes simple spike generation in Purkinje cells. These occur continuously at rates of 50 to 150 per second and resemble conventional brief action potentials seen in other neurons. Each **climbing fiber** arising in the inferior olive makes extensive connections onto the soma and proximal dendrite of 1 to 10 Purkinje cells. Climbing fibers cause powerful excitation of Purkinje cells,[97] and produce large plateau potentials that lead to complex spikes.[98] This activity involves calcium action potentials in the dendrites (see Chapter 8), leading to a calcium influx.[99,100]

Functions of the Cerebellum

Experiments with trained monkeys, including lesion experiments, and clinical disorders have shown that the cerebellum plays a key role in planning and performing coordinated movements, in motor learning, and even in higher cognitive function.[101,102] However, the precise nature of these roles is obscure. Several individuals have been studied who have virtually no cerebellum as the result of developmental defects. They are able to live more or less normal lives, without severe motor impairment and no apparent sensory defects.[103]

Most lesions of the cerebellum in individuals, whether due to disease or development, are diffuse rather than focal, with signs and symptoms that relate to balance and motor control.[104] As one might expect from their connections to the vestibular system, localized lesions of the nodulus and flocculus give rise to disturbances in equilibrium and eye movements as well as to disordered movements of the trunk. A common feature of cerebellar lesions is an intention tremor during a movement, say of the hand, in which small,

[96] Rokni, D., Llinas, R., and Yarom, Y. 2008. *Front. Syst. Neurosci.* 2: 192–198.

[97] Ito, M., and Simpson, J. I. 1971. *Brain Res.* 31: 215–219.

[98] Foust, A. et al. 2009. *Neuroscience* 162: 836–851.

[99] Miyakawa, H. et al. 1992. *J. Neurophysiol.* 68: 1178–1189.

[100] Zagha, E. et al. 2010. *J. Neurophysiol.* 103: 3516–3525.

[101] Strick, P. L., Dum, R. P., and Fiez, J. A. 2009. *Annu. Rev. Neurosci.* 32: 413–434.

[102] Thach, W. T. 2007. *Cerebellum* 6: 163–167.

[103] Boyd, C. A. R. 2010. *Brain* 133: 941–944.

[104] Dietrichs, E. 2008. *Acta Neurol. Scand. Suppl.* 188: 6–11.

rhythmical, and purposeless trembling begins and becomes stronger. This tremor is different from that occurring at rest with disorders of the basal ganglia (see the next section).

The Basal Ganglia

The nuclei that constitute the basal ganglia play an essential role in motor control. Whereas the cerebellum is primarily concerned with phasic movements of the body (for example, eye saccades and finger pointing), a principal function of the basal ganglia is to regulate posture, counteract tremor, and maintain steady muscular contractions. Neurons in basal ganglia can activate agonists and antagonists together—a mechanism appropriate for stabilizing a joint, such as the knee.[105] Basal ganglia also cooperate in terminating movements and in motor learning. Here we provide only a brief summary and guide to the vast literature that deals with the structure and functions of the basal ganglia (see for example[106–108]).

The basal ganglia consist of nuclear masses situated beneath the outer cortical layers of the cerebral hemispheres. Key structures are the **caudate nucleus** and the **putamen** (known together as the **neostriatum**), and the external and internal divisions of the **globus pallidus** (Figure 26.27). Two midbrain structures, the **substantia nigra** and the **subthalamic nucleus**, have afferent and efferent connections with the basal ganglia and are part of the circuit. Dopaminergic neurons in the substantia nigra (see Chapter 14) project to the striatum (the nigrostriatal pathway). Nigral neurons release dopamine, which inhibits some neurons and excites others; the overall effect of dopamine on the striatum is excitatory.[109] The gas nitric oxide (NO), which functions as a local neurotransmitter in the basal ganglia and reaches its targets by diffusion in solution, inhibits dopamine release.[110]

The striatum receives widespread inputs from the cerebral cortex, particularly from the precentral gyrus and the thalamus. Major outputs of the basal ganglia from the globus pallidus are directed to the ventrolateral and ventroanterior nuclei of the thalamus (overlapping with regions receiving input from the cerebellum) and back to the cortex. The basal ganglia modulate motor output through this complex feedback circuitry.[111]

[105] Mink, J. W., and Thach, W. T. 1991. *J. Neurophysiol.* 65: 330–351.

[106] Graybiel, A. M. 2008. *Annu. Rev. Neurosci.* 31: 359–387.

[107] Kreitzer, A. C., and Malenka, R. C. 2008. *Neuron* 60: 543–554.

[108] Kreitzer, A. C. 2009. *Annu. Rev. Neurosci.* 32: 127–147.

[109] Surmeier, D. J. et al. 2007. *Trends Neurosci.* 30: 228–245.

[110] Del-Bel, E. et al. 2011. *Curr. Pharm. Des.* 17: 471–488.

[111] Mink, J. W., and Thach, W. T. 1993. *Curr. Opin. Neurobiol.* 3: 950–957.

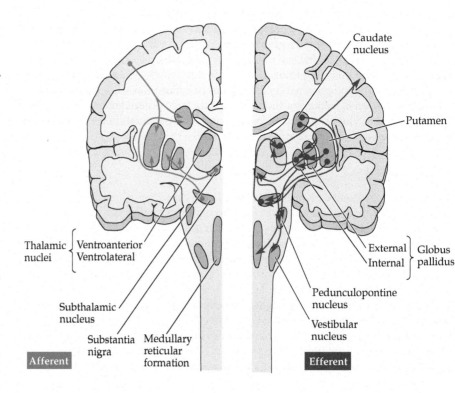

FIGURE 26.27 The Basal Ganglia. Coronal section through the cerebral hemispheres, continued as a longitudinal section of the brainstem and spinal cord. Basal ganglia include the caudate nucleus, putamen, and globus pallidus (external and internal divisions). Two additional nuclei, the substantia nigra and the subthalamic nucleus, have extensive interconnections with the basal ganglia and are sometimes included with them. The predominant input to the basal ganglia is from the cortex (left side, blue). Outputs from the basal ganglia go to the ventroanterior and ventrolateral nuclei of the thalamus, which in turn project to cortex (right side, red), completing a cortical feedback circuit. Additional output pathways project to the vestibular nucleus and medullary reticular formation through the pedunculopontine nucleus.

Circuitry of the Basal Ganglia

The caudate and putamen function as the input stage of the basal ganglia (Figure 26.28). The putamen receives its input from the sensorimotor strip surrounding the central sulcus, so its activity relates most directly to motor activity. The caudate is innervated by frontal cortex and is involved in higher-order cognitive processing. This parallel arrangement underlies the role of the basal ganglia in cognition and affect as well as in motor processing. GABAergic neurons of the caudate and putamen project to the globus pallidus and inhibit its activity. Neurons of the globus pallidus are also inhibitory;[112] they release GABA onto thalamic neurons in the ventroanterior and ventrolateral nuclei. Since neurons in the globus pallidus fire tonically, they continuously inhibit the flow of excitation from thalamus to cortex.[105] The firing rates of individual neurons in the globus pallidus concerned with wrist movements are relatively unaffected by the wrist's position, the velocity of movement, or the load on the wrist. The strongest stimulus for such neurons is instead a sudden movement, which causes a pronounced increase in frequency after a delay. Mink and Thach have proposed that pallidal cell discharges are associated with the release of holding mechanisms responsible for joint fixation, thereby allowing the movement to occur.[105] An analogy for the delayed firing is that of starting a car on a hill: The hand brake is released only after power has been applied to the wheels.

Projections running from the thalamus to the striatum, named thalamostriatal projections, also contribute to the control of movement. Experiments using optogenetic inhibition of neurons from the thalamostriatal projections and recordings from neurons of animals trained for certain tasks showed that the projections from the parafascicular and ventroposterior regions of the thalamus contribute to the initiation of trained behaviors, but only the ventroposterior projection contributes to the execution of the learned sequences of movements.[113]

Diseases of the Basal Ganglia

The importance of the basal ganglia in motor control is emphasized by the devastating consequences of neurodegenerative diseases that affect their function.[114] James Parkinson described the "shaking palsy" in 1817. **Parkinson's disease** is characterized by a continuous tremor at rest ("pill rolling"), an increased tone due to simultaneous activation of antagonist muscles, difficulty in initiating or finishing movements, and slowness of movement once begun. Deficits are prominent in tasks that involve switching from one action to another.

A factor in the development of Parkinson's disease is the degeneration of dopaminergic neurons of the substantia nigra. However, dopamine cannot be given to individuals to counteract the deficit because it cannot cross the blood–brain barrier (see Chapter 10) and has devastating peripheral side effects. Instead, the standard therapy is oral administration of a dopamine precursor, which does cross the barrier and typically is used by substantia nigra neurons to synthesize dopamine. In brief, the loss of dopamine in Parkinson's disease reduces striatal activity. As a result, there is less inhibition of the globus pallidus, and its increased firing inhibits neurons in the thalamus. They, in turn, provide a lower level of excitatory input to the motor cortex. The result is the hypokinesis that is a dominant deficit of this disease.

As the disease progresses, complications appear in the response to L-DOPA treatment. These include muscle spasms and involuntary movements, together known as L-DOPA-induced dyskinesia. There is evidence that NO modulates the activity of L-DOPA to shift the balance between excitation and inhibition and reduce L-DOPA-induced dyskinesia.[115]

Another clinically important disorder of the basal ganglia is the genetically determined **Huntington's disease**, the hallmark of which is the appearance of spontaneous, disruptive movements that give this disease its other name, Huntington's chorea (from the Greek word meaning "dance").[116] Individuals typically develop symptoms and signs in their twenties or thirties, as a result of degeneration of striatal neurons supplying the external globus pallidus.

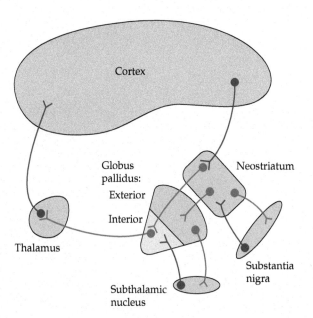

FIGURE 26.28 Functional Circuits of the Basal Ganglia. Glutamatergic neurons in cortex excite GABAergic cells of the neostriatum (caudate and putamen). Striatal neurons project to the external globus pallidus (the indirect pathway) and internal globus pallidus (the direct pathway) to inhibit GABAergic neurons in those nuclei. GABAergic neurons of the internal globus pallidus project to and inhibit the thalamus. Dopaminergic neurons of the substantia nigra produce net excitation of the striatum. Glutamatergic neurons of the subthalamic nucleus are inhibited by the projection from the external globus pallidus and excite GABAergic neurons of the internal globus pallidus. Excitatory neurons are shown in red and inhibitory neurons in blue.

[112] Rav-Acha, M. et al. 2005. *Neuroscience* 135: 791–802.

[113] Díaz-Hernández, E. et al. 2018. *Neuron* 100: 739–752.

[114] DeLong, M., and Wichmann, T. 2009. *Parkinsonism Relat. Disord.* 15: S237–240.

[115] Bortolanza, M. et al. 2016. *Neurotox Res.* 30: 88–100.

[116] Gil, J. M., and Rego, A. C. 2008. *Eur. J. Neurosci.* 27: 2803–2820.

Although lesions and diseases of the nervous system lead to behavioral changes that provide essential clues about normal functions, they do not reveal mechanisms. That the basal ganglia and cerebellum organize, coordinate, and take part in the learning of movements is certain, but how they do so is still not known.

Interactions between the Cerebellum and Basal Ganglia

The cerebellum and the basal ganglia have long been considered to be separate subcortical systems, each with its own distinct connections to thalamic nuclei and hence to the neocortex. However, recent data have shown that they are heavily interconnected.[117] The subthalamic nucleus in the basal ganglia sends a dense projection to the cerebellar cortex, and the dentate nucleus in the cerebellum is the source of a dense projection to the striatum. Thus, the cerebellum and basal ganglia, rather than acting separately, form an integrated network with the cerebral cortex. In addition, the network is topographically organized so that the functional territories of each component are interconnected, and discrete events in one component can have network-wide effects.

Concluding Remarks

We know far less about the mechanisms that allow us to point to an object than about the steps that occur as we see the object. For coordinated movements, numerous anatomical structures and complex connections need to be considered, each involved in feedback and feedforward control. In addition, lesions to structures such as the cerebellum and the cortex have not provided definitive explanations of what these areas of the brain do or how they do it. But there is good news. First, new methods for recording from large groups of nerve cells individually and at once are becoming available at an ever more rapid pace. Second, the eager investigator who enters the field of neurobiology can see at once that there are abundant, fascinating problems about motor systems still begging to be explored, let alone solved.

[117] Bostan, A. C., and Strick, P. L. 2018. *Nat. Rev. Neurosci.* 19: 338–350.

SUMMARY

- A motor unit consists of a single α motor neuron and the skeletal muscle fibers it innervates.

- Muscle spindle afferents diverge to make synaptic contacts onto all the motoneurons innervating the muscle of origin.

- Muscular contraction begins with small motor units and progresses to large motor units (the size principle of motor recruitment).

- The stretch reflex excites agonist muscles, and inhibits antagonists through inhibitory interneurons.

- Flexor reflexes initiated by painful stimuli comprise elements of interlimb coordination essential for locomotion.

- The muscle spindle's sensitivity to stretch is modulated by activation of γ efferent (fusimotor) fibers that cause the intrafusal muscle fibers to contract.

- Co-activation of α and γ motoneurons continuously adjusts the spindle to maintain its sensitivity during programmed movements.

- Respiration and locomotion provide examples of motor programs arising from pattern generators in the CNS.

- Medial and lateral pools of spinal motoneurons innervate the muscles of the trunk and distal limbs, respectively.

- The primary motor cortex (M1) lies anterior to the central sulcus and is somatotopically mapped.

- Many neurons in M1 are grouped in columns according to their direction selectivity.

- The planning of coordinated movements includes anticipatory adjustments to take account of the effects of muscular contractions on feedback mechanisms.

- The cerebellum plans and executes motor commands through feedback with the cortex and via descending commands through the red nucleus and brainstem nuclei. Lesions of the cerebellum disrupt coordination.

- The basal ganglia provide negative feedback to the cerebral cortex. The consequences of basal ganglia disease reflect the complex pattern of feedback loops that underlie their function.

Suggested Reading

General Reviews

Benagiano, V., Rizzi, A., Lorusso, L., Flace, P., Saccia, M., Cagiano, D., Ribatti, D., Roncali, L., and Ambrosi, G. 2018. The functional anatomy of the cerebrocerebellar circuit: A review and new concepts. *J. Comp. Neurol.* 526: 769–789.

Bostan, A. C., and Strick, P. L. 2018. The basal ganglia and the cerebellum: nodes in an integrated nework. *Nature Rev. Neurosci.* doi: 10.1038/s41583-018-0002-7

Briggman, K. L., and Kristan, W. B. 2008. Multifunctional pattern-generating circuits. *Annu. Rev. Neurosci.* 31: 271–294.

Cattaneo, L., and Rizzolatti, G. 2009. The mirror neuron system. *Arch. Neurol.* 66: 557–560.

Georgopoulos, A. P., and Stefanis, C. N. 2007. Local shaping of function in the motor cortex: motor contrast, directional tuning. *Brain Res. Rev.* 55: 383–389.

Hultborn, H. 2006. Spinal reflexes, mechanisms and concepts: from Eccles to Lundberg and beyond. *Prog. Neurobiol.* 78: 215–242.

Kreitzer, A. C. 2009. Physiology and pharmacology of striatal neurons. *Annu. Rev. Neurosci.* 32: 127–147.

Lemon, R. N. 2008. Descending pathways in motor control. *Annu. Rev. Neurosci.* 31: 195–218.

Pearson, K. G. 2008. Role of sensory feedback in the control of stance duration in walking cats. *Brain Res. Rev.* 57: 222–227.

Sherrington, C. S. 1906. *The Integrative Action of the Nervous System*, 1961 ed. Yale University Press, New Haven, CT.

Taccola, G., and Nistri, A. 2006. Oscillatory circuits underlying locomotor networks in the rat spinal cord. *Crit. Rev. Neurobiol.* 18: 25–36.

Thach, W. T. 2007. On the mechanism of cerebellar contributions to cognition *Cerebellum* 6: 163–167.

Vandermeeren Y, Bastings, E., Good, D., Rouiller, E., and Oliver, E. 2003. Plasticity of motor maps in primates: recent advances and therapeutical perspectives. *Rev. Neurol. (Paris)* 159: 259-275.

Original Papers

Bannatyne, B. A., Liu, T. T., Hammar, I., Stecina, K., Jankowska, E., and Maxwell, D. J. 2009. Excitatory and inhibitory intermediate zone interneurons in pathways from feline group I and II afferents: differences in axonal projections and input. *J. Physiol.* 587: 379–399.

Durbaba, R., Taylor, A., Ellaway, P. H., and Rawlinson, S. 2003. The influence of bag$_2$ and chain intrafusal muscle fibers on secondary spindle afferents in the cat. *J. Physiol.* 550: 263–278.

Eugenin, J., Nicholls, J. G., Cohen, L. B., and Muller, K. J. 2006. Optical recording from respiratory pattern generator of fetal mouse brainstem reveals a distributed network. *Neuroscience* 137: 1221–1227.

Georgopoulos, A. P., Merchant, H., Naselaris, T., and Amirikian, B. 2007. Mapping of the preferred direction in the motor cortex. *Proc. Natl. Acad. Sci. USA* 104: 11068–1072.

Henneman, E., Somjen, G., and Carpenter, D. O. 1965. Functional significance of cell size in spinal motoneurons. *J. Neurophysiol.* 28: 560–580.

Kuffler, S. W., Hunt, C. C., and Quilliam, J. P. 1951. Function of medullated small-nerve fibers in mammalian ventral roots: Efferent muscle spindle innervation. *J. Neurophysiol.* 14: 29–51.

Meier, J. D., Aflalo, T. N., Kastner, S., and Graziano, M. S. A. 2008. Complex organization of human primary motor cortex: a high-resolution fMRI study. *J. Neurophysiol.* 100: 1800–1812.

Rochat, M. J., Caruana, F., Jezzini, A. et al. 2010. Responses of mirror neurons in area F5 to hand and tool grasping observation. *Exp. Brain Res.* 204: 605–616.

Xerri, C., Coq, J. O., Merzenich, M. M., and Jenkins, W. M. 1996. Experience-induced plasticity of cutaneous maps in the primary somatosensory cortex of adult monkeys and rats. *J. Physiol. (Paris)* 90: 277–287.

Young, N. A., Vuong, J., and Teskey, G. C. 2012. Development of motor maps in rats and their modulation by experience. *J. Neurophysiol.* 108: 1309–1317.

PART VI

Development and Regeneration of the Nervous System

A question that naturally arises from reading about neuronal signaling, sensory perception, and motor functions concerns the way in which the nervous system is formed during development and how it is modified by experience and injury. Chapter 27 deals with the way in which the nervous system develops in an embryo, in terms of cellular and molecular mechanisms that give rise to highly complex structures. Selected examples are used to show how key molecules play crucial roles in the formation of the central and peripheral nervous systems.

A logical question concerns the role of experience in the formation of the brain after an animal is born. In Chapter 28 we describe the progress that has been made in understanding how visual, auditory, and olfactory experiences in the first months of life influence not merely the performance of the nervous system but its very structure.

A related question of obvious importance concerns the ability of the nervous system to repair itself after injury. In Chapter 29 we show that nerve fibers in the periphery can regenerate to restore function after they have been damaged. By contrast, axons in the central nervous system are unable to do so, for reasons that are not yet known.

CHAPTER 27

Development of the Nervous System

During development, cells acquire specific neuronal or glial identities, and establish orderly and precise synaptic connections, under the influence of factors intrinsic to the cells (genotype, gene expression patterns) and of extrinsic factors in the embryonic environment (inductive and trophic interactions among cells, cues that guide cell migration and axon outgrowth, specific cell–cell recognition, and activity-dependent refinement of connections).

The scope of all the topics problems relating to vertebrate neural development is too great to be described in a single chapter, particularly for readers unfamiliar with basic principles of embryonic development (for more comprehensive reviews see[1–3]). In this chapter we discuss general principles about vertebrate neural development and describe selected experiments to illustrate underlying cellular and molecular mechanisms. Our aim is to provide a concise, coherent account of neural development of the sort that might be delivered in three or four lectures. Selected topics are discussed in developmental sequence.

[1] Gilbert, S. F. and Barresi, M. J. F. 2016. *Developmental Biology*, 11th ed. Oxford University Press/Sinauer, Sunderland, MA.

[2] Sanes, D. H., Reh, T. A., and Harris, W. A. 2019. *Development of the Nervous System*, 4th ed. Academic Press, Burlington, VT.

[3] Price, D. J. et al. 2011. *Building Brains: An Introduction to Neural Development*, Wiley Blackwell, Oxford, UK.

Development: General Considerations

Generating the correct numbers and types of neurons, at the appropriate positions and forming the right synaptic connections with one another and with peripheral tissues, is a prerequisite for normal function of the nervous system. How do precursor cells acquire their identities? What cues guide cells to their correct positions? Which mechanisms enable a neuron to extend an axon to a particular target, among myriad possible choices, and form a synapse?

First of all, the assemblage of 10^{10}–10^{12} cells and an almost uncountable number of synapses is established with fewer than 30,000 genes, suggesting that cell identities and synaptic connections are specified in a combinatorial manner. Moreover, the overall wiring plan requires that flexibility be maintained during critical periods in development, and even in the adult (see Chapter 28).

Somatic cell nuclear transfer experiments, pioneered by John Gurdon in the frog,[4] allowed the cloning of whole animals from individual adult differentiated cells,[5,6] and demonstrated that differentiated cells all contain the same genes and that the primary sequence of their genome remains equivalent to that of a fertilized egg. It follows that the biochemical, morphological, and functional differences underlying the variety of neurons and glia reflect qualitative and quantitative differences in the expression levels of specific genes among the various cell types. The acquisition of adult cell identities is therefore the result of a developmental **gene regulatory network** determining differential gene expression.[7] This molecular barcode defines the unique molecular "ground state" of each cell type of the brain, which can now be measured by cell-type and single-cell transcriptomics.[8] During development, the ground state identifying neuronal identity is reached by the sequential and hierarchical expression of many different transcription factors.

The transcription factors control gene expression by acting on promoter and enhancer DNA genomic sequences, which are the same in every cell. However, any given enhancer can regulate different genes in different cells or tissue, depending on which transcription factor it binds. The same transcription factor, in conjunction with other factors, can regulate different promoters in different cells. Thus, **combinatorial transcriptional codes** determine the cell-type specific expression of a given gene and allow the encoding of a large set of cell identities by a limited number of transcription factors.[9,10]

A few functional categories illustrate the general principles by which transcription factors generate and maintain cellular diversity during development. Among these, the importance of pioneer [11] and master transcription factors is highlighted by the work that led Shinya Yamanaka to obtain induced pluripotent stem cells (iPSCs) from adult differentiated somatic cells (Box 27.1). Pioneer transcription factors engage with silent chromatin and open it up to initiate transcriptional programs that lead to cell fate change. Another class of transcription factors, called **terminal selectors**,[9] are responsible for maintaining the identities of differentiated neurons.

Some transcription factors, instead of regulating cell-autonomous pathways in the same cell in which they are expressed, activate signaling pathways that, in turn, regulate gene expression in neighboring cells. Cell-to-cell communication plays a crucial role in shaping embryonic development, by local and long-range signaling molecules that are either secreted or positioned in the cell's membrane, as shown later in the chapter, in the section Proneural Genes and Lateral Inhibition. Local signaling is carried out via membrane receptors that bind directly to a membrane protein on the neighboring cell (such as the Notch and Delta signaling proteins), in a process called **juxtacrine signaling**. The Notch-Delta pathway plays a critical role in cell fate determination in the neural plate, by a process called lateral inhibition.

Another important mechanism governing cell fate specification during development involves longer-range **paracrine signaling** by molecules secreted in the extracellular environment, forming morphogenetic gradients. Among the secreted gradient-forming morphogens relevant for the nervous system's development are retinoic acid (RA), fibroblast growth factors (FGFs), Sonic hedgehog (Shh), Wingless/Int-1 (Wnt), and bone morphogenetic proteins (BMPs). How the receiver cells "read" morphogen concentration gradients is a subject of intense research.

These signaling pathways are remarkably conserved throughout the animal kingdom and are used over and over again in development, often with different functional roles at different times and places, in the embryos of diverse species. Often there are multiple versions of each pathway within a single species. A systematic description of these pathways is out of the scope of this chapter. We recommend that students consult comprehensive reviews.[1,2]

[4] Gurdon, J. B., and Melton, D. A. 2008. *Science* 322: 1811–1815.

[5] Eggan, K. et al. 2004. *Nature* 428: 44–49.

[6] Wilmut, I. et al. 1997. *Nature* 385: 810–813.

[7] Fishell, G. and Heintz, N. 2013. *Neuron* 80: 602–612.

[8] Tasic, B. 2018. *Curr. Op. Neurobiol.* 50: 242–249.

[9] Allan, D. W., and Thor, S. 2015. *WIREs Dev. Biol.* 2015: 4: 505–528.

[10] Jessel, T. M. 2000. *Nat. Rev. Genet.* 1: 20–29.

[11] Iwafuchi-Doi, M., and Zaret, K. S. 2014. *Genes Dev.* 28: 2679–2692.

BOX 27.1   Induced Pluripotent Stem Cells

Somatic cell nuclear transplant experiments in animals showed that the genome of a differentiated somatic cell remains equivalent to that of a fertilized egg (principle of genomic equivalence)[12] and that development and cellular differentiation do not cause an irreversible genetic loss.

John Gurdon's research taught us that the nucleus of a mature, specialized cell can return to an immature, pluripotent state. However, it remained unclear to what extent the epigenetic changes imposed on the genome by development are reversible. Some studies had shown that lineage-associated *master transcription factors* can switch one somatic cell type into another,[13] but the generality of this finding was uncertain. Might it be possible to **reprogram** somatic differentiated cells into embryonic pluripotent stem cells (running the developmental clock in the reverse direction)?

To address this question, in 2006 Takahashi and Yamanaka[14] devised a screen for transcription factors that could reactivate, in differentiated cells, a dormant selectable reporter gene (providing resistance to a killing drug) driven by an embryonic stem cell–specific promoter (Figure). This selection approach allowed screening for factors able to induce the expression of the dormant selectable gene, when introduced into differentiated somatic cells (reprogramming factors). The approach ensured that rare reprogrammed cells would survive and that non-reprogrammed colonies would be eliminated. This led to the identification of a minimal core of four transcription factors able to reprogram adult mouse fibroblasts (and any other cell in the adult mouse) into **induced pluripotent stem cells (iPSCs)**, displaying the pluripotency of embryonic stem cells. The identified genes were *Sox2*, *Oct4*, *c-Myc*, and *Klf4*, collectively known as Yamanaka factors. Like embryonic stem cells, iPSCs can be propagated indefinitely and can be made to differentiate into cell types of all three germ layers. Within a short time, other research groups reported that the same or a similar cocktail of transcription factors could induce pluripotency in a variety of differentiated human cells.

Most important, entire mice could be generated from single iPSCs, thus fulfilling the most stringent criterion for pluripotency. Shinya Yamanaka shared the 2012 Nobel Prize in Physiology or Medicine with John Gurdon "for the discovery that mature cells can be reprogrammed to become pluripotent."

iPSCs open new windows for direct investigation of the mechanisms of human brain development[15] and allow experimentation on diseased human tissue while avoiding the complications of using human embryonic stem cells. Two different medically relevant research approaches are currently being pursued with iPSCs:[16] (1) deriving patient-specific iPSCs for studying disease pathology mechanisms (the "disease in a dish" approach); importantly, in the case of genetic diseases, the disease-causing mutation can be repaired by gene targeting in the patients' iPSCs, providing control cell lines with exactly the same genetic background; and (2) using differentiated cells derived from patient-derived iPSCs for drug screening. In perspective, in some cases patient-specific iPSC-derived progenitor cells might be considered for autologous cell transplants in patients, without the complications of immune rejection.

The basis for modeling diseases is the ability to differentiate iPSCs into the cell type that is affected in the patient and to recapitulate in a petri dish the cell-autonomous abnormalities as they are seen in patients. For example, patient-specific iPSCs have been differentiated into dopaminergic neurons to model Parkinson's disease,[17] and into motor neurons to establish a spinal motor atrophy culture model.[18]

---

[12] Gurdon, J. 1962. *J. Embryol. Exp. Morphol.* 10: 622.

[13] Davis, R. L. et al. 1987. *Cell* 51: 987–1000.

[14] Takahashi, K. and Yamanaka, S. 2006. *Cell* 126: 663.

[15] Suzuki, I. K., and Vanderhaeghen, P. 2015. *Development* 142: 3138.

[16] Hochedlinger, K. and Jaenisch, R. 2015. *Cold Spring Harb. Perspect. Biol.* A019448.

[17] Soldner, F. et al. 2011. *Cell* 146: 318.

[18] Ebert, R. et al. 2009. *Nature* 457: 277.

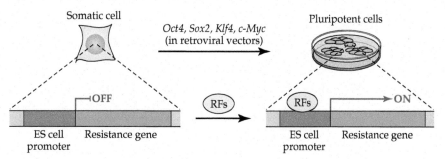

Schematic representation of the genetic assay system used by Yamanaka to screen for reprogramming factors (RFs) that could transcribe a dormant drug-resistance allele, integrated into an embryonic stem (ES) cell-specific genomic locus. Candidate reprogramming transcription factors were inserted into the reporter cell by viral infection. Cells were treated with a killing drug. Successful reprogramming to pluripotency (iPSCs) allowed the expression of the resistance gene. (After K. Hochedlinger and R. Jaenisch, 2015. *Cold Spring Harb. Perspect. Biol.* 7: a019448.)

A good starting point for many studies of development is the question of when and where the diverse cell types of interest arise during embryogenesis. The process of answering such questions is called **cell fate mapping**, or lineage tracing.[19] To assess and identify the intrinsic and extrinsic influences on cell fate, one experimental strategy that has proved useful is to transplant labeled progenitor cells into different cellular environments, at different developmental times (**heterochronic transplantation**). Recently, lineage tracing with sophisticated multicolored reporter constructs and live-cell imaging (see Chapter 1) has provided great insights into neural development.

Studies on invertebrates, such as the fruit fly, have uncovered many widely shared developmental mechanisms and general principles. Investigations of the cell and regional specification of neural tissue of the vertebrate brain were aided immensely by the finding that in *Drosophila* most developmental regulatory genes (which often encode transcription factors) have vertebrate homologues that usually serve similar functions. One vertebrate preparation that is very convenient for developmental studies is the zebrafish (*Danio rerio*), which was introduced by Streisinger.[20] The embryo is transparent, and the adult animal reproduces rapidly; throughout embryogenesis, individual cells can be observed under the microscope as they divide and grow. Mutations in developmental regulatory genes can be readily induced and their effects studied.[21]

Early Morphogenesis of the Nervous System

Neural Induction

Early in vertebrate embryogenesis, the region of the gastrula that will give rise to the nervous system is a sheet of cells on the outer surface of the embryo called ectoderm.[1] The three basic layers of the embryo—the endoderm, mesoderm and ectoderm—arise during gastrulation:[1] Cells ingress from the surface ectoderm into the interior of the embryo, to give rise to the mesodermal and endodermal germ layers. Cell ingression occurs in amphibians through the *blastopore*, and in amniotes (birds, reptiles, mammals) through the *primitive streak* (Figure 27.1). It is in this embryonic period that a specific region of the ectoderm becomes fated to generate neural tissue, forming what is called the **neural plate**.

To study the induction of the neural plate, in 1924 Hans Spemann and his student Hilde Mangold[22] transplanted the dorsal lip of a blastopore from a pigmented amphibian embryo to the interior of a nonpigmented host embryo, so they could identify host and donor tissue on the basis of the color. The blastopore lip was grafted in the region that would normally become ventral epidermis. The transplanted embryo was allowed to develop into a tadpole. Spemann and Mangold found that an entire second nervous system, made mostly of nonpigmented cells, developed from the place where they had grafted the new blastopore, indicating that it came from the host blastula and not from the transplanted dorsal lip. Thus, they concluded that the grafted blastopore cells (known as the **Spemann organizer**

[19] Kretschmar, K. and Watt. F. M. 2012. *Cell* 148: 33-45.

[20] Streisinger, G. et al. 1981. *Nature* 291: 293-296.

[21] Nusslein-Volhard, C. 2012. *Development* 139: 4099-4103.

[22] Spemann, H. and Mangold, H. 1924. *Arch. Mikr. Anat. Entw. Mech.* 100: 599-638.

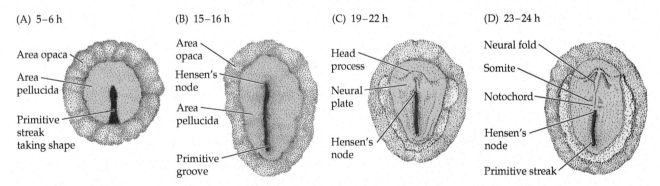

(A) 5–6 h — Area opaca, Area pellucida, Primitive streak taking shape

(B) 15–16 h — Area opaca, Hensen's node, Area pellucida, Primitive groove

(C) 19–22 h — Head process, Neural plate, Hensen's node

(D) 23–24 h — Neural fold, Somite, Notochord, Hensen's node, Primitive streak

FIGURE 27.1 Early Morphogenesis in the Vertebrate Embryo. Dorsal views of the first day in the development of a chick embryo. (A) 5-6 hours: formation and elongation of the primitive streak. (B) 15-16 hours: formation of the primitive groove and Hensen's node. (C) 19-22 hours: formation of the head process and neural plate. (D) 23-24 hours: formation of the neural fold, notochord, and mesodermal somites. (After S. F. Gilbert, 2000. *Developmental Biology*, 6th ed. Oxford University Press/Sinauer, Sunderland, MA; based on B. M. Patten, 1951. *Early Embryology of the Chick*, 4th ed., pp. 70-85. The Blakiston Company: Philadelphia.)

in amphibian, **Hensen's node** in chick, and the **node** in mammalian embryos) have the capacity to *induce* neural tissues in a region of the ectoderm that would normally not produce a nervous system (such as the neighboring dorsal ectoderm). In the absence of this influence, such as in the ventral region, the ectoderm differentiates instead into epidermis.

What is the molecular nature of the inducer? On the basis of Spemann and Mangold's seminal experiments, in the following decades the search for neural inducers was dominated by the idea that neural induction depends on a positive signal from the organizer, which would convert the ectoderm into the neural plate. However, it turned out that scientists were looking for the wrong mechanism.

Molecular studies eventually led to the opposite conclusion: The ectoderm secretes proteins that induce it to become epidermal tissue. These proteins were identified as belonging to the BMP family (part of the transforming growth factor TGF-β superfamily). The organizer, however, secretes a panel of BMP-inhibiting molecules, which prevent the ectoderm from becoming epidermis. As a result of BMP inhibition, this region becomes the neural plate.[23,24] Functional expression-cloning screens, whereby cDNAs prepared from organizer tissue are expressed in ectodermal explants and screened for neural induction, led to the identification of the neural inducers Noggin, Chordin, and follistatin.[25] These factors have in common that they all bind proteins of the TGF-β superfamily (Noggin and Chordin bind BMP4, while follistatin binds activin, another member of the TGF-β superfamily) in the extracellular space, preventing their interactions with BMP membrane receptors (Figure 27.2). Experiments with *Xenopus* ectodermal explants showed that neural tissue is induced when cells of the explant are dissociated or when dominant negative inhibitors of BMP or of activin receptors are expressed in the ectoderm (see Figure 27.2). This led to the view that, in amphibians, neural induction is a default developmental program that unfolds in the region of the ectoderm where the action of BMPs is inhibited via secreted BMP antagonists (see Figure 27.2).[26] Experiments with chick embryos and other amniotes have suggested that additional neural inducers are involved, one of which is a member of the FGF family.[19,27]

The **default model for neural induction**, with high BMP activity defining epidermis and absence of BMP specifying neural plate, illustrates a key principle of

[23] Hemmati-Brivanlou, A. and Melton, D. A. 1997. *Cell* 88: 13-17.

[24] Wilson, S. I. and Edlund, T. 2001. *Nat. Neurosci. Suppl.* 4: 1161-1168.

[25] Hemmati-Brivanlou, A., and Melton, D. 1997. *Annu. Rev. Neurosci.* 20: 43-60.

[26] Ozair, M. Z. et al 2013. *Wiley Interdiscip. Rev. Dev. Biol.* 2: 479-498.

[27] Stern, C. D. 2007. *Development* 132: 2007.

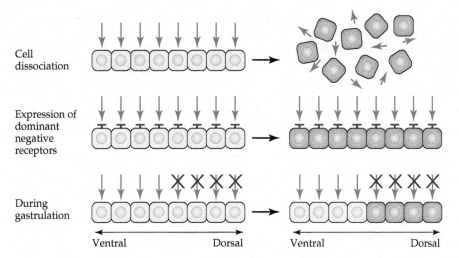
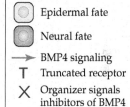

FIGURE 27.2 Neural Induction. The default model of neuralization in the amphibian embryo. Top: In ectodermal explants, BMP4 (blue arrows) secreted by the ectodermal cells induces an epidermal fate and inhibits the neural fate. Upon dissociation of the cells, the secreted epidermal inducer (and neural inhibitor) is diluted, and the "default" neural fate is unveiled by derepression. Middle: Experimental expression of truncated (inactive) BMP or activin receptors (dominant negative inhibitors) interferes with the cells' ability to receive the BMP4 signal. The epidermal fate can no longer be induced and the default neural fate can unfold. Bottom: In the embryo, the ectoderm has a ventral-dorsal polarity. Factors secreted by the underlying organizer, such as Noggin and Chordin, block BMP4, which cannot induce the epidermal fate. As a consequence, neural tissue forms on the dorsal side. (After A. Hemmati-Brivanlou and D. Melton, 1997. *Cell* 88: 13-17.)

development: The signals promoting the specification of one cell type often also block the specification of an alternative cell type.

After binding to their receptors, BMPs and Activin activate intracellular signaling pathways leading to the phosphorylation of SMAD transcription factors. Phosphorylated SMADs repress the expression of neural progenitor transcription factors, needed for the ectodermal cells to become neural tissue. Inhibition of SMAD phosphorylation by BMP antagonists allows the proneural transcriptional program to unfold.[19,27]

This mechanism of neural induction is conserved between invertebrates and vertebrates: The *Drosophila dpp* (*decapentaplegic*) gene is homologous with vertebrate BMP genes, while the *sog* (*short gastrulation*) gene is homologous with the vertebrate BMP inhibitor *chordin*. In *sog* null mutants, the epidermis expands and the neurogenic region is reduced, whereas *dpp* mutations induce an expansion of the neurogenic region.

Proneural Genes and Lateral Inhibition

After the specification of the neural plate, a class of master regulator genes known as **proneural genes** regulate the formation of neuroblasts (i.e., progenitor cells that will generate the nervous system).[28] Studies in insects have highlighted the role of Notch-Delta juxtacrine signaling in the mechanism of action of proneural genes.[29] In insects, the initial formation of neuroblasts occurs in small domains called *proneural clusters*, distributed across the surface of the neurogenic region of the ectoderm. Only one cell per cluster becomes a neuroblast (Figure 27.3A). The newly formed neuroblasts separate from the ectoderm by a process known as delamination: The neuroblasts enlarge, relative to the surrounding ectodermal cells, and are forced to squeeze out of the epithelium and into the inside of the embryo where they divide and differentiate, to form the insect nervous system.

Studies of mutations in genes involved in the early stages of neural development in *Drosophila* led to the identification of genes that also turned out to be critical for early neurogenesis in higher organisms. Among these, the *Achaete scute* (*Asc*) and the *Neurogenin* (*Ngn*) gene families are the prototypical proneural genes. In flies mutant for proneural genes, no neuroblast forms, whereas flies overexpressing these genes have additional ectopic neurons. The proneural genes code for transcription factors, which activate genes involved in neural differentiation pathways and in inhibition of glial differentiation.

By contrast, in flies with mutations in the class of genes called **neurogenic genes**, which includes *Notch* and *Delta*, more neuroblasts undergo delamination at the positions where only a single neuroblast would develop in wild-type individuals. Proneural genes and neurogenic genes are functionally connected: The *Asc* proneural gene upregulates the expression of the neurogenic gene *Delta* (*Dlx*) (a Notch ligand).

The mechanisms by which one cell, from the original cluster, is singled out to become the neuroblast involves the Notch-Delta signaling pathway, in a process known as **lateral inhibition** (see Figure 27.3B).[30] Notch and Delta are transmembrane proteins that symmetrically connect adjacent cells of the proneural cluster, all of which also express *Asc* proneural genes (see Figure 27.3B). The binding of Delta to Notch leads to its proteolytic cleavage, releasing the Notch intracellular domain, which enters the nucleus and turns on the expression of *E(spl)* (*Enhancer of split*), a repressor of *Asc* transcription (see Figure 27.3B, top). Remember that *Asc* upregulates the expression of Delta. If a particular cell in the cluster, by a random fluctuation, expresses a higher level of *Asc* than its neighbors (see Figure 27.3B, middle), this will increase Delta expression in that cell, which will then activate the Notch pathway more strongly in neighboring cells. This will increase *E(spl)* and lower *Asc* and Delta levels in the neighboring cells. This lateral inhibitory loop among the cells of the proneural cluster ensures that the first cell (with higher levels of *Asc*) will be singled out as the neural progenitor of that proneural cluster, while the others become epidermal cells (see Figure 27.3B, bottom).

The Notch-Delta juxtacrine signaling pathway is an evolutionary conserved *symmetry-breaking mechanism,* by which neighboring identical cells become different via lateral inhibition.[29,30] Proneural genes in organisms as different as fly and mouse have remarkably similar functions, with the difference[28] that, in *Drosophila*, proneural genes are first expressed in ectodermal cells with both epidermal and neuronal potential. In vertebrates, by contrast, proneural genes are first expressed in neuroepithelial cells that are already specified for a neural fate.

[28] Bertrand, N. et al. 2002. *Nat. Rev. Neurosci.* 3: 517-530.

[29] Kunisch, M. et al. 1994. *Proc. Natl. Acad. Sci. USA* 91: 10139-10143.

[30] Sjöqvist, M. and Andersson, E. R. 2019. *Dev. Biology* 447: 58-70.

(A)

(a)   (b)

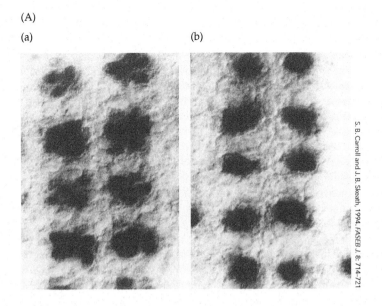

S. B. Carroll and J. B. Skeath, 1994. FASEB J. 8: 714–721

(B)

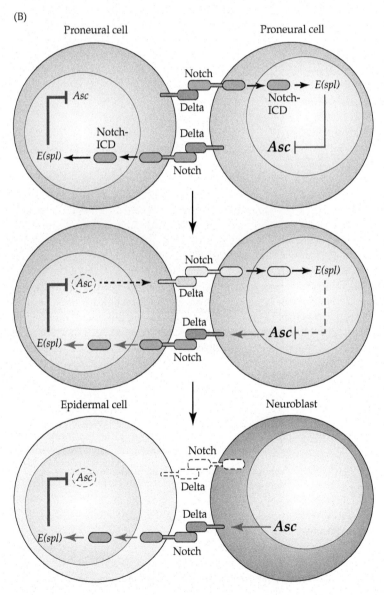

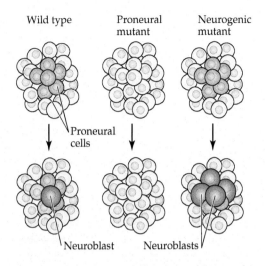

FIGURE 27.3 Proneural Genes and Lateral Inhibition via Notch-Delta Signaling. (A) Left: Proneural clusters in the developing nervous system of a Drosophila embryo, stained with an antibody against Asc protein, before (a) and after (b) delamination. A single neuroblast develops from each cluster and continues to express Asc, while the adjacent cells downregulate the Asc gene and become epidermal cells. Right: Scheme showing the effects of mutations in proneural (middle) and neurogenic (bottom) genes in Drosophila. In the wild-type embryo (top), a given cluster of proneural cells in the ectoderm gives rise (arrow) to only one neuroblast (red). In flies mutant for proneural genes (middle; such as Achaete scute), no neuroblast forms (arrow), whereas in flies mutant for neurogenic genes (bottom) (like Notch and Delta) many neuroblasts form (arrow), instead of only one. (B) Lateral inhibition mechanism between adjacent progenitor cells, symmetrically connected by Notch-Delta signaling proteins. If the cell on the top right expresses by chance a higher level of Asc than its neighbor on the left, this will increase the expression of Delta, which will activate the Notch pathway more strongly, which will inhibit the expression of Asc and of Delta in the neighboring cells. This inhibitory loop ensures that only a single cell in the proneural cluster becomes a neuroblast. Asc = Achaete scute gene; E(spl) = Enhancer of split complex; Notch-ICD = intracellular domain of Notch. (After D. Sanes et al., 2019. *Development of the Nervous System*, 4th ed. Academic Press: Cambridge, MA.)

Transforming the Neural Plate into a Closed Tube

After neural induction, the vertebrate brain and spinal cord start their development as a flat plate of elongated neuroepithelial cells (the neural plate) that folds up along most of its length to form a tube, in a process called neurulation. The edges of the neural plate region of the ectoderm thicken and move upward to produce neural folds. The folds fuse at the midline to give rise to a hollow neural tube (Figure 27.4), which separates from the rest of the ectoderm. Some of the cells at the lips of the neural fold (the point of fusion of the

(A)

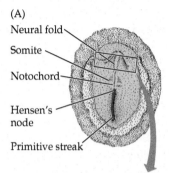

Neural fold
Somite
Notochord
Hensen's node
Primitive streak

FIGURE 27.4 Formation of the Neural Tube in the Chick Embryo.
(A) Diagram of neurulation. (B–E) Scanning electron micrographs of neural tube formation. (B) Neural plate, formed by elongated cells in the dorsal region of the ectoderm. (C) Neural groove formed by elongated neuroepithelial cells and surrounded by mesenchymal cells. (D) Neural folds, covered by flattened epidermal cells. (E) Neural tube covered by presumptive epidermis and flanked on the sides by somites and on the bottom by the notochord. Folding of the neural tube is driven by cell-shape changes at medial and dorsolateral hinge points (MHP and DLHP, respectively). (After S. F. Gilbert, 2000. *Developmental Biology*, 6th ed. Oxford University Press/Sinauer, Sunderland, MA, based on J. L. Smith and G. C. Schoenwolf, 1997. *Trends Neurosci.* 20: 510–517.)

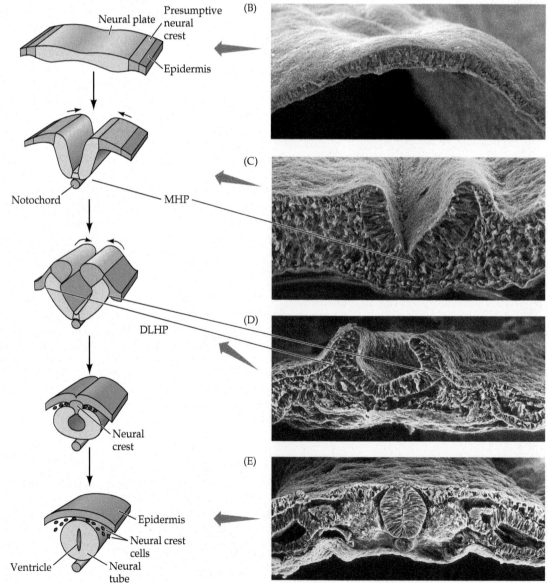

Neural plate
Presumptive neural crest
Epidermis

(B)

Notochord
MHP

(C)

DLHP

(D)

Neural crest

(E)

Epidermis
Neural crest cells
Ventricle
Neural tube

neural tube) come to lie between the neural tube and the overlying ectoderm, forming the neural crest (see section Lineage of Neural Crest Cells later in this chapter).

Folding of the flat neural plate into a cylinder requires bending a sheet of epithelial cells. This occurs through a coordinated shape change of the individual epithelial cells in three pivotal hinge points, the *medial hinge point*, creating the neural groove with a V-shaped cross section, and the two *dorsolateral hinge points*, generating longitudinal furrows that bring the neural fold tips toward each other in the dorsal midline (see Figure 27.4).[31] At these hinge points, the rectangular cells of the flat epithelium acquire a wedge-shaped morphology along the apicobasal axis (wider basally than apically). These cellular changes at the hinge points are induced and regulated by morphogens.[32]

The closure of the neural tube occurs in an anterior-to-posterior fashion, by a progressive "zipping up" from the initial closure site(s). The mechanisms that rule the zipping up and closure of the neural tube are still being investigated.[32,33] After closing into a hollow cylinder, the neural tube separates from the surface ectoderm, by shifting the expression of *homophilic adhesion molecules*, from the epithelial E-cadherin to the neuronal N-cadherin form. As a result, the ectoderm and neural tube tissues beneath it no longer adhere to each other and separate.

The two open ends of the neural tube cylinder, called the anterior and posterior neuropores, also undergo regulated closing. Failure to close the posterior neuropore, in the caudal spinal cord, gives rise to a clinical condition known as spina bifida, whereas failure to close the anterior neuropore, resulting in the forebrain remaining in contact with the amniotic fluid, causes anencephaly. The failure of the entire neural tube to close over the body axis is called craniorachischisis. In humans, closure defects of the neural tube occur in about 1 in every 1000 live births, and can result from both genetic and environmental causes. Dietary factors such as folic acid are crucial for correct human neural tube closure.

[31] McShane et al. 2015. *Dev. Biol.* 404: 113-124.

[32] Nikolopoulou, E. et al. 2017. *Development* 144: 552-566.

[33] Hashimoto, H. et al. 2015. *Develop. Cell* 32: 241-255.

[34] Chambers, S. M. et al. 2009. *Nat. Biotech.* 27: 275-280.

Patterning along the Anteroposterior and Dorsoventral Axes

The brain shows regional differences along both the anteroposterior and dorsoventral axes. Although the basic developmental principles are similar, different steps are needed to create a cerebellum, the cortex, a spinal cord, or an eye. As development proceeds, the anterior (or rostral) portion of the neural tube undergoes a series of swellings, constrictions, and flexures that form anatomically defined regions of the brain. The caudal portion of the neural tube retains a relatively simple tubular structure and forms the spinal cord.

An anterior or rostral identity constitutes the "primitive" regional identity, established by default after neural induction. A subsequent caudalizing step (i.e., a step determining the acquisition of a caudal neural character), by anteroposterior morphogen gradients (Wnts, FGFs, and retinoic acid) in the neural plate, specifies these anterior-fated neural cells to more posterior fates, such as midbrain, hindbrain, and spinal cord (Figure 27.5). Thus, in the absence of instructive signals, the ectoderm will form neural tissue with forebrain character. Regional patterning of the nervous system is then induced by posteriorizing instructive signals.

The in vivo developmental processes of neural induction and of regional patterning and specification can be mimicked in vitro. A dual inhibition of SMAD signaling (combined inhibition of BMPs and of activin signaling), in the absence of

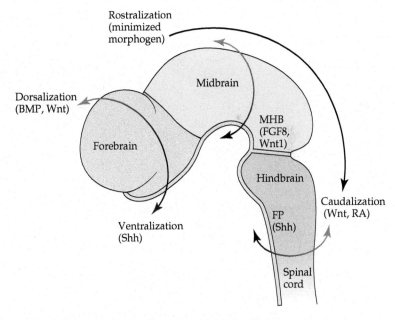

FIGURE 27.5 **Regional Patterning of CNS in the Mouse Embryo.** Following rostral neural fate acquisition, the regional identities within the CNS are determined along the rostrocaudal and dorsoventral axes through the action of the indicated morphogens, derived from various organizing centers (including those indicated in yellow). Morphogens induce the expression of regional patterning genes, such as *Emx2* (forebrain), *Pax2* (hindbrain), *Otx2* (expressed from the MHB to the most anterior part of the brain), and *Gbx2* (from the posterior end of the embryo to the MHB). FP = floor plate; MHB = midbrain-hindbrain boundary; RA = retinoic acid; Shh = Sonic hedgehog. (After I. K. Suzuki and P. Vanderhaegen, 2015. *Development* 142: 3138-3150. CC BY 3.0.)

any added growth factor and morphogens, is the first step in experimental neuralization protocols in vitro.[34] Under these conditions, neural progenitors derived from embryonic stem cells or from induced pluripotent stem cells (see Box 27.1) acquire, by default, a rostral identity. This "primitive" identity can be further converted to more caudal fates, in vitro, by the combinatorial or sequential addition of the same morphogens acting in vivo (see Figure 27.5), allowing one to custom derive, from pluripotent stem cells, a diverse set of neurons in culture, with a large spectrum of regional identities.[35]

Anteroposterior Patterning and Segmentation in the Hindbrain

The vertebrate hindbrain provides examples of how developing nervous systems are patterned along the anteroposterior axis. Unlike the rest of the vertebrate brain, the embryonic hindbrain (**rhombencephalon**) has a conspicuously segmented structure. Each segment (called a rhombomere) exhibits the same general pattern of neuronal differentiation, but from segment to segment the pattern is modified in specific ways (Figure 27.6). Several genes have been identified whose anterior-to-posterior pattern of expression at early developmental stages correlates with segmental boundaries of the hindbrain.[36] Among these,

[35] Bertacchi, M. 2013. *Cell Mol. Life Sci.* 70: 1095-1111.

[36] Lumsden, A., and Krumlauf, R. 1996. *Science* 274: 1109-1115.

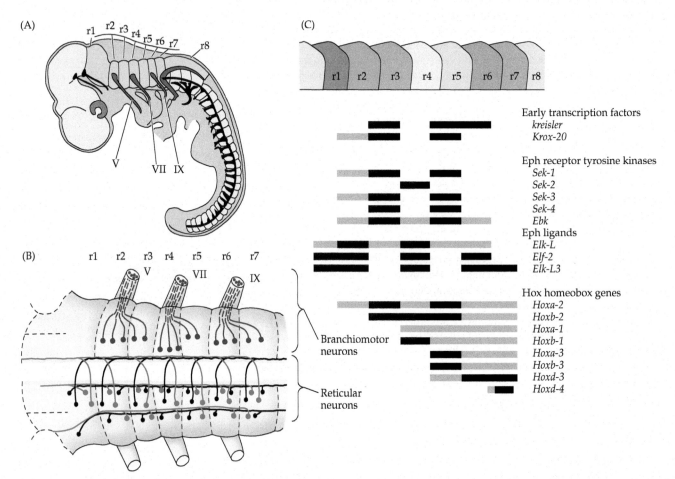

FIGURE 27.6 The Vertebrate Hindbrain Develops as a Conspicuously Segmented Structure. (A) Diagram of a 3-day chick embryo (lateral view), illustrating the segmental arrangement of rhombomeres (r1–r8) in the hindbrain. (B) Pattern of cell organization in rhombomeres r1 to r7 of the 3-day chick embryonic hindbrain (dorsal view). Reticular neurons (blue and black) and branchiomotor neurons (red) occur in a segmentally repeating pattern. Motor neurons send their axons into cranial nerves V, VII, and IX. (C) Segmental expression of genes in rhombomeres r1 to r8 of the vertebrate hindbrain. Gray bars indicate in which rhombomeres and how strongly individual genes are expressed; black bars indicate a high level of expression. Early transcription factors, Eph family receptor tyrosine kinases, and Eph ligands establish the segmental pattern of rhombomeres. The Hox homeobox genes determine the fate of cells within each rhombomere in a segmentally specific way. Data from chick and mouse. (A after R. Keynes and A. Lumsden, 1990. *Neuron* 4: 1-9; B,C after A. Lumsden and R. Krumlauf, 1996. *Science* 274: 1109-1115.)

genes belonging to the highly conserved Hox family play a key role in assigning regional identities along the anteroposterior axis.

Hox genes were first characterized in *Drosophila* as **homeotic genes**[37]—genes that, when mutated, cause one body part to be changed so as to resemble another body part (**homeosis**).[38] For example, one homeotic mutation in *Drosophila* called *proboscipedia* causes an antenna to resemble a leg; another, *antennapedia,* causes the transformation of a leg into an antenna. Studies in *Drosophila* revealed that several homeotic genes occur as a tandem array along the chromosome, reflecting ancient gene duplications. All homeotic genes share a DNA sequence called a **homeobox**, encoding a 60-amino acid DNA-binding motif named the **homeodomain**.[39] In vertebrates, 39 Hox genes are distributed across four genomic clusters. Each Hox gene is expressed in discrete rostrocaudal domains within the hindbrain and spinal cord. Remarkably, the pattern of Hox gene expression along the rostrocaudal axis is directly correlated with its position within the cluster along the chromosome: Hox genes located at the 3′ end of a cluster are expressed earlier and at more rostral levels of the neuraxis, whereas 5′genes are activated later and more caudally. This colinearity is also conserved across species.[40]

The segmental pattern of Hox gene expression observed in the chick, zebrafish, and rodent hindbrain indicates that Hox genes act as patterning *master regulator genes* in the development of rhombomere identity. Evidence from cell transplantation, gene knockout, and gene misexpression studies suggests that Hox genes create structures appropriate to particular anteroposterior positions in the embryonic hindbrain.[41,42] Accordingly, mutations of Hox and other patterning genes in humans give rise to malformations of the corresponding CNS regions.[43,44]

What determines the pattern of Hox gene expression? Different mechanisms contribute.[45,46] A combination of rostrocaudal morphogen signaling gradients establish initial patterns of Hox gene expression (see Figure 27.5).[45] Although the activity of these morphogen signals is transient, it has a lasting effect on the pattern of Hox gene expression that is maintained for the rest of embryonic development. Epigenetic changes in the state of the chromatin are responsible for this and spread along the chromosome in the region of the Hox cluster, to stabilize sequentially activated Hox gene transcription,[46,47] in response to transient rostrocaudal patterning signals.[48]

Hox gene expression stops sharply at the midbrain–hindbrain boundary. Two other homeodomain transcription factors, Emx and Otx, regulate the development and regional identity in the more anterior parts of the brain. Emx2 is expressed in the region that will give rise to forebrain, Otx2 from the midbrain–hindbrain border into the forebrain. Mutations in *emx* give rise to gross defects in the structure of the cortex.

The homeodomain transcription factors Otx2 and Gbx2 are necessary for the division between the forebrain and the hindbrain.[49] Gbx2-expressing cells extend from the posterior end of the brain up to the midbrain–hindbrain border, with a regional expression pattern that is complementary to that of Otx2. Deletion of the *Otx2* gene in mice results in animals without a brain anterior to rhombomere 3,[50] whereas mice without the *Gbx2* gene lack the hindbrain region. Otx2 and Gbx2 cross-repress each other, creating a sharp expression border between them.[50,51]

Cross-repression of transcription factors in progenitor cells, expressed in adjacent domains, is a widely used mechanism for the generation of sharp boundaries between expression domains in the embryo (see also next section).

Dorsoventral Patterning in the Spinal Cord

The vertebrate nervous system is also patterned along the dorsoventral axis. In the adult spinal cord, the dorsal region receives input from sensory neurons, whereas the ventral region is where the motoneurons reside. In the middle are numerous interneurons that relay information between the sensory and the motor neurons. Along the ventral midline of the developing neural tube lies a band of specialized glial cells, called the **floor plate**.

The different cell types, organized along the dorsoventral axis of the presumptive spinal cord, arise from progenitor domains, defined by the expression of specific transcription factors, which specify progeny to differentiate into specific cell types.[10,52,53]

The dorsoventral domains of the neural tube are induced by opposing gradients of morphogen signals originated ventrally from the notochord (which secretes sonic

[37] Lewis, E. B.1978. *Nature* 76: 565-570.

[38] Bateson, W. 1894. *Materials for the Study of Variation: Treated with Special Regard to Discontinuity in the Origin of Species.* Macmillan and Co., New York.

[39] McGinnis, W. et al 1984. *Nature* 308: 428-433.

[40] Duboule, D. 2007. *Development* 134: 2549-2560.

[41] Capecchi, M. R. 1997. *Cold Spring Harb. Symp. Quant. Biol.* 62: 273-281.

[42] Morrison, A. D. 1998. *BioEssays* 20: 794-797.

[43] Boncinelli, E., Mallamaci, A., and Broccoli, V. 1998. *Adv. Genet.* 38: 1-29.

[44] Mallamaci, A. 2011. *Prog. Brain Res.* 189: 37-64.

[45] Philippidou, P. and Dasen, J. S. 2013. *Neuron* 80: 12.

[46] Mallo, M. and Alonso, C. R. 2013. *Development* 140: 3951-3963.

[47] Tschopp, P., and Duboule, D. 2011. *Dev. Biol.* 351: 288-296.

[48] Mazzoni, E. O. et al. 2013. *Nat. Neurosci.* 16: 1191-1198.

[49] Joyner, A. L. et al. 2000. *Curr. Opin. Cell Biol.* 12: 736-741.

[50] Acampora, D. et al. 1995. *Development* 121: 3279-3290.

[51] Glavic, A. et al. 2002. *Development* 129: 1609-1621.

[52] Wilson, L., and Maden, M. 2005. *Dev. Biol.* 282: 1-13.

[53] Briscoe, J. 2009. *EMBO J.* 28: 457-465.

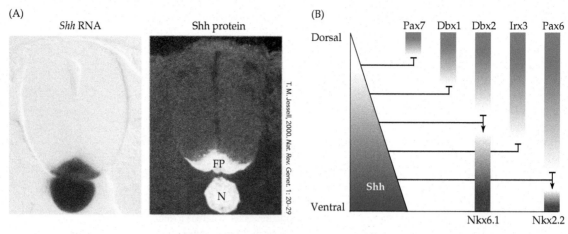

(A) *Shh* RNA · Shh protein

Dorsal · Ventral · Shh · Pax7 · Dbx1 · Dbx2 · Irx3 · Pax6 · Nkx6.1 · Nkx2.2 · FP · N

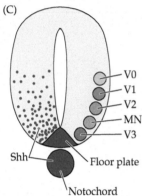

(C) V0 · V1 · V2 · MN · V3 · Shh · Floor plate · Notochord

FIGURE 27.7 **Generation of Neuronal Subtypes in the Ventral Spinal Cord in Response to a Sonic Hedgehog Gradient.** (A) Cross section through embryonic day-18 chick spinal cord showing the expression of *Sonic hedgehog* (*Shh*) RNA and Shh protein by the notochord (N) and floor plate (FP). (B) Left: Shh gradient (shaded triangle) (ventral [V] = high concentration, D [dorsal] = low concentration) defines a homeodomain protein code. Right: Two classes of homeodomain transcription factors are regulated by Shh gradient in ventral progenitors: Class I (Pax7, Dbx1, Dbx2, Irx3, and Pax6) are repressed by Shh; class II (Nkx6.1 and Nkx2.2) require Shh for their expression. The transcription factor pairs Pax6-Nkx2.2 and Dbx2-Nkx6.1 have similar Shh concentration thresholds for repression and activation of their expression, respectively, and repress each other's expression. This sharpens the borders between adjacent domains. (C) Distinct neuronal subtypes generated along the dorsoventral axis in response to graded Shh signaling (blue dots): V0-V3 (different classes of ventral interneurons) and motor neurons (MN). N = notochord; FP = floor plate. (B after T. M. Jessell, 2000. *Nat. Rev. Genet.* 1: 20-29; C after J. Briscoe and B. G. Novitch, 2008. *Phil. Trans. Royal Soc. B* 363: 57-70.)

hedgehog [Shh]) and dorsally from the epidermis (which secretes BMPs).[54] In this view, the pattern of cellular differentiation is a direct readout of a concentration gradient. Progenitor cells integrate both the spatial and temporal distributions of morphogen signals to ultimately determine their fates[55]

Shh is initially secreted by cells of the notochord, just ventral to the neural tube. In response, ventral cells of the neural tube are induced to become floor plate cells, which then become a secondary Shh signaling center.[56] As a result, a ventrodorsal gradient of Shh is established in the neural tube (Figure 27.7A). Cells experiencing different levels of Shh protein are induced to express different transcription factors, which specify five ventral progenitor domains (Figure 27.7B,C).[10,52,53] Each progenitor domain generates a distinct class of postmitotic neurons, including motoneurons. Consistently, transplanting an extra notochord (i.e., an extra source of Shh) produces an extra floor plate (Figure 27.8A,B), and vice versa: In the absence of a notochord, the floor plate and the motoneurons, which require the highest levels of Shh, fail to develop (Figure 27.8C,D).[57] Similarly, the disruption of domain borders, by ectopically expressing a progenitor domain transcription factor in another domain, leads to mis-specification of progenitor cell identity and mis-localization of postmitotic neurons (e.g., motoneurons in dorsal position and interneurons in ventral position).[10,52,53]

The general motoneuron identity is therefore specified according to the dorsoventral axis. Motoneurons, however, are not all equivalent one to the other and are organized into motor columns. Motoneurons of the lateral columns innervate limb muscles, while those of the medial column innervate trunk muscles. The motoneurons of the different motor columns express distinct combinations of LIM homeodomain transcription factors that further specify their muscle projection patterns.[10,58]

In parallel to the ventrodorsal Shh gradient, the dorsal fates of the neural tube are established by a dorsoventral countergradient of BMPs, emanating from the **roof plate** cells of the neural tube, which determines the differentiation of the dorsal (i.e., sensory) regions of the developing spinal cord.[10,53,54]

[54] Roelink, H. et al. 1995. *Cell* 81: 445-455.

[55] Balaskas, N. et al. 2012. *Cell* 148: 273-284.

[56] Placzek, M. et al. 1991. *Development* 113 (Suppl. 2): 105-122.

[57] Yamada, T. et al. 1991. *Cell* 64: 635-647.

[58] Appel, B. et al. 1995. *Development* 121: 4117-4125.

(A)　　　　　　　　　　　(B)　　　　　　　　　　　(C)

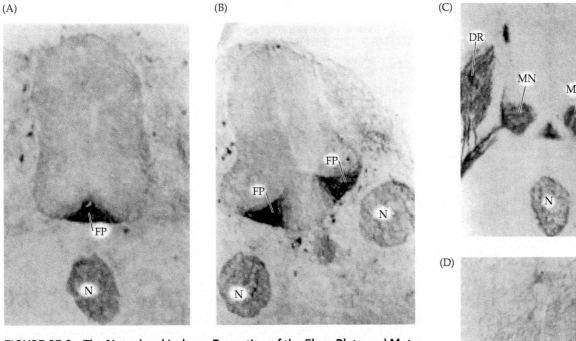

All photos from M. Placzek et al., 1991. *Development* 113: 105-122

(D)

FIGURE 27.8　The Notochord Induces Formation of the Floor Plate and Motor Neurons during development of the spinal cord. (A,B) Specific labeling with an antibody that recognizes floor plate cells (FP). (A) Normal chick embryo. (B) Addition of a second notochord (N) induces a second FP. (C,D) Specific labeling with an antibody that recognizes floor plate cells, motor neurons (MN), and dorsal root ganglion cells (DR). In the absence of notochord (dashed circle), the floor plate and motor neurons are absent, and dorsal roots are displaced ventrally.

The example of hindbrain segmentation illustrates a general principle: Different combinations of morphogen cues along the anteroposterior and dorsoventral axes of the embryo establish a *coordinate system*, providing positional cues specifying the expression of particular combinations of transcription factors and, hence, cells to assume specific fates appropriate to their location (Figure 27.9). Any one factor can induce quite different effects, depending on where in the embryo it is expressed.

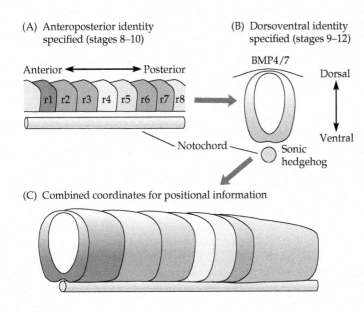

(A) Anteroposterior identity specified (stages 8–10)

Anterior ⟷ Posterior

r1　r2　r3　r4　r5　r6　r7　r8

Notochord

(B) Dorsoventral identity specified (stages 9–12)

BMP4/7

Dorsal

Ventral

Notochord　Sonic hedgehog

(C) Combined coordinates for positional information

FIGURE 27.9　Coordinate System of Positional Information in the Vertebrate Hindbrain is established in two steps. (A) First, anteroposterior position is encoded—for example, by Hox gene expression. (B) Subsequently, dorsoventral position is encoded by opposing gradients of midline signals, such as Sonic hedgehog and BMP4/7. (C) The resulting two-dimensional coordinate system of positional information restricts the repertoire of cell fates available to pluripotent precursor cells. (B,C after A. Lumsden and R. Krumlauf, 1996. *Science* 274: 1109-1115.)

Development of Cerebral Cortex

The cerebral cortex contains millions (mouse) or billions (human) of neurons and glial cells, organized into multiple layers (see Chapter 3) and tangentially subdivided in different functional areas. Information processing in the cortex requires a sophisticated circuitry that is established, during development, through the coordinated production, migration, and positioning of distinct excitatory and inhibitory neuronal subtypes.

The wall of the neural plate and of the early neural tube is initially composed of a single layer of rapidly dividing cells (*germinal neuroepithelium*). Neuroepithelial cells, the first multipotent neural stem cells of the embryo, undergo a massive proliferation and extend a process spanning the full width of the neuroepithelium (from the ventricular border to the external, or pial, surface).

As a proliferating neuroepithelial cell progresses through the cell cycle, its nucleus moves back and forth through the cytoplasm between the ventricular and the pial surfaces, a process known as *interkinetic nuclear migration*. Once the nucleus arrives back at the ventricular surface, the cell divides. The function of interkinetic nuclear migration is still unclear.[59]

As a result of the stem cell proliferation, the newly formed neural tube expands into a three-layered configuration, along the apicobasal axis: the innermost **ventricular zone** (where proliferation occurs), the **intermediate** (or **mantle**) **zone** (containing the cell bodies of the migrating neurons), and the **marginal zone** (composed of the elongating axons of the underlying neurons). This three-layered structure characterizes the spinal cord and medulla development. In the cerebrum, instead, the first wave of neurons migrates toward the pial basal surface and accumulates to form a new layer, the **cortical plate**, which eventually matures into the six layers of adult cortex, in successive waves of neuron migration (see Figure 27.15).

Radial Glia: Transport Highways and Neural Stem Cells

At the time when cortical neurogenesis begins, around embryonic day 9–10 (E9–10) in the mouse, neuroepithelial stem cells begin to acquire features associated with glial cells (glycogen storage granules, expression of the astrocytic intermediate filaments GFAP and of GLAST) and generate the radial glial cells. As the walls of the neural tube thicken, through the continued division of cells in the ventricular layer, the processes of the radial glial cells become elongated and span the apicobasal axis of the expanding neural tube, while their cell bodies are retained within the ventricular zone.

Radial glial cells have long been known to provide a mechanical scaffolding transport highway, guiding neural progenitor cell migration from the inner region to the outer zones of the neural tube.[60] From light- and electron-microscopic studies, Pasko Rakic deduced that developing neurons move along this scaffolding of radial glial cells to reach their appropriate positions in the cortex (Figure 27.10).[61] The migrating neurons wrap around radial glia processes as if climbing up a pole. According to the radial unit hypothesis of neocortical development, the clonal relationship of precursor cells migrating along shared radial glial fiber guides determines the adult radial cortical columns.[61]

Therefore, it came as a surprise to find out that radial glial cells, in addition to their function as a transport highway for new cortical neurons, can generate neurons themselves, constituting the major neural stem cell pool throughout embryonic development.[62,63] This discovery led to a paradigm shift in our views on the developmental origins of adult neurons and glial cells.[64]

Magdalena Goetz and her colleagues[62] isolated radial glial cells from a transgenic mouse in which green fluorescent protein (GFP) was placed under the control of the glial fibrillary acidic promoter (Figure 27.11A) and performed in vitro clonal analysis of the sorted cells (Figure 27.11B). While freshly isolated cells (from E14 cortex) had a clear radial glial phenotype, surprisingly, after 7 days in culture almost 70% of the sorted cells were neurons, showing that radial glial cells generate neurons at this stage. When radial glial cells were isolated from an E18 cortex, the progeny were mostly astrocytes (see Figure 27.11).

Following this evidence, the neurogenic role of radial glial cells was demonstrated in vivo.[63] Kriegstein and his colleagues performed intraventricular injections of a retrovirus

[59] Miyata, T. et al. 2015. *Front. Cell Neurosci.* 8: 473.

[60] Rakic, P. 1972. *J. Comp. Neurol.* 145: 61–84.

[61] Rakic, P. 1988. *Science* 241: 170–176.

[62] Malatesta, P. et al. 2000. *Development* 157: 5253–5263.

[63] Noctor, S. C. et al. 2001. *Nature* 409: 714–720.

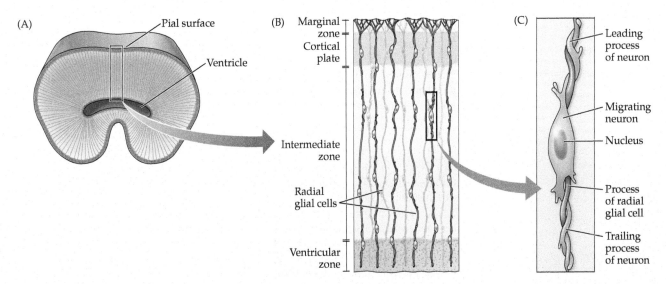

FIGURE 27.10 Developing Cortical Neurons Migrate along Radial Glia Fibers. (A) Scheme of a coronal section of the Golgi-impregnated telencephalon of a 97-day monkey embryo, at the parieto-occipital level. (B) Enlargement of the portion of cortex indicated by the box in (A), showing the radial glial cells, with their fibers extending from the ventricular zone to the pial surface, and neurons crawling along the radial glial fibers. The rectangle in (B) is enlarged in (C). (C) Reconstruction of a neuron migrating along radial glia fibers, at the level of the intermediate zone. (After P. Rakic, 1972. *J. Comp. Neurol.* 145: 61–84.)

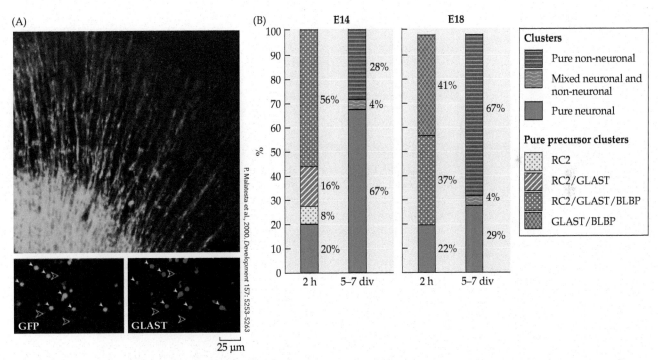

P. Malatesta et al., 2000. *Development* 157: 5253-5263

FIGURE 27.11 Clonal Analysis of Single Radial Glial Cells Reveals a Neuronal Lineage. (A) Top: Green fluorescent radial glial cells from the embryonal cortex (E16) of transgenic mice expressing green fluorescent protein (GFP) under the control of a glial promoter. Pial surface is upwards. Bottom: Acutely dissociated cells from E14 cortex double-stained for GFP (green) and for the glial marker GLAST (red). Filled arrowheads: double-positive cells. Open arrowheads: double-negative cells. GFP is localized in GLAST-positive precursor cells with radial glia morphology. (B) GFP-positive radial glial cells were isolated by fluorescence-activated cell sorting. The cellular composition of radial glial cells, isolated at E14 and E18, was analyzed after 5–7 days in vitro (div) with cell-type-specific antibodies (β-tubulin III as neuronal and RC2, GLAST, and BLBP as precursor markers). Neurons: blue; precursor cells: green. Most sorted precursor cells (2 h) are immunoreactive for GLAST. The large number of neuronal clusters generated from radial glial cells isolated at E14 suggests that most GLAST-positive radial glia generate neurons at this stage. In contrast, when radial glial cells were isolated at E18, the progeny were mostly astrocytes. (After P. Malatesta et al., 2000. *Development* 157: 5253-5263.)

encoding GFP to label proliferating precursor cells in the E15 mouse cortex, and followed their clonal progeny by time-lapse observation in vivo (Figure 27.12A). Labeled clones, examined 1–3 days later, comprised mitotic radial glia and postmitotic neurons (Figure 27.12B). Radial glial cells underwent interkinetic nuclear migration, similarly to neuropithelial cells but confined to the ventricular zone (Figure 27.12C). Time-lapse images

(A)

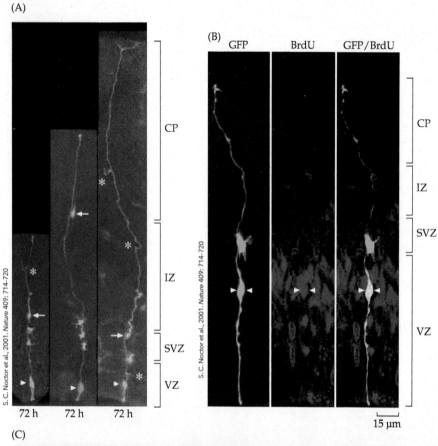

S. C. Noctor et al, 2001. *Nature* 409: 714–720

FIGURE 27.12 Radial Glia Are Neurogenic. A retroviral vector encoding GFP was injected in the E15 mouse cortex. (A) Radial clonal units 72 hours after retroviral infection comprise one bipolar radial glial cell (arrowheads), contacting both pial and ventricular surfaces, and one to four migrating neurons (arrows), distributed along the radial process of the radial glial cell. Asterisks = blood vessels. CP = cortical plate; IZ = intermediate zone; SVZ = subventricular zone; VZ = ventricular zone. (B) Mitotically active S-phase clonal cell members were labeled with bromodeoxyuridine (BrdU) in utero after viral infection. All GFP-positive clone members that double-labeled with BrdU had radial glial morphology. (C) Time-lapse video-microscopy of radial glial cell division. A single radial glial cell at 24 hours after infection (t = 0), with an end foot at the ventricular surface and a radial process extending to the pia. The soma of the radial glial cell descends to the ventricular surface, divides, and translocates to the top of the VZ, while its daughter cell begins radial migration. Times are indicated in minutes.

(C)

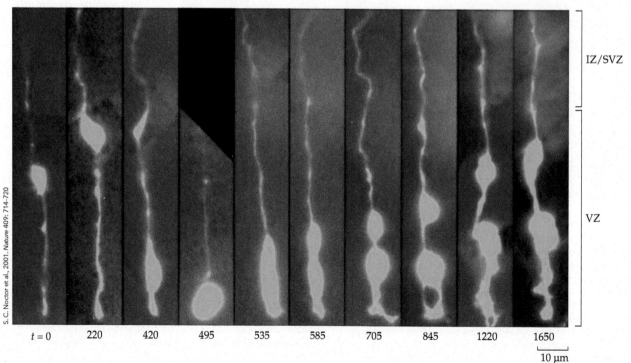

S. C. Noctor et al, 2001. *Nature* 409: 714–720

showed that proliferative radial glia generated neurons and also acted as migrational guides for their clonally related neuronal progeny (see Figure 27.12C). This *dual function of radial glia* provides a parsimonious mechanism by which local clonal relationships in the embryonic ventricular zone can be translated into functional columnar units in the adult neocortex (integrating the *radial unit hypothesis* by Rakic).[61]

Intriguingly, the long apicobasal process of radial glial cells is not lost during mitosis, but remains in place and is inherited asymmetrically by one of the two daughter cells.[65] This permits proliferative radial glia to provide a migration guidance role for the daughter cells they generate during division.

Altogether, these results demonstrated that radial glia are neural stem cells during development,[65] including in the human cerebral cortex.[66]

Radial glial cells at first divide *symmetrically*, thus increasing the pool of stem cells (self-renewing divisions).[64] Subsequently, they switch to an *asymmetrical* cell division, contributing to neurogenesis while maintaining the progenitor pool. In addition to generating neurons directly, radial glia also do so indirectly, by generating other intermediate cell types, the outer radial glia (radial glia lacking apical attachment) and the intermediate progenitor cells (which are not anchored to either the apical or the basal cortical surface) (Figure 27.13). These cells act as *transit-amplifying cells*, undergoing limited proliferation (often only a single division) before dividing symmetrically to produce two neurons (symmetrical differentiation division). The cell-type potency becomes more restricted in the progression from neuroepithelial cell to radial glia cell, to outer radial glia and intermediate progenitor cell. After neurogenesis is complete, neural progenitors shift to a gliogenic mode (see Figure 27.13).[64]

[64] Kriegstein, A. and Alvarez-Buylla, A. 2009. *Annu. Rev. Neurosci.* 32: 149–84.

[65] Miyata, T. et al. 2001. *Neuron* 31: 727–741.

[66] Hansen, D. V. et al. 2010. *Nature* 464: 554–561.

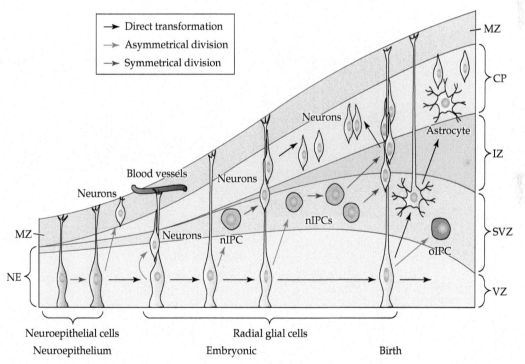

FIGURE 27.13 Generation of Cortical Cells by Radial Glia. Following the early period of development (left) during which neurons arise primarily from neuroepithelial cells (brown cells, left), cortical cells (neurons and glia) derive, directly or indirectly, from radial glia (light blue cells, center). Some neurons arise as the direct descendants of radial glia. In other cases, the immediate progeny of the radial glia act as neuron intermediate progenitor cells (nIPCs), which undergo a few additional rounds of division. After neurogenesis is complete, neural progenitors generate astrocytes and oligodendrocytes (right). CP = cortical plate; IZ = intermediate zone; MZ = marginal zone; NE = neuroepithelium; oIPC = oligodendrocyte intermediate progenitor cell; SVZ = subventricular zone; VZ = ventricular zone. (After A. Kriegstein and A. Alvarez-Buylla, 2009. *Annu. Rev. Neurosci.* 32: 149–184.)

Cerebral Cortex Histogenesis: Assembling the Cortex

To address the histogenesis of the layered structure of the cortex, we must study the birth date and fate of newly generated cells derived from the neuroepithelial and radial glia stem cells. One technique to determine where and when a cell was born is to apply a pulse of a thymidine analogue (such as tritiated ^{3}H-thymidine or bromodeoxyuridine [BrdU]) into the live embryo.[67] The molecule is incorporated into the DNA of cells that were in the DNA synthesis S phase of the cell cycle at the time of exposure. Postmitotic cells are not labeled, and in cells that continue to divide after the pulse, the label is diluted during subsequent rounds of DNA synthesis. However, cells that undergo their final round of DNA synthesis during the pulse, to become postmitotic neurons, will remain heavily labeled. Thus, by examining tissues (by autoradiography or anti-BrdU immunohistochemistry) soon after the injection, it is possible to determine where and when cell divisions are taking place; that information, combined with observations made at later times after the injection, permits one to infer where the labeled cells have migrated.[68]

Such experiments show that cortical neurogenesis begins with the early birth of deeper projection neurons (composed of corticofugal neurons innervating thalamus, brainstem, or spinal cord) and continues with successive generation of layer 4 neurons, and then of superficial projection neurons (which project ipsilaterally or to contralateral cortical hemisphere). Characteristically, cortical development proceeds in successive waves, in an inside-out fashion[68]

[67] Angevine, J. B., Jr., and Sidman, R. L. 1961. *Nature* 192: 766-768.

[68] Rakic, P. 1974. *Science* 183: 425-427.

(A)

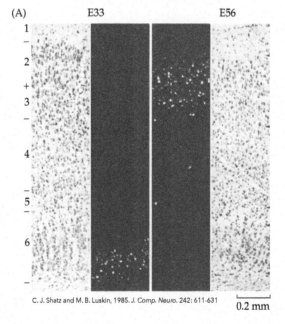

C. J. Shatz and M. B. Luskin, 1985. *J. Comp. Neuro.* 242: 611-631

0.2 mm

FIGURE 27.14 Neurogenesis of Cat Cortex. (A) Autoradiographs of sections of the adult cat visual cortex that had been injected with ^{3}H-thymidine on E33 or E56. Bright-field micrographs of the same sections stained with cresyl violet indicate that labeled cells are located in layer 6 after the E33 injection and in layers 2 and 3 after E56 injection.
(B) Layer distribution of cells labeled on various days between E30 and E56 illustrates the inside-out pattern of neurogenesis in the visual cortex. (After C. J. Shatz and M. B. Luskin, 1985. *J. Comp. Neuro.* 242: 611-631.)

(B)

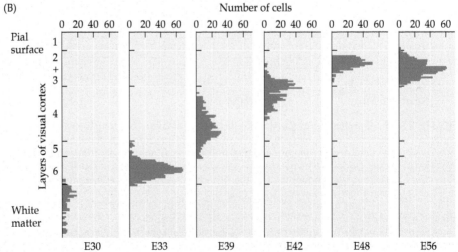

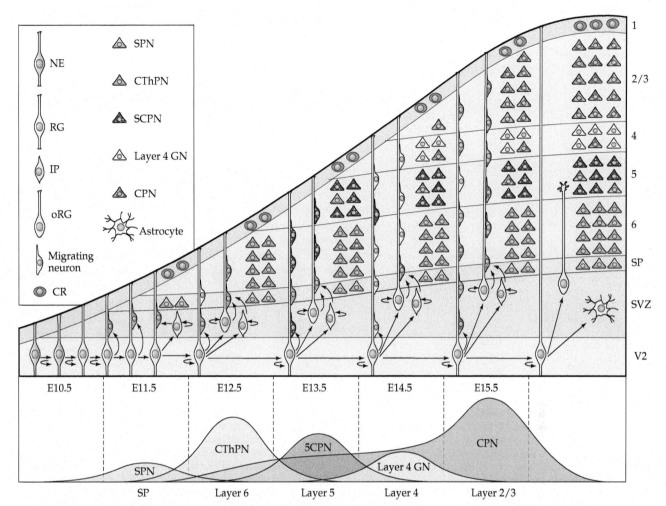

FIGURE 27.15 Sequential Inside-Out Generation of Neocortical Projection Neurons and their migration to appropriate layers during mouse development. (A) Radial glia (RGs) in the ventricular zone (VZ) begin to produce projection neurons around E11.5. At the same time, radial glia generate intermediate progenitors (IPs) and outer radial glia (oRGs), which establish the subventricular zone (SVZ) and act as transit-amplifying cells to increase neuronal production. Cajal-Retzius (CR) cells migrate tangentially into neocortical layer 1 from noncortical locations, whereas other projection neurons are born in the neocortical VZ or SVZ and migrate radially along radial glial processes to reach their final laminar destinations. CPN = callosal projection neurons; CThPN = corticothalamic projection neurons; GN = layer 4 granular neurons; NE = neuroepithelial cell; oRG = outer radial glia; SCPN = subcerebral projection neurons; SPN = subplate neurons. (B) Distinct projection neuron subtypes are born in sequential waves. Peak sizes reflect the approximate number of neurons of each subtype born on each day. SP = subplate. (After L. F. Custo-Greig et al., 2013. *Nat. Rev. Neurosci.* 14: 755–769.)

(Figures 27.14 and 27.15). The neurons with the earliest birth dates form the deepest cortical layers, closest to the ventricle. Neurons that are born later migrate radially along the radial glial progenitor processes, past the cells positioned in the deeper layers, to occupy the more superficial layers of the developing cortex. Neurons that occupy the same radial position are generated within the same time window and share common projection targets (see Figure 27.15).

Regional Specification of the Cortex

In addition to its radial organization in six layers, the cerebral cortex is organized tangentially into several regions (more than 40 in the human cerebral cortex). Major tangential cortical areas are the motor (M1), somatosensory (S1), auditory (A1), and visual (V1) cortical areas. How do these distinct cortical areas attain their identity during corticogenesis? Is such regional cortical specification (named arealization) already prespecified in the ventricular region?

Cortical arealization is initiated by morphogen gradients, which generate different **positional identities** along the anteroposterior and mediolateral axes of the dorsal

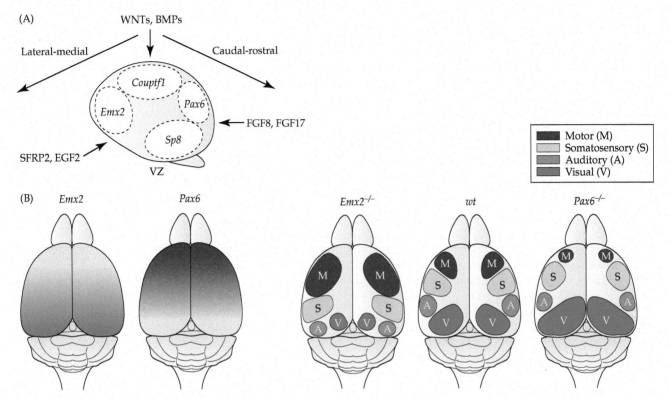

FIGURE 27.16 Patterning the Cerebral Cortex: Regional Identity of Cortical Areas. (A) Arealization of the cerebral cortex is initiated by diffusible morphogens secreted from opposing sides of the neocortical boundaries (WNTs, BMPs, FGFs, EGFs, SFRP2). Morphogens induce complementary gradients of transcription factor expression (Pax6-Emx2 and Sp8-Couptf1), shown in a schematized flat-mount view of the ventricular zone (VZ). (B) Left: *Emx2* and *Pax6* countergradients. Right: Area identity shifts in cerebral cortices of perinatal *Emx2-/-* and *Pax6-/-* brains, with respect to the cortex of control mice (wt), dorsal views. Loss of *Pax6* causes an expansion of *Emx2*'s domain of expression, such as the visual cortex, and a severe reduction of the motor cortex. Loss of *Emx2* causes the *Pax6*-expressing domain to expand, resulting in an expansion of the motor cortx. A = auditory; M = motor; S = somatosensory; V = visual. (A after L. F. Custo-Greig et al., 2013. *Nat. Rev. Neurosci.* 14: 755–769; B after L. Muzio and A. Mallamaci, 2003. *Cereb. Cortex* 13: 641–647.)

telencephalon, by establishing expression domains of key transcription factors (e.g., Pax6, Sp8, Emx2, Couptf1) in ventricular zone (VZ) progenitors (Figure 27.16A). These transcription factors, in turn, specify the relative size and position of cortical areas.[69,70] Pax6 is expressed most highly rostrolaterally, in opposition to Emx2, which is higher caudomedially (Figure 27.16B). Similarly, Sp8 is expressed most highly rostrolaterally, in opposition to Couptf1, which is higher caudolaterally. These countergradients of transcription factor expression define a set of coordinates in the VZ. Progenitors located at different mediolateral and rostrocaudal coordinates express specific levels of these transcription factors, which *combinatorially establish a fate "proto-map" of cortical areas in the VZ*, which is later translated into a definitive area map in the cortical plate. Experimental interference with VZ transcription factor expression results in dramatic changes in the size and position of cortical areas.[69,70] Good examples are provided by Pax6 and Emx2 (see Figure 27.16B).[71,72]

In conclusion, intrinsic genetic programs and local morphogens establish an initial regional proto-map of the future cortex.[69,70]

Radial and Tangential Migration

Two distinct modes of radial migration by newly born neurons are observed. During early cortical development, when the luminal and pial surfaces are relatively close, a newly born neuron extends basal filopodia toward the pial surface. By shortening the process attached to the pial surface, the cell body is pulled from the apical to the basal region of the cell, using a spring-like mechanism, and no actual cell migration occurs (somal translocation).[73] During later development, however, progenitor cells actively migrate along the radial glial cell's basal process.[74]

[69] Custo Greig, L. et al. 2013. *Nat. Rev. Neurosci.* 14: 755–769.

[70] Cadwell, C. R. et al. 2019. *Neuron* 103: 980–1004.

[71] Bishop, K. M. et al. 2000. *Science* 288: 344–349.

[72] Mallamaci, A. et al. 2000. *Nat. Neurosci.* 3: 679–686.

[73] Miyata, T. and Ogawa, M. 2007. *Curr. Biol.* 17: 146.

[74] Marin, O. et al. 2010. *Cold Spring Harb. Perspect. Biol.* 2: a001834.

How do radially migrating neurons "know" when to stop? The mutant mouse *reeler* (so called because of the uneven gait it displays) demonstrates how a neuron's final position can be determined by an extracellular signal. In the developing cortex of *reeler* mice, neurons fail to migrate past one another.[75] Therefore, their relative positions in the adult are inverted: Neurons born at early times end up in the most superficial layers, whereas those born later end up in deeper layers. The product of the *reeler* gene is a large extracellular matrix glycoprotein called Reelin.[76,77] It is secreted by Cajal–Retzius cells, a transient population of cells that migrate tangentially into the developing cortex prior to the first radial wave of migration and are situated superficially, in the outer marginal zone of the cortex (see Figure 27.15).[78] Reelin, secreted by these superficial cells, forms a diffusive gradient down the depth of the developing cortex. Migrating neurons express membrane receptors for Reelin (a member of the low-density lipoprotein receptor family), whose signaling depends on the levels of Reelin. Low to moderate Reelin levels, as are found by migrating neurons at the beginning of their journey, support migration and induce N-cadherin expression on the migrating neurons, allowing them to stay attached to radial glial cells, also expressing N-cadherin. High levels of Reelin, encountered once the migrating neurons reach the layer where the Cajal–Retzius cells are located, induce neurons to lose their cell adhesion molecules and stop ("All passengers, step down from the radial glia here, please").[79]

Neurons can also migrate tangentially, without crawling along radial glial cells.[80] For example, the cortical inhibitory GABAergic interneurons (and some cortical oligodendrocytes) originate in the subcortical zone known as the medial ganglionic eminence in the ventral telencephalon (subpallium) and migrate long distances tangentially to the cortical surface[81,82] (Figure 27.17). The clonal relationship of migrating GABAergic interneurons has been directly visualized by fluorescent labeling and DNA barcoding of the pre-migratory population in the medial ganglionic eminence and by tracking their migration to the cerebral cortex.[83,84] Clonal analysis has revealed that only a minority of medial ganglionic eminence–derived clones in the cortex are found to be clustered, while the majority disperse over large areas. Lineage relationships do not appear to determine interneuron allocation to particular cortical regions.[83,84] Interestingly, laminar positioning of interneurons is altered by changes in projection neuron identity and location, suggesting that projection neurons play an important role in guiding interneurons to their appropriate radial destinations.[85]

Another remarkable example of migration without radial glia is provided by a population of neurons expressing gonadotropin-releasing hormone (GnRH). These precursors migrate from the periphery into the CNS.[86] The GnRH cells travel from the olfactory pit (an

[75] Caviness, V. S., Jr. 1982. *Dev. Brain Res.* 4: 293–302.

[76] D'Arcangelo, G. et al. 1997. *J. Neurosci.* 17: 23–31.

[77] Förster, E. et al. 2010. *Eur. J. Neurosci.* 31: 1511–1518.

[78] Meyer, G. 2010. *J. Anat.* 217: 334–343.

[79] Zhao, S., and Frotscher, M. 2010. *Neuroscientist* 16: 421–434.

[80] O'Rourke, N. A. et al. 1995. *Development* 121: 2165–2176.

[81] Corbin, J. G. et al. 2001 *Nat. Neurosci.* 4: 1177–1182.

[82] Marin, O. 2013. *Eur. J. Neurosci.* 38: 2019–2029.

[83] Mayer, C. et al. 2015. *Neuron* 87: 989–998.

[84] Harwell, C. C. et al. 2015. *Neuron* 87: 999–1007.

[85] Lodato, S. et al. 2011. *Neuron* 69: 763–779.

[86] Wray, S. et al. 1989. *Proc. Natl. Acad. Sci. USA* 86: 8132–8136.

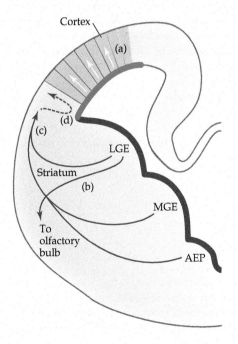

FIGURE 27.17 Tangential Migration. The schema shows a coronal slice of the telencephalon at midembryonic stage. While cortical projection neurons migrate radially from the dorsal ventricular zone (a) (thick blue line), GABAergic interneurons originate from subpallium structures (LGE, MGE, and AEP; thick red line) and migrate tangentially into striatum and the olfactory bulb (b) or to the cortex (c and d). When cortical interneuron precursors reach the cortex, they are divided in two streams. Some of them migrate directly into the cortical marginal zone (c), while others move toward the ventricular zone before radially migrating into the cortex (dashed red line) (d). AEP = anterior entopeduncular area; LGE = lateral ganglionic eminence; MGE = medial ganglionic eminence. (After R. Ayala et al., 2007. *Cell* 128: 29–43.)

ectodermal derivative, or placode, that gives rise to the nasal epithelium) into the hypothalamus along a previously established axon tract (axophilic migration). Individuals suffering from a condition known as Kallmann syndrome (a genetic disorder of the olfactory placode) display a defective sense of smell and also sterility.[87,88] The cause is a failure of migration of olfactory precursors and of GnRH cells to their destinations within the hypothalamus.

Adult Neurogenesis

Despite early autoradiographic evidence for ^{3}H-thymidine incorporation into neuronal DNA in the adult rat brain by Altman[89] and the demonstration of adult neurogenesis in songbirds by Nottebohm and colleagues,[90] the dogma that "no new neurons are made in the adult mammalian brain" held for decades.

In songbirds, Nottebohm and his colleagues demonstrated neuronal proliferation throughout adult life. In canary brains, the high vocal center (HVC) nucleus plays a crucial role in the acquisition and retention of song—a uniquely male behavior.[91] This area of the brain, more developed in males than in females, is under hormonal control (Figure 27.18) and recruits newborn neurons (in males), peaking in the fall and spring following periods of neuronal death. This recruitment period is just when males modify their song for the next breeding season. The period of neuronal death coincides with a drop in testosterone levels, and recruitment peaks when testosterone levels rise. Administration of testosterone to females causes an increase in the recruitment of new HVC neurons and induces the females to sing. The HVC nucleus and other structures associated with song production become enlarged in such androgenized females. New HVC neurons in males and females receive appropriate synaptic input and project axons to the proper targets. These remarkable observations indicate not only that new neurons arise in the adult songbird brain, but also that they can be assimilated into complex circuits so as to provide the substrate for the remodeling of a behavior as intricate as birdsong.

At the turn of the twenty-first century a flurry of investigations demonstrated the continued appearance of new neurons in the adult mammalian brain,[92,93] arising from self-renewing neural stem cells (NSCs) in two neurogenic niches, the subventricular zone, lining the walls of the lateral ventricles, and the subgranular zone, within the dentate gyrus of the adult hippocampus.[94][95] Such cells can give rise to differentiated neurons, oligodendrocytes, and astrocytes. NSCs from both niches have long processes that allow them to contact the vasculature, but only NSCs of the subventricular zone maintain contact with the cerebrospinal fluid.

Sustained neurogenesis throughout life requires a tight balance between NSC proliferation and the number of differentiated progeny produced. This is regulated by the microenvironment of the neurogenic niche.[96] Signaling systems, such as Notch-Delta, involved in developmental neurogenesis, also ensure the maintenance of the NSC pool in the adult neurogenic niches.[96] Adult neurogenesis is also regulated by extrinsic influences, such as stress, physical exercise, diet, and enriched environment, and by endocrine signals delivered through the vasculature that infiltrates the niche.

Despite the similarities in neurogenesis in the developing and adult brain, there are key differences.[97] Embryonic neurogenesis takes place in an environment where neurogenesis is the default fate and gliogenesis is inhibited, whereas adult neurogenesis occurs in a gliogenic environment, hence requiring adult-specific, different mechanisms of neuronal fate specification and maintenance.

The functional roles of adult subventricular zone and subgranular zone neurogenesis remain an open, and fascinating, question.[98,99]

[87] Wray, S. 2010. *J. Neuroendocrinol.* 22: 743-753.

[88] Sarfati, J. et al. 2010. *Front. Horm. Res.* 39: 121-132.

[89] Altman, J., and Das, G. D. 1965. *J. Comp. Neurol.* 124: 319-335.

[90] Nottebohm, F. 1989. *Sci. Am.* 260: 74-79.

[91] Adar, E. et al. 2008. *J. Neurosci.* 28: 5394-5400.

[92] Kornack, D. R., and Rakic, P. 1999. *Proc. Natl. Acad. Sci. USA* 96: 5768-5773.

[93] Reynolds, B. A., and Weiss, S. 1996. *Dev. Biol.* 175: 1-13.

[94] Bond, A. M. et al. 2015. *Cell Stem Cell* 17: 385.

[95] Goncalves, J. T. et al. 2016. *Cell* 167: 897-914.

[96] Fuentealba, L. C. et al. 2012. *Cell Stem Cell* 10: 698.

[97] Goetz, M. et al. 2016. *Cold Spring Harb. Perspect. Biol.* doi: 10.1101/cshperspect.a018853.

[98] Lazarini, F., and Lledo, P. M. 2011. *Trends Neurosci.* 34: 20-30.

[99] Aimone, J. B. et al. 2014. *Physiol. Rev.* 94: 991-1026.

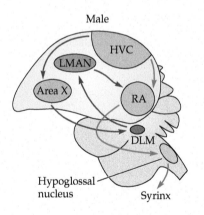

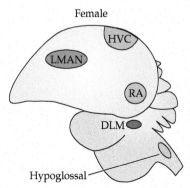

FIGURE 27.18 Sexual Dimorphism in an Avian Brain. Schematic diagram of the major brain areas and pathways involved in production of song in songbirds. The higher vocal center (HVC), robust nucleus of the archistriatum (RA), and hypoglossal nucleus form the posterior, vocal motor pathway (green arrows). The HVC, area X, medial dorsolateral nucleus of the thalamus (DLM), and lateral magnocellular nucleus of the anterior neostriatum (LMAN) form the anterior pathway (red arrows). The HVC, hypoglossal nucleus, and RA are significantly larger in male birds; area X has not been observed in brains of female finches.

Evidence for Adult Neurogenesis in the Human Brain

A question of obvious importance is whether new neurons are also added to the adult human brain. Addressing this question is challenging, because currently human adult neurogenesis cannot be imaged in a noninvasive way and can only be investigated in postmortem brains.

A study by Gage and his colleagues provided the first evidence for adult neurogenesis in humans.[100] They analyzed postmortem brains of terminal patients afflicted with localized carcinomas, with no spread to the brain, who received a single intravenous infusion of BrdU for diagnostic purpose (to assess the proliferative activity of the tumor cells). The postmortem analysis of five brains showed that BrdU-labeled neurons could be detected by antibody labeling, demonstrating neurogenesis in the adult human dentate gyrus.[100]

Using an ingenious approach (*retrospective birth-dating*)[101–103] (Figure 27.19), Frisen and his colleagues made use of the fact that during the nuclear weapons tests of 1955–1963, ^{14}C in the environment increased sharply and was incorporated into the food supply. After the test ban treaty of 1963, levels of ^{14}C in the environment fell sharply (see Figure 27.19B). The ^{14}C level in our bodies reflects that of the atmosphere. Consequently, when a cell divides, newly synthesized DNA integrates a trace amount of ^{14}C that is proportional to the environmental

[100] Eriksson, P. et al., 1998. *Nat. Med.* 4: 1313.

[101] Bhardwaj, R. D. et al. 2006. *Proc. Natl. Acad. Sci. USA* 103: 12564–12568.

[102] Spalding, K. L. et al. 2013. *Cell* 153: 1219-1227.

[103] Kheirbek, M. A. and Hen, R. 2013. *Cell* 153: 1183.

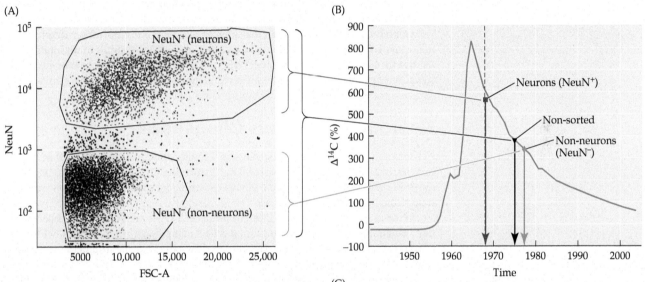

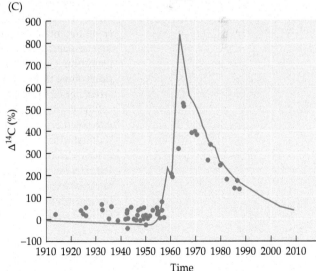

FIGURE 27.19 Retrospective Birth Dating of Adult Human Neurons. (A) ^{14}C radioactivity was measured in cell nuclei of neurons identified by high levels of the NeuN marker (NeuN+, red) and non-neuronal cells (NeuN-, green) isolated by flow cytometry from postmortem human cortex. FSC-A = forward scatter channel-A (a measure of relative size in arbitrary units). (B) In 1955-1963 the levels of ^{14}C in the atmosphere increased dramatically as a result of nuclear weapons tests and subsequently declined (blue line). One can infer the time of birth of cells by first relating the level of ^{14}C in their DNA to that in the atmosphere (guidelines from A to B), and then reading the age of the cells off the x-axis (vertical arrows). The age of the individual is given by the dashed line. The average age of all cells in the cortex (neuronal and non-neuronal) is less than the age of the individual (black circle and arrow), indicating overall cell turnover. Non-neuronal cells (glial and endothelial cells) (green circle and arrow) are younger, whereas cortical neurons (red circle and arrow) are as old as the individual. (C) Hippocampal neurogenesis in adult humans. Individually measured ^{14}C concentrations in genomic DNA of human hippocampal neurons from individuals between 19 and 92 years of age correspond to the concentration in the atmosphere after the date of birth of the individual, demonstrating postnatal generation of hippocampal neurons. Note that ^{14}C levels above or below the atmospheric ^{14}C curve (blue line), for individuals born before or after the onset of nuclear bomb tests, respectively, indicate cell turnover, hence adult neurogenesis.

Δ [14]C = measured ^{14}C levels in relation to a universal standard and corrected for radioactive decay. (A,B after R. D. Bhardwaj et al., 2006. *Proc. Natl. Acad. Sci. USA* 103: 12564-12568. © 2006 National Academy of Sciences, USA; C after K. L. Spalding et al., 2013. *Cell* 153: 1219-1227.)

level at the time of mitosis. Because DNA is stable after a neuron has gone through its last cell division, the radioactivity of a cell nucleus can be used as a time stamp of the cell's genesis, and the measured ^{14}C level in DNA can be used to retrospectively birth date cells in humans, after comparison with the atmospheric levels. Data points above the atmospheric radioactivity curve for subjects born before the bomb peak and below the bomb curve for subjects born after the nuclear tests indicate cell turnover. Data points on the atmospheric curve show the absence of turnover. Measurements showed that ^{14}C levels in the genomic DNA of human cortical or olfactory bulb neurons corresponded to the atmospheric ^{14}C levels at the time when the individual was born (see Figure 27.19A,B).[102] This showed that few if any new neurons had been produced in these regions of adult human brains. However, the ^{14}C levels in genomic DNA of hippocampal neurons corresponded to the ^{14}C concentration in the atmosphere at times *after the birth* of the individual (see Figure 27.19C),[103] showing that new neurons were generated in the adult human hippocampus. The oldest studied individuals had higher ^{14}C concentrations in neuronal DNA than were present in the atmosphere before 1955 (see Figure 27.19C). This established that new neurons had been generated after 1955 (the oldest individual was 42 years old in 1955). Altogether, these data proved that in the human hippocampus neurogenesis occurs at significant levels through adulthood. A similar study demonstrated neuronal turnover in the adult human striatum.[104] Postnatally generated striatal neurons are preferentially depleted in patients with Huntington's disease.[104]

Two recent, well-controlled studies, based on the analysis of neuroblast marker proteins in postmortem human brains, showed thousands of newborn neurons in the hippocampal dentate gyrus from neurologically healthy humans, up to the ninth decade of life, while a significant neurogenesis decline was observed in individuals with Alzheimer's disease.[105,106]

Neurogenesis versus Gliogenesis

Neurons and glia acquire their identities in a multistep sequential process that involves both intrinsic and extrinsic influences. This "nature and nurture" question has been studied by a combination of in vitro and in vivo experimental approaches, lineage tracing, cell transplants, and single clone analysis.

In the vertebrate retina, the different retinal cell types are born in a histogenetic order: Ganglion, amacrine, and horizontal cells and cones are the first born, while rods, bipolar cells, and the Müeller glia are produced last. Cell-lineage studies in the rat retina were performed by infecting a few early retinal progenitors with a retrovirus encoding β-galactosidase and observing the adult stained retina (Figure 27.20A). The resultant clones had a mixed cellular composition comprising different cell types, in multiple layers of the retina[107] (Figure 27.20B,C). When progenitors were labeled at a later developmental stage, they gave rise to clones of only late types of cells, suggesting that, with time, progenitors lose competence to produce early cell types. Studies in which labeled retinal progenitors from different stages of development were placed in an environment of a different age likewise suggested that the competence of retinal progenitors to produce early cell types becomes restricted as development proceeds, leaving late progenitors largely capable of producing only late cell types.[108]

Likewise, in the cortex a key question is whether the production of different types of neurons and of glia is the result of (1) a progressive competence-restriction mechanism, in which common progenitors progressively restrict their outcomes, or (2) a predetermined fate-restriction mechanism, by which different progenitors are pre-committed to generate distinct cell types. In the first case, analysis of the cellular output of single identified clones should reveal a mixed population of different neuronal types and of glia, while in the second case only pure homogeneous clones should be observed.

Experiments in the 1990s addressed these questions at the cell population level, by *heterochronic transplantation* of progenitors.[109,110] By transplanting cortical progenitors between fetal and neonatal ferrets, McConnell and colleagues found that when fetal pre-migratory neurons (which would normally become layer 6, deep cortical neurons) were transplanted into older neonatal hosts, many of the transplanted cells ended up in superficial cortical layers 2 and 3, and changed their projection patterns, suggesting that these young cortical neurons are flexible with regard to fate. The reverse transplant gave

[104] Ernst, A. et al., 2014. *Cell* 156: 1072-1083.

[105] Boldrini, M. et al., 2018. *Cell Stem Cell* 22: 589.

[106] Moreno-Jimenez, E. P. et al. 2019. *Nat. Med.* 25: 55.

[107] Turner, D., and Cepko, C. 1987. *Nature* 328: 131-136.

[108] Livesey, F. J., and Cepko, C. L. 2001. *Nat. Rev. Neurosci.* 2: 109.

[109] McConnell, S. K. 1995. *Neuron* 15: 761-768.

[110] Desai, A. R., and McConnell, S. K. 2000. *Development* 127: 2863-2872.

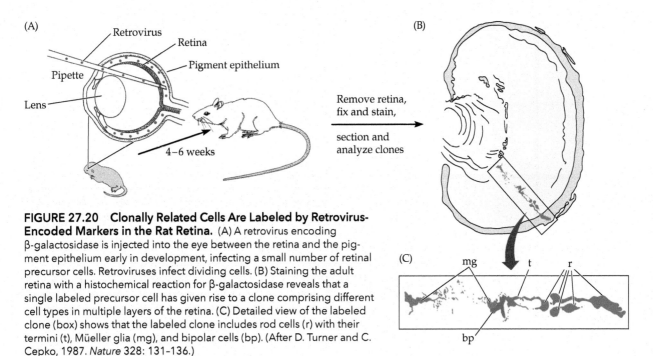

FIGURE 27.20 Clonally Related Cells Are Labeled by Retrovirus-Encoded Markers in the Rat Retina. (A) A retrovirus encoding β-galactosidase is injected into the eye between the retina and the pigment epithelium early in development, infecting a small number of retinal precursor cells. Retroviruses infect dividing cells. (B) Staining the adult retina with a histochemical reaction for β-galactosidase reveals that a single labeled precursor cell has given rise to a clone comprising different cell types in multiple layers of the retina. (C) Detailed view of the labeled clone (box) shows that the labeled clone includes rod cells (r) with their termini (t), Müeller glia (mg), and bipolar cells (bp). (After D. Turner and C. Cepko, 1987. *Nature* 328: 131–136.)

different results. When precursors from neonatal cortex were transplanted into embryonic hosts, they all differentiated into superficial layer 2 and 3 neurons, suggesting they had lost the competence to differentiate as deep cortical layer cells. Thus, early cortical progenitors are multipotent, whereas late cortical progenitors, even when exposed to a younger environment, are unable to produce the earlier neuronal fates. These results suggest that the competence of these precursors becomes progressively restricted over time.

Studies in vitro revealed an intrinsic timing mechanism that recapitulates the in vivo developmental steps of corticogenesis. When cultured in vitro, mouse cortical stem cell clones, individually followed by time-lapse video-microscopy to construct family trees of the cells generated from individual progenitors, sequentially generate neurons before glia[111] (Figure 27.21A). These data reveal that the order in which individual progenitors generate neurons and glia is intrinsically determined. Is a similar intrinsic mechanism operating during the sequential generation of neurons destined for different neocortical layers, which occurs in vivo?[112,113] Mouse embryonic stem cells, allowed to differentiate in culture at low density, autonomously recapitulate the sequential generation of neuronal subtypes that are characteristic of corticogenesis in vivo, as determined with layer-specific markers, and sequentially give rise to successive "waves" of deep-layer neurons, followed by upper-layer neurons, before starting gliogenesis (Figure 27.21B).[113] When grafted into the mouse brain, progenitor-derived cortical neurons develop layer characteristics and axonal projections corresponding to their cortical layer identity acquired in vitro.[113]

These results demonstrate that, as early as E10.5, neocortical progenitors contain an intrinsic program that specifies cortical identity and the order in which different cortical cells develop, in the absence of external influence from the developing brain.[112,113]

In vivo clonal studies in the mouse support the *progressive competence-restriction* model of corticogenesis.[114] Lineage progression of single radial glial cells was investigated in the developing cortex in vivo by a technique that allows sister cells derived from a common radial glia progenitor to be permanently labeled with different colors, in a time-controlled way. All clones labeled in green or red (progeny of siblings of a radial glia progenitor) at early stages (E10–E12) contained both superficial- and deep-layer neurons. Mixed clones, containing both neurons and glia, were also frequently found. No clone with only glial cells was observed. Instead, when radial glial cells were labeled at later stages (E15), 92% of the clones contained only superficial-layer neurons. Consistent with the inside-out sequence of neocortical neurogenesis, a gradual shift of labeled neurons in the clones from deep layers to superficial layers was observed, as a function of labeling induction time.[114]

[111] Qian, X. et al. 2000. *Neuron* 28: 69–80.

[112] Shen et al. 2006. *Nat. Neurosci.* 9: 743.

[113] Gaspard, N. et al. 2008. *Nature* 455: 351.

[114] Gao, P. et al. 2014. *Cell* 159: 775–788.

(A)

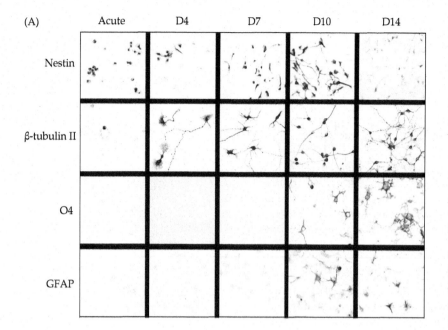

(B)

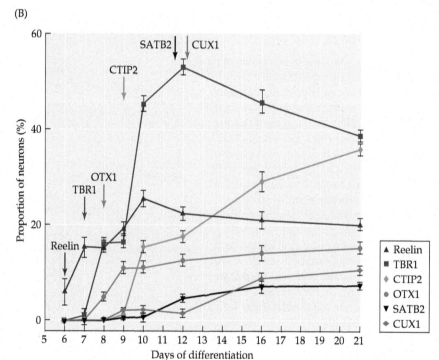

FIGURE 27.21 Mouse Embryonic Stem Cells Recapitulate In Vitro the Major Milestones of Cortical Development In Vivo. (A) E10.5 mouse embryonic cortical stem cells (nestin-positive) were grown in culture under clonal conditions, from 1–4 hours after plating (acute) to 14 days (D14). Neurons (indicated by β-tubulin marker) appear early, before glial astrocytes (GFAP marker) and oligodendrocytes (O4 marker). (B) Pyramidal neurons of different layers can be identified in vivo by a repertoire of cortical layer-specific molecular markers: Reelin and TBR1 for subplate and Cajal-Retzius neurons, CTIP2, OTX1 and TBR1 for deep-layer neurons, SATB2 and CUX1 for upper-layer neurons. Mouse embryonic stem cell–derived cortical progenitors were cultured in vitro and the expression of their layer-specific cortical markers was followed in time. First markers for subplate neurons and Cajal-Retzius neurons (Reelin [violet], TBR1 [red]) appeared, followed by deep-layer neuron markers (CTIP2 [green], OTX1 [light blue], TBR1 [red]), and, finally, upper-layer neuron markers (SATB2 [black], CUX1 [orange]). The sequential generation in vitro of the different subtypes of cortical neurons follows the same order as that observed in vivo, and is encoded within single cell lineages. Colored arrows indicate the first day of appearance of each marker. Data are represented as mean +/– SEM. (A after X. Qian et al., 2000. *Neuron* 28: 69–80; B after N. Gaspard et al., 2008. *Nature* 455: 351–357.)

Determination of Neuronal Phenotype

In the developing brain, neurogenesis and cell migration are closely coupled and most neurons end up some distance from where they were generated. The mature neuronal architecture depends on cells getting to the right place at the right time. Once there, neurons differentiate, grow dendrites and axons, and acquire their characteristic morphology and synaptic phenotype (in terms of neurotransmitter released and receptors expressed). The following paragraphs deal with some of the steps that establish the phenotype of a differentiated neuron once it has reached its final destination.

The genesis, migration, and differentiation of the cells of the neural crest provide a fascinating system to address such questions.

Lineage of Neural Crest Cells

The vertebrate neural crest arises along the lateral edges of the neural plate and joins together dorsally as the neural tube closes, migrating along different streams, to become distinct types of peripheral cells: (1) neurons and glia of the sensory dorsal root ganglia, of the sympathetic and parasympathetic autonomic nervous system, and of the gastric mucosal plexus, (2) the epinephrine-producing (medulla) adrenal chromaffin cells, (3) melanocytes, and (4) many of the skeletal and connective tissue components of the head.

Given the wide diversity of cells generated by the neural crest, a key question is whether the cells leaving the neural crest are multipotent or are a heterogeneous population of restricted progenitors, each already fated to a particular cell type, before leaving the neural tube.

The lineage of individual trunk neural crest precursor cells, each genetically labeled with different colors, was traced in the mouse embryo, revealing that the majority of individual neural crest clones are multipotent and contribute to multiple sites and cell types in the trunk and spinal cord: dorsal root ganglia, sympathetic ganglia, Schwann cells, and melanocytes.[115]

Neurotransmitter Choice in the Peripheral Nervous System

The fate of sympathetic neurons, including the decision to secrete a particular transmitter, for example acetylcholine or norepinephrine, has been studied in chick and quail.[116–118]

Neural crest cells at different positions along the neuraxis give rise to different cell types of the peripheral nervous system (Figure 27.22A). To investigate whether the differentiated phenotype of cells derived from the neural crest was fixed early in development

[115] Baggiolini, A. et al. 2015. *Cell Stem Cell* 16: 314–322.

[116] Weston, J. 1970. *Adv. Morphogenesis* 8: 41–114.

[117] Teillet, M. A. et al. 2008. *Methods Mol. Biol.* 461: 337–350.

[118] Le Douarin, N. M. et al. 2008. *Cell Cycle* 7: 1013–1019.

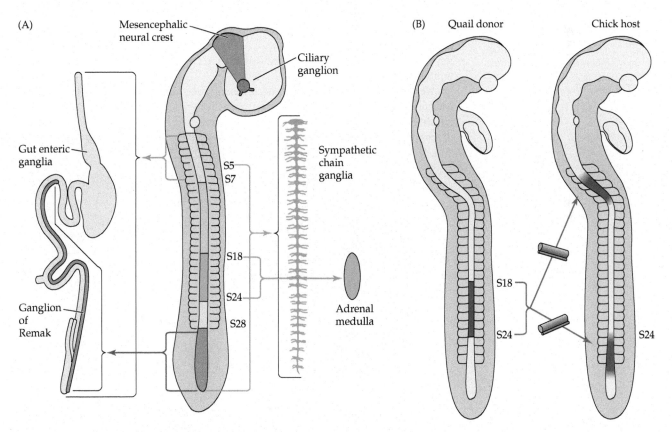

FIGURE 27.22   The Fate of a Neural Crest Cell is determined by environmental cues. (A) Neural crest cells give rise to a variety of peripheral ganglia. The ciliary ganglion is formed by migrating cells from the mesencephalic neural crest. The ganglion of Remak and the enteric ganglia of the gut are formed by cells from the vagal (somites 1-7) and lumbosacral (caudal to S28) regions of the neural crest. The ganglia of the sympathetic chain are derived from all regions of the neural crest caudal to S5. The adrenal medulla is populated by crest cells from S18-S24. (B) If crest cells from S18-S24, which are destined to form the adrenal medulla, are transplanted from a quail donor to the vagal or lumbosacral region of a host chick embryo, they will adopt the fate appropriate to their new location and populate the ganglion of Remak and the enteric ganglia of the gut. (After N. M. Le Douarin, 1986. *Science* 231: 1515-1522.)

or could be altered at a later date, in classic experiments Nicole Le Douarin and her colleagues transplanted pre-migratory crest cells from quail embryos into host chick embryos (Figure 27.22B).[119] The transplanted cells could be recognized by cytological differences between quail and chick cells. When donor cells from one region of the neural crest were transplanted to a different region of a host embryo, the donor cells assumed the fate appropriate to their new position in the host. For example, the normal destiny of a cell situated in segment 12 is to become a sympathetic ganglion cell and secrete norepinephrine as its transmitter. When transplanted to a region of segments 18–24, however, cells from segment 12 became chromaffin cells and secreted epinephrine.[119] Several transplantation experiments, showing similar switching of phenotypes, demonstrated that neural crest cells display great flexibility in fate choice, which appears to be largely determined by local environmental cues.

Changes in the choice of neurotransmitter also occur during normal development.[120] For example, in the peripheral nervous system sympathetic neurons that innervate sweat glands initially synthesize norepinephrine, but during the second and third weeks of life they are induced to synthesize acetylcholine by factors associated with their target.[121] Sympathetic ganglion cells in culture have been used to explore the mechanism by which neurotransmitters are switched. Neurons dissociated from the superior cervical ganglia of newborn rats and grown in culture in the absence of other cell types contain tyrosine hydroxylase and synthesize catecholamines.[122] However, neurons that are grown together with heart muscle cells or sweat glands cease synthesizing catecholamines and begin synthesizing choline acetyltransferase and acetylcholine. To establish unequivocally that this change occurs in individual cells, single neurons were cultured on micro-islands of heart cells (Figure 27.23).[123] The neuron rapidly extended neurites and established synaptic contact with the heart cells. Initially, these synapses were purely adrenergic, but over several days the cell began to release both acetylcholine and norepinephrine. Finally, transmission became purely cholinergic. A factor that induces cholinergic differentiation of sympathetic neurons was identified from heart-conditioned medium as leukemia inhibitory factor (LIF).[124]

Neurotransmitter switching also occurs during development of CNS neurons.[120] One example is provided by the hippocampal mossy fibers–CA3 principal cell synapses. In the immediate postnatal period the axons of dentate gyrus granule cells release GABA as the only neurotransmitter, which exerts onto targeted cells a depolarizing and excitatory action (see

[119] Le Douarin, N. M. et al. 1975. *Proc. Natl. Acad. Sci USA* 72: 728-732.

[120] Spitzer, N. 2017. *Annu Rev. Neurosci.* 40: 1-19.

[121] Francis, N. J., and Landis, S. C. 1999. *Annu. Rev. Neurosci.* 22: 541-566.

[122] Mains, R. E., and Patterson, P. H. 1973. *J. Cell Biol.* 59: 329-345.

[123] Furshpan, E. J. et al. 1976. *Proc. Natl. Acad. Sci. USA* 73: 4225-4229.

[124] Yamamori, T. et al. 1989. *Science* 246: 1412-1416.

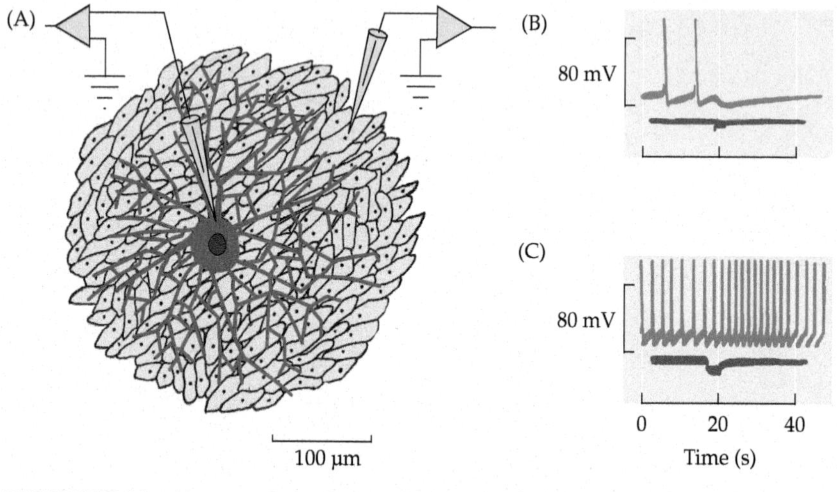

FIGURE 27.23 Neurons from Sympathetic Ganglia Can Release Both Acetylcholine (ACh) and Norepinephrine at synapses on heart cells in culture. (A) A microculture containing a single sympathetic neuron is grown on an island of cardiac muscle cells. (B) A brief train of impulses in the neuron (10 Hz, deflection of lower trace) produced inhibition of spontaneous myocyte activity due to release of ACh (upper trace). (C) Addition of atropine (10^{-7} M) blocked the inhibitory cholinergic response, revealing an excitatory effect, which is due to the release of norepinephrine. (After E. J. Furshpan et al., 1976. *Proc. Natl. Acad. Sci. USA* 73: 4225-4229.)

the following section), before switching to glutamate in adulthood.[125] In adulthood, markers of the GABAergic phenotype disappear but they can be transiently expressed during seizures.

In the embryonic *Xenopus* spinal cord, Spitzer and his colleagues showed that altering the frequency of spontaneous calcium spike activity in vivo causes homeostatic replacement of one transmitter with another.[126] Silencing neurons caused a decrease in the number of inhibitory glycinergic and GABAergic neurons, in parallel with an increase of neurons expressing excitatory transmitters, acetylcholine and glutamate (Figure 27.24A).

[125] Safiulina, V. F. et al. 2006. *J. Neurosci.* 26: 597–608.

[126] Borodinsky, L. N. et al. 2004. *Nature* 429: 523–530.

(A)

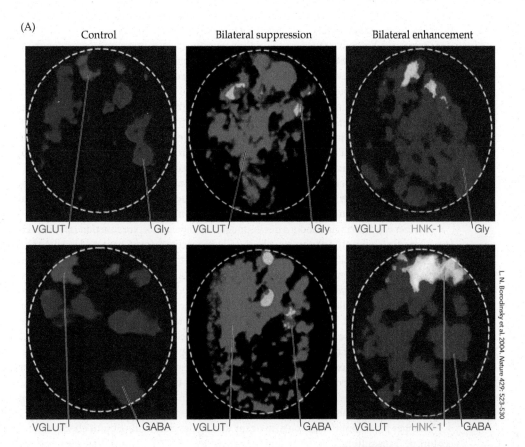

L. N. Borodinsky et al. 2004. *Nature* 429: 523–530

(B)

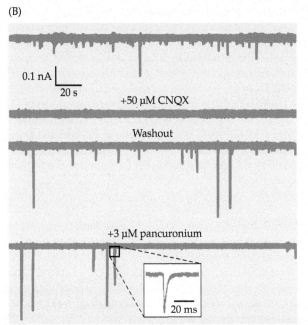

FIGURE 27.24 Neurotransmitter and Receptor Switching in the Xenopus Neural Tube. (A) Neurotransmitter switching. Neural tube sections (white dashed oval) from Xenopus embryos double-stained for vesicular glutamate transporter (VGLUT: red, excitatory) plus glycine (Gly) or GABA (purple, inhibitory). Left: Control embryos. Middle: Embryos in which spontaneous spike activity was bilaterally suppressed, by expressing an inwardly rectifying K+ channel. Pink: co-expression of excitatory and inhibitory transmitters. Right: Embryos in which spike activity was bilaterally enhanced, by expression of a Na channel. A marker of sensory neurons was added (HNK-1 green). Light blue: co-expression of HNK-1 and inhibitory transmitter; white: co-expression of HNK-1 and both excitatory and inhibitory transmitters. (B) Matching of transmitter and receptor. Whole-cell recordings from a larval Xenopus muscle cell of the axial musculature of 3-day spike-suppressed larva in which motor neurons express glutamate. Glutamatergic (noncholinergic) miniature post-synaptic currents were recorded and pharmacologically identified with AMPA receptor and nicotinic ACh receptor antagonists (CNQX and pancuronium, respectively). A single miniature post-synaptic current is shown on an expanded time base to illustrate its kinetics. (After L. N. Borodinsky and N. C. Spitzer, 2007. *Proc. Natl. Acad. Sci. USA* 104: 335–340. © 2007 National Academy of Sciences, USA.)

Symmetrically, enhancing spike activity increased the number of neurons expressing inhibitory transmitters (see Figure 27.24A). GABA or glycine expression was observed in neurons that also expressed markers for sensory or motor neurons, implying replacement of excitatory transmitters with inhibitory ones in these neurons.[120,126]

Changes in Receptors during Development

One would expect that when the neurotransmitter changes, there would be matching switches in postsynaptic receptor composition, in order to ensure continuity of synaptic function. This is what has been observed.[127,128]

Embryonic *Xenopus* striated muscle cells in vivo normally co-express receptors for glutamate, GABA, and glycine as well as for acetylcholine. As maturation progresses, acetylcholine receptor expression prevails, matching the incoming cholinergic innervation, and the other neurotransmitter receptors disappear. The developmental receptor selection is altered when spontaneous neuronal activity is perturbed. Remaining receptors parallel changes in transmitter phenotype. For instance, after suppressing spike activity (as in Figure 27.24A, middle), glutamatergic non-cholinergic excitatory currents could be recorded from the skeletal muscle (Figure 27.24B).[127,128] The results indicate that early neuronal activity ensures matching of transmitters and their receptors and regulates the identity of newly formed synapses.

Neurons may also change the expressed receptors during development independently of switching transmitters. One example is provided by the nicotinic ACh receptors. Arrival of the motor nerve induces a change in their subunit composition (see Chapter 28).

Another way of bringing about a developmental change in receptor function is **RNA editing**, as exemplified by the glutamate AMPA (GluA) receptors (see Chapter 11). All AMPA receptor subunits contain a critical glutamine (Q) residue that contributes to the channel's ion selectivity. AMPA receptors translated from unedited GluA mRNAs show significant calcium permeability.[129] However, beginning during embryonic development and continuing into adulthood, the **RNA editing enzyme** ADAR2 (adenosine deaminase on RNA) modifies the GluA2 mRNA so that it is translated with an arginine (R) residue instead of asparagine at the critical site.[130] The presence of even one Q-to-R-edited GluA subunit drastically reduces the calcium permeability of the receptor complex. The developmental functions of this particular way of regulating the ion permeability of AMPA receptors are still unclear,[131–133] but they may have pathological consequences. A Q-R defect in the editing of the mRNA encoding the GluA2 subunit of glutamate AMPA receptors was found in the spinal motor neurons, but not in other neurons, of individuals with amyotrophic lateral sclerosis.[134]

Changes in transmitter action also occur during development without changes in receptors or transmitters. Cherubini and his colleagues[135,136] have shown that at early postnatal stages GABA released by hippocampal interneurons acts as an excitatory transmitter. Only at about 12 days in rats does GABA cause hyperpolarization and inhibition as in the adult (Figure 27.25). In this case, neither the receptors nor the transmitter change. Instead, the critical difference is that the intracellular chloride level is higher in immature postsynaptic neurons than in mature neurons, owing to the presence of an *inwardly* directed chloride transporter NKCC1 in the immature neurons (see Chapter 9).[137] With high intracellular Cl⁻, opening GABA-gated channels leads to outward movement of Cl⁻ and depolarization of the cell. Later in development, NKCC1 in these neurons is replaced by an *outward* chloride transporter, KCC2. As a result, intracellular Cl⁻ becomes lower inside the cell and the hyperpolarizing response to GABA appears. There is evidence that excitation and firing produced by GABA play a part in the formation of connections while circuits are being established.[138]

Migration of Neural Crest Cells

The neural crest cells are a collectively migrating population.[139] No other cell type undergoes such extensive migration during development.

In preparation for leaving the neural tube, neural crest cells undergo an epithelial-to-mesenchymal transition.[140] In this process, they lose their epithelial characteristics, such as the tight junctions and the adhesion proteins that tie them together in the epithelium, and acquire mesenchymal properties, typical of loosely packed cells, usually of

[127] Borodinsky, L. N. and Spitzer, N. 2007. *Proc. Natl. Acad. Sci USA* 104: 335–340.

[128] Dulcis, D. et al. 2013. *Science* 340: 449–453.

[129] Hollmann, M., Hartley, M., and Heinemann, S. 1991. *Science* 252: 851–853.

[130] Rueter, S. M. et al. 1995. *Science* 267: 1491–1494.

[131] Kask, K. et al. 1998. *Proc. Natl. Acad. Sci. USA* 95: 13777–13782.

[132] Brusa, R. et al. 1995. *Science* 270: 1677–1680.

[133] Higuchi, M. et al. 2000. *Nature* 406: 78–81.

[134] Kwak, S., and Kawahara, Y. 2005. *J. Mol. Med.* 83: 110–120.

[135] Cherubini, E., Gaiarsa, J. L., and Ben-Ari, Y. 1991. *Trends Neurosci.* 14: 515–519.

[136] Lagostena, L. et al. 2010. *J. Neurosci.* 30: 885–893.

[137] Tyzio, R. et al. 2011. *J. Neurosci.* 31: 34–45.

[138] Cherubini, E. et al. 2011. *Mol. Neurobiol.* 43: 97–106.

[139] Szabo, A., and Mayor, R. 2018. *Annu. Rev. Genet.* 52: 43–63.

[140] Kuriyama, S., and Mayor, R. 2008. *Philos. Trans. R Soc. Lond. Ser B Biol. Sci.* 363: 1349–1362.

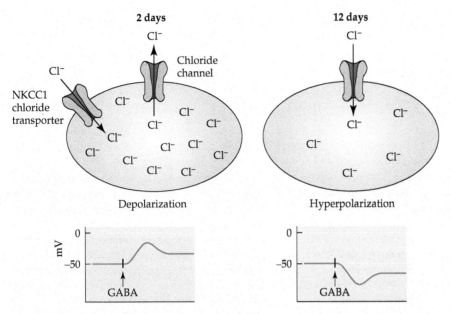

FIGURE 27.25 GABA as a Depolarizing Transmitter during Development.
Two days after birth, CA3 neurons in the rat hippocampus are depolarized by GABA
and by inhibitory synaptic inputs. At early stages, the opening of chloride channels by
γ-aminobutyric acid (GABA) allows the negatively charged ion to exit. By 12 days, the effects
of GABA and inhibitory inputs have reversed and, as in the adult, give rise to hyperpolarization (inward movement of Cl⁻) at the normal resting potential. The change to hyperpolarization is caused by a decrease in intracellular chloride concentration. At 2 days the concentration is high owing to the activity of an inward chloride transporter (NKCC1), which virtually
disappears by day 12. (After E. Cherubini et al., 1991. *Trends Neurosci.* 14: 515-519.)

mesodermal origin, that move around the body. This transition allows neural crest cells
to leave the epithelium.

Most neural crest cells migrate collectively, as a large coherent flock of cells, via different collective migratory streams. The separate migratory streams are kept apart by inhibitory chemorepellent guidance signals (similar to those involved in growth cone guidance;
see the next section) expressed on migrating neural crest cells of different flocks, which
create "migration corridors" and restrict cells from wandering outside of their stream. Experimentally blocking the repulsion signals causes the separate migratory streams to mix.

Long-range gradients of chemoattracting factors contribute to guiding the migrating
neural crest flock through the embryonic environment toward their targets, which in the
developing embryo may be moving targets.[141] The collective migration of cranial neural
crest cells toward placodal cells, an epithelial tissue that contributes to sensory organs, is described by a *chase-and-run model.*[142] Neural crest cells "chase" placodal cells by chemotaxis,
while placodal cells "run" when contacted by neural crest cells.[142]

Axon Outgrowth and Growth Cone Navigation

The Growth Cone

There is a deep analogy between migrating cells and growth cones of migrating axons. Both
undertake similar environment sensing and navigation tasks and use similar chemorepellent and chemoattractive signaling molecules. Because of this, the growth cone has been
called a "neural crest on a leash." The axon of a cell can extend up to a meter or more (far
more in a giraffe or a whale) to form synapses on appropriate cells in a region that contains
many potential targets. During development, cues in the environment guide the navigation
of axons along specific pathways.

Ramón y Cajal was the first to recognize the **growth cone** as the region at the tip of
an axon responsible for navigation toward a target (Figure 27.26). Growth cones extend and
retract broad membranous sheets, called lamellipodia, and slender spike-like protrusions,

141 Thevenau, E. et al. 2013. *Nat. Cell Biol.* 15: 763-772.

142 Scarpa, E., and Mayor, R. 2016. *J. Cell Biol.* 212: 143-155.

(A)

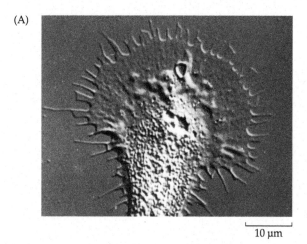

(B)

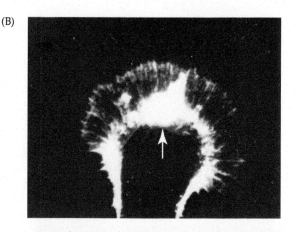

(C)

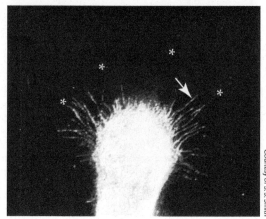

10 μm

FIGURE 27.26 Morphology of Growth Cones.
(A) Growth cone observed by differential interference contrast microscopy. (B) Fluorescence micrograph showing the distribution of filamentous actin visualized with rhodamine-conjugated phalloidin. Actin filaments align with filopodia, or microspikes, in the periphery of the growth cone; randomly oriented filaments are often concentrated near the central domain (arrow). (C) Microtubule distribution visualized with antitubulin antibodies and fluorescein-conjugated secondary antibodies. Microtubules are concentrated in the axon. Most terminate in the central domain of the growth cone; some (arrow) extend toward the growth cone margin (asterisks).

P. Forscher, S. J. Smith. 1988. *J. Cell Bio* 107: 1505-1516. Courtesy of S. J. Smith

termed filopodia, sampling the substrate in every direction for distances of tens of micrometers.[143,144] Filopodia may adhere to the substrate, in which case the retraction serves to pull the growth cone in that direction. Both lamellipodia and filopodia are rich in filamentous actin; actin polymerization inhibitors, such as the fungal toxin cytochalasin B, immobilize growth cones. Dynamics of the actin cytoskeleton are responsible for producing protrusion and retraction of lamellipodia and filopodia as well as for the forward movement of the body of the growth cone. Transient, localized increases in cytoplasmic calcium levels, triggered by extracellular guidance cues, are important in regulating motility of the growth cone.[145]

Growth Cone Guidance Mechanisms

The guidance cues for axonal navigation toward the target can function at short or long ranges, and can be either attractive or repulsive.[146] Different classes of molecules mediate growth cone navigation: (1) cell adhesion molecules, which allow one neuron to grow along another, (2) extracellular matrix molecules, which allow selective adhesion of axons to a substrate, and are either permissive for growth or not, and (3) diffusible factors, forming concentration gradients.[146]

As more and more neurons start sending their axons out into the developing nervous system, the axonal surfaces of the first pioneering neurons become increasingly available for navigation, a *labeled-line mechanism* first demonstrated in studies of the embryonic grasshopper nervous system.[147]

Ramón y Cajal originally proposed a *chemoattractant model* of axon guidance, whereby the growth cone navigates along a gradient of molecules released by its target. Nerve growth factor (NGF)[148] was the first identified chemotactic factor in vivo[149] and in vitro.[150] Axons of cultured sensory neurons rapidly turn toward the tip of a micropipette that ejects NGF, creating a local concentration gradient. As the NGF pipette is moved, the axon reorients its growth.[150] These chemotactic (neurotropic) activities of NGF are

[143] Lowery, L. A., and Van Vactor, D. 2009. *Nat. Rev. Mol. Cell. Biol.* 10: 332-343.

[144] Gallo, G., and Letourneau, P. C. 2004. *J. Neurobiol.* 58: 92-102.

[145] Hutchins, B. I., and Kalil, K. 2008. *J. Neurosci.* 28: 143-153.

[146] Kolodkin, A. L., and Tessier-Lavigne, M. 2010. *Cold Spring Harb. Perspect. Biol.* 3: doi: 10.1101/cshperspect.a001727.

[147] Goodman, C. S. et al. 1983. *Progr. Brain Res.* 58: 283-304.

[148] Levi-Montalcini, R. 1987. *Science* 237: 1154-1162.

[149] Menesini-Chen, M. L., Chen, J. S., Levi-Montalcini, R. 1978. *Arch. Ital. Biol.* 116: 53-84.

[150] Gundersen, R. W. and Barret, J. N. 1979. *Science* 206: 1079-1080.

distinct from its neurotrophic survival actions (see section Nerve Growth Factor and Neurotrophins later in this chapter).

Lumsden and Davies[151] studied the growth of axons from the trigeminal ganglion in the head of the mouse embryo into the adjacent epithelial tissue (the maxillary pad epithelium), at a distance of about 1 mm. (These axons ultimately give rise to the sensory innervation of the whiskers; see Chapter 21). If the developing trigeminal ganglion is placed in culture near explants from several peripheral tissues, neurites grow from the ganglion only toward their appropriate target, ignoring other tissues. Explants of target epithelium have this effect on axon outgrowth only if they are taken from embryos at the stage when innervation normally occurs, when they release a chemoattracting factor, which was identified as a combination of the two neurotrophins BDNF and NT-3.[152]

In contrast, the ability of spinal motor axons to grow to the appropriate region in the limb seems not to depend on the presence of their target muscles. This was shown by removing the tissues that give rise to limb musculature, early in development.[153,154] Motor axons extended normally from the spinal cord, grew into the limb, and formed the appropriate pattern of muscle nerves—all in the absence of muscle. Thus, the factors that guide motor axons in the initial steps toward their destinations in the limb are not supplied by the muscles that the axons ultimately innervate.[153]

Navigation via Guidepost Cells and Intermediate Targets

As axons extend over very long distances toward their final targets, sequential responses to guidance cues found en route allow for complex navigation pathways. This requires that neurons extinguish their responses to certain cues and acquire responsiveness to others, by changing the expression of guidance receptors, in coincidence with navigation decision points.

When the distance from a neuron to its target is more than several hundred microns, the pathway may be marked with intermediate targets. For example, growth cones arising from sensory cells in the limbs of developing grasshoppers make abrupt changes in direction as they extend toward the CNS (Figure 27.27). The turns occur when the growth cones contact so-called *guidepost cells*,[155,156] which are often immature neurons responsible for redirecting the growth cones, acting like stepping-stones for the pioneer axons. If the guidepost cells are removed by laser ablation before the growth cone arrives, the appropriate change in trajectory is not made.

Synaptic interactions can occur with guidepost cells. For example, axons arising from the lateral geniculate nucleus of the mammalian visual system reach the developing cortical plate before their synaptic targets (i.e., the pyramidal cells of layer 4) have been born. The geniculate axons form synaptic connections with the subplate neurons, which are produced

151 Lumsden, A. G. S., and Davies, A. M. 1986. *Nature* 323: 538-539.

152 O'Connor, R., and Tessier-Lavigne, M. 1999. *Neuron* 24: 165-178.

153 Bonanomi, D., and Pfaff, S. L. 2010. *Cold Spring Harb. Perspect. Biol.* 2: a001735.

154 Phelan, K. A., and Hollyday, M. 1990. *J. Neurosci.* 10: 2699-2716.

155 Bentley, D., and Caudy, M. 1983. *Cold Spring Harb. Symp. Quant. Biol.* 48: 573-585.

156 Shen, K., Fetter, R. D., and Bargmann, C. I. 2004. *Cell* 116: 869-881.

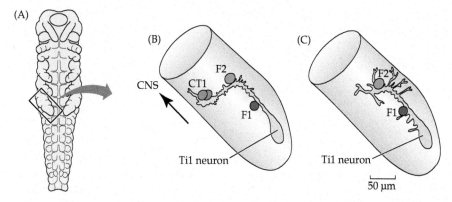

FIGURE 27.27 Growth Cones of Peripheral Neurons Rely on Guidepost Cells to navigate through the limb of the grasshopper (A). (B) In normal embryos, the axon of the Ti1 neuron encounters a series of guidepost cells on its route to the central nervous system: F1, F2, and two CT1 cells. (C) If the CT1 cells are killed early in development, the Ti1 neuron forms several axonal branches at the site of cell F2, with growth cones extending in abnormal directions. (After D. Bentley and M. Caudy, 1983. *Cold Spring Harb. Symp. Quant. Biol.* 48: 573-585.)

early, lie beneath the developing cortical plate, and disappear shortly after birth.[157,158] After a few weeks, when layer 4 pyramidal cells have reached their position in the cortex, geniculate axons abandon their connections with subplate neurons and invade the cortex to establish the adult pattern of innervation. If the subplate neurons are eliminated early in development by local application of neurotoxins, lateral geniculate nucleus axons grow past the developing visual cortex, and ocular dominance columns fail to form.[159]

A good example of intermediate targets is provided by the navigation of commissural interneurons in the vertebrate spinal cord. Early in development these sensory interneurons, which lie in the dorsal part of the spinal cord, extend axons that grow ventrally, cross the midline, and then run longitudinally along the spinal cord toward their targets in the brainstem and thalamus (see Chapter 21).[160]

Axons of such commissural interneurons are initially attracted to the ventral midline by the protein netrin-1, a diffusible chemoattractant released by the floor plate cells that form the ventral midline of the spinal cord (Figure 27.28A).[161] Growing axons express a netrin-1 receptor (DCC) that steers their navigation up the dorsoventral concentration gradient of netrin-1.

The existence of a chemoattractant produced by the floor plate was demonstrated by culturing explants of dorsal spinal cord either alone or with pieces of floor plate.[160,161] As shown in Figure 27.29, axons of commissural interneurons specifically grew toward the floor plate, even when the tissues were separated by several hundred microns. This distance is too great to be spanned by a filopodium from a growth cone. Commissural interneurons were similarly attracted to cell aggregates that secreted netrin-1 (see Figure 27.29, middle panel) but not to non-secreting control cells (right panel).

After being attracted in the direction of the floor plate, the commissural axon growth cones cross the ventral midline to the contralateral side (Figure 27.28B,C). Crossing is facilitated by the interaction of two cell surface adhesive molecules: TAG-1, which is expressed on the surface of commissural axons, and NrCAM, expressed on the floor plate cells. As the axons cross, they receive signals from floor plate cells to stop synthesizing TAG-1 and start synthesizing a protein called roundabout (robo). Robo is the receptor for another protein, called slit, which is also released by floor plate cells.[162,163] The slit–robo interaction *repels* commissural interneuron growth cones. The loss of the TAG-1–NrCAM contact attraction

[157] Shatz, C. J., and Luskin, M. B. 1986. *J. Neurosci.* 6: 3655-3658.

[158] Luskin, M. B., and Shatz, C. J. 1985. *J. Neurosci.* 5: 1062-1075.

[159] Kanold, P. O., and Shatz, C. J. 2006. *Neuron* 51: 627-638.

[160] Tessier-Lavigne, M. et al. 1988. *Nature* 336: 775-778.

[161] Kennedy, T. E. et al. 1994. *Cell* 78: 425-435.

[162] Dickson, B. J., and Gilestro, G. F. 2006. *Annu. Rev. Cell Dev. Biol.* 22: 651-675.

[163] Brose, K. et al. 1999. *Cell* 96: 795-806.

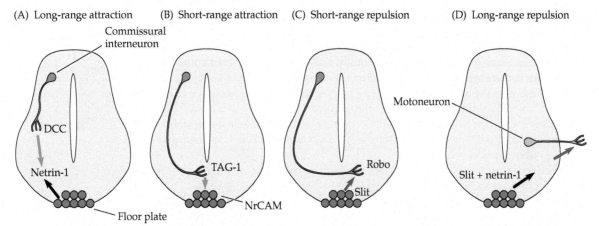

FIGURE 27.28 Long- and Short-Range Chemoattraction and Chemorepulsion guide developing axons in the vertebrate spinal cord. (A) Netrin-1, acting as a long-range chemoattractant, secreted by cells of the floor plate (blue), diffuses (black arrow) and binds to its receptor (DCC) on the growth cones of commissural interneurons (orange), attracting them (green arrow). (B) Transient axonal glycoprotein-1 (TAG-1) on commissural axon growth cones binds to neuronal cell adhesion molecules (NrCAM) on floor plate cells. This short-range chemoattraction (green arrow) facilitates extension of commissural axon growth cones across the floor plate. (C) As the commissural axons cross the midline, the TAG-1 on their growth cones is replaced by roundabout (robo), which binds to slit on floor plate cells. This short-range chemorepulsion (red arrow) prevents the axons from recrossing the floor plate. (D) Slit and netrin-1 diffuse from the floor plate (black arrow), interact with receptors on growth cones of motor neurons (blue), and repel them (red arrow). This long-range chemorepulsion helps direct the growth of motor axons away from the cord.

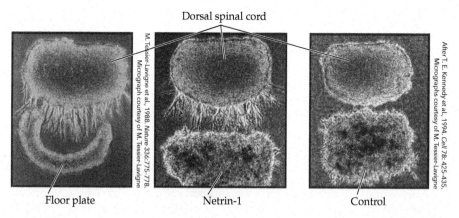

Dorsal spinal cord

Floor plate   Netrin-1   Control

FIGURE 27.29 Netrins and Netrin Receptors function in long-range attraction and repulsion. (A) Micrographs of pieces of dorsal spinal cord from embryonic rats (top in each panel) cultured with a piece of floor plate tissue (left), an aggregate of cells secreting recombinant netrin-1 (middle), or control cells (right). The floor plate and netrin-1 both elicit the profuse and directed outgrowth of bundles of commissural axons from the dorsal spinal cord tissue.

and the acquisition of slit–robo short-range repulsion prevent commissural axons from turning back and recrossing the midline. (The gene name *Robo* comes from the mutation in *Drosophila* that knocks out the function of this receptor.[164] In mutant embryos, the repulsive signal is lost and the growth cones in the developing nerve cord cross and recross the midline. The thickened commissural nerves come to resemble a traffic circle, or *roundabout*.[164]) Netrin-1, while attracting commissural interneuron growth cones, acts in concert with slit to instead repel growth cones of motoneurons. These repulsive interactions direct motor axons away from the cord toward the periphery (Figure 27.28D).[160,161]

Semaphorins are another family of secreted chemorepellent proteins,[165] acting via their Neuropilin receptors.[166]

Growth Cone Navigation and Axonal Protein Synthesis

During navigation, growth cones make rapid turning decisions, in response to environmental guidance cues. Following early evidence suggesting axonal mRNA translation,[167,168] local protein synthesis in the growth cone has emerged as a mechanism responsible for the rapid turning responses during axonal navigation (see also Chapter 17).[169,170] Growth cones still navigate correctly when the axon has been mechanically separated from the cell body.[171]

In isolated retinal growth cones, an external gradient of netrin-1 increases the translation of β-actin mRNA on the near side of the gradient,[172,173] leading to a rapid polarized increase in β-actin protein that helps axon turning toward the gradient source. Isolated growth cones fail to turn in a chemotropic gradient of netrin-1 or Semaphorin 3A (Sema3A) when translation is inhibited.[174]

Different guidance cues elicit the translation of specific subsets of mRNAs at growth cones.[175,176] β-actin mRNA translation is triggered by netrin-1 but not by Sema3A, whereas *RhoA* and *cofilin* mRNA translation is induced by Sema3A but not by netrin-1. This suggests the *differential translation model*, whereby translation-dependent repulsive and attractive turning responses in growth cones depend on the differential translation of mRNAs involved in assembly or disassembly of the actin cytoskeleton[175,176] (Figure 27.30).

We saw earlier (see Figure 27.28) that in the developing spinal cord, after crossing the midline, the axons of commissural interneurons undergo a drastic switch in responsiveness: They are now repelled by the floor plate and gain responsiveness to cues that guide the next step of their journey. One mechanism for this responsiveness switch is provided by the local translation of axonal guidance receptors, such as ephrin and *ROBO3.2*, within navigating commissural interneuron growth cones.[177,178] Interestingly, the abrupt upregulation of *ROBO3.2* translation, upon crossing the floor plate, was accompanied by a subsequent downregulation of its mRNA, determining a brief pulse of ROBO3.2 protein synthesis.[178] The translation-dependent degradation of *ROBO3.2* mRNA occurs by a mechanism known as *nonsense mediated decay*, similar to what has been described for *Arc* mRNA in synaptic plasticity (see Chapter 17).[179]

[164] Seeger, M. et al 1993. *Neuron* 19: 409-426.

[165] Derijck, A. A., Van Erp, S., and Pasterkamp, R. J. 2010. *Trends Cell Biol.* 20: 568-576.

[166] Fujisawa, H. 2004. *J. Neurobiol.* 59: 24-33.

[167] Giuditta, A. et al. 1968. *Proc. Natl. Acad. Sci. USA* 59: 1284-1287.

[168] Thoenen, H. et al. 1970. *Proc. Natl. Acad. Sci USA* 65: 58-62.

[169] Lin, A. C., and Holt, C. E. 2007. *EMBO J.* 26: 3729-3736.

[170] Jung, H. et al. 2012. *Nat. Rev. Neurosci.* 13: 308.

[171] Harris WA et al. 1987. *Development* 101: 123-133.

[172] Leung, K. M. et al. 2006. *Nat. Neurosci.* 9: 1247-1256.

[173] Yao, J. et al. 2006. *Nat. Neurosci.* 9: 1265-1273.

[174] Campbell, D. S., and Holt, C. E. 2001. *Neuron* 32: 1013-1026.

[175] Piper, M. et al. 2006. *Neuron* 49: 215-228.

[176] Wu, K.Y. et al. 2005. *Nature* 436: 1020-1024.

[177] Brittis, P. A., Lu, Q., and Flanagan, J. G. 2002. *Cell* 110: 223-235.

[178] Colak, D. et al. 2013. *Cell* 153: 1252-1265.

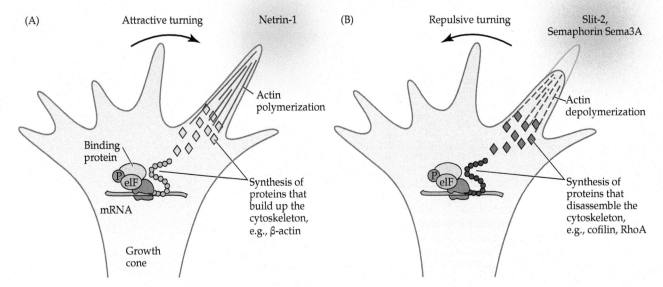

(A) Attractive turning   Netrin-1   (B) Repulsive turning   Slit-2, Semaphorin Sema3A

Actin polymerization

Binding protein

mRNA

Growth cone

Synthesis of proteins that build up the cytoskeleton, e.g., β-actin

Actin depolymerization

Synthesis of proteins that disassemble the cytoskeleton, e.g., cofilin, RhoA

FIGURE 27.30 Differential mRNA Translation in Growth Cones exposed to gradients of attractive or repulsive guidance cues. (A) A lateral gradient of an attractive guidance cue, such as netrin-1, induces asymmetrical activation of mRNA translation in the growth cone, causing asymmetrical translation of proteins (e.g., β-actin) that build up the cytoskeleton, leading to attractive turning. (B) A lateral gradient of a repulsive guidance cue, such as slit2 or Sema3A, induces similar asymmetrical activation of translation of different mRNAs, causing asymmetrical translation of proteins (e.g., cofilin and RhoA) that disassemble the cytoskeleton, which leads to repulsive turning. RhoA is a small GTPase that mediates growth cone collapse, while cofilin disassembles actin microfilaments. P-eIF = phosphorylated translation initiation factor. Binding protein in (A) indicates a generic protein of the translation initiation complex. (After A. C. Lin and C. E. Holt, 2008. *Curr. Op. Neurobiol.* 18: 60–68.)

Growth Factors and Survival of Neurons

Cell Death in the Developing Nervous System

During nervous system development, many cells die. In invertebrates, for example, the sweeping changes that occur during metamorphosis include the programmed cell death (**apoptosis**) of many neurons.[180] However, in developing invertebrate and vertebrate nervous systems, cell death also occurs in the absence of such gross morphological changes.[181] Overproduction of neurons followed by a period of cell death is a common pattern throughout development. Some of the neurons that die may not have made any synapses or may have innervated an inappropriate target. Most, however, appear to have reached and innervated their correct targets. An important finding was that inhibitors of mRNA or protein synthesis prevented the normal death of neurons.[182] Thus, apoptosis is a process that activates an intrinsic suicide machinery in a cell, involving synthesis or activation of families of proteolytic enzymes called **caspases**.[183]

The extent of neuronal apoptosis in vertebrate embryos depends also on the size of the target tissue.[184] When synaptic connections are first formed on myofibers in developing limbs, many of the motoneurons that had sent axons into the limb have died. Implantation of a supernumerary limb reduces the fraction of motoneurons that die, while removal of the limb bud exacerbates the death of motoneurons.[184]

In addition to cell death, another process, called synaptic reorganization, refines the pattern of innervation after axons reach their targets and make synaptic connections. Synaptic reorganization entails a reduction in the number of axons and synapses, accompanied by a reorganization of surviving connections, to achieve the adult pattern.

Cell death and synaptic reorganization often involve competition for limited supplies of target-derived neurotrophic factors, such as those described in the following section.

Nerve Growth Factor and Neurotrophins

The first identified neurotrophic substance was nerve growth factor (NGF), a target-derived survival and differentiating factor for sensory and sympathetic neurons, as well as for basal forebrain cholinergic neurons.[148] The discovery of NGF (Box 27.2) is a saga that mixes scientific breakthroughs with personal life events, in the tragedy of the racial

[179] Giorgi C et al. 2007. *Cell* 130, 179–191.

[180] Truman, J. W., Thorn, R. S., and Robinow, S. 1992. *J. Neurobiol.* 23: 1295–1311.

[181] Buss, R. R., Sun, W., and Oppenheim, R. W. 2006. *Annu. Rev. Neurosci.* 29: 1–35.

[182] Martin, D. P. et al. 1988. *J. Cell Biol.* 106: 829–844.

[183] Ryan, C. A., and Salvesen, G. S. 2003. *Biol. Chem.* 384: 855–861.

[184] Hollyday, M., and Hamburger, V. 1976. *J. Comp. Neurol.* 170: 311–320.

BOX 27.2   The Discovery of the Nerve Growth Factor

While investigating the effects of limb bud ablation in the chick embryo, Viktor Hamburger had observed a dramatic decline in the number of nerve cells in spinal ganglia.[185] He attributed this decline to a failure of neural induction of nerve cell precursors to proliferate and differentiate. Rita Levi-Montalcini, a medical graduate at the University of Turin (Italy), reinvestigated the effects of limb bud extirpation, in a clandestine makeshift laboratory she had set up in her bedroom while hiding with her family from the Nazi fascists during World War II. By performing a detailed time course after the limb bud ablation and following the fate of sensory neurons, Levi-Montalcini proposed that the severe hypoplasia of nerve centers deprived of their fields of innervation resulted from *death of already differentiated neurons*[186,187] and not from a failure of neural induction, as proposed by Hamburger. In 1947 Hamburger, who had come across Levi-Montalcini's wartime papers,[186,187] invited her to join him at Washington University. There the scientific controversy was settled, when new experiments demonstrated that nerve cell death after limb bud ablation was caused by the absence of a survival factor for differentiated neurons.[188] The subsequent finding that sarcoma tumors grafted in the chick embryo produce a diffusible factor that promotes neuron growth[189,190] set the stage for identifying this mysterious factor. Levi-Montalcini developed an in vitro bioassay based on sensory ganglia explanted from chick embryos in proximity to fragments of mouse sarcoma. As result there was growth of a dense "halo" of nerve fibers on the side facing the tumor.[191] Armed with this bioassay, Levi-Montalcini and biochemist Stanley Cohen (who later discovered the epidermal growth factor and shared with Levi-Montalcini the 1986 Nobel Prize in Physiology or Medicine) succeeded in partially purifying, from mouse sarcoma supernatant, proteins and nucleic acids that replicated in culture the halo produced by the growing tumor (Figure).[192] To determine whether the "factor" was a protein or a nucleic acid, they incubated it with snake venom, known to be a rich source of phosphodiesterase, an enzyme that degrades nucleic acids. To their huge surprise, the snake venom not only did not destroy the nerve growth-promoting effect of the tumor extract, but rather turned out to be an extremely rich source of the factor.[193] This serendipitous observation allowed them

to use snake venom to purify *nerve growth factor* (*NGF*), a protein that, when injected in chick embryos, induced overgrowth of sensory and sympathetic ganglia and nerve fibers.[194] Despite the dramatic growth-promoting activity of purified NGF, its unusual sources—tumors, snake venom, and later mouse salivary glands— left the question about

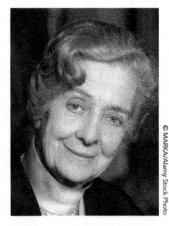

Rita Levi-Montalcini

the physiological relevance of NGF. To address this question, Cohen and Levi-Montalcini prepared an antiserum against purified NGF and injected it into newborn mice and several other species. The treatment resulted in the almost complete destruction of the sympathetic nervous system (*immunosympathectomy*).[195] Such results proved conclusively that the endogenous NGF is responsible for the survival of sympathetic neurons in vivo. The immunosympathectomy experiment also provided a technical and conceptual breakthrough in the quest to validate the function of biological molecules.[196]

[185] Hamburger, V. 1934. *J. Exp. Zool.* 68: 449–494.
[186] Levi-Montalcini, R., and Levi, G. 1942. *Arch. Biol. (Liege)* 53: 537–545.
[187] Levi-Montalcini, R., and Levi, G. 1943. *Arch. Biol. (Liege)* 54: 189–206.
[188] Hamburger, V., and Levi-Montalcini, R. 1949. *J. Exp. Zool.* 111: 457–501.
[189] Levi-Montalcini, R. 1952. *Ann. NY Acad. Sci.* 55: 330–344.
[190] Levi-Montalcini., R., and Hamburger, V. 1953. *J. Exp. Zool.* 123: 233–287.
[191] Levi-Montalcini, R., Meyer, H., and Hamburger, V. 1954. *Cancer Res.* 14: 49–57.
[192] Cohen, S., Levi-Montalcini, R., and Hamburger, V. 1954. *Proc. Natl. Acad. Sci. USA* 40: 1014–1018.
[193] Cohen, S., and Levi-Montalcini, R. 1956. *Proc. Natl. Acad. Sci. USA* 42: 571–574.
[194] Levi-Montalcini, R., and Cohen, S. 1956. *Proc. Natl. Acad. Sci. USA* 42: 695–699.
[195] Levi-Montalcini, R., and Booker, B. 1960. *Proc. Natl. Acad. Sci. USA* 46: 384–391.
[196] Cattaneo, A. 2013. *Proc. Natl. Acad. Sci. USA* 110: 4877.

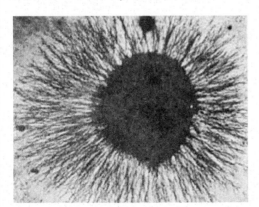

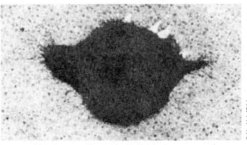

The NGF "halo." Chick embryo sensory ganglion cultured with a purified preparation of nerve growth factor (left) and with control medium (right).

prosecutions by fascism during World War II, and has been beautifully narrated by Rita Levi-Montalcini in her autobiography.[197]

NGF is a homodimer that interacts with two distinct receptors, the so-called p75NTR,[198] shared by all members of the neurotrophin family (see later in this paragraph), and tropomyosin-related kinase A (TrkA), a tyrosine kinase receptor.[199,200] The receptor p75NTR does not contain a cytoplasmic catalytic motif and activates distinct intracellular signaling pathways. The NGF homodimer induces TrkA dimerization and trans-autophosphorylation, followed by activation of intracellular signaling cascades and receptor internalization. p75NTR is a co-receptor for TrkA, increasing its affinity for NGF and enhancing its specificity against other neurotrophins.[201] The formation of a trimolecular signaling complex between NGF, TrkA, and p75NTR at the plasma membrane has been proposed, but its demonstration is currently debated.[202–204]

NGF is released in limiting amounts by the target tissue so that axons innervating the target compete for it. NGF is taken up and retrogradely transported via the axon to the cell body,[205,206] ultimately influencing transcriptional events in the nucleus. When sympathetic neurons are grown in three-compartment culture chambers (Figure 27.31), the central compartment in which the neurons are placed must initially contain NGF for the cells to survive (see Figure 27.31A).[207] However, after neurites have reached the side compartments, NGF can be removed from the central compartment and the cells will remain alive, so long as the side compartments contain NGF (not shown). Removal of NGF from one side compartment causes neurites on that side to degenerate (see Figure 27.31B). These trophic effects of NGF are mediated by signals evoked in growing terminals that activate the CREB transcription factor in the nucleus. Considerable evidence supports the view that *signaling endosomes* that contain internalized NGF–TrkA complexes are essential carriers of retrograde NGF signals to the nucleus,[206,208] but retrograde signaling supporting neuronal survival, without retrograde transport of NGF, has been suggested to act in parallel.[209] Intriguingly, in presynaptic terminals of sympathetic neurons NGF induces local translation of the transcription factor CREB, which is then retrogradely transported to the nucleus, where it induces survival.[210]

NGF-mediated interactions through p75NTR and Trk receptors frequently have opposing consequences. For example, NGF activation of TrkA receptors usually promotes neuronal survival and differentiation, while engagement of p75NTR often promotes cell death by apoptosis. In the developing chick retina, endogenous NGF induces via p75NTR

[197] Levi-Montalcini, R. 1989. *In Praise of Imperfection.* Sloan Foundation Science Series.

[198] Chao, M. V. et al. 1986. *Science* 232: 518-521.

[199] Kaplan, D. R. et al. 1991. *Science* 252: 554-558.

[200] Klein, R. et al. 1991. *Cell* 65: 189-197.

[201] Chao, M. V. 2003. *Nat. Rev. Neurosci.* 4: 299-309.

[202] Barker, P. A. 2007. *Neuron* 53: 1-4.

[203] Marchetti, L. et al. 2019. *Proc. Natl. Acad. Sci. USA.* doi: 10.1073/pnas.1902790116.

[204] Chao, M. V. 2019. *Proc. Natl. Acad. Sci. USA.* doi: 10.1073/pnas.1914583116.

[205] Hendry, I. A. et al. 1974. *Brain Res.* 68: 103-121.

[206] Howe, C. L., and .Mobley, W. C. 2005. *Curr. Opin. Neurobiol.* 15: 40-48.

[207] Campenot, R. B. 1977. *Proc. Natl. Acad. Sci. USA* 74: 4516-4519.

[208] Zweifel, L. S., Kuruvilla, R., and Ginty, D. D. 2005. *Nat. Rev. Neurosci.* 6: 615-625.

[209] MacInnis, B. L., and Campenot, R. B. 2002. *Science* 295: 1536-1539.

[210] Cox, J. J. et al. 2008. *Nat. Cell Biol.* 10: 149-59.

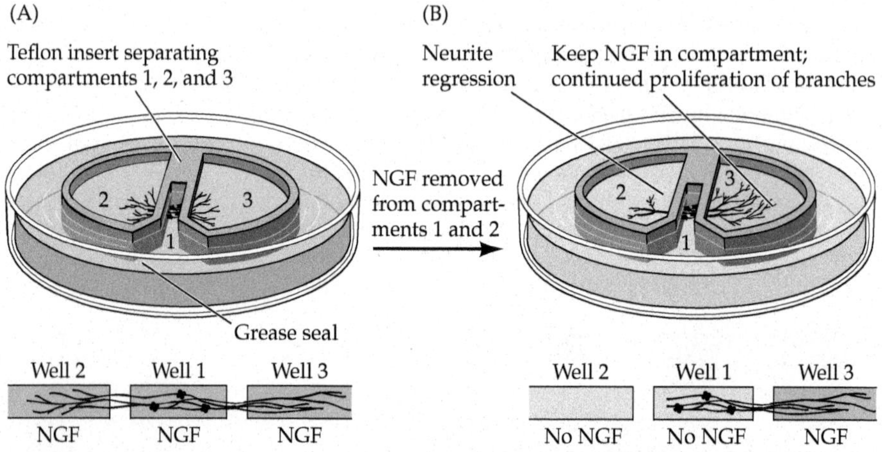

FIGURE 27.31 Nerve Growth Factor (NGF) and the Survival of Axon Branches from sympathetic ganglion cells grown in cell culture. (A) Neurons dissociated from neonatal sympathetic ganglia plated in the central compartment send neurites under a Teflon divider and into the adjacent compartments; all compartments contain NGF. (B) After initial outgrowth has occurred, removal of NGF from compartment 1 and 2 causes the neurites entering compartment 2 to degenerate, while those in compartment 3, containing NGF, remain. On the other hand, removal of NGF only from compartment 1 for 20 days has no effect, as neurons are maintained by NGF transported retrogradely from their terminals in the side compartments (not shown) (After R. B. Campenot, 1982. *Dev. Biol.* 93: 1-12.)

the developmentally regulated cell death of retinal ganglion cells.[211] This might provide a means to refine the correct target innervation during development.

NGF is translated as a longer polypeptide (pro-NGF) that is subsequently cleaved to the mature form. In the brain, pro-NGF is the predominant form. While mature NGF promotes cell survival and differentiation, pro-NGF usually promotes apoptosis.[212,213] The ratio of TrkA and p75 receptors, as well as that of NGF and pro-NGF, is therefore important in dictating the outcome of neurotrophin signaling.

NGF actions are not unique to the peripheral nervous system. In the brain, NGF is a survival factor for the cholinergic neurons in the basal forebrain.[214] Their axons innervate the cerebral cortex and hippocampus. Much research is in progress to assess defects in NGF signaling that might give rise to neurodegeneration[215,216] such as Alzheimer's disease, in which death of basal forebrain cholinergic neurons typically occurs. Thus, disruption of the homeostatic balance between NGF and pro-NGF in the adult brain can lead to neurodegeneration.[215,216] In the CNS, microglial cells, too, are a target of NGF,[217] that exerts an anti-inflammatory action on these cells. Altogether, this provides a strong rationale for ongoing efforts at developing NGF-based therapies for neurodegenerative diseases.[218]

The discovery of NGF prompted the search for other neurotrophic factors. One notable example is provided by brain-derived neurotrophic factor (BDNF), which was purified by Barde and Thoenen[219] as a survival factor for neuronal populations not responsive to NGF, such as nodose ganglia and trigeminal mesencephalic sensory neurons. BDNF has a high degree of sequence and structural homology with NGF. Together, NGF and BDNF defined a protein family called neurotrophins. Other members of the family are NT-3, NT-4/5, and NT-6 (in fish). Different neurotrophins bind distinct members of the Trk family (for instance, NGF binds TrkA, and BDNF binds TrkB), while all neurotrophins bind the shared p75NTR.[201,220] In the adult nervous system, BDNF is a key effector of synaptic plasticity (see Chapter 17).

In addition to the neurotrophins, several other neurotrophic factors have been identified. They include insulin-like growth factors (IGF-1 and IGF-2), ciliary neurotrophic factor (CNTF), cholinergic differentiation factor (CDF, also called leukemia inhibitory factor (LIF)), glial cell line-derived neurotrophic factor (GDNF).

Formation of Connections

Establishment of the Retinotectal Map

Even after the growth cones have guided axons to their broad destinations, the problem of matching each axon with its particular target cells remains. The growth of retinal ganglion cell axons to their targets provides a good example. Roger Sperry proposed the chemoaffinity hypothesis to explain the topographic projections of retinal axons onto the optic tectum, postulating the existence of *cytochemical tags* expressed in corresponding gradients on both the retina and the tectum.[221] This hypothesis prompted the search for molecules expressed in gradients along either the anteroposterior or dorsoventral axis of the retina and the tectum.

During development, axons from ganglion cells in the temporal part of the chick retina grow to innervate neurons in the anterior part of the tectum, while those arising from nasal retina innervate posterior neurons (Figure 27.32A). Experiments by Bonhoeffer and his colleagues demonstrated that axons sort out their territories through repulsive interactions that prevent growth cones of temporal axons from penetrating into the posterior tectum.[222,223] Retinal ganglion cells in culture were allowed to grow into parallel lanes whose surfaces were coated with membranes purified from either the anterior or the posterior tectum. Axons from neurons in the nasal retina grew equally well on both membranes (Figure 27.32B). Temporal axons, however, preferred to grow on lanes coated with anterior membranes (Figure 27.32C). However, when posterior membranes were denatured by heat treatment, temporal axons no longer showed any preference (Figure 27.32D). Thus, their preference for the anterior lanes was not due to attraction by the anterior membranes, but rather to repulsion by the posterior membrane. Curiously, when not offered a choice of membranes, retinal axons elongated rapidly on either substrate.

The molecules responsible for this repulsive interaction in the optic tectum (or superior colliculus in mammals) are members of a family of receptor tyrosine kinases

[211] Frade, J. M., Rodriguez-Tebar, A., and Barde, Y. A. 1996. *Nature* 383: 166-168.

[212] Lee, R. et al. 2001. *Science* 294: 1945-1948.

[213] Nykjaer, A. et al. 2004. *Nature* 427: 843-848.

[214] Hefti, F. 1986. *J. Neurosci.* 6: 2155-2162.

[215] Capsoni, S. et al. 2010. *Proc. Natl. Acad. Sci. USA* 107: 12299-12304.

[216] Iulita, M. F., and Cuello, A. C. 2014. *Trends Pharmacol. Sci.* 35: 338-348.

[217] Rizzi, C. et al. 2018. *Glia* doi: 10.1002/glia.23312.

[218] Cattaneo, A. and Capsoni, S. 2018. *Pharmacol. Res.* doi.org/10.1016/j.phrs.2018.10.028.

[219] Barde, Y. A. et al. 1982 *EMBO J.* 1: 549-553.

[220] Huamg, E. J. and Reichardt, L. F. 2001 *Annu. Rev. Neurosci.* 246: 77-136.

[221] Sperry, R. 1963. *Proc. Natl. Acad. Sci. USA* 50: 703-710.

[222] Walter, J. et al. 1987. *Development* 101: 685-696.

[223] Walter, J., Henke-Fahle, S., and Bonhoeffer, F. 1987. *Development* 101: 909-913.

(A)

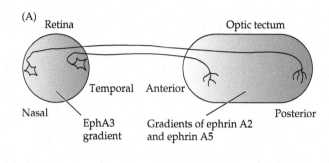

(B) Nasal axons

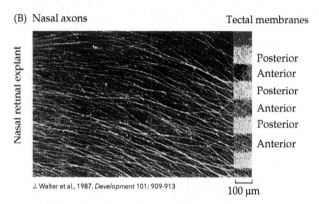

(C) Temporal axons

(D) Temporal axons

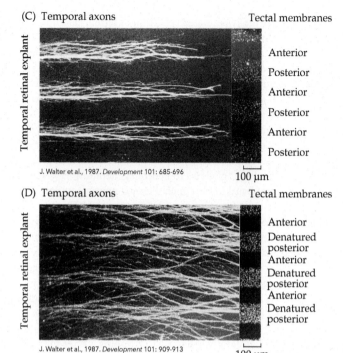

FIGURE 27.32 Repulsive Interactions in Innervation of the optic tectum in the chick. (A) Ganglion cells in the nasal retina innervate neurons in the posterior tectum; ganglion cells in the temporal retina innervate neurons in the anterior tectum. There is a nasotemporal gradient of the EphA3 receptor tyrosine kinase in retinal ganglion cells and anteroposterior gradients of the Eph receptor ligands ephrin A2 and ephrin A5 in the tectum. Axons of temporal ganglion cells are prevented from entering the posterior tectum by the repulsive interaction of Eph receptors and ligands. (B) In cell culture, axons from neurons in the nasal retina grow equally well on lanes coated with membranes isolated from anterior or posterior tectum. (C) Axons from neurons in the temporal retina prefer to grow on anterior membranes. (D) Axons from temporal retina grow equally well on intact anterior membranes and denatured posterior membranes, indicating that normally they are repelled by heat-sensitive components of the posterior membranes.

(known as Eph kinases) and their ligands (called ephrins).[224] Ephrin A2 and ephrin A5 are expressed in the tectum when retinotectal connections are being formed, and their concentration increases in a graded manner from anterior to posterior. The EphA3 receptor is expressed on retinal axons in a corresponding nasotemporal gradient. When incorporated into lipid vesicles and added to the medium in which temporal retinal axons are growing, ephrins A2 and A5 cause the growth cones to detach from the substrate and retract.[225]

The other axis of the topographic projection maps the dorsoventral positions in the retina to mediolateral positions in the tectum. Here, patterning is achieved by a different family of ligands and receptors, the ephrin B ligands and EphB kinase receptors. The molecular logic that underlies the dorsoventral and mediolateral mapping is more complex.[226]

Synapse Formation

Synapse formation starts after a growth cone contacts its postsynaptic target and undergoes differentiation from a migratory structure to a presynaptic terminal. Likewise, on growth cone contact, the postsynaptic target neuron begins to differentiate, generating the specialized postsynaptic region of the membrane.

The vertebrate skeletal neuromuscular junction provides a favorable preparation for studying the mechanisms of synapse formation. The first steps in synapse formation occur rapidly. As the growth cone of a motor axon approaches a myotube (i.e., an immature muscle fiber), depolarizing potentials arise due to the release of ACh from the growth cone (Figure 27.33).[227] Upon contact, the rate of spontaneous release of quanta of ACh rapidly increases, as does the size of the synaptic potential evoked by stimulating the axon. Thus, within minutes a functional synaptic connection is established. In Chapter 29 we give an account of **agrin**, which is released from the motor nerve axon as it

[224] Feldheim, D. A., and O'Leary, D. D. 2010. *Cold Spring Harb. Perspect. Biol.* 2: a001768.

[225] Cox, E. C. et al. 1990. *Neuron* 4: 31-37.

[226] Pittman, A., and Chien, C. B. 2002 *Neuron* 35: 409-411.

[227] Evers, J. et al. 1989. *J. Neurosci.* 9: 1523-1539.

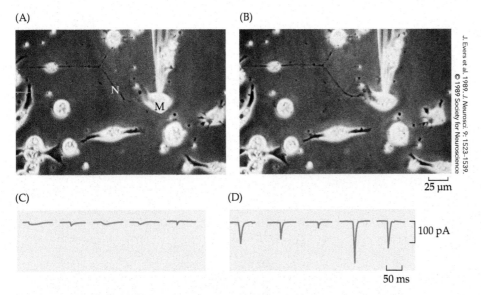

J. Evers et al. 1989. J. Neurosci. 9: 1523-1539. © 1989 Society for Neuroscience

FIGURE 27.33 Rapid Formation of Functional Synaptic Connections between motor axons and muscle cells. (A,B) Phase-contrast photographs of a growing neurite (N) and a spindle-shaped myocyte (M) in a *Xenopus* neuron-muscle cell culture at the beginning (A) and end (B) of electrical recording. (C,D) Whole-cell patch clamp records from the myocyte. Spontaneous synaptic currents can be recorded within 1 minute of contact (C) and have increased in strength several-fold by 18 minutes (D). (After J. Evers et al. 1989. *J. Neurosci.* 9: 1523-1539. © 1989 Society for Neuroscience.)

approaches the muscle fiber. Agrin causes postsynaptic structures to be formed and ACh receptors to accumulate at the motor end plate.[228]

In the CNS, two families of interacting cell adhesion transmembrane proteins, **neuroligins** and **neurexins**, have emerged as key players in the functional development of CNS synapses.[229,230] Neuroligins are located in the postsynaptic membrane and interact trans-synaptically with their presynaptic neurexin binding partners to mediate synapse formation and function.[231]

Neuroligins presented to neurons by expression in co-cultured non-neuronal cells, or linked to beads, induce the formation of presynaptic specializations in the neurons, and similar presentation of neurexins (which share extracellular domains similar to those of agrin) induce the formation of postsynaptic specializations, an assay referred to as *artificial synapse formation.*

Neuroligins are expressed from four genes (*Nlgn1–4*), with Nlgn1 expressed exclusively at excitatory synapses, Nlgn2 at inhibitory synapses, and Nlgn3 at both excitatory and inhibitory synapses. Thus, the spatial location of inhibitory or excitatory synapses on the dendritic tree of a pyramidal neuron might be determined also by the subcellular distribution of the appropriate neuroligin on the postsynaptic membrane.

The mammalian genome harbors three neurexin genes, each of which directs transcription of α- and β-neurexins from independent promoters. Extensive alternative splicing generates thousands of neurexin isoforms.[232] Conceptually, this enormous diversity could specify a combinatorial "code" of neuroligin–neurexin trans-synaptic interacting pairs specifying circuit formation during development.[231,232]

Pruning and the Removal of Polyneuronal Innervation

Once synapses have formed and the population of neurons innervating a target has been restricted through cell death, axons of surviving neurons compete with one another for synaptic territory. This competition typically results in the loss of some of the terminal branches and synapses made initially—a process referred to as **pruning**.[233] Pruning ensures appropriate and complete innervation of a target and, in some cases, also provides a mechanism for correcting mistakes.

A clear example of competitive pruning occurs in developing skeletal muscle. In the adult, each motor neuron innervates a group of up to 300 muscle fibers, forming a motor

228 Reist, N. E., Werle, M. J., and McMahan, U. J. 1992. *Neuron* 8: 865-868.

229 Craig, A. M., and Kang, Y. 2007. *Curr. Opin. Neurobiol.* 17: 43-52.

230 Sudhof, T. 2008. *Nature* 455: 903-911.

231 Sudhof, T. 2017. *Cell* 171: 745.

232 Schreiner, D. et al. 2014. *Neuron* 84: 386.

233 Luo, L., and O'Leary, D. D. 2005. *Annu. Rev. Neurosci.* 28: 127-156.

FIGURE 27.34 Polyneuronal Innervation and Its Elimination at the vertebrate skeletal neuromuscular junction. (A) During embryonic development, motor axons branch to innervate many muscle fibers, and each muscle fiber is innervated by several motor axons (polyneuronal innervation). (B) Fluorescence micrograph of a neuromuscular junction of an E18 mouse showing the distribution of terminals of two axons, each labeled with a lipophilic probe (DiI in red, DiA in green). During the period of polyneuronal innervation, the terminal arbors of all motor axons innervating a particular muscle fiber interdigitate at a single synaptic site. (C) After birth, polyneuronal innervation is eliminated as axon branches retract, leaving each muscle fiber innervated by a single motor axon. (D) Fluorescence micrograph of a mouse neuromuscular junction during the period of removal of polyneuronal innervation. Two axons innervating the junction were labeled as in (B). All terminals of one axon (green) have been eliminated, and the axon is being withdrawn.

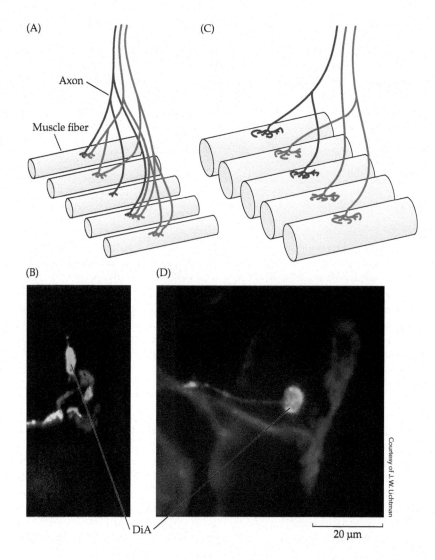

unit (see Chapter 24), but each muscle fiber is innervated by only one axon. In developing muscle, however, motor neurons branch extensively so that each muscle fiber comes to be innervated by axons from several motor neurons (Figure 27.34)—a phenomenon called **polyneuronal innervation**.[234,235] On each developing muscle fiber, the synaptic endings of multiple axons are interspersed at a single site and are juxtaposed to aggregates of ACh receptors and other components of the postsynaptic apparatus. As development progresses, axon branches are eliminated until the adult pattern is formed. This process does not involve neuronal cell death (which occurs at an earlier developmental stage), only a reduction in the number of muscle fibers innervated by each motor neuron.

The pruning of exuberant synaptic connections during CNS development might also involve microglial cells.[236]

Neuronal Activity and Synapse Elimination

Neuronal activity plays a role in synapse elimination, influencing both the rate and outcome of the competition between axon terminals. Stimulation of the nerve to a muscle with 100-Hz bursts via implanted electrodes increases the rate of synapse elimination, whereas the same number of stimuli presented continuously at 1 Hz does not.[237] If activity is reduced, by applying tetrodotoxin a cuff around the nerve to block action potentials or by inhibiting synaptic transmission, synapse elimination is slowed.[238] In muscles that receive input from axons that run in two different nerves, one can block impulses in one nerve and not the other.[239] In such cases, inactive axons are at a competitive disadvantage, as axons

[234] Redfern, P. A. 1970. *J. Physiol.* 209: 701–709.

[235] Brown, M. C., Jansen, J. K., and Van Essen, D. 1976. *J. Physiol.* 261: 387–422.

[236] Thion, M.S. et al. 2018. *Science* 362: 185–189.

[237] Thompson, W. 1983. *Nature* 302: 614–616.

[238] Brown, M. C., Hopkins, W. G., and Keynes, R. J. 1982. *J. Physiol.* 329: 439–450.

[239] Ribchester, R. R., and Taxt, T. 1983. *J. Physiol.* 344: 89–111.

in the blocked nerve innervate smaller than normal motor units (i.e., they innervate fewer muscle fibers) and those in the active nerve innervate more fibers than usual.

Activity-dependent competition extends to the level of branches of a single motor axon.[240] If a small region of an adult junction is inactivated by focal application of α-bungarotoxin, the inactive region of the junction is eliminated. If the entire junction is silenced, no elimination occurs.

Similar competition for synaptic targets occurs during the development of CNS pathways. One example is the formation of the ocular dominance columns in visual cortex (see Chapter 28).

What Makes Us Human: The Development of the Human Brain

The cerebral cortex underwent a considerable increase in size and complexity over the last millions of years of hominid evolution.[241,242] One significant developmental aspect that distinguishes humans is the retention of fetal neuronal growth rate after birth and the extension of postnatal brain development for several years. A fivefold increase in brain weight accompanies this postnatal development, during which approximately 250,000 neurons per minute are added and the number of synapses increases at the astronomical rate of approximately 0.5 million synapses per second.[243] Human cortex is highly folded (gyrencephalic) compared with rodent brain, which completely lacks folds (lissencephalic).

Attention has focused on human-specific mechanisms of cortical neurogenesis, such as expansion of cortical progenitors and higher neuronal production. In humans, radial glial cells go through an increased number of divisions compared with nonhuman-primates or rodents and a specific class of progenitors, the outer radial glia, is expanded.

Several human- and hominid-specific gene duplications have been found, whereby an ancestral gene is duplicated in the genome, resulting in two related paralogous genes.[244,245] Among these, one family of paralogs of *NOTCH2* genes (named *NOTCH2NL*), specifically expressed in radial glial cells, was shown to promote self-renewal of human radial glia, ultimately increasing neuronal output.[244,245]

A transcriptomic study identified the human-specific *ARHGAP11B* gene, expressed specifically in human radial glial cells (and not in mature cortical neurons).[246] When the *ARHGAP11B* gene is electroporated in the developing mouse cortex (which is normally lissencephalic), it promotes neural progenitor generation and self-renewal and increases cortical plate area, inducing gyrification, which mice normally lack.[246]

The recent evolutionary emergence of *NOTCH2NL* and *ARHGAP11B* gene duplications makes them attractive candidates as players in human brain evolution, by facilitating an extended period of neurogenesis and a larger neuronal output during development.

Whether the increased proliferative potential of neural progenitors is directly responsible for the expansion of the human cerebral cortex and for its convoluted organization remains, however, difficult to test, because of the inaccessible nature of the developing human cortex.

Recent advances in human pluripotent stem cell technology (see Box 27.1) and 3D organoid culture systems (Box 27.3) have opened new avenues to address these questions and to investigate human cortical development in vitro.[247,248]

General Considerations of Neural Specificity and Development

Considerable progress has been made in understanding how nerve cells acquire their identity, differentiate, find their targets, and establish synaptic contacts. However, when one contemplates the number and specificity of the fate decisions that must be made and connections that must be formed when wiring up the nervous system, the challenges seem daunting. A commonplace analogy may be encouraging. Let us assume that we are ignorant about the workings and design of the postal system. A chapter from a book on the nervous system, without its illustrations, is posted in Trieste, Italy, and addressed to Sunderland, Massachusetts, USA, where it arrives a few days later. How does it get there? The writer

[240] Balice-Gordon, R. J., and Lichtman, J. W. 1994. *Nature* 372: 519–524.

[241] Lui et al. 2011. *Cell* 146: 18.

[242] Sousa, A. M. M. et al. 2017. *Cell* 170: 226–247.

[243] Changeux, J. P. 2017. *Trends Cog. Sci.* doi: 10.1016/j.tics.2017.01.004.

[244] Fiddes et al. 2018. *Cell* 173: 1356.

[245] Suzuki et al. 2018. *Cell* 173: 1370.

[246] Florio, M. et al. 2015. *Science* 347: 1465–1470.

[247] Suzuki, I. K., and Vanderhaeghen, P. 2015. *Development* 142: 3138–3150.

[248] Van den Ameele, J. et al. 2014. *Trends Neurosci.* 37: 334–342.

BOX 27.3 3D Brain Organoids: A Brain in a Dish?

Induced pluripotent stem cells (iPSCs) (see Box 27.1) can be used to investigate cell-autonomous mechanisms of human development and disease at the cellular level, but they are not suitable to study the cell-to-cell signals in a developing brain. Following the pioneering work by Yoshiki Sasai, researchers have now been able to grow rudimentary brain regions from pluripotent stem cells, called brain 3D organoids, exploiting a remarkable self-organizing capacity of embryonic stem cells (ESCs) when grown in a "multicellular society."[249] (Figure A).

Building on the default model of neural induction, Sasai's team developed a three-dimensional culture system in which aggregates of mouse and human ESCs spontaneously self-organized to recapitulate a three-dimensional architecture, forming apicobasally polarized cortical tissue, with neuronal layering reminiscent of early cerebral cortical development.[250,251] These aggregates could be further patterned to different fates by the addition of morphogens. This was followed by the striking

(Continued)

(A) Blastocyst

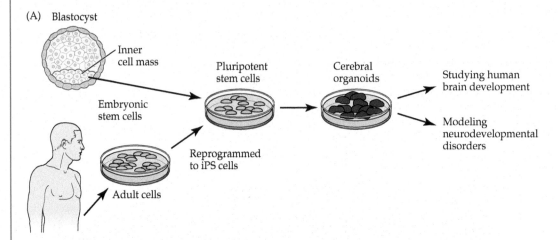

(B)

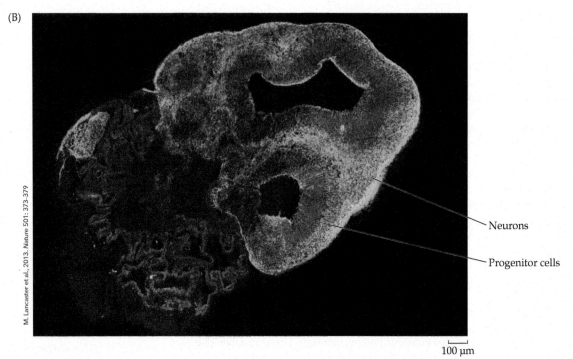

M. Lancaster et al., 2013. *Nature* 501: 373-379

100 μm

(A) Organoid generation from human pluripotent stem cells, either as embryonic stem (ES) cells or induced pluripotent stem (iPS) cells (see Box 27.1). (B) Image of an organoid, labeled for neurons (green) and progenitor cells (magenta).

The morphology of the upper-right region matches that of the cerebral cortex, and the region in the lower left has a similar morphology to that of the choroid plexus. (A after O. Brüstle, 2013. *Nature* 501: 319-320.)

| BOX **27.3** | 3D Brain Organoids: A Brain in a Dish? (continued) |

demonstration that mouse and human ESCs could be forced into making an eyecup in a dish, with a well-organized mouse or human retina (see Figure 1.16).[252,253] Current protocols to grow brain organoids involve an initial aggregation of mouse or human stem cells (ESCs or iPSCs), to form embryoid body aggregates, which are then placed into droplets of Matrigel (a matrix made from solubilized basement membrane) to provide a three-dimensional architecture, and then grown into a media-filled spinning bioreactor. The gentle movement of the growing organoid in this three-dimensional matrix serves to increase nutrient uptake. Cultures are exposed to a general neural induction, with brief periods of exposure to specific morphogens for region-specific patterning and growth factor stimulation, followed by an extended period in growth-factor-free medium to favor cell-cycle exit and differentiation. Different types of brain organoids can be obtained, depending on the conditions and the added patterning morphogens, to direct specific regional identites. Using minimalistic culture media, cerebral organoids with tissue architecture reminiscent of the human cerebral cortex have been generated[254] (Figure B). Cerebral organoids have been generated from iPSCs derived from patients affected by various developmental disorders.[254,255]

Human brain organoids are becoming powerful research tools to understand and mimic normal and abnormal human brain development and to address developmental questions that have been difficult or impossible to answer using traditional techniques. Moreover, the ability to generate "personalized" organoids from patient-specific iPSCs has opened new frontiers for disease modeling and drug discovery. Notwithstanding this potential, a key question that we should ask is to what extent organoids mimic the in vivo counterpart. Ultimately, brain organoids should not be taken as a system that reproduces comprehensively and faithfully the developing brain, but instead as a model for specific aspects of human brain development that would otherwise be difficult to investigate.

[249] Sasai, Y. 2013. *Cell Stem Cell* 12: 520.
[250] Eiraku, M. et al. 2008. *Cell Stem Cell* 3: 519-532.
[251] Mariani, J. and Vaccarino, F. M. 2019. *Cell Stem Cell* 24: 837.
[252] Eiraku, M. et al. 2011. *Nature* 472: 51-56.
[253] Nakano, T. et al., 2012. *Cell Stem Cell* 10: 771-785.
[254] Lancaster, M. et al. 2013. *Nature* 501: 373.
[255] Klaus, J. et al. 2019. *Nat. Med.* 25: 561-568.

knows only the closest mailbox and is unaware even of the post office in his district. The postal worker who empties the mailbox knows the post office; there the clerk who handles the mail may not know where Sunderland is but does know how to direct the package to the airport, and so on, to the right country, city, street, building, and eventually the correct person. If this were not enough, the illustrations that complement the chapter are posted separately from Berkeley and Baltimore to the same destination, where they arrive almost simultaneously with the chapter from Trieste. All the while, other mail is moving through the same mailboxes and post offices in different directions to different destinations.

The comforting feature of this analogy is that, although the problem seems altogether baffling at first sight, one can solve the postal puzzle by following the mail step by step to its destination. This would reveal some of the logic and design of postal organization (albeit without disclosing the identity of the designer). At any one step, only a limited number of instructions are followed and a limited number of mechanisms operate.

Some aspects of neural specificity may not be too different. A retinal ganglion cell sends its axon toward the back of the eye, where it makes a turn to enter the optic nerve together with fibers from other regions of the retina. The optic chiasm presents the next choice point, where the decision to enter the optic tract, leading either to the left or the right lateral geniculate nucleus, may be made based on local chemical signals. Within the lateral geniculate nucleus, retinal axons may arrange themselves and innervate their targets according to gradients of repulsive molecules. Axons of geniculate neurons likewise follow a fairly simple path to their targets in the cortex, stopping along the way to form transient connections with subplate neurons. Thus, the seemingly complex task of forming specific connections between retinal ganglion cells and neurons in the visual cortex can be broken down into a series of relatively simple, independent events, each of which shapes the next event. This general principle also applies to the even more complex question of how retinal ganglion cells, and all the many other types of neurons and non-neuronal cells, are generated in the proper numbers and places as the organism develops from the fertilized egg.

SUMMARY

- During development, cells acquire specific neuronal identities and establish orderly synaptic connections under the influence of intrinsic and extrinsic factors.

- Cell identity is the result of differential gene expression.

- The unique set of genes that each cell type expresses is determined by a combinatorial code of transcription factors.

- Cell-to-cell communication by local and longer-range signaling plays a crucial role in development.

- During vertebrate neural induction, BMP inhibitor proteins diffuse from the Spemann organizer, and a default neural developmental program can unfold.

- A class of master regulator genes, known as proneural genes, regulates the formation of neuroblasts, by a lateral inhibition process regulated by the Notch-Delta neurogenic signaling.

- The edges of the neural plate fold to form a closed neural tube.

- In the vertebrate CNS, the fates of developing neurons are specified according to anteroposterior position and dorsoventral position.

- Hox genes determine anteroposterior identity in the hindbrain.

- Dorsoventral neural fates in the spinal cord are induced by opposing gradients of BMP and Sonic hedgehog.

- Cells divide rapidly at the ventricular surface of the neural tube neuroepithelium, which undergoes a thickness expansion in a multilayered configuration.

- When cortical neurogenesis begins, neuroepithelial stem cells acquire features associated with glial cells and generate the radial glial cells.

- Radial glial cells carry out a dual function: (1) They provide a mechanical scaffolding, guiding radial migration of neural progenitor cells, and (2) they constitute a major neural stem cell pool for the brain.

- In mammalian cerebral cortex, development proceeds in an inside-out fashion. Neurons of the deepest cortical layers are born first.

- The regional specification of cortical areas is initiated by gradients of diffusible morphogens that establish expression domains of key transcription factors.

- Neural stem cells in specialized niches of the CNS of adult birds and mammals (including humans) continually produce new neurons.

- Lineage progression during cortical development is the result of a progressive competence-restriction mechanism. Gliogenesis consistently occurs after neurogenesis.

- Neural crest cells migrate away from the neural tube to form the peripheral nervous system, pigment cells, and bones of the head. The phenotype adopted by neural crest cells is determined by signals from the environment.

- Growing axons tipped with growth cones explore the environment during navigation toward their target. Growth cone navigation is controlled by short- and long-range attractive and repulsive cues.

- Local protein synthesis of axonally transported mRNAs allows rapid turning responses of growing axons.

- When a motoneuron growth cone contacts a muscle cell, functional synaptic transmission is established within minutes.

- Axonal projections made during development are often more extensive than those in the adult.

- Neurons rely on target-derived trophic factors for survival and differentiation.

- Programmed neuronal death (apoptosis) is a common feature of neural development and is regulated by competition for trophic substances.

- The evolution of the human brain has been linked to the expansion of cortical progenitors (such as outer radial glia) and to a higher neuronal production.

- Recent advances in human induced pluripotent stem cell technologies and in 3D organoid culture systems have opened new avenues to investigate human brain development in vitro.

Suggested Reading

General Reviews

Allan, D. W., and Thor, S. 2015. Transcriptional selectors, masters and combinatorial codes: regulatory principles of neural subtype specification. *WIREs Dev. Biol.* 4: 505–528. doi: 10.1002/wdev.191.

Bergmann, O., Spalding, K. L., and Frisén, J. 2015. Adult neurogenesis in humans *Cold Spring Harb. Perspect. Biol.* 7: a018994. doi: 10.1101/cshperspect.a018994.

Bertrand, N., Castro, D. S., and Guillemot, F. 2002. Proneural genes and the specification of neural cell types *Nat. Rev. Neurosci.* 3: 517–530.

Bond, A. M., Ming, G. L., and Song, H. 2015. Adult mammalian neural stem cells and neurogenesis: five decades later. *Cell Stem Cell* 17: 385.

Briscoe, J. 2000. A homeodomain protein code specifies progenitor cell identity and neuronal fate in the ventral neural tube. *Cell* 101: 435–445.

Buss, R. R., Sun, W., and Oppenheim, R. W. 2006. Adaptive roles of programmed cell death during nervous system development. *Annu. Rev. Neurosci.* 29: 1–35.

Cadwell, C. R. et al. 2019. Development and arealization of the cerebral cortex. *Neuron* 103: 980–1004.

Chao, M. V. 2003. Neurotrophins and their receptors: A convergence point for many signaling pathways. *Nat. Rev. Neurosci.* 4: 299–309. doi: 10.1038/nrn1078.

Crispino, M., Chun, J. T., Cefaliello, C., et al. 2013. Local gene expression in nerve endings. *Dev. Neurobiol.* 74: 279–291. doi: 10.1002/dneu.22109.

Custo Greig, L. F., Woodworth, M. B., Galazo, M. J., et al. 2013. Molecular logic of neocortical projection neuron specification, development and diversity. *Nat. Rev. Neurosci.* 14: 755–769.

Dimou, L., and Goetz, M. 2014. Glial cells as progenitors and stem cells: new roles in the healthy and diseased brain. *Physiol. Rev.* 94: 709–737.

Fishell, G. and Heintz, N. 2013. The neuron identity problem: form meets function. *Neuron* 80: 602–612.

Gehring, W. J., Kloter, U., and Suga, H. 2009. Evolution of the *Hox* gene complex from an evolutionary ground state. *Curr. Top. Dev. Biol.* 88: 35–61.

Gilbert, S. F. and Barresi, M. J. F. 2016. *Developmental Biology*, 11th Ed. Oxford University Press/Sinauer, Sunderland, MA.

Goncalves, J. T., Schafer, S. T., and Gage, F. H. 2016. Adult neurogenesis in the hippocampus: from stem cells to behavior *Cell* 167: 897–914.

Gurdon, J. 2012. The egg and the nucleus: a battle for supremacy (Nobel Lecture). *Development* 140: 2449–2456.

Gurdon, J. B., and Melton, D. A. 2008. Nuclear reprogramming in cells. *Science* 322: 1811–1815.

Hochedlinger, K., and Jaenisch, R. 2015. Induced pluripotency and epigenetic reprogramming *Cold Spring Harb. Perspect. Biol.* A019448.

Jessel, T. M. 2000. Neuronal specification in the spinal cord: inductive signal and transcriptional codes. *Nat. Rev. Genet.* 1: 20–29.

Kiecker, C., and Lumsden, A. 2005. Compartments and their boundaries in vertebrate brain development. *Nat. Rev. Neurosci.* 6: 553–564.

Kriegstein, A., and Alvarez-Buylia, A. 2009. The glial nature of embryonic and adult neural stem cells. *Annu. Rev. Neurosci.* 32: 149–84.

Le Douarin, N. M. 2008. Developmental patterning deciphered in avian chimeras. *Dev. Growth Differ.* 50(Suppl. 1): S11–28.

Levi-Montalcini, R. 1982. Developmental neurobiology and the natural history of nerve growth factor. *Annu. Rev. Neurosci.* 5: 341–362.

Levi-Montalcini, R. 1987 The Nerve Growth Factor thirty-five years later. Nobel Lecture) *Science* 237: 1154–62.

Lin, A. C., and Holt, C. E. 2007. Local translation and directional steering in axons. EMBO J. 26: 3729–3736.

Lodato, S. and Arlotta, P. 2015. Generating neuronal diversity in the mammalian cerebral cortex. *Annu. Rev. Cell Dev. Biol.* 31: 11.1–11.22.

Lowery, L. A., and Van Vactor, D. 2009. The trip of the tip: understanding the growth cone machinery. *Nat. Rev. Mol. Cell Biol.* 10: 332–343.

Mallo, M. and Alonso, C. R. 2013. The regulation of Hox gene expression during animal development. *Development* 140: 3951–3963.

Marin, O. 2013. Cellular and molecular mechanisms controlling the migration of neocortical interneurons. *Eur. J. Neurosci.* 38: 2019–2029.

Nikolopoulou, E., Galea, G. L., Rolo, A., Greene, N. D. E., and Copp, A. J. 2017. Neural tube closure: cellular, molecular and biomechanical mechanisms. *Development* 144: 552–566. doi: 10.1242/dev.145904.

Philippidou, P., and Dasen, J. S. 2013. Hox genes: Choreographers in neural development, architects of circuit organization. *Neuron* 80: 12–34.

Rakic, P. 2009. Evolution of the neocortex: a perspective from developmental biology. *Nat. Rev. Neurosci.* 10: 724–735.

Reichardt, L. 2006. Neurotrophin-regulated signalling pathways. *Phil. Trans. R. Soc. Lond. B Biol.* 36: 1545–1564.

Sidhaye, J., and Knoblich, J. A. 2020 Brain organoids: an ensemble of bioassays to investigate human neurodevelopment and disease. *Cell Death and Diff.* https://doi.org/10.1038/s41418-020-0566-4.

Spitzer, N. C. 2017. Neurotransmitter switching in the developing and adult brain. *Ann. Rev. Neurosci.* https://doi.org/10.1146/annurev-neuro-072116-031204.

Stern, C. D. 2005. Neural induction: old problem, new findings, yet more questions. *Development* 132: 2007–2021.

Suzuki, I. K., and Vanderhaeghen, P. 2015. Is this a brain which I see before me? Modeling human neural development with pluripotent stem cells. *Development* 142: 3138–3150.

Szabó, A., and Mayor, R. 2018. Mechanisms of neural crest migration. *Ann. Rev. Genetics* 52: 43–63.

Thion, M. S., Ginhoux, F., and Garel, S. 2018. Microglia and early brain development: An intimate journey, *Science* 362: 185–189. doi: 10.1126/science.aat0474.

van den Ameele, J., Tiberi, L., Vanderhaeghen, P., and Espuny-Camacho, I. 2014. Thinking out of the dish: what to learn about cortical development using pluripotent stem cells. *Trends Neurosci.* 37: 334–342.

Original Papers

Adar, E., Nottebohm, F., and Barnea, A. 2008. The relationship between nature of social change, age, and position of new neurons and their survival in adult zebra finch brain. *J. Neurosci.* 28: 5394–5400.

Baggiolini, A. et al. 2015. Premigratory and migratory neural crest cells are multipotent in vivo. *Cell Stem Cell* 16: 314–322.

Briscoe, J., Pierani, A., Jessell, T. M., and Ericson, J. 2000. A homeodomain protein code specifies progenitor cell identity and neuronal fate in the ventral neural tube. *Cell* 101: 435–445.

Brittis, P. A., Lu, Q., and Flanagan, J. G. 2002. Axonal protein synthesis provides a mechanism for localized regulation at an intermediate target. *Cell* 110: 223–235.

Campenot, R. B. 2009. NGF uptake and retrograde signaling mechanisms in sympathetic neurons in compartmented cultures. *Results Probl. Cell. Differ.* 48: 141–158.

Capsoni, S., Ugolini, G., Comparini, A., Ruberti, F., Berardi, N., and Cattaneo, A. 2000. Alzheimer-like neurodegeneration in aged antinerve growth factor transgenic mice. *Proc. Natl. Acad. Sci USA* 97: 68266831. doi: 10.1073/pnas.97.12.6826.

Colak, D., Ji, S. J., Porse, B. T., and Jaffrey, S. R. 2013. Regulation of axon guidance by compartmentalized nonsense-mediated mRNA decay. *Cell* 153: 1252–1265.

Cox, E. C., Muller, B., and Bonhoeffer, F. 1990. Axonal guidance in the chick visual system: Posterior tectal membranes induce collapse of growth cones from the temporal retina. *Neuron* 4: 31–47.

Cox, L. J., Hengst, U., Gurskaya, N. G., Lukyanov, K. A., and Jaffrey, S. R. 2008. Intraaxonal translation and retrograde trafficking of CREB promotes neuronal survival. *Nat. Cell Biol.* 10: 149–159. doi: 10.1038/ncb1677.

De Nadai, T., Marchetti, L., Di Rienzo, C., et al. 2015. Precursor and mature NGF live tracking: one *versus* many at a time in the axons *Scientif. Rep.* 6: 20272 | DOI: 10.1038/srep20272.

Desai, A. R., and McConnell, S. K. 2000. Progressive restriction in fate potential by neural progenitors during cerebral cortical development. *Development* 127: 2863–2872.

Drescher, U., Kremoser, C., Handwerker, C., Loschinger, J., Noda, M., and Bonhoeffer, F. 1995. In vitro guidance of retinal ganglion cell axons by RAGS, a 25 kDa tectal protein related to ligands for Eph receptor tyrosine kinases. *Cell* 82: 359–370.

Evers, J., Laser, M., Sun, Y-A., Xie, Z-P., and Poo, M-M. 1989. Studies of nerve–muscle interactions in *Xenopus* cell culture: Analysis of early synaptic currents. *J. Neurosci.* 9: 1523–1539.

Fiddes, I. T., et al. 2018. Human-specific NOTCH2NL genes affect notch signaling and cortical neurogenesis. *Cell* 173: 1356–1369.

Florio, M., Albert, M., Taverna, E., et al. 2015. Human-specific gene ARHGAP11B promotes basal progenitor amplification and neocortex expansion, *Science* 347: 1465–1470 doi: 10.1126/science.aaa1975.

Gallo, G., and Letourneau, P. C. 2004. Regulation of growth cone actin filaments by guidance cues. *J. Neurobiol.* 58: 92–102.

Gao, P. et al. 2014. Deterministic progenitor behavior and unitary production of neurons in the neocortex. *Cell* 159: 775–788.

Gaspard, N., Bouschet, T., Dimidschstein, J., et al. 2008. An intrinsic mechanism of corticogenesis from embryonic stem cells. *Nature* 455: 351.

Gundersen, R. W. and Barret, J. N. 1979 Neuronal chemotaxis: Chick dorsal root axons turn toward high concentrations of nerve growth factor. *Science* 206: 1079–1080.

Kennedy, T. E., Serafini, T., de la Torre, J. R., and Tessier-Lavigne, M. 1994. Netrins are diffusible chemotropic factors for commissural axons in the embryonic spinal cord. *Cell* 78: 425–435.

Lumsden, A. G. S., and Davies, A. M. 1986. Chemotropic effect of specific target epithelium in the developing mammalian nervous system. *Nature* 323: 538–539.

Malatesta, P., Hartfuss, E., and Gotz, M. 2000. Isolation of radial glial cells by fluorescent-activated cell sorting reveals a neuronal lineage. *Development* 157: 5253–5263.

Miyata, T., Kawaguchi, A., Okano, H., and Ogawa, M. 2001. Asymmetric inheritance of radial glial fibers by cortical neurons. *Neuron* 31: 727–741.

Moreno-Jiménez, E. P., Flor-García, M., Terreros-Roncal, J., Rábano, A., Cafini, F., Pallas-Bazarra, N., Ávila, J., and Llorens-Martín, M. 2019. Adult hippocampal neurogenesis is abundant in neurologically healthy subjects and drops sharply in patients with Alzheimer's Disease. *Nat. Med.* 25: 55.

Noctor, S. C., Flint, A. C., Weissman, T. A., Dammerman, R. S., and Kriegstein, A. R. 2001. Neurons derived from radial glial cells establish radial units in neocortex. Nature 409:

Rakic, P. 1974. Neurons in rhesus monkey visual cortex: Systematic relationship between time of origin and eventual disposition. *Science* 183: 425–427.

Shen, Q., Wang, Y., Dimos, J. T., Fasano, C. A., Phoenix, T. N., Lemischka, I. R., Ivanova, N. B., Stifani, S., Morrisey, E. E., and Temple, S. 2006. The timing of cortical neurogenesis is encoded within lineages of individual progenitor cells. *Nature Neurosci.* 9: 743.

Smith, R.S., Kenny, C.J., Ganesh, V., Jang, A., Borges-Monroy, R., Partlow, J.N., Hill, R.S., Shin, T., Chen, A.Y., Doan, R.N., et al. 2018. Sodium channel SCN3A (Na$_V$1.3) regulation of human cerebral cortical folding and oral motor development. *Neuron* 99: 905–913.e7.

Spalding, K. L., Bergmann, O., Alkass, K., Bernard, S., Salehpour, M., Huttner, H. B., Boström, E., Westerlund, I., Vial, C., Buchholz, B. A., Possnert, G., Mash, D. C., Druid, H., and Frisén, J. 2013. Dynamics of hippocampal neurogenesis in adult humans. *Cell* 153: 1219–1227.

Suzuki, I. K., Gacquer, D., Van Heurck, R., Kumar, D., Wojno, M., Bilheu, A., Herpoel, A., Lambert, N., Cheron, J., Polleux, F., Detours, V., and Vanderhaeghen, P. 2018. Human-specific *NOTCH2NL* genes expand cortical neurogenesis through delta/notch regulation. *Cell* 173: 1370–1384.

Thompson, W. 1983. Synapse elimination in neonatal rat muscle is sensitive to pattern of muscle use. *Nature* 302: 614–616.

Vitali, I. et al. 2018. Progenitor hyperpolarization regulates the sequential generation of neuronal subtypes in the developing neocortex. *Cell* 174: 1264–1276.e15.

CHAPTER 28

Critical Periods in Sensory Systems

The development of neural circuits can be shaped by experience and by environmental inputs. Experience-dependent changes have been best studied in sensory systems, showing that early sensory experience determines the way in which sensory circuits are consolidated during early postnatal life. The capacity to undergo experience-dependent changes in neural circuits is not constant throughout life, and there are phases of greatly enhanced plasticity during specific time-windows (called critical periods) of early postnatal life.

This chapter describes the effects of use and disuse on the visual systems of monkeys, kittens, and mice, as well as on other sensory systems. Experiments made by Wiesel and Hubel have shown that visual input in early life plays an essential role in developing the structure and function of neurons in the visual cortex. In monkeys, at the time of birth the receptive fields of neurons in the retina, lateral geniculate nucleus (LGN), and visual cortex resemble those of adults. However, if one eye receives greater visual input during early life—the critical period—it takes over the territory of the other eye in the cortex. Closure of the lids of one eye during the critical period leads to loss of that eye's ability to drive cortical cells. Columns in the visual cortex and the geniculate axons supplied by the deprived eye shrink, while those supplied by the normal, non-deprived eye expand. These results suggest that there is competition for territory in early life. Lid closure in adult animals has no effect on columnar architecture or responses to visual stimuli.

Evidence for competition between the two eyes is provided by experiments in which both eyes were deprived by lid closure shortly after birth or in which an ocular muscle was cut in a newborn so as to produce a squint (strabismus). When neither eye has an advantage, normal columnar structure develops; however, each neuron in the cortex is driven by only one eye. The role of impulse activity in competition was shown by blocking impulse traffic in both optic nerves by application of tetrodotoxin (TTX). Under these conditions, ocular dominance columns desegregate.

Appropriate sensory input is also essential in the development of the auditory system. Barn owls localize their prey by sight and sound. The visual and auditory maps of the outside world are normally aligned in the optic tectum at birth. When the visual input is displaced by applying prisms to the two eyes, young owls adapt to this mismatch in auditory and visual maps of the outside world. The receptive fields of auditory neurons in the tectum shift over days and weeks to fit the displaced visual map. Once the prisms are removed, the visual fields again shift abruptly, while the auditory fields move back slowly over time. After a critical period, such shifts in auditory receptive fields no longer occur. In owls brought up in an enriched environment with enhanced sensory experience, the critical period during which maps can be brought into register is prolonged.

Sensory deprivation experiments are significant for considering the development of higher brain functions. The opening and closure of the critical periods correlate with the maturation of inhibitory circuits, with the activity of long-distance neuromodulatory systems, and with epigenetic processes. Interfering with these mechanisms can result in prolonging or reopening the time-window for plasticity in the adult brain.

In previous chapters we have emphasized that highly specific connections are necessary for the nervous system to function properly. This chapter shows that development and fine-tuning of connections between neurons are not complete at birth. For example, kittens—unlike monkeys, which that are able to see at birth—are born with their eyes closed. If the lids are opened and light is shone into an eye, the pupil constricts but the animal appears to be completely blind.[1] By 10 days kittens show evidence of vision and thereafter begin to recognize objects and patterns. When kittens are brought up in total darkness, the pupillary reflex continues to function but they remain blind. However, adult cats that have been kept in darkness for prolonged periods can see immediately when exposed to light. Such results suggest that there is a critical period of vulnerability in early life. One might intuit that circuits, such as those used for spinal cord or pupillary reflexes, should be genetically determined, whereas the development of circuits controlling complex functions might require continuous interaction with the environment. What are the relative contributions of genetic factors and experience for cortical development? What mechanisms ensure that cortical circuits become stabilized when development is complete?

In this chapter we show that the visual systems of the kitten and newborn monkey are first established in utero by intrinsic, genetically driven neuronal differentiation. Then, for a brief, well-defined period, visual experience refines neuronal circuits for optimal operation in the growing animal. We start by focusing on work that follows logically from the material presented in Chapters 2 and 3. Studies of the role of experience in forming the immature visual system set the stage for analyzing plasticity in other sensory circuits, notably the auditory system in birds and mammals.

The Visual System in Newborn Monkeys and Kittens

A good deal is known about the organization of the connections that underlie visual perception in the adult cat and monkey. A simple cell in the cortex selectively recognizes one well-defined type of visual stimulus, such as the movement of a narrow bar of light oriented vertically, in a particular region of the visual field of either eye. Such responses are possible because of the precise and orderly connections made to cortical cells from the retina by way of the lateral geniculate nucleus (LGN; see Chapters 2 and 3). It is natural to wonder whether cells and connections of this type are already present in the newborn animal or whether they develop as a result of visual experience, in which case visual stimuli in early life would direct or refine a set of preexisting connections.

To study visually naïve animals, monkeys were taken immediately after natural birth or after delivery by cesarean section, with care being taken to avoid exposure to light. To prevent form vision until animals were old enough to be studied, the lids were either sutured or the cornea was covered by a translucent occluder, which blurs images but allows light to pass. Other visually naïve animals, such as kittens, rats, and ferrets, have also been examined during the first weeks after birth.[2-6]

Receptive Fields and Response Properties of Cortical Cells in Newborn Animals

A newborn monkey appears visually alert and is able to fixate. The responses of cortical neurons in many ways resemble those of the adult animal. For example, recordings made from individual cells in primary visual cortex (V1) show that the cells are not driven by diffuse illumination. As in a mature animal, they fire best when light or dark bars with a particular orientation are shone onto a particular region of the retina.[2] In recordings

[1] Riesen, A. H., and Aarons, L. 1959. *J. Comp. Physiol. Psychol.* 52: 142–149.

[2] Wiesel, T. N., and Hubel, D. H. 1974. *J. Comp. Neurol.* 158: 307–318.

[3] Hubel, D. H., and Wiesel, T. N. 1963. *J. Neurophysiol.* 26: 994–1002.

[4] Crair, M. C., Gillespie, D. C., and Stryker, M. P. 1998. *Science* 279: 566–570.

[5] Chapman, B., Stryker, M. P., and Bonhoeffer, T. 1996. *J. Neurosci.* 16: 6443–6453.

[6] Katz, L. C. and Crowley J. C. 2002. *Nat. Rev. Neurosci.* 3: 34–42.

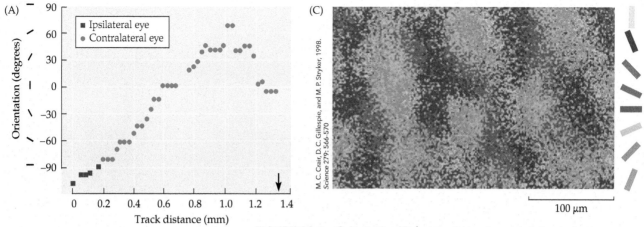

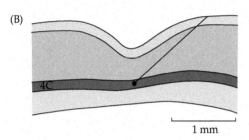

FIGURE 28.1 Orientation Columns in the absence of visual experience. (A) Axis orientation of receptive fields encountered by an electrode during an oblique penetration through the cortex of a 17-day-old baby monkey whose eyes had been sutured closed on the second day after birth. The receptive field orientation changes progressively as columns are traversed, indicating that normal orientation columns are present in the visually naïve animal. Red squares are from the ipsilateral eye, blue dots from the contralateral eye. The black arrow marks the end of the electrode track in layer 4. (B) The black dot marks the lesion made at the end of the electrode track in (A). (C) Orientation columns displayed by imaging in a 14-day-old kitten with lids sutured at birth. Colored bars (right) represent the orientation of the stimulus. Note that pinwheels are already present. (A,B after T. N. Wiesel and D. H. Hubel, 1974. *J. Comp. Neurol.* 158: 307-318.)

made in animals lacking prior visual experience, the range of orientations cannot be distinguished from that in adults. The receptive fields are also organized into antagonistic "on" and "off" areas that are driven by both eyes. Moreover, with oblique penetrations, the preferred orientation changes in a regular sequence as the electrode moves through the cortex, as shown in Figure 28.1. The figure also shows that orientation preference maps with characteristic pinwheels (see Chapter 3) are already evident, with all orientations represented equally at the time of birth.[4]

Ocular Dominance Columns in Newborn Monkeys and Kittens

In monkeys, at birth most cells in all layers of V1 are already driven by both eyes—some better by one eye, some by the other, and some equally well by both. Figure 28.2 shows ocular dominance—the distribution of responses of neurons distributed throughout all cortical layers according to eye preference—in a newborn and an adult monkey.

The degree of ocular dominance is expressed in the histograms by grouping neurons into seven categories according to the discharge frequency with which they responded to stimulation of one or the other eye (see Chapter 3). The majority of cells respond to appropriate illumination of either eye. Cells in groups 1 and 7 in Figure 28.2 were driven only by visual stimuli applied to one eye, while cells in groups 2 through 6 responded to both eyes. The histograms in Figure 28.2A,B appear similar, with a range of eye preferences for cells throughout the cortical layers. What these data fail to show, however, is a striking and important difference in the properties of cells in layer 4. In that layer, cells in the newborn monkey are driven by both eyes; after 6 weeks of development, however, cells in layer 4 are driven by only one eye.[7] Outside of layer 4, cortical cells in newborn monkeys appear similar in their responses to those in adults, except that in some cells discharges are less vigorous or absent.

Compared with that of monkeys, the visual system of kittens is less developed at birth. Kittens open their eyes around postnatal day 10 and cells of the visual cortex (V1) start responding like adult cells at about 3 to 4 weeks of age, when they clearly show an ocular dominance distribution.[8] In kittens, as in newborn monkeys, cells in all cortical layers, including layer 4, are more markedly binocular than in the adult, reflecting the ongoing gradual development of ocular dominance columns.

[7] Wiesel, T. N. 1982. *Nature* 299: 583-591.

[8] Shatz, C. J., and Stryker, M. P. 1978 *J. Physiol.* 281: 267-283.

FIGURE 28.2 Ocular Dominance Distribution in the visual cortex of a normal adult monkey (A) and a normal newborn monkey (B). Cells in groups 1 and 7 of the histograms are driven by one eye only (ipsilateral or contralateral). All other cells have input from both eyes. In groups 2, 3, 5, and 6, one eye predominates. In group 4, both eyes have equal influence. (After T. N. Wiesel and D. H. Hubel, 1974. *J. Comp. Neurol.* 158: 307–318.)

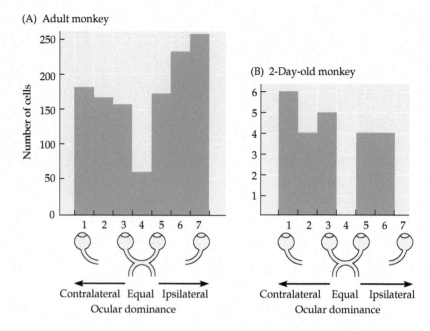

9 LeVay, S., Wiesel, T. N., and Hubel, D. H. 1980. *J. Comp. Neurol.* 191: 1–51.

10 LeVay, S., Stryker, M. P., and Shatz, C. J. 1978. *J. Comp. Neurol.* 179: 223–24.

Initial Development of Ocular Dominance Columns

The time of initial formation of ocular dominance columns has been the subject of intense discussions. Transneuronal anterograde transport of tritiated amino acids (3H-proline) or sugars (3H-fucose), injected in one eye, made it possible to directly visualize ocular dominance columns at the anatomical level and study their initial development. LeVay, Wiesel, and Hubel[9] found a striking difference between adult and newborn monkeys. The newborn cortex showed an anatomical and a physiological mixing of left- and right-eye inputs to layer 4, even if the basic columnar pattern was evident. By 6 weeks of age an adult degree of columnar segregation was established (Figure 28.3A,B). In kittens, transneuronal labeling in the cortex appeared homogeneous before 3 weeks of age.[10]

FIGURE 28.3 Age Dependence of Ocular Dominance Columns and of Branching Patterns of Axons from Lateral Geniculate Nucleus. (A) Dark-field micrograph of autoradiographic labeling pattern in the striate cortex of a normal 6 day-old monkey, ipsilateral to the eye that had been injected with 3H-fucose 5 days earlier. This is a single section that grazes layer 4C tangentially in the central oval region. Silver grains are distributed continuously over layer 4C, but there are bands of alternating higher and lower grain density, indicating that afferents for the two eyes are already in the process of columnar segregation. (B) Autoradiographic montage from a 6-week-old normal monkey, ipsilateral to the injected eye. The labeled bands are as sharply defined as they would be in adults. (C) Ending in layer 4, labeled by injection with horseradish peroxidase, of an axon of a 17-day-old kitten. The axon spreads over a large uninterrupted territory in layer 4 of the visual cortex. (D) In the adult cat, the geniculate axon ends in two discrete tufts, interrupted by unlabeled fibers coming from the other eye. (C,D from T. N. Wiesel, 1982. *Nature* 299: 583–591.)

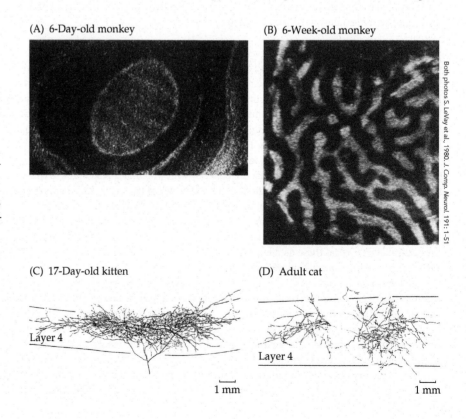

Both photos S. LeVay et al., 1980. *J. Comp. Neurol.* 191: 1–51

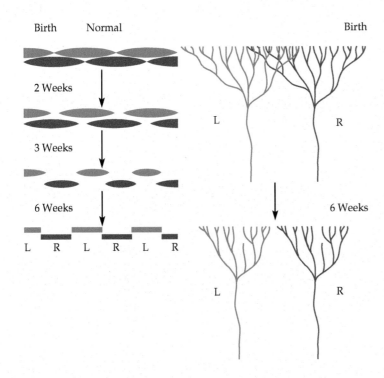

Birth   Normal   Birth

2 Weeks

L   R

3 Weeks

6 Weeks   6 Weeks

L   R   L   R   L   R

L   R

FIGURE 28.4   Retraction of Lateral Geniculate Nucleus Axons in Layer 4, from Birth to 6 Weeks. The figure shows the overlap of inputs from the right (R) and left (L) eyes present at birth and the subsequent segregation during the first 6 weeks of life into separate clusters corresponding to ocular dominance columns. The overlap at birth is greater in kittens than in monkeys. (After D. H. Hubel and T. N. Wiesel, 1977. *Proc. R. Soc. Lond., B, Biol. Sci.* 198: 1-59.)

This result has a correlate at the single-neuron level: In contrast to the well-segregated geniculate terminals in the adult, arborizations of geniculate fibers ending in layer 4 overlap extensively in newborn kittens (Figure 28.3C,D). As a result of the overlap in territories supplied by each eye, the immature neurons in layer 4 respond to stimulation of both eyes rather than just one. Similarly, during the first 6 weeks of a monkey's life, the axons of geniculate cells in layer 4 retract to form smaller arborizations, as though pruned. In this way, separate domains of cortex in layer 4 become established, each supplied exclusively by one or the other eye (Figure 28.4). However, it was later recognized that anterogradely transported tracer injected into one eye could leak and "spill over" into inappropriate eye-specific layers of the LGN.[6] This undermined the conclusion that the initial establishment of ocular dominance columns requires visual experience. Indeed, earlier work with macaque monkeys indicated that thalamocortical afferents begin to segregate into stripes before birth and are arranged into functional columns before birth, in the absence of visual experience.[11-13] Subsequent work in the ferret (and cat) visual system, using direct injection of tracers into the eye-specific layers of developing LGN instead of into the eye, demonstrated that ocular dominance columns are already segregated weeks before eye opening and before the onset of visual experience[14] (Figure 28.5). In addition, monocular enucleation prior to the onset of the critical period (next paragraph), but after LGN axons have arrived in V1 layer 4, does not cause a corresponding change in the size of ocular dominance columns (see Figure 28.5).[14]

There is now a consensus that the *initial establishment* of ocular dominance columns takes place before the onset of visual experience and can be separated from the *critical period for ocular dominance column plasticity*, which relies on visually evoked neuronal activity.[6,15] The initial formation of ocular dominance columns may involve innate intrinsic molecular cues, or activity-dependent mechanisms not related to visual experience, such as spontaneous impulse activity or waves in the retina.[16,17] Shadows cast on the cortex by retinal blood vessels have been proposed to play a role in this process.[18]

Surprisingly, if both eyes are removed early in life (P0 in the ferret), before the layers of LGN have segregated (and well before LGN afferents have reached the cortex), normally segregated columns of layer-specific LGN afferents still form in the cortex.[19] Molecular cues, or correlated spontaneous activity in LGN neurons, instead of retinal activity, might be involved. Comparable changes during development occur at the preceding stage in the LGN of the visual pathway.[20,21]

As optic nerve fibers from the two eyes grow into the LGN, their arborizations overlap extensively before they separate into distinct layers. This segregation depends on retinal

[11] Rakic, P. 1976. *Nature* 261: 467-471.

[12] Des Rosiers, M. H. et al. 1978. *Science* 200: 447-449.

[13] Kuljis, R. O., and Rakic, P. 1990. *Proc. Natl. Acad. Sci. USA* 87: 5303-5306.

[14] Crowley, J. C., and Katz, L. C. 2000. *Science* 290: 1321-1324.

[15] Crowley, J. C., and Katz, L. C. 2002. *Curr. Op. Neurobiol.* 12: 104-109.

[16] Galli, L., and Maffei, L. 1988. *Science* 242: 90-91.

[17] Meister, M. et al. 1991. *Science* 252: 939-943.

[18] Adams, D. L., and Horton, J. C. 2002. *Science* 298: 572-576.

[19] Crowley, J. C. and Katz, L. C. 1999. *Nat. Neurosci.* 2: 1125-1130.

[20] Rakic, P. 1977. *Philos. Trans. R. Soc. Lond., B, Biol. Sci.* 278: 245-260.

[21] Shatz, C. J. 1996. *Proc. Natl. Acad. Sci. USA* 93: 602-608.

FIGURE 28.5 Early Appearance of Ocular Dominance Columns and Their Resistance to Monocular Enucleation. (A) Ocular dominance (OD) columns in ferret V1 are viewed after transneuronal transport of tritiated amino acids injected into eye-specific LGN layers. OD columns appear before the onset of the critical period and are resistant to imbalances of retinal influence during this time. Both panels represent coronal sections and show three patches of labeled (dark) geniculocortical axons in layer 4 of V1, corresponding to OD columns. The top panel is from a normal postnatal-day-18 (P18) ferret. The bottom panel is from a P18 ferret that was monocularly enucleated (ME) at P14. The size, spacing, and general appearance of the columns from the two animals are similar. Scale bar applies to both panels. (B) Timeline of ferret OD column development. The emergence of OD columns as revealed by direct LGN injections precedes the critical period for monocular deprivation (MD), the appearance of segregation by transneuronal transport, the opening of the eyes, and the onset of visual responses in the cortex. The appearance of segregated columns occurs while LGN axons are arriving and forming synapses in layer 4 of V1. The sequence of events in the developing cat cortex (not shown) is the same. The equivalent ages for the cat can be roughly determined by subtracting 21 days from the ferret (e.g., P21 in the ferret is ~P0 in the cat; P0 is equivalent to cat embryonic day 44). (B after J. C. Crowley and L. C. Katz, 2000. *Science* 290: 1321–1324.)

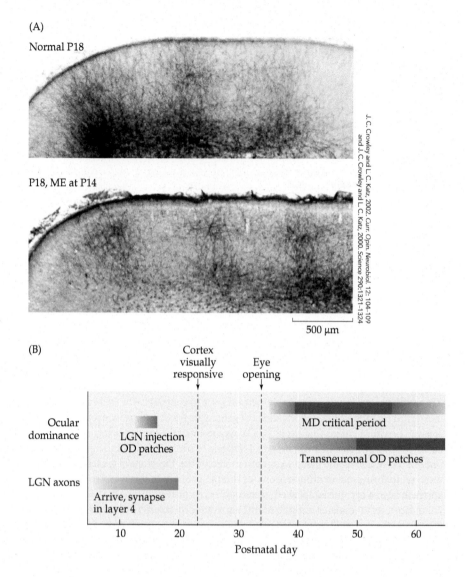

(A)

Normal P18

P18, ME at P14

500 μm

J. C. Crowley and L. C. Katz, 2002. *Curr. Opin. Neurobiol.* 12: 104–109 and J. C. Crowley and L. C. Katz, 2000. *Science* 290:1321–1324

(B)

[22] Sretavan, D. W., and Shatz, C. J. 1986. *J. Neurosci.* 6: 234–251.

[23] Penn, A. A. et al. 1998. *Science* 279: 2108–2112.

[24] Hubel, D. H. 1988. *Eye, Brain and Vision.* Scientific American Library, New York.

activity: Blockade by tetrodotoxin (TTX) or by agents that block retinal waves prevents retinal axons from developing their layer-specific arborization in the LGN.[22,23]

In animals reared in total darkness, the early postnatal development of ocular dominance columns and geniculate layers that starts before birth proceeds normally.

Effects of Abnormal Visual Experience in Early Life

After the initial establishment of ocular dominance columns, the visual system enters into a plastic phase, corresponding to the critical period, that relies on patterned neural activity. Initial establishment of ocular dominance columns and ocular dominance plasticity can thus be separated one from another.

This section describes three types of experiments, many of them first performed by Hubel and Wiesel, in which animals were deprived of normal visual stimuli.[7,24] Hubel and Wiesel studied the effects on the physiological responses of nerve cells and the structure of the visual system after (1) closing the lids of one or both eyes; (2) preventing patterned vision, but not access of light to the eye; and (3) leaving light and form vision intact, but producing an artificial strabismus (squint) in one eye. These procedures cause remarkable abnormalities in the function and anatomy of the cortex.

Blindness after Lid Closure

When the lids of one eye were sutured during the first 2 weeks of life, causing monocular deprivation, monkeys and kittens still developed normally and used their unoperated eye. At the end of 1 to 3 months, however, when the operated eye was opened and the normal one was closed (a procedure called **reverse suture**; see Figure 28.9), it was clear that the animals were practically blind in their previously deprived eye (a condition called amblyopia). For example, kittens would bump into objects and fall off tables.[7,25] There was no gross evidence of a physiological defect in the eyes—pupillary reflexes appeared normal and so did the electroretinogram, which is an index of the average electrical activity of the eye. Records made from retinal ganglion cells in deprived animals showed no changes in their responses, and their receptive fields appeared normal. Thus, the monkey and cat retinas are immune to the effects of lid closure. This may not be the case for the rodent retina, in which retinal alterations are induced by dark rearing[26] and contribute to experience-dependent changes in the visual cortex.[27]

Responses of Cortical Cells after Monocular Deprivation

Although responses of cells in the LGN appeared relatively unchanged after monocular deprivation,[28] there were major changes in the responses of cortical cells.[7,29,30] When electrical recordings were made in the visual cortex, very few cells could be driven by the eye that had been closed. The majority of the cells that did respond had abnormal receptive fields. Responses of cells driven by the non-deprived eye were normal. Figure 28.6 shows ocular dominance histograms obtained from the cells examined in a monkey raised with closure of one eye during the early weeks of life.

Relative Importance of Diffuse Light and Form for Maintaining Normal Responses

The results described so far indicate that if one eye is not used normally in the first weeks of life, its power wanes and it ceases to be effective in the visual cortex. These far-reaching changes are produced by the relatively minor procedure of closing the lids, without cutting any nerves. What is the important condition for maintaining and developing proper visual responses? Is diffuse light adequate?

Lid closure reduces the level of light that reaches the retina but does not completely exclude it. A series of experiments in newborn kittens demonstrated that form vision, rather than the mere presence of light, is required to prevent abnormal development of cortical connections. A plastic occluder (such as a table tennis ball) was placed over the cornea instead of closing the eyelids; the occluder prevented form vision but admitted light. All of these cats were blind in the deprived eye.[25] Furthermore, cortical cells were no longer driven by the deprived eye. Neither retinal nor geniculate responses were noticeably changed under such conditions.

Morphological Changes in the Lateral Geniculate Nucleus after Visual Deprivation

Cells in the LGN of the cat and monkey are arranged in layers, each supplied predominantly by one or the other eye (see Chapter 2). In the same animals that showed marked abnormalities in the cortex after lid closure, the geniculate cells seemed at first to be normal. However, after lid closure of one eye, it was found that cells were noticeably smaller than in the layers supplied by the non-deprived eye.[28] The reduction in size depended on the duration of lid closure. Surprisingly, the shrunken cells showed little physiological deficit. Several lines of evidence suggest that the size of the LGN cells may reflect the extent of their arborization in the cortex.[31,32]

Morphological Changes in the Cortex after Visual Deprivation

The morphological consequences of eye closure are particularly conspicuous in layer 4 of V1, where geniculate fibers terminate in an orderly manner.[9,33] Changes in the morphology

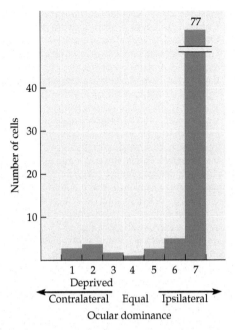

FIGURE 28.6 Damage Produced by Closure of One Eye. Ocular dominance distribution in a monkey whose right eye was closed from 21 to 30 days of age. In spite of a subsequent 4 years of binocular vision, most cortical neurons were unresponsive to stimulation of the deprived eye. (After S. LeVay et al., 1980. *J. Comp. Neurol.* 191: 1-51.)

[25] Wiesel, T. N., and Hubel, D. H. 1963. *J. Neurophysiol.* 26: 1003-1017.

[26] Tian, N., and Copenhagen, D.R. 2003. *Neuron* 39: 85-96.

[27] Mandolesi, G. et al. 2005. *Curr. Biol.* 15: 2119.

[28] Wiesel, T. N., and Hubel, D. H. 1963. *J. Neurophysiol.* 26: 978-993.

[29] LeVay, S., Stryker, M. P. and Shatz, C. J. 1978. *J. Comp. Neurol.* 179: 223-244.

[30] Wiesel, T. N. and Hubel, D. H. 1965. *J. Neurophysiol.* 28: 1029-1040.

[31] Guillery, R. W. and Stelzner, D. J. 1970. *J. Comp. Neurol.* 139: 413-421.

[32] Humphrey, A. L. et al. 1985. *J. Comp. Neurol.* 233: 159-189.

[33] Hubel, D. H., Wiesel, T. N., and LeVay, S. 1977. *Philos. Trans. R. Soc. Lond., B, Biol. Sci.* 278: 377-409.

FIGURE 28.7 Ocular Dominance Columns in Layer 4 after Closure of One Eye. (A) Normal adult monkey. The right eye had been injected with a radioactive proline-fucose mixture 10 days earlier. Layer 4 displays alternating light and dark stripes of equal width. Radioactively labeled geniculate axons in layer 4 of the right hemisphere appear as fine white granules forming columns. Intervening dark bands correspond to the other eye. This image was made as a photomontage reconstruction from parallel sections of layer 4 with autoradiography. (B) Reconstruction of layer 4 in an 18-month-old monkey whose right eye had been closed at the age of 2 weeks. Radioactive material was injected into the normal left eye. White grains demonstrate columns in layer 4 from the non-deprived eye, which are larger than normal. Columns supplied by the eye that had been closed (black) are narrower than normal. (C) Cortical arborization of labeled geniculate axons ending in layer 4 of a kitten in which one eye had been closed for 33 days. The terminal arborization of the geniculate axon from the deprived eye shows a dramatic reduction of branches compared with that from the non-deprived eye. (C after A. Antonini and M. P. Stryker, 1993. *Vis. Neurosci.* 15: 401–409.)

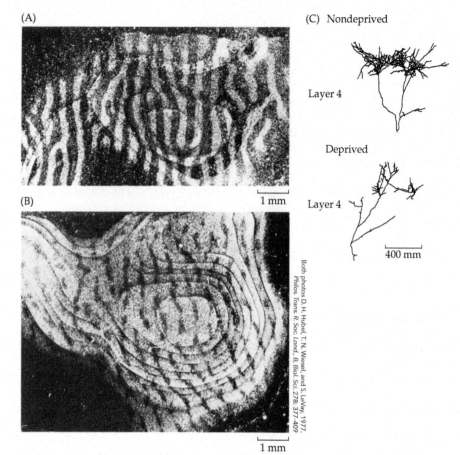

(A)

(B)

1 mm

1 mm

(C) Nondeprived

Layer 4

Deprived

Layer 4

400 mm

Both photos D. H. Hubel, T. N. Wiesel, and S. LeVay, 1977. *Philos. Trans. R. Soc. Lond., B, Biol. Sci.* 278: 377–409

of ocular dominance columns following lid closure in monkeys have been revealed by autoradiography of the cortex after injection of radioactive tracers into one eye. After lid closure, there is a marked reduction in the width of ocular dominance columns receiving projections from the occluded eye. At the same time, the columns with inputs from the normal eye show a corresponding increase in width. The shrinkage of ocular dominance columns is evident in Figure 28.7, in which the normal columns can be compared with columns in animals in which one eye had been closed at 2 weeks and left closed for 18 months. The changes indicate that geniculate axons activated by the normal eye retained or captured territory in the cortex lost by their weaker, visually deprived neighbors. These results are consistent with physiological observations made by recording from cells in layer 4. Almost all cells were driven only by the eye that had *not* been deprived. Certain features of the cortex, such as the alternating striped pattern of cytochrome oxidase staining in secondary visual cortex (V2),[34] are less vulnerable to deprivation than layer 4 in V1.[35]

Critical Period for Susceptibility to Lid Closure

When the lids of one eye are closed in an adult cat or monkey, no abnormal consequences are seen.[7,9] Even if an eye is closed for more than a year, the cells in the cortex continue to be driven normally by both eyes and display the normal ocular dominance histogram. Moreover, after one eye has been completely removed in an adult monkey, the structure of layer 4 remains normal when observed with autoradiography or other staining methods, even though there is atrophy in the LGN. This finding indicates a remarkable resistance to change in layer 4 of the adult animal when compared with the changes seen in the immature animal.

In monkeys, the greatest sensitivity to lid closure is during the first 6 weeks of life.[6,7,20] At any time during that period, with a peak at 1 week of age,[36] substantial changes in eye preference and columnar architecture develop if one eye is closed for a few days. During the subsequent months (up to about 12–16 months), several weeks of closure are required to

[34] Horton, J. C. and Hocking, D. R. 1998. *Vis. Neurosci.* 15: 289–303.

[35] Hensch, T. K. 2004. *Annu. Rev. Neurosci.* 27: 549–579.

[36] Horton, J. C. and Hocking, D. R. 1997. *J. Neurosci.* 17: 3684–3709.

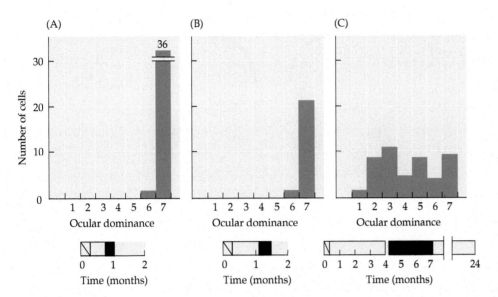

FIGURE 28.8 Critical Period in Kittens. Histograms showing eye preference in the visual cortex of kittens that were littermates, in which the right eye was closed at different ages. The period during which the eye was closed is indicated under the histograms. (A) Eyelids sutured for 6 days at 23 days of age. (B) Eyelids sutured for 9 days at 30 days of age. (C) The right eye was open the first 4 months, closed for 3 months, and then kept open until 2 years of age, when the recordings were made. (After D. H. Hubel and T. N. Wiesel, 1970. *J. Physiol.* 206: 419-436.)

produce obvious changes in ocular dominance histograms or the width of columns in layer 4. At later times, changes do not develop even after surgical removal of one eye.

The period of greatest susceptibility to lid closure in kittens has been narrowed down to weeks 4 and 5 after birth.[37,38] During the first 3 weeks or so of life, eye closure has little effect. This is not surprising, since the kittens' eyes are normally closed for the first 10 days. But abruptly, during weeks 4 and 5, sensitivity increases. Closure at that age for as little as 3 to 4 days leads to a sharp decline in the number of cells that can be driven by the deprived eye. An experiment in which littermates are compared is shown in Figure 28.8. In this example, 6- and 9-day closures starting at the age of 23 and 30 days (see Figure 28.8A,B) caused about as great an effect as 3 months of monocular deprivation from birth. The susceptibility to lid closure declines after the critical period has passed and eventually disappears by about 3 months of age (see Figure 28.8C). The critical period can, however, be prolonged by rearing kittens in the dark.[39,40] In that situation, susceptibility to monocular closure can still be demonstrated at 6 months of age, as though stimulus-driven activity is required to complete eye-specific cortical contacts. However, there is evidence that even a brief exposure of the kitten to light for a few hours may be sufficient to prevent such extension of the critical period.

In conclusion, the sensitivity of the visual cortex to lid closure (monocular deprivation) defines a time-window in early life when the cortical neural circuitry can be robustly restructured in response to visual experience. Collectively, these changes have been termed ocular dominance plasticity, and unlike the initial formation of ocular dominance columns, they depend strongly on patterned visual activity and competition between the two eyes (discussed in a forthcoming section).

Recovery during the Critical Period

To what extent is recovery possible after lid closure during the critical period? Even if the deprived eye in an adult cat or monkey is subsequently opened for months or years, the damage remains, with little or no recovery. Thus, the animal continues to be blind in that eye, with shrunken columns and skewed ocular dominance histograms. In animals with monocular closure, experiments have been made with reverse suture, in which the lids are opened in the deprived eye and closed over the normal eye (Figure 28.9). This procedure leads to a recovery of vision, provided it is carried out during the critical period.[9,41,42] Monkeys and kittens not only begin to see again with the initially deprived eye, but they become blind in the other eye. Accompanying these changes, the ocular dominance histograms switch; that is, the newly opened eye drives most cells, while the eye that had been open for the first weeks (now closed) cannot. Moreover, the anatomical pattern in layer 4 revealed by autoradiography shows a corresponding change: The shrunken regions supplied by the initially closed eye expand at the expense of the initially open (but then closed) eye (see Figure 28.9C).

[37] Malach, R., Ebert, R., and Van Sluyters, R. C. 1984. *J. Neurophysiol.* 51: 538-551.

[38] Hubel, D. H., and Wiesel, T. N. 1970. *J. Physiol.* 206: 419-436.

[39] Cynader, M., and Mitchell, D. E. 1980. *J. Neurophysiol.* 43: 1026-1040.

[40] Daw, N. W. et al. 1995. *Ciba Found. Symp.* 193: 258-276; discussion 322-254.

[41] Blakemore, C., and Van Sluyters, R. C. 1974. *J. Physiol.* 237: 195-216.

[42] Kim, D. S., and Bonhoeffer, T. 1994. *Nature* 370: 370-372.

FIGURE 28.9 Effects of Reverse Suture on Ocular Dominance in a Monkey. (A) Experimental procedure. The right eye was closed from days 2 to 21 after birth, after which it was opened while the left eye was closed from day 21 for 9 months. (B) The ocular dominance histogram shows that almost all cells were driven exclusively by the right eye, which had been initially deprived. Virtually no cortical cells were driven by the left eye. (Had both eyes been kept open at 21 days, the histogram would be reversed.) Accordingly, fibers driven by the right eye recaptured cortical cells they had previously lost. (C) Tangential section of cortex passing through layers 4Cβ and 4Cα. The bands labeled by the right eye are expanded in layer 4Cβ even though it had been deprived of light for 19 days. During those first days, the columns supplied by the right eye had shrunk before expanding. Recovery did not occur equally well in other layers, such as 4Cα. (After S. LeVay et al., 1980. *J. Comp. Neurol.* 191: 1-51.)

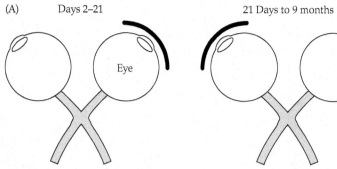

Days 2–21 / 21 Days to 9 months

Right eye closed from day 2 to day 21.

Right eye opened, left eye closed from day 21 for 9 months.

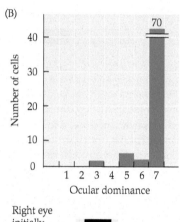
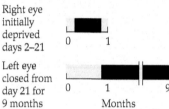
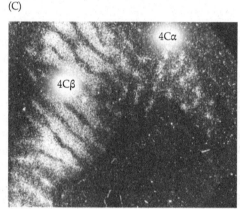

The conclusions from these experiments are that: (1) during the critical period in a normal animal, geniculate fibers supplying layer 4 of the cortex retract so that each eye supplies areas of comparable extent; (2) lid closure of one eye during the critical period leads to unequal retraction; and (3) reverse suture during the critical period produces "sprouting" of the geniculate axons so that an eye can recapture the cells it had lost (Figure 28.10).[30]

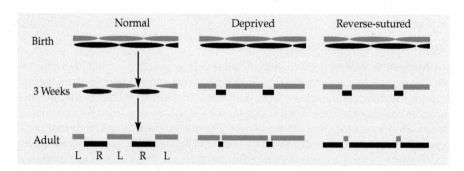

FIGURE 28.10 Summary of Effects of Eye Closure. In a normal monkey, ocular dominance columns start being clearly segregated at 3 weeks and have become well defined in layer 4 of the cortex by 6 weeks. Lid closure causes excessive retraction of geniculate fibers supplied by the deprived eye. Fibers supplied by the open eye retract less than usual, so their columns in layer 4 of the cortex are larger than normal in the adult. After reverse suture during the critical period, the initially deprived eye can recapture the territory it had lost in layer 4. (After D. H. Hubel and T. N. Wiesel, 1977. *Proc. R. Soc. Lond., B, Biol. Sci.* 198: 1-59.)

If postponed until adulthood, reverse suture is without effect. For example, in a monkey in which the reverse suture was performed at 1 year of age, the labeled columns for the initially deprived eye remained shrunken.

Requirements for Maintenance of Functioning Connections in the Visual System

At this stage one might be tempted to conclude that simple loss of activity in the visual pathways is the main factor that disrupts normal responses of cortical neurons. After all, cortical cells are driven not by diffuse illumination but by shapes and forms, so in the absence of form vision, cortical activity ceases. The following discussion shows that there must be additional causes that are more subtle than loss of activity.

Binocular Lid Closure and the Role of Competition

The first clue that loss of visually evoked activity cannot on its own account for the changed performance of neurons is shown by the following experiments. Both eyes were closed in newborn monkeys that were either born at term or delivered prematurely by cesarean section.[2,7] Surprisingly, after binocular closure for 17 days or longer, most cortical cells could still be driven by appropriate illumination, and the receptive fields of simple and complex cells appeared largely normal. The columnar organization for orientation was similar to that in controls (see Figure 28.1). The principal abnormality was the appearance of a substantial fraction of the cells that could not be driven binocularly. In addition, some spontaneously active cells could not be driven at all, and others did not require specifically oriented stimuli. However, the areas of cortex supplied by each eye were equal, and the pattern resembled that seen in normal adult monkeys—that is, in layer 4, cells were driven by one eye only, and columns were well defined when marked by autoradiography or by cytochrome oxidase. Binocular closure in kittens led to similar effects, except that a larger fraction of cortical cells continued to be binocularly driven.[30] The arborizations of lateral geniculate axons in layer 4 were not shrunken.[43] At the same time, cells in the lateral geniculate body showed atrophy (a decrease in size of approximately 40%) in all layers.

The conclusion from these experiments is that some, but not all, of the ill effects expected from closing one eye are reduced or averted by closing both eyes. It is as though inputs from the two eyes are in competition for representation in cortical cells, and with one eye closed, the contest becomes unequal.

Effects of Strabismus (Squint)

The abnormal effects described in the preceding discussion were produced by suturing eyelids or by using translucent diffusers, implicating loss of form vision. Following the clue that cross-eyed children (i.e., those with strabismus or squint) or wall-eyed children can become blind in one eye, Hubel and Wiesel produced artificial strabismus in kittens and newborn monkeys by cutting an eye muscle.[7,44] The optical axis of that eye was thereby deflected from normal. Under such conditions, illumination and pattern stimulation for each eye remained unchanged but the visual fields were not aligned.

The results at first seemed disappointing because after several months vision in both eyes of the operated animals appeared normal, and individual cortical cells had normal receptive fields and responded briskly to precisely oriented stimuli. However, *almost every cell responded to only one eye*; some cells were driven only by the ipsilateral eye and others only by the contralateral, but almost none were driven by both. The cells were, as usual, grouped in columns with respect to eye preference and orientation preference.[45] As expected, no atrophy occurred in the LGN, and the columnar architecture of layer 4 was unchanged. The critical period for displaced images to produce changes was comparable to that for monocular deprivation.

These experiments provide an example in which all the usual parameters of light are normal—the amount of illumination and form and pattern stimuli. The only change consists of a failure of the images to fall on corresponding regions of the two retinas. The factor that seems important for the loss of binocular convergence of geniculate projections to the cortex is lack of congruity of input from the two eyes. It is as though the homologous

[43] Antonini, A. et al. 1998. *J. Neurosci.* 18: 9896-9909.

[44] Hubel, D. H., and Wiesel, T. N. 1965. *J. Neurophysiol.* 28: 1041-1059.

[45] Lowel, S., and Singer, W. 1992. *Science* 255: 209-212.

receptive fields in both eyes must be in register with one another, so that excitation will be simultaneous. The following experiment further supports this idea.

During the first 3 months of its life, the eyes of a kitten were occluded with an opaque plastic cover that was switched on alternate days from one eye to the other, so that the two eyes received the same total experience but at different times.[44] The result was the same as in the cross-eyed experiments, namely that cells were driven predominantly by either one eye or the other, but not equally by both. The maintenance of normal binocularity therefore depends not only on the amount of impulse traffic but also on the appropriate spatial and temporal overlap of activity in the different incoming fibers.

Changes in Orientation Preference

A logical question to ask is whether raising animals in an environment in which they see only one orientation can change the orientation preference of cortical cells. An experimental approach that involved both competition and deprivation was used by Carlson, Hubel, and Wiesel.[46] The lids of one eye were sutured in a newborn monkey. The animal was kept in darkness except when it placed its head in a holder (Figure 28.11). Then, with the head held vertically, it would see vertical stripes with the unsutured eye. Since the monkey received orange juice each time it placed its head in the holder correctly, it performed this maneuver frequently. Thus, during the critical period one eye received no visual input, while the other saw only vertical stripes. After 57 hours of experience, occurring between 12 and 54 days after birth, normal levels of cortical activity were found, with cells of all orientations arranged as usual in columns. As expected, the open eye tended to dominate. However, when tests were made for orientation preference, the results shown in Figure 28.11 were obtained. Both eyes could drive cells well when horizontal lines were the

[46] Carlson, M., Hubel, D. H., and Wiesel, T. N. 1986. *Brain Res.* 390: 71–81.

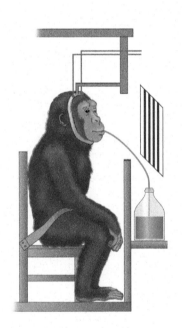

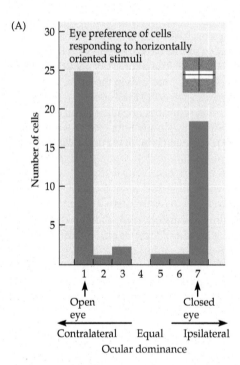

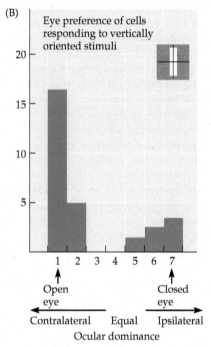

FIGURE 28.11 Orientation Preferences of Cortical Cells in a monkey with altered visual experience. The monkey was kept in a dark room. At 12 days, the right eye was closed. Whenever the monkey placed its head in a holder (to ensure that the head was not tilted), it received orange juice. At that time, it also saw vertical stripes with its left eye. For a total of 57 hours of exposure between 12 and 54 days, the only visual experience was an image of vertical lines seen by the left eye. The right eye saw nothing. (A) After 54 days the right eye was reopened and horizontally oriented light stimuli shone onto the screen stimulated cortical cells driven by the left eye or the right eye equally well. In this histogram, no deprivation is apparent for horizontal orientation, except for a lack of binocular cells. (B) With vertically oriented stimuli, the left eye, which had been kept open to view vertical stripes, was much more effective in driving cortical cells. This histogram resembles that seen after monocular deprivation. The results suggest that competition was equal for horizontal stimuli that neither eye had ever seen, and unequal for vertical stimuli (favored by the left, open eye). (After M. Carlson et al., 1986. *Brain Res.* 390: 71–81.)

stimulus, but the left (open) eye produced more effective responses to vertical stripes. The probable explanation for this result is that neither eye saw horizontal bars or edges during the critical period. Hence, the stimulation for horizontality was analogous to binocular closure; that is, the competition was equal. For the vertical input, however, the open eye had an enriched experience and, in a sense, captured cells in vertical orientation columns that had previously been supplied by the deprived eye. Similar results (stimulus-selective response potentiation, or SRP) have been observed by Bonhoeffer and his colleagues in kittens reared in a striped environment[47] and by Bear and colleagues in mice exposed to repeated presentations of grating stimuli of a single orientation.[48]

Segregation of Visual Inputs without Competition

In the experiments described so far, an underlying principle has been that the two eyes compete for connections and territory in the LGN and in layer 4 of V1, starting with roughly equal opportunity. However, Rakic and his colleagues have shown that during development, cells in the magnocellular (M) and parvocellular (P) systems (see Chapters 2 and 22) sort out their terminal formation *without* competition.[49] The two systems occupy distinct layers in the LGN and in visual cortex. By staining individual M and P axons, as they grew into the LGN Rakic and his colleagues showed that from the outset axons arrive in the correct M and P layers, where they form characteristic, nonoverlapping arborizations. M fibers end only in geniculate layers 1 and 2, while P fibers end only in layers 3, 4, 5, and 6, with no spillover. Thus, the connections in the M and P systems develop according to principles in which competition is not of the essence. Other examples of connections that form without signs of competition are the formation of blobs and of stripes in V2[34] and the alignment of orientation maps in the visual cortex of the kitten.[50]

Effects of Impulse Activity on the Developing Visual System

The role of impulse activity in shaping synaptic connections has been studied in experiments on kittens. When the lids are closed or the animal is brought up in complete darkness, impulse traffic in the visual pathways does not stop entirely. Neurons can fire spontaneously, providing the activity necessary for the development of LGN layers and of ocular dominance columns.

Experiments by Stryker, Shatz, and their colleagues[50,51] have shown that this presumably equal spontaneous activity from the two eyes is important for normal development. They injected TTX into both eyes of newborn kittens, thereby blocking impulse conduction in the visual pathways from the retina through the geniculate to the cortex. Several days later the toxin was removed and impulse conduction was restored. However, in the LGN, inputs from the two eyes had failed to segregate into separate layers (Figure 28.12).[52]

[47] Sengpiel, F., Stawinski, P., and Bonhoeffer, T. 1999. *Nat. Neurosci.* 2: 727-732.

[48] Frenkel, M. Y. et al. 2006. *Neuron* 51: 339-349.

[49] Meissirel, C. et al. 1997. *Proc. Natl. Acad. Sci. USA* 94: 5900-5905.

[50] Godecke, I., and Bonhoeffer, T. 1996. *Nature* 379: 251-254.

[51] Stryker, M. P., and Harris, W. A. 1986. *J. Neurosci.* 6: 2117-2133.

[52] Sretavan, D. W., Shatz, C. J., and Stryker, M. P. 1988. *Nature* 336: 468-471.

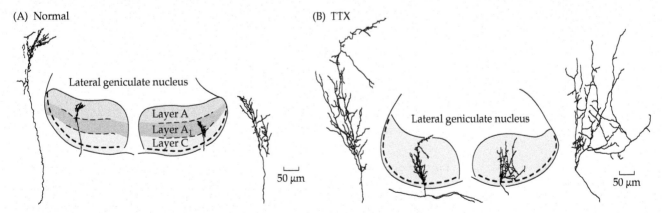

(A) Normal

Lateral geniculate nucleus

Layer A
Layer A₁
Layer C

50 μm

(B) TTX

Lateral geniculate nucleus

50 μm

FIGURE 28.12 Effect of Abolition of Electrical Activity by Tetrodotoxin (TTX) on arborization of optic nerve fibers terminating in the lateral geniculate nucleus. (A) In a normal kitten, the terminals of optic nerve fibers labeled with horseradish peroxidase are restricted to the single layer where they end. (B) After application of TTX for 16 days during embryonic life, labeled axons show much larger arborizations that are not restricted to individual layers. (After D. W. Sretavan et al., 1988. *Nature* 336: 468-471, based on D. W. Sretavan and C. J. Shatz. 1986. *J. Neurosci.* 6: 234-251.)

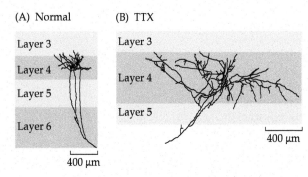

(A) Normal

(B) TTX

Layer 3
Layer 4
Layer 5
Layer 6

Layer 3
Layer 4
Layer 5

400 μm

400 μm

400 μm

FIGURE 28.13 Increased Arborization of Lateral Geniculate Fibers ending in layer 4 of visual cortex after application of tetrodotoxin (TTX) to both eyes. (A) Normal arborization of a labeled geniculate axon in layer 4 (30-day-old animal). (B) Labeled geniculate axon in a kitten in which TTX had been applied to the eyes for 12 days (29-day-old animal). The axons of this neuron cover a much larger area of cortex. (After A. Antonini and M. P. Stryker, 1993. *J. Neurosci.* 13: 3549-3573. © 1993 Society for Neuroscience.)

Moreover, cells in layer 4 of the visual cortex were still driven by both eyes as in the newborn animal, and the ocular dominance columns revealed by autoradiography resembled the neonatal pattern, with extensive overlap and no clear boundaries. Thus, in the absence of *all* firing, optic nerve fibers failed to segregate in the geniculate, and geniculate fibers failed to retract normally in layer 4 of the cortex.

The effects of lid closure on ocular dominance columns can also be modified by blocking impulse activity within the cortex itself (Figure 28.13). To demonstrate this, TTX was infused into the visual cortex of a kitten during the critical period while one eye was deprived of form and light.[53] After the TTX was removed, cortical cells were responsive to stimuli in both eyes, even though one had been deprived. Again, in the absence of activity, retraction failed to occur. Stryker and his colleagues performed similar experiments, using agents that inhibited firing of cortical neurons but left geniculate axons functional.[54] Retraction was also inhibited under these conditions, indicating that it is not simply the amount of incoming activity that is important but also whether that activity successfully drives cortical neurons.

Synchronized Spontaneous Activity in the Absence of Inputs during Development

The experiments with TTX suggest that action potential activity in the visual pathway is necessary for the sorting of axons to their appropriate targets. Without ongoing activity, axons remain spread across layers in the LGN and across boundaries of ocular dominance columns in the cortex. Yet as we have seen, much of the development has already proceeded by the time of birth. In the darkness of the womb, before a kitten or a monkey has seen anything and before photoreceptors have become functional, the layers of the LGN and the cortical columns are recognizable. Does this mean there is intrinsic impulse activity in the system that guides development? Elegant experiments by Galli and Maffei demonstrated that this is indeed the case, showing that synchronous bursts of action potential do, in fact, propagate along the rat optic nerve in utero.[16,55]

Consistent with these results, Meister, Baylor, and their colleagues showed that in retinas isolated from immature ferrets and fetal kittens, ganglion cells exhibit periodic, synchronized discharges.[17] Retinas were placed in a chamber over an array of 61 electrodes; from each electrode, it was possible to identify the discharges of as many as four different ganglion cells. The recordings revealed an ordered pattern of activity sweeping across the retina from ganglion cell to ganglion cell. An example is shown in Figure 28.14. Small black dots represent the positions of retinal ganglion cells, larger blue dots show the location of

[53] Reiter, H. O., Waitzman, D. M., and Stryker, M. P. 1986. *Exp. Brain Res.* 65: 182-188.

[54] Hata, Y., Tsumoto, T., and Stryker, M. P. 1999. *Neuron* 22: 375-381.

[55] Maffei, L., and Galli-Resta, L. 1990. *Proc. Natl. Acad. Sci. USA* 87: 2861-2864.

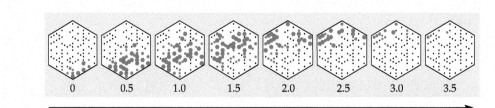

0   0.5   1.0   1.5   2.0   2.5   3.0   3.5

Time (s)

FIGURE 28.14 Wave of Impulse Activity Spreading across Isolated Retina of a neonatal ferret. The isolated retina was placed on recording electrodes, embedded in a regular array in the dish. The position of each of 82 retinal neurons is represented by a small black spot. Electrically active neurons are marked by larger blue spots, the sizes of which are proportional to the firing rates. Each frame represents the activity averaged over successive 0.5-second (s) intervals. During the time represented by the eight frames (3.5 s), action potentials begin with one small group of cells and spread slowly across the retina. A new wave begins shortly thereafter, and then another, each spreading in a different direction. At this stage of development, photoreceptors in the ferret are not responsive to light. (After M. Meister et al., 1991. *Science* 252: 939-943.)

action potential discharges, and the size of the dot indicates discharge frequency. Successive frames were taken at 0.5-second intervals. The wave of activity spread across the retina over a period of about 3 seconds. Typically, such waves recurred repeatedly, separated by silent periods on the order of 2 seconds in duration. Wong[56] has reported a similar wavelike spread of transient changes in intracellular calcium concentration and suggested that these play a role in synchronization of the electrical activity. There is evidence that cholinergic neurons, starburst amacrine cells, and electrical coupling play a part in the generation of the coordinated firing of ganglion cells in the immature retina.[57,58,59] We will show later in the chapter that waves of intrinsic activity also occur in the developing cochlea.

Triggers and Brakes Regulate the Critical Period in the Visual System

What are the physiological mechanisms that control the opening and closing of the critical period for ocular dominance plasticity? While earlier studies on the critical period for ocular dominance plasticity were carried out in mammals such as cats, ferrets, and monkeys, much of our current knowledge regarding the mechanistic regulation of critical period opening and closing is based on experiments on the rodent visual system. The practical advantages of working with rodents (among them, the possibility of using molecular biology and genetics methods) compensate for the fact that mice and rats are poorly visual animals.

The rodent visual cortex lacks segregated ocular dominance columns, but most neurons in the binocular region of the visual cortex receive input from both eyes and differ distinctly in their ocular dominance. In juvenile mice around postnatal day 30, eyelid suture in one eye for 1 to 3 days produces a depression of deprived eye responses without affecting the responses to stimulation of the open eye. By contrast, 7 days of monocular deprivation yields both deprived-eye depression and potentiation of open-eye responses.

Neurotrophins Regulate Visual Cortical Plasticity

The experience-driven mechanisms that shape the formation and maintenance of geniculo-cortical synapses might reflect a competition between left- and right-eye LGN terminals for a target-derived neurotrophic factor providing activity-dependent trophic support to the incoming fibers. Maffei and his colleagues provided experimental evidence for this idea, showing that exogenous supply of the neurotrophin nerve growth factor (NGF) prevents the effects of monocular lid closure in the developing rat visual system,[60,61] whereas blockade of endogenous NGF action with antibodies severely interferes with development of the cortical ocular dominance distribution[62] and delays the critical period closure.[63]

The brain-derived neurotrophic factor (BDNF) also plays a significant role in activity-dependent visual cortical plasticity. Light strongly activates BDNF mRNA expression[64] and dendritic localization[65] in the rat visual cortex. Blockade of signaling by endogenous BDNF inhibited formation of ocular dominance columns in the cat,[66] while transgenic overexpression of cortical BDNF in mice hastened the formation of intracortical inhibitory synapses and accelerated the onset and closure of the ocular dominance critical period.[67,68]

The site of action of neurotrophins on visual cortical plasticity is not necessarily represented by the LGN afferent fibers. Thus, NGF likely regulates ocular dominance plasticity by acting on the neuromodulatory cholinergic input to the cortex, while BDNF regulates it by inducing the maturation of inhibitory synapses on pyramidal cortical cells, in addition to participating directly in the plasticity of the excitatory synapses (see Chapter 17). Thus, a purely homosynaptic mechanism involving only the thalamocortical afferents provides an incomplete insight into the competitive mechanism for ocular dominance plasticity, and local circuits in the visual cortex must be taken into account.

The Maturation of Inhibitory Circuits Controls the Time Course of the Critical Periods

The refinement of ocular dominance columns involves interactions between excitatory thalamocortical inputs and GABAergic inhibitory cortical interneurons.[69,70] The experience-dependent maturation of GABA-mediated inhibition in the cortex is regulated by BDNF[67,68] and determines the opening of the critical period for plasticity in the visual

[56] Wong, R. O. 1999. *Annu. Rev. Neurosci.* 22: 29-47.

[57] Feller, M. B. 2009. *Neural Dev.* 4: 24.

[58] Zhou, Z. J. 1998. *J. Neurosci.* 18: 4155-4165.

[59] Brivanlou, I. H., Warland, D. K., and Meister, M. 1998. *Neuron* 20: 527-539.

[60] Domenici, L. et al. 1991. *Proc. Natl. Acad. Sci. USA* 88: 8811-8815.

[61] Maffei, L. et al. 1992. *J. Neurosci.* 12: 4651-4662.

[62] Berardi, N. et al.1994. *Proc. Natl. Acad. Sci. USA* 91: 684-688.

[63] Domenici, L. et al. 1994. *Neuroreport* 5: 2041-2044.

[64] Castrén, E., Zafra, F., Thoenen, H., and Lindholm, D. 1992. *Proc. Natl. Acad. Sci. USA* 89: 9444-9448.

[65] Capsoni, S. et al. 1999. *Neuroscience* 88: 393-403.

[66] Cabelli, R. J., Shelton, D. L., Segal, R. A., and Shatz, C. J. 1997. *Neuron* 19: 63-76.

[67] Huang, Z. J. et al. 1999. *Cell* 98: 739-755.

[68] Hanover, J. L., Huang, Z. J., Tonegawa, S., and Stryker, M. P. 1999. *J. Neurosci.* 19: RC40.

[69] Hensch, T. K., and Stryker, M. P. 2004. *Science* 303: 1678-1681.

[70] Hensch, T. K. et al. 1998. *Science* 282: 1504-1508.

system.[69,70] Chronic infusion of cat visual cortex with diazepam, a positive modulator of GABA$_A$ receptors, reduced the binocularity of cortical neurons and broadened anatomically defined ocular dominance columns.[69] Downregulation of GABA$_A$ receptors produced opposite effects. Similarly, knock-out mice lacking the GABA-synthesizing enzyme glutamic acid decarboxylase 65 (GAD$_{65}$) lacked ocular dominance plasticity, and plasticity was restored by cortical infusion of diazepam.[70] Cortical plasticity may involve a specific subtype of GABAergic interneuron. Synapse formation on pyramidal cells in the visual cortex by parvalbumin-positive (PV+) GABAergic neurons is influenced by visual experience during early postnatal life.[71] Remarkably, transplantation of embryonic inhibitory neurons into mouse visual cortex (at postnatal day 10) extended the period of ocular dominance plasticity to postnatal day 43; this is 2 weeks beyond the normal close of the critical period on postnatal day 28.[72]

The transcription factor Otx2 is transported from the retina to the visual cortex in an activity-dependent way, is selectively captured and internalized by PV+ GABAergic interneurons, and controls their maturation, thereby regulating the onset of visual cortical plasticity.[73]

We can conclude that inhibitory interneurons are important for opening and maintaining the period for development of ocular dominance. The levels of intracortical GABA inhibition therefore cross two thresholds: The first threshold allows ocular dominance plasticity to be expressed, thereby opening the critical period; as postnatal development proceeds, the inhibitory tone further increases and crosses a second threshold, after which inhibition drastically reduces the potential for plasticity, closing the critical period.[74]

Reopening the Critical Period and Promoting Adult Ocular Dominance Plasticity

The waning of cortical plasticity and the closure of the critical period for visual plasticity are carried out by the activation of molecular "brakes" that prevent plasticity in the adult brain. Removing these brakes can reopen the critical period in adulthood and promote adult plasticity. The identification of specific processes and molecules that actively suppress plasticity in the adult visual cortex may inform strategies for pharmacological interventions to reopen the critical period.

In normal adult animals, in which inhibitory processes have completed their maturation, a brief reduction of GABAergic inhibition is sufficient to reopen a window of plasticity in the visual cortex, well after the normal closure of the critical period.[75]

While a single well-defined developmental event appears to be linked to the opening of the critical period (i.e., the maturation of PV+ interneuron-mediated inhibition), the mechanisms responsible for the closure of the critical period seem more diverse. One pathway that has been postulated is the developmental switch in the subunits that make up the *N*-methyl-d-aspartate (NMDA) receptor, from the NR2B subunit in young animals to the NR2A subunit in adults. It has been proposed that the shortening of NMDA receptor currents, by NR2A subunit insertion, delimits the critical period for experience-dependent refinement of circuits in visual cortex, but whether this switch plays a causal role in the closure of the critical period is still debated.

The importance of inhibitory interneurons for closure of the critical period received additional support from the role of extracellular matrix (ECM) in synapse stabilization and plasticity.[76] Large perineuronal nets (PNNs) of specific components of the ECM, including the chondroitin sulphate proteoglycans, develop into tightly woven nets around fast-spiking PV+ interneurons at the end of the ocular dominance critical period. Pizzorusso and his colleagues have shown that enzymatic degradation of the molecular lattice of PNNs with chondroitinase ABC reactivates ocular dominance plasticity in the adult visual cortex.[77] This established PNN as a structural brake that limits experience-dependent plasticity, restricting the extent to which neural circuits can undergo plastic changes during late postnatal development, a fact of general relevance for strategies aimed at reopening plasticity in the adult nervous system.[78] PNNs facilitate the internalization of the Otx2 transcription factor in PV+ interneurons, thereby promoting their maturation. In turn, Otx2 modifies PNN structure and composition, indicating a positive feedback loop between PNN and somatic inhibition by PV+ interneurons during the critical period.

Plasticity is accompanied by the regulation of gene expression. Epigenetic mechanisms appear to regulate the expression of genes that control the opening and closure of the critical period. Accumulating evidence suggests that the cortex responds to sensory stimuli via

[71] Chattopadhyaya, B. et al. 2004. *J. Neurosci.* 24: 9598-9611.

[72] Southwell, D. G. et al. 2010. *Science* 327: 1145-1148.

[73] Sugiyama, S. et al. 2008. *Cell* 134: 508-520.

[74] Fagiolini, M., and Hensch, T. 2000 *Nature* 404: 183-186.

[75] Harauzov A. et al. 2010. *J. Neurosci.* 30: 361-371.

[76] Fawcett, J. 2009. *Prog. Brain Res.* 175: 501-509.

[77] Pizzorusso, T. et al. 2002. *Science* 298: 1248-1251.

[78] Sorg, B. A. et al. 2016. *J. Neurosci.* 36: 11459-11468.

dynamic epigenetic changes in DNA methylation and histone post-translation modifications. Accordingly, histone deacetylase inhibition reinstates plasticity in adult visual cortex, allowing for recovery of the effects of amblyopia,[79,80] a disorder of sight in which the visual cortex fails to process inputs from one eye and over time favors inputs from the other eye. Also, monocular deprivation modulated the expression of factors controlling DNA methylation. Inhibition of DNA methyltransferase (DNMT) blocked molecular and functional effects of monocular deprivation.[81] The downstream target genes of histone acetylation, and of DNA methylation, as well as the cells in which transcription of these genes is occurring, have yet to be identified. This will require the study of epigenetic modifications in specific cells of the visual cortex.

What are the structural underpinnings of adult ocular dominance cortical plasticity? Spine dynamics (see Chapter 17) have been investigated using two-photon laser scanning microscopy on apical dendrites of pyramidal neurons in the adult mouse visual cortex, during plasticity of eye-specific responses to repeated closure of one eye (Figure 28.15A).[82] The

[79] Putignano, E. et al. 2007. *Neuron* 53: 747-759.

[80] Baroncelli, L. et al. 2016. *J. Neurosci.* 36: 3430-3440.

[81] Tognini, P. et al. 2015. *Nat. Neurosci.* 18: 956-958.

[82] Hofer, S. B. et al. 2009. *Nature* 457: 313-317.

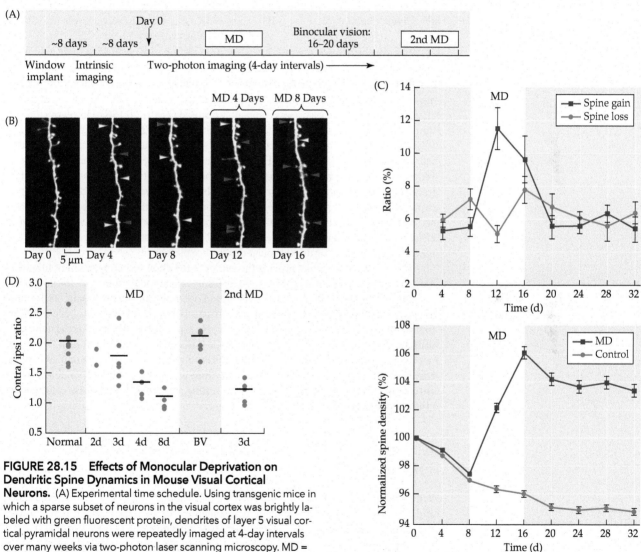

FIGURE 28.15 Effects of Monocular Deprivation on Dendritic Spine Dynamics in Mouse Visual Cortical Neurons. (A) Experimental time schedule. Using transgenic mice in which a sparse subset of neurons in the visual cortex was brightly labeled with green fluorescent protein, dendrites of layer 5 visual cortical pyramidal neurons were repeatedly imaged at 4-day intervals over many weeks via two-photon laser scanning microscopy. MD = monocular deprivation. (B) High-magnification view of a layer 5 apical dendrite. Arrows point to spines appearing (solid red) or disappearing (open blue) compared with the previous imaging session. Monocular deprivation increases the rate of new spine formation in layer 5 neurons in the binocular portion of visual cortex. (C) Percentage of spines appearing (spine gain) and disappearing (spine loss) on layer 5 visual cortex pyramidal neurons imaged at 4-day intervals. Already after a few days of eye closure, more new spines appeared (top graph). Surprisingly, even after the eye was reopened and neurons recovered their normal binocular responses (see part D), many of the new spines persisted and the spine density remained elevated (bottom graph). Error bars are standard error of the mean. (D) Ocular dominance shifts during contralateral eye monocular deprivation, 1-2 weeks after eye reopening (BV, binocular vision) and during a second monocular deprivation episode, measured by intrinsic optic signal imaging and shown as the ratio of contralateral-eye (contra) to ipsilateral-eye (ipsi) response strength. Circles and squares depict data from individual mice; horizontal lines indicate mean values. (After S. B. Hofer et al., 2009. *Nature* 457: 313-317.)

FIGURE 28.16 Time Course of the Critical Period for Ocular Dominance Plasticity in Response to Monocular Deprivation in Rodents. Developmental increase of brain GABAergic inhibition levels is paralleled by a progressive reduction of experience-dependent plasticity. An arbitrary measure of ocular dominance plasticity is plotted against developmental time, normalized to its peak level during the critical period. Onset of the critical period can be anticipated by increasing intracortical inhibition through benzodiazepine treatment or polysialic acid (PSA) removal (blue arrow pointing left). Conversely, the end of the critical period can be delayed by preventing the maturation of GABAergic inhibition through dark rearing from birth (red arrow pointing right). The effects of dark rearing can be counteracted by concomitant environmental enrichment. BDNF overexpression promotes a faster maturation of GABAergic interneurons, acting both on the opening and closure of the critical period, thus shifting leftward the entire developmental plasticity curve. (After A. Sale et al. 2010. *Front. Cell Neurosci.* 4: 10.)

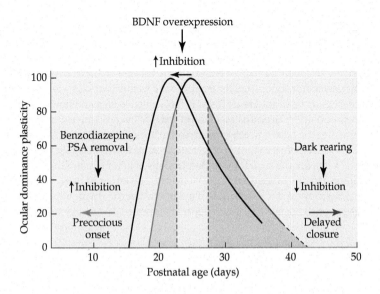

first monocular deprivation episode doubled the rate of new spine formation, thereby increasing the density of dendritic spines in the visual cortex (Figure 28.15B). This increase persisted after normal binocular vision was completely restored (Figure 28.15C). However, closure of the eye a second time did not produce further spine addition. This absence of structural plasticity stands out against the robust changes of eye-specific responses that occur even faster on repeated deprivation (Figure 28.15D). Thus, spines added during the first monocular deprivation episode may provide a structural basis for subsequent functional shifts, a structural trace of prior experience.[82] The increase in dendritic spine dynamics induced by monocular deprivation can be mimicked by degradation of the ECM with the tissue-type plasminogen activator (tPA)/plasmin proteolytic cascade. Monocular deprivation occludes a subsequent effect of ECM degradation on spine dynamics, suggesting that matrix degradation mediates the structural remodeling during ocular dominance plasticity.[83]

Altogether, these results provide the evidence for a common regulation of functional plasticity and specific structural synaptic rearrangements and go some way toward providing a mechanistic explanation of critical period opening and closure. Figure 28.16 shows a schematic representation of the different triggers and brakes that have been described to modulate opening and closure of the critical period, by anticipating or delaying these transitions. Among these, a central player is the intracortical inhibitory system.[69,70,75]

Understanding in detail the local circuits involved in the regulation of plasticity will represent the next step in this investigation. Thus, while it is clear that PV+ interneurons are a central hub controlling critical period timing, the way in which these cells perform critical period gating remains elusive.

Critical Periods in Somatosensory and Olfactory Systems

Whisker barrels constitute a prominent feature of the somatosensory cortex in rodents and correspond exactly in number and arrangement to the large whisker follicles on the rodent snout (see Chapter 23). The whisker-specific patterning of thalamocortical terminals emerges during the 3 days after birth, first with the formation of rows and then with the development of individual whisker follicle representations. Barrels fail to develop if a whisker is ablated in early life.[84] However, such peripheral lesions no longer alter cortical barrels after postnatal day 4,[85] revealing a sensitive period for structural plasticity in the trigeminal pathway.[86] One might expect that fundamental processes such as the formation of somatotopic maps would be driven by intrinsic cues and rely less on sensory experience for direction. Indeed, blockade of peripheral action potentials with TTX does not disrupt cortical barrel formation.[87] At the same time, although overall cortical structure appears normal, rats that have had their whiskers trimmed for the first 3 days of life (but not later)

[83] Oray, S., Majewska, A. and Sur, M. 2004. *Neuron* 44: 1021–1030.

[84] Van der Loos, H., and Woolsey, T. A. 1973. *Science* 179: 395–398.

[85] Rebsam, A., Seif, I., and Gaspar, P. 2005. *J. Neurosci.* 25: 706–710.

[86] Erzurumlu, R. S. 2010. *Exp. Neurol.* 222: 10–12.

[87] Henderson, T. A., Woolsey, T. A., and Jacquin, M. F. 1992. *Brain Res. Dev. Brain Res.* 66: 146–152.

show changes in dendritic structure within the barrels and have both impaired sensory discrimination and reduced social interaction as adults.[88] It is not yet known how such early changes might relate to plasticity in the synaptic organization of the adult barrel cortex.[89] The critical period concept for the whisker-barrel pathway was inspired by the ocular dominance plasticity studies and shares mechanistic aspects with them, such as the dependence on GABAergic inhibition and regulation by perineuronal nets. Such similitudes exist in spite of the differences between the sensory deprivation paradigms used to study both systems—occlusion of an eye by lid suture versus whisker follicle lesions.[90]

Yet another system in which sensory input is required for the development of normal structure is olfaction. The olfactory system remains plastic throughout life because of continuous neurogenesis of olfactory sensory neurons (OSNs; see Chapter 21). Maintaining the precision of the glomerular map in the olfactory bulb, in the presence of continuous lifelong regeneration, poses a particular challenge.

In immature mice, each glomerulus in the bulb is supplied by axons of OSNs that express a variety of distinct olfactory receptor proteins. In the adult, however, each glomerulus is supplied by a group of axons that express the same unique odorant receptor.[91]

Closure of a nostril in the immature rat prevents the normal development of olfactory glomeruli.[92] In contrast, olfactory glomeruli develop normally in mice in which the odorant-activated cyclic nucleotide-gated channel is missing and whose OSNs are electrically inactive.[93] The role of neuronal activity in the formation of olfactory topographic maps is therefore still unclear. Despite the fact that the topography of the olfactory bulb depends on odorant receptor identity, odor-evoked neuronal activity does not appear to have a significant impact on the formation of the sensory map. An additional role of the odorant receptors might provide a clue. Thus, in addition to being present on the cilia of OSNs in the nasal epithelium, where they detect odors, odorant receptors are also present on the axonal terminals of OSNs, where they have been postulated to act as axon guidance molecules.[91] Evidence for a role of olfactory receptors as axon guidance molecules came from recent experiments showing that odorant receptors on axonal terminals bind and respond to ligand molecules expressed in the olfactory bulb.[94] The distinct mechanisms of activation and signaling of the odorant receptors expressed at the opposite locations in OSNs, at the cilia and at the axon terminal, link the specificity of odor perception with the formation of the topographic map in the olfactory bulb.

Evidence for a critical period in the formation of the sensory map in the olfactory bulb was reported by interfering with the developing OSNs in defined time-windows.[95] The convergence of OSNs axons that express the same olfactory receptor onto the same glomerulus can be disrupted, and subsequently recover, during a critical period (before postnatal day 7), but map organization then becomes immutable after critical period closure.

Sensory Deprivation and Critical Periods in the Auditory System

Auditory processing and language acquisition provide familiar examples of the role of sensory experience in development. It is common knowledge that language is most easily acquired in the first years of life. In fact, there is an early loss of perceptual sensitivity to some phonetic distinctions that are not part of the native language; for example, Japanese-speaking infants lose their initial ability to distinguish between "R" and "L" sounds.[96] From clinical studies there is a clear correlation between speech or language delays in hard-of-hearing children and the severity of their hearing loss.[97] The profound importance of human language gives further impetus to studies of developmental plasticity in the auditory system.

Studies in animals have focused on manipulation of the tonotopic map of the cortex by over- or under exposure to selected sound frequencies, with expansion or contraction of related cortical (A1 cortex) representations.[98] For example, exposure of young rats to a continuous pure tone expanded cortical representation for that frequency[99] (Figure 28.17). Plasticity of the tonotopic cortical map (for near threshold tones) is restricted to a brief period from postnatal days 11 to 13,[100] but sensitive periods for more complex acoustic features, such as tuning bandwidth and temporal coding, occur progressively later.[101] The

[88] Lee, L. J. et al. 2009. *Exp. Neurol.* 219: 524-532.

[89] Lebedev, M. A. et al. 2000. *Cereb. Cortex.* 10: 23-31.

[90] Erzurumlu, R. S., and Gaspar, P. 2012. *Eur. J. Neurosci.* 35: 1540-1553.

[91] Wang, F. et al. 1998. *Cell* 93: 47.

[92] Zou, D. J. et al. 2004. *Science* 304: 1976-1979.

[93] Lin, D. M. et al. 2000. *Neuron* 26: 69-80.

[94] Zamparo, I. et al. 2019. *Cell Rep.* 29: 4334-4348.

[95] Tsai, L., and Barnea, G. 2014. *Science* 344: 197.

[96] Werker, J. F., and Tees, R. C. 2005. *Dev. Psychobiol.* 46: 233-251.

[97] Schonweiler, R., Ptok, M., and Radu, H. J. 1998. *Int. J. Pediatr. Otorhinolaryngol.* 44: 251-258.

[98] Sanes, D. H., and Bao, S. 2009. *Curr. Opin. Neurobiol.* 19: 188-199.

[99] Han, Y. K. et al. 2007. *Nat. Neurosci.* 10: 1191-1197.

[100] de Villers-Sidani, E. et al. 2007. *J. Neurosci.* 27: 180-189.

[101] Insanally, M. N. et al. 2009. *J. Neurosci.* 29: 5456-5462.

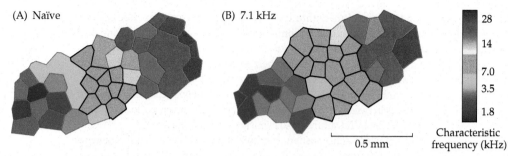

(A) Naïve (B) 7.1 kHz

0.5 mm

Characteristic frequency (kHz)

FIGURE 28.17 **Plasticity of the Tonotopic Map in Auditory Cortex of Young Rats.** Representative cortical tonotopic maps from a naïve rat and a rat that had been exposed to 7.1-kHz tone pips from postnatal days 9 to 30. Each polygon corresponds to a recording site and to the color codes for the characteristic frequency of the recorded neurons. The gray areas had characteristic frequencies in a range of 7.1 kHz ± 0.2 octaves. Note the enlarged representation of frequencies near 7.1 kHz in the tone-exposed animal. (After D. H. Sanes and S. Bao, 2009. *Curr. Opin. Neurobiol.* 19: 188–199, modified from Y. K. Han et al., 2007. *Nat. Neurosci.* 10: 1191–1197.)

[102] Barkat T. R., Polley, D. B. and Hensch T. K. 2011 *Nat. Neurosci.* 14: 1189–1194.

[103] Lippe, W. R. 1994. *J. Neurosci.* 14: 1486–1495.

[104] Jones, T. A. et al. 2007. *J. Neurophysiol.* 98: 1898–1908.

[105] Walsh, E. J., and McGee, J. 1987. *Hear. Res.* 28: 97–116.

[106] Tritsch, N. X. et al. 2007. *Nature* 450: 50–55.

locus of change for the tonotopic plasticity in A1 has been found to be in spine maturation on layer 4 pyramidal cell dendrites.[102]

Studies on the development of lower levels of the auditory pathway have revealed similarities to events in the visual system. As in the developing retina, spontaneous bursting of primary afferent neurons occurs in the immature cochlea before the onset of hearing.[103-105] Bergles and colleagues have delineated the cellular mechanisms underlying this early spontaneous activity and have shown that it depends on transmitter release from sensory hair cells (Figure 28.18).[106] The sensory hair cells in turn are depolarized not by sound (the middle ear remains blocked until postnatal day 12), but rather by release of ATP from nearby supporting cells. As in the retina, waves of excitation spread along the cochlea, causing

(A)

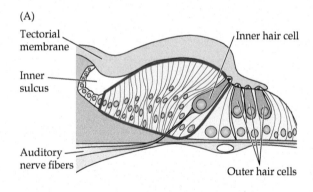

Tectorial membrane
Inner hair cell
Inner sulcus
Auditory nerve fibers
Outer hair cells

(B)

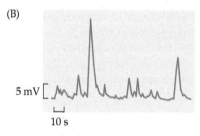

5 mV
10 s

(C)

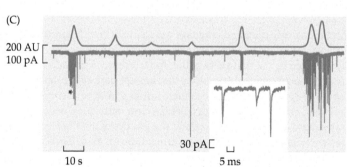

200 AU
100 pA
*
30 pA
10 s
5 ms

FIGURE 28.18 **Spontaneous Purinergic Signaling in the Developing Cochlea.** (A) Drawing of the organ of Corti in a young rat (postnatal day 7). Kölliker's organ (outlined in red) temporarily fills much of the space that will become the inner sulcus. Inner hair cells are activated by ATP released from surrounding cells. (B) Slow changes in membrane potential recorded from a supporting cell in the postnatal-day-7 rat cochlea. (C) ATP-driven slow waves in supporting cells (upper trace, arbitrary units [AU] optical density) excite hair cells to release glutamate onto afferent nerve fibers. The lower trace is a voltage clamp recording from an afferent dendrite showing bursts of glutamatergic synaptic currents elicited from the inner hair cell by ATP released from supporting cells. Inset: Details of synaptic currents from region marked by asterisk (*). (After N. X. Tritsch et al., 2007. *Nature* 450: 50–55.)

intracellular calcium to rise and ATP to be released, exciting neighboring supporting cells. Thus, ATP-mediated excitation causes neighboring hair cells and their postsynaptic afferents to coordinate their activity. The spontaneously active supporting cells make up a transient epithelium called Kölliker's organ that disappears by the onset of hearing, as does the spontaneous bursting of cochlear afferents.[107]

The influence of sensory activity on synaptic structure in brainstem neurons has been studied in congenitally deaf cats by Ryugo, Niparko, and colleagues using cochlear implants to restore hearing (Box 28.1).[108] They focused their attention on the end bulb of Held—a large contact made by cochlear afferent fibers on cells in the cochlear nucleus in the brainstem (see Chapter 13). In young deaf cats (less than 6 months of age), the end bulbs had fewer synaptic vesicles than normal and exhibited expanded postsynaptic densities. When functional hearing was restored with cochlear implants, these morphological changes were reversed (Figure 28.19). Cochlear implants also have reversed the shrinkage of cells in the cochlear nucleus that occurs in deaf animals.[109]

A strong motivation to study the mechanisms of cortical plasticity is to determine whether the adult cortex retains or can regain elements of plasticity for the purpose of repair, or to correct developmental disorders. Comparative studies of birds have provided considerable insight regarding brain plasticity, ranging from learning by songbirds[110] to determination of conditions for plasticity in the auditory system of adult barn owls.

[107] Tritsch, N. X., and Bergles, D. E. 2010. *J. Neurosci.* 30: 1539-1550.

[108] Ryugo, D. K., Kretzmer, E. A., and Niparko, J. K. 2005. *Science* 310: 1490-1492.

[109] Lustig, L. R. et al. 1994. *Hear. Res.* 74: 29-37.

[110] Mooney, R. 2009. *Curr. Opin. Neurobiol.* 19: 654-660.

BOX **28.1**   The Cochlear Implant

Hearing loss is the most common sensory deficit experienced by humans.[111] Exposure to ototoxic compounds, damaging levels of sound (in the workplace or elsewhere), and age-related hearing loss (presbycusis) contribute to significantly elevated hearing thresholds in approximately 25% of people over 50 years of age. Also, 1 to 3 children in 1000 are born with significant hearing loss, 40% of which qualify as profoundly deaf,[112] with a genetic basis for half of these.[113] External hearing aids can relieve partial hearing loss, but until the late twentieth century profound deafness was essentially untreatable. This picture changed dramatically with the advent of the cochlear implant.[114] By December 2012, approximately 324,200 people had received cochlear implants worldwide.[115] Today cochlear implants represent the standard of therapy of congenital deafness in childhood.[115] Cochlear implants have revealed a critical period for therapy of prelingual (congenital) deafness.[116]

In the best cases, a cochlear implant can provide impressive functional recovery, such as telephone use for those who lost hearing as adults or age-appropriate schooling for deaf children implanted in the first year or two of life.

The cochlear implant consists of an array of electrodes inserted into the cochlear coil. An external microphone and analyzer decomposes sound into its frequency components and converts energy within each frequency band into a series of electrical pulses on one of the implant's electrodes. Each electrode activates nearby spiral ganglion neurons–mimicking the frequency-labeled lines provided in the hearing

Low-frequency syllable "ah"   High-frequency syllable "choo"

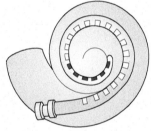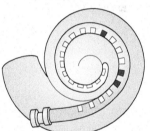

cochlea by synapses with sensory hair cells. The figure shows activation of a cochlear implant by two distinct syllables, "ah" and "choo." "Ah," a vowel sound, activates electrodes farther along the implant, toward low-frequency locations in the cochlea. "Choo" begins with high-frequency frictives (i.e., consonant sounds) and so activates electrodes nearer to the insertion point at the high-frequency base of the cochlea.

[111] Lustig, L. R. 2010. In *The Oxford Handbook of Auditory Science: The Ear.* Oxford University Press, New York. pp. 15-47.

[112] Smith, R. J. et al. 2005. *Lancet* 365: 879-890.

[113] Morton, N. E. 1991. *Ann. N Y Acad. Sci.* 630: 16-31.

[114] Moller, A. R. 2006. *Adv. Otorhinolaryngol.* 64: 1-10.

[115] NIDCC Fact Sheet: Cochlear Implants. National Institute on Deafness and Other Communication Disorders. Publication No. 00-4798 , February 2016. (www.nidcd.nih.gov/sites/default/files/Documents/health/hearing/Cochlear Implants.pdf)

[116] Kral, A. 2013. *Neuroscience* 247: 117-133.

(A) Normal hearing cat

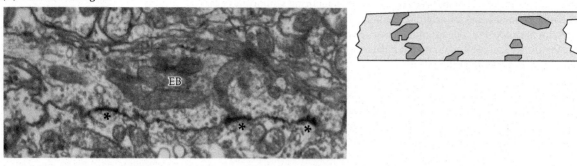

(B) Congenitally deaf cat, untreated

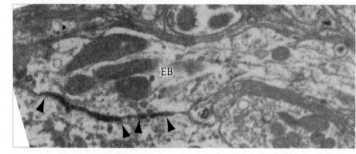

(C) Congenitally deaf cat, cochlear implant

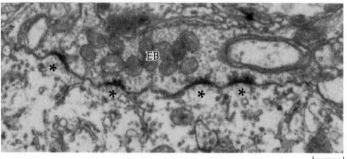

All three photos D. K. Ryugo et al., 2005.
Science 310: 1490–1492.

0.5 μm

0.5 μm

FIGURE 28.19   Synaptic Plasticity in the Cochlear Nucleus.
Electron micrographs of end bulb (EB) synapses from a normal
hearing cat (A), a congenitally deaf cat that was untreated (B), and
a congenitally deaf cat that received 3 months of electrical stimulation from a cochlear implant (C). All micrographs were collected
from cats that were 6 months of age. The hearing and treated cats
exhibit synapses that are punctate, curved, and accompanied by
nearby synaptic vesicles (asterisks). In contrast, the synapses from
the untreated deaf cat are large, flattened, and mostly void of synaptic vesicles (arrowheads). Postsynaptic densities from end bulbs
of Held, indicative of release sites, were reconstructed through
serial sections using three-dimensional software and then rotated
(illustrations on right). These views present the surface of the
bushy plasma membrane that lies under the auditory nerve ending. The shaded regions represent the reconstructed synapses.
The untreated congenitally deaf cat exhibited hypertrophied
synapses, whereas the treated congenitally deaf cat exhibited synapses having normal shapes and distributions. (After D. K. Ryugo
et al., 2005. *Science* 310: 1490–1492.)

Critical Periods in the Auditory System of Barn Owls

During the critical period, neural organization is particularly sensitive to environmental experience; beyond that time, equivalent sensory exposure does not produce an equivalent change
in brain circuitry. The critical period serves to form an animal's nervous system in a way that
is optimally adapted to the environment, and accordingly, one would expect the changes to
be relatively permanent. However, emerging evidence indicates that even fundamental aspects of established circuitry can be modified if required by an altered environment.[117] This
adaptability has been illustrated by the experiments of Knudsen and his colleagues on barn
owls.[118] Early experience shapes the auditory spatial localization of neurons in the barn owl's

[117] Keuroghlian, A. S., and Knudsen, E. I.
2007. *Prog. Neurobiol.* 82: 109–121.

[118] Knudsen, E. I. 1999. *J. Comp. Physiol.
A* 185: 305–321.

optic tectum in a frequency-dependent manner.[119] The resulting auditory space map must be aligned with the visual world for the owl to locate and capture mice with optimum efficiency. The following account shows how altered visual input influences the representation of the auditory system in the owl's brain, a remarkable example of cross-modal plasticity.

Barn owls are able to locate sound sources with exceptional accuracy.[120] Horizontal location is achieved by turning the head until the interaural time difference (see Chapter 24) is zero. Vertical localization is enabled by the fact that asymmetrical earflaps collect sound from above for one ear and from below for the other. So the head is tilted up or down until the sound intensity is equal in the two ears. The owl's eyes provide another index of the position and path taken by mice. Figure 28.20A shows that in normal adult owls the neural maps for

[119] Gold, J. I., and Knudsen, E. I. 1999. *J. Neurophysiol.* 82: 2197-2209.

[120] Moiseff, A. 1989. *J. Comp. Physiol. A* 164: 637-644.

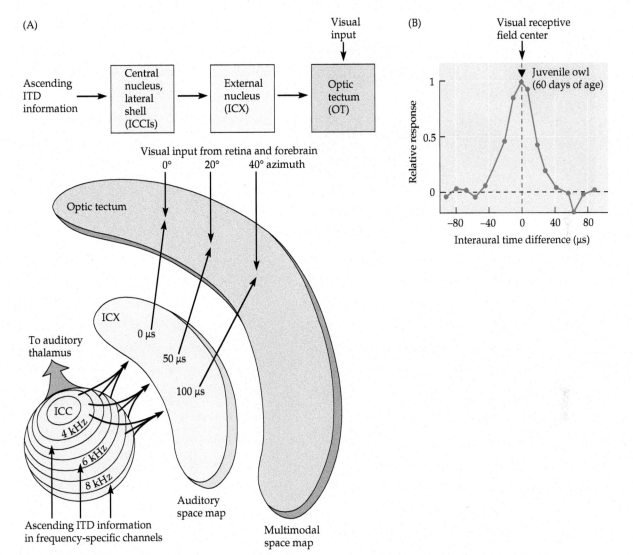

FIGURE 28.20 Superimposition of Auditory and Visual Space Maps in the Optic Tectum of a Barn Owl. (A) Ascending auditory pathway to the optic tectum. Auditory neurons in the nuclei of the internal inferior colliculus (ICC) and external inferior colliculus (ICX) are tonotopically arranged. They project to the optic tectum, maintaining an orderly sequence. The auditory space map depends on the time difference of the arrival of sounds in the two ears. Auditory and visual space maps are in register with each other. Thus, neurons that one records from the position marked "0 μs" respond to visual and auditory stimuli that are directly in front of the bird. ITD = interaural time difference. (B) Graph of responses by a neuron to interaural time differences plotted in a juvenile owl 60 days of age. The time difference between the two sounds indicates the position to the left or to the right. The neuron that responds to the time value of a 0-μs interval in interaural time difference fires best when the stimulus is directly in front of the animal, corresponding to a receptive field position at the center of the visual field. Sounds coming from the left or the right of the owl reach the ears with a delay, activating neurons with different response curves, peaks being displaced from 0 μs and in register with optical stimuli. (A after E. I. Knudsen, 1999. *J. Comp. Physiol. A* 185: 305-321; B after D. E. Feldman and E. I. Knudsen,1997. *J. Neurosci.* 17: 6820-6837. © 1997 Society for Neuroscience.)

visual and auditory space are precisely aligned in one layer of the optic tectum (which corresponds to the superior colliculus in mammals). Such maps were produced by measuring responses evoked in individual neurons in the tectum by sound stimuli from different locations and by light presented in different parts of the visual field (Figure 28.20B).

Baby owls were raised with visual fields displaced by 23° to the left or the right by prisms placed over their eyes (Figure 28.21A).[121,122] As a result, the image of the visual field on the retina and hence on the tectum was shifted so that the visual and auditory maps were no longer in alignment (Figure 28.21B,C). Over the next 6 to 8 weeks, the auditory space map shifted until it once again came into exact register with the new, displaced visual map. As a result, the owl became able to orient its eyes toward sounds in spite of the prisms. When the prisms were removed, the visual and auditory maps were again out of register. Provided that the owls were less than 200 days old, the auditory map shifted a second time

[121] Knudsen, E. I., and Knudsen, P. F. 1990. *J. Neurosci.* 10: 222-232.
[122] Feldman, D. E., and Knudsen, E. I. 1997. *J. Neurosci.* 17: 6820-6837.

(A)

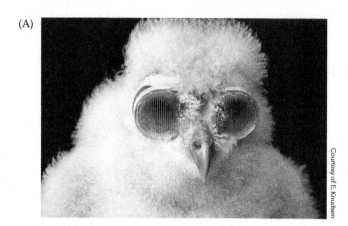

Courtesy of E. Knudsen

(B)

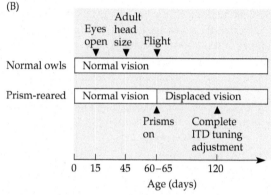

(C)

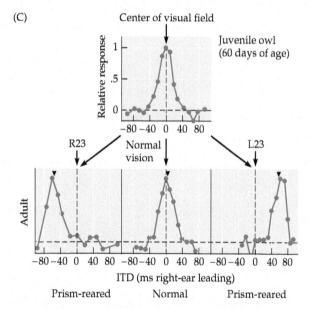

(D) Time course of correction of auditory maps at various ages

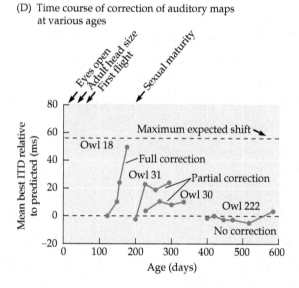

FIGURE 28.21 Shift of Auditory Receptive Fields after Application of Prisms during the Critical Period.
(A) A baby owl with glasses consisting of prisms that offset its visual field by 23° to the right (or left, depending on the spectacles). (B) Stages at which prisms were placed on owl eyes. (C) Tuning curves showing responses to sounds with different interaural time differences (ITDs). In the normal juvenile owl at 60 days, the response of the neurons resemble that in Figure 28.20B in which an ITD value of 0 µs corresponds to the center of the visual field. After rearing with prisms for 6-8 weeks, the tuning curves of owls (120 days old) were shifted. Visual

receptive fields were displaced to the left or the right by 23°. Now the best responses (small arrowheads) of the auditory neurons occurred at ITDs that corresponded to the displaced visual fields. The auditory and visual maps were again in register. (D) Time course of shift in auditory tuning curves in three juvenile owls and one adult. The adult (owl 222) showed no correction. (B,C after D. E. Feldman and E. I. Knudsen,1997. *J. Neurosci.* 17: 6820-6837; © 1997 Society for Neuroscience; D after M. S. Brainard and E. I. Knudsen, 1998. *J. Neurosci.* 18: 3929-3942. © 1998 Society for Neuroscience.)

to align in register with the original visual map (Figure 28.21D). In other tests, it was shown that owls that had once learned to adapt to prisms in early life could reestablish these connections as adults, unlike animals that had no such experience beforehand.[123]

Effects of Enriched Sensory Experience in Early Life

Since the flexibility of connections and structure in early life make the brain vulnerable to sensory deprivation, it is natural to wonder whether enrichment and a fuller early life during the critical period could enhance cortical function. Tests to assess this outcome have been pioneered by Rosenzweig, who initiated the so-called enriched environment (EE) approach.[124] EE consists of wide cages in which animals are reared in large social groups and in the presence of a variety of stimulating objects, which are changed regularly to stimulate explorative behavior, curiosity, attentional processes, and voluntary physical exercise. EE has long been exploited to investigate the influence of the environment on structure and function in sensory systems. Recently, EE has been shown to accelerate the development of the visual system, to reverse the effects of dark rearing, and to enhance visual cortex plasticity in adulthood.[125] EE appears to stimulate the same class of molecular and cellular mediators that control the opening and closure of visual cortical plasticity (including BDNF and the GABAergic inhibitory system), as well as the insulin-like growth factor 1 (IGF-1) signaling pathway.

An interesting and unexpected effect of enrichment in early life was found by Brainard and Knudsen[126] in barn owls, using the visual field displacements already mentioned. In a second set of experiments, they repeated their earlier procedures, with one important difference in the way the young owls were brought up. Instead of the young owl being confined on its own in a cage (as in the earlier experiments), it spent the first weeks of life in an aviary where it lived with other owls and was able to fly around. In these owls with enriched experience, Brainard and Knudsen confirmed that, as before, the effect of a visual field displacement in early life was corrected in the tectum by realignment of the auditory field onto the new position of the visual field. And as before, when the prisms were removed from the young animals the auditory field moved back to its original mapping in the cortex, thereby allowing auditory and visual responses to be matched. However, in contrast to the earlier experiment, now this realignment could occur after periods longer than 200 days, at times when the owl had matured and become adult. Thus, the richer early environment lengthened the period of adaptability in the auditory system.

Behavioral relevance also can have profound influences on brain plasticity, even in adults.[127] Ordinarily, adult owls never adapt to the effect of displacing prisms. However, adult owls that had to hunt live mice (rather than simply receiving dead mice) adapted

[123] Knudsen, E. I. 1998. *Science* 279: 1531–1533.

[124] Rosenzweig, M. R., and Bennet, E. L. 1996. *Behav. Brain Res.* 78: 57–65.

[125] Sale, A. et al. 2014. *Physiol. Rev* 94: 189–234.

[126] Brainard, M. S., and Knudsen, E. I. 1998. *J. Neurosci.* 18: 3929–3942.

[127] Bergan, J. F. et al. 2005. *J. Neurosci.* 25: 9816–9820.

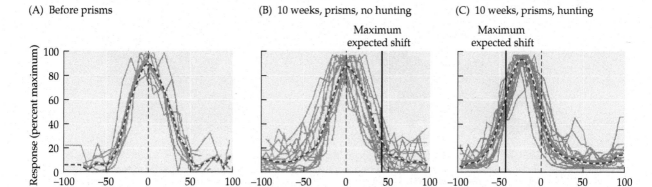

FIGURE 28.22 Effect of Prism Experience, with and without hunting, on interaural time difference (ITD) tuning in the optic tectum of an adult barn owl. Negative ITDs designate left-ear leading ITDs. Shown are ITD tuning curves derived from all sites sampled in the same bird. Gray lines are curves from individual sites; red dashed lines are population averages. (A) Data collected before prism experience. (B) Data collected from the same owl after 10 weeks of experience with rightward-shifting prisms and no hunting. (C) Data collected from the same owl after 10 weeks of experience with leftward-shifting prisms and hunting. The shifts in ITD tuning were larger and more consistent when the owl had to hunt live prey. (After J. F. Bergan et al., 2005. *J. Neurosci.* 25: 9816–9820. © 2005 Society for Neuroscience.)

partially to prisms over the eyes that displaced the visual fields (Figure 28.22). Interaural time differences measured in the optic tectum were essentially unchanged after 10 weeks of displacing prisms in adult owls that were fed dead mice. However, when adult owls with displacing prisms were required to hunt live mice for 10 weeks, interaural time differences in the optic tectum were shifted approximately half the expected maximum (somewhat less than in juveniles). What is particularly striking here is that all the adult birds had otherwise identical experiences, including flight in an open aviary. The additional impact of hunting was to couple a reward (food) with the desired change in circuitry, emphasizing that motivation is an important parameter in brain plasticity.

The impact of behavioral conditioning has also been shown in mapping of the rat auditory cortex. The usual sensitive period for frequency representation in rat primary auditory cortex is from postnatal days 11 to 13.[100] However, reward conditioning can alter frequency mapping in the adult.[128] When adult rats were trained to distinguish either specific frequencies or specific intensities of sounds, substantial shifts were produced in the representation of those parameters in auditory cortex (Figure 28.23). Although all

128 Polley, D. B., Steinberg, E. E., and Merzenich, M. M. 2006. *J. Neurosci.* 26: 4970–4982.

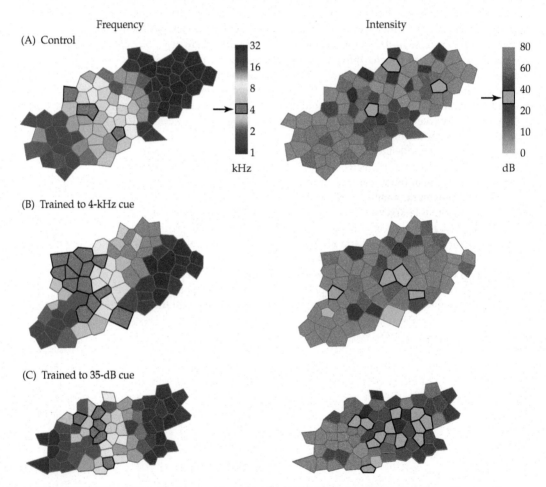

FIGURE 28.23 Task-Specific Reorganization of Cortical Maps in Primary Auditory Cortex of Rats. Adult rats were trained to respond to either a specific tone frequency or specific tone intensity. Multi-unit recordings were made to characterize the best frequency and best intensity level throughout primary auditory cortex. Each polygon represents a single recording site. (A) The resulting control maps are shown for frequency (left) and intensity (right). Four gray polygons responded to 4 kHz; three blue polygons were selective for the 35-decibel (dB) intensity. Color scales are shown on the right. (B) Rats trained to the 4-kHz frequency cue showed expanded representation of that frequency (left, gray polygons), but no increase in representation of the 35-dB or best-intensity frequency (right, blue polygons). (C) Rats trained to the 35-dB intensity cue showed expansion of that best intensity (right, blue polygons) but no major change in representation of the 4-kHz frequency (left, gray polygons). Note as well that much of the cortex responds best to 80-dB sound (right panels, green polygons), while the effect of training to 35 dB has greatly reduced the 80-dB best area (right panel, bottom row). (After D. B. Polley et al., 2006. *J. Neurosci.* 26: 4970–4982. © 2006 Society for Neuroscience.)

animals received identical sound exposures, only the rewarded (i.e., motivated) component gained cortical representation.

The ability to alter the adult cortex has potential significance for overcoming lesions or combating degenerative and developmental disorders. Evidence continues to accumulate that experience-dependent plasticity extends to greater ages for higher-order cortical functions. One can expect that different molecular and cellular mechanisms will be responsible at different times, but that a core mechanism might be shared.

Common Molecular Pathways Controlling Critical Periods in Different Systems

How generally might these same mechanisms apply to critical periods in other parts of the brain? Investigations on the critical periods for plasticity in different brain systems allow us to identify common pathways. Neurotrophins, neuromodulators (cholinergic and serotoninergic), inhibitory interneurons, and PNN components of the extracellular matrix are established factors that control cortical plasticity in different sensory systems. For instance, PNNs are causally linked to the closure of the critical period not only in the visual[77] and the barrel cortex[129] but also in the zebra finch brain in relation to song learning.[130] In rodents, conditioned fear can be eliminated during early life by extinction training but is protected from erasure in adulthood. A developmental progression of PNN formation around PV+ cells coincides with this switch, and enzymatic degradation of PNNs in the adult amygdala reopens a critical period during which fear memories are once again fully erased by extinction training.[131]

Still more candidates are emerging as transcriptomic strategies are used to examine gene expression during development and after altered experience, providing candidate targets for plasticity modulation.[132–134] A candidate identified from transcriptomic screens was Lynx, an endogenous inhibitor of nicotinic acetylcholine receptors (nAChRs), which promotes nAchR desensitization and acts as a cholinergic brake that actively limits plasticity in the adult visual cortex.[135] Knocking out Lynx1 extends the critical period into adulthood.[99] Lynx1 likely modulates excitatory and inhibitory (E/I) balance, because treatment with diazepam in Lynx1 knock-out mice abolishes adult plasticity by restoring this balance to normal adult levels.

The small noncoding microRNAs (miRNAs; see Chapter 17) are emerging as new players in the control of critical periods in cortical plasticity, via a fine-tuning of the translation and degradation of their target mRNAs. Among these, the experience-dependent miR-132 is important for ocular dominance plasticity. Surprisingly, manipulating miR-132 in vivo, by either increasing[136] or decreasing its levels,[137] completely blocks ocular dominance plasticity during the critical period, suggesting that among its target mRNAs there are positive and negative effectors of plasticity, whose levels need to be carefully tuned.

In conclusion, investigations into the visual system of rodents have discovered several new mechanisms relevant for the opening and closure of the critical period for cortical plasticity. The relevance of studying the visual system of mice and rats has been the object of discussions,[138] because rodents are poorly visual animals and view the world at a very low resolution. However, most of the proposed pathways appear to be involved also in the regulation of the critical period in other sensory systems, and many have also been confirmed in other more visual species, thus validating the generality of the conclusions reached.

Critical Periods in Humans, and Clinical Consequences

The susceptibility of cortical development in animals during early life is reminiscent of clinical observations made in humans. It has long been known that removal of a clouded or opaque lens (or cataract) in adults can lead to a restoration of vision, even though the individual has been blind for many years. In contrast, a cataract developed in a newborn or premature baby in the past often led to blindness. Before Hubel and Wiesel's experiments, cataracts were removed from children at a late stage, when they were considered to be ready for the operation. The result was that blindness was permanent, without the possibility of recovery.[139] More recently, cataracts in newborn babies are removed by surgery as early as possible, with

[129] McRae, P.A. et al. 2007 *J. Neurosci.* 27: 5405-5413.

[130] Balmer, T. S. et al.2009 *J. Neurosci.* 29: 12878-12885.

[131] Gogolla, N., Caroni, P., Luethi, A., and Herry, C. 2009 *Science* 325: 1258.

[132] Tropea, D., Van Wart, A., and Sur, M. 2009. *Philos. Trans. R. Soc. Lond., B, Biol. Sci.* 364: 341-355.

[133] Lyckman, A. W. et al. 2008. *Proc. Natl. Acad. Sci. USA* 105: 9409-9414.

[134] Majdan, M., and Shatz, C. J. 2006 *Nat. Neurosci.* 9: 650-659.

[135] Morishita, H. et al.2010 *Science* 33: 1238-1240.

[136] Tognini, P. et al. 2011. *Nat. Neurosci.* 14: 1237-1239.

[137] Mellios, N. et al. 2011. *Nat. Neurosci.* 14: 1240-1242.

[138] Seabrook, T. A. et al. 2017. *Annu. Rev. Neurosci.* 40: 499-538.

[139] Francois, J. 1979. *Ophthalmology* 86: 1586-1598.

excellent prospects for full vision.[140,141] Another clinical example is the modification of treatment of cross-eyed or wall-eyed children. Routinely, the good eye used to be patched for prolonged periods in order to encourage use of the weaker eye. This can lead to loss of acuity in the patched eye, depending on the child's age at the time and the duration of patching.[142] Such prolonged patching is no longer routinely practiced. Clinical observations suggest that the greatest sensitivity occurs in babies during the first year but that the critical period may vary in length for different aspects of vision.[143] The brain's intrinsic potential for plasticity is not lost with age but instead is actively constrained, beyond critical periods, by a set of plasticity "brakes." Learning how to remove these "brakes" in order to unmask plasticity in adulthood will lead to targeted therapeutic strategies to promote amblyopia recovery.[144]

The parallel with experiments in animals extends to anatomical studies of postmortem human brain tissue. Cytochrome oxidase staining of layer 4 of the visual cortex in postmortem human brains has shown that monocular deprivation causes changes in ocular dominance columns similar to those in monkeys or kittens. Horton and Hocking[34] have studied the patterns of staining in the primary visual cortex of people that had grown up after having had one eye surgically removed at 1 week of age because of a tumor. In the postmortem brains, as expected, the staining in layer 4C was uniform instead of displaying clear territories for each eye, as in people with normal vision or in people who have had one eye removed in adult life. Again as predicted from animal studies, a long-term strabismus in an individual who developed a squint in the second year of life (after closure of the critical period) showed no changes in column width postmortem at the age of 79.[145]

The development of cochlear implants illustrates the enormous benefit that can accrue by tapping into the brain's ability to reorganize with altered sensory input. These prosthetic devices can restore functional hearing after the loss of sensory hair cells. The implant consists of a series of electrodes inserted into the cochlear duct (see Box 28.1). An external pickup converts sound waves into their component frequencies and applies electrical signals **tonotopically** to the inserted electrodes, which in turn activate nearby spiral ganglion neurons. Although these devices continue to improve, even the optimum performance is exceedingly limited compared with the selective signaling of the thousands of hair cells they replace. Nonetheless, cochlear implants can enable speech comprehension (even on the telephone) for deaf adults with previously developed spoken language.[146] Still more impressive is the performance achieved by profoundly deaf children provided with implants early in life—some of whom achieve age-appropriate language skills.[147] Longitudinal studies of children given cochlear implants between 18 months and 5 years of age show that the earlier the implant is received, the better is the development of language comprehension and expression. The outcome of cochlear implantation in prelingually (i.e., congenitally) deaf children is optimal only in early implantations (within the first 1–3 years of life), indicating the existence of a critical period for the therapy of human prelingual deafness.[115,148]

Also, as predicted from animal studies on enriched environment paradigms, better outcomes are correlated with more extensive parent–child interactions and socioeconomic status. Even apparently minor levels of hearing loss can have long-term consequences. For example, chronic middle ear infections in childhood can result in long-lasting binaural hearing deficits.

A wealth of literature related to other complex behavioral processes, in a variety of animals, also shows periods of susceptibility. Behavioral studies in dogs indicate that if they are handled by humans during a critical period of 4 to 8 weeks after birth, they are far more tractable and tame than animals that have been isolated from human contact.[149] Imprinting is another well-known example. Lorenz[150] has shown that a duck will follow any moving object, provided it is presented during the first day after hatching, and will act throughout life as if that object were its mother. Similarly, birdsongs, such as produced by zebra finches, depend on the tutorial songs that the juvenile birds hear during a critical period.[116] Birds of a particular species will remember and reproduce appropriate (but not inappropriate) melodies that they hear in early life, although they might be exposed to multiple song models, try out different ones, and even preserve memories of discarded songs.[151]

Infantile amnesia, the inability of adults to recollect early episodic memories, is associated with the rapid forgetting that occurs in childhood. Although early memories are inaccessible to adults, early-life events, such as neglect or aversive experiences, can greatly affect adult behavior and may predispose individuals to various psychopathologies. The long-lasting

[140] Lloyd, I. C. et al. 2007. *Eye (Lond)*. 21: 1301-1309.

[141] Hamill, M. B., and Koch, D. D. 1999. *Curr. Opin. Ophthalmol.* 10: 4-9.

[142] Daw, N. W. 1998. *Arch. Ophthalmol.* 116: 502-505.

[143] Lewis, T. L., and Maurer, D. 2005. *Dev. Psychobiol.* 46: 163-183.

[144] Hensch, T. K., and Quinlan, E. M. 2018 *Vis. Res.* 35: E024.

[145] Horton, J. C., and Hocking, D. R. 1996. *Vis. Neurosci.* 13: 787-795.

[146] Fallon, J. B., Irvine, D. R., and Shepherd, R. K. 2008. *Hear Res.* 238: 110-117.

[147] Niparko, J. K., and Marlowe, A. 2010. In *The Oxford University Handbook of Auditory Science: The Ear*. Oxford University Press, New York. pp. 409-436.

[148] Niparko J. K. et al. 2010 *JAMA* 303: 1498-1506.

[149] Fuller, J. L. 1967. *Science* 158: 1645-1652.

[150] Lorenz, K. 1970. *Studies in Animal and Human Behavior*. Harvard University Press, Cambridge, MA.

[151] Prather, J. F. et al. 2010. *J. Neurosci.* 30: 10586-10598.

influence of episodic infantile experiences poses a paradox: How can episodes that are rapidly forgotten, and of which there is no recollection in adulthood, exert a lifelong effect on the brain? Cristina Alberini and her colleagues, using a model of episodic contextual fear memory in rats, showed that an experience learned during the infantile amnesia period (postnatal day 17) is stored as a latent memory trace for a long time; indeed, reminders later in life reinstate a robust, context-specific, and long-lasting memory.[152] The formation and storage of this latent memory occur through mechanisms typical of developmental critical periods, including the switch of NMDA receptor subunits from 2B to 2A in the hippocampus, which is dependent on BDNF and metabotropic glutamate receptor 5 (mGluR5). Activating mGluR5 or increasing BDNF in the hippocampus closes the infantile amnesia period and accelerates the acquisition of hippocampal functional competence. These data highlight a developmental critical period, for learning to learn and to remember.[153]

The critical period in an animal's development seems to correspond to a time during which a significant sharpening of senses or faculties occurs. Why should plasticity in early life be so pronounced? The developing brain must not only form itself but must be able to represent the outside world, the body, and its movements.[154] The eye, for example, must grow to be the right size for distant objects to be in focus on the retina through the relaxed lens. And the two eyes, separated by different distances in different newborn babies, must act together. As if this were not enough, gross changes occur in limb length, skull diameter, and therefore body image in the first months and years of life. At all times, the maps in the brain for different functions must be in register, as in the owl experiments of Knudsen and his colleagues.

Will lessons from animal studies of brain plasticity guide future therapeutic strategies? This is certainly to be hoped for, since deficits in communication and social behavior can have such debilitating consequences.[155] Indeed, it is tempting to speculate about the effects of deprivation on higher functions in humans. Neglect and early adversities can interfere with brain development and wiring, leading to severe psychopathologies such as depression and anxiety, as well as to learning and cognitive disabilities and neuropsychiatric disorders, as demonstrated by the Bucharest Early Intervention Project—the first randomized controlled trial of a foster care intervention for infants and young children who were exposed to early psychosocial adversity.[156,157] Orphans and neglected children need to be placed with caring foster families before 2 years of age in order to develop cognitive, social, and intellectual skills, as they are not able to recover normal function if they are placed later in similar foster homes. Comparable effects are seen for the development of the primary sensory systems. Critical periods in infancy and childhood are developmental windows of opportunity and vulnerability, and what happens in those periods imposes long-term effects that persist into adulthood.

Why is the brain able to recover function early in life, but loses this ability with maturity? Can we recreate the plasticity of the immature brain later in life and eventually recover proper function? We have seen in this chapter that a precise balance of cortical excitatory and inhibitory (E/I) neurotransmission gates entry and exit of critical period plasticity and that manipulating this balance allows reopening of cortical plasticity. Accumulating evidence suggests that neurodevelopmental and neuropsychiatric disorders, including schizophrenia, autism spectrum disorders, and intellectual disabilities, may result from disruption of this E/I balance early in life, due to a combination of genetic or environmental causes.[158] It is tempting to speculate that neuropsychiatric and neurodevelopmental disorders may result from disruption of the expression or timing of critical periods across brain regions[159-161] and that manipulation of the triggers and brakes that control critical periods might help in developing new and much-needed therapeutic interventions.

One can imagine, as Hubel has said,

> Perhaps the most exciting possibility for the future is the extension of this type of work to other systems besides sensory. Experimental psychologists and psychiatrists both emphasize the importance of early experience on subsequent behavior patterns—could it be that deprivation of social contacts or the existence of other abnormal emotional situations early in life may lead to a deterioration or distortion of connections in some yet unexplored parts of the brain?[162]

To find a physiological basis for such behavioral questions seems a distant, but not impossible, goal.

[152] Travaglia, A. et al. 2016 *Nat. Neurosci.*19: 1225-1233.

[153] Alberini, C., and Travaglia, A. 2017 *J. Neurosci.* 37: 5783-5795.

[154] Singer, W. 1995. *Science* 270: 758-764.

[155] Blakemore, S. J. 2010. *Neuron* 65: 744-747.

[156] Zeanah, C. H. et al. 2009 *Am J. Psychiatry* 166: 777-785.

[157] Nelson C. A. et al. 2007 *Science* 318: 1937-1940.

[158] Marin, O. 2012. *Nat. Rev. Neurosci.* 10: 7834.

[159] Marin, O. 2016. *Nat. Med.* 22: 1229-1238.

[160] LeBlanc, J. J., and Fagiolini, M. 2011 *Neural Plast.* Epub 2011: 921680.

[161] Cameron, J. L. et al. 2017 *J. Neurosci.* 37: 10783-10791.

[162] Hubel, D. H. 1967. *The Physiologist* 10: 17-45.

SUMMARY

- Receptive fields and cortical architecture in newborn monkeys and kittens resemble those of adults in many respects.

- In layer 4 of the cortex, however, incoming axons from the lateral geniculate nucleus overlap and cells are driven by both eyes instead of just one during the first 6 weeks of life.

- A critical period of about 3 months exists after birth, during which closure of the lids of one eye causes changes in structure and function.

- Closure of the lids of one eye leads to blindness in that eye. Cortical cells are no longer driven by the deprived eye, and its ocular dominance columns shrink.

- After the critical period, closure of lids does not change cortical architecture.

- Binocular lid closure or induction of squint during the critical period does not cause changes in ocular dominance columns but does prevent binocular responses. Such results suggest that the two eyes compete for cells in the visual cortex.

- Endogenous spontaneous activity of the sensory periphery shapes cortical organization before the onset of sensory function.

- Inhibitory cortical parvalbumin-positive interneurons are key players in opening and maintaining cortical critical periods.

- Perineuronal nets are extracellular matrix structures that wrap around GABAergic interneurons and limit plasticity.

- The closure of the critical period for visual plasticity is carried out by the emergence of molecular "brakes" that actively prevent plasticity in the adult brain. Removing these brakes can reopen the critical period in adulthood and promote adult plasticity.

- In adult barn owls the neural maps for visual and auditory space are precisely aligned in the optic tectum.

- In baby owls raised with prisms placed over their eyes, the visual field is displaced and the auditory space map adjusts to the misalignment, bringing the visual and auditory maps into register again.

- The plasticity of visual-auditory integration in barn owls is enhanced by enrichment in early life or behavioral motivation.

- In rodent models for infantile amnesia, a critical period for hippocampal learning has been observed.

Suggested Reading

General Reviews

Adams, D. L., and Horton, J. C. 2009. Ocular dominance columns: Enigmas and challenges. *Neuroscientist* 15: 62–77.

Alberini, C., and Travaglia, A. 2017. Infantile Amnesia: A critical period of learning to learn and remember *J. Neurosci.* 37: 5783–5795.

Crowley, J. C., and Katz, L. C. 2002. Ocular dominance columns revisited. *Curr. Op. Neurobiol.* 12: 104–109.

Daw, N. 2006. *Visual Development,* 2nd ed. Springer, New York.

Erzurumlu, R. 2010. Critical period for the whisker-barrel system. *Exp. Neurol.* 222: 10–12.

Hanganu-Opatz, I. 2010. Between molecules and experience: role of early patterns of coordinated activity for the development of cortical maps and sensory abilities. *Brain Res. Rev.* 64: 160–176.

Hensch, T. K. 2004. Critical period regulation. *Annu. Rev. Neurosci.* 27: 549–579.

Hofer, S. B., Mrsic-Flogel, T. D., Bonhoeffer, T., and Hübener, M. 2008 Experience leaves a lasting structural trace in cortical circuits. *Nature* 457: 313–317.

Hooks, B. M., and Chen, C. 2007. Critical periods in the visual system: changing views for a model of experience-dependent plasticity. *Neuron* 56: 312–326.

Hubel, D. H., and Wiesel, T. N. 2005. *Brain and Visual Perception.* Oxford University Press, New York.

Huebener M., and Bonhoeffer, T. 2014. Neuronal plasticity: Beyond the critical period. *Cell* 159: 727–737.

Katz, L. C. and Crowley J. C. 2002 Development of cortical circuits: lessons from ocular dominance columns. *Nat. Rev. Neurosci.* 3: 34–42.

LeBlanc J. J., and Fagiolini, M. 2011 Autism: A "critical period" disorder? *Neural Plast.* doi: 10.1155/2011/921680.

Keroughlian, A., and Knudsen, E. 2007. Adaptive auditory plasticity in developing and adult animals. *Prog. Neurobiol.* 82: 109–121.

Morin, O. 2016, Development timing and critical windows for the treatment of psychiatric disorders. *Nature Med.* 22: 1229–1238.

Sanes, D., and Bao, S. 2009. Tuning up the developing auditory CNS. *Curr. Opin. Neurobiol.* 19: 188–199.

Schreiner C. E., and Polley D. B. 2014 Auditory map plasticity: diversity in causes and consequences. *Curr. Op. Neurobiol.* 24: 143–156

Sorg, B. A., Berretta, S., Blacktop, J. M., Fawcett, J. W., Kitagawa, H., Kwok, J. C. F., and Miquel, M. 2016 Casting a wide net: role of perineuronal nets in neural plasticity. *J. Neurosci.* 36: 11459–11468.

Takesian A. E. and Hensch T. K. 2013 balancing Plasticity/stability across brain development. *Prog. Brain Res.* 207: 3–33.

Trachtenberg J.T. 2015 Competition, inhibition, and critical periods of cortical plasticity. *Curr. Op. Neurobiol.* 35: 44–48.

Tropea, D., Van Wart, A., and Sur, M. 2009. Molecular mechanisms of experience-dependent plasticity in visual cortex. *Philos. Trans. R. Soc. Lond., B, Biol. Sci.* 364: 341–355.

Wiesel, T. N. 1982. The postnatal development of the visual cortex and the influence of environment. Nature 299: 583–591.

Original Papers

Antonini, A., Gillespie, D. C., Crair, M. C., and Stryker, M. P. 1998. Morphology of single geniculocortical afferents and functional recovery of the visual cortex after reverse monocular deprivation in the kitten. *J. Neurosci.* 18: 9896–9909.

Bergan, J. F., Ro, P., Ro, D., and Knudsen, E. I. 2005. Hunting increases adaptive auditory map plasticity in adult barn owls. *J. Neurosci.* 25: 9816–9820.

Brainard, M. S., and Knudsen, E. I. 1998. Sensitive periods for visual calibration of the auditory space map in the barn owl optic tectum. *J. Neurosci.* 18: 3929–3942.

Carlson, M., Hubel, D. H., and Wiesel, T. N. 1986. Effects of monocular exposure to oriented lines on monkey striate cortex. *Brain Res.* 390: 71–81.

Chattopadhyaya, B., Di Cristo, G., Higashiyama, H., Knott, G. W., Kuhlman, S. J., Welker, E., and Huang, Z. J. 2004. Experience and activity-dependent maturation of perisomatic GABAergic innervation in primary visual cortex during a postnatal critical period. *J. Neurosci.* 24: 9598–9611.

Crowley, J. C., and Katz, L. C. 2000. Early development of ocular dominance columns. *Science* 290: 1321–1324.

de Villers-Sidani, E., Chang, E. F., Bao, S., and Merzenich, M. M. 2007. Critical period window for spectral tuning defined in the primary auditory cortex (A1) in the rat. *J. Neurosci.* 27: 180–189.

Fagiolini, M., and Hensch, T. 2000. Inhibitory threshold for critical-period activation in primary visual cortex. *Nature* 404: 183–186.

Galli, L., and Maffei, L. 1988. Spontaneous impulse activity of rat retinal ganglion cells in prenatal life. *Science* 242: 90–91.

Hensch, T. K., and Stryker, M. P. 2004. Columnar architecture sculpted by GABA circuits in developing cat visual cortex. *Science* 303: 1678–1681.

Horton, J. C., and Hocking, D. R. 1996. An adult-like pattern of ocular dominance columns in striate cortex of newborn monkeys prior to visual experience. *J. Neurosci.* 16: 1791–1807.

Hubel, D. H., and Wiesel, T. N. 1965. Binocular interaction in striate cortex of kittens reared with artificial squint. *J. Neurophysiol.* 28: 1041–1059.

Hubel, D. H., Wiesel, T. N., and LeVay, S. 1977. Plasticity of ocular dominance columns in monkey striate cortex. *Philos. Trans. R. Soc. Lond., B, Biol. Sci.* 278: 377–409.

Knudsen, E. I., and Knudsen, P. F. 1990. Sensitive and critical periods for visual calibration of sound localization by barn owls. *J. Neurosci.* 10: 222–232.

LeVay, S., Wiesel, T. N., and Hubel, D. H. 1980. The development of ocular dominance columns in normal and visually deprived monkeys. *J. Comp. Neurol.* 191: 1–51.

Lebedev, M. A., Mirabella, G., Erchova, I., and Diamond, M. E. 2000. Experience-dependent plasticity of rat barrel cortex: redistribution of activity across barrel-columns. *Cereb. Cortex* 10: 23–31.

Meissirel, C., Wikler, K. C., Chalupa, L. M., and Rakic, P. 1997. Early divergence of magnocellular and parvocellular functional subsystems in the embryonic primate visual system. *Proc. Natl. Acad. Sci. USA* 94: 5900–5905.

Meister, M., Wong, R. O., Baylor, D. A., and Shatz, C. J. 1991. Synchronous bursts of action potentials in ganglion cells of the developing mammalian retina. *Science* 252: 939–943.

Pizzorusso, T., Medini, P., Berardi, N., Chierzi, S., Fawcett, J. W., and Maffei, L. 2002. Reactivation of ocular dominance plasticity in the adult visual cortex. *Science* 298: 1248–1251.

Popescu, M. V., and Polley, D. B. Monaural deprivation disrupts development of binaural selectivity in auditory midbrain and cortex. *Neuron* 65: 718–731.

Ryugo, D. K., Kretzmer, E. A., and Niparko, J. K. 2005. Restoration of auditory nerve synapses in cats by cochlear implants. *Science* 310: 1490–1492

Sale A, Berardi N and Maffei L 2014 Environment and brain plasticity: towards an endogenous pharmacotherapy. *Physiol. Rev.* 94: 189–234.

Tritsch, N. X., Yi, E., Gale, J. E., Glowatzki, E., and Bergles, D. E. 2007. The origin of spontaneous activity in the developing auditory system. *Nature* 450: 50–55.

Wiesel, T. N., and Hubel, D. H. 1963. Single-cell responses in striate cortex of kittens deprived of vision in one eye. *J. Neurophysiol.* 26: 1003–1017.

Yang, J. W., Hanganu-Opatz, I. L., Sun, J. J., and Luhmann, H. J. 2009. Three patterns of oscillatory activity differentially synchronize developing neocortical networks in vivo. *J. Neurosci.* 29: 9011–9025.

CHAPTER 29

Regeneration and Repair of Synaptic Connections after Injury

When an axon in the vertebrate nervous system is severed, the distal portion degenerates. Over time, changes occur in its cell body and its targets. The changes result from the interruption of axonal transport of molecules that control neuronal differentiation and survival and from alterations in the pattern of electrical activity. In the peripheral nervous system (PNS) of adult mammals, damaged axons regrow to restore sensory and motor functions. They are guided back to skin and muscle by Schwann cells and the basal lamina. Agrin, a large protein secreted by motor nerve terminals during regeneration and during development, triggers differentiation of postsynaptic specializations in muscle cells.

The ability of damaged central nervous system (CNS) axons to grow and innervate appropriate targets varies widely among species. In invertebrates, such as the leech, and in lower vertebrates, such as frogs, axons in the CNS can regenerate and reconnect precisely with their original synaptic partners after injury. By contrast, in the adult mammalian CNS, regeneration and repair fail to occur. CNS neurons sprout new axons and form new synapses only over short distances. They can, however, extend axons for long distances through peripheral nerve grafts to establish synaptic connections. In fetal and neonatal mammals, the CNS does regenerate axons and connections, but after a critical period the capacity for regeneration is lost.

The different ability of PNS and CNS neurons to regenerate after injury naturally prompted the question: Do CNS neurons lack the intrinsic capability of regeneration or are there extrinsic factors that influence their inability to regenerate? In this chapter we will show that both intrinsic and extrinsic factors come into play to explain the failure of spinal cord neurons to regenerate after axotomy. We shall also discuss whether the reactivation of developmental processes can elicit axon regeneration in the injured CNS.

There is not a single reason why regeneration of CNS neurons fails. It is therefore unlikely that there will be a single intervention that is appropriate for all forms of incomplete or anatomically complete spinal cord injury.

Embryonic neurons and neural stem cells grafted into the adult CNS differentiate, extend axons, and can become integrated appropriately into the existing synaptic circuitry. The aim of this repair strategy is that the grafted cells will form relay stations to restore functional circuit connectivity across the lesion. The in situ reprogramming of scar-forming astrocytes in the injured spinal cord lesion, to become neurons, is being actively investigated as a therapeutic approach.

In many animals the nervous system has a remarkable ability to reestablish with a high degree of specificity synaptic connections that have been disrupted by trauma. The regenerative powers of neurons in the CNS were first investigated by Matthey, who in the 1920s sectioned the optic nerve of a newt and found that vision was restored within a few weeks.[1] Beginning in the 1940s, Sperry, Stone, and their colleagues took advantage of this regenerative capacity to explore how specific connections form within the nervous system. Their experiments on regenerating retinotectal connections in frogs and fish provided support for the idea that neurons selectively reinnervate their targets during regeneration, rather than making connections at random that are subsequently reorganized[2] (see Chapter 27). Later, studies in leeches, crickets, and crayfish demonstrated that, after being severed, axons of individual identified neurons in invertebrates can reconnect precisely with their original synaptic partners, avoiding a multitude of other potential targets.[3] In contrast, regeneration of severed connections in the adult mammalian nervous system is typically incomplete or absent altogether.[4]

This chapter begins with the sequence of events after a peripheral axon is damaged. The connections of motoneurons to skeletal muscle fibers are particularly useful for this. We then consider why regeneration typically fails in the adult mammalian CNS and the current attempts to solve the problem.

[1] Matthey, R. 1925. *C. R. Soc. Biol.* 93: 904-906.

[2] Sperry, R. W. 1963. *Proc. Natl. Acad. Sci. USA* 50: 703-710.

[3] Anderson, H., Edwards, J. S., and Palka, J. 1980. *Annu. Rev. Neurosci.* 3: 97-139.

[4] Mladinic, M., Muller, K. J., and Nicholls, J. G. 2009. *J. Physiol.* 587: 2775-2782.

Regeneration in the Peripheral Nervous System

Wallerian Degeneration and Removal of Debris

After a sensory or motor axon in a vertebrate peripheral nerve is severed, a characteristic sequence of changes occurs (Figure 29.1). The distal portion of the axon degenerates, by a characteristic and orderly process called **Wallerian degeneration**, after the

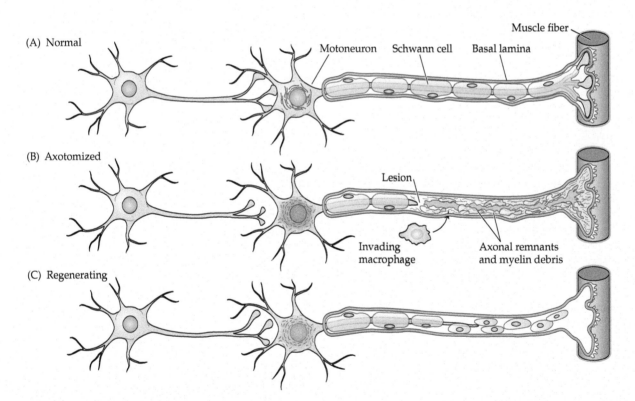

FIGURE 29.1 Degenerative Changes after Axotomy.
(A) A typical motoneuron in an adult vertebrate. (B) After axotomy, both the nerve terminal (i.e., the distal segment of the axon) and a short length of the proximal segment of the axon degenerate. Schwann cells de-differentiate, proliferate, and together with invading microglial cells and macrophages, phagocytize the axonal and myelin remnants. The axotomized neuron undergoes chromatolysis, presynaptic terminals retract, and degenerative changes may occur in pre- and postsynaptic cells. (C) The axon regenerates along the column of Schwann cells within the endoneurial tube and sheath of basal lamina that had surrounded the original axon. (After S. Rotshenker, 2009. *J. Mol. Neurosci.* 39: 99-103.)

nineteenth-century anatomist Augustus Waller, who first described it.[5,6] The endoplasmic reticulum breaks down, the neurofilaments are degraded, the mitochondria swell, and the axon breaks up into fragments that are phagocytosed. Wallerian degeneration occurs in both peripheral and central nervous system neurons, when a trauma, a vascular accident, or other insults injure axons locally.

Because severing of the axon (axotomy) cuts off the supply of proteins from the cell body, it has long been thought that the disconnected axon degenerates as a result of "starvation." However, the discovery of a spontaneous mutation in mice, called *Wallerian degeneration slow* (*Wld^s*), suggests that this type of degeneration is an active process. In these mice, Wallerian degeneration in the PNS and CNS is greatly slowed and the distal portion of a transected *Wld^s* axon remains viable and conducts action potentials for up to 3 weeks.

Axonal degeneration is followed by degradation of the myelin sheath and infiltration by macrophages. The Schwann cells that had formed the myelin sheath of the distal segment of the nerve de-differentiate and proliferate together with macrophages that are recruited from the blood stream to the site of injury. There they scavenge and remove debris, including myelin. The cell body and its nucleus swell, the nucleus moves from its typical position in the center of the cell soma to an eccentric location, and the ordered arrays of endoplasmic reticulum, called **Nissl substance**, disperse. Since the Nissl substance stains prominently with commonly used basic dyes, its dispersal following axotomy causes a decrease in intensity, which is referred to as **chromatolysis**. Chromatolysis also occurs after axons are severed in the CNS.

New axonal sprouts emerge from near the tip of the proximal stump and begin regenerating within a few hours. After a regenerating peripheral axon successfully reestablishes contact with a target, the cell body regains its original appearance. If regeneration of the peripheral nerve fails, many motor and dorsal root ganglion sensory neurons die. Autonomic ganglion cells that survive become less sensitive to acetylcholine (ACh) and shrink in size. In the adult mammalian CNS (discussed later in the chapter), the responses of neurons that fail to reestablish contact with their targets are variable. Thus, retinal ganglion cells rapidly die if their axons in the optic nerve are severed,[7,8] whereas motoneurons survive axotomy.

A different form of axonal degeneration is the so called dying back. Here, the axon of an unhealthy neuron progressively degenerates, over weeks or months, beginning distally and spreading toward the cell body. This process is often observed in peripheral nerve diseases caused by a variety of toxic, metabolic, and infectious insults.

Retrograde Trans-Synaptic Effects of Axotomy

Axotomy can also cause changes in the presynaptic neurons that provide inputs to the damaged cell. For example, after axotomy of an autonomic ganglion cell in a chick, rat, mouse, or guinea pig, synaptic inputs onto the ganglion cell become less effective.[9,10] This is due in part to a decrease in the sensitivity of the axotomized cell to the neurotransmitter ACh. In addition, retrograde trans-synaptic effects cause many of the presynaptic terminals to retract from the axotomized cell and the remaining terminals to release fewer quanta of transmitter (Figure 29.2).[11] Thus, damage to a neuron alters its ability to keep its presynaptic inputs. Rotshenker has shown an additional, retrograde trans-synaptic effect in motoneurons in the frog and the mouse.[12] When a motor nerve is cut on one side of the animal, a signal spreads from the axotomized neurons, crosses the spinal cord, and influences undamaged motoneurons on the other side of the animal. The axon terminals of those intact motor neurons sprout new branches and form additional synapses on their muscle. Motoneurons innervating other muscles are not affected.

Certain effects of axotomy—chromatolysis, atrophy, and cell death—result from the loss of trophic substances that are normally produced by the target tissue and transported retrogradely along the axon to the cell body.[13] Clear examples come from studies of the effects of nerve growth factor (NGF) on sensory and sympathetic neurons, as discussed in Chapter 27. Thus, in guinea pig autonomic ganglia the effects of axotomy are mimicked by injecting antibodies to NGF subcutaneously for several days or by blocking retrograde transport in postganglionic nerves. Conversely, the effects of axotomy are largely prevented by application of NGF to the ganglion.[14]

[5] Coleman, M. P., and Freeman, M. R. 2010. *Annu. Rev. Neurosci.* 33: 245–267.

[6] Rotshenker, S. 2009. *J. Mol. Neurosci.* 39: 99–103.

[7] Aguayo, A. J. et al. 1996. *Ciba Found. Symp.* 196: 135–144.

[8] McKernan, D. P., and Cotter, T. G. 2007. *J. Neurochem.* 102: 922–930.

[9] Brenner, H. R., and Martin, A. R. 1976. *J. Physiol.* 260: 159–175.

[10] Simões, G. F., and Oliveira, A. L. 2010. *Neuropathol. Appl. Neurobiol.* 36: 55–70.

[11] Matthews, M. R., and Nelson, V. H. 1975. *J. Physiol.* 245: 91–135.

[12] Rotshenker, S. 1988. *Trends Neurosci.* 11: 363–366.

[13] Campenot, R. B. 2009. *Results Probl. Cell. Differ.* 48: 141–158.

[14] Nja, A., and Purves, D. 1978. *J. Physiol.* 277: 55–75.

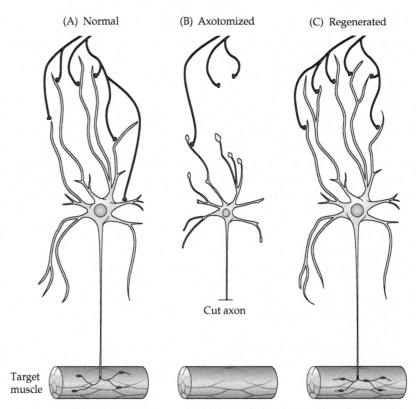

(A) Normal (B) Axotomized (C) Regenerated

Cut axon

Target muscle

FIGURE 29.2 Axotomized Autonomic Ganglion Cells Atrophy and Lose Presynaptic Inputs. (A) Normal neuron. (B) Within a few days after axotomy, neurons atrophy and many dendrites show large varicosities. Many presynaptic terminals retract from dendrites; those that remain release less transmitter. (C) If the postganglionic axon regenerates and reinnervates its peripheral target, the cell and synaptic inputs recover. (After D. Purves, 1975. *J. Physiol.* 252: 429–463.)

Effects of Denervation on Postsynaptic Cells

The Denervated Muscle Membrane

Toward the end of the nineteenth century, it was found that denervated skeletal muscles show certain clear-cut changes, such as spontaneous, asynchronous contractions called **fibrillation**. Fibrillation is initiated by the muscle membrane, not by ACh,[15] although most of the spontaneous action potentials producing fibrillation originate in the region of the former end plate.[16] The onset of fibrillation may be as early as 2 to 5 days after denervation in rats, guinea pigs, and rabbits and well over a week in monkeys and humans.

Before or at the start of fibrillation, mammalian muscle fibers become supersensitive to a variety of chemicals. This means that the concentration of a substance required to excite a muscle is reduced by a factor of several hundred to 1000. For example, a denervated mammalian skeletal muscle is about 1000 times more sensitive to ACh, applied either directly in the bathing fluid or injected into an artery supplying the muscle, than is a normally innervated muscle.[17] The action potential in denervated muscles also changes, becoming more resistant to tetrodotoxin (TTX), the puffer fish poison that blocks sodium channels (see Chapter 7). This change is due to the reappearance of TTX-resistant sodium channels that are the prevailing form in immature muscle.[18] Other changes occur in denervated muscle, such as a gradual atrophy, or wasting, of muscle fibers.[19]

Appearance of New ACh Receptors after Denervation or Prolonged Inactivity of Muscle

Supersensitivity of muscle to acetylcholine is explained by an increase in number and a change in the distribution of ACh receptors (AChRs) in denervated muscles. This effect was

[15] Purves, D., and Sakmann, B. 1974. *J. Physiol.* 239: 125–153.

[16] Belmar, J., and Eyzaguirre, C. 1966. *J. Neurophysiol.* 29: 425–441.

[17] Brown, G. L. 1937. *J. Physiol.* 89: 438–461.

[18] Kallen, R. G. et al. 1990. *Neuron* 4: 233–342.

[19] Guth, L. 1968. *Physiol. Rev.* 48: 645–687.

demonstrated by applying ACh to small regions of the muscle surface by ionophoretic release from an extracellular micropipette while recording the membrane potential. In a normally innervated frog, snake, or mammalian muscle, only the end plate region—where the nerve fiber makes a synapse—is sensitive to ACh; the rest of the muscle membrane has a very low sensitivity (see Chapter 11). After denervation, the area sensitive to ACh increases until the surface of the muscle is almost uniformly sensitive to ACh (Figure 29.3).[20] In mammals this process takes about a week; in frog muscle the changes are smaller and take longer to develop.[21]

The receptors that appear in extrasynaptic areas have not simply drifted away from the original end plate. This was first shown in experiments by Katz and Miledi in which frog muscles were cut in two; nucleated fragments that were physically separated from the original end plate survived and developed increased sensitivity to ACh.[22] Thus, new receptors are synthesized in extrajunctional regions of denervated muscles.

Synthesis and Degradation of Receptors in Denervated Muscle

A valuable technique for studying the distribution and turnover of AChRs is to label them with radioactive α-bungarotoxin, which binds to them strongly and with high specificity. Bathing normal and denervated muscles in toxin and measuring binding at end plate and end-plate-free areas confirmed that the number and distribution of binding sites are changed after denervation.[23,24] In normal muscle there are approximately 10^4 binding sites per square micrometer (μm^2) in the postsynaptic membrane, compared with fewer than 10/μm^2 in end-plate-free areas. After denervation, receptor sites in the extrasynaptic regions increase to about $10^3/\mu m^2$, with little change in density in the synaptic region.

The increase in the number of receptors in denervated muscle is attributable to enhanced receptor synthesis.[23,25] Thus, the rate of appearance of new AChRs increases markedly after denervation, and substances that block mRNA and protein synthesis (e.g., actinomycin and puromycin respectively) prevent the increase in extrasynaptic receptor density

[20] Axelsson, J., and Thesleff, S. 1959. *J. Physiol.* 147: 178–193.

[21] Miledi, R. 1960. *J. Physiol.* 151: 1–23.

[22] Katz, B., and Miledi, R. 1964. *J. Physiol.* 170: 389–396.

[23] Fambrough, D. M. 1979. *Physiol. Rev.* 59: 165–227.

[24] Salpeter, M. M., and Loring, R. H. 1985. *Prog. Neurobiol.* 25: 297–325.

[25] Scheutze, S. M., and Role, L. M. 1987. *Annu. Rev. Neurosci.* 10: 403–457.

(A)

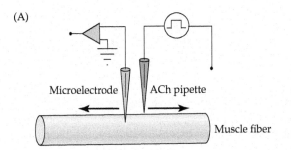

Microelectrode ACh pipette

Muscle fiber

FIGURE 29.3 New Acetylcholine Receptors (AChRs) Appear after Denervation in cat muscle. (A) Pulses of ACh are applied from an ACh-filled pipette at different positions along the surface of a muscle fiber, while the membrane potential is recorded with an intracellular microelectrode. (B) In a muscle fiber with intact innervation, a response is seen only in the vicinity of the end plate. (C) After 14 days of denervation, a muscle fiber responds to ACh along its entire length. (B,C after J. Axelsson and S. Thesleff, 1959. *J. Physiol.* 147: 178–193.)

(B) Normal

Visible end plate region

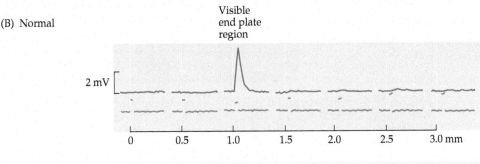

2 mV

0   0.5   1.0   1.5   2.0   2.5   3.0 mm

(C) 14 days denervated

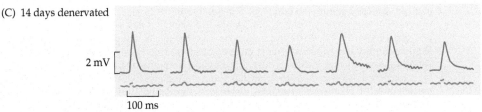

2 mV

100 ms

in muscles maintained in organ culture. Northern blot analysis and in situ hybridization demonstrate that in normal muscle, only those few nuclei located immediately beneath the end plate are transcribing AChR-subunit mRNAs; in contrast, AChR mRNAs are transcribed by nuclei all along the length of denervated muscle fibers (Figure 29.4).[26]

Denervation also affects the subunit composition and rate of degradation of AChRs. In mature muscle, junctional and extrajunctional AChRs contain an ε-subunit and have a half-life of about 10 days.[27,28] Following denervation, the half-life of ε-subunit–containing receptors remaining at the end plate decreases to 3 days. Turnover can be slowed again by reinnervation or by an increase in intracellular cAMP and consequent activation of protein kinase A.[29]

New receptors synthesized in denervated adult muscle are found all over the surface of the myofiber (synaptic or extrasynaptic) and resemble those in embryonic muscle (see Chapter 5 and Figure 29.4C). They contain a γ- instead of an ε-subunit and turn over with a half-life of 1 day.[30,31,32]

Role of Muscle Inactivity in Denervation Supersensitivity

How does sectioning of a nerve lead to the appearance of new receptors? Lømo and Rosenthal[33] investigated this problem by blocking conduction in rat nerves. A local anesthetic or diphtheria toxin was applied through a cuff to a short length of the nerve some distance from the muscle. With this technique, the muscles became inactive because

[26] Fontaine, B., and Changeux, J.-P. 1989. *J. Cell Biol.* 108: 1025–1037.

[27] Salpeter, M. M., and Marchaterre, M. 1992. *J. Neurosci.* 12: 35–38.

[28] Sala, C. et al. 1997. *J. Neurosci.* 17: 8937–8944.

[29] Xu, R., and Salpeter, M. M. 1995. *J. Cell. Physiol.* 165: 30–39.

[30] Mishina, M. et al. 1986. *Nature* 321: 406–411.

[31] Shyng, S.-L., Xu, R., and Salpeter, M. M. 1991. *Neuron* 6: 469–475.

[32] O'Malley, J., Moore, C. T., and Salpeter, M. M. 1997. *J. Cell Biol.* 138: 159–165.

[33] Lømo, T., and Rosenthal, J. 1972. *J. Physiol.* 221: 493–513.

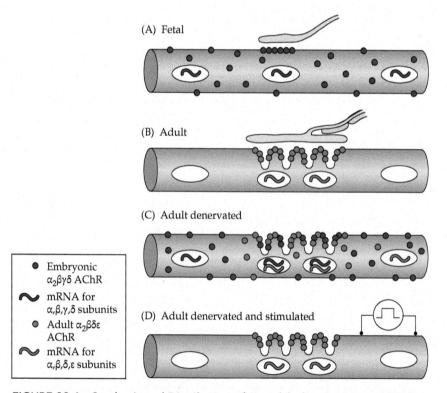

FIGURE 29.4 Synthesis and Distribution of Acetylcholine Receptors (AChRs) in rat muscle. (A) In fetal muscles, mRNAs for the α-, β-, γ-, and δ-subunits of the AChR are expressed in nuclei all along the length of the myofiber. The embryonic $\alpha_2\beta\gamma\delta$ form of the receptor is found over the entire surface of the myofiber and accumulates at the site of innervation. (B) In adult muscles, mRNAs for the α-, β-, δ-, and ε-subunits are expressed only in nuclei directly beneath the end plate. The adult form of the receptor is highly localized to the crests of the junctional folds. (C) In denervated adult muscles, nuclei directly beneath the end plate express α-, β-, γ-, δ-, and ε-subunits; all other nuclei reexpress the fetal pattern of subunits. Embryonic AChRs are found all over the surface of the myofiber (producing denervation supersensitivity), including the postsynaptic membrane; the adult form of the receptor is restricted to the end plate region. (D) If denervated muscles are stimulated directly, the pattern of AChR expression resembles that in innervated myofibers. (After V. Witzemann et al., 1991. *J. Cell Biol.* 114: 125–141.)

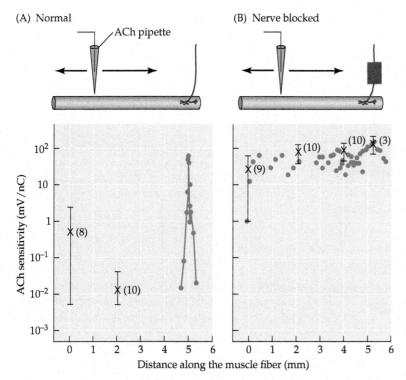

FIGURE 29.5　New Acetylcholine Receptors (AChRs). These receptors appear after block of nerve conduction in rat muscle. (A) In the normal muscle, ACh sensitivity is restricted to the end plate region (near the 5-mm position along the muscle fiber). (B) After the nerve to the muscle is blocked for 7 days by a local anesthetic, ACh sensitivity is distributed over the entire muscle fiber surface. Sensitivity is expressed numerically in millivolts of depolarization (mV) per nanocoulomb (nC) of charge ejected from the pipette (see Chapter 9). The crosses and bars represent the mean and range of sensitivities of a number (in parentheses) of adjacent muscle fibers. (From T. Lømo and J. Rosenthal, 1972. *J. Physiol.* 221: 493–513.)

motor impulses failed to conduct past the cuff. Test stimulation of the nerve distal to the block produced a twitch of the muscle as usual, and miniature end plate potentials still occurred normally, showing that synaptic transmission was intact. And yet, after 7 days of nerve block, the muscle had become supersensitive (Figure 29.5). Other experiments demonstrated that new extrajunctional receptors appeared when neuromuscular transmission was blocked by long-term application of curare or α-bungarotoxin to a muscle. These results show that denervation supersensitivity is produced by the loss of synaptic activation of the muscle.[34,35]

The importance of muscle activity itself as a factor in controlling supersensitivity was confirmed in experiments in which denervated muscles in the rat were stimulated directly through permanently implanted electrodes. Repetitive, direct stimulation of muscles over several days caused the sensitive area to become restricted, so that once again only the synaptic region was sensitive to ACh (Figure 29.6; see also Figure 29.4D).[33] The frequency of spontaneous activity in fibrillating muscle is too low to reverse the effects of denervation on the distribution of AChRs.[15]

Role of Calcium in Development of Supersensitivity in Denervated Muscle

What is it about the lack of muscle activity that causes supersensitivity to develop? Changes in intracellular calcium appear to be the key factor (Figure 29.7).[36] Electrical activity of innervated muscle results in the influx of calcium through voltage-activated calcium channels. Increased intracellular calcium activates protein kinase C, which in turn phosphorylates and inhibits a molecule known as myogenin. Myogenin is a transcription factor that induces the expression of AChR-subunit genes and also regulates other aspects of muscle

[34] Berg, D. K., and Hall, Z. W. 1975. *J. Physiol.* 244: 659–676.

[35] Witzemann, V., Brenner, H.-R., and Sakmann, B. 1991. *J. Cell Biol.* 114: 125–141.

[36] Sakuma, K., and Yamaguchi, A. 2010. *J. Biomed. Biotechnol.* 2010: 721219.

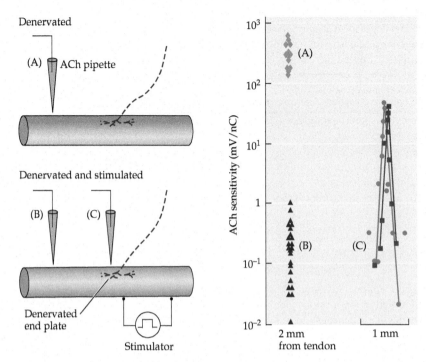

Denervated

(A) ACh pipette

Denervated and stimulated

(B) (C)

Denervated
end plate

Stimulator

FIGURE 29.6 Reversal of Supersensitivity in a denervated rat muscle by direct stimulation of the muscle fibers. (A) Increased sensitivity in the extrasynaptic portion of a muscle fiber after 14 days of denervation. (B) Sensitivity in the extrasynaptic region of a muscle that had been denervated for 7 days without stimulation and then stimulated intermittently for another 7 days. This treatment reversed the denervation supersensitivity. (C) Acetylcholine (ACh) sensitivity in two stimulated fibers of the same muscle near their denervated end plate regions. The high sensitivity is confined to this region in the stimulated muscle. (From T. Lømo and J. Rosenthal, 1972. *J. Physiol.* 221: 493–513.)

differentiation.[37] Thus, in innervated muscle, calcium influx inhibits AChR gene expression and thereby keeps overall AChR levels low. (Additional signals that specifically induce AChR expression in the few muscle nuclei immediately beneath the postsynaptic membrane are discussed later.) In inactive muscle, calcium influx is reduced; this removes the inhibition of myogenin and leads to an increase in AChR expression.

[37] Macpherson, P. C., Cieslak, D., and Goldman, D. 2006. *Mol. Cell. Neurosci.* 31: 649–660.

FIGURE 29.7 Control of Acetylcholine Receptor (AChR) Synthesis by Calcium and Neural Factors. In extrasynaptic regions of a vertebrate skeletal muscle fiber, influx of calcium through voltage-activated calcium channels activates protein kinase C (PKC), which phosphorylates and inactivates myogenin. At the synapse, agrin (see Figure 29.14) is released from nerve terminals and interacts with agrin receptors. This activates phosphatidylinositol 3-kinase (PI3K) and Ras/mitogen-activated protein kinase (Ras-MAPK) pathways, leading to expression of AChR α-, β-, γ-, δ-, and ε-subunits. Other neural signals suppress expression of the γ-subunit. (After K. Sakuma and A. Yamaguchi, 2010. *J. Biomed. Biotech.* 2010: 721219. CC BY-3.0.)

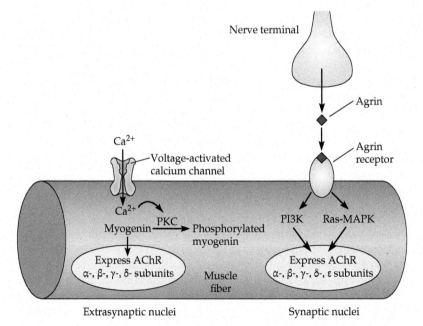

Nerve terminal

Agrin

Agrin receptor

Ca^{2+}

Voltage-activated calcium channel

Ca^{2+}

PI3K   Ras-MAPK

Myogenin $\xrightarrow{\text{PKC}}$ Phosphorylated myogenin

Express AChR
α-, β-, γ-, δ- subunits

Express AChR
α-, β-, γ-, δ-, ε subunits

Muscle
fiber

Extrasynaptic nuclei

Synaptic nuclei

The changes in AChR half-life that occur in denervated muscle are also a consequence of reduced muscle activity. The rate of receptor degradation increases to a similar extent in muscles paralyzed by denervation and in those made inactive by continuous application of TTX to the nerve. Conversely, direct electrical stimulation of denervated muscle restores the turnover rate of AChRs at synaptic sites to normal levels. Again, influx of calcium through voltage-activated calcium channels plays an important role.[31,36,38]

Activity is not the only factor that maintains the normal complement of receptors in skeletal muscles. Experiments in which slowly developing changes occur without activity per se playing an obvious role have been made on partially denervated muscles. Fibers in the frog sartorius muscle are innervated at more than one site along their length. If the muscle is partially denervated by cutting intramuscular branches of the nerve, supersensitivity develops in the denervated portions of the muscle fibers. Yet these fibers have not been inactive, but have kept contracting all along.[21]

Supersensitivity of Peripheral Nerve Cells after Removal of Synaptic Inputs

The effect of denervation on the distribution of transmitter receptors in neurons has been studied in autonomic ganglion cells in frogs and chicks. In the living frog heart, parasympathetic neurons can be seen in the transparent interatrial septum, greatly facilitating application of ACh to discrete spots on the cell surface. The cells have no dendrites; synapses are made on the cell soma (Figure 29.8A). Like skeletal muscle fibers, these neurons are sensitive to the transmitter ACh at selected spots on their surfaces (i.e., immediately under the presynaptic terminals).[39] When the distribution of AChRs was assessed by immunofluorescence microscopy, each ganglion cell was found to have approximately 30 large, dense AChR clusters located at synaptic sites and more than 100 small extrasynaptic clusters spread over the cell surface (Figure 29.8B).[40] Approximately 20% of the receptors were at extrasynaptic sites.[41]

[38] Caroni, P. et al. 1993. *J. Neurosci.* 13: 1315–1325.

[39] Harris, A. J., Kuffler, S. W., and Dennis, M. L. 1971. *Proc. R. Soc. Lond., B, Biol. Sci.* 177: 541–553.

[40] Wilson Horch, H. L., and Sargent, P. B. 1996. *J. Neurosci.* 16: 1720–1729.

[41] Sargent, P. B., and Pang, D. Z. 1989. *J. Neurosci.* 9: 1062–1072.

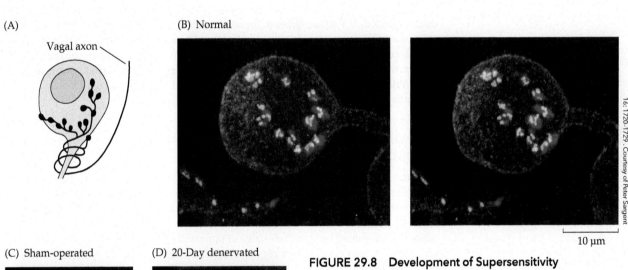

(A)

Vagal axon

(B) Normal

10 µm

All photos H. L. Horch, and P. B. Sargent, 1996. *J. Neurosci.* 16: 1720-1729. Courtesy of Peter Sargent

(C) Sham-operated

(D) 20-Day denervated

10 µm

FIGURE 29.8 Development of Supersensitivity in parasympathetic nerve cells in frog heart after denervation. (A) Parasympathetic ganglion cells are innervated by axons in the vagus nerve, which form terminal boutons scattered over the cell surface. (B) Stereo pair immunofluorescence micrographs of a ganglion cell in a normal animal, labeled with antibodies to acetylcholine receptors (AChRs; green) and to synaptic vesicles (red). Large, dense clusters of AChRs are located at synaptic sites; more than 100 small extrasynaptic clusters are spread over the rest of the cell surface. (C,D) Images of sham-operated (C) and 20-day denervated (D) ganglion cells labeled with antibodies to AChRs. Denervation causes a decrease in the number of synaptic clusters and a marked increase in small extrasynaptic clusters, producing supersensitivity.

To study the effects of denervation, the two vagus nerves to the heart were cut, and the frog was left to recover.[42,43] Synaptic transmission between vagal nerve terminals and ganglion cells failed rapidly, starting on the second day after denervation. At the same time, the area of the neuronal surface membrane sensitive to ACh increased. By days 4 to 5, ACh caused a membrane depolarization when applied anywhere on the cell surface. In other respects, the cells were normal. It was not the number of AChRs that changed, rather it was the distribution (Figure 29.8C,D).[44] Denervation reduced the number of synaptic clusters by 90% and caused a two- to threefold increase in the number of small extrasynaptic clusters spread over the cell surface. Denervation also caused a decrease in the level of acetylcholinesterase. Thus, the sensitivity to ACh was increased. If the original nerve was allowed to grow back, the sensitive area became restricted once more to synaptic sites.[43] In certain other chick and frog ganglia, denervation has little or no effect on the number or distribution of surface AChRs.[45]

Susceptibility of Normal and Denervated Muscles to New Innervation

In adult mammals and frogs, an innervated muscle fiber will not accept innervation by an additional nerve.[46] Thus, if a cut motor nerve is placed on an innervated muscle, it will not form additional new end plates on the muscle fibers. In contrast, nerve fibers do grow out and form end plates on denervated or injured muscle fibers. Unlike the situation during development, in which growth cones contact muscle fibers at random sites[47] (but see also Kummer et al.[48]), reinnervation usually occurs at the site of the original end plate. Regenerating axons appear to be guided to the original synaptic sites by the endoneurial tubes of the former axons (see Figure 29.1) and by processes extended by the Schwann cells that had capped the former axon terminal (see Chapter 10).[49] However, if a cut nerve is placed far enough away from the denervated end plate, then an entirely new end plate can be formed on a muscle. This means that nerve fibers can form synapses in a region that had never been innervated, and there they induce both pre- and postsynaptic specializations.

Similarly, after rat muscles are made supersensitive by blocking impulse transmission in the nerve or by application of botulinum toxin, foreign nerves are able to form additional distant synapses.[46,49] After release of the block, each of the two nerves can give rise to synaptic potentials and evoke contractions. Conversely, when a denervated muscle is stimulated directly, its ability to accept extra innervation is lost together with its supersensitivity. It is not, however, a prerequisite that the muscle be supersensitive to ACh for innervation to occur. Thus, reinnervation occurs in denervated rat and *Xenopus* muscles when AChRs are blocked by α-bungarotoxin or curare.[50,51]

Role of Schwann Cells and Microglia in Axon Outgrowth after Injury

Schwann cells of the PNS provide an environment conducive to axon regeneration.[52] Moreover, they proliferate after injury. If a peripheral nerve is crushed rather than cut, the endoneurial tubes and Schwann cell basal lamina that surround the axons remain intact (see Figure 29.1). Under such conditions, axons regenerate within their parent tubes and are guided back to their original targets. If the endoneurial tubes are disrupted, as when a nerve is cut, then regenerating axons enter tubes in the distal portion of the nerve at random; frequently, the regenerating axons are guided to inappropriate targets. The growth-promoting activity of Schwann cells is due to secretion of trophic factors, surface expression of cell adhesion molecules and integrins, and production of extracellular matrix components such as laminin.[53] For example, experiments in which the sciatic nerve is lesioned have shown that as the peripheral portion of the axon degenerates, proliferating Schwann cells synthesize high levels of brain-derived neurotrophic factor (BDNF) and NGF (Figure 29.9).[54] Thus, Schwann cells temporarily supply regenerating motor, sensory, and sympathetic axons with BDNF and NGF as they grow back to their peripheral targets. It is interesting that such denervated Schwann cells also express large numbers of low-affinity NGF/BDNF receptors on their surface, perhaps to hold the NGF and BDNF they produce along the path that regenerating axons should

[42] Kuffler, S. W., Dennis, M. J., and Harris, A. J. 1971. *Proc. R. Soc. Lond., B, Biol. Sci.* 177: 555-563.

[43] Dennis, M. J., and Sargent, P. B. 1979. *J. Physiol.* 289: 263-275.

[44] Sargent, P. B. et al. 1991. *J. Neurosci.* 11: 3610-3623.

[45] Wilson Horch, H. L., and Sargent, P. B. 1995. *J. Neurosci.* 15: 7778-7795.

[46] Jansen, J. K. S. et al. 1973. *Science* 181: 559-561.

[47] Lin, S. et al. 2008. *J. Neurosci.* 28: 3333-3340.

[48] Kummer, T. T., Misgeld, T., and Sanes, J. R. 2006. *Curr. Opin. Neurobiol.* 16: 74-82.

[49] Son, Y. J., and Thompson, W. J. 1995. *Neuron* 14: 125-132.

[50] Cohen, M. W. 1972. *Brain Res.* 41: 457-463.

[51] Van Essen, D., and Jansen, J. K. 1974. *Acta Physiol. Scand.* 91: 571-573.

[52] Fawcett, J. W., and Keynes, R. J. 1990. *Annu. Rev. Neurosci.* 13: 43-60.

[53] Madduri, S., and Gander, B. 2010. *J. Peripher. Nerv. Syst.* 15: 93-103.

[54] Meyer, M. et al. 1992. *J. Cell Biol.* 119: 45-54.

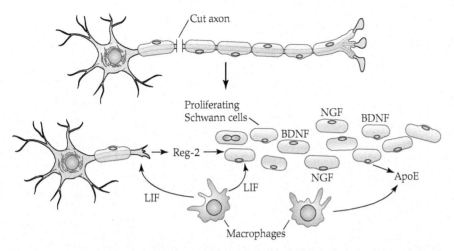

FIGURE 29.9 Schwann Cells Promote Axon Regrowth in the vertebrate peripheral nervous system. After axotomy, the distal portion of the axon and the myelin degenerate and are phagocytized. Schwann cell proliferation is stimulated by two cytokines: leukemia inhibitory factor (LIF) from macrophages and Reg-2 from axon terminals. Expression of Reg-2 is enhanced by LIF. Proliferating Schwann cells synthesize two neurotrophic factors, brain-derived neurotrophic factor (BDNF) and nerve growth factor (NGF), which are held on the cell surface by low-affinity BDNF and NGF receptors and help sustain regenerating axons and guide them to their targets. Schwann cells and macrophages also synthesize apolipo-protein E (ApoE), which may help promote neuron survival and axon regrowth.

take. As regeneration progresses, the Schwann cells cease production of NGF and BDNF and once again ensheathe the axons.

Apolipoprotein E (ApoE), synthesized by Schwann cells and macrophages, also accumulates in the distal portion of damaged peripheral nerves and becomes associated with the Schwann cell basal lamina (see Figure 29.11).[55,56] ApoE promotes the health and survival of neurons by virtue of its protective effects against oxidative damage; it also promotes neurite outgrowth and adhesion. Factors that promote Schwann cell proliferation include cytokines, leukemia inhibitory factor, and mitogens.[57] Microglial cells (discussed in Chapter 10) also contribute to repair after a lesion.[58] They migrate rapidly to the site of an injury, where they remove debris and provide growth-promoting molecules to axons.[59]

Denervation-Induced Axonal Sprouting

Not only are denervated muscles amenable to innervation, but also they actively induce undamaged nerves to sprout new terminal branches. After a muscle is partially denervated, the remaining axon terminals sprout and innervate the denervated muscle fibers (Figure 29.10).[60] As with regulation of AChR synthesis and degradation, muscle inactivity triggers this process. Sprouting and hyperinnervation occur if muscle activity is prevented (by blocking action potential propagation in the nerve with a cuff impregnated with TTX) or if neuromuscular transmission is blocked (with botulinum toxin or α-bungarotoxin). The terminal Schwann cell plays an important role in the regulation of axon terminal sprouting (see Chapter 10).[61–63] Axons of sensory cells other than motoneurons can also sprout to supply denervated territories. In the leech, for example, the killing of a particular sensory neuron, by injecting it with pronase, induces axon sprouting into the denervated area of skin. However, only axons of cells that have the same sensory modality grow into the denervated area.[64]

Appropriate and Inappropriate Reinnervation

For complete recovery of function, regenerating axons must reestablish connections with their original targets. Classic experiments of Langley demonstrated that regenerating mammalian preganglionic autonomic axons can reinnervate the appropriate postganglionic neurons. One mechanism for reestablishing connections selectively is competition between axons; in salamander muscles that have been innervated by inappropriate axons,

[55] Skene, J. H. P., and Shooter, E. M. 1983. *Proc. Natl. Acad. Sci. USA* 80: 4169–4173.

[56] Fullerton, S. M., Strittmatter, W. J., and Matthew, W. D. 1998. *Exp. Neurol.* 153: 156–163.

[57] Banner, L. R., and Patterson, P. H. 1994. *Proc. Natl. Acad. Sci. USA* 91: 7109–7113.

[58] Gitik, M., Reichert, F., and Rotshenker, S. 2010. *FASEB J.* 24: 2211–2221.

[59] Samuels, S. E. et al. 2010. *J. Gen. Physiol.* 136: 425–452.

[60] Brown, M. C., Holland, R. L., and Hopkins, W. G. 1981. *Annu. Rev. Neurosci.* 4: 17–42.

[61] Son, Y. J., and Thompson, W. J. 1995. *Neuron* 14: 133–141.

[62] Love, F. M., Son, Y. J., and Thompson, W. J. 2003. *J. Neurobiol.* 54: 566–576.

[63] Hayworth, C. R. et al. 2006. *J. Neurosci.* 26: 6873–6884.

[64] Blackshaw, S. E., Nicholls, J. G., and Parnas, I. 1982. *J. Physiol.* 326: 261–268.

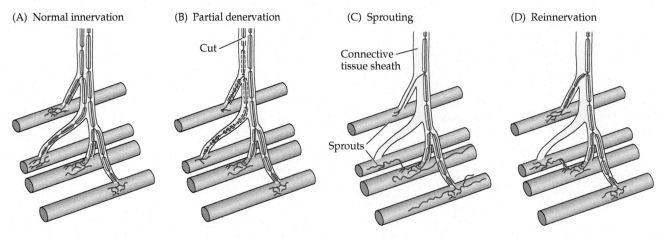

(A) Normal innervation (B) Partial denervation (C) Sprouting (D) Reinnervation

Cut

Connective tissue sheath

Sprouts

FIGURE 29.10 Nerve Terminals Sprout in Response to Partial Denervation of a mammalian skeletal muscle. (A) Normal pattern of innervation. (B) Some fibers are denervated by cutting a few of the axons innervating the muscle. (C) Axons sprout from the terminals and from nodes along the preterminal axons of undamaged motoneurons to innervate the denervated fibers. (D) After 1 or 2 months, sprouts that have contacted vacant end plates are retained, while other sprouts disappear. (After M. C. Brown et al., 1981. *Annu. Rev. Neurosci.* 4: 17–42.)

the foreign synapses are eliminated after the normal nerve reestablishes its connection.[65] In adult mammals, foreign nerves can be as effective as the original ones in innervating muscle fibers, if they manage to reach them.[52,66] Observations concerning the consequences of inappropriate contacts date back to 1904, when Langley and Anderson made the remarkable observation that muscles of the cat could become innervated by cholinergic preganglionic sympathetic fibers,[67] which normally make synapses on nerve cells in ganglia. (At that time, it was of course not known that ACh was the transmitter used by preganglionic fibers or even that transmitters existed!) Similar synapses have been shown to be formed by autonomic nerves on frog and rat skeletal muscle.[68] In such experiments, many of the properties of the nerve and muscle were found to remain unchanged, despite the abnormal innervation.

By contrast, the properties of muscles can become markedly changed by foreign innervation. Slow and fast skeletal muscle fibers in the frog have quite different properties. Slow fibers are diffusely innervated, have a characteristic fine structure, and do not give regenerative impulses or twitches. After denervation, slow fibers can become reinnervated by nerves that normally innervate twitch muscles at discrete end plates. Under these conditions, slow fibers become able to give conducted action potentials and twitches.[69] Eccles, Eccles, Buller, and their colleagues[70] cut and interchanged the nerves to rapidly and slowly contracting skeletal muscles in kittens and rats. Both of these types of mammalian muscle fibers produce propagating action potentials and are called slow-twitch and fast-twitch fibers. After the muscles were reinnervated by the inappropriate nerves, the slow-twitch muscles became faster and the fast-twitch ones slower.[71,72] A major factor in the transformation is the pattern of impulses in the nerve and the resulting muscle contractions—the motoneurons innervating slow- and fast-twitch muscle fibers tend to fire at different frequencies.[73]

Basal Lamina, Agrin, and the Formation of Synaptic Specializations

The best example available at present to show how a nerve causes a synapse to form on its target is provided by the neuromuscular junction. There it has been shown that a structure that plays a key role in the regeneration of neuromuscular synapses is the **synaptic basal lamina**, which lies between the nerve terminal and the muscle membrane. The synaptic basal lamina constitutes a densely staining extracellular matrix made up of proteoglycans and glycoproteins. As shown in Figure 29.11A, basal lamina surrounds the muscle, the nerve terminal, and the Schwann cell, and dips into the folds in the postsynaptic membrane.

[65] Dennis, M. J., and Yip, J. W. 1978. *J. Physiol.* 274: 299–310.

[66] Bixby, J. L., and Van Essen, D. C. 1979. *Nature* 282: 726–728.

[67] Langley, J. N., and Anderson, H. K. 1904. *J. Physiol.* 31: 365–391.

[68] Grinnell, A. D., and Rheuben, M. B. 1979. *J. Physiol.* 289: 219–240.

[69] Miledi, R., Stefani, E., and Steinbach, A. B. 1971. *J. Physiol.* 217: 737–754.

[70] Buller, A. J., Eccles, J. C., and Eccles, R. M. 1960. *J. Physiol.* 150: 417–439.

[71] Close, R. I. 1972. *Physiol. Rev.* 52: 129–197.

[72] Pette, D. 2001. J. Appl. Physiol. 90: 1119–1124.

[73] Salmons, S., and Sreter, F. A. 1975. *J. Anat.* 120: 412–415.

McMahan, Wallace, and their colleagues made systematic and elegant studies of the effects of the synaptic basal lamina on the differentiation of nerve and muscle.[74-77] The key to their analysis was to use an easily accessible, very thin muscle in the frog, called the cutaneous pectoris, in which the position of the end plates is highly ordered and easily seen in a living muscle. As a first step, cells in the region of innervation were killed by cutting the nerve and muscle fibers or by repeated application of a brass bar cooled in liquid nitrogen (Figure 29.11B). Within days the portion of the muscle fibers in the damaged region, together with the nerve terminals, degenerated and were phagocytized, but the basal lamina sheaths remained intact (Figure 29.11C). The location of the original neuromuscular junctions could still be recognized by the distinctive morphology of the basal lamina sheaths of the muscle and Schwann cell at the junctional sites and by the presence of cholinesterase. The enzyme remained concentrated in the basal lamina of the synaptic cleft and folds for weeks following the operation.

Two weeks after damage to the muscles, new myofibers had formed within the basal lamina sheaths and were contacted by regenerated axon terminals, which evoked muscle twitches when the nerves were stimulated. Nearly all of the regenerated synapses were located precisely at original synaptic sites, as marked by cholinesterase. Thus, signals associated with the synaptic basal lamina had specified where regenerating synapses were to be formed.

[74] Sanes, J. R., Marshall, L. M., and McMahan, U. J. 1978. *J. Cell Biol.* 78: 176-198.

[75] Burden, S. J., Sargent, P. B., and McMahan, U. J. 1979. *J. Cell Biol.* 82: 412-425.

[76] McMahan, U. J., and Slater, C. R. 1984. *J. Cell Biol.* 98: 1453-1473.

[77] Anglister, L., and McMahan, U. J. 1985. *J. Cell Biol.* 101: 735-743.

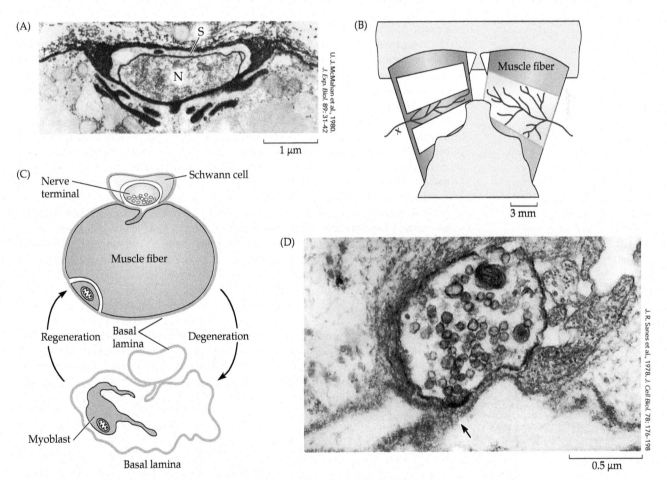

FIGURE 29.11 Basal Lamina and Regeneration of Synapses. (A) Electron micrograph of a normal neuromuscular synapse in the frog, stained with ruthenium red to show the basal lamina that dips into the postsynaptic folds and surrounds the Schwann cell (S) and nerve terminal (N). (B) Diagram of the cutaneous pectoris muscle, showing the region frozen (right) or cut away (left) to damage muscle fibers. (C) Freezing causes all cellular elements of the neuromuscular junction to degenerate and be phagocytized, leaving only the basal lamina sheath of the muscle fiber and Schwann cell intact. New neuromuscular junctions are restored by regenerating axons and muscle fibers. (D) Nerve and muscle were damaged, and regeneration of muscle fibers was prevented by x-radiation. In the absence of muscle fibers, axons regenerated; contacted original synaptic sites, marked by the tongue of basal lamina that had extended into the junctional fold (arrow); and formed active zones. (B after J. R. Sanes et al., 1978. *J. Cell Biol.* 78: 176-198; C after S. J. Burden et al., 1979. *J. Cell Biol.* 82: 412-425.)

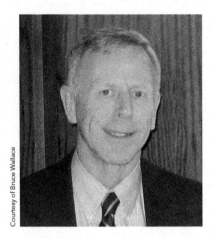

Bruce Wallace, codiscoverer of agrin and coauthor of previous editions of *From Neuron to Brain*.

To investigate further the nature of the signals associated with the synaptic basal lamina, muscles were damaged and the nerve was crushed, but muscle fiber regeneration was prevented by x-radiation. Regenerating axons grew to the former synaptic sites on the basal lamina, as marked by cholinesterase, and formed active zones for release precisely opposite portions of the basal lamina that had projected into the junctional folds—all this without a postsynaptic target (Figure 29.11D).

In a parallel series of experiments, it was shown that synaptic basal lamina in the adult frog contains a factor that triggers differentiation of postsynaptic specializations in regenerating myofibers. Muscles were damaged as described, but reinnervation was prevented by removing a long segment of the nerve. When new muscle fibers regenerated within the basal lamina sheaths, they formed junctional folds and aggregates of AChRs and acetylcholinesterase precisely at the point where they came in contact with the original synaptic basal lamina (Figure 29.11D). Thus, signals stably associated with synaptic basal lamina can trigger the formation of synaptic specializations in both regenerating myofibers and nerve terminals.

Identification of Agrin

In order to identify the molecule in synaptic basal lamina that triggers postsynaptic differentiation, McMahan, Wallace, and their colleagues prepared basal lamina–containing extracts from the electric organ of the marine ray *Torpedo californica*.[78] The electric organ, which generates large currents that are used to stun animals, is a tissue derived embryologically from muscle that receives very dense cholinergic innervation. It resembles a giant array of motor end plates. There would be no chance of isolating the relevant molecule from normal skeletal muscle fibers because the area of the end plate is so small compared with the whole surface of the muscle. When added to myofibers in culture, purified extracts from torpedo mimicked the effects of synaptic basal lamina on regenerating muscle fibers; that is, they induced the formation of specializations at which AChRs accumulated, together with several other components of the postsynaptic apparatus[78,79] (Figures 29.12 and 29.13). The active component in the extracts, called **agrin**, was purified and characterized, and cDNAs encoding it were cloned from chick, rat, and ray.[79]

Results of in situ hybridization and immunohistochemical studies demonstrate that agrin is synthesized by motor neurons, transported down their axons, and released to induce differentiation of the postsynaptic apparatus at developing neuromuscular junctions.[80] Agrin itself becomes incorporated into the synaptic basal lamina, where it helps maintain the postsynaptic apparatus in the adult and triggers its differentiation during regeneration.

[78] McMahan, U. J., and Wallace, B. G. 1989. *Dev. Neurosci.* 11: 227–247.

[79] Bowe, M. A., and Fallon, J. R. 1995. *Annu. Rev. Neurosci.* 18: 443–462.

[80] McMahan, U. J. 1990. *Cold Spring Harb. Symp. Quant. Biol.* 50: 407–418.

(A)

(B)

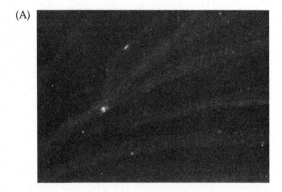

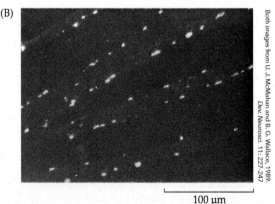

100 μm

Both images from U. J. McMahan and B. G. Wallace, 1989. *Dev. Neurosci.* 11: 227–247

FIGURE 29.12 Agrin Causes Aggregation of Acetylcholine Receptors (AChRs), seen here in chick myotubes in culture. The images are fluorescence micrographs of myotubes labeled with rhodamine-conjugated α-bungarotoxin to mark AChRs.

(A) Receptors are distributed over the surface of control myotubes at low density. (B) Overnight incubation with agrin causes the formation of patches at which AChRs accumulate, together with other components of the postsynaptic apparatus.

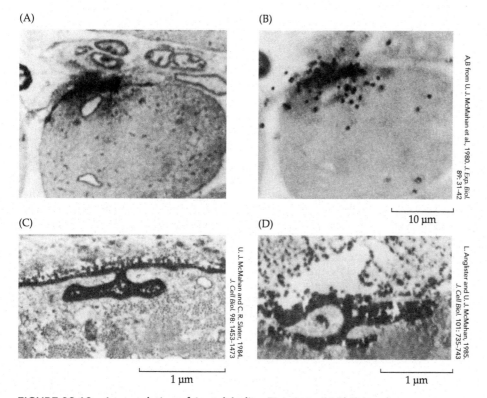

(A) (B)

A,B from U. J. McMahan et al., 1980. *J. Exp. Biol.* 89: 31-42.

10 µm

(C) (D)

U. J. McMahan and C. R. Slater, 1984. *J. Cell Biol.* 98: 1453-1473.

L. Anglister and U. J. McMahan, 1985. *J. Cell Biol.* 101: 735-743.

1 µm   1 µm

FIGURE 29.13   Accumulation of Acetylcholine Receptors (AChRs) and Acetylcholinesterase at original synaptic sites, seen here on muscle fibers regenerating in the absence of nerve. The muscle was frozen as in Figure 29.11B, but the nerve was prevented from regenerating. New muscle fibers formed within the basal lamina sheaths. (A,B) Light-microscope autoradiography of a regenerated muscle stained for cholinesterase to mark the original synaptic site (in focus in A) and incubated with radioactive α-bungarotoxin to label AChRs (silver grains in focus in B). (C) Electron micrograph of the original synaptic site in a regenerated muscle labeled with horseradish peroxidase (HRP)-α-bungarotoxin. The distribution of AChRs is indicated by the dense HRP reaction product, which lines the muscle fiber surface and the junctional folds. (D) Electron micrograph of the original synaptic site in a regenerated muscle stained for cholinesterase. The original cholinesterase was permanently inactivated at the time the muscle was frozen. Thus, the dense reaction product is due to cholinesterase synthesized and accumulated at the original synaptic site by the regenerating muscle fiber.

The Role of Agrin in Synapse Formation

Additional evidence for the role of agrin in synapse formation is provided by comparisons made between developing and regenerating neuromuscular synapses. Early in development, AChRs are distributed diffusely over the surface of non-innervated myotubes, as in denervated muscle. When the growth cone of a motoneuron approaches a myotube, depolarizing potentials arise due to the release of ACh.[81,82] A functional synaptic connection is established within hours. AChRs and acetylcholinesterase accumulate beneath the axon terminal.[83] Detailed morphological and physiological experiments demonstrate that motor axons contact the developing muscle cells at random positions on their surface, rather than at preexisting AChR clusters.[47,84] Over time, the γ-subunit of the AChR is replaced by an ε-subunit (see Figure 29.4 and Chapter 5), and the density of receptors in nonsynaptic portions of the muscle fiber decreases.[35]

The signal that produces these changes is not ACh. Acetylcholine receptors still accumulate beneath axon terminals in cultures grown in the presence of curare or α-bungarotoxin, which block the interaction of ACh with its receptor. During normal development, as in the reinnervation of denervated muscle, it is agrin, released by motor nerve terminals, that triggers the accumulation of receptors, cholinesterase, and other components of the postsynaptic apparatus at synaptic sites.[78] Among other proteins that accumulate in agrin-induced specializations is ARIA, a member of the neuregulin protein family, and the receptor proteins ErbB-2,

[81] Evers, J. et al. 1989. *J. Neurosci.* 9: 1523-1539.

[82] Dan, Y., Lo, Y., and Poo, M. M. 1995. *Prog. Brain Res.* 105: 211-215.

[83] Sanes, J. R., and Lichtman, J. W. 1999. *Annu. Rev. Neurosci.* 22: 389-442.

[84] Anderson, M. J., and Cohen, M. W. 1977. *J. Physiol.* 268: 757-773.

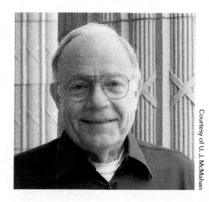

Courtesy of U. J. McMahan

U. J. McMahan

ErbB-3, and ErbB-4.[85] It was originally proposed that activation of ErbB receptors in muscle might be the mechanism responsible for accumulation of AChR subunits. However, mice in which *Aria* genes have been deleted can still form normal neuromuscular synapses.[86,87]

In other experiments by McMahan and his colleagues, denervated rat soleus muscles were transfected with cDNA encoding neural agrin. After transfection, extrajunctional regions of the muscle fibers expressed and secreted neural agrin. Moreover, they formed typical postsynaptic specializations, including membrane infoldings and aggregates of AChRs at sites far distant from the original synapse.[88]

Mechanism of Action of Agrin

Agrin occurs in several isoforms that arise from a single gene by alternative splicing.[81] Motoneurons, muscle cells, and Schwann cells all express agrin, but only motoneurons express the isoform that is potent in inducing postsynaptic differentiation. Agrin is a large heparan sulfate proteoglycan, with domains that interact with its receptor (Lrp4), and with laminin, heparin-binding proteins, α-dystroglycan, heparin, and integrins (Figure 29.14).[89]

The ability to induce the formation of postsynaptic specializations resides in the C-terminal domain (Figure 29.15). The essential role of agrin in the formation of the neuromuscular junction is evident in mice in which agrin expression is prevented by homologous recombination.[90,91] In such agrin gene knockouts, myofibers appear normally and axons grow into the developing muscles, but neuromuscular junctions fail to form. (The agrin knock-out animals die because of failure of respiration.) A similar phenotype is seen in mice in which the

[85] Fischbach, G. D., and Rosen, K. M. 1997. *Annu. Rev. Neurosci.* 20: 429–458.

[86] Escher, P. et al. 2005. *Science* 308: 1920–1923.

[87] Rimer, M. 2010. *J. Biol. Chem.* 285: 32370–32377.

[88] Cohen, I. et al. 1997. *Mol. Cell. Neurosci.* 9: 237–253.

[89] Denzer, A. J. et al. 1998. *EMBO J.* 17: 335–343.

[90] Gautam, M. et al. 1996. *Cell* 85: 525–535.

[91] Burgess, R. W. et al. 1999. *Neuron* 23: 33–44.

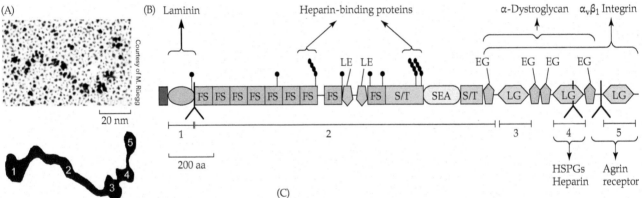

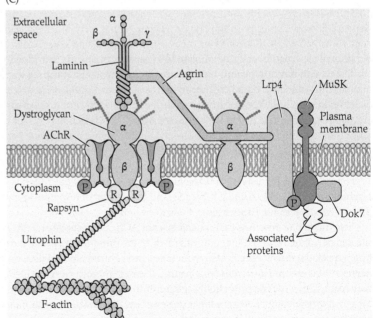

FIGURE 29.14 Agrin Is a Large Heparan Sulfate Proteoglycan (400–600 kDa) with domains that interact with laminin, heparan sulfate proteoglycans (HSPGs), heparin, α-dystroglycan, integrin, heparin-binding proteins, and the agrin receptor (Lrp4) that causes acetylcholine receptor (AChR) aggregation. (A) Electron micrographs of agrin after rotary shadowing. (B) Schematic diagram of the structural and binding domains of chick agrin. Binding regions are indicated, as are globular (1, 3–5) and extended (2) regions of the molecule that can be recognized in part (A). (C) Diagram showing the relation of agrin to the receptor Lrp4 and downstream molecules. Agrin, after binding to its Lrp4 receptor, activates MuSK and induces tyrosine phosphorylation of the β subunit of nearby AChR, leading to AChR clustering and its linkage to the cytoskeleton at the nascent synapse. EG = epidermal growth-factor-like domain; FS = follistatin-like domain; LE = laminin EGF-like domain; LG = laminin G-like domain; SEA = motif found in sea urchin sperm protein, enterokinase, and agrin; S/T = serine- and/or threonine-rich domain. (B after A. J. Denzer et al., 1998. *EMBO J.* 17: 335–343; C courtesy of M. Rüegg.)

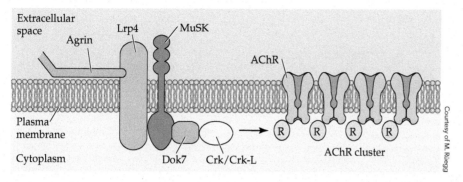

Courtesy of M. Ruegg

FIGURE 29.15 Molecules Genetically Proved to Be Critical for the formation of neuromuscular synaptic structure and for aggregation of acetylcholine receptors at the motor end plate.

muscle-specific receptor kinase (MuSK) is knocked out.[92] The lack of presynaptic specializations in agrin- and MuSK-deficient mutant mice suggests that during development presynaptic differentiation is triggered by retrograde signals released by muscle cells in response to agrin.[93]

The sequence of events initiated by agrin is as follows: First, agrin binds to its Lrp4 receptor and thus stimulates MuSK. This leads to phosphorylation of both proteins.[94,95] Phosphorylated MuSK then interacts with the adapter protein Dok7.[96] Mutation of the agrin Lrp4 receptor, MuSK, or Dok7 prevents agrin from inducing AChR clusters to form in cultured muscle cells and prevents the formation of neuromuscular junctions in embryonic mice.[92,96,97] While there is evidence that another adapter protein, Crk, interacts with MuSK, the downstream signal pathways of the Lrp4/MuSK/Dok7 complex remain unclear.[98] Ultimately, rapsyn[99] recruits the aggregation of AChRs. Much less is known about differentiation of the presynaptic nerve terminal in regenerating motor axons, even though it has been shown that molecules stably associated with the synaptic basal lamina in adult muscle can induce the formation of active zones in regenerating axons (see Figure 29.11).[78]

Regeneration in the Mammalian CNS

The adult mammalian CNS has limited capacity for regeneration. Transection of major axon tracts is not followed by axon regrowth and restitution of function. Nevertheless, it has become apparent that after tracts in the CNS are severed, axons can, under suitable circumstances, regrow for some distance and form synapses with appropriate targets,[100–103] depending on the severity and the type of lesion. Spinal cord injury (SCI) in people is currently untreatable. SCI lesions can vary considerably in size, complexity, and functional consequences. Anatomically incomplete SCI spares at least some neural connectivity across the lesion, either directly from supraspinal sources or indirectly through propriospinal relay circuits, which may lead to varying degrees of spontaneous functional recovery. By contrast, anatomically complete SCI results in the complete absence of neural connectivity across the lesion level and therefore in a complete loss of function.

Glial Cells and CNS Regeneration

Of importance for limiting axonal regeneration in the CNS is the immediate environment provided by CNS glial cells (see Chapter 10). Clues to an inhibitory role of CNS glial cells are provided by several experiments. First, although axons severed in the CNS typically do not regrow, motor neurons (whose cell bodies lie within the spinal cord) can regenerate severed peripheral axons (Figure 29.16). Likewise, axons of sensory neurons regrow to their targets in the periphery but fail to regenerate when severed within the CNS. Indeed, after a dorsal root is cut, sensory axons regenerate toward the spinal cord but stop growing when they reach the astrocytic processes that delimit the surface of the CNS. Moreover, axons in the periphery will not enter an optic nerve graft, which consists of CNS glial cells.[104] These findings suggest that CNS glial cells actively inhibit growth.

[92] DeChiara, T. M. et al. 1995. *Cell* 83: 313–322.

[93] Noakes, P. G. et al. 1995. *Nature* 374: 258–262.

[94] Kim, N. et al. 2008. *Cell* 135: 334–342.

[95] Zhang, B. et al. 2008. *Neuron* 60: 285–297.

[96] Okada, K. et al. 2006. *Science* 312: 1802–1805.

[97] Weatherbee, S. D., Anderson, K. V., and Niswander, L. A. 2006. *Development* 133: 4993–5000.

[98] Hallock, P. T. et al. 2010. *Genes Dev.* 24: 2451–2461.

[99] Moransard, M. et al. 2003. *J. Biol. Chem.* 278: 7350–7359.

[100] Dusart, I. et al. 2005. *Brain Res. Brain Res. Rev.* 49: 300–316.

[101] Bunge, M. B. 2008. *J. Spinal Cord Med.* 31: 262–269.

[102] Afshari, F. T., Kappagantula, S., and Fawcett, J. W. 2009. *Expert Rev. Mol. Med.* 11: e37.

[103] Huebner, E. A., and Strittmatter, S. M. 2009. Results Probl. *Cell Differ.* 48: 339–351.

[104] Aguayo, A. J. et al. 1978. *Neurosci. Lett.* 9: 97–104.

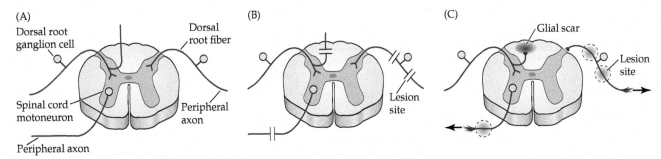

FIGURE 29.16 Axons of Sensory and Motor Neurons Regenerate in the Periphery but Not in the CNS.
(A) Motoneurons, dorsal root ganglion sensory neurons, and their axonal processes in the mammalian nervous system. (B) Sites of axon lesions. (C) Extent of regeneration. Axons of dorsal root ganglion neurons and motoneurons regenerate through lesion sites in peripheral nerves and dorsal roots (blue). However, regenerating dorsal root fibers stop when they reach the astrocytic processes that delimit the surface of the spinal cord. Axons of dorsal root ganglion sensory neurons also do not regenerate through glial scars that form at lesion sites in the CNS (red).

However, when dorsal root ganglion neurons are injected into CNS white matter tracts in such a way as to minimize trauma, they frequently extend axons for long distances in the white matter, invade gray matter, and form terminal arbors.[105] Thus, when there is no trauma-induced glial reaction, regeneration of axons by adult neurons is not prevented by contact with CNS glial cells.

SCI lesions are not homogeneous and exhibit three lesion compartments: the non-neural (stromal) lesion core, glial scar borders, and spared neural tissue that is reactive. Mechanisms in different SCI compartments contribute to regeneration failure. When tracts in the CNS are lesioned, astrocytes, microglial cells, meningeal cells, and oligodendrocyte precursor cells accumulate at the site of the lesion to form a glial scar. These cells produce a variety of molecules that have been shown to inhibit axon growth, including free radicals, nitric oxide, arachidonic acid derivatives, and a variety of proteoglycans.[106,107]

In addition, it has been shown that oligodendrocytes from the mature CNS have a protein on their surface, known as Nogo-A, which is a member of the reticulon family of genes.[108] Nogo binds to a specific receptor (Nogo-66 receptor), induces long-lasting collapse of growth cones, and inhibits neurite outgrowth in vitro.[103,109] Application of a monoclonal antibody that neutralizes this activity allows axons to regenerate across a spinal cord lesion. Partial locomotor function can be restored, although the extent of regeneration under such conditions is still meager.[110]

Such observations led to the suggestion that failure of CNS neurons to regenerate might be due to the action of Nogo and other proteins in mature myelin (such as myelin associated glycoprotein [MAG], oligodendrocyte myelin glycoprotein [OMgp], and myelin basic protein). It seems unlikely that the actions of these inhibitors on their own could be the complete explanation for regeneration failure,[111,112] Indeed, regeneration still fails in transgenic animals in which three growth inhibitory myelin proteins (Nogo, MAG, and OMgp) have been genetically deleted, either singly or collectively.[111,113]

Components of the extracellular matrix, and particularly chondroitin sulfate proteoglycans (CSPGs) produced by astrocytes and forming structures called perineuronal nets (PNNs), have been proposed as a principal cause for regeneration failure.[114] Enzymatic digestion of the inhibitory glycan chains by chondroitinase, which promotes adult plasticity (see Chapter 28), has been shown to induce some benefit in rat and, more recently, in rhesus monkey SCI models.[115,116]

A problem for regeneration that is commonly considered is the glial scar produced by astrocytes days and weeks after a spinal cord lesion.[105,117] The injury-induced glial cells are called reactive glial cells, and they facilitate the formation of a defensive barrier to prevent the spread of injury and "inflammatory soup." The idea that astrocytic scars are one main barrier to CNS axon regrowth[117] has recently been challenged by experiments in which preventing astrocyte scar formation, or ablating chronic astrocytic scars 5 weeks after the spinal cord lesion, exacerbated the injury and failed to enhance regeneration.[118] Reactive glial cells are therefore a double-edged sword, releasing not only neurotrophic and neuroprotective factors but also neural inhibitory factors that inhibit axonal regeneration. Thus,

[105] Davies, S. J. A. et al. 1997. *Nature* 390: 680–683.

[106] Camand, E. et al. 2004. *Eur. J. Neurosci.* 20: 1161–1176.

[107] Kuzhandaivel, A. et al. 2010. *Neuroscience* 169: 325–338.

[108] Schwab, M. E., and Caroni, P. 1988. *J. Neurosci.* 8: 2381–2393.

[109] Fournier, A. E., GrandPre, T., and Strittmatter, S. M. 2001. *Nature* 409: 341–346.

[110] Schnell, L., and Schwab, M. E. 1990. *Nature* 343: 269–272.

[111] Silver, J. 2010. *Neuron* 66: 619–621.

[112] Hu, F., and Strittmatter, S. M. 2004. *Semin. Perinatol.* 28: 371–378.

[113] Lee, J. K. et al. 2010. *Neuron* 66: 663–670.

[114] Fawcett, J. W. 2015. *Progr. Brain Res.* 218: 213–226.

[115] Bradbury, E. J. et al. 2002. *Nature* 416: 636–640.

[116] Rosenzweig, E. S. et al. 2018. *Nat. Neurosci.* 22: 1269–1275.

[117] J. M., et al. 2014. *Exp. Neurol.* 253: 197–207.

[118] Anderson, M. A. et al 2016 *Nature* 532: 195–200.

in the fashion of a drawbridge, reactive scar astrocytes can be either a barrier or, on occasion, a roadway depending on the conditions present normally or created experimentally inside or outside the lesion penumbra, as well as on time after the lesion.[119,120] Indeed, time after lesion is important: Reactive gliosis and glial scars are initially protective in restricting further spreading of damage, but in the longer term they act as both a physical and biochemical barrier to neuronal regeneration. It is clear that growth of damaged axons starts to occur within hours after the lesion has been made. In the CNS, this initial growth ends within a few micrometers unless it is somehow enhanced. Hence, after SCI the scar might be a *consequence* of failure of regeneration rather than the main obstacle to growth.[120]

Peripheral Nerve Bridges, Cell Transplants, and Regeneration

Schwann cells produce a favorable environment for the growth of axons of CNS neurons. For example, when segments of peripheral nerves are grafted between the cut ends of the spinal cord in a mouse or rat, fibers grow across and fill the gap.[121] The graft is composed of Schwann cells and connective tissue; the peripheral axons degenerate. Similarly, cultures of Schwann cells implanted into the spinal cord promote growth. This effect can be enhanced by genetically engineering the Schwann cells to produce supra-normal amounts of neurotrophic factors.[122]

Ensheathing glial cells are found only in the olfactory system, where new neurons are born and extend axons into the CNS throughout adulthood. Olfactory ensheathing glial cells form a conduit that guides the growing axons of the olfactory receptor neurons. For this reason, olfactory ensheathing cells have been investigated as candidates for cell transplant experiments, as it is hypothesized that they might assist growth and regeneration of axons in the injured spinal cord as they do in the constantly regenerating olfactory system. Injection of olfactory ensheathing glial cells either into the stumps of a transected spinal cord or at the site of an electrolytic lesion in the corticospinal tract likewise enhances regeneration of axons.[123,124] However, it has been challenged whether olfactory ensheathing cells promote corticospinal axon regeneration.[125,126]

In a seminal approach, Aguayo and his colleagues observed a dramatic effect by the use of bridges of the type shown in Figure 29.17.[18,29,127] One end of a segment of sciatic nerve is implanted into the spinal cord, the other into a higher region of the nervous system (upper spinal cord, medulla, or thalamus). Bridges have even been made to extend from cortex to another part of the CNS or to muscle. After several weeks or months, the graft resembles a normal nerve trunk filled with myelinated and unmyelinated axons. These neurons fire impulses and are electrically excited or inhibited by stimuli applied above or below the sites of implantation. By cutting the bridge and dipping the cut ends into horseradish peroxidase or other markers, the cells of origin become labeled and their distribution can be mapped (see Figure 29.17B). Such experiments show that axons in the bridge, which have grown over distances of several centimeters, arise from neurons whose cell bodies lie within the CNS. Usually only those neurons with somata that are not more than a few millimeters from the bridge send axons into it. Similarly, axons leaving the bridge to enter the CNS grow only a short distance before terminating.

[119] Silver, J. 2016. *Exp. Neurol.* 286: 147–149.

[120] Rolls, A., Shechter, R., and Schwartz, M. 2009. *Nat. Rev. Neurosci.* 10: 235–241.

[121] Richardson, P. M., McGuinness, U. M., and Aguayo, A. J. 1980. *Nature* 284: 264–265.

[122] Menei, P. et al. 1998. *Eur. J. Neurosci.* 10: 607–621.

[123] Li, Y., Field, P. M., and Raisman, G. 1998. *J. Neurosci.* 18: 10514–10524.

[124] Raisman, G. 2007. *C. R. Biol.* 330: 557–560.

[125] Lu, P. et al. 2006. *J. Neurosci.* 26: 11120–11130.

[126] Steward, O. et al. 2006. *Exp. Neurol.* 198: 483–499.

[127] David, S., and Aguayo, A. J. 1981. *Science* 214: 931–933.

FIGURE 29.17 Bridges between Medulla and Spinal Cord enable CNS neurons to grow for prolonged distances. The grafted bridge consists of a segment of adult rat sciatic nerve in which axons have degenerated, leaving Schwann cells. The bridges act as a conduit along which central axons can grow. (A) Sites of insertion of the graft. (B) Neurons are labeled by cutting the graft and applying horseradish peroxidase (HRP) to the cut ends. Positions of 1472 neuronal cell bodies were labeled by retrograde transport of HRP in seven grafted rats. Most of the cells sending axons into the graft are situated close to its points of insertion. (After S. David and A. J. Aguayo, 1981. *Science* 214: 931–933.)

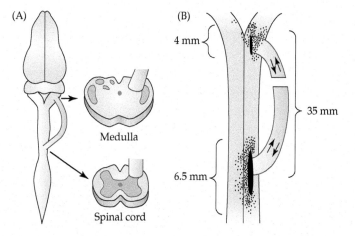

Not all CNS neurons extend axons into permissive environments. For example, if the axons of cerebellar Purkinje cells are severed in the adult, the cells survive indefinitely but no axonal regrowth occurs,[128,129] even if pieces of embryonic cerebellum are grafted adjacent to the severed axons. Axons of other cerebellar cells readily innervate such grafts. Thus, regeneration depends both on growth-permissive, or growth-promoting, conditions and on the intrinsic properties of the neuron. The inability of Purkinje cells to regrow severed axons is correlated with their failure to upregulate proteins involved in axon growth in response to axotomy and not with the presence of myelin.[130]

The seminal experiments by Aguayo and his colleagues demonstrated that some CNS axons are capable of regeneration given a permissive environment, without axon growth-inhibitory processes. In addition to being limited by the environmental inhibitory factors associated with myelin, extracellular matrix, and astrocytic scars, axonal growth after SCI is limited by the reduced intrinsic growth capacity of mature CNS neurons. Cell-autonomous intrinsic factors controlling axon regeneration include transcription factors (Krüppel-like factor[131]) and signaling proteins such as PTEN[132,133] and SOCS3.[134] Genetic deletion of either PTEN, a negative regulator of the mTOR signaling pathway, or of SOCS3, a negative regulator of the JAK/STAT pathway, promotes significant optic nerve regeneration in adult mice, but such regrowth tapers off 2 weeks after the injury. Remarkably, simultaneous deletion of both PTEN and SOCS3 enables robust and sustained axon regeneration.[134] PTEN and SOCS3 regulate two independent intrinsic pathways that act synergistically to promote enhanced axon regeneration and might be negatively regulated by the inhibitory extracellular factors at the lesion site.

Formation of Synapses by Axons Regenerating in the Mammalian CNS

Can axons regenerating in the CNS of mammals locate their usual targets and make functional synapses? Experiments on regenerating retinal ganglion cell axons indicate that, under the right circumstances, the answer can be yes.[135] If the optic nerve is cut and a peripheral nerve bridge is inserted between the eye and the superior colliculus, retinal ganglion cell axons that grow through the bridge can extend into the target, arborize, and form synapses (Figure 29.18). The regenerated synapses are formed on the correct regions of their target cells, have a normal structure when visualized by electron

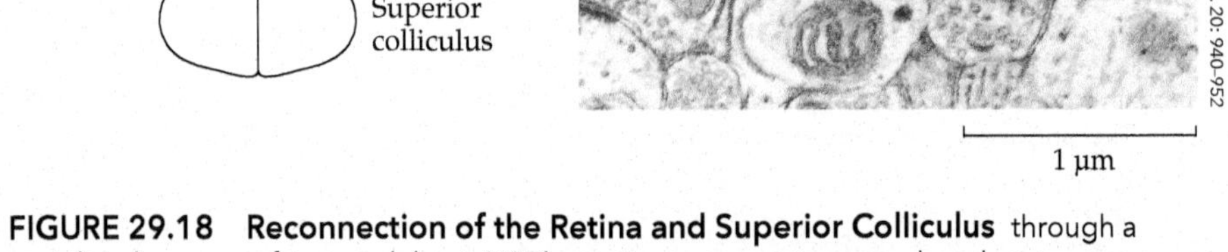

[128] Zagrebelsky, M. et al. 1998. *J. Neurosci.* 18: 7912-7929.

[129] Carulli, D., Buffo, A., and Strata, P. 2004. *Prog. Neurobiol.* 72: 373-398.

[130] Bouslama-Oueghlani, L. et al. 2003. *J. Neurosci.* 23: 8318-8329.

[131] Moore, et al. 2009. *Science* 326: 298-301.

[132] Park, et al. 2008 *Science* 322: 963-966.

[133] Liu, et al. 2010. *Nat. Neurosci.* 13: 1075-1081.

[134] Sun, et al. 2011. *Nature* 480: 372-375.

[135] Bray, G. M. et al. 1991. *Ann. NY Acad. Sci.* 633: 214-228.

FIGURE 29.18 Reconnection of the Retina and Superior Colliculus through a peripheral nerve graft in an adult rat. (A) The optic nerves were severed, and one was replaced by a 3- to 4-cm segment of the peroneal nerve (yellow). Regeneration was tested by injecting anterograde tracers into the eye or by recording responses of superior colliculus neurons to light flashed onto the retina. (B) Electron microscope autoradiogram of a regenerated retinal ganglion cell axon terminal in the superior colliculus. 3H-labeled amino acids were injected into the eye 2 days before the brain was fixed and sectioned; silver grains exposed by radiolabeled proteins transported from the injected eye identify ganglion cell axon terminals. The regenerated terminal resembles those seen in control animals; it is filled with round synaptic vesicles and forms asymmetrical synapses.

microscopy, and are functional in that the postsynaptic cells can be electrically driven by illumination of the eye. Nevertheless, in spite of occasional reports to the contrary, very few axons actually succeed in growing through the graft to their targets, and it remains unclear the extent to which axons induced to regenerate can form functional synapses with their presumptive targets. A promising approach for optic nerve lesions is the transplant of retinal ganglion cells in the mature retina of the mouse,[136] which integrate into host retinal circuits, making functional synapses and responding to light. In some cases, axons from grafted ganglion cells extend within the host optic nerve and optic tract and terminate into the lateral geniculate and superior colliculus.[136]

The combined genetic deletion of PTEN and SOCS3 in both juvenile and adult mice, or delivery of a growth factor cocktail, induces regrowth of retinal axons and formation of functional synapses, but no significant recovery of visual function.[137] Regenerated axons fail to conduct action potentials from the eye to the superior colliculus, due to the lack of myelination. Administration of voltage-gated potassium channel blockers restores conduction and results in increased visual function. Thus, enhancing both the intrinsic mechanisms for axon regeneration and electrical conduction might effectively improve the formation of synapses and visual function after retinal axon injury.[137]

Regeneration in Immature versus Adult Mammalian CNS

Compared with that of the adult, the immature mammalian CNS provides a favorable environment for regeneration.[4,130] If the spinal cord of a neonatal opossum is crushed or cut, axons grow across the lesion and conduction through the damaged region is restored within a few days, even when the spinal cord is removed from the animal and maintained in culture (Figures 29.19 and 29.20).[138–140] Similar results have been obtained in embryonic rat and mouse spinal cord in culture. Even after complete transection of the spinal cord in a newborn opossum, prolonged survival leads to substantial and precise regeneration and excellent functional recovery. For example, sensory axons reestablish direct synaptic connections onto motor neurons (see Figure 29.20), and the animal can walk, swim, and climb in a coordinated manner.

There is a **critical period** in early life during which regeneration can occur. The spinal cord of a 9-day-old opossum regenerates after a lesion has been made, while that of a 12-day-old animal does not. The very narrow time-window separating the regenerating from the non-regenerating epochs is a distinctive advantage, because it limits the confounding factor of developmental changes. A striking feature of the opossum spinal cord at 9 days of age is the absence of myelin and the small number of glial cells it contains. As in opossums, neurons in the CNS of embryonic chicks regenerate if the spinal cord is transected prior to the onset of myelination.[141]

The newborn opossum offers advantages for identifying molecules that are responsible for promoting or inhibiting spinal cord regeneration since RNA expression can be compared in spinal cords that can (9 days) and cannot (12 days) regenerate. Mladinic and her colleagues[142,143] have measured changes in mRNA expression between 9 and 12 days. Growth-promoting molecules and their receptors are overexpressed in cords that regenerate.

[136] Venugopalan, P. et al. 2016. *Nat. Commun.* 7: 10472.

[137] Bei, F. et al. 2016 *Cell* 164: 219-232.

[138] Nicholls, J., and Saunders, N. 1996. *Trends Neurosci.* 19: 229-234.

[139] Varga, Z. M. et al. 1995. *Eur. J. Neurosci.* 7: 2119-2129.

[140] Saunders, N. R. et al. 1998. *J. Neurosci.* 18: 339-355.

[141] Keirstead, H. S. et al. 1995. *J. Neurosci.* 15: 6963-6974.

[142] Mladinic, M. et al. 2005. *Cell. Mol. Neurobiol.* 25: 405-424.

[143] Mladinic, M. et al. 2010. *Brain Res.* 1363: 20-39.

(A)
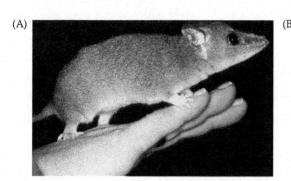

(B)
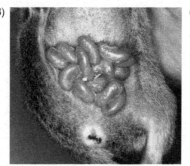

(C)
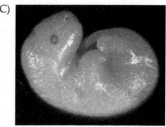

J. G. Nicholls and N. Saunders, 1996. *Trends Neurosci.* 19: 229-234.

FIGURE 29.19 The South American Opossum (*Monodelphis domestica*) (A) is born in an immature state (B,C) corresponding roughly to a 15.16-day mouse embryo. The entire CNS can be removed and maintained in culture for more than 1 week.

(A)

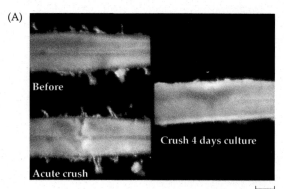

Before

Acute crush

Crush 4 days culture

0.5 mm

(B)

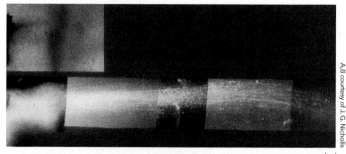

A,B courtesy of J. G. Nicholls

100 µm

(C)

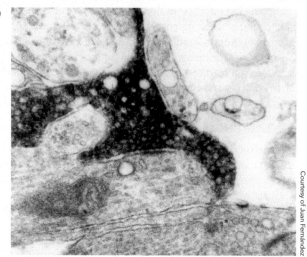

Courtesy of Juan Fernández

100 nm

FIGURE 29.20 Regeneration of Axons after Spinal Cord Lesions in isolated CNS of an 8-day-old opossum. (A) Whole mount of opossum spinal cord in culture before and after lesioning one side. After 4 days, the lesion becomes hard to detect. (B) Growth of axons labeled by the fluorescent dye DiI 5 days after injury, bright field (above) and fluorescence microscopy (below). Note the large number of fibers and their extensive and rapid growth through and beyond the lesion. (C) Horseradish peroxidase (HRP)-labeled sensory axon that formed a synapse on a motoneuron 6 days after injury.

[144] Lane, M. A. et al. 2007. *Eur. J. Neurosci.* 25: 1725–1742.

[145] Fink, K. L. et al. 2017. *Cell Rep.* 18: 2687–2701.

[146] Belin, S. et al. 2015. *Neuron* 86: 1000–1014.

[147] Chandran, V. et al. 2016. *Neuron* 89: 956–970.

[148] Sekine, Y. et al. 2018 *Cell Rep.* 23: 415–428.

By contrast, inhibitory molecules and their receptors appear at 12 days, when regeneration is no longer possible. The lists of molecules are long, which is not surprising since during the period between 9 and 12 days after birth extensive developmental changes are occurring.[144] Candidate molecules overexpressed at 9 days include cytokines, mitogen-activated protein kinases (MAPKs), and laminin receptors, to name only a few, all of which can promote neurite survival or outgrowth. Those overexpressed at 12 days include inhibitory molecules or molecules inducing cell death, such as myelin basic protein, reticulon, annexins, semaphorins, and ephrins.[143] A next step will be to test these molecules separately or in combination to determine whether transfection with a growth-promoting molecule allows regeneration to occur after 12 days or, conversely, whether an inhibitor prevents it at less than 9 days. At present, it is not known which molecules or how many different molecules are involved in the initiation and prevention of neurite outgrowth across a lesion.

Following the gene-expression studies in opossum, gene-expression profiling has been used extensively in various systems to evaluate changes in mRNA or proteomic expression in spinal cords that can and cannot regenerate after injury.[145–147] These expression surveys have identified a large number of injury-associated genes whose expression changes are correlated with, but not necessarily functionally linked to, regeneration. To search for functionally validated genes linked to regeneration failure, an unbiased genome-wide assessment of mammalian genes whose loss of function allows axonal sprouting and regeneration in mouse cortical neurons in vitro was recently performed.[148] More than 400 mRNAs were found to affect regeneration after injury. Surprisingly, this functional screen identified genes largely distinct from genes identified by expression surveys after axon injury, and not previously linked to axonal regeneration or neuronal repair. This would suggest that inhibition of regeneration is mediated largely by genes that are constitutively expressed rather than by injury-induced genes.

The heterogeneity of the lesions and the diversity of cells involved in the lesion exacerbate the problem of identifying single-gene candidates responsible for the intrinsic inability to grow. The major differences in regenerative potential between regenerating and quiescent adult CNS neurons may reflect differences in injury-related transcriptional networks controlling multiple regeneration-associated signaling pathways. A coordinated global transcriptional program, rather than individual gene candidates, distinguishes the regenerating-supportive from the non-regenerating phenotypes.[149]

This global transcriptional regulation is achieved through epigenetic mechanisms (see Appendix D). For instance, peripheral nerve regeneration after injury depends on the activation of a gene-expression program in Schwann cells that supports axonal regeneration. The reprogramming of the Schwann cell transcriptome after injury was found to depend on an epigenomic pathway leading to the collective demethylation of histones at the promoters of all injury-activated genes.[150] Epigenetic mechanisms play a role also in the diminished axon growth potential in adult sensory dorsal root ganglion neurons.[151] This was demonstrated in the conditioning lesion paradigm: The central branch of dorsal root ganglion neurons, which are normally refractory to regeneration, can be triggered into a growth state if the peripheral branch is axotomized first (the so-called conditioning lesion). The conditioning effect involves the transcription of many regeneration-associated genes, and the central branch can take advantage of the genes induced by the peripheral injury-induced genes. In this paradigm, the peripheral, but not the central, axotomy strongly increases the acetylation of Histone 4, both globally and on the promoters of regeneration-activated genes.[153] Inhibitors of histone deacetylases induce regeneration-activated genes in dorsal root ganglion neurons and enhance regeneration of the central sensory axon.[153]

How Function Could Be Restored: Repair Strategies

Regeneration of injured adult CNS axons is regulated at multiple levels and fails for several different reasons, including both cell-autonomous intrinsic and extrinsic mechanisms (Figure 29.21). The former regulate the regeneration-gene-expression program in the neuron whose axon was cut, while the latter occur in the complex environment of the lesion site.

As for intrinsic mechanisms, finding ways to reactivate the intrinsic axon growth program, active during development, through a modulation of the underlying epigenetic mechanisms, is a promising approach for the future.

As for extrinsic mechanisms, regeneration or repair could be promoted by influencing different mechanisms in different lesion compartments (see Figure 29.21). Also, repair strategies will depend crucially on the extent and the type of the lesion. It is unlikely that

[149] Fawcett, J. W., and Verhaagen, J. 2018. *Dev. Neurobiol.* 78: 890–897.

[150] Ma, K. H. et al 2016 *J. Neurosci.* 36: 9135–9147.

[151] Finelli, M. J. et al. 2013. *J. Neurosci.* 33: 19664–19676.

[152] Weidner, et al. 2001. *Proc. Natl. Acad. Sci. USA* 98: 3513–3518.

[153] Bareyre, et al. 2004. *Nat. Neurosci.* 7: 269–277.

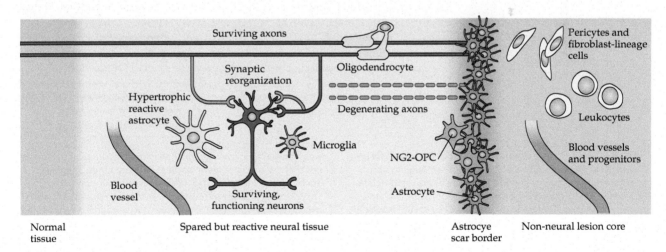

FIGURE 29.21 How SCI Lesions Are Organized.
SCI lesions are not homogenous and exhibit distinct tissue compartments: Non-neural (stromal) lesion core, astrocyte scar border (ASB), spared but reactive neural tissue. The mechanisms underlying regeneration failure vary in different SCI lesion compartments and also at different times after the injury. These compartments consist of different cell types that have entirely different roles in repair and regeneration. The different cell biology and molecular mechanisms in each compartment influence axon growth or regrowth in different ways. NG2-OPC are reactive oligodendrocyte progenitor cells that express chondroitin sulfate proteoglycan 4 (also known as NG2). (After T. M. O'Shea et al. 2017. *J. Clin. Invest.* 127: 3259–3270.)

there will be a single intervention that is appropriate for all forms of incomplete or of anatomically complete SCI. Different recovery and repair strategies can be envisaged.

RECOVERY VIA REORGANIZATION OF SPARED CIRCUITS   Incomplete SCI lesions in humans and experimental animals are often associated with varying degrees of spontaneous functional recovery during the first months after injury.[152,153] Such recovery is widely attributed to axons spared from the injury that descend from the brain and bypass incomplete lesions, or to synapse remodeling and axon sprouting in spared neural tissue. A spontaneous reorganization of preexisting circuits to convey functional information past lesions could create detour, or relay, pathways (Figure 29.22A). Propriospinal axons, originating from neurons in the spinal cord and projecting inter-segmentally to terminate at other spinal levels, are uniquely suited for injury-induced plasticity.[153] After unilateral hemisection SCI, locomotor function recovers spontaneously on the injured side, enabled by interactions with the normally functioning contralateral limb and muscle spindle feedback.[154,155] Long-tract axons descending from the mouse brain were cut by opposite-side staggered lateral hemisections of the spinal cord at the T7 (cervical) and T12 (lumbosacral) segments (Figure 29.22B). For successful recovery of weight-bearing locomotor function

[154] Courtine, G. et al. 2008. *Nat. Med.* 14: 69–74.

[155] Takeoka, A. et al. 2014. *Cell* 159: 1626–1639.

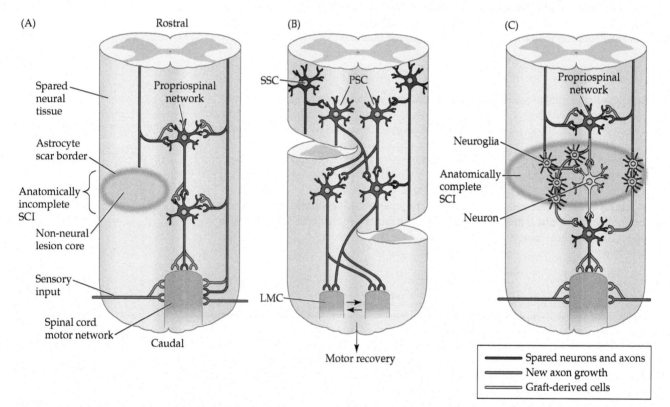

FIGURE 29.22 How Function Could Be Restored: Repair Strategies. (A) Axon growth and synapse remodeling occur spontaneously in spared neural tissue, which, after incomplete SCI, can lead to circuit reorganization and formation of detour, or relay, pathways. Therapies to augment such circuit reorganization could improve functions. (B) Spontaneous recovery from incomplete SCI. All long-tract axons descending from the mouse brain (supraspinal connections, SSCs) were cut using opposite-side staggered lateral hemisections of the spinal cord at the T7 (cervical, forelimb) and T12 (lumbosacral, hindlimb) segments. The remaining propriospinal connections (PSC) could indirectly relay motor information from the brain to lumbar motor circuits (LMC) involved in coordinated hindlimb stepping. PS axons originate from neurons within the spinal cord and project intersegmentally to terminate at other spinal levels. PSCs restored full,

weight-bearing locomotor function in the hindlimbs of these mice, but only if the lesions were made at different times. This demonstrates that the adult CNS, while unable to support regeneration, remains capable of reorganizing existing neurons into novel circuits and using these connections in a functional way, bridging the lesion. (C) Anatomically complete SCI requires therapeutic approaches that attempt to restore connectivity across lesions by (i) facilitating the regrowth of host propriospinal or supraspinal axons across damaged tissue or (ii) grafting neural stem cells to create relays of propriospinal neurons that receive host afferents and project past damaged tissue into spared neural tissue. The neuronal relay strategy uses grafts to function as novel interneurons between the injured axons and denervated neurons distal to the injury. (A,C after T. M. O'Shea et al., 2017. *J. Clin. Invest.* 127: 3259–3270; B after D. J. Stelzner, 2008. *Nat. Med.* 14: 19.)

in these mice, these lesions had to occur at different times, with the more rostral (T7) lesion made many weeks after the more caudal lesion (T12). When the lesions were made at the same time, no spontaneous recovery was seen.[154] The findings suggest that the remaining intact supraspinal connections (SSCs), present before the second lesion was made, are necessary for this lesion-induced plasticity to occur in propriospinal connections (PSCs). Notably, function can also return after simultaneous bilateral injuries if limb use is enabled and trained by neuro-prosthetic rehabilitation and circuit activation,[156] demonstrating that training-mediated use is required to establish detour circuits after complete SCI.

Thus, the adult CNS—while unable to regenerate—remains capable of *reorganizing existing neurons into novel circuits* and using these connections in a functionally meaningful way. Experimental enhancement of spontaneous plasticity after incomplete SCI lesions may be useful in promoting further recovery (see Figure 29.22B). After incomplete SCI, spontaneous synapse remodeling and circuit reorganization can be aided by modulating growth-inhibitory signals such as Nogo or chondroitin sulfate proteoglycans,[114,157,158] by increasing neuron-intrinsic growth potential in supraspinal afferent projection areas in the cerebral cortex and brainstem,[134,158] or by rehabilitative training combined with activation of spared circuits.[156]

RECOVERY VIA NEW CIRCUITS FORMED ACROSS ANATOMICALLY COMPLETE LESIONS   Repair of anatomically complete SCI requires formation of new circuits that connect across non-neural lesion cores and their scar borders. Recapitulating connectivity precisely as it was before injury may not be required to restore meaningful function, and establishing short-distance axon growth across complete SCI that connects into spared propriospinal networks may instead be sufficient. In principle, there are two strategies to form such new connections (Figure 29.22C):

1. Achieve regrowth of endogenous supraspinal descending or propriospinal axons across lesions that connect with spared circuits, or

2. Graft appropriate cells to repopulate the lesion core with neurons that provide a bridging relay station, receiving inputs from, and sending inputs to, host circuits on either side of lesions, to restore circuit connectivity across the lesion

One alternative strategy to address the medical problem of SCI, without dealing directly with the regeneration failure, is to bypass the spinal cord lesion using neuro-technologies based on brain–spine neuroprosthetic interfaces (Box 29.1).

Neuronal and Stem Cell Transplants: The Neuronal Relay Strategy

Cell therapy by grafting embryonic neurons and stem cells is a promising strategy being actively investigated for repair after SCI[159,160] (see Figure 29.22C), as well as for CNS lesions of a different nature, including stroke and neurodegenerative diseases. Among the most devastating of human diseases are those resulting from the spontaneous progressive degeneration of CNS neurons, such as Parkinson's disease, Alzheimer's disease, and Huntington's disease. In the adult, most nerve cells are postmitotic; at present, no physiological mechanisms are known for replacing neurons that have been lost. One approach to cell replacement has been to transplant embryonic nerve cells into the adult brain.[161] Unlike neurons from the adult CNS, which die following transplantation, cells taken from fetal or neonatal animals can survive and grow after being inserted into the gray matter of the adult CNS (Figure 29.23). There they differentiate, extend axons, and release transmitters.

An early example of such transplantation, pioneered by Olle Lindvall and Anders Björklund, is provided by experiments in which dopaminergic neurons from the developing ventral mesencephalon were transplanted into the basal ganglia of rats after destruction of dopamine-containing neurons in the substantia nigra—a loss that mimics in some ways the deficits caused by Parkinson's disease in humans (see also Chapters 14 and 24).[162] In normal animals, the dopaminergic neurons in the substantia nigra (a region in the midbrain) innervate cells in the basal ganglia (a region involved in programming movements; see Chapter 24 and Appendix C). If a lesion of this dopamine pathway is made on one side of a rat, a disorder of movement results in which the animal turns toward the side

[154] van den Brand, et al. 2012. *Science* 336: 1182-1185.

[157] Schwab, M. E., and Strittmatter, S. M. 2014. *Curr. Op. Neurobiol.* 27: 53-60.

[158] Hollis, R. E. 2016. *Nat. Neurosci* 19: 697-705.

[159] Sahni, V., and Kessler, J. A. 2010. *Nat. Rev. Neurol.* 6: 363-372.

[160] Rossi, S. L., and Keirstead, H. S. 2009. *Curr. Opin. Biotechnol.* 20: 552-562.

[161] Björklund, A. 2000. *Novartis Found. Symp.* 231: 7-15.

[162] Thompson, L. H., and Björklund, A. 2009. *Prog. Brain Res.* 175: 53-79.

BOX 29.1 Neuroprosthethic Approaches to Treating Spinal Cord Injury

Spinal cord injury disrupts the bidirectional communication between the brain and the spinal circuits that orchestrate movement. Neurotechnologies based on brain-spine neuroprosthetic interfaces represent an alternative approach that is being pursued to solve the SCI medical problem without dealing directly with regeneration failure. The goal of the neuroprosthetic approach to SCI is to bypass the lesion with a neuro-electronic interface.

Courtine and his colleagues interfaced leg motor cortex activity with epidural electrical stimulation proto-

cols to establish a brain-spine interface that alleviated gait deficits after a partial SCI in rhesus monkeys.[163] The conceptual and technological design of the brain-spine interface is shown in the figure. The implantable components of the brain-spine interface are approved for investigational applications in similar human research. This brain-spine neurotechnology, while still in its infancy, is being tested in human patients with SCI.[164]

[163] Capogrosso, M. et al. 2016. *Nature* 539: 284-288.
[164] Wagner, F. B. et al. 2018. *Nature* 563: 65-71.

Brain–spine interface

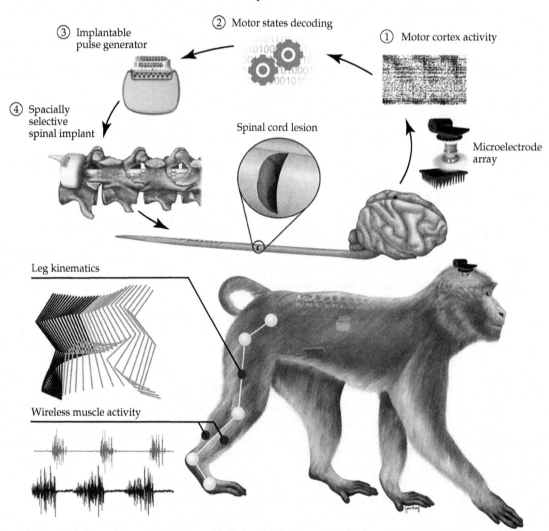

③ Implantable pulse generator
② Motor states decoding
① Motor cortex activity
④ Spacially selective spinal implant
Spinal cord lesion
Microelectrode array
Leg kinematics
Wireless muscle activity

Monkeys were implanted with a microelectrode array into the leg area of the left motor cortex. During recordings, a wireless module transmitted neural signals to a control computer. (1) Raster plot recorded over three successive gait cycles. Each line represents spiking events identified from one electrode; the horizontal axis indicates time. (2) A decoder running on the control computer identified motor states from these neural signals. (3) These motor states triggered electrical spinal cord stimulation protocols. For this, the monkeys were implanted with

a pulse generator featuring real-time triggering capabilities. (4) The stimulator was connected to a spinal implant targeting specific dorsal roots of the lumbar spinal cord. Electromyographic signals of an extensor (gray) and a flexor (black) muscle acting at the ankle recorded over three successive gait cycles are shown together with a stick diagram decomposition of leg movements during the stance (gray) and swing (black) phases of gait. (From M. Capogrosso et al., 2016. *Nature* 539: 284-288. © Jemère Ruby 2016.)

of the lesion in response to stress or certain drug treatments. This asymmetry of movement disappears after dopamine-containing neurons from the substantia nigra of immature animals are transplanted into the basal ganglia on the lesioned side. Ultrastructural studies have shown that the transplanted neurons extend axons into the surrounding region and form synapses with host neurons. This replacement therapy approach using embryonic dopaminergic neuroblasts was extended to clinical studies in people, for restoration of dopamine function in Parkinson's disease patients, showing that fetal ventral mesencephalon grafts can survive and grow in the brain and provide mixed but encouraging clinical improvements.[165,166] When the postmortem brains of some patients were examined 20 years after the implant, the grafted dopaminergic cells were found to contain Lewy bodies, a hallmark of Parkinson's disease.[166] This provided evidence that the neurodegeneration can propagate from the host to the graft, highlighting, more generally, the importance of the host local environment. The degree of functional recovery following grafts depends on the extent to which synaptic connections are reestablished.

A remarkable example of effective transplantation is the appropriate integration of transplanted embryonic cerebellar Purkinje cells in the adult *pcd* (*Purkinje cell degeneration*) mouse—a mutant whose cerebellar Purkinje cells degenerate shortly after birth (Figure 29.24).[167] Sotelo and his colleagues grafted either dissociated cells or solid pieces of the cerebellar primordium into the cerebellum of the adult mutant mouse. Donor Purkinje cells migrated out of the graft to the positions originally occupied by the degenerated Purkinje cells. They did so along the host Bergmann radial glial cells, which were induced by the graft to reexpress proteins involved in guiding Purkinje cells. Within 2 weeks, many transplanted cells formed dendritic arbors that resembled those of normal Purkinje cells, climbing fibers formed synapses (first on the cell body, then on the proximal dendrites), and parallel fibers innervated the distal dendrites. Characteristic synaptic potentials were recorded following stimulation of the climbing-fiber and mossy-fiber inputs. However, the implanted cells rarely succeeded in establishing synaptic connections with their normal targets in the deep cerebellar nuclei of the host, instead innervating nearby donor deep nuclear neurons that survived in the remnant of the graft. Nevertheless, such experiments demonstrate that transplanted cells can become incorporated into the synaptic circuitry of an adult host to a remarkable extent.

The use of human fetal tissue and embryo-derived stem cells is limited, however, by ethical issues. Many attempts are being made to repair SCI by implantation of stem cells of different origin.[168,169]

In the context of SCI, grafted cells could provide a combination of mechanisms cooperating to facilitate axonal regrowth: They might replace lost neurons and glia or secrete growth factors or attenuate the glial scar and restrain the production of inhibitory proteoglycans. Since the first attempts at cell transplantation for SCI repair,[170–172] using segments of fetal spinal cord, several cell types have been used, including Schwann cells,[101,173] olfactory ensheathing cells,[174] and more recently, neural stem cells.[168,169]

The transplant of non-neuronal cells can only provide, at best, structural and trophic support to the injury site and may counteract the toxic environment of the lesion site. On the other hand, the transplant of neural stem cells aims to form a novel relay circuit between injured axons in the spinal cord and distal targets (see Figure 29.22C), circumventing the inhibitory environment of the lesion that hinders regeneration. While regeneration of the severed axonal fibers across the lesion would be a highly desirable outcome, it has proven difficult if not impossible to achieve. Relay formation by grafted neural stem cells is a different potential strategy for SCI repair, one that does not rely on long-distance regeneration across the lesion site. Moreover, relay formation would have the advantage of using developmentally young neurons that are intrinsically primed for growth. Along these lines, Tuszynski and his colleagues[175,176] have grafted dissociated GFP-expressing multipotent neural progenitor cells, derived from either rat embryonic spinal cord or embryonic stem cells, into the rat spinal cord after a complete spinal transection (at T3 thoracic level). To

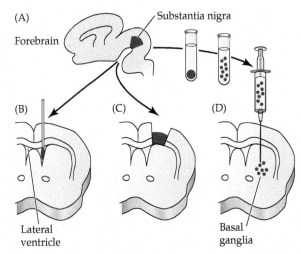

FIGURE 29.23 Procedures for Transplanting Embryonic Tissue into Adult Rat Brain. Tissue rich in cells containing dopamine is dissected from the substantia nigra (A) and is injected into the lateral ventricle (B) or grafted into a cavity in the cortex overlying the basal ganglia (C). Alternatively, a suspension of dissociated substantia nigra cells can be injected directly into the basal ganglia (D). Such embryonic cells survive, sprout, and secrete transmitter. (After S. B. Dunnett et al., 1983. *Trends Neurosci.* 6: 266-270.)

[165] Barker, R. A. et al. 2015. *Nat. Rev. Neurol.* 11: 492-503.

[166] Björklund, A. and Lindvall, O. 2017. *J. Parkinson's Dis.* 7: S21-S31.

[167] Sotelo, C. et al. 1994. *J. Neurosci.* 14: 124-133.

[168] Assinck, P. et al. 2017. *Nat. Neurosci.* 20: 637.

[169] Goldman, S. A. 2016. *Cell Stem Cell* 18: 174-188.

[170] Bregman, B. S., and Reier, P. J. 1986. *J. Comp. Neurol.* 244: 86-95.

[171] Wictorin, K., and Bjorklund, O. 1992. *Neuroreoport* 3: 1045-1048.

[172] Reier, P. J. et al. 1992. *Exp. Neurol.* 115: 177-188.

[173] Bunge, M. B. 2016. *J. Physiol.* 594: 3533-3538.

[174] Raisman, G. 2007. *C. R. Biol.* 330: 557-560.

[175] Lu, P. et al. 2012. *Cell* 150: 1264-1273.

[176] Lu, P. et al. 2014. *Neuron* 83: 789-796.

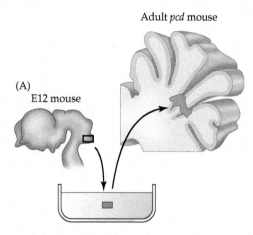

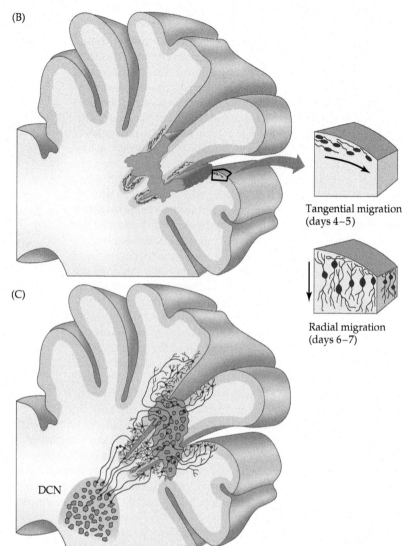

Tangential migration
(days 4–5)

Radial migration
(days 6–7)

DCN

FIGURE 29.24 Reconstruction of Cerebellar Circuits by transplantation of embryonic cerebellar tissue (outlined in black) into an adult *Purkinje cell degeneration* (*pcd*) mouse—a mutant in which Purkinje cells degenerate shortly after birth. (A) Solid pieces of cerebellar primordium from a 12-day embryo (E12) are injected into the cerebellum of a 2- to 4-month-old *pcd* mouse. (B) By 4 to 5 days after transplantation, Purkinje cells have migrated out of the graft tangentially along the cerebellar surface. During days 6 and 7 after transplantation, Purkinje cells migrate radially inward along Bergmann glial cells, penetrating the host molecular layer. (C) Donor Purkinje cells that lie within 600 mm of the host deep cerebellar nuclei (DCN) extend axons into the DCN and make synaptic contacts on their specific targets. Donor Purkinje cells farther from the host DCN make contact with donor DCN cells in the graft remnant. (A,C after C. Sotelo and R. M. Alvarado-Mallart, 1991. *Trends Neurosci.* 14: 350–355; B after C. Sotelo et al., 1990. *J. Comp. Neurol.* 295: 165–187.)

enhance survival of the graft, the cells are embedded in a fibrin matrix containing a growth factor cocktail. The grafted cells grow robust axons over remarkably long distances (more than 25 mm in each direction) and form connections with host neurons (Figure 29.25A). Moreover, host supraspinal axons locally regenerate into the neural stem cell grafts (but not beyond). This reciprocal axonal growth supports a functional improvement, as demonstrated by the recovery of electrophysiological transmission across the lesion and by the improvement of hindlimb locomotion (Figure 29.25B, top). The functional recovery is abolished by spinal re-transection immediately rostral to the lesion and by pharmacological inhibition of excitatory synaptic transmission in the graft, showing that the recovery depends on synaptic transmission through the graft (Figure 29.25B, bottom). These findings demonstrate the ability of novel neural bridging relays created by grafted neural stem cells to support functional recovery even after complete spinal transection of rat spinal cord. Subsequent experiments showed that human neural stem cells (either embryonic neural stem cells or induced pluripotent stem cells; see Chapter 27) grafted into the spinal cord lesion exhibit axonal growth properties and functional recovery similar to those observed with rodent stem cells.[176,177]

Grafts of rodent or human multipotent neural progenitor cells into the spinal cord lesion enable the extensive local sprouting of severed corticospinal axons into the graft at the lesion, which form connections with grafted neurons (a phenomenon called bridging regeneration).[177] This sprouting of corticospinal afferents into the neural progenitor cell graft, together with the extensive axonal growth of neural progenitor cells past the lesion and toward caudal targets, enables functional improvement in a skilled forelimb reaching task.[177]

[177] Kadoya, K. et al. 2016. *Nat. Med.* 22: 479–487.

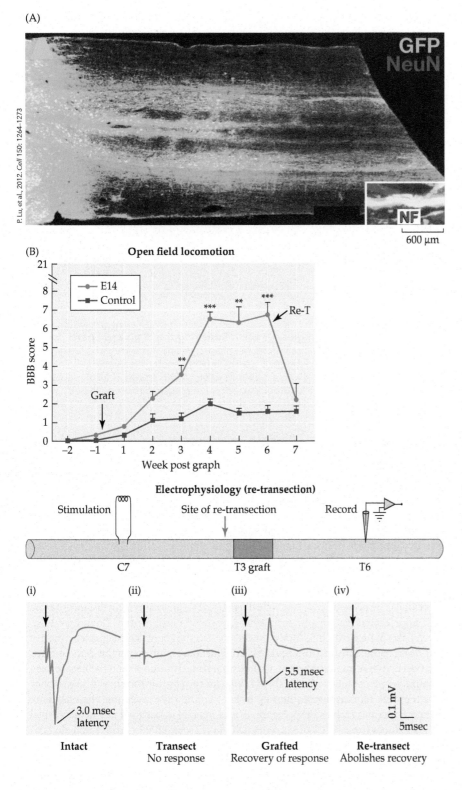

(A)

(B) **Open field locomotion**

Electrophysiology (re-transection)

(i) **Intact** — 3.0 msec latency

(ii) **Transect** No response

(iii) **Grafted** Recovery of response — 5.5 msec latency

(iv) **Re-transect** Abolishes recovery

FIGURE 29.25 Long-Distance Axonal Outgrowth and Connectivity of Neural Stem Cell Grafts after Complete Spinal Cord Injury. (A) GFP-expressing rat fetal (E14) neural stem cell grafts robustly extend axons into the host spinal cord (white matter and gray matter) rostral and caudal to the T3 complete transection site (caudal shown). Inset: GFP-labeled projections arising from grafts express neurofilament (NF), confirming their identity as axons. NeuN = mature neuronal marker. (B) Functional and electrophysiological improvement after T3 complete transection. (Top) Functional scores for locomotion (BBB, open field 21-point locomotion rating scale), show significant improvement in rats that received neural stem cell graft. Re-transection (Re-T arrow) at the rostral interface of the graft abolishes functional improvements (mean ± SEM; [**p<0.01, ***p<0.001]). Red: lesioned untreated control group; E14: lesioned grafted group. (Bottom) A stimulating electrode was placed in the dorsal C7 spinal cord and recordings were made at T6. The figure shows electrophysiological transmission across the T3 complete lesion site. (i) In intact animals, stimulation at C7 evoked a short-latency, large-amplitude response at T6. (ii) Transection of the cord at T3 completely abolished this response. (iii) In lesion-and-grafted animals, recovery of an evoked response was observed. (iv) Re-transection of the spinal cord at T3 (blue arrow), just rostral to the graft (green bar), abolished the recovered evoked response. (After P. Lu et al., 2012. *Cell* 150: 1264–1273.)

This neural stem cell grafting approach has been extended to a non-human primate model of SCI. Multipotent neural progenitor stem cells derived from human spinal cord have been grafted in rhesus monkeys after a hemisection of the spinal cord.[178] Monkey axons regenerated into grafts where they formed synapses. More than 150,000 human axons extended out from grafts through monkey white matter and formed synapses in distal gray matter. Grafts gradually matured and improved forelimb function beginning several months after grafting.[178]

[178] Rosenzweig, E. S. et al. 2018. *Nat. Med.* 24: 484–490.

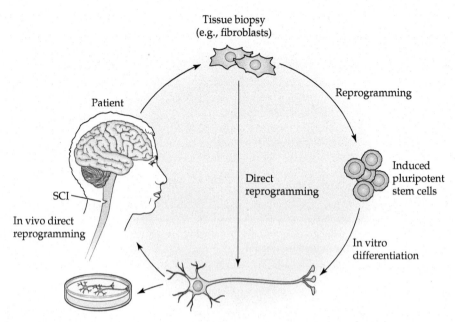

FIGURE 29.26 Potential Strategies Aimed at Repairing the Brain and Spinal Cord after Injury or Disease. Somatic cells (from the patient) can be reprogrammed to neurons in vitro, either deriving induced pluripotent stem cells (iPSCs) or by direct reprogramming. These reprogrammed neurons are a source of cells to be grafted. In vivo direct reprogramming uses endogenous glial cells for the in situ reprogramming into neurons, thereby avoiding host-to-graft immune rejection associated with exogenous cell sources. (After O. Torper and M. Götz, 2017. *Prog. Brain Res.* 230: 69-97.)

This promising therapeutic strategy for SCI justifies the search for improved sources of stem cells for cell transplant (Figure 29.26), exploiting the rapid progress in the field of stem cell biology and cell reprogramming (see Chapter 27).

Induced pluripotent stem cells (iPSCs)[179,180] are being investigated for their ability to improve neural function after spinal cord injury.[181,182] Using iPSCs overcomes the ethical and resource limitations of using human embryonic stem cells and allows for autologous cell grafting and replacement strategies, thus reducing the risk of immune-rejection of the graft when using heterologous embryonic stem cells.[179,180]

In Vivo Direct Reprogramming of Astrocytes to Neurons for Brain and Spinal Cord Repair

In addition to being derived from the iPSC method, new neurons can be derived from differentiated somatic cells directly, without passing through a stem cell stage (see Chapter 27), a process referred to as **direct lineage reprogramming**.[183,184] Astrocytes can be effectively reprogrammed into neurons. Forcing the expression of neurogenic transcription factors (such as Pax6, Neurog2, and Mash1) in cultured postnatal cortical astrocytes induces them to acquire a neuronal identity, based on markers and electrophysiological properties.[185,186]

Despite these advances, grafting externally reprogrammed autologous cells, be they iPSCs or in vitro directly reprogrammed neurons, into the CNS still faces huge hurdles. First, the time required to prepare these cells for autologous transplantation is much longer than the therapeutically optimal time-window after injury. Second, the risk of tumorigenesis induced by residual non-differentiated stem cells at the injury site must be evaluated.[187]

For this reason, the direct reprogramming of endogenous non-neuronal cells in vivo is being investigated as a promising strategy for treating CNS injuries in the future.[188,189] For example, endogenous glial cells and NG2 precursors (see Chapter 10) can be converted in situ into functional mature neurons (see Figure 29.26) without passing through a progenitor state, and therefore represent a potential pool of local progenitor cells that can

[179] Okano, and Yamanaka: 2014. *Mol. Brain.* 7: 22.

[180] Hochedlinger, K., and Jaenisch, R. 2015. *Cold Spring Harb. Perspect. Biol.* 7: a019448.

[181] Dell'Anno, M. T. et a.l 2018. *Nat. Comm.* 9: 3419.

[182] Kumamaru, H. et al. 2018. *Nat. Methods* 15: 723-731.

[183] Masserdotti, G. et al. 2016. *Development* 143: 2494-2510.

[184] Xu, J., Du, Y., and Deng, H. 2015. *Cell Stem Cell* 16: 119-134.

[185] Heins, N. et al. 2002. *Nat. Neurosci.* 5: 308-315.

[186] Berninger, B. et al. 2007. *J. Neurosci.* 27: 8654-8224.

[187] Steward, O. et al. 2014. *Cell* 156: 385.

[188] Grade, S. and Goetz, M. 2017. *NPJ Regen.* Med. 2: 29.

[189] Srivastava, D. and DeWitt, N. 2016. *Cell* 166: 1386-1396.

be directed toward neurogenesis.[190] One successful way of doing this is through the ectopic expression of a cocktail of neurogenic transcription factors, or even of a single factor, such as NeuroD1 or Ascl1.[191–193] Reactive astrocytes in a lesion seem to be facilitated in their ability to be converted into neurons, when compared with their responses in non-lesioned tissue. Retroviruses that infect dividing cells can be targeted to reactive glial cells or NG2 precursors after injury with neurogenic transcription factors.[194] Guo and his colleagues have efficiently converted in vivo cortical astrocytes and NG2 precursors into glutamatergic and GABAergic neurons by the in situ retroviral-mediated expression of the neurogenic transcription factor NeuroD1.[191] Cortical slice recordings revealed both spontaneous and evoked synaptic responses in NeuroD1-converted neurons, suggesting that they are functionally integrated into local neural circuits. By using a viral-based system to specifically target and convert resident glia at high efficiency, Torper and colleagues showed that striatal NG2 glia can be converted to GABAergic and glutamatergic neurons that remain stable over a long period of time and display electrophysiological properties of functional neurons. The newly reprogrammed neurons integrate into local circuitry in an efficient manner.[195] This seems a promising strategy to be adapted to other neurons. Dopaminergic or cholinergic neurons are immediate candidates for therapeutic possibilities in Alzheimer's and Parkinson's diseases. Here it is enough to say that the timing of the reprogramming effects is of major interest. Reactive astrocytes gradually lose their beneficial functions to become harmful at later stages. It may be ideal to design protocols in which a timed targeting of reactive astrocytes restores the neuronal population and simultaneously eliminates the inhibitory astrocytes. It remains to be seen whether the direct reprogramming of astrocytes in the injured adult spinal cord[196] can induce the functional recovery in SCI animal models.

Prospects for Developing Treatment of Spinal Cord Injury in Humans

Dating from the sixteenth century BCE, the Edwin Smith Papyrus from Thebes (Egypt) is the oldest known medical text on trauma (Figure 29.27).[197] One of the 48 cases in the scroll (Case 31) concerns a dislocation of a vertebra in the neck and concludes: "if you examine a man with a neck injury….and find he is without sensation in both arms and both legs and unable to move…..and find he is without sensation in both arms and both

[190] Dimou, L. and Goetz, M. 2014. *Physiol. Rev.* 94: 709-737.

[191] Guo, Z. et al. 2014. *Cell Stem Cell* 14: 188-202.

[192] Liu, Y et al. 2015. *J. Neurosci.* 35: 9336-9355.

[193] Heinrich, C. et al. 2014. *Stem Cell Reports* 3: 1000-1014.

[194] Dimou, L., and Gallo, V. 2015. *Glia* 63: 1429-1451

[195] Torper, O. et al. 2015. *Cell Rep* 12: 474-481.

[196] Su, Z. et al. 2014. *Nat. Comm.* 5: 3338.

[197] van Middendorp, J. J. et al. 2010. *Eur. Spine J.* 19: 1815-1823.

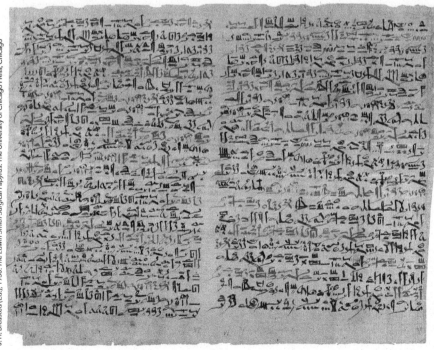

J. H. Breasted (Ed.), 1930. *The Edwin Smith Surgical Papyrus*. The University of Chicago Press, Chicago

FIGURE 29.27 The Edwin Smith Papyrus (1550 BCE): Instructions on a Case of Spinal Cord Injury. "If you examine a man with a neck injury…and find he is without sensation in both arms and both legs, and unable to move them, and he is incontinent of urine…it is due to the breaking of the spinal cord caused by the dislocation of a cervical vertebra. This is a condition that cannot be treated." *Edwin Smith Surgical Papyrus*, Case 31.

legs, and unable to move them, and he is incontinent of urine…it is due to the breaking of the spinal cord caused by the dislocation of a cervical vertebra. This is a condition that cannot be treated."[197]

Despite the intense research in the past decades, sadly this statement still holds true, for most serious cases of SCI. However, we have witnessed a tremendous advancement in our knowledge on several aspects and complexities of the problem. It is still not known what causes the failure of regeneration that is so evident after most CNS lesions. Extrinsic inhibitor factors and intrinsic mechanisms both contribute to the failure of CNS neurons to regenerate. Identifying ways to suppress endogenous growth-inhibiting factors is an active area of research, as is the development of neural stem cell lines that offer the potential of providing a readily available source of glial cells and neurons whose properties can be manipulated by genetic engineering. Such advances, combined with improved transplantation techniques, may provide hope for the amelioration of functional deficits resulting from CNS lesions by a neuronal relay strategy. A promising approach for treating CNS lesions and SCI in the future is to induce the in situ conversion of patients' endogenous glial cells to neurons. This strategy might face fewer obstacles to clinical applications than other approaches, since exogenous cells and transplantation are not required. However, the current reprogramming efficiency and the number of converted neurons are low. Also, the best anatomical site for direct reprogramming remains to be ascertained—the lesion or the site where the cell bodies of the projecting neurons are located? Further studies are necessary to enhance the reprogramming process and to define a precise strategy to generate subtype-specific and region-specific neurons that are required for functional recovery after SCI.

Two important provisos must be borne in mind—important because they are of vital interest to patients who have suffered SCI. We mention them here because many of the papers referred to in this chapter end on an optimistic note and suggest that new and effective treatments are just around the corner. First, if and when an effective therapy is developed, it will almost certainly be applicable only for repair of acute SCI. It is beyond reasonable hope to imagine that walking and sensation could be restored in a person whose spinal cord had been transected, say, 2 years (or perhaps 2 months) earlier. By that time, the distal part of the spinal cord will have undergone major degenerative changes. Moreover, as with every therapy, there may well be side effects, perhaps serious ones. Second, while it is natural that optimism should drive research, no one can predict how long it will take until a reliable therapy becomes available. No one (not even the enthusiastic scientists who make the predictions) can say for sure whether it will take weeks, months, years, decades, or longer. To repair a spinal cord is literally millions of times more difficult than repairing a computer. While time is not of the essence for a research worker, it is for the patient. False hopes aroused in paraplegics can (and often do) lead to failure to adapt themselves to their new circumstance as well as they could otherwise. Neurologists testify that, if a cure seems to be imminent, there is a temptation for SCI patients to avoid the intensive, continuous physical and mental rehabilitation that is required if the fullest possible life is to be led for all the years ahead.

SUMMARY

- When an axon is severed in the vertebrate peripheral and nervous system, the distal portion degenerates. The axotomized cell body may undergo chromatolysis or die.

- Many of the presynaptic terminals innervating an axotomized neuron retract.

- In denervated skeletal muscle fibers, new ACh receptors are synthesized and inserted in extrasynaptic regions, making the muscle supersensitive to ACh. Denervated neurons also become supersensitive to the transmitters released by damaged presynaptic axons.

- Muscle activity is an important factor determining receptor number and distribution. Muscle activity also influences the rate at which ACh receptors are degraded and replaced.

- In adult mammals and frogs, an innervated muscle will not accept innervation by an additional nerve. In contrast, nerve fibers will form new synapses on denervated or injured muscle fibers.

- In the peripheral nervous system, Schwann cells provide an environment conducive to axonal regrowth.

- Partially denervated muscles and neurons cause nearby undamaged nerves to sprout new branches and form new synapses.

- The synaptic portion of the basal lamina sheath that surrounds muscle fibers is associated with a molecule known as agrin—a proteoglycan synthesized by motor neurons and released from their axon terminals. Agrin induces the formation of postsynaptic specializations.

- The adult mammalian CNS has limited capacity for regeneration. Regeneration occurs instead in the CNS of immature mammals.

- Components of the extracellular matrix produced by astrocytes have been proposed as a cause for regeneration failure.

- Glial scars produced days and weeks after a spinal cord lesion are commonly regarded as a main barrier to CNS axon regrowth, but they can also have a beneficial role.

- Time after lesion is important: Reactive gliosis and glial scars are initially protective but in the longer term are deleterious, acting as barriers to neuronal regeneration.

- Schwann cells, in the form of a peripheral nerve graft or injected as a cell suspension at the site of a lesion, produce a favorable environment for regrowth of axons of mammalian CNS neurons.

- Regeneration or repair could be promoted by influencing different mechanisms in different lesion compartments: (i) recovery via reorganization of spared circuits, in the case of incomplete lesions or (ii) recovery via new circuits formed across anatomically complete lesions.

- Neurons from fetal or neonatal animals as well as neurons and glial cells derived from neural stem cell lines can survive and grow when transplanted into the adult mammalian CNS. The aim is that these cells will form relay stations, to restore circuit connectivity across the lesion.

- Transplanted stem cells can become incorporated into the existing synaptic circuitry and partially restore normal function.

- The in situ direct reprogramming in vivo of endogenous non-neuronal cells, such as scar-forming astrocytes, into neurons in the lesioned adult spinal cord is emerging as a new therapeutic approach for treating CNS injuries. In this approach, endogenous glial cells are directly converted in situ into functional mature neurons, thus obviating the need for grafting cells.

Suggested Reading

General Reviews

Assinck, P., Duncan, G. J., Hilton, B. J., Plemel, J. R., and Tetzlaff, W. 2017. Cell transplantation therapy for spinal cord injury. *Nat. Neurosci.* 20: 637.

Berninger, B. and Jessberger, S. 2016. Engineering of adult neurogenesis and gliogenesis. *Cold Spring Harbour Perspect. Biol.* 8: a018861.

Bonner, J. F., and Steward, O. 2015. Repair of Spinal Cord injury with neuronal relays: From fetal grafts to neural stem cells. *Brain Res.* 1619: 115–123.

Bradbury, E. J., Burnside, E. R. 2019. Moving beyond the glial scar for spinal cord repair. *Nat. Comm.* 10: 3879.

Deller, T., Haas, C. A., Freiman, T. M., Phinney, A., Jucker, M., and Frotscher, M. 2006. Lesion-induced axonal sprouting in the central nervous system. *Adv. Exp. Med. Biol.* 557: 101–121.

Dusart, I., Ghoumari, A., Wehrle, R., Morel, M. P., Bouslama-Oueghlani, L., Camand, E., and Sotelo, C. 2005. Cell death and axon regeneration of Purkinje cells after axotomy: challenges of classical hypotheses of axon regeneration. *Brain Res. Brain Res. Rev.* 49: 300–316.

Fawcett, J. W., and Verhaagen, J. 2018. Intrinsic determinants of axon regeneration. *Dev. Neurobiol.* 78: 890– 97.

Griffin, J. M., and Bradke, F. 2020. Therapeutic repair for spinal cord injury: combinatory approaches to address a multifaceted problem. *EMBO Mol. Med.* 12: e11505.

He, Z., and Jin, Y. 2016. Intrinsic control of axon regeneration. Neuron 90: 437–451

Hedong, L., and Gong, C. 2016. In vivo reprogramming for CNS repair: Regenerating neurons from endogenous glial cells. *Neuron* 91: 728–738.

Heinrich, C., Spagnoli, F. M., and Berninger, B. 2015. In vivo reprogramming for tissue repair *Nat. Cell Biol.* 17: 294–211.

Hilton, B. J., and Bradke, F. 2017. Can injured adult CNS axons regenerate by recapitulating development? *Development* 144: 3417–3429.

Huebner, E. A., and Strittmatter, S. M. 2009. Axon regeneration in the peripheral and central nervous systems. *Results Probl. Cell Differ.* 48: 339–351.

Madduri, S., and Gander, B. 2010. Schwann cell delivery of neurotrophic factors for peripheral nerve regeneration. *J. Peripher. Nerv. Syst.* 15: 93–103.

Mladinic, M., Muller, K. J., and Nicholls. J. G. 2009. Central nervous system regeneration: from leech to opossum. *J. Physiol.* 587: 2775–2782.

McMahan, U. J. 1990. The agrin hypothesis. *Cold Spring Harb. Symp. Quant. Biol.* 50: 407–418.

Schaffran, B., and Bradke, F. 2019. Reproducibility: The key towards clinical implementation of spinal cord injury treatments? *Exp. Neurol.* 313: 135–136.

Sofroniew, M. V. 2018 Dissecting spinal cord regeneration. *Nature* 557: 343–350.

Steward, O., Zheng B. and Tessier-Lavigne, M. 2003 False resurrections: Distinguishing regenerated from spared axons in the injured nervous system. *J. Comp. Neurol.* 459: 1–8.

Steward, O., Popovich, P. G., Dietrich, W. D., and Kleitman, N. 2012. Replication and reproducibility in spinal cord injury research. *Exp. Neurol.* 233: 597–605.

Torper, O., and Goetz, M. 2017. Brain repair from intrinsic cell sources: turning reactive glia into neurons. *Progr, Brain Res.* 230: 69–97.

Tuszynski, M. H., and Steward, O. 2012 Concepts and methods for the study of axonal regeneration in the CNS. *Neuron* 74: 777–791.

Wang, L. L. and Zhang, C. L. 2018. Engineering new neurons: in vivo reprogramming in the mammalian brain and spinal cord. *Cell Tissue Res.* 37: 201–212.

Wictorin, K., Brundin, P., Gustavii, B., Lindvall, O., and Björklund, A.1990. Reformation of long axon pathways in adult rat central nervous system by human forebrain neuroblasts. *Nature* 347: 556–558.

Original Papers

Björklund, A., Dunnett, S. B., Stenevi, U., Lewis, N. E., and Iversen, S. D. 1980. Reinnervation of the denervated striatum by substantia nigra transplants: Functional consequences as revealed by pharmacological and sensorimotor testing. *Brain Res.* 199: 307–333.

Bunge, M. B. 2016. Efficacy of schwann cell (SC) transplantation for spinal cord repair is improved with combinatorial strategies. *J. Physiol. (Lond.)* 594: 3533–3538.

Burden, S. J., Sargent, P. B., and McMahan, U. J. 1979. Acetylcholine receptors in regenerating muscle accumulate at original synaptic sites in the absence of the nerve. *J. Cell Biol.* 82: 412–425.

Courtine, G., Song, B., Roy, R. R., Zhong, H., Herrmann, J. E., Ao,Y., Qi, J., Edgerton, V. R., and Sofroniew, M. V. 2008. Recovery of supraspinal control of stepping via indirect propriospinal relay connections after spinal cord injury *Nat. Med.* 14: 69–74.

David, S., and Aguayo, A. J. 1981. Axonal elongation into peripheral nervous system "bridges" after central nervous system injury in adult rats. *Science* 214: 931–933.

Kim, N., Stiegler, A. L., Cameron, T. O., Hallock, P. T., Gomez, A. M., Huang, J. H., Hubbard, S. R., Dustin, M. L., and Burden, S. J. 2008. Lrp4 is a receptor for agrin and forms a complex with MuSK. *Cell* 135: 334–342.

Fournier, A. E., GrandPre, T., and Strittmatter, S. M. 2001. Identification of a receptor mediating Nogo-66 inhibition of axonal regeneration. *Nature* 409: 341–346.

Guo, Z., Zhang, L., Wu, Z., Chen, Y., Wang, F., and Chen, G. 2014. In vivo direct reprogramming of reactive glial cells into functional neurons after brain injury and in an Alzheimer's disease model. *Cell Stem Cell* 14: 188–202.

Kadoya, K., Lu, Pl, Nguyen, K., Lee-Kubli, C., Kumamaru, H., Yao, L., Knackert, J., Poplawski, G., Dulin, J. N., Strol, H., Takashima, Y., Biane, J., Conner, J., Zhang, S.-C., and Tuszynski, M. H. 2016. Spinal cord reconstitution with homologous neural grafts enables robust corticospinal regeneration *Nat. Med.* 22: 479–487.

Karow, M., Camp, J. G., Falk, S., Gerber, T., Pataskar, A., Gac-Santel, M., Kageyama, J., Brazovskaja, A., Garding, A., Fan, W., Riedemann, T., Casamassa, A., Smiyakin, A., Schichor, C., Götz, M., Tiwari, V. K., Treutlein, B., and Berninger, B. 2018. Direct pericyte-to-neuron reprogramming via unfolding of a neural stem cell-like program. *Nat. Neurosci.* 21: 932–940.

Lin, S., Landmann, L., Rüegg, M. A., and Brenner, H. R. 2008. The role of nerve- versus muscle-derived factors in mammalian neuromuscular junction formation. *J. Neurosci.* 28: 3333–3340.

Liu, Y., Wang, X., Li, W., Zhang, Q., Li, Y., Zhang, Z., Zhu, J., Chen, B., Williams, P. R., Zhang, Y., Yu, B., Gu, X., and He, Z. 2017. A sensitized IGF1 treatment restores corticospinal axon-dependent functions. *Neuron* 95: 817–833.

Lømo, T., and Rosenthal, J. 1972. Control of ACh sensitivity by muscle activity in the rat. *J. Physiol.* 221: 493–513.

Love, F. M., Son, Y. J., and Thompson, W. J. 2003. Activity alters muscle reinnervation and terminal sprouting by reducing the number of Schwann cell pathways that grow to link synaptic sites. *J. Neurobiol.* 54: 566–576.

Lu, P., Lu, P., Wang, Y., Graham, L., McHale, K., Gao, M., Wu, D., Brock, J., Blesch, A., Rosenzweig, E. S., Havton, L. A., Zheng, B., Conner, J. M., Marsala, M., and Tuszynski, M. H. 2012 Long-distance growth and connectivity of neural stem cells after severe spinal cord injury. *Cell* 150: 1264–1273.

Niu, W., Zang, T., Smith, D. K., Vue, T. Y., Zou, Y., Bachoo, R., Johnson, J. E., and Zhang, C. L. 2015. SOX2 reprograms resident astrocytes into neural progenitors in the adult brain. *Stem Cell Reports* 4: 780–794.

Rosenzweig, E. S.., Salegio, E A.., Liang, J. J., Weber, J. L., Weinholtz, C. A., Brock, J. H., Moseanko, R., Hawbecker, S., Pender, R., Cruzen C. L., et al. 2019. Chondroitinase improves anatomical and functional outcomes after primate spinal cord injury. *Nat. Neurosci.* 22: 1269–1275.

Rotshenker, S. 2009. The role of Galectin-3/MAC-2 in the activation of the innate-immune function of phagocytosis in microglia in injury and disease. *J. Mol. Neurosci.* 39: 99–103.

Samuels, S. E., Lipitz, J. B., Dahl, G., and Muller, K. J. 2010. Neuroglial ATP release through innexin channels controls microglial cell movement to a nerve injury. *J. Gen. Physiol.* 136: 425–452.

Saunders, N. R., Kitchener, P., Knott, G. W., Nicholls, J. G., Potter, A., and Smith, T. J. 1998. Development of walking, swimming and neuronal connections after complete spinal cord transection in the neonatal opossum, *Monodelphis domestica*. *J. Neurosci.* 18: 339–355.

Schwab, M. E., and Caroni, P. 1988. Oligodendrocytes and CNS myelin are nonpermissive substrates for neurite growth and fibroblast spreading in vitro. *J. Neurosci.* 8: 2381–2393.

Su, Z., Niu, W., Liu, M.-L., Zou, Y., and Zhang, C.-L. 2014. in vivo conversion of astrocytes to neurons in the injured adult spinal cord. *Nat. Comm.* 5: 3338.

Warren, P. M., Steiger, S. C., Dick, T. E., MacFarlane, P. M., Alilain, W. J., and Silver, J. 2018. Rapid and robust restoration of breathing long after spinal cord injury. *Nat. Comm.* 9: 4843.

PART VII

Conclusion

CHAPTER 30

Open Questions

With each new edition of *From Neuron to Brain*, our understanding of how nerve cells produce electrical signals, how they communicate with one another, how they act in concert, and how they become connected during development has become deeper. In the last years, major advances have been obtained through novel molecular biological, genetic, and imaging techniques. For example, we now have detailed knowledge of the intimate structural changes that mediate the opening, closing, and inactivation of channels (see Chapter 5). The visualization and localization of individual molecules associated with exocytosis have provided us with an essential understanding of the process of synaptic transmission (see Chapter 13). We have gained significant knowledge of the way in which repetitively stimulated synapses are modified by activity-dependent regulation of local and cell-wide gene expression (see Chapter 17), and how these changes may underlie perception and memory. Mechanisms of transmitter release outside synapses and how extrasynaptic release adapts the responses of neuronal circuits and behavior are now better understood (Chapter 18). Progress has also been made toward understanding the molecular events and the logic that control the development of the diverse neuronal cell types that make up the neocortex (see Chapter 27).

What can one predict today about novel concepts that might be incorporated into the next edition of this book? One reasonable guess is that more intensive collaboration among basic scientists working at the cellular and molecular levels, cognitive neuroscientists, computational scientists, and clinical neurologists will be important for understanding integrative and higher brain functions relating to perception, movement, and memory. One can hope also that an increase in fundamental knowledge of the nervous system will lead to better hypotheses about the causes, prevention, and alleviation of diseases of the nervous system that arise from unknown causes and that cannot yet be treated effectively.

Many open questions about the nervous system and the brain are more apparent than those in physics, or chemistry, or even biology in general. A layperson outside science is aware that we do not know the mechanisms underlying higher functions such as consciousness, learning, the production of coordinated movements, or even how one initiates the bending of a finger as an act of will. The same person, even if highly sophisticated and well educated, would probably have much more difficulty in pointing out what one still needs to know about relativity, particle physics, chemical reactions, or genetics. It is this wealth of obvious, unsolved, and important human questions in neuroscience that makes it so appealing today.

To illustrate one everyday example of our present ignorance of how the brain performs its functions, consider a sport such as table tennis, already mentioned in Chapter 18. An expert player sees his opponent hit the ball. He can compute rapidly where it will land and how high it will bounce. The ball may be traveling at 80 km/hr, but he can rush to the right spot, arm extended, and hit the ball in the center of the paddle, with exactly the right force to send it exactly onto the line in the other court (exploiting the remembered weakness of his opponent's backhand), all in fractions of seconds.

We could just as well have picked as examples the way in which a pelican dives for a fish, a frog catches a fly with its tongue, or a bee drinks from a particular flower. In each of these examples, objects must be recognized against a rich background, and highly coordinated movements must be planned, initiated, regulated, and brought to fulfillment. And all the necessary neuronal connections for perception, planning, and execution of the movement must have been already formed.

In this chapter we consider selected problems in neuroscience that might become more approachable in the future, particularly in relation to the topics emphasized in this book.

Object Recognition and Memory Formation

In the pursuit of problems of high interest, such as the neural mechanisms underlying perception, and the relation of long-term potentiation and long-term depression to learning and memory, several detailed experiments have begun to reveal essential information.

One important contribution to our ideas about perception has been the emergence of studies on cells in the medial temporal lobe of the brain that respond exclusively to particular visual images. Of special interest are studies on such cells in awake humans with recording electrodes implanted in their brains for the purpose of monitoring neuronal activity during surgical treatment for epilepsy (for a review see Quian Quiroga, 2013).[1] Many such cells are silent but respond vigorously with a burst of action potentials when a specific visual stimulus is presented to the patient on a computer screen—for example, a picture of a particular person or place that the patient recognizes. In one experiment a neuron in the hippocampus fired strongly when the patient was presented with any one of several different pictures of the actress Pamela Anderson, but not at all to any of 80 other pictures, including other faces. Interestingly, the response could be evoked with other stimulus modalities, for instance by reading Anderson's name on a screen (Figure 30.1). In another patient, a neuron responded to pictures of Luke Skywalker (from the *Star Wars* movies) and also to a picture of Yoda, another *Star Wars* character. So the cell discharges were associated not only with the particular images, but also with some wider conceptual framework, such as a written name or a related image. Such neurons have been designated **concept cells**.[1]

Do the neuronal responses always coincide with the perceptions of the patient? Quian Quiroga and his colleagues approached this problem by studying responses to images that were presented for periods as short as one-thirtieth of a second, near the threshold time for visual recognition.[2] Patients were shown a random sequence of images, one of which elicited a response in the concept cell under study. At this short duration, patients recognized the test image in about half of the trials. The striking result was that presentation of the image resulted in recognition by the patient only if the concept cell also responded. If the concept cell did not respond to the image, then neither did the patient. In other words, the cell discharge was an essential component of the recognition process.

As noted in Chapter 25, the idea that the neuronal activity of a group of concept cells is causally related to visual perception is supported by other experiments on neurons in the inferior temporal lobe of monkeys that respond preferentially to facial images. Monkeys were presented with blurred images of faces which they were required to categorize

[1] Quian Quiroga, R. 2013. *Acta Neurobiol. Exp.* 73: 463–471.

[2] Quian Quiroga, R. et al. 2008. *Proc. Natl. Acad. Sci. USA* 105: 3599–3604.

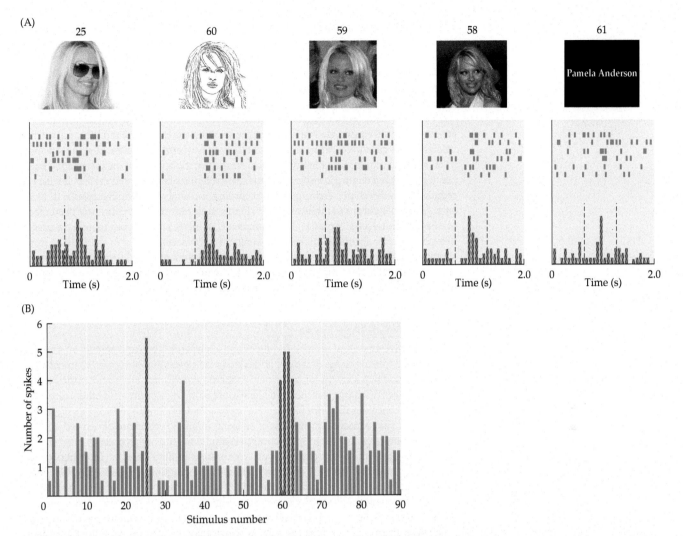

FIGURE 30.1 Neuronal Representation of a Concept in Human Hippocampus. Responses of a single unit in the right posterior hippocampus of a human neurosurgical patient. (A) The neuron fired when pictures of the actress Pamela Anderson were presented with and without sunglasses—and even as a caricature. Blue bars represent the times of neuronal action potentials across single stimulus presentations; the histograms below are the action potentials summated in time bins. Vertical dashed lines are the start and end of stimulus presentation. The fact that the neuron fired when the written letter string was presented as a stimulus indicates that the neuron's activity is part of the representation of the concept of Pamela Anderson, not just the visual likeness. (B) Vertical bars show the number of spikes fired by the same neuron for 87 different stimuli. Those stimuli related to Pamela Anderson (red patterned bars) evoked the largest response. The neuron fired for other stimuli, so its selectivity was not absolute. (After R. Quian Quiroga et al., 2005. *Nature* 435: 1102–1107.)

as "face" or "non-face," depending on how they perceived the image.[3] When the blurred image presentations were accompanied by discrete electrical stimulation of clusters of face-selective neurons, the fraction of responses designated "face" increased. So stimulation of face-selective neurons facilitated perception of a facial image.

It is generally accepted that a neuron that responds to a particular image or concept is not acting on its own. Instead it is one member of a large ensemble, each member of which responds to the same stimulus. The size of such an ensemble is not known, but is thought to be at least tens of thousands, possibly hundreds of thousands of neurons.[1] Also, a given neuron belongs to more than one ensemble, probably a very large number. For example, the Luke Skywalker neuron also responded to a picture of Yoda, and might have responded to other images related to the *Star Wars* movies.

Recognition of a face or other object involves memory recall; in other words, the object in view is compared with an image previously stored in memory. One model proposed for memory allocation is the neuronal activation model, in which an ensemble of neurons is

[3] Afraz, S. R. et al. 2006. *Nature* 442: 692–695.

activated during memory formation to serve as the physical representation of the memory trace in the brain (see Chapter 17). In this model, a subset of dendritic synapses in each participating neuron is potentiated during the learning process so that it responds regularly when activated by the relevant synaptic input. As proposed for the face-recognition cells, any given neuron might belong to a large number of separate ensembles, each with its own subset of synapses representing a unique memory trace.

To explore the neuronal activation model further, and to understand how memories are created and are associated with each other, we will have to understand the mechanisms whereby such ensembles are assembled and how they overlap and interact at the synaptic level. This will require new methods to achieve the genetic tagging of the presynaptic partner of potentiated dendritic spines,[4] and the manipulation of potentiated spines.[5] It will also require highly developed techniques for recording and analyzing simultaneous activity of large groups of neurons in the awake brain. Remarkable technical advances have been made in this direction (see Chapter 1). For example, R. A. Silver and his colleagues have used a two-photon laser scanning microscope to record fluorescent activity in multiple neurons simultaneously in the brains of awake mice.[6] Records were obtained from a population of cells throughout a 250-μm cube of tissue with a spatial resolution sufficient to resolve the fine structure of cerebellar pyramidal cells, including dendritic spines.

Consciousness

A more elusive goal is an understanding of consciousness. The experiments on concept cells revealed that discharge of the cell under study (and presumably of many of its cohorts) was an absolute requirement for conscious recognition of the image. This raises the issue of whether the cell discharge was the immediate cause of the recognition—in other words, the cause of the conscious memory recall.

The idea that conscious awareness of an event might be generated by a specific nerve discharge pattern is consistent with an observation made during an entirely different experiment on generation and execution of a motor task. In the 1980s Ben Libet performed studies on movement that were designed specifically to examine the relation between neuronal activity underlying voluntary movement, and conscious awareness (see Chapter 26).[7] He used electroencephalography to record readiness potentials that preceded voluntary movements. Individuals were asked to make a spontaneous movement, such as lifting a finger, and afterward to report the time at which they decided to make the movement. When the decision time was compared with the time of occurrence of the readiness potential, the onset of cerebral activity preceded the reported time of intent by several hundred milliseconds. In other words, the neuronal activity underlying the movement began before the individuals were aware that they intended to move, so the neural processing required for planning and execution of the movement began without conscious input. These observations have been confirmed repeatedly, most recently by recording brain activity with functional magnetic resonance imaging (fMRI).[8] Again, this observation raises the possibility that conscious awareness of an event (the decision to move) might be generated by a particular nerve discharge pattern associated with the event itself.

These experiments suggest that perception and decision making are subconscious functions of the brain, and that conscious awareness of such events is generated by their associated neuronal activity. The idea that a conscious experience is generated in some such manner seems apparent—what likely mechanism other than neuronal activity does the brain have? However, the details of how a particular neuronal firing pattern might be transduced into a specific conscious event remain obscure.

Development and Regeneration

In spite of remarkable progress, it is still not known how growing neurons select their precise targets. One can now approach problems such as directed neurite outgrowth toward targets, termination of growth, and the refinement of connections by selective pruning and cell death in molecular terms. At the same time, we can only wonder how the extraordinary precision of connections is achieved, for example by terminals of muscle spindle afferent fibers on motoneurons in the spinal cord. With several thousand neurons in each cubic millimeter of tissue,

[4] Choi, J. H. et al. 2018. *Science* 360: 430-435.

[5] Gobbo, F. et al. 2017. *Nat. Comm.* 8: 1629.

[6] Nadella, K. M. et al. 2016. *Nat. Meth.* 13: 1001-1004.

[7] Libet, B. 1983. *Brain* 106: 623.

[8] Bode, S. et al. 2011. *PLOS ONE* 6: e21612.

how are the appropriate motor cells selected and innervated at the appropriate sites? And through what mechanisms does the same sensory cell form synapses with quite different release characteristics on specific neurons in the medulla? Understanding in detail the development of the human brain is an open question of the utmost importance, but it has been challenging to explore because of the inherent experimental difficulties.[9,10,11]

As for the failure of regeneration after injury to the mammalian CNS, the reasons are still not known, in spite of considerable advances in our understanding of the intrinsic and extrinsic molecular mechanisms that promote and inhibit axonal growth (see Chapter 29).[12,13] It seems likely that a combination of treatments—one for making the inhibitory environment more permissive and a second to increase the intrinsic regenerative ability of axons—could be the key to a future clinically relevant regeneration or repair breakthrough.[14] Because long-distance regeneration of injured axons of central neurons is still unattainable, an actively pursued repair strategy is the transplant of neural stem cells into the lesion site, to form relay stations that provide transmission continuity across the lesion.[15] The direct conversion of resident reactive glial cells to neurons in vivo, by the targeted expression of reprogramming transcription factors, is an alternative strategy for the future that would avoid the problems of cell grafting.[16,17,18] If carefully timed, the direct in situ reprogramming strategy may "kill two birds with one stone," allowing the reactive astrocytes to perform their protective actions acutely after the injury, followed by their reprogrammed conversion into neurons before exerting their adverse effects.

An exciting question for the future, inspired by the epigenetic methods to reprogram cell identity into different types,[19,20] is whether we can identify combinations of transcription factors that are capable of reprogramming CNS neurons into a pro-regenerative transcriptional state, rejuvenating their pro-regeneration gene expression program, without altering their cell identity. The possibility of treatment with genetically engineered cells is now being intensively investigated in muscular dystrophy, Parkinson's disease, and spinal cord lesions, and gene therapies are being developed for retinal and neurological diseases.

Genetic Approaches to Understanding the Nervous System

It is hard to predict the consequences of the revolution in genetic and genomic techniques for understanding brain function. The present use of transgenic animals in which identified genes have been altered or deleted provides a powerful tool, but one still hampered by difficulties of interpretation owing to redundancy of function and unexpected side effects. Since the completion of the Human Genome Project, the advent of next-generation sequencing (NGS) platforms, for DNA and RNA sequencing, has provided the opportunity to examine genome-wide gene expression, even at the single cell level. A huge number of candidate genes and molecules that are altered in disease and development are becoming known. To analyze this large array of information and separate the important from the incidental constitutes an immense task that requires sophisticated bioinformatic and computational approaches.

The scope of the problem of defining the biological function of a protein is illustrated by the study of inherited diseases, such as Huntington's disease, in which the altered gene can be identified by linkage analysis of the affected families.[21] Yet although the altered sequences of the Huntington's disease gene were identified long ago, the function of the protein remains unknown.[22,23] Similarly, mutations in genes coding for voltage-gated calcium channels are associated with familial hemiplegic migraine and cerebellar ataxia.[24] But again, there is no clear link in terms of mechanisms. Even for a molecule as important as the prion protein, which is abundant in the normal brain and which, when transformed, gives rise to transmissible spongiform encephalopathies (of which bovine spongiform encephalopathy, or mad cow disease, is the best known), there is no known normal function, nor is there complete information about the mechanism by which cortical tissue becomes infected through eating infected brains.[25]

Another example is provided by the amyloid precursor protein (APP). Biochemical and genetic evidence establishes a central role of APP in Alzheimer's disease pathogenesis. Despite the huge efforts devoted to understanding the biological functions of APP since its cloning in 1988, the underlying mechanisms remain largely undefined and often controversial.[26] Two major obstacles complicate the analysis of functions of APP in vivo: (1) APP is subject to complex proteolytic processing that generates several polypeptides, each of

[9] Sidhaye, J. and Knoblich, J. A. 2020. *Cell Death Differ.* doi: 10.1038/s41418-020-0566-4.

[10] Qian, X. et al. 2019. *Development* 146: dev166074.

[11] Lancaster, M. A. and Knoblich, J. A. 2014 *Science* 345: 1247125.

[12] Mahar, M. and Cavalli, V. 2018. *Nat. Rev. Neurosci.* 19: 323-337.

[13] Fawcett, J. W. 2020. *Neurochem. Res.* 45: 144-158.

[14] Griffin, J. M. and Bradke, F. 2020. *EMBO Mol. Med.* 12: e11505.

[15] Fischer, I. et al. 2020. *Nat. Rev. Neurosci.* https://doi.org/10.1038/s41583-020-0314-2.

[16] Su, Z. et al. 2014. *Nat. Comm.* 5: 3338.

[17] Wang, L. L. and Zhang, C. L. 2018. *Cell Tissue Res.* 371: 201-212.

[18] Li, H. and Chen, G. 2016. *Neuron* 91: 728-738.

[19] Hochedlinger, K. and Jeanisch, R. 2015. *Cold Spring Harb. Perspect. Biol.* 7: a019448.

[20] Guo C, Morris SA. 2017. *Curr. Opin. Genet. Dev.* 46: 50-57.

[21] Ross, C. A., and Tabrizi, S. J. 2011. *Lancet Neurol.* 10: 83-98.

[22] Ha, A. D., and Fung, V. S. 2012. Huntington's disease. *Curr. Opin. Neurol.* 25: 491-498.

[23] Sadou, F. and Humbert, S. 2016. *Neuron* 89: 910.

[24] Pietrobon, D. 2010. *Pflügers Arch.* 460: 375-393.

[25] Weissmann, C. 2009. *Folia Neuropathol.* 47: 104-113.

[26] Mueller, U. C. and Zheng, H. 2012. *Cold Spring Harb. Perspect. Med.* 4: a006288.

which likely performs specific and distinct functions, and (2) APP is part of a gene family with partially overlapping functions.

Deciphering the function of proteins remains a daunting task, as no single approach can provide the answer. The complexity of the proteome outnumbers the complexity of the genome, due to RNA splicing, proteolytic processing, post-translational modifications, conformational variants, complex quaternary associations, cell localization, and context. As sophisticated as the genetic methods targeting the gene or the RNA encoding a protein may be, they cannot, by definition, address these post-transcriptional and post-translational complexities.

A long-term hope is that genetic therapies will be developed for neurological and neurodegenerative diseases,[27] as well as for certain conditions that cause degeneration of the retina.[28] At present, genetic therapies are being clinically tested in patients suffering from macular degeneration and retinitis pigmentosa.[29,30] Nevertheless, it is worth commenting that the slow progress in devising treatments for Huntington's disease and other long-established monogenic diseases (such as cystic fibrosis,[31] a defect in an epithelial anion transporter, the genetic cause for which was discovered more than 30 years ago[32]) suggests that developing effective gene therapy may take a long time.

On the positive side, the study of human (and animal) genetic mutations, coupled with information yielded by the Human Genome Project, has provided important advances in basic neuroscience. An example is the discovery of the entire orexin (hypocretin) system for controlling sleep and appetite described in Chapter 14. On a smaller scale, it was only through genetic analysis of inherited human epilepsies that the molecular structure of the M-channel became known.[33] It is clear that application of known genetic information will continue to provide new information about the function of individual proteins, through the inhibition of their expression by use of small-interfering RNAs, of site-specific DNA recombinases (such as Cre recombinase),[34,35] and of the CRISPR toolkit for genome editing,[36] as well as by methods to interfere selectively with the post-translationally modified pool of a given protein.[34] Genetic knowledge can also yield big advances in technology, for example the possibility of color-coding individual neurons,[37] stimulating or silencing them, and recording their activity in the brain in situ.[38] These techniques are already enabling cell-type-specific imaging, neurophysiological, and perturbation studies and are becoming valuable for sorting out the brain's functional wiring.[39,40]

Sensory and Motor Integration

A serious deficiency in our knowledge concerns the enormous numbers of neurons with no obvious function, particularly unmyelinated fibers, which greatly outnumber myelinated fibers. One example from this book is how the various amacrine cell types (about 40) contribute to processing in the retina. Another is the role of Group II afferents from muscle spindles in spinal cord function. Traditionally, the diversity of cell identities in the nervous system has been categorized through the use of classical descriptors such as shape, electrophysiological properties, and immunomarkers. It is now possible to collect RNA sequence (RNA-seq) data from large numbers of individual neurons (single-cell transcriptomics), providing a molecular barcode, or signature, for the classification of cell identities in the brain,[41] and thereby identifying a large number of different cell types in the cortex,[42,43] retina,[44] and several other brain regions. The multimodal integration of these data within the experimental armamentarium of neuroscientists opens endless opportunities to ask new questions about the development, evolution, physiology, and pathology of the brain.

Mechanisms for the initiation and control of coordinated movements represent problems that have seen progress but still remain open. Thanks to noninvasive techniques for imaging and stimulation, one can now obtain detailed images of brain activity. Yet more than 75 years ago, in remarkably prescient comments, Adrian pointed out (see Chapter 26) that once you have learned to write your name, you can do it at once by holding the pencil between your toes.[45] For our ability to transfer such programs from one effector system to another, we have no explanation.

In addition to these obvious gaps in our knowledge, the mechanisms for the precise control of body temperature, blood pressure, and intestinal functions remain black boxes. Interactions of the brain with the immune system and with the microbiome represent another major field of active research that is still at an early stage, with many open questions.

[27] Deverman, B. E. et al. 2018. *Nat. Rev. Drug Discov.* 17: 641.

[28] Petit, L. et al. 2016. *Human Gene Ther.* 27: 563.

[29] Russel, S. et al. 2017. *Lancet* 390: 849.

[30] Cehajic-Kapetanovic, J. et al. 2020. *Nat. Med.* 26: 354-359.

[31] Yan, Z. et al. 2019. *Hum. Mol. Genetics* 28: R88-R94.

[32] Kerem, B. et al. 1989. *Science* 245: 1073-1080.

[33] Jentsch, T. J. 2000. *Nat. Rev. Neurosci.* 1: 21-30.

[34] Cattaneo, A. and Chirichella, M. 2019. *Trends Biotech.* 37: 578.

[35] Branda, C. S. and Dymecki, S. M. 2004. *Dev. Cell 6*: 7-28.

[36] Adli, M. 2018. *Nat. Comm.* 9: 1911.

[37] Livet, J. et al. 2007. *Nature* 450: 56-62.

[38] Knöpfel, T. et al. 2010. *J. Neurosci.* 30: 14998-15004.

[39] Gradinaru, V. et al. 2009. *Science* 324: 354-359.

[40] Luo, L. et al. 2018. *Neuron* 98: 256-281.

[41] Tasic, B. 2018. *Curr. Op. Neurobiol.* 50: 242-249.

[42] Zeisel, A. et al. 2015. *Science* 347: 1138-1142.

[43] Tasic, B. et al. 2016. *Nat. Neurosci.* 19: 335-346.

[44] Menon, M. et al. 2019. *Nat. Comm.* 10: 4902.

[45] Adrian, E. D. 1946. *The Physical Background of Perception.* Clarendon, Oxford, England.

Rhythmicity

Neuronal rhythms considered in this book include respiration and circadian rhythms as well as the periodicity of firing by neurons in the cerebellum, hippocampus, thalamus, and spinal cord. Except in a few examples, such as the stomatogastric ganglion of the lobster and the swimming of the leech, we have no detailed information about the mechanisms that underlie the genesis or the regularity of firing patterns. Moreover, it is not at all clear what functions are played by current oscillations in well-known phenomena such as theta waves or the alpha and delta waves of the electroencephalogram.[46] While information about circadian rhythms is becoming available at the molecular level (thanks largely to work on *Drosophila*), the precise role of sleep and the way it arises are still obscure, as are the mechanisms by which anesthetics produce their effects.

Input from Clinical Neurology to Studies of the Brain

For many years neurology was not only inseparable from neurobiology but provided the only method for studying higher functions in relation to brain structure. A triumph of the early neurologists was their application of nature's own experiments to describe functions of various brain areas from careful correlation of symptoms with lesions. Their achievements are all the more remarkable because the use of lesions to assess function is fraught with pitfalls. With techniques now available, such as fMRI and positron emission tomography (PET), the neurologist is able to locate and observe lesions directly, to follow their progress in the living brain, and to make inferences about areas of brain related to higher cortical functions.

The dramatic story of Phineas Gage emphasizes the advantages and pitfalls of lesions and deficits as a means of analyzing brain function.[47] In 1848, at the age of 25, Phineas Gage suffered a massive lesion to the brain while working as a construction foreman on a railway in Vermont. As he pushed on a tamping iron to place a charge of gunpowder into a rock, the gunpowder exploded and blew the iron rod clear through the front of his skull. Gage lost consciousness only briefly and could soon sit up and speak. What astounded the doctor was that Gage recovered rapidly and was able to lead a relatively normal life for more than 12 years. Gage's personality, however, underwent a major change. From being a well-liked, quiet, sober, industrious, and careful worker, he changed into a loud-mouthed, boastful, impatient, and restless braggart. At a time when nothing was known of sensory, motor, visual, or auditory cortex, the neurological investigation showed that the prefrontal area was associated with the very highest functions of human conduct and personality.

Other examples of neurological observations made in the nineteenth century that defined specific brain areas involved in higher functions were those of Broca and Wernicke, who correlated defects in speech with the areas of cortex that had been damaged by vascular accidents or tumors. Even when precise areas are not known, clinicians and neuropsychologists can reliably define and separate processes such as long- and short-term memory. Patient H.M. had a severe memory impairment, which resulted from experimental neurosurgery to control seizures, and was the subject of study for five decades by Brenda Milner, until his death in December 2008. Work with H.M. established fundamental principles about how memory functions are organized in the brain.[48]

Highly counterintuitive and difficult to comprehend at first sight are effects of lesions to the parietal lobe on one side, usually the right. Patients with such lesions may no longer recognize that there are two sides to the body and to the outside world. The left side of the body ceases to exist, so a patient will not recognize his left hand as his own. When such patients with a lesion of the right parietal lobe are asked to draw a daisy, all the petals are on the right; likewise, all the spokes of a bicycle wheel are drawn on the right.[49] A drawing of a cat made by a right-handed, 61-year-old patient with a parietal lesion is shown in Figure 30.2. It is important to emphasize that these are true neurological defects, not hysterical reactions of the patient. Such clinical observations show that our inner world, which seems so complete, so unitary, and so perfect, is composed of elementary components welded together to form a continuum.

As information becomes available from brain scans and from sophisticated tests of language and performance, one can expect the exploration of higher functions to depend ever more on input from cognitive neuroscience and neurology. Moreover, even as knowledge

[46] Lisman, J. E. et al. 2010. *Biol. Psychiat.* 68: 17-24.

[47] Harlow, J. M. 1868. *Publ. Mass. Med. Soc.* 2: 328-334.

[48] Squire, L. R. 2009. *Neuron* 61: 6-9.

[49] Driver, J., and Halligan, P. W. 1991. *Cogn. Neuropsychol.* 8: 475-496.

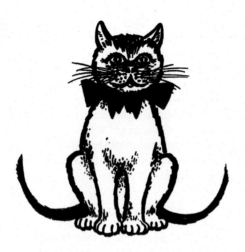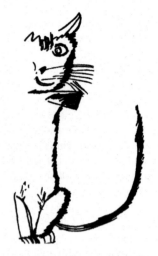

Figure 30.2   Drawing of a Cat. The drawing (right) was made by a patient who had a large lesion of the right parietal lobe. Only the right side of the drawing was copied. All details on the left were overlooked. Such deficits are commonly seen following lesions of this type. (After J. Driver and P. W. Halligan, 1991. *Cogn. Neuropsychol.* 8: 475–496; drawing provided by J. Driver.)

of human brain advances, it is clear from the work of Kravitz and his colleagues that genetic studies of lower animals, such as lobsters and flies, can shed light on higher functions such as the role of specific molecules in aggressive behavior.[50]

Input from Basic Neuroscience to Neurology

There clearly exists a two-way street between basic and applied neuroscience. Molecular biological and genetic techniques are already playing a role in the diagnosis of several neurological conditions. Genome-wide association studies (GWAS) are contributing to our understanding of the genetic underpinnings of human neurological, neurodevelopmental, and neuropsychiatric disorders, providing the first step in elucidation of the biological mechanisms responsible for the onset of disease, which will eventually lead to their translation into clinical practice. Basic neuroscience will continue to identify and validate gene candidates and targets for drug development and biomarkers of diagnostic relevance.

Sophisticated electrophysiological techniques are used by neurosurgeons for recording from individual neurons, for implanting electrodes (as for control of the bladder), for noninvasive stimulation, and for devising prostheses to replace lost functions. It is now commonplace to implant electrodes in humans for long periods to selectively stimulate neurons for the relief of pain. Furthermore, progress has been made in interception of signals from the nervous system to initiate coordinated movements in paralyzed muscles, and to produce accurate and reproducible movements in prosthetic limbs.

One example from experiments described in this book can illustrate how research in basic neuroscience can help provide new treatments for serious conditions. As a result of the work of Hubel and Wiesel on sensory deprivation in newborn kittens and monkeys, it became evident that a newborn baby that suffers from a cataract should have it removed as soon as possible. Such procedures have prevented countless cases of blindness. This was not an outcome that the investigators had in mind at the time they were doing their initial experiments on receptive fields in the visual cortex.

For most diseases of the nervous system that afflict humanity (e.g., Alzheimer's disease and amyotrophic lateral sclerosis), we have little or no knowledge of the root cause for the sporadic forms and no effective treatment. Will a cure for Alzheimer's disease come from targeting the molecular endpoints of the disease, such as the Aβ peptide or Aβ oligomers or the microtubule-associated protein tau, or from the study of the basic mechanisms of memory formation and recall or of other basic neurobiological processes? It is hard to predict, but supporting good curiosity-driven neuroscience will undoubtedly be rewarding and deliver results. It might be argued that it would be better to invest the money used for

---

[50] Miczek, K. A. et al. 2007. *J. Neurosci.* 27: 11803–11806.

basic neuroscience in applied science or neurology. Surely it would be better to find cures for the diseases directly rather than trying to find out how the nervous system works? In instances in which applied research has been emphasized over basic biological research, the results have been disappointing, to say the least. For example, the Soviet Union established and supported massive institutes for applied research in physiology and pharmacology, each with hundreds of research workers. (The type of research in which the investigator followed a scientific problem for its interest and its beauty was considered to be "bourgeois" and was not permitted.) Yet during the existence of the Soviet Union, not one new drug was developed there that came into routine clinical use.

In fact, the best reason for studying neuroscience is really to find out how the nervous system works, in both people and in animals. If through this we get a better understanding of what goes wrong in disease states and how to cure them, that is a wonderful bonus. Of course, a desire to treat horrible diseases is a noble motive for a scientist, but it is rarely successful in the absence of basic knowledge. To cite just one example, the revolutionary experiments of Katz and his colleagues on neuromuscular transmission in the frog were not initially stimulated by a desire to cure myasthenia gravis. An obvious inference from history is that approaches to the treatment of diseases often arise unexpectedly from experiments devoted to quite different questions. For example, understanding of the mechanism of myasthenia gravis came unexpectedly from incidental observations by Steve Heinemann and his colleagues, who injected mice with enriched fractions of acetylcholine receptors to produce antibodies for isolation of receptors. Injected mice developed the symptoms of myasthenia as they formed antibodies against receptor. Helmholtz, often quoted in this book, stated in 1862, "Whoever, in the pursuit of science, seeks after immediate practical utility may rest assured that he seeks in vain."[51]

Conclusions

When one is faced with the fantastic range of animal behavior, from navigation by an ant to the reading of a textbook by a student, it is clear that understanding how the nervous system works is a fascinating, open-ended task of first-order interest in its own right. An increase of natural knowledge on its own is a worthy objective, for without it, logical approaches to prevention and treatment of neurological problems can be only partially realized. In this context, it is almost impossible to define the "relevance" of any particular project at the time it is undertaken. Indeed, when asked about the "significance" of a research plan, complete honesty usually requires a very simple answer: "Don't know!"

Quite apart from the treatment of disease, the dividends that can accrue for society as a result of understanding the development and the functions of the nervous system are beyond today's imagination.

Suggested Reading

Adams, R. D., Victor, M., and Ropper, A. H. 2009. *Principles of Neurology*, 9th ed. McGraw-Hill, New York.

Hawkins, J., and Blakeslee, S. 2004. *On Intelligence*. Times Books, New York.

imaging in awake behaving animals. *Nat. Meth.* 13: 1001–1004.

Kravitz, E. A., and Fernandez, M. P. 2015. Aggression in Drosophila. *Behav. Neurosci.* 129: 549–563. doi: 10.1037/bne0000089.

Nadella, K. M., Roš, H., Baragli, C., et al. 2016. Random-access scanning microscopy for 3D

Pietrobon, D. 2010. CaV2.1 channelopathies. *Pflügers Arch.* 460: 375–393.

Quian Quiroga, R. 2013. Gnostic cells in the 21st century. *Acta Neurobiol. Exp.* 73: 463–471.

Ross, C. A., and Tabrizi, S. J. 2011. Huntington's disease: From molecular pathogenesis to clinical treatment. *Lancet Neurol.* 10: 83–98.

Weissmann, C. 2009. Thoughts on mammalian prion strains. *Folia Neuropathol.* 47: 104–113. https://play.hbonow.com/page/urn:hbo:page:home

[51] Brasch, F. E. 1922. *Science* 55: 405-408.

APPENDIX A

Current Flow in Electrical Circuits

A few basic concepts are required to understand the electrical circuits used in this presentation. For our purposes it is sufficient to describe the properties of circuit elements and explain how they work when connected together in ways that correspond to the circuits described for nerves. The difficulties sometimes encountered on first reading accounts of electrical circuits often stem from the apparently abstract nature of the forces and movements involved. It is reassuring, therefore, to realize that many of the original pioneers in the field must have been faced with similar problems, since the terms devised in the last century are mainly related to the movement of fluids. Thus, the words *current*, *flow*, *potential*, *resistance*, and *capacitance* apply equally well to both electricity and hydraulics. The analogy between the two systems is illustrated by the fact that complex problems in hydraulics may be solved by using solutions to equivalent electrical circuits.

The analogy between a simple electrical circuit and its hydraulic equivalent is illustrated in Figure A.1. The first point to be made is that a source of energy is required to keep the current flowing. In the hydraulic circuit, it is a pump; in the electrical circuit, a battery. The second point is that neither water nor electrical charge is created or lost within such a system. Thus, the flow rate of water is the same at points a, b, and c in the hydraulic circuit, since no water is added or removed between them. Similarly the electrical current in the equivalent circuit is the same at the three corresponding points. In both circuits, there are a number of *resistances* to current flow. In the hydraulic circuit, such resistance is offered by narrow tubes; similarly, thinner wires offer greater resistance to electrical current flow.

Terms and Units Describing Electrical Currents

The unit used to express rate of flow is to some extent a matter of choice; one can measure flow of water through a pipe in cubic feet per minute, for example, although in some other situation milliliters per hour might be more suitable. Electrical current flow is conventionally measured in **coulombs/sec** or **amperes** (abbreviated A). One coulomb is equal to the charge carried by 6.24×10^{18} electrons. In electrical circuits and equations, current is usually designated by I or i. As with flow of water, flow of current is a vector quantity, which is just a way of saying that it has a specified direction. The direction of flow is often indicated by arrows, as in Figure A.1, current always being assumed to flow from the positive to the negative pole of a battery.

What do *positive* and *negative* mean with regard to current flow? Here the hydraulic analogy does not help. It is useful instead to consider the effects of passing current through a chemical solution. For example, suppose two copper wires are dipped into a solution of copper sulfate and connected to the positive and negative poles of a battery. Copper ions in solution are repelled from the positive wire, move through the solution, and are deposited from the solution onto the negative wire. In short, positive ions move in the direction conventionally designated for current: from positive to negative in the circuit. At the same time, sulfate ions move in the opposite direction and are deposited onto the positive wire. The direction specified for current, then, is the direction in which positive charges move in the circuit; negative charges move in the reverse direction.

To explain the energy source for current flow and the meaning of **electrical potential**, the hydraulic analogy is again useful. The flow of fluid depicted in Figure A.1 depends on a pressure difference, the direction of flow being from high to low. No net movement occurs between two parts of the circuit at the same pressure. The overall pressure in the circuit is supplied by expenditure of

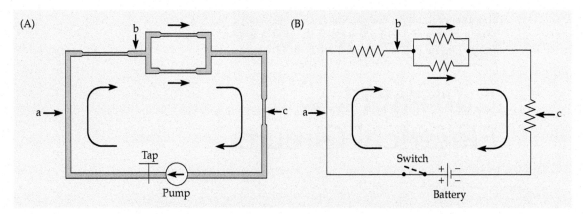

FIGURE A.1   Hydraulic and Electrical Circuits. (A,B) Corresponding circuits for the flow of water and of electrical current. A battery is analogous to a pump that operates at constant pressure, the switch to a tap in the hydraulic line, and resistors to constrictions in the tubes. The letters "a," "b," and "c" indicate equivalent points in the two currents.

energy in driving the pump. In the electrical circuit shown here, the electrical "pressure" or *potential* is provided by a *battery* in which chemical energy is stored. Hydraulic pressure is measured in gm/cm^2; electrical potential is measured in *volts*.

Symbols used in electrical circuit diagrams and arrangements of circuit elements in series and in parallel are illustrated in Figure A.2. As the names imply, a *voltmeter* measures electrical potential and is equivalent to a pressure gauge in hydraulics; an *ammeter* measures current flowing in a circuit and is equivalent to a flowmeter.

Ohm's Law and Electrical Resistance

In hydraulic systems, at least under ideal circumstances, the amount of current flowing through the system increases with pressure. The factor that determines the relation between pressure and flow rate is an inherent characteristic of the pipes, their *resistance*. Small-diameter, long pipes have greater resistances than large-diameter, short ones. Similarly, current flow in electrical circuits depends on the resistance in the circuit. Again, small, long wires have larger resistances than large, short ones. If current is being passed through an ionic solution, the resistance of the solution will increase as the solution is made more dilute. This is because there are fewer ions available to carry the current. In conductors such as wires, the relation between current and potential difference is described by Ohm's law, formulated by Ohm in the 1820s. The law says that the amount of current (I) flowing in a conductor is related to the potential difference (V) applied to it, $I = V/R$. The constant R is the resistance of the wire. If I is in amperes and V is in volts, then R is in units of *ohms* (Ω).

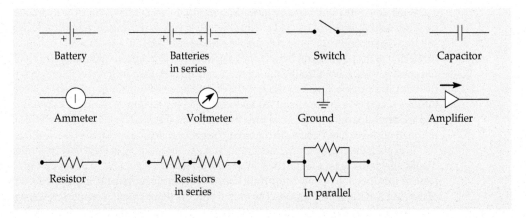

FIGURE A.2   Symbols in Electrical Circuit Diagrams

The reciprocal of resistance is called conductance, and is a measure of the ease with which current flows through a conductor. Conductance is indicated by $g = 1/R$; the units of conductance are **siemens** (S). Thus, Ohm's law may also be written $I = gV$.

Use of Ohm's Law in Understanding Circuits

Ohm's law holds whenever the graph of current against potential is a straight line. In any circuit or part of a circuit for which this is true, any one of the three variables in the equation may be calculated if the other two are known. For example,

1. We can pass a known current through a nerve membrane, measure the change in potential, and then calculate the membrane resistance ($R = V/I$).

2. If we measure the potential difference produced by an unknown current and know the membrane resistance, we can calculate the applied current ($I = V/R$).

3. If we pass a known current through the membrane and know its resistance, then we can calculate the change in potential ($V = IR$).

Two additional simple, but important, rules (Kirchoff's laws) should be mentioned:

1. The algebraic sum of all the battery voltages is equal to the algebraic sum of all the IR voltage drops in a loop. An example of this is shown in Figure A.3B: $V = IR_1 + IR_2$ (this is a statement of the conservation of energy).

2. The algebraic sum of all the currents flowing toward any junction is zero. For example, at point a in Figure A.4, $I_{total} + I_{R1} + I_{R3} = 0$, which means that I_{total} (arriving) $= -I_{R1} - I_{R3}$ (leaving) (this is merely a statement that charge is neither created nor destroyed anywhere in the circuit).

We can now examine in more detail the circuits of Figures A.3 and A.4, which are needed to construct a model of the membrane. Figure A.3A shows a battery (V) of 10 V connected to a resistance (R) of 10 Ω. The switch S can be opened or closed, thereby interrupting or establishing current flow. The voltage applied to R is 10 V; therefore the current measured by the ammeter, I, is, by Ohm's law, 1.0 A. In Figure A.3B, the resistor is replaced by two resistors, R_1 and R_2, *in series*. By the first of Kirchoff's laws, the current flowing into point b must be equal to that leaving. Therefore, the same current, I, must flow through both the resistors. By the second of Kirchoff's laws, then, $IR_1 + IR_2 = V$ (10 V). It follows that the current, $I = V/(R_1 + R_2) = 0.5$ A. The voltage at b, then, is 5 V positive to that at c and a is 5 V positive to b. Note that because there is only one path for the current, the total resistance, R_{total}, seen by the battery is simply the sum of the two resistors; that is,

$$R_{total} = R_1 + R_2$$

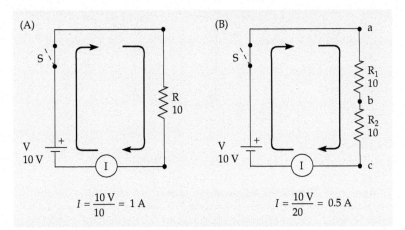

$$I = \frac{10\ V}{10} = 1\ A$$

$$I = \frac{10\ V}{20} = 0.5\ A$$

FIGURE A.3 Ohm's Law Applied to Simple Circuits. (A) Current I = (10 V)/(10 Ω) = 1 A. (B) Current = (10 V)/(20 Ω) = 0.5 A, and the voltage across each resistor is 5 V.

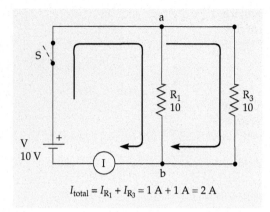

$$I_{total} = I_{R_1} + I_{R_3} = 1\,A + 1\,A = 2\,A$$

FIGURE A.4 Parallel Resistors. When R_1 and R_3 are in parallel, the voltage drop across each resistor is 10 V and the total current is 2 A.

What happens if, as shown in Figure A.4, we add a second resistor, also of 10 Ω, in parallel rather than in series? In the circuit, the two resistors R_1 and R_3 provide two separate pathways for current. Both have a voltage V (10 V) across them, so the respective currents will be

$$I_{R_1} = V/R_1 = 1\,A$$

$$I_{R_3} = V/R_3 = 1\,A$$

Therefore, to satisfy the first of Kirchoff's laws, there must be 2 A arriving at point a and 2 A leaving point b. The ammeter, then, will read 2 A. Now the combined resistance of R_1 and R_3 is $R_{total} = V/I = (10\,V)/(2\,A) = 5\,Ω$, or half that of the individual resistors. This makes sense if one thinks of the hydraulic analogy: Two pipes in parallel will offer less resistance to flow than one pipe alone. In the parallel electrical circuit the conductances add: $g_{total} = g_1 + g_3$, or $1/R_{total} = 1/R_1 + 1/R_3$.

If we now generalize to any number (n) of resistors, resistances in series simply add:

$$R_{total} = R_1 + R_2 + R_3 + \bullet \ \bullet \ \bullet + R_n$$

and in parallel their reciprocals add:

$$1/R_{total} = 1/R_1 + 1/R_2 + 1/R_3 + \bullet \ \bullet \ \bullet + 1/R_n$$

Applying Circuit Analysis to a Membrane Model

Figure A.5A shows a circuit similar to that used to represent nerve membranes. Notice that the two batteries drive current around the circuit in the same direction and that the resistors R_1 and R_2 are in series. What is the potential difference between points b and d (which represent the outside and inside of the membrane)? The total potential across the two resistors between a and c is 150 mV, a being positive to c. Therefore, the current flowing between a and c through the resistors is 150 mV/100,000Ω = 1.5 μA. When 1.5 μA flows across 10,000 Ω, as between a and b, a potential drop of 15 mV is produced, a being positive with respect to b. The potential difference between the inside and the outside is therefore

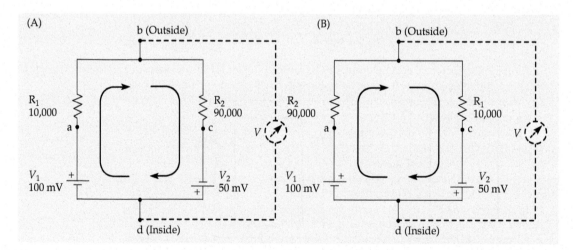

FIGURE A.5 Analogue Circuits for Nerve Membranes. In A and B the resistors R_1 and R_2 are reversed; otherwise the circuits are the same. The batteries V_1 and V_2 are in series. In (A), point b (the "outside" of the membrane) is positive with respect to d (the "inside") by 85 mV; in (B) it is negative by 35 mV. These circuits illustrate how changes in resistance can give rise to membrane potential changes even though the batteries (which represent ionic equilibrium potentials) remain constant.

100 mV – 15 mV = 85 mV. We can obtain the same result by considering the voltage drop across R_2 (1.5 μA × 90,000 Ω = 135 mV) and adding it to V_2 (135 mV – 50 mV = 85 mV). This *must* be so, as the potential between b and d must have a unique value.

In Figure A.5B, R_1 and R_2 have been exchanged. As the total resistance in the circuit is the same, the current must be the same, 1.5 μA. Now the potential drop across R_2, between a and b, is 90,000 Ω × 1.5 μA = 135 mV, a being positive to b. Now the potential across the membrane is 100 mV – 135 mV = –35 mV, *outside negative*; the same result can, of course, be obtained from the current through R_1. This simple circuit illustrates an important point about membrane physiology: *The potential across a membrane can change as a result of resistance changes while the batteries remain unchanged.* A general expression for the membrane potential in the circuit shown in Figure A.5A can be derived simply, as follows:

$$V_m = V_1 - IR_1$$

As $I = (V1 + V2)/(R1 + R2)$:

$$V_m = V_1 - \frac{(V_1 + V_2)R_1}{R_1 + R_2}$$

On rearranging:

$$V_m = \frac{V_1 R_2/R_1 - V_2}{1 + R_2/R_1}$$

Electrical Capacitance and Time Constant

In the circuits described in Figures A.3 and A.4, closing or opening the switch produces instantaneous and simultaneous changes in current and potential. Capacitors introduce a time element into the consideration of current flow. They accumulate and store electrical charge, and, when they are present in a circuit, current and voltage changes are no longer simultaneous. A capacitor consists of two conducting plates (usually of metal) separated by an insulator (air, mica, oil, or plastic). When voltage is applied between the plates (Figure A.6A), there is an instantaneous displacement of charge from one plate to the other through the external circuit. Once the capacitor is fully charged, however, there is no further current, as none can flow across the insulator. The **capacitance** (C) of a capacitor is defined by how much charge (q) it can store for each volt applied to it:

$$C = q/V$$

The units of capacitance are coulombs/volt or **farads** (*F*). The larger the plates of a capacitor and the closer together they are, the greater its capacitance. A one-farad capacitor is very large; capacitances in common use are in the range of microfarads (μF) or smaller.

When the switch in Figure A.6A is closed, then, there is an instantaneous charge separation at the plates. The amount of charge stored in the capacitor is proportional to its capacitance and to the magnitude of the applied voltage (V_0). When the switch is opened, as in Figure A.6B, the charge on the capacitor remains, as does the voltage (V) between the plates. (One can sometimes get a surprising shock from electronic apparatus after it has been turned off because some of the capacitors in the circuits may remain charged.) The capacitor can be discharged by shorting it with a second switch, as in Figure A.6C. Again, the current flow is instantaneous, returning the charge and the voltage on the capacitor to zero. If, instead, the capacitor is discharged through a resistor (R, Figure A.6D), the discharge is no longer instantaneous. This is because the resistor limits the current flow. If the voltage on the capacitor is V, then by Ohm's law the maximum current is $I = V/R$. With no resistor in the circuit, the current becomes infinitely large and the capacitor is discharged in an infinitesimal time period; if R is very large, the discharge process takes a very long time. The rate of discharge at any given time, dq/dt, is the current flowing at that particular time. In other words, $dq/dt = -V/R$ (negative because the charge is decreasing with time), where

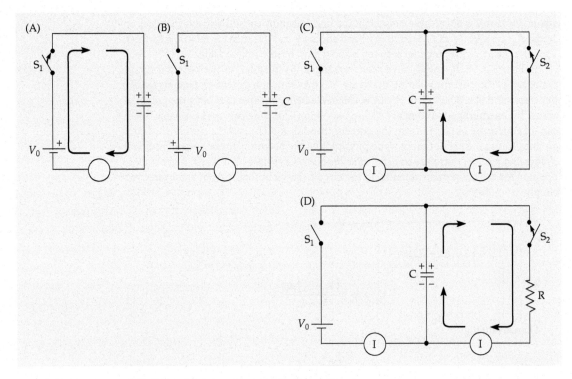

FIGURE A.6 Capacitors in Electrical Circuits. A, B, and C are idealized circuits having no resistance. When S_1 is closed in (A), the capacitor is charged instantaneously to voltage V_0. If S_1 is then opened (B), the potential remains on the capacitor. Closing switch S_2 (C) discharges the capacitor instantaneously. In (D) the capacitor is discharged through resistor R. The maximum discharge current is $I = V_0/R$.

V initially is equal to the battery voltage and decreases as the capacitor is discharged. As $q = CV$, $dq/dt = CdV/dt$, and we can then write $CdV/dt = -V/R$, or

$$dV/dt = -V/RC$$

The equation says that the rate of loss of voltage from the capacitor is proportional to the voltage remaining. Thus, as the voltage decreases, the rate of discharge decreases. The constant of proportionality, $1/RC$, is the *rate constant* for the process: RC is its *time constant*. This kind of process arises over and over again in nature. For example, the rate at which water drains from a bathtub decreases as the depth, and hence the pressure at the drain, decreases. In this kind of situation, the discharge process is described by an exponential function:

$$V = V_0\,e^{-t/\tau}$$

where V_0 is the initial charge on the capacitor and the time constant $\tau = RC$. Similarly, when the capacitor is charged through a resistor, as in Figure A.7, the charging process takes a finite time. The voltage between the plates increases with time until the battery voltage is reached and no further current flows. The charging process is now a rising exponential, with a time constant $\tau = RC$:

$$V = V_0(1 - e^{-t/\tau})$$

These examples illustrate another property of a capacitor. Current flows into and out of the capacitor only when the potential is changing:

$$I_c = dQ/dt = CdV/dt$$

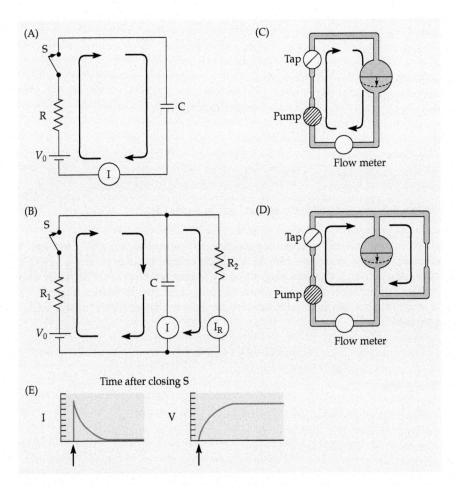

FIGURE A.7   Charging a Capacitor. In (A) the capacitor is charged at a rate limited by the resistor, the initial rate being $I = V_0/R$. In (B) the charging rate depends on both resistors in the circuit. In (E) the capacitive current and the voltage across the capacitor are shown as functions of time. The voltage reaches its final value only when the capacitor is fully charged, i.e., when no more current flows into the capacitor. (C) and (D) are hydraulic analogues of the circuits in A and B.

When the voltage across the capacitor is steady ($dV/dt = 0$), the capacitative current, Ic, is zero. In other words, the capacitance has an "infinite resistance" for a steady potential difference and a "low resistance" for a rapidly changing potential. Figure A.7B shows a circuit in which current flows through a resistor and capacitor in parallel and Figure A.7E the time courses of the capacitative current and voltage.

The properties of a capacitor in a circuit can be illustrated by the slightly more elaborate hydraulic analogy shown in Figure A.7C. The capacitor is represented by an elastic diaphragm that forms a partition in a fluid-filled chamber. When the tap is opened, fluid is pumped from one side of the chamber to the other. The pressure generated by the pump causes the diaphragm to bulge. Fluid continues to flow until, because of its elasticity, the diaphragm provides an equal and opposite pressure; then there is no more fluid flow and the chamber is fully charged. If a tube is placed alongside, as in Figure A.7D, some fluid flows through the tube and some is used to expand the diaphragm. The rate of expansion depends on the resistance of the tube, and on the capacity of the chamber. If the tube is of high resistance, then for a given flow the pressure difference between its two ends will be relatively large. In that case, the distention of the diaphragm will be large and take a relatively long time to achieve. Similarly, if the capacity of the chamber is larger, more fluid is diverted during the filling (or "charging") process and a longer time is required to reach a steady state. Thus, the characteristic time constant of the system is determined by the product of resistance and capacitance.

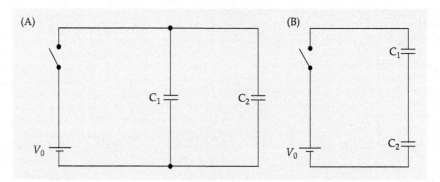

FIGURE A.8 Capacitors in Parallel (A) and in Series (B)

When capacitors are arranged in parallel, as in Figure A.8A, the total capacitance is increased. The total charge stored is the sum of the charges stored in each: $q_1 + q_2 = C_1 V_0 + C_2 V_0$ or $q_{total} = C_{total} V_0$, where $C_{total} = C_1 + C_2$. In contrast, capacitance decreases when capacitors are arranged in series (Figure A.8B). It turns out that the relation is the same as for resistors in parallel: their reciprocals sum. In summary, for a number (n) of capacitors in parallel:

$$C_{total} = C_1 + C_2 + C_3 + \bullet \quad \bullet \quad \bullet + C_n$$

and in series,

$$1/C_{total} = 1/C_1 + 1/C_2 + 1/C_3 + \bullet \quad \bullet \quad \bullet + 1/C_n$$

APPENDIX B

Metabolic Pathways for the Synthesis and Inactivation of Low-Molecular-Weight Transmitters

The figures on the following pages summarize the predominant metabolic pathways for the low-molecular-weight transmitters acetylcholine, GABA, glutamate, dopamine, norepinephrine, epinephrine, 5-HT, and histamine. Glycine, purines, NO, and CO are not included; there appear to be no special neuronal pathways for their synthesis or degradation. Pathways for endocannabinoid synthesis and degradation are still under investigation (see Chapter 15). For each metabolic step, the portion of the molecule being modified is highlighted in color. Further information can be found in several comprehensive texts:

Berg, J. M., Tymoczko, T., and Stryer, L. B. (Eds.) 2011. *Biochemistry*, 7th ed. W. H. Freeman, New York.

Brunton, L. L., Chabner, B. S., and Knollmann, B. C. (Eds.) 2011. *Goodman and Gilman's The Pharmacological Basis of Therapeutics*, 12th ed. McGraw-Hill, New York.

Siegel, J., Albers, R. W., Brady, S. T., and Price, D. L. (Eds.) 2006. *Basic Neurochemistry: Molecular, Cellular, and Medical Aspects*, 7th ed. Elsevier Academic Press, Burlington, MA.

FIGURE B.1

ACETYLCHOLINE (ACH)

Synthesis

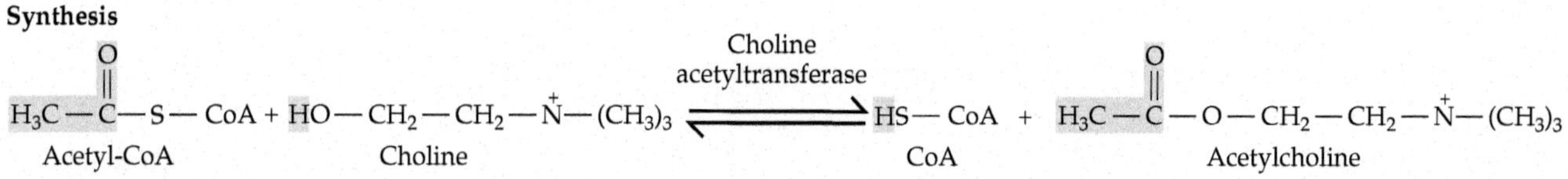

Degradation

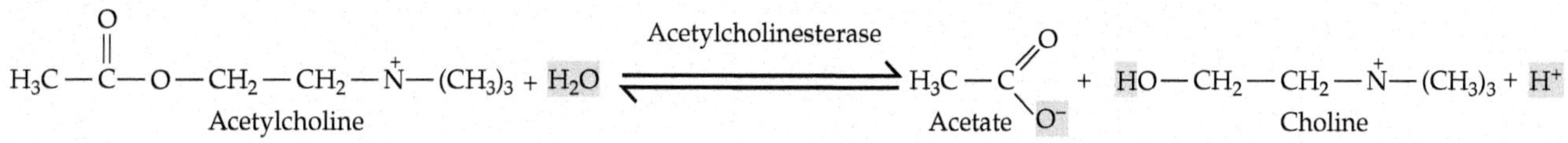

FIGURE B.2

γ-AMINOBUTYRIC ACID (GABA)

Synthesis

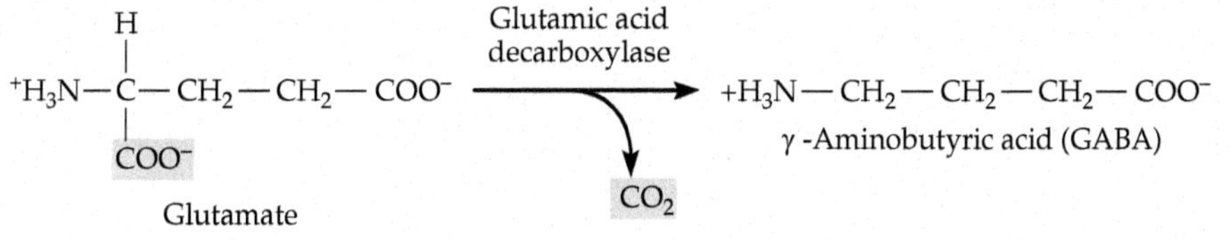

Degradation

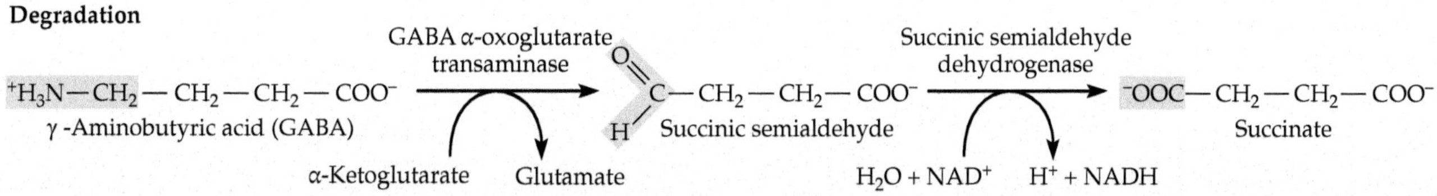

FIGURE B.3

GLUTAMATE

Synthesis

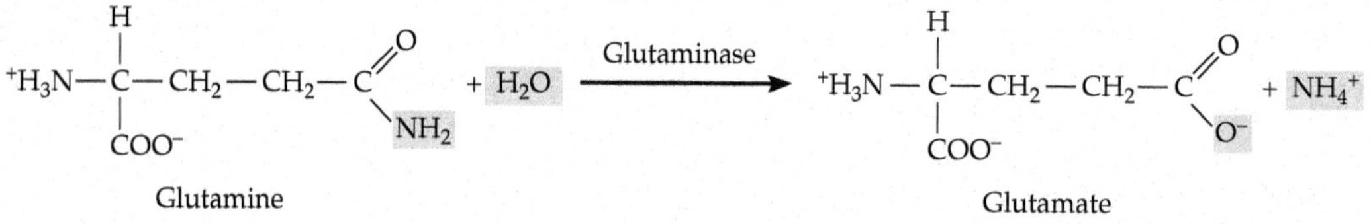

Glutamine + H_2O → (Glutaminase) → Glutamate + NH_4^+

Degradation

Glutamate + NH_4^+ → (Glutamine synthetase, ATP → ADP + P_i) → Glutamine + H^+

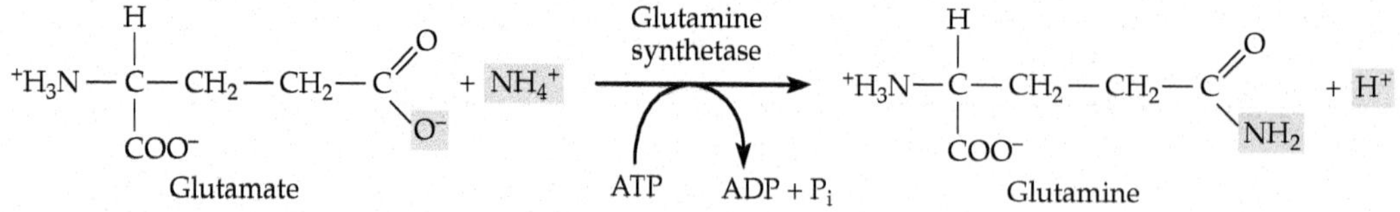

FIGURE B.4

CATECHOLAMINES: DOPAMINE

Synthesis

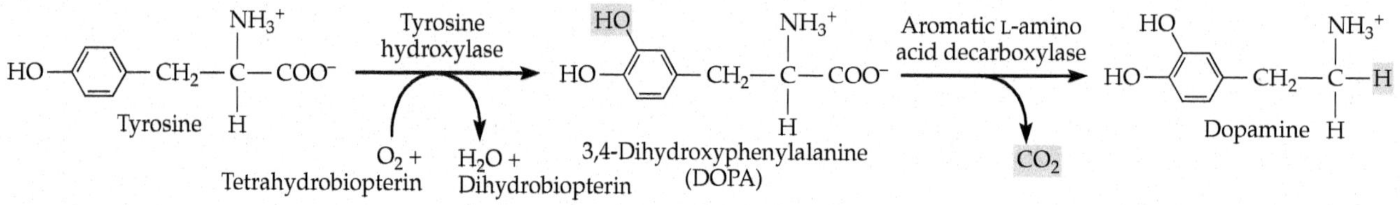

Tyrosine → (Tyrosine hydroxylase; O_2 + Tetrahydrobiopterin → H_2O + Dihydrobiopterin) → 3,4-Dihydroxyphenylalanine (DOPA) → (Aromatic L-amino acid decarboxylase; CO_2) → Dopamine

Degradation

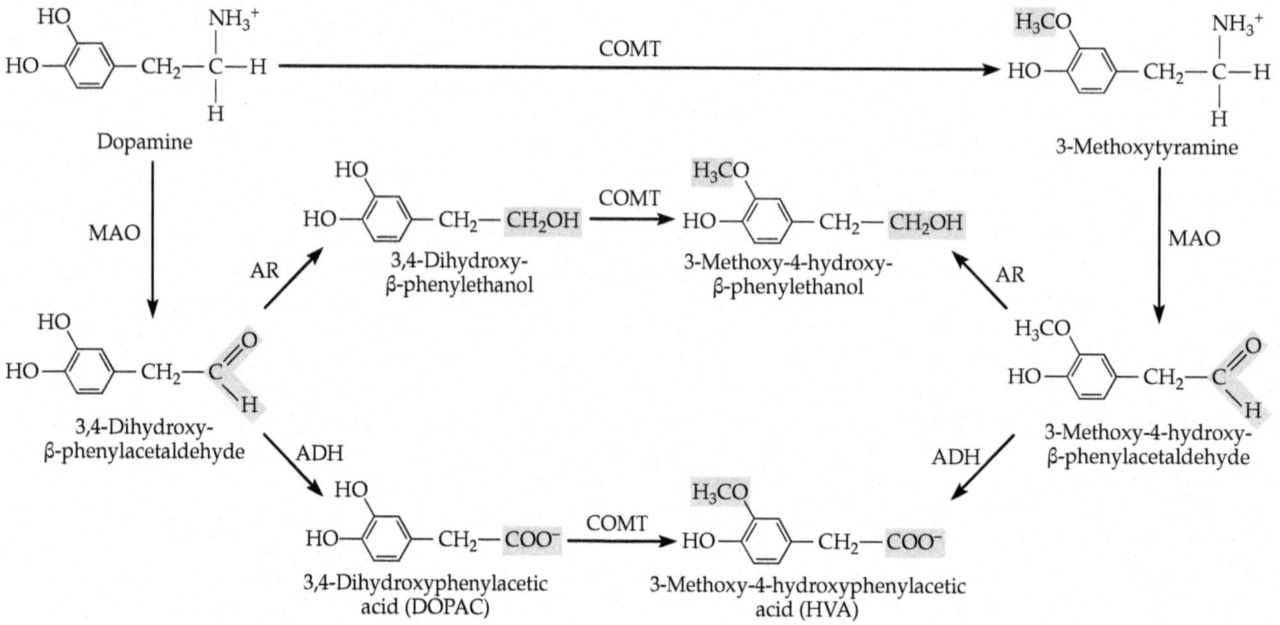

Dopamine → (COMT) → 3-Methoxytyramine

Dopamine → (MAO) → 3,4-Dihydroxy-β-phenylacetaldehyde

3,4-Dihydroxy-β-phenylacetaldehyde → (AR) → 3,4-Dihydroxy-β-phenylethanol → (COMT) → 3-Methoxy-4-hydroxy-β-phenylethanol

3,4-Dihydroxy-β-phenylacetaldehyde → (ADH) → 3,4-Dihydroxyphenylacetic acid (DOPAC) → (COMT) → 3-Methoxy-4-hydroxyphenylacetic acid (HVA)

3-Methoxytyramine → (MAO) → 3-Methoxy-4-hydroxy-β-phenylacetaldehyde → (AR) → 3-Methoxy-4-hydroxy-β-phenylethanol

3-Methoxy-4-hydroxy-β-phenylacetaldehyde → (ADH) → 3-Methoxy-4-hydroxyphenylacetic acid (HVA)

FIGURE B.5

CATECHOLAMINES: NOREPINEPHRINE AND EPINEPHRINE

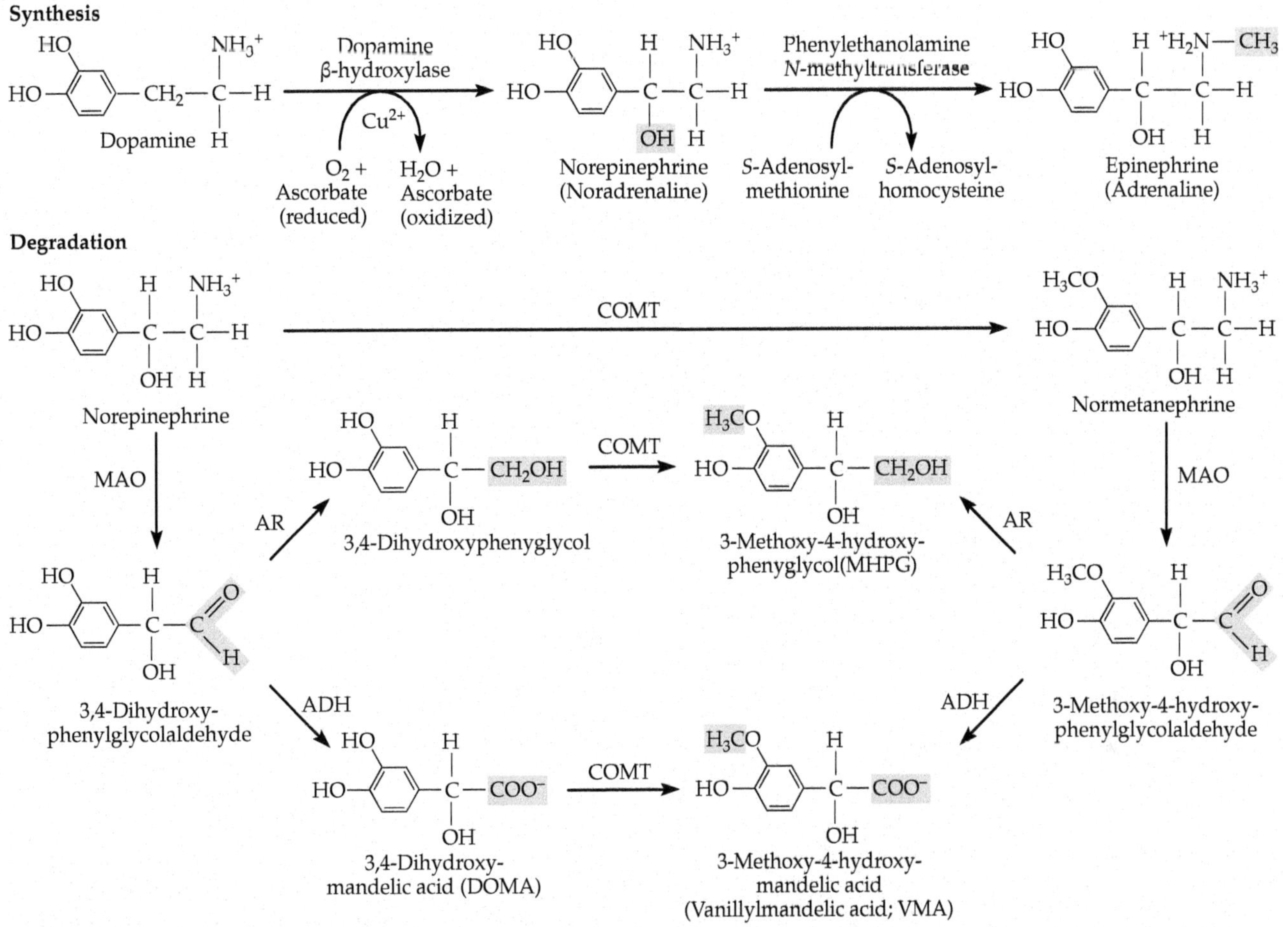

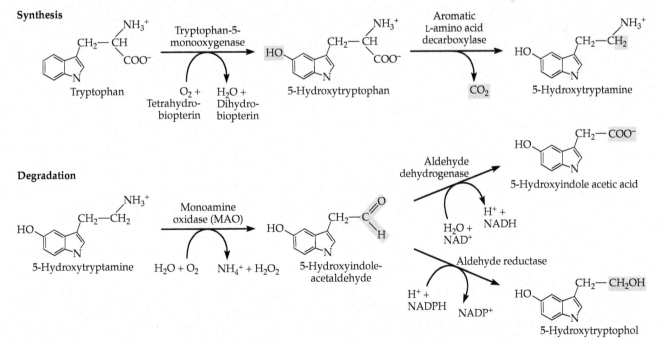

FIGURE B.6

5-HYDROXYTRYPTAMINE (5-HT; SEROTONIN)

FIGURE B.7

HISTAMINE

Synthesis

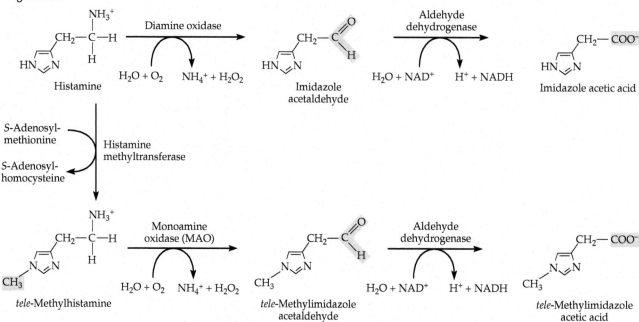

Degradation

FIGURE B.8

DEGRADATION OF BIOGENIC AMINES

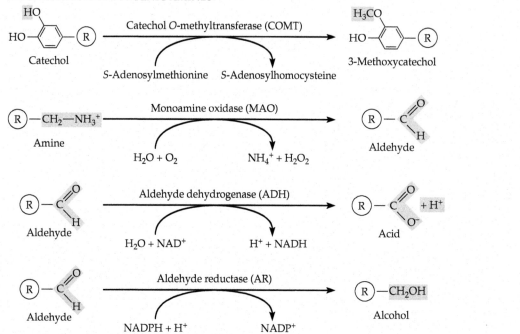

APPENDIX C

Structures and Pathways of the Brain

The following figures show the brain viewed from different aspects and cut in different sections. The aim is to provide a visual equivalent of a glossary relating to material in the text, rather than to present a full atlas. Consequently, only key landmarks and structures are illustrated. Further anatomical information can be found in a number of comprehensive texts:

Carpenter, M. B. 1991. *Core Text of Neuroanatomy*, 4th ed. Williams and Wilkins, Baltimore.

Martin, J. H. 2003. *Neuroanatomy: Text and Atlas*, 3rd ed. Mcgraw-Hill Medical, New York.

Nolte, J. 2008. *The Human Brain: An Introduction to Its Functional Anatomy*, 6th ed. Mosby-Year Book, St. Louis.

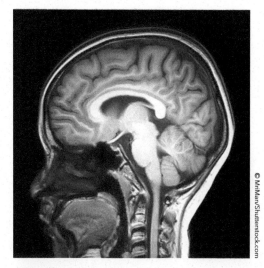

FIGURE C.1   Magnetic resonance image of a living human brain (sagittal section).

FIGURE C.2

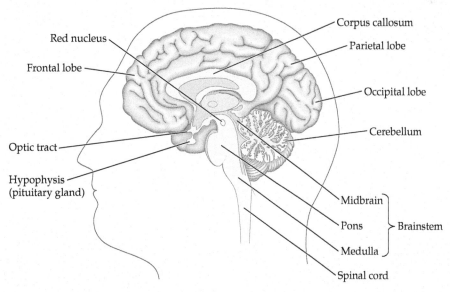

Red nucleus

Frontal lobe

Optic tract

Hypophysis (pituitary gland)

Corpus callosum

Parietal lobe

Occipital lobe

Cerebellum

Midbrain
Pons } Brainstem
Medulla

Spinal cord

FIGURE C.3

SIDE VIEW

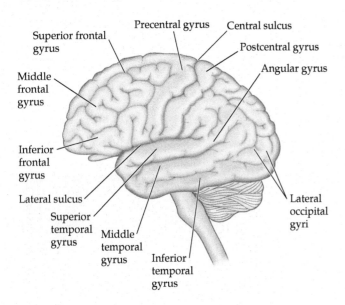

FIGURE C.4

FROM ABOVE

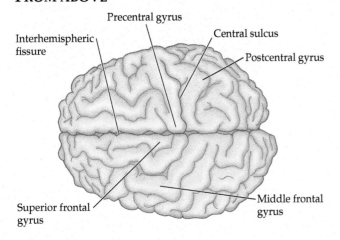

FIGURE C.5

FROM BELOW

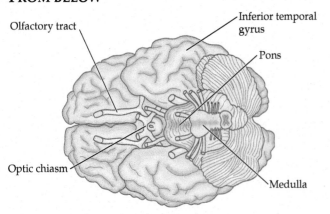

FIGURE C.6

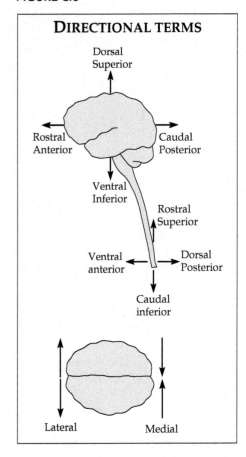

DIRECTIONAL TERMS

FIGURE C.7

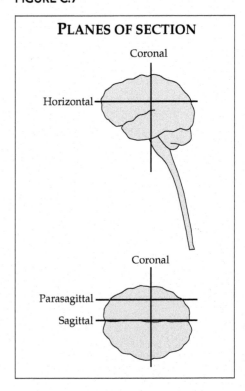

PLANES OF SECTION

FIGURE C.8

NUMBERED ANATOMICAL AREAS
OF THE CEREBRAL CORTEX
(BRODMANN'S AREAS)

LOCALIZATION OF MOTOR AND
SENSORY FUNCTIONS

LATERAL VIEW

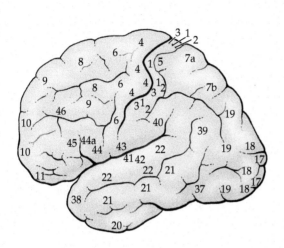
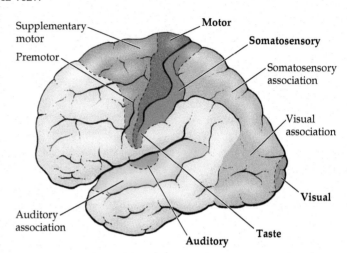

SAGITTAL VIEW

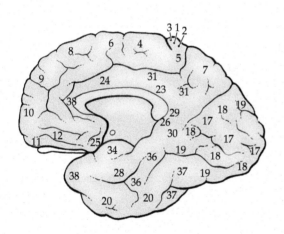
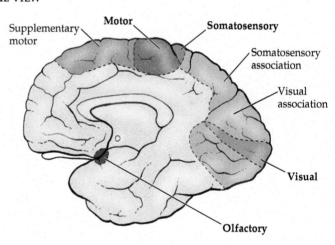

FIGURE C.9

SAGITTAL SECTIONS

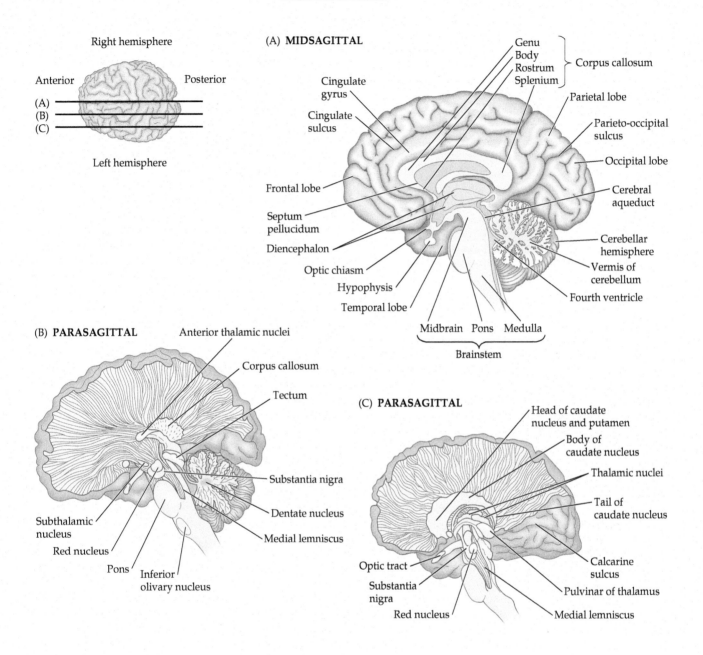

FIGURE C.10

HORIZONTAL SECTIONS

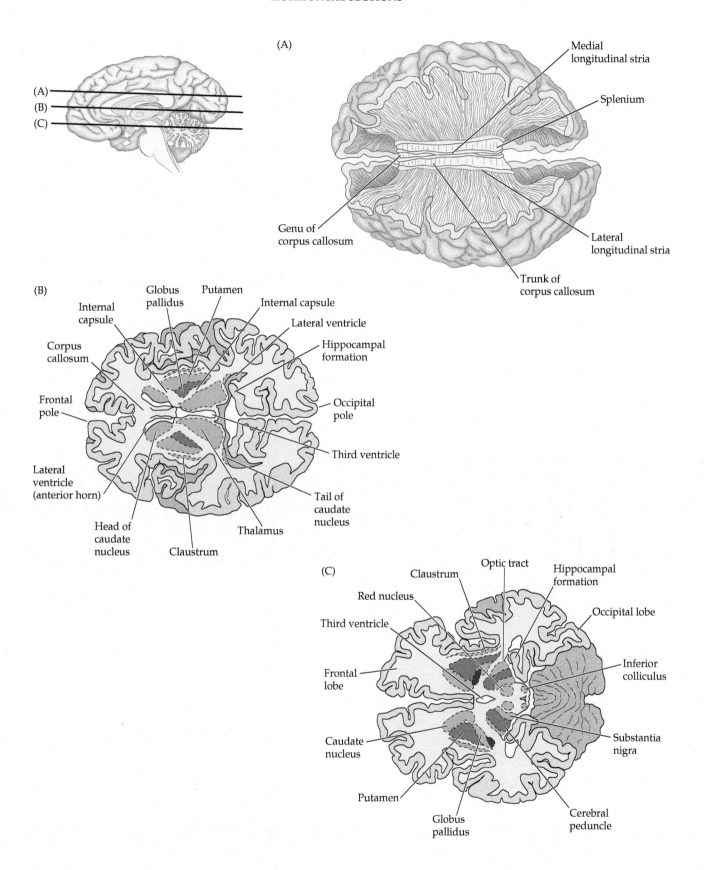

FIGURE C.11

CORONAL SECTIONS

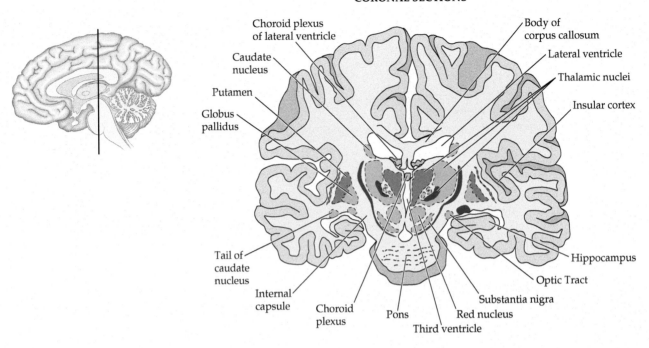

Choroid plexus of lateral ventricle
Caudate nucleus
Putamen
Globus pallidus
Body of corpus callosum
Lateral ventricle
Thalamic nuclei
Insular cortex
Tail of caudate nucleus
Internal capsule
Choroid plexus
Pons
Third ventricle
Red nucleus
Substantia nigra
Optic Tract
Hippocampus

FIGURE C.12

THE CEREBELLUM

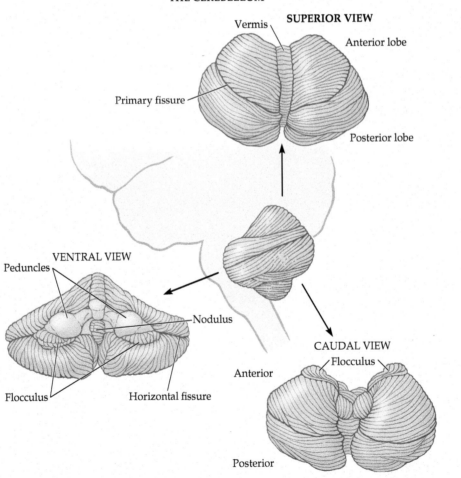

SUPERIOR VIEW
Vermis
Anterior lobe
Primary fissure
Posterior lobe

VENTRAL VIEW
Peduncles
Nodulus
Flocculus
Horizontal fissure

CAUDAL VIEW
Flocculus
Anterior
Posterior

FIGURE C.13

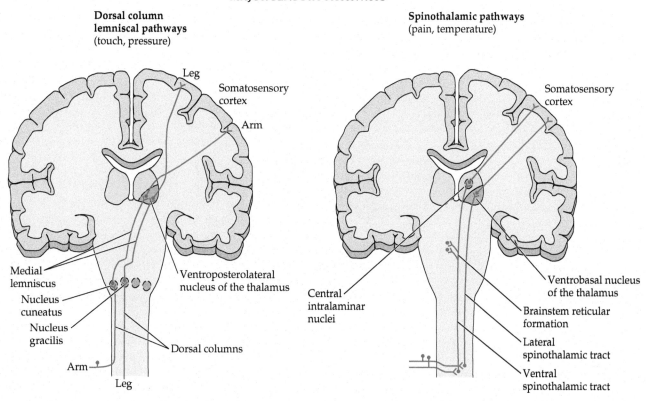

MAJOR SENSORY PATHWAYS

Dorsal column
lemniscal pathways
(touch, pressure)

Spinothalamic pathways
(pain, temperature)

FIGURE C.14

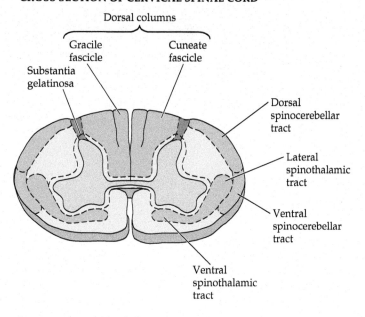

CROSS SECTION OF CERVICAL SPINAL CORD

FIGURE C.15

MAJOR MOTOR PATHWAYS

Tracts descending to the spinal cord

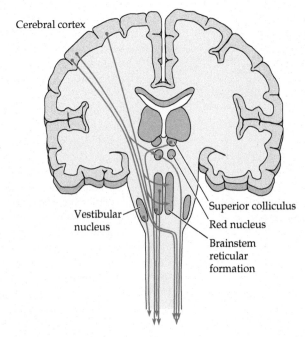

Cross section of cervical spinal cord

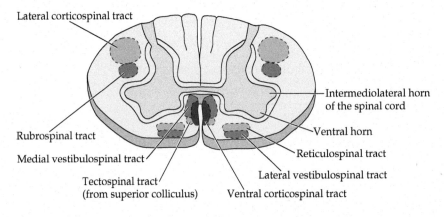

Glossary

The definitions below apply to the terms used in the context of this book. Thus, *excitation*, *adaptation*, and *inhibition* all have additional meanings that are not included.
For structural formulae of transmitters see Appendix B.
For anatomical terms see Appendix C.

A

absolute refractory period The time following an action potential during which a stimulus cannot elicit a second action potential. [7]

action potential A brief regenerative, all-or-nothing electrical potential that propagates along an axon or muscle fiber. [1, 4]

activated 1. An action potential that has been initiated. 2. Increased probability that an ion channel will open. [4]

active transport The movement of ions or molecules against an electrochemical gradient. [9]
    primary active transport Active transport that uses metabolic energy, specifically the hydrolysis of ATP. [9]
    secondary active transport Active transport that uses energy provided by the electrochemical gradient for another ion (usually sodium). [9]

active zone (AZ) A location within the presynaptic terminal where synaptic vesicles fuse with the presynaptic plasma membrane to discharge their neurotransmitters into the synaptic cleft. [11, 13]

activity The effective concentration of an ion in solution. [4]

adaptation procedure Repetition of a class of stimuli in order to generate reduced responsiveness of neurons selective to that class of stimuli. [25]

adaptation Resetting of the response of a sensory neuron to the amplitude of a maintained stimulus. [21]

adaptive optics ophthalmoscopy Optical technique that measures and compensates optical imperfections of the eye to visualize and provide optical access of individual retinal cells in living eyes. [22]

adequate stimulus The form of stimulus energy to which a sensory receptor neuron is most sensitive. [21]

afterdepolarizing potential (ADP) Depolarization following one or more action potentials due to persistent changes in membrane conductance. [7]

afterhyperpolarizing potential (AHP) Hyperpolarization following one or more action potentials due to persistent changes in membrane conductance. [7]

agonists 1. Molecules that activate receptors. 2. The coordinated contraction of groups of muscles that work together. [11, 26]

agrin A protein secreted by motoneurons that becomes embedded in extracellular matrix at the motor end plate and give rise to postsynaptic specialization. [27, 29]

amacrine cells Group of retinal neurons that contribute to diverse visual functions through synaptic and extrasynaptic communication with other types of retinal cells. [22]

amacrine type II (AII cell) Special type of amacrine cell that connects the rod to the cone pathways. [22]

ampere Coulombs/second. See *coulomb*. [App. A]

antagonists 1. Molecules that prevent activation of receptors. 2. Muscles that oppose agonist muscles. [11, 26]

apoptosis Also known as programmed cell death. Extracellular or intracellular stimuli trigger a cell to destroy itself by a defined cascade of proteases. [27]

association cortex Regions of cortex that represent the external world through the combination of inputs from primary sensory cortical regions, creating responses that encode real-life stimulus properties more so than elemental features of stimuli. [25]

associative LTD LTD in which depression of one synapse is produced by activation of another. [16]

associative LTP LTP in which potentiation of one synapse is produced by activation of another. [16]

astrocytes One of four classes of glial cells found in the vertebrate CNS. [10]

asymmetry currents See *gating currents*. [7]

augmentation An increase in evoked transmitter release from nerve terminals, following a brief train of repetitive stimuli. Augmentation can last for several seconds. [16]

axon The process or processes of a neuron that conduct impulses, usually over long distances. [1]

axonal transport The movement of proteins, intracellular particles, and organelles along axons. [15]

axoplasmic flow The bulk movement of axoplasm along the axon. One form of axonal transport. [15]

B

ball-and-chain model A proposed mechanism for inactivation of voltage-activated channels whereby a ball of amino acids, tethered by an amino acid chain, swings into the mouth of an open channel to block its pore. [7]

barrelette A cluster of neurons in the brainstem of rats and mice associated with a single whisker on the face. It receives input from sensory receptor neurons and projects to a barreloid in the thalamus. [23]

barreloid A cluster of neurons in the somatosensory thalamus of rats and mice associated with a single whisker on the face. It receives input from a barrelette and projects to a cortical barrel. [23]

barrels Columnar organization of somatosensory cortex related to facial whiskers. [23]

basal lamina An extracellular, glycoprotein- and proteoglycan-containing matrix that ensheaths many tissues in the body, including nerves and muscle fibers. [11]

basilar membrane The acellular sheet upon which rests the organ of Corti and whose vibration by sound drives motion of the hair cells stereocilia. [24]

basket cells Inhibitory interneurons in the cerebellar cortex whose cell bodies are located in the Purkinje cell layer and whose axons make basketlike terminal arbors around Purkinje cell bodies, providing lateral inhibition that focuses the spatial distribution of Purkinje cell activity. [26]

binocular fusion Merging of slightly different images from the two eyes, arising from binocular disparity, into a single stereoscopic perception. [2]

binomial distribution Discrete probability distribution of the number of successes in a sequence of n independent units participating in a process with a probability p of success. [13]

bipolar cell A neuron with two major processes arising from the cell body; in the vertebrate retina, bipolar cells are interposed between photoreceptors and ganglion cells. They integrate the on and off visual fields. [1, 22]

blood oxygen level-dependent (BOLD) Signal that reveals the change in the oxygenation level of blood as a result of consumption by neuronal metabolism. [25]

boutons Small terminal expansions of the presynaptic nerve fiber at a synapse; sites of transmitter release. [11]

C

calcium ATPase A molecule that transports calcium across a cell membrane against its electrochemical gradient, using energy derived from the hydrolysis of ATP. [9]

calcium-sensitive (Ca^{2+}-gated) Channels whose opening is determined by the concentration of Ca^{2+}. [24]

capacitance Electrical charge that can be stored and separated, usually measured in microfarads per square cm (μF/cm^2). [App. A]

capacitative current A transient current that flows across a cell membrane in response to a voltage change, thereby recharging the membrane capacitance to the new membrane potential. [7]

caspases Caspases (cysteine-aspartic proteases or cysteine-dependent aspartate-directed proteases) are a family of proteolytic enzymes essential for programmed cell death. Their name is due to their specific cysteine protease activity—a cysteine in its active site nucleophilically attacks and cleaves a target protein only after an aspartic acid residue. [27]

catecholamine A general term referring to molecules having both a catechol ring and an amino group; typically dopamine, norepinephrine, and epinephrine. [15]

caudate nucleus One of the three major components of the basal ganglia (the other two are the putamen and nucleus accumbens). [26]

cell-attached patch A small segment of cell membrane attached to the cell and sealed inside a micropipette tip. [4]

cell body Also called *soma*, the compartment of neurons that contains the nucleus. Dendrites and axons usually extend from the cell body. [1]

cell fate mapping A method to determine when and where the diverse cell types of the brain (or more generally of the organism) arise during development. Also called *lineage tracing*. [27]

center–surround Visual field in the retina in which a center that responds to light is surrounded by a periphery that is inhibited by light, or vice versa. [22]

central nervous system (CNS) The brain and spinal cord of vertebrates (by analogy, the central nerve cord and ganglia of invertebrates). [1]

central pattern generators Oscillatory spinal cord or brainstem circuits responsible for programmed, rhythmic movements such as locomotion. [26]

channel conductance Ability of a membrane channel to pass charged ions down an electrical membrane gradient; the inverse of channel resistance. [4]

channel permeability Ability of a channel to pass ions or molecules down an electrochemical gradient. [4]

chemical synaptic transmission Transmission that occurs via the secretion of specific chemical signals (neurotransmitters). [11]

chemoreceptor molecule Molecules that produce a physiological effect on specific binding of a chemical substance. [1]

chemotransduction Conversion of the binding of molecular compounds into nerve signals. [21]

choice probability index A method to quantify how accurately behavioral responses can be predicted from single neuronal responses. When the index measured for one neuron is high, it is likely that that neuron contributes to the behavioral outcome. [25]

cholinergic Referring to a neuron that releases acetylcholine as a transmitter or sometimes to a synapse using acetylcholine as a transmitter. [14]

chord conductance The difference in current passed through a cell membrane at two different membrane potentials per volt dfference in potential. [4]

choroid plexus Network of cells that produces the cerebrospinal fluid. [18]

chromatolysis Disappearance and dispersal of Nissl bodies following axotomy. [29]

climbing fiber An axon that originates in the inferior olivary nuclei, ascends through the inferior cerebellar peduncle, and makes terminal arborizations that invest the proximal dendritic trees of Purkinje cells. Climbing fibers induce complex spikes and long-term depression in cerebellar Purkinje cells. [26]

cochlea The bony canal containing the sensory apparatus for hearing. [21]

combinatorial transcriptional codes The transcriptional effects of any given transcription factor depend on its combination with other transcription factors and cofactors. [27]

command neuron A single neuron that can initiate or orchestrate a particular behavioral response in an animal. [20]

complementary DNA (cDNA) DNA synthesized by reverse transcriptase using mRNA as a template. [5]

completion phenomenon Seeing a figure as complete when part of it falls in a blind area of the visual field. [2]

concept cell Any one of a large number of cells that discharges when the subject is presented with a particular concept, for example a person's face, a movie, or a particular place. [30]

cones Retinal photoreceptors that discriminate colors. [1, 22]

connexon A membrane channel bridging the space between two adjacent cells, connecting the cytoplasm of one to that of the other. See *gap junction*. [11]

constant field equation An equation used to calculate membrane potential in the presence of multiple ions and that takes into account individual ion concentrations both outside and inside the cell, and membrane permeability to each ion. Sometimes called the *GHK equation* (for its three originators). [6]

contextual fear conditioning A form of associative learning whereby pairing a footshock (unconditioned stimulus) with a certain spatial context (conditioned stimulus), determined a fear response (freezing) on re-exposure of the mouse to the conditioning context. [17]

contrast adaptation Adaptation of visual neurons to a large range of luminance levels to enhance contrast discrimination. [22]

contrast gain control Capacity of visual neurons to modify the amplitude of their responses to contrasting luminance levels. [22]

corpus callosum The large medial fiber bundle that connects the cortices of the two cerebral hemispheres. [3]

cortical plate Region of the developing cortex where the first wave of migrating neurons accumulate, and which eventually matures into the six-layered structure, as successive waves of migrating neurons pass by. [27]

coulomb Unit of electrical charge. [App. A]

coupling ratio The degree of electrical coupling between cells. [11]

critical period A time during nervous system maturation when activity permanently shapes connectivity. [29]

Cys-loop receptors A large superfamily of channel-forming receptors, the subunits of which all have a pair of disulfide-bonded cysteines separated by 13 amino acid residues. Includes (among many others) receptors for serotonin, glycine, and γ-aminobutyric acid. [5]

D

deactivated The response of a channel to a stimulus that reduces the probability that the channel will open. [4]

default model for neural induction An influential model postulating that ectodermal cells will become neurons if they receive no signals at all, but that this is normally inhibited in prospective epidermal cells by the action of bone morphogenetic proteins. [27]

delayed rectifier A type of potassium channel activated by membrane depolarization after a brief delay. [7]

dendrite The process of a neuron that receives inputs from other neurons. In some neurons, dendrites also produce and conduct impulses and release transmitters. [1]

depolarization Reduction in magnitude of the resting membrane potential toward zero. [4]

depolarization-induced suppression of inhibition (DSI) A phenomenon in which depolarization of the postsynaptic cell reduces the synaptic inhibition of that cell by afferent inhibitory nerve fibres. [12]

depolarize To reduce the magnitude of the resting membrane potential toward zero. [1]

desensitization Reduction of the response of a receptor to a ligand after prolonged or repeated exposure. [4]

detection task A common psychophysical measure of the sensitivity of a perceptual system, where the individual must indicate on each trial whether a stimulus did or did not occur. [25]

direct chemical inhibitory synapses Presynaptic nerve terminals at which postsynaptic inhibition is mediated by the release of an inhibitory chemical transmitter. [11]

direct lineage reprogramming The direct transformation of differentiated cell types from one lineage to another lineage without passing through an intermediate pluripotent state or progenitor cell type. [29]

dishabituation A form of behavior in which the recovery of sensitivity to a weak stimulus is brought about by exposure to a stronger stimulus. [20]

DNA methylation DNA methylation (forming 5'-methylcytosine) of genomic DNA is an epigenetic mark responsible for the constitutive silencing of genome regions, occurring preferentially at cytosine-guanine dinucleotide sequences (so called CpG islands). [17]

dopaminergic Referring to a neuron that releases dopamine as a transmitter, or a synapse using dopamine as a transmitter. [14]

dorsal cochlear nucleus A processing stage along the auditory pathway whose neurons project to the inferior colliculus. [24]

dorsal pathway The cortical visual processing pathway that runs from the occipital cortex to the parietal cortex, and involves the spatial properties of visual scenes. [25]

driving force The difference between the membrane potential and the equilibrium potential for movement of an ion species through a membrane channel. [4]

duplex theory The distinct, separate sensory processing of coarsely and finely textured surfaces. [23]

E

electrical coupling The spread of a potential change from one cell to another, usually by current flow through gap junctions. [8]

electrical potential changes to the neuron's membrane potential that do not lead directly to the generation of new current by action potentials. [App. A]

electrical synapse A synapse that transmits information via the direct flow of electrical current through gap junctions. [11]

electrochemical gradient The transmembrane difference in potential energy of an ion arising from the combined electrical and diffusional forces acting on it. [4]

electrogenic Capable of generating an electrical current; usually applied to membrane transporters that create electrical currents while translocating ions. [6, 9]

electromotility The change in shape of outer hair cells in response to depolarization and hyperpolarization. [24]

electrotonic potentials Localized, graded, subthreshold potentials produced by artificially applied currents, and characterized by the passive electrical properties of cells. [8]

end inhibition A decrease in the response of a neuron as the length of an image increases. Also called *end stopping*. [2]

end plate potential (EPP) Depolarization of the motor end-plate caused by the action potential-induced release of transmitter from the motor nerve terminal. A *miniature end-plate potential (mEPP)* is the depolarization of the motor end-plate produced by the spontaneous release of a single quantum of transmitter from the motor nerve terminal. [11]

end stopping See *end inhibition*. [2]

endorphins Endogenous peptides with chemical structure resembling that of opiates, that function as neurotransmitters. [23]

engram A persistent change in the brain that results from a specific learning experience and can be re-activated and recalled, yielding a memory experience. The operational definition of an engram requires to perform necessity (loss-of-function), sufficiency (gain-of-function) and mimicry experiments. [17]

enkephalins Small neuropeptides that comprise five amino acids and act on opioid receptors. [14]

enteric nervous system A division of the autonomic nervous system containing millions of nerve cells arranged in the wall of the intestine as sensory neurons, interneurons, and motor neurons. [19]

ependymal cells Cells in the CNS that line the cerebral ventricles and central canal of the spinal cord and that contribute to the flow of cerebrospinal fluid. [10]

excitatory postsynaptic current (EPSC) Inward (depolarizing) postsynaptic ionic current produced by the action of an excitatory neurotransmitter released from the presynaptic nerve terminal. [11]

excitatory postsynaptic potential (EPSP) Depolarization of the postsynaptic membrane of a neuron produced by an excitatory transmitter released from presynaptic terminals. [11]

excitatory synaptic potentials Synaptic potentials that increase the probability that a postsynaptic cell will generate an action potential. [1]

exocytosis The process whereby synaptic vesicles fuse with presynaptic terminal membrane and empty transmitter molecules into the synaptic cleft. [11, 13]

EXP-1 A $GABA_A$ receptor that functions as an excitatory cation channel in invertebrates. [5]

extensor muscles Muscles that open or extend the joints. [26]

extracellular microelectrode Electrical conductor that serves to collect the extracellular electrical activity of neurons, or to stimulate extracellularly a neuron or groups of neurons. [1]

extrasynaptic release In the nervous system, the release of transmitter occurring from the cell body, dendrites, and axon in the absence of synaptic structures. Release occurring outside synapses. [1, 18]

Eyring rate theory model A model of a channel's ability to pass an ion or molecule, based on the internal structure of the channel. [4]

F

5-HT_3 receptors A serotonin receptor, belonging to the large superfamily of Cys-loop receptors. [5]

farad Unit of capacitance; more commonly used is microfarad ($\mu F = 10^{-6}F$). [App. A]

feedback inhibition A mechanism for controlling the rate of synthesis of substances in cells, whereby the rate-limiting step in a biosynthetic pathway is inhibited by the final product. [15]

fibrillation Denervated skeletal muscles undergo spontaneous asynchronous contractions. [29]

final common path The information-processing pathway consisting of all the motor neurons in the body. Motor neurons are known by this collective term because they receive and integrate all motor signals from the brain and then direct movement accordingly. [26]

flexor muscles Muscles that close or flex the joints and pull the limbs toward the body. [26]

flexor reflex A limb-withdrawal reflex characterized by two consistent features: (1) Movement of the affected limb is primarily flexion and is directed away from the offending stimulus; and (2) if necessary, weight is transferred to the contralateral limb. [26]

floor plate A specialized glial structure located on the ventral midline of the embryonic neural tube and that spans the anteroposterior axis from the midbrain to the tail regions. [27]

formants Frequency components of basic speech elements. [24]

free nerve ending A sensory fiber that terminates in the skin and is not encapsulated by any accessory structure. [23]

frequency-labeled lines The property of the afferent auditory pathway whereby each neuron is excited by a restricted frequency range as a result of the place along the basilar membrane from which it receives input. [24]

functional magnetic resonance imaging (fMRI) A method developed in the 1990s for measuring the changes in blood oxygenation related to neuronal activity in the brain or spinal cord of humans and other animals. [1]

fusimotor fibers Motoneurons supplying muscle fibers in a muscle spindle. [21]

G

G protein A receptor-coupled protein that binds guanine nucleotides and activates intracellular messenger systems. [12]

G protein-coupled receptors (GPCRs) A large family of metabotropic receptors that are characterized by seven transmembrane domains and that produce their effects by first interacting with G proteins in the cell membrane. [12]

$GABA_A$ receptors γ-aminobutyric acid receptors. [5]

γ-aminobutyric acid (GABA) An inhibitory neurotransmitter. [14]

ganglia Discrete collections of nerve cells. [11]

ganglion cells Neurons located in a ganglion. In the visual system, ganglion cells are the output of the retina; their axons carry information to other central regions along the optic nerve. [1, 22]

gap junction The region of contact between two cells in which the space between adjacent membranes is reduced to about 2 nm and is bridged by connecting channels called connexons. See *connexon*. [11]

gate The mechanism whereby a channel is opened and closed. [4]

gating currents Currents produced by movement of charge within a cell membrane, associated with the opening or closing of a channel. Also called *asymmetry currents*. [7]

gating spring The structure that is hypothesized to block the ion channels at top of the hair cell cilium; the gate is opened when pulled by the tip link, and then springs shut. [21]

gene regulatory network A network of molecular inter-actions that control the spatial and temporal expression of genes to determine cell fate. [27]

glia See *neuroglial cells*.

glial cells See *neuroglial cells*.

globus pallidus The principal component of the pallidum. The external division is involved with the indirect path-way from striatum to pallidum. The internal division provides major output from the basal ganglia to motor circuits in the thalamus and brainstem. [26]

glutamate An amino acid that serves as a major excitatory neurotransmitter. [14]

glutamate-gated chloride receptor (GluCl) Receptor found in invertebrates belonging to the large super-family of Cys-loop receptors. [5]

glycine receptor (GlyR) Any molecule that binds glycine. [5]

glycine A transmitter liberated at many inhibitory synapses in the spinal cord and brain stem. [14]

Golgi cells Inhibitory interneurons in the granular cell layer of the cerebellar cortex that provide inhibitory feedback from parallel fibers to granule cells, regulat-ing the temporal properties of the granule cell input to the Purkinje cells. [26]

Golgi tendon organs Sensory elements in muscle tendons that are activated by muscle stretch or contraction. [26]

granule cell A type of small nerve cell. [26]

growth cone The expanded tip of a growing axon. [27]

H

habituation A form of behavior characterized by a de-creasing response to repeated applications of a given stimulus. [20]

hair cells Sensory cells in which bending of stereocilia ("hairs") causes a change in membrane potential; responsible for auditory transduction, transduction of vestibular stimuli, and vibratory transduction in lateral line organs of fish. [21, 24]

hair follicle Richly innervated skin structure in which a hair is rooted. [23]

Hebbian-type plasticity A form of synaptic plasticity based on the coincidence of activity in the pre-synaptic and the post-synaptic neuron. [17]

hemodynamic lag The time that passes between the increase in activity in a neuronal population and the consequent increase in blood flow. [25]

hemodynamic response The release of oxygen from blood preferentially to neuronal populations that require more oxygen due to their ongoing high activity level. [25]

Hensen's node The equivalent of the Spemann organizer in chick and in mammalian embryos, respectively. [27]

heterochronic transplantation Transplant of donor cells into hosts embryos of different developmental stage. Allows testing for the flexibility of intrinsic cell fate de-termination in response to stage-dependent environ-mental cues. [27]

heterosynaptic LTD Prolonged depression of synaptic transmission produced by previous activity in a differ-ent afferent pathway to the same cell. [16]

homeobox The DNA sequence in homeotic genes en-coding the DNA-binding homeodomain. [27]

homeodomain A 60-amino acid DNA-binding domain, encoded by a DNA sequence in homeotic genes called a homeobox. [27]

homeosis The transformation of one organ into another, arising from mutation in or misexpression of certain developmentally critical genes, specifically homeotic genes. [27]

homeotic genes Genes that regulate downstream gene networks involved in body patterning and determin-ing the developmental fate of an entire segment of an animal. Mutations in these genes drastically alter the characteristics of the body segment (as when wings grow from a fly body segment that should have pro-duced legs). [27]

homosynaptic LTD Prolonged depression of synaptic transmission produced by previous repetitive activity in the same pathway. [16]

homosynaptic LTP Prolonged increase in synaptic trans-mission produced by previous repetitive activity in the same pathway. [16]

homunculus A maplike representation of regions of the body in the brain. [23]

horizontal cells Retinal neurons that integrate responses of photoreceptors and determine the size of the visual field. [22]

Huntington's disease An autosomal dominant genetic disorder in which a single gene mutation results in personality changes, progressive loss of control of vol-untary movement, and eventually death. Primary target early in the disease is medium spiny neurons of the striatum that participate in the indirect pathway. [26]

hyperpolarization Increased negativity of the resting membrane potential, tending to reduce excitability. [4]

hyperpolarize To increase the negativity of the resting membrane potential, tending to reduce excitability. [1]

I

inactivate In reference to ion channels, the process of entering a state that no longer allows the passage of ions through the pore. [5]

inactivation Removal of the ability of a voltage-activated channel to respond to a change in membrane potential. [4, 7]

indirect transmission Chemical transmission in which the transmitter binds to a metabotropic receptor and produces a slow, long-lasting postsynaptic effect by inducing a cascade of intracellular changes. [12]

induced pluripotent stem cells (iPSCs) Adult somatic terminally differentiated cells reprogrammed by the expression of some embryonic transcription factor to become pluripotent stem cells. [27]

inhibition The effect of one neuron on another that tends to prevent it from initiating impulses. [12]

inhibitory postsynaptic potential (IPSP) The potential change (usually hyperpolarizing) in a neuron produced by an inhibitory transmitter released from presynaptic terminals. [11]

inhibitory synaptic potentials Synaptic potentials that decrease the probability that a postsynaptic cell will generate an action potential. [1]

inner hair cells Cilated cells that transduce sound-induced vibrations in the fluids of the cochlea into afferent electrical signals. [24]

input capacitance (c_{input}) The capacitance of a whole cell. [8]

input resistance (r_{input}) The resistance measured by injecting current into a cell or fiber; in a cylindrical fiber, $r_{input} = 0.5(r_m r_i)^{1/2}$. [8]

input specificity A property of homosynaptic LTP in which only the stimulated synapse is potentiated. [16]

input time constant The time constant of a whole cell (input capacitance × input resistance). [8]

inside-out patch A small segment of cell membrane removed from the cell, sealed inside a micropipette tip with the cytoplasmic side facing the extracellular solution. [4]

integration The process whereby a neuron sums the various excitatory and inhibitory influences converging on it and synthesizes a new output signal. [2]

intermediate mantle zone Region containing the cell bodies of the migrating neurons. [27]

intracellular microelectrode Electrical conductor that is used to collect electrical activity inside the neuron. [1]

inward rectifier A type of potassium channel that allows potassium ions to move inward, but not outward, across the cell membrane. [4]

ion channels Integral membrane proteins possessing pores that allow only certain ions to diffuse across cell membranes, thereby conferring selective ionic permeability. [4]

ionophoresis The ejection of ions caused by passing current through a micropipette; used for applying charged molecules with a high degree of temporal and spatial resolution. Also spelled *iontophoresis*. [11]

J

juxtacrine signaling Signaling between two adjacent cells connected by a ligand-receptor pair positioned on the membrane of the two cells. [27]

K

kiss-and-run A mechanism of transmitter release in which vesicles combine briefly with the membrane, forming a transient pore through which transmitter leaks out. Vesciles then return to the cytoplasm. [13]

koniocellular (K) cell In the visual system, a third type of ganglion cell that carries information about space and blueish contrasts. [22]

L

L-type channels A type of high voltage-dependent calcium channels with a long-lasting current, resistant to inactivation. There are four types of L-type channels known as Cav1.1, Cav1.2, Cav1.3, Cav1.4. [13]

lateral corticospinal tract The spinal portion of the corticospinal tract in the lateral column of the spinal cord derived from the contralateral motor cortex; governs skilled movements of the extremities. Also called the *pyramidal tract*. [26]

lateral inhibition A general contrast-enhancing mechanism, whereby an activated neuron reduces the activity of its neighbor(s). [27]

lateral superior olive A structure in the auditory brainstem that aids in sound localization by computing interaural intensity differences. [24]

lateral system Sensory pathways involved in generating discriminative aspects of somatosensory experience. [23]

law of mass action The proposition that the rate of a chemical reaction is proportional to the products of the concentrations of the reactants; and further that the equilibrium the ratio between the concentrations of the reactants and products of the reaction is constant. [15]

leak current A small steady current through resting ion channels, seen when the cell membrane is displaced from its resting potential. [6, 7]

length constant (λ) The distance (usually in millimeters) over which a localized graded potential decreases to $1/e$ of its original size in an axon or a muscle fiber. [8]

ligand-activated channels A channel that is activated by binding an ion or molecule to an external or internal receptor region of the channel. [4]

local autocrine loop A positive feedback loop, whereby a secreted growth factor acts back on its receptors located in spatial proximity of the same cell. [17]

local graded potential Small voltage signal that is produced in terminals of receptor cells or at synapses in response to transmitters. [1]

locus coeruleus A small nucleus in the brainstem that innervates widespread regions of the brain and spinal cord; important in the governance of sleep and waking. [14]

long receptors Sensory receptors that generate action potentials, which are transmitted over long distances where the synapse is made with the next neuron. [21]

long-term depression (LTD) A decrease in the size of a synaptic potential lasting hours or more, produced by previous synaptic activation. [16]

long-term potentiation (LTP) An increase in the size of a synaptic potential lasting hours or more, produced by previous synaptic activation. [16]

M

M-channel A voltage-activated potassium channel that is inactivated by acetylcholine through muscarinic receptors. [12, 19]

magnocellular (M) cell In the visual system, large retinal ganglion cells and lateral geniculate cells that project to discrete cortical areas, particularly sensitive to movement and small changes in contrast. [3, 22]

magnocellular division In the visual system, the two ventral layers of larger cells in the lateral geniculate nucleus to which the M ganglion cells project; concerned with movement and small changes in contrast. [2]

marginal zone Region comprising the elongating axon terminals of the underlying neurons and the Cajal-Retzius neurons. [27]

mean open time (τ) The average time spent in the open state by a membrane channel. [4]

mechanoreceptor channels Channels specialized to sense mechanical forces. [4]

mechanotransduction Conversion of the impingement of mechanical energy into nerve signals. [21]

medial nucleus of the trapezoid body (MNTB) A structure that provides inhibitory input to the lateral superior olive. [24]

medial superior olive A structure in the auditory brainstem that aids in sound localization by computing interaural time differences. [24]

medial system Sensory pathways involved in generating emotional, affective aspects of somatosensory experience. [23]

Meissner's corpuscle Rapidly adapting mechanoreceptor in superficial skin. [23]

melatonin A hormone secreted by the pineal gland. [19]

memory allocation Neurons that are more active at the time of a learning experience are more likely to be incorporated in the memory trace for that experience. This property can be used to allocate a subset of neurons into a memory trace, by experimentally increasing their activity. [17]

Merkel's disk Slowly adapting mechanoreceptor in superficial skin. [23]

metabotropic glutamate receptors (mGluRs) Receptors that are activated by neurotransmitters or other extracellular signals, and that subsequently induce an intracellular or intramembrane biochemical change, typically through the aegis of a G-protein (G protein-coupled receptors). [14]

metabotropic receptors Neurotransmitter receptors that interact with another membrane protein, such as a G protein, to produce their effect on a neuron. [12]

microdomain Calcium signal produced when a cluster of calcium channels open. [13]

microglial cells One of four classes of glial cells found in the vertebrate CNS; these wandering, macrophage-like cells accumulate at sites of injury and scavenge debris. [10]

microneurography A method to measure electrical activity arising in the skin of human subjects by insertion of metal microelectrodes into nerve fascicles, usually in the arm. [23]

mirror neurons Neurons in the posterior frontal and inferior parietal lobes that respond during the execution of goal-oriented action and the observation of the same actions, even when such actions are not executed. [26]

MOD-1 receptors A serotonin receptor, belonging to the large superfamily of Cys-loop receptors. [5]

mossy fibers Afferent axons to the cerebellum from all sources except for the inferior olivary nuclei; the vast majority enter the cerebellum via the inferior and middle cerebellar peduncles. [26]

motor end plate Region of the skeletal muscle fiber membrane specialized for attachment of the motor nerve terminal and reception of its chemical transmitter. [11]

motor pool All the motor neurons that innervate a particular muscle. [26]

motor unit A single motoneuron and the muscle fibers it innervates. [26]

multielectrode array An array that contains multiple electrodes usually used to collect the activity of multiple neurons simultaneously. [1]

multivesicular body Intracellular membrane compartment filled with vesicles and material retrieved on endocytosis. [18]

muscarinic acetylcholine receptors (mAChR) G protein-coupled acetylcholine receptor that is selectively activated by muscarine. A membrane protein that binds ACh. Activated by muscarine, contains a single protein molecule coupled by a G protein to one or more intracellular second messenger systems. See *acetylcholine receptor*. [11, 12]

muscle spindles Fusiform (spindle-shaped) structures in skeletal muscles containing small muscle fibers and sensory receptors activated by stretch. [26]

myelin The coiled membranes of glial cells forming an isolating sheath around an axon. [1]

N

N2G cells Glia-related cells (named for expressing NG2 proteoglycan) that form oligodendrocytes and astrocytes in the adult CNS. NG2 cells form synaptic-like connections with neurons and can produce action potentials. [10]

nanodomain Calcium signal that occurs when a calcium channel opens. [13]

narcolepsy A chronic sleep disorder characterized by repeated periods of extreme daytime sleepiness (sleep attacks), and in some cases, sudden loss of muscle tone that results in collapse (cataplexy). [14]

neostriatum A major component of the basal ganglia, comprising the caudate nucleus and the putamen. [26]

Nernst equation A mathematical formula that predicts the electrical potential generated ionically across a membrane at electrochemical equilibrium. [4]

neural plate The thickened region of the dorsal ectoderm of a neurula that gives rise to the neural tube. [27]

neurexins A family of transmembrane pre-synaptic proteins that bind post-synaptic proteins including neuroligins, and regulate the formation and maintenance of synapses between central neurons. [27]

neuroepigenetics The set of epigenetic mechanisms implicated in long term gene expression regulation and chromatin remodeling in the nervous system. An epigenetic molecular mark in an adult neuron can be long-lasting, permanent, and self-regenerating but cannot be inherited by a daughter cell since the neuron does not divide. [17]

neurogenic genes Mutations in neurogenic genes (such as the *Notch* and *Delta* genes) determine an excess of neuroblast formation. [27]

neuroglial cells Non-neuronal cells in the nervous system that surround and support neurons. In the CNS, includes oligodendrocytes, astrocytes, radial glial cells, and microglial cells; in the PNS, Schwann cells. Also called *glial cells* or *glia*.

neuroligins Cell adhesion proteins on the postsynaptic membrane that mediate the formation and maintenance of synapses between central neurons. Neuroligins act as ligands for β-neurexins. Neuroligins also mediate trans-synaptic modulation of synaptic transmission. [27]

neuromuscular transmission Transmission from a motor nerve to a skeletal muscle fiber via the motor end plate. See *motor end plate*. [11]

neuropeptides Peptides present in the nervous system that act as neurotransmitters or neurohormones. [14]

nicotinic acetylcholine receptor (nAChR) Activated by nicotine, consists of five polypeptide subunits that form a cation channel when activated. [5]

Nissl substance Granules made of ordered arrays of rough endoplasmic reticulum and ribosomes. [29]

nocebo A sham or simulated medical intervention, opposite of the **placebo**, in which the patient, due to pessimistic expectations, experiences a substantial increase in pain sensation without administration of pharmacologically active substances. [23]

noise analysis Analysis of the frequency components of a record in order to determine the the magnitude and time course of underlying channel activity. [4]

non-adrenergic, non-cholinergic (NANC) Transmission that is mediated by some chemical other that acetylcholine or a catecholamine, such as nitric oxide or ATP. The term also applies to the fibers containing these transmitters. [12]

O

ocular dominance columns Vertically stacked columns of neurons in the primary visual cortex (V1) that are grouped according to which eye, right or left, influences them more strongly. [3]

Ohm's law Relates current (I) to voltage (V) and resistance (R); $I = V/R$. [App. A]

oligodendrocytes One of four classes of glial cells found in the vertebrate CNS; their primary function is to form myelin. [10]

open channel block Block of ion flow through an open channel by a physical obstruction, such as a large molecule in the channel mouth. [4]

optogenetics A field of research that uses genetic tools to induce neurons to become sensitive to light, such that experimenters can excite or inhibit a cell by exposing it to light. [1]

orexins Hypothalmic neuropeptides that regulate sleep and feeding. Also called *hypocretins*. [14]

organ of Corti The sensory epithelium of the cochlea. [24]

orientation columns Vertically stacked columns of neurons in the primary visual cortex (V1) that respond only to specific line orientations, such as vertical, oblique, or horizontal. [3]

ossicles The bones of the middle ear. [24]

otolithic membrane An acellular gelatinous matrix enclosing calcium carbonate crystals to mass-load hair cells in the saccule and utricle. [21]

otolithic organs Another term for the saccule and utricle, structures whose function depends on forces applied to tiny masses of calcium carbonate crystals (liths, or stones). [24]

outer hair cells Cilated cells that receive efferent signals from the brain and change shape to control the gain of the sensory signal. [24]

outside-out patch A small segment of cell membrane removed from the cell, sealed inside a micropipette tip with the extracellular side facing the extracellular solution. [4]

P

Pacinian corpuscle A rapidly adapting mechanoreceptor sensitive to vibration; found in deep skin and other tissues. [23]

paracrine signaling Signaling by a diffusible ligand secreted by a source cell, forming a concentration gradient, and acting on receiver cells at some distance. [27]

paracrine transmission Chemical transmission that occurs via the secretion of hormone-like agents whose effects are mediated locally rather than by the general circulation. In the brain, this type of diffuse signaling is called *volume transmission*. [12]

parahippocampal place area (PPA) Medial-most gyral structure in the inferior temporal lobe; part of the medial temporal lobe memory system that generates cognitive maps in spatial frameworks that facilitate the acquisition of episodic and declarative memory. [25]

parallel fibers The bifurcated axons of cerebellar granule cells that extend along the length of the folia in the molecular layer of the cerebellar cortex, where they synapse on dendritic spines of Purkinje cells. [26]

parasympathetic division A division of the autonomic nervous system arising from the cranial and sacral segments of the CNS. [19]

Parkinson's disease A progressive neurodegenerative disease of the substantia nigra pars compacta that results in a characteristic tremor at rest and a general paucity of movement. [14, 26]

parvocellular (P) cell In the visual system, smaller retinal ganglion cells and lateral geniculate cells that project to discrete areas of the visual cortex; concerned with color detection and fine discrimination. [3, 22]

parvocellular division In the visual system, the four dorsal layers of smaller cells in the lateral geniculate nucleus to which the P ganglion cells project; concerned with color detection and discrimination of fine detail at high contrast. [2]

patch clamp recording A technique whereby a small patch of membrane is sealed to the tip of a micropipette, enabling currents through single membrane channels to be recorded. [4]

perforated patch A small segment of cell membrane attached to the cell, sealed inside a micropipette tip and made permeable to biological materials by one or more molecules in the micropipette solution. [4]

perisynaptic release Release from vesicles, usually dense-core vesicles, in extrasynaptic sites of boutons. [18]

phasic firing Repetitive firing of a cell at regular intervals interspersed with silent periods. [19]

phonemes Basic sound element of speech. [24]

photoreceptors The specialized neurons in the eye—rods and cones—that are sensitive to light. [1, 22]

placebo A sham or simulated medical intervention in which the patient, due to optimistic expectations, experiences a substantial relief of symptoms without administration of pharmacologically active drugs or effective surgery. [23]

plasticity Temporary changes in synaptic efficacy between that neuron and its target. [1]

Poisson distribution Discrete probability distribution in which the number n of participants is large and the probability p of occurrence is low. [13]

polyneuronal innervation A state in which neurons or muscle fibers receive synaptic inputs from multiple, rather than single, axons. [27]

pontine Referring to the pons. [26]

positional identities Differences in cell position in the embryo correspond to distinct developmental fates, in response to environmental gradient cues. [27]

post-tetanic potentiation (PTP) An increase in evoked transmitter release from nerve terminals, following a prolonged train of presynaptic action potentials. PTP can last for several minutes. [16]

post-translational modifications of histone proteins Histone tails protruding from the nucleosome subunits are sites of numerous posttranslational modifications, including lysine acetylation and methylation. In general, histone acetylation loosens histone-DNA interactions, facilitating the association between transcription factors and DNA, thereby activating transcription. Histone methylation usually represses transcription. [17]

posterior fusiform Region of human visual cortex, homologous with the IT in monkeys, where neurons are excited specifically by the viewing of faces. [25]

postjunctional folds Infolding of the plasma membrane within the motor end plate. [11]

postsynaptic terminal The terminal of a dendritic spine or shaft or a location on a cell body that is specialized for transmitter reception; downstream at a synapse. [1]

potassium equilibrium potential (E_K) The membrane potential at which there is no net passive movement of a permeant ion species into or out of a cell. The potential that just balances the potassium concentration gradient. [4, 6]

predictive coding Theory according to which the brain generates and updates mental models of the environment, to which sensory information is compared. [22]

presynaptic inhibition The process in which a chemical transmitter acts on the presynaptic nerve ending to reduce the amount of neurotransmitter released. [11]

presynaptic terminal The terminal of an axon at a synapse specialized for transmitter release; upstream at a synapse. [1]

primary auditory cortex (A1) The target of neurons of the thalamic medial geniculate nucleus and thus the first cortical processing stage of auditory signals. [24]

primary endings The terminations of Group Ia afferents in the muscle spindle. [21, 26]

primary somatosensory cortex (S1) Functional division of the cerebral cortex in the postcentral gyrus, corresponding to Brodmann's areas 3, 1, and 2, that receives somatosensory projections from the ventral posterior complex of thalamic nuclei; processes somatosensory information from the body surface, subcutaneous tissues, muscles, and joints. [23]

proneural genes Genes that encode master regulator transcription factors that are necessary and sufficient, in the context of the ectoderm, to initiate the development of neuronal lineages and to promote the generation of progenitors that are committed to neuronal differentiation. [27]

prosopagnosia A type of agnosia in which the ability to recognize faces is impaired, while the ability to recognize other objects remains normal. See *agnosia*. [25]

pruning The process of synapse elimination during development. [27]

Purkinje cell A type of large nerve cell in the cerebellar cortex. [26]

putamen One of the three major components of the basal ganglia (the other two are the caudate nucleus and the nucleus accumbens). Also called *putamen nuclei*. [26]

pyramidal tract See *lateral corticospinal tract*. [26]

Q

quanta (sing: quantum) Packages with a fixed number of molecules of neurotransmitter released from a vesicle. [13]

quantal size The number of molecules in a quantum. [13]

quantum content The number of quanta in a synaptic response. [13]

quantum hypothesis The hypothesis that the single quantal events represent the building blocks for the synaptic potentials. [13]

R

radial glial cells One of four classes of glial cells found in the vertebrate CNS; they play an essential role in the developing CNS, forming filaments along which developing neurons migrate to their final destinations, and also act as stem cells for neurogenesis. [10]

raphe nuclei A chain of serotonergic nuclei on the midline of the brainstem that innervate wide areas of the brain and extend down the spinal cord; important in the governance of sleep and waking. [14]

rapidly adapting Neurons that rapidly reset their level of excitability in the face of a maintained stimulus are known as rapidly adapting (RA). [21]

receptive field The area of the periphery whose stimulation influences the firing of a neuron. For cells in the visual pathway, the area on the retina where illumination influences the activity of a neuron. [2, 22]

simple receptive field Receptive field of simple cells in the visual cortex. [2]

complex receptive field Receptive field of complex cells in the visual cortex. [2]

receptor complex Nerve termination together with the specialized filtering structure surrounding it. [23]

receptor potential Graded, localized potential change in a sensory receptor initiated by the appropriate stimulus; the electrical sign of the transduction process. [21]

receptor 1. A nerve terminal or accessory cell associated with sensory transduction. 2. A molecule in the cell, usually a transmembrane protein that initiates a response when combined with a specific chemical. [1]

reciprocal innervation Interconnections of neurons arranged so that pathways exciting one group of muscles inhibit the antagonistic motoneurons. [26]

recruitment Addition of more and more inputs, for example when stimulus strength is increased. [26]

rectification The property of a membrane, or membrane channel, that allows it to conduct ion current more readily in one direction than in the other. [11]

refractory period

absolute refractory period The time following an action potential during which a stimulus cannot elicit a second action potential.

relative refractory period The time following the absolute refractory period when the threshold for initiation of a second action potential is increased. [7, 8]

reprogram The process by which somatic cells are converted into different cell types (and in particular into pluripotent stem cells) by the expression of a small set of transcription factors. [27]

resting membrane potential The inside-negative electrical potential that is normally recorded across all cell membranes. [4]

resting potential The steady electrical potential across the cell membrane in the quiescent state. [1]

reticulospinal tract A tract of axons arising from the brainstem reticular formation and descending to the spinal cord to modulate movement. [26]

retinal Chromophore that in photoreceptors binds to an opsin protein to form rhodopsin. On photon absorption, retinal changes configuration and initiates phototransduction. [22]

retrograde synaptic signaling Signaling that travels "backward," that is, from the postsynaptic cell to the presynaptic terminal. [12]

retrograde transport Axonal transport in the direction from the axon terminal toward the cell body. [15]

reversal potential (V_r) The value of the membrane potential at which a chemical transmitter produces no change in potential. [11]

reverse suture Deprivation of the previously open eye and opening of the previously deprived eye. [28]

rhombencephalon The caudal part of the brain between the mesencephalon and the spinal cord, derived from the embryonic hindbrain vesicle; includes the pons, cerebellum, and medulla. Also known as the *hindbrain*. [27]

ribbon synapses The active zone of hair cells and retinal cells specialized for continuous transmitter release. [24]

RNA editing Replacement of one codon by another in messenger RNA after transcription. [5, 27]

RNA editing enzyme Enzyme that catalyzes the RNA editing process. [27]

rods Retinal photoreceptors sensitive to dim light. [1, 22]

roof plate The dorsalmost medial region of the vertebrate neural tube, where the two edges of the neuroectoderm fuse during neurulation. The roof plate produces secreted signals that control the specification and differentiation of dorsal cell types in the neural tube, as well as the neural crest. [27]

rubrospinal tract In non-human mammals, the pathway from the magnocellular divisions of the red nucleus of the midbrain to the spinal cord; participates with the lateral corticospinal tract in governing the distal extremities. In humans, however, the corticospinal tract serves this function and the rubrospinal tract is vestigial (perhaps even nonexistent). [26]

Ruffini's corpuscle Slowly adapting mechanoreceptor found deep in skin. [23]

S

saccades Ballistic, conjugate eye movements that change the point of foveal fixation. [22, 26]

saturated disk An area on the postsynaptic membrane in which the average occupancy of the postsynaptic receptors by the transmitter during synaptic transmission equals 100%. [15]

scala media A fluid-filled compartment of the cochlea. [24]

scala tympani A fluid-filled compartment of the cochlea. [24]

scala vestibuli A fluid-filled compartment of the cochlea. [24]

Schwann cells Glial cells in the vertebrate PNS that form myelin. [10]

second messenger A molecule forming part of a second-messenger system. [12]

second-messenger system A series of intracellular molecular reactions initiated by occupation of extracellular receptor sites and leading to a functional response, such as opening or closing of membrane channels. [12]

secondary ending The terminations of Group II afferents in the muscle spindle. [21]

secondary somatosensory cortex (S2) Functional division of the cerebral cortex in the parietal operculum just posterior to the postcentral gyrus; processes somatosensory information received from the primary somatosensory cortex. [23]

selectivity filter Structure within an ion channel that allows selected ions to permeate, while rejecting other types of ions. [4]

selectivity A measure of how effectively a receptor is shielded from forms of energy that are not the adequate stimulus. [21]

semicircular canal Fluid-filled loop in the vestibular apparatus associated with detection of head rotation. [21]

sensitivity A measure of how tiny a quantity of energy is required to excite the receptor. [21]

sensitization Increased responses to a standard weak stimulus following an initial exposure to a much stronger stimulus. [20]

sensory ending The termination of the nerve fiber within the sensory organ, the site of transduction. [21]

sensory receptor A cell that responds to external physical stimuli. [1]

short receptors Sensory receptors that transmit signals to the next neuron through graded neurotransmitter release, which is proportional to the energy transduced. [21]

siemens (S) Unit of conductance; reciprocal of ohm. [App. A]

silent synapses Synapses that are devoid of receptors and thus do not respond to presynaptic stimulation, making them incapable of releasing transmitter. [16]

size principle The orderly recruitment of motor units of increasing size as the strength of a muscle contraction increases. [26]

slope conductance Change in current produced per volt change in membrane potential at a particular potential of the membrane. [4]

slowly adapting Neurons that gradually reset their level of excitability in the face of the maintained stimulus are known as slowly adapting (SA). [21]

SNARE Soluble *N*-ethylmaleimide-sensitive factor *A*ttachment protein *RE*ceptor. [13]

sodium-potassium ATPase The molecule responsible for transport in the sodium–potassium exchange pump. For every molecule of ATP hydrolyzed, sodium-potassium ATPase carries three sodium ions out of the cell and two potassium ions in. [9]

sodium-potassium exchange pump An ATPase pump in the cell membrane of most cells that keeps intracellular sodium and potassium concentrations constant by transporting three sodium ions out across the cell membrane for every two potassium ions carried in. [9]

spatial buffering A mechanism by which glial cells regulate their concentration of extracellular potassium. [10]

specific capacitance The capacitance of 1 square centimeter of cell membrane. [8]

specific resistance 1. The resistance of 1 square centimeter of cell membrane. 2. The resistance of a volume of cytoplasm 1 square centimeter in cross section and 1 centimeter in length. [8]

Spemann organizer The group of cells in the dorsal lip of the blastopore that are responsible for the induction of neural tissue during development in amphibian embryos. [27]

spillover Leak of transmitter from synaptic connection on increases in presynaptic release. [18]

steady state In reference to a cell, the state in which the passive gain or loss of solutes is exactly balanced by active transport processes, so that the composition of the cytoplasm remains constant. [6]

stellate cells Small star-shaped cells in the molecular layer of the cerebellum. [26]

stick and slip Irregular, jerky motion caused by friction between two interacting objects. [23]

stria vascularis Specialized epithelium lining the cochlear duct that maintains the high potassium concentration of the endolymph. [24]

substantia nigra A bipartite gray matter structure in the ventral midbrain; contains a pallidal division, called the pars reticulata, defined by a network (reticulum) of cells that provide inhibitory (GABAergic) output from the basal ganglia to the thalamus and brainstem, and a compact division, called the pars compacta, comprising densely packed neurons that synthesize and release dopamine in the caudate and putamen. [26]

subthalamic nucleus A nucleus in the ventral thalamus that receives input from the cerebral cortex and external segment of the globus pallidus and sends excitatory (glutamatergic) projections to the internal segment of the globus pallidus. A component of the indirect pathway from striatum to pallidum. [26]

superfamily A group of gene families, each of whose ancestral genes arose by duplication and divergence from a yet more ancient ancestral gene. [5]

surround receptive field The skin area adjacent to the center, providing weaker input. [23]

sympathetic division A division of the autonomic nervous system arising from the thoracic and lumbar segments of the CNS. [19]

synapse Site at which neurons make functional contact; a term coined by Sherrington. [1, 11]

synaptic basal lamina A layer of extracellular matrix connecting the different elements of a synapse. [29]

synaptic cleft The space between the membranes of the pre- and postsynaptic cells at a chemical synapse, across which transmitter diffuses. [11]

synaptic delay The time between a presynaptic nerve impulse and a postsynaptic response. [11, 13]

synaptic depression A decrease in evoked release of transmitter from nerve terminals, due to previous synaptic activity. Depression can persist for several seconds. [16]

synaptic facilitation An increase in evoked release of transmitter from nerve terminals, due to previous synaptic activity. Facilitation can last for several hundred milliseconds. [16]

synaptic ribbon An intracellular organelle that tethers large numbers of vesicles near the active zone in the presynaptic terminal. [13]

synaptic vesicles Small membrane-enclosed sacs in presynaptic nerve terminals that contain neurotransmitters. [11]

syncytium A group of cells interconnected by protoplasmic bridges. [11]

T

tag-and-manipulate An experimental strategy to study engrams, whereby neurons active during a learning experience are genetically tagged to express an actuator (for instance a chemogenetic or an optogenetic protein) that can be used to negatively or positively manipulate the activity of those neurons at a later time point. [17]

tectorial membrane An acellular gelatinous sheet that lies over the organ of Corti and contacts the hair cells stereocilia. [24]

tectospinal tract A group of nerve fibers running from the superior colliculus (tectum) to the spinal cord. [26]

terminal selectors Transcription factors that induce and maintain the expression of the genes that characterize the identity and the properties of terminally differentiated neuron types. [27]

threshold for excitation The level of membrane potential at which an action potential is generated. [7]

threshold 1. The critical value of membrane potential or depolarization at which an impulse is initiated. 2. The minimal stimulus required for a sensation. [1]

tip links Fine extracellular fiber connecting the tips of adjacent stereocilia on hair cells. [21]

tonic firing Repetitive firing of a cell. [19]

tonotopic map Brain representation of acoustic frequencies where neighboring positions in the map are excited by neighboring frequencies. [24]

tonotopically According to a tonotopic organization, whereby there is a relationship between position on the cochlea and frequency response. Different regions of the cochlea are stimulated by different frequencies of the incoming sound stimulus. [28]

top-down inputs Pathways from high-order levels of the cortical processing stream in the direction of the primary sensory cortical region. Top-down inputs can modulate sensory responses at earlier stages of processing according to learning, attention, memory, and expectation. [25]

topographic map Point-to-point correspondence between neighboring regions of the sensory periphery (e.g., the visual field or the body surface) and neighboring neurons within the central components of the system (e.g., in the brain and spinal cord). [23]

trans-synaptic regulation Regulation of events on one side of a synapse by events on the other side. It can be anterograde (from presynaptic to postsynaptic) or retrograde (from postsynaptic to presynaptic) and can be through multiple synapses. [15]

transcranial direct-current stimulation (tDCS) Stimulation of brain regions or neurons by inserting an extracellular electrode to pass direct current across the cranium. [1]

transcranial magnetic stimulation (TMS) Localized, noninvasive stimulation of cortical neurons through the induction of electrical current by the application of strong, focal magnetic fields. [1]

transcriptional profiles All the mRNA transcripts expressed by a given cell type, plus their relative abundances. [20]

transcriptome All of the mRNA transcripts, plus their relative abundances, expressed by a cell in a particular developmental state or physiological condition. [1]

transcriptomics The study of transcriptomes. [1]

transducin The G protein that mediates phototransduction. [22]

transport molecules Molecules involved in the translocation of other molecules or ions across cell membranes in biological systems. [4]

tuning curve A plot that reveals the best frequency of cochlear afferent neurons by depicting the amplitude of sound that is required to excite the neuron across the frequency dimension. [24]

tympanic membrane The eardrum. [24]

V

ventral cochlear nucleus A processing stage along the auditory pathway whose neurons project both ipsilaterally and contralaterally to the superior olivary complex in the brainstem. [24]

ventral corticospinal tract The group of nerve fibers running from the cerebral cortex down the spinal cord in the ventral spinal column. [26]

ventral pathway The cortical visual processing pathway that runs from the occipital cortex to the anterior tip of the inferior temporal lobe, and involves object recognition. [25]

ventricular zone Region adjacent to the lumen of the neural tube (future ventricle) in the developing vertebrate neuroepithelium where cell proliferation occurs. [27]

vestibulospinal tract The group of nerve fibers running from the vestibular nucleus to the spinal column. [26]

visual agnosia Loss of ability to recognize real-world things (for instance, objects, persons, sounds, shapes, or smells) in spite of preserved capacities in sensing the elemental properties of things. [25]

voltage clamp A technique for displacing membrane potential abruptly to a desired value and keeping the potential constant while measuring currents across the cell membrane; devised by Cole and Marmont. [7]

voltage-gated potassium (BK) Channels whose opening is determined by the concentration of membrane voltage. [24]

voltage-sensitive sodium channel A sodium channel that is activated or inactivated by changes in membrane potential. [4]

volume transmission Chemical transmission in the brain that occurs via the secretion of hormone-like agents whose effects are mediated locally rather than by the general circulation. Elsewhere in the body, this type of diffuse signaling is called *paracrine transmission*. [12, 18]

W

Wallerian degeneration When an axon is cut, the isolated distal segment undergoes Wallerian degeneration. [29]

whisker barrels Columnar organization of somatosensory cortex related to facial whiskers. [28]

whole-cell patch recording Recording of membrane currents of an intact cell with a patch clamp electrode, through an opening in the cell membrane. [1, 4]

Z

ZAC A receptor activated by ionic zinc. [5]

Bibliography

Abbott, N. J., Patabendige, A. A., Dolman, D. E., et al. 2010. Structure and function of the blood-brain barrier. *Neurobiol. Dis.* 37: 13–25. [10]

Abbracchino, M. P., Burnstock, G., Verkhratsky, A., and Zimmerman, H. 2009. Purinergic signalling in the nervous system: An overview. *Trends Neurosci.* 32: 19–29. [5, 14]

Abbracchio, M. P., Burnstock, G., Boeynaems, J.-M., et al. 2006. International Union of Pharmacology. Update and subclassification of the P2Y G protein-coupled nucleotide receptors: From molecular mechanisms and pathophysiology to therapy. *Pharmacol. Rev.* 58: 281–341. [14]

Abdou, K., et al. 2018. Synapse-specific representation of the identity of overlapping memory engrams. *Science* 360: 1227–1231. [17]

Abe, H., Honma, S., Ohtsu, H., and Honma, K. 2004. Circadian rhythms in behavior and clock gene expressions in the brain of mice lacking histidine decarboxylase. *Mol. Brain Res.* 124: 178–187. [14]

Abraham, W. C., and Williams, J. M. 2003. Properties and mechanisms of LTP maintenance. *Neuroscientist* 9: 463–474. [16]

Acampora, D., et al. 1995. Forebrain and midbrain regions are deleted in Otx2-/- mutants due to a defective anterior neuroectoderm specification during gastrulation. *Development* 121: 3279–3290. [27]

Accili, E. A., Proenza, C., Baruscotti, M., and DiFrancesco. D. 2002. From funny current to HCN channels: 20 years of excitation. *News Physiol. Sci.* 17: 32–37. [12]

Ache, B. W., and Zhainazarov, A. 1995. Dual second-messenger pathways in olfactory transduction. *Curr. Opin. Neurobiol.* 5: 461–466. [21]

Acklin, S. E. 1988. Electrical properties and anion permeability of doubly rectifying junctions in the leech central nervous system. *J. Exp. Biol.* 137: 1–11. [11]

Adams, D. J., Dwyer, T. M., and Hille, B. 1980. The permeability of endplate channels to monovalent and divalent metal cations. *J. Gen. Physiol.* 75: 493–510. [11]

Adams, D. L., and Horton, J. C. 2002. Shadows cast by retinal blood vessels mapped in primary visual cortex. *Science* 298: 572–576. [28]

Adams, D. L., and Zeki, S. 2001. Functional organization of macaque V3 for stereoscopic depth. *J. Neurophysiol.* 86: 2195–2203. [3]

Adams, D. L., Sincich, L. C., and Horton, J. C. 2007. Complete pattern of ocular dominance columns in human primary visual cortex. *J. Neurosci.* 27: 10391–10403. [3]

Adams, J. P., and Dudek, S. M. 2005. Late-phase long-term potentiation: getting to the nucleus. *Nat Rev. Neurosci.* 6: 737–743. [17]

Adams, P. R., and Brown, D. A. 1975. Actions of gamma-aminobutyric acid on sympathetic ganglion cells. *J. Physiol.* 250: 85–120. [11]

Adams, P. R., and Brown, D. A. 1980. Luteinizing hormone-releasing factor and muscarinic agonists act on the same voltage-sensitive K⁺-currents in bullfrog sympathetic neurones. *Brit. J. Pharmacol.* 68: 353–355. [12, 19]

Adams, S. R., Kao, J. P. Y., Grynkiewicz, G., et al. 1988. Biologically useful chelators that release Ca²⁺ upon illumination. *J. Am. Chem. Soc.* 110: 3212–3220. [13]

Adar, E., Nottebohm, F., and Barnea, A. 2008. The relationship between nature of social change, age, and position of new neurons and their survival in adult zebra finch brain. *J. Neurosci.* 28: 5394–5400. [27]

Adler, E. M., Augustine, G. J., Duffy, S. N., and Charlton, M. P. 1991. Alien intracellular calcium chelators attenuate neurotransmitter release at the squid giant synapse. *J. Neurosci.* 11: 1496–1507. [13]

Adler, E., Hoon, M. A., Mueller, K. L., et al. 2000. A novel family of mammalian taste receptors. *Cell* 100: 693–702. [21]

Adrian, E. D. 1946. *The Physical Background of Perception.* Clarendon, Oxford, England. [1, 26, 30]

Adrian, E. D. 1953. Sensory messages and sensation; the response of the olfactory organ to different smells. *Acta Physiol. Scand.* 29: 5–14. [21]

Adrian, E. D. 1959. *The Mechanism of Nervous Action.* University of Pennsylvania Press, Philadelphia. [26]

Adrian, E. D., and Zotterman, Y. 1926. The impulses produced by sensory nerve-endings: Part II. The response of a Single End-Organ. *J. Physiol.* 61: 151–171. [21]

Afraz, S., Kiani, R., and Esteky, H. 2006. Microstimulation of inferotemporal cortex influences face categorization. *Nature* 442: 692–695. [25, 30]

Afshari, F. T., Kappagantula, S., and Fawcett, J. W. 2009. Extrinsic and intrinsic factors controlling axonal regeneration after spinal cord injury. *Expert Rev. Mol. Med.* 11: e37. [29]

Aghajanian, G. K., Foote, W. E., and Sheard, M. H. 1968. Lysergic acid diethylamide: Sensitive neuronal units in the midbrain raphe. *Science* 161: 706–708. [18]

Aghajanian, G. K., and VanderMaelen, C. P. 1982. Alpha 2-adreno-ceptor-mediated hyperpolarization of locus coeruleus neurons: Intracellular studies in vivo. *Science* 215: 1394–1396. [14]

Aghajanian, G. K., Cedarbaum, J. M., and Wang, R. Y. 1977. Evidence for norepinephrine-mediated collateral inhibition of locus coeruleus neurons. *Brain Res.* 136: 570–577. [14]

Agnati, L. F., Fuxe, K., Zoli, M., et al. 1986. A correlation analysis of the regional distribution of central enkephalin and β-endorphin immunoreactive terminals and of opiate receptors in adult and old male rats. Evidence for the existence of two main types of communication in the central nervous system: The volume transmission and the wiring transmission. *Acta Physiol. Scand.* 128: 201–207. [18]

Aguayo, A. J., Clarke, D. B., Jelsma, T. N., et al. 1996. Effects of neurotrophins on the survival and regrowth of injured retinal neurons. *Ciba Found. Symp.* 196: 135–144. [29]

Aguayo, A. J., Dickson, R., Trecarten, J., et al. 1978. Ensheathment and myelination of regenerating PNS fibres by transplanted optic nerve glia. *Neurosci. Lett.* 9: 97–104. [29]

Agulhon, C., Fiacco, T. A., and McCarthy, K. D. 2010. Hippocampal short- and long-term plasticity are not modulated by astrocyte Ca²⁺ signaling. *Science.* 327: 1250–1254. [10]

Ahern, P., Klyachko, V. A., and Jackson, M. B. 2002. cGMP and S-nitrosylation: Two routes for modulation of neuronal excitability by NO. *Trends Neurosci.* 25: 510–517. [12]

Ahlquist, R. P. 1948. A study of the adrenotropic receptors. *Am. J. Physiol.* 153: 586–600. [19]

Ahmed, M. S., and Siegelbaum, S A. 2009. Recruitment of N-Type Ca²⁺ channels during LTP enhances low release efficacy of hippocampal CA1 perforant path synapses. *Neuron* 63: 372–385. [16]

Aiba, A., Chen, C., Herrup, K., et al. 1994. Reduced hippocampal long-term potentiation and context-specific deficit in associative learning in mGluR1 mutant mice. *Cell* 79: 365–375. [14]

Aimone J. B., et al. 2014. Regulation and function of adult neurogenesis: From genes to cognition. *Physiol. Rev.* 94: 991–1026. [27]

Aimone, J. B., Deng, W., and Gage, F. H. 2010. Adult neurogenesis: Integrating theories and separating functions. *Trends Cogn. Sci.* 14: 325–337. [29]

Airaksinen, M. S., and Saarma, M. 2002. The GDNF family: Signalling, biological functions and therapeutic value. *Nat. Rev. Neurosci.* 3: 383–394. [27]

Akaaboune, M., Grady, R. M., Turney, S., et al. 2002. Neurotransmitter receptor dynamics studied in vivo by reversible photo-unbinding of fluorescent ligands. *Neuron* 34: 865–876. [11]

Aksoy-Aksel et al. 2014. MicroRNAs and synaptic plasticity—a mutual relationship. *Phil. Trans. R. Soc. B* 369: 20130515. [17]

Alabi, A. A., and Tsien, R. W. 2013. Perspectives on kiss-and-run: Role in exocytosis, endocytosis and neurotransmission. *Annu. Rev. Physiol.* 785: 393–422. [13]

Alberini, C. M. 2009. Transcription factors in long-term memory and synaptic plasticity. *Physiological Rev.* 89: 121–145. [17]

Alberini, C. M., and LeDoux J. E. 2013. Memory reconsolidation. *Curr. Biol.* 23: R746. [17]

Alberini, C. M., and Travaglia, A. 2017. *J. Neurosci.* 37: 5783–5795. [28]

Albillos, A., Dernick, G., Horstmann, H., et al.1997. The exocytotic event in chromaffin cells revealed by patch amperometry. *Nature* 389: 509–512. [13]

Albrecht, J., Sonnewald, U., Waagepetersen, H. S., and Schousboe, A. 2007. Glutamine in the central nervous system: Function and dysfunction. *Front Biosci.* 12: 332–343. [15]

Albright, T. D. 1984. Direction and orientation selectivity of neurons in visual area MT of the macaque. *J. Neurophysiol.* 52: 1106–1130. [25]

Albus, H., Vansteensel, M. J., Michel, S., et al. 2005. A GABAergic mechanism is necessary for coupling dissociable ventral and dorsal regional oscillators within the circadian clock. *Current Biology* 15: 886–893. [19]

Alfano et al. 2014. Postmitotic control of sensory area specification during neocortical development. *Nature Commun.* 5: Article number: 5632. [27]

Alkadhi, K. A., Alzoubi, K. H., and Aleisa, A. M. 2005. Plasticity of synaptic transmission in autonomic ganglia. *Prog. Neurobiol.* 75: 83–108. [16]

Allan, D. W., and Thor, S. 2015. Transcriptional selectors, masters and combinatorial codes: Regulatory principles of neural subtype specification. *WIREs Dev. Biol.* 4: 505–528. doi: 10.1002/wdev.191. [27]

Allen, N. J., and Barres, B. A. 2005. Signaling between glia and neurons: Focus on synaptic plasticity. *Curr. Opin. Neurobiol.* 15: 542–548. [10]

Allen, R. D., Allen, N. S., and Travis, J. L. 1981. Video-enhanced differential interference contrast (AVEC-DIC) microscopy: A new method capable of analyzing microtubule-related movement in the reticulopodial network of *Allogromia laticollaris. Cell Motil.* 1: 291–302. [15]

Allen, T. G., and Brown, D. A. 1993. M_2 muscarinic receptor-mediated inhibition of the Ca^{2+} current in rat magnocellular cholinergic basal forebrain neurones. *J. Physiol.* 466: 173–189. [14]

Allen, T. G., and Brown, D. A. 1996. Detection and modulation of acetylcholine release from neurites of rat basal forebrain cells in culture. *J. Physiol.* 492: 453–466. [14]

Allen, T. G., Abogadie, F. C., and Brown, D. A. 2006. Simultaneous release of glutamate and acetylcholine from single magnocellular "cholinergic" basal forebrain neurons. *J. Neurosci.* 26: 1588–1595. [14, 15]

Allen, T. J., Ansems, G. E., and Proske, U. 2008. Evidence from proprioception of fusimotor coactivation during voluntary contractions in humans. *Exp. Physiol.* 93: 391–398. [26]

Alonso, J. M. 2002. Neural connections and receptive field properties in the primary visual cortex. *Neuroscientist* 8: 443–456. [2]

Alonso, J. M. 2009. My recollections of Hubel and Wiesel and a brief review of functional circuitry in the visual pathway. *J. Physiol.* 587: 2783–2790. [2]

Alonso, J. M., Yeh, C. I., Weng, C., and Stoelzel, C. 2006. Retinogeniculate connections: A balancing act between connection specificity and receptive field diversity. *Prog. Brain Res.* 154: 3–13. [2]

Altaf, M. A., and Sood, M. R. 2008. The nervous system and gastrointestinal function. *Dev. Disabil. Res. Rev.* 14: 87–95. [19]

Altman, J., and Das, G. D. 1965. Autoradiographic and histological evidence of postnatal hippocampal neurogenesis in rats. *J Comp Neurol.* 124: 319–335. [27]

Alvarez-Castelao, B., and Schuman, E. M. 2015. The regulation of synaptic protein turnover. *J. Biol. Chem.* 290: 28623–28630. [17]

Alvarez-Maubecin, V., García-Hernández, F., Williams, J. T., and Van Bockstaele E. J. 2000. Functional coupling between neurons and glia. *J. Neurosci.* 20 : 4091–4098. doi: 10.1523/jneurosci.20-11-04091.2000. [10]

Amanzio, M., and Benedetti, F. 1999. Neuropharmacological dissection of placebo analgesia: Expectation-activated opioid systems versus conditioning-activated specific subsystems. *J. Neurosci.* 19: 484–494. [23]

Amar, A. P., and Weiss, M. H. 2003. Pituitary anatomy and physiology. *Neurosurg. Clin. N. Am.* 14: 11–23. [19]

Amitai, Y., Gibson, J. R., Beierlein, M., et al. 2002. The spatial dimensions of electrically coupled networks of interneurons in the neocortex. *J. Neurosci.* 22: 4142–4152. [11]

An et al. 2008. Distinct role of long 3′ UTR BDNF mRNA in spine morphology and synaptic plasticity in hippocampal neurons. *Cell* 134: 175–187. [17]

Anderson, C. R., and Stevens, C. F. 1973. Voltage clamp analysis of acetylcholine-produced end-plate current fluctuations at frog neuromuscular junction. *J. Physiol.* 235: 665–691. [4]

Anderson, H., Edwards, J. S., and Palka, J. 1980. Developmental neurobiology of invertebrates. *Annu. Rev. Neurosci.* 3: 97–139. [29]

Anderson, M. A., Burda, J. E., Ren, Y., et al. 2016. Astrocyte scar formation aids central nervous system axon regeneration. *Nature* 532: 195–200. [29]

Anderson, M. J., and Cohen, M. W. 1977. Nerve-induced and spontaneous redistribution of acetylcholine receptors on cultured muscle cells. *J. Physiol.* 268: 757–773. [29]

Andres, F. L., and van der Loos, H. 1985. From sensory periphery to cortex: The architecture of the barrelfield as modified by various early manipulations of the mouse whiskerpad. *Anat. Embryol. (Berl.)* 172: 11–20. [23]

Angelaki, D. E., and Cullen, K. E. 2008. Vestibular system: The many facets of a multimodal sense. *Annu. Rev. Neurosci.* 31: 125–150. [24]

Angelaki, D. E., Klier, E. M., and Snyder, L. H. 2009. A vestibular sensation: Probabilistic approaches to spatial perception. *Neuron* 64: 448–461. [24]

Angevine, J. B., Jr., and Sidman, R. L. 1961. Autoradiographic study of cell migration during histogenesis of cerebral cortex in the mouse. *Nature* 192: 766–768. [27]

Angleson, J. K., and Betz, W. J. 1997. Monitoring secretion in real time: Capacitance, amperometry and fluorescence compared. *Trends Neurosci.* 20: 281–287. [13]

Anglister, L., and McMahan, U. J. 1985. Basal lamina directs acetylcholinesterase accumulation at synaptic sites in regenerating muscle. *J. Cell Biol.* 101: 735–743. [29]

Annunziato, L., Pignatoro, G., and DiRenzo, G. F. 2004. Pharmacology of brain Na^+/Ca^{2+} exchanger: From molecular biology to therapeutic perspectives. *Pharmacol. Rev.* 56: 633–654. [9]

Antonini, A., and Stryker, M. P. 1993. Development of individual geniculocortical arbors in cat striate cortex and effects of binocular impulse blockade. *J. Neurosci.* 13: 3549–3573. [28]

Antonini, A., and Stryker, M. P. 1993. Rapid remodeling of axonal arbors in the visual cortex. *Vis. Neurosci.* 15: 401–409. [28]

Antonini, A., Gillespie, D. C., Crair, M. C., and Stryker, M. P. 1998. Morphology of single geniculocortical afferents and functional recovery of the visual cortex after reverse monocular deprivation in the kitten. *J. Neurosci.* 18: 9896–9909. [28]

Antunes, G., and Simoes de Souza, F. M. 2016. Olfactory receptor signaling. *Methods Cell Biol.* 132: 127–145. [21]

Apkarian, A. V., Bushnell, M. C., Treede, R. D., and Zubieta, J. K. 2005. Human brain mechanisms of pain perception and regulation in health and disease. *Eur. J. Pain* 9: 463–484. [23]

Appel, B., Korzh, V., Glasgow, E., et al. 1995. Motoneuron fate specification revealed by patterned LIM homeobox gene expression in embryonic zebrafish. *Development* 121: 4117–4125. [27]

Arabzadeh, E., Panzeri, S., and Diamond, M. E. 2006. Deciphering the spike train of a sensory neuron: Counts and temporal patterns in the rat whisker pathway. *J. Neurosci.* 26: 9216–9226. [23]

Arabzadeh, E., Zorzin, E., and Diamond, M. E. 2005. Neuronal encoding of texture in the whisker sensory pathway. *PLOS Biol.* 3: e17. [23]

Arbuthnott, E. R., Boyd, I. A., and Kalu, K. U. 1980. Ultrastructural dimensions of myelinated peripheral nerve fibres in the cat and their relation to conduction velocity. *J. Physiol.* 308: 125–157. [8]

Arakawa, H., Suzuki, A., Zhao, S., et al., 2014. Thalamic NMDA receptor function is necessary for patterning of the thalamocortical somatosensory map and for sensorimotor behaviors. *J. Neurosci.* 34: 12001–12014. doi: 10.1523/JNEUROSCI.1663-14.2014. [23]

Armentano, M., Chou S. J., Tomassy, G. S., et al. 2007. COUP-TFI regulates the balance of cortical patterning between frontal/motor and sensory areas. *Nat. Neurosci.* 10: 1277–86. [27]

Armstrong-James, M., Fox, K., and Das-Gupta, A. 1992. Flow of excitation within rat barrel cortex on striking a single vibrissa. *J. Neurophysiol.* 68: 1345–1358. [23]

Armstrong, C. M. 1981. Sodium channels and gating currents. *Physiol. Rev.* 61: 644–683. [7]

Armstrong, C. M., and Bezanilla, F. 1974. Charge movements associated with the opening and closing of the activation gates of sodium channels. *J. Gen. Physiol.* 63: 533–552. [7]

Armstrong, C. M., and Bezanilla, F. 1977. Inactivation of the sodium channel II. Gating current experiments. *J. Gen. Physiol.* 70: 567–590. [7]

Armstrong, C. M., and Hille, B. 1972. The inner quaternary ammonium ion receptor in potassium channels of the node of Ranvier. *J. Gen. Physiol.* 59: 388–400. [7]

Armstrong, C. M., and Hille, B. 1998. Voltage-gated ion channels and electrical excitability. *Neuron* 20: 371–380. [7]

Arnth-Jensen, N., Jabaudon, D., and Scanziani, M. 2002. Cooperation between independent hippocampal synapses is controlled by glutamate uptake. *Nat. Neurosci.* 5: 325–331. [18]

Arrang, J. M., Garbarg, M., and Schwartz, J. C. 1983. Auto-inhibition of brain histamine release mediated by a novel class (H_3) of histamine receptor. *Nature* 302: 832–837. [14]

Art, J. J., and Fettiplace, R. 1984. Efferent desensitization of auditory nerve fibre responses in the cochlea of the turtle *Pseudemys scripta elegans*. *J. Physiol.* 356: 507–523. [24]

Art, J. J., and Fettiplace, R. 1987. Variation of membrane properties in hair cells isolated from the turtle cochlea. *J. Physiol.* 385: 207–242. [24]

Art, J. J., Crawford, A. C., Fettiplace, R., and Fuchs, P. A. 1985. Efferent modulation of hair cell tuning in the cochlea of the turtle. *J. Physiol.* 360: 397–421. [24]

Art, J. J., Fettiplace, R., and Fuchs, P. A. 1984. Synaptic hyperpolarization and inhibition of turtle cochlear hair cells. *J. Physiol.* 356: 525–550. [24]

Art, J. J., Wu, Y. C., and Fettiplace, R. 1995. The calcium-activated potassium channels of turtle hair cells. *J. Gen. Physiol.* 105: 49–72. [24]

Arunlakshana, O., and Schild, H. O. 1959. Some quantitative uses of drug antagonists. *Brit. J. Pharmacol. Chemother.* 14: 48–58. [11]

Asada, H., Kawamura, Y., Maruyama, K., et al. 1997. Cleft palate and decreased brain γ-aminobutyric acid in mice lacking the 67-kDa isoform of glutamic acid decarboxylase. *Proc. Natl. Acad. Sci. USA* 94: 6496–6499. [15]

Ashmore, J. 2008. Cochlear outer hair cell motility. *Physiol. Rev.* 88: 173–210. [24]

Ashmore, J. F. 1987. A fast motile response in guinea-pig outer hair cells: The cellular basis of the cochlear amplifier. *J. Physiol.* 388: 323–347. [24]

Ashraf et al. 2006. Synaptic protein synthesis associated with memory is regulated by the RISC pathway in *Drosophila*. *Cell* 124: 191–205. [17]

Assad, J. A., Shepherd, G. M., and Corey, D. P. 1991. Tip-link integrity and mechanical transduction in vertebrate hair cells. *Neuron* 7: 985–994. [21]

Assinck, P., Duncan, G. J., Hilton, B. J., et al. 2017. Cell transplantation therapy for spinal cord injury. *Nat. Neurosci.* 20: 637. [29]

Attwell, D., Barbour, B., and Szatkowski, M. 1993. Nonvesicular release of neurotransmitter. *Neuron* 11: 401–407. [9]

Attwell, D. et al. 2010. Glial and neuronal control of brain blood flow. *Nature* 468: 232–243. [18]

Atwood, H. L., and Morin, W. A. 1970. Neuromuscular and axoaxonal synapses of the crayfish opener muscle. *J. Ultrastruct. Res.* 32: 351–369. [11]

Atwood, H. L., ed. 1982. *Biology of Crustacea*. Academic Press, New York. [20]

Aubert, A., Costalat, R., Magistretti, P. J., and Pellerin L. 2005. Brain lactate kinetics: Modeling evidence for neuronal lactate uptake upon activation. *Proc. Natl. Acad. Sci. USA* 102: 16448–16553. [10]

Avidan, G., Levy, I., Hendler, T., et al. 2003. Spatial vs. object specific attention in high-order visual areas. *Neuroimage* 19: 308–318. [25]

Awapara, J., Landua, A. J., Fuerst, R., and Seale, B. 1950. Free γ-aminobutyric acid in brain. *J. Biol. Chem.* 187: 35–39. [14]

Axelrod, J. 1971. Noradrenaline: Fate and control of its biosynthesis. *Science* 173: 598–606. [15]

Axelsson, J., and Thesleff, S. 1959. A study of supersensitivity in denervated mammalian skeletal muscle. *J. Physiol.* 147: 178–193. [11, 29]

Ayala, R., et al. 2007. Trekking across the Brain: The journey of neuronal migration. *Cell* 128: 29–43. [27]

Azevedo, F. A., Carvalho, L. R., Grinberg, L. T., et al. 2009.Equal numbers of neuronal and nonneuronal cells make the human brain an isometrically scaled-up primate brain. *J. Comp. Neurol.* 513: 532–541. doi: 10.1002/cne.21974. [1]

Azouz, R., Jensen, M. S., and Yaari, Y. 1996. Ionic basis of spike afterdepolarization and burst generation in adult rat hippocampal CA1 pyramidal cells. *J. Physiol.* 492: 211–223. [7]

Baader, A. P., and Kristan, W. B., Jr. 1995. Parallel pathways coordinate crawling in the medicinal leech, *Hirudo medicinalis*. *J. Comp. Physiol. A* 176: 715–726. [20]

Baas, P. W., and Brown, A. 1997. Slow axonal transport: The polymer transport model. *Trends Cell Biol.* 7: 380–384. [15]

Baca, S. M., Marin-Burgin, A., Wagenaar, D. A., and Kristan, W. B., Jr. 2008. Widespread inhibition proportional to excitation controls the gain of a leech behavioral circuit. *Neuron* 57: 276–289. [20]

Bacci, A., Huguenaard, J. and Prince, D.A. 2004. Long-lasting self-inhibition of neocortical interneurons mediated by endocannabinoids. *Nature* 431: 312–316. [12]

Baccus, S. A. 2007. Timing and computation in inner retinal circuitry. *Annu. Rev. Physiol.* 69: 271–290. [22]

Baccus, S. A., and Meister, M. 2002. Fast and slow contrast adaptation in retinal circuitry. *Neuron* 36: 909–919. [22]

Baccus, S. A., Burrell, B. D., Sahley, C. L., and Muller, K. J. 2000. Action potential reflection and failure at axon branch points cause stepwise changes in EPSPs in a neuron essential for learning. *J. Neurophysiol.* 83: 1693–1700. [8]

Baccus, S. A., Olveczky, B. P., Manu, M., and Meister, M. 2008. A retinal circuit that computes object motion. *J. Neurosci.* 28: 6807–6817. [2, 22]

Bach, F. W., and Yaksh, T. L. 1995. Release into ventriculo-cisternal perfusate of beta-endorphin- and Met-enkephalin-immunoreactivity: effects of electrical stimulation in the arcuate nucleus and periaqueductal gray of the rat. *Brain Res.* 690: 167–176. [18]

Baggiolini, A., et al. 2015. Premigratory and migratory neural crest cells are multipotent in vivo. *Cell Stem Cell* 16: 314–322. [27]

Bailey, C. H., Kandel, E. R., and Si, K. 2004. The persistence of long-term memory: A molecular approach to self-sustaining changes in learning-induced synaptic growth. *Neuron* 44: 49–57. [20]

Baird, R. A., Desmadryl, G., Fernandez, C., and Goldberg, J. M. 1988. The vestibular nerve of the chinchilla. II. Relation between afferent response properties and peripheral innervation patterns in the semicircular canals. *J. Neurophysiol.* 60: 182–203. [24]

Baj, G., et al. 2011. Spatial segregation of BDNF transcripts enables BDNF to differentially shape distinct dendritic compartments. *Proc. Natl. Sci. USA* 108: 16813–16818. [17]

Baker, M. W., Kauffman, B., Macagno, E. R., and Zipser, B. 2003. *In vivo* dynamics of CNS sensory arbor formation: A time-lapse study in the embryonic leech. *J. Neurobiol.* 56: 41–53. [20]

Baker, M. W., Peterson, S. M., and Macagno, E. R. 2008. The receptor phosphatase HmLAR2 collaborates with focal adhesion proteins in filopodial tips to control growth cone morphology. *Dev. Biol.* 320: 215–223. [27]

Baker, P. F., Blaustein, M. P., Keynes, R. D., et al. 1969. The ouabain-sensitive fluxes of sodium and potassium in squid giant axons. *J. Physiol.* 200: 459–496. [9]

Baker, P. F., Hodgkin, A. L., and Ridgeway, E. B. 1971. Depolarization and calcium entry in squid giant axons. *J. Physiol.* 218: 709–755. [6, 9]

Baker, P. F., Hodgkin, A. L., and Shaw, T. I. 1962. Replacement of the axoplasm of giant squid fibres with artificial solutions. *J. Physiol.* 164: 330–354. [6]

Balaban, C. D. 1999. Vestibular autonomic regulation (including motion sickness and the mechanism of vomiting). *Curr. Opin. Neurol.* 12: 29–33. [24]

Balaskas, N., Ribeiro, A., Panovska, J., et al. 2012. Gene regulatory logic for reading the Sonic hedgehog signaling gradient in the vertebrate neural tube *Cell* 148: 273–284. [27]

Balasubramanian, V., and Sterling, P. 2009. Receptive fields and functional architecture in the retina. *J. Physiol.* 587: 2753–2767. [2, 22]

Baldassi, C., Borgs, C., Chayes, J. T., et al. 2016. Unreasonable effectiveness of learning neural networks: From accessible states and robust ensembles to basic algorithmic schemes. *Proc. Natl. Acad. Sci. USA* 113: e7655–e7662. [25]

Balice-Gordon, R. J., and Lichtman, J. W. 1994. Long-term synapse loss induced by focal blockade of postsynaptic receptors. *Nature* 372: 519–524. [27]

Ballanyi, K., Grafe, P., and ten Bruggencate, G. 1987. Ion activities and potassium uptake mechanisms of glial cells in guinea-pig olfactory cortex slices. *J. Physiol.* 382: 159–174. doi: 10.1113/jphysiol.1987. sp016361. [10]

Ballerini, L., Galante, M., Grandolfo, M., and Nistri, A. 1999. Generation of rhythmic patterns of activity by ventral interneurones in rat organotypic spinal slice culture. *J. Physiol.* 517: 459–475.Bampton, E. T., and Taylor, J. S. 2005. Effects of Schwann cell secreted factors on PC12 cell neuritogenesis and survival. *J. Neurobiol.* 63: 29–48. [10]

Balmer, T. S., Carels, V. M., Frisch, J. L. and Nick, T. A. 2009. Modulation of perineuronal nets and parvalbumin with developmental song learning. *J. Neurosci.* 29: 12878–12885. [28]

Baluk. P., and Fujiwara, T. 1984. Macro- and microstructure of the superior cervical ganglion in dogs, cats and horses during maturation. *Neurosci. Lett.* 51: 265–270. [18]

Bandettini, P. A. 2009. What's new in neuroimaging methods? *Ann. N Y Acad. Sci.* 1156: 260–293. [1]

Banerjee, S., Neveu, P., Kosik, K. S., et al. 2009. A coordinated local translational control point at the synapse involving relief from silencing and MOV10 degradation. *Neuron* 64: 871–884. [17]

Banks, G. B., Fuhrer, C., Adams, M. E., and Froehner, S. C. 2003. The postsynaptic submembrane machinery at the neuromuscular junction: Requirement for rapsyn and the utrophin/dystrophin-associated complex. *J. Neurocytol.* 32: 709–726. [11]

Bannatyne, B. A., Liu, T. T., Hammar, I., et al.2009. Excitatory and inhibitory intermediate zone interneurons in pathways from feline group I and II afferents: Differences in axonal projections and input. *J. Physiol.* 587: 379–399. [26]

Banner, L. R., and Patterson, P. H. 1994. Major changes in the expression of the mRNAs for cholinergic differentiation factor/leukemia inhibitory factor and its receptor after injury to adult peripheral nerves and ganglia. *Proc. Natl. Acad. Sci. USA* 91: 7109–7113. [29]

Bao, H., Hakeem, A., Henteleff, M., et al. 1999. Voltage-insensitive gating after charge-neutralizing mutations in the S4 segment of *Shaker* channels. *J. Gen. Physiol.* 113: 139–151. [5]

Bao, L. et al. 2003. Activation of delta opioid receptors induces receptor insertion and neuropeptide secretion. *Neuron* 37: 121–133. [18]

Barchi, R. L. 1997. Ion channel mutations and diseases of skeletal muscle. *Neurobiol. Dis.* 4: 254–264. [6]

Barchi, R. L. 1983. Protein components of the purified sodium channel from rat skeletal muscle sarcolemma. *J. Neurochem.* 40: 1377–1385. [5]

Barco, A., et al. 2002. Expression of constitutively active CREB protein facilitates the late phase of long-term potentiation by enhancing synaptic capture. *Cell* 108: 689–703. [17]

Barde, Y. A. 1989. Trophic factors and neuronal survival. *Neuron* 2: 1525–1534. [27]

Barde, Y. A., Edgar, D., and Thoenen, H. 1982. Purification of a new neurotrophic factor from mammalian brain. *EMBO J.* 1: 549–553. [27]

Bareyre, F. M., Kerschensteiner, M., Raineteau, O., et al. 2004. The injured spinal cord spontaneously forms a new intraspinal circuit in adult rats. *Nat. Neurosci.* 7: 269–277. [29]

Barkat T. R., Polley, D. B. and Hensch T. K. 2011. A critical period for auditory thalamocortical connectivity. *Nat. Neurosci.* 14: 1189–1194. [28]

Barker, P. A. 2007. High affinity not in the vicinity? *Neuron,* 53: 1–4. [27]

Barker, R. A., Drouin-Ouellet, J., and Parmar, M. 2015. Cell-based therapies for Parkinson's disease: Past insights and future potential. *Nat. Rev. Neurol.* 11: 492–503. [29]

Barlow, H. B. 1953. Summation and inhibition in the frog's retina. *J. Physiol.* 119: 69–88. [2]

Barlow, H. B., Blakemore, C., and Pettigrew, J. D. 1967. The neural mechanism of binocular depth discrimination. *J. Physiol.* 193: 327–342. [2, 3]

Barlow, H. B., Hill, R. M., and Levick, W. R. 1964. Retinal ganglion cells responding selectively to direction and speed of image motion in the rabbit. *J. Physiol.* 173: 377–407. [2]

Barnes, N. M., and Sharp, T. 1999. A review of central 5-HT receptors and their function. *Neuropharmacology* 38: 1083–1152. [14]

Barnes, N. M., Hales, T. G., Lummis, S. C., and Peters, J. A. 2009. The 5-HT$_3$ receptor—the relationship between structure and function. *Neuropharmacology* 56: 273–284. [14]

Baroncelli, L., Scali, M., Sansevero, G., et al. 2016. Experience affects critical period plasticity in the visual cortex through an epigenetic regulation of histone post-translational modifications. *J. Neurosci.* 36: 3430–3440. [28]

Barres, B. A. 2008. The mystery and magic of glia: A perspective on their roles in health and disease. *Neuron* 60: 430–440. [10]

Barres, B. A., Chun, L. L., and Corey, D. P. 1988. Ion channel expression by white matter glia: I. Type 2 astrocytes and oligodendrocytes. *Glia* 1: 10–30. [10]

Barrett, E. F., and Barrett, J. N. 1976. Separation of two voltage-sensitive potassium currents, and demonstration of tetrodotoxin-resistant calcium current in frog motoneurones. *J. Physiol.* 255: 737–774. [7]

Barrionuevo, G., and Brown, T. H. 1983. Associative long-term potentiation in hippocampal slices. *Proc. Natl. Acad. Sci. USA* 80: 7347–7351. [16]

Barrionuevo, P. A., and Cao, D. 2014. Contributions of rhodopsin, cone opsins, and melanopsin to postreceptoral pathways inferred from natural image statistics. *J. Opt. Soc. Am. A Opt. Image Sci. Vis.* 31: A131–A139. doi: 10.1364/JOSAA.31.00A131. [22]

Barron, H. C., et al. 2017. Inhibitory engrams in perception and memory. *Proc. Natl. Acad. Sci. USA* 114: 6666–6674. [17]

Barry, M. F., Vickery, R. M., Bolsover, S. R., and Bindman, L. J. 1996. Intracellular studies of heterosynaptic long-term depression (LTD) in CA1 hippocampal slices. *Hippocampus* 6: 3–8. [16]

Bartlett, S. E., Reynolds, A. J., and Hendry, I. A. 1998. Retrograde axonal transport of neurotrophins: Differences between neuronal populations and implications for motor neuron disease. *Immunol. Cell Biol.* 76: 419–423. [15]

Bartel, D. P. 2009. MicroRNAs: target recognition and regulatory functions. *Cell* 136: 215–233. [17]

Bartol, T. M., Land, B. R., Salpeter, E. E., and Salpeter, M. M. 1991. Monte Carlo simulation of miniature endplate current generation in the vertebrate neuromuscular junction. *Biophys. J.* 59: 1290–1307. [15]

Basbaum, A. I., Bautista, D. M., Scherrer, G., and Julius, D. 2009. Cellular and molecular mechanisms of pain. *Cell* 139: 267–284. [21]

Basheer, R., Strecker, R. E., Thakkar, M. M., and McCarley, R. W. 2004. Adenosine and sleep-wake regulation. *Prog. Neurobiol.* 73: 379–396. [14]

Bassell, G. J., and Warren, S. T. 2008. Fragile X syndrome: Loss of local mRNA regulation alters synaptic development and function. *Neuron* 60: 201–214. [17]

Basu, A., Lagier, S., Vologodskaia, M., et al.2016. Direct mechanical stimulation of tip links in hair cells through DNA tethers. *Elife* 5: e16041. doi: 10.7554/eLife.16041. [21]

Bateson, W. 1894. Materials for the Study of Variation: Treated with Special Regard to Discontinuity in the Origin of Species. Macmillan and Co., New York. [27]

Baumgartner, T., Heinrichs, M., Vonlanthen, A., et al. 2008. Oxytocin shapes the neural circuitry of trust and trust adaptation in humans. *Neuron.* 58: 639–650. [14]

Bautista, D. M., Wilson, S. R., and Hoon, M. A. 2014. Why we scratch an itch: The molecules, cells and circuits of itch. *Nature Neurosci.* 178: 175–182. [21]

Bayazitov, I. T., Richardson, R. J., Fricke, R. G., and Zakharenko, S. S. 2007. Slow presynaptic and fast postsynaptic components of compound long-term potentiation. *J Neurosci.* 27: 11510–11521. [16]

Baylis, G. C., Rolls, E. T., and Leonard, C. M. 1987. Functional subdivisions of the temporal lobe neocortex. *J. Neurosci.* 7: 330–342. [25]

Baylor, D. A. 1987. Photoreceptor signals and vision. Proctor lecture. *Invest. Ophthalmol. Vis. Sci.* 28: 34–49. [22]

Baylor, D. 1996. How photons start vision. *Proc. Natl. Acad. Sci. USA* 93: 560–565. [22]

Baylor, D. A., and Burns, M. E. 1998. Control of rhodopsin activity in vision. *Eye (Lond).* 12 (Pt 3b): 521–525. [22]

Baylor, D. A., and Fettiplace, R. 1977. Transmission from photoreceptors to ganglion cells in turtle retina. *J. Physiol.* 271: 391–424. [1]

Baylor, D. A., and Fettiplace, R. 1979. Synaptic drive and impulse generation in ganglion cells of turtle retina. *J. Physiol.* 288: 107–127. [1]

Baylor, D. A., and Fuortes, M. G. F. 1970. Electrical responses of single cones in the retina of the turtle. *J. Physiol.* 207: 77–92. [6, 22]

Baylor, D. A., and Nicholls, J. G. 1969. Chemical and electrical synaptic connexions between cutaneous mechanoreceptor neurones in the central nervous system of the leech. *J. Physiol.* 203: 591–609. [11]

Baylor, D. A., Fuortes, M. G., and O'Bryan, P. M. 1971. Receptive fields of cones in the retina of the turtle. *J. Physiol.* 214: 265–294. [22]

Baylor, D. A., Lamb, T. D., and Yau, K. W. 1979. The membrane current of single rod outer segments. *J. Physiol.* 288: 589–611. [22]

Baylor, D. A., Nunn, B. J., and Schnapf, J. L. 1984. The photocurrent, noise and spectral sensitivity of rods of the monkey *Macaca fascicularis. J. Physiol.* 357: 575–607. [22]

Bazan, N. G. 2006. Eicosanoids, platelet-activating factor and inflammation. In G. J. Siegel, B. W. Agranoff, R. W. Albers, S. K. Fisher, and M. D. Uhler (Eds.), *Basic Neurochemistry: Molecular, Cellular and Medical Aspects*, 7th ed. Lippincott-Raven, Philadelphia, pp. 731–741. [12]

Bazemore, A., Elliott, K. A., and Florey, E. 1956. Factor I and γ-aminobutyric acid. *Nature* 178: 1052–1053. [14]

Beadle, D. J., Lees, G., and Kater, S. B. 1988. *Cell Culture Approaches to Invertebrate Neuroscience.* Academic Press, London. [20]

Bean, B. P. 1989. Neurotransmitter inhibition of neuronal calcium currents by changes in channel voltage dependence. *Nature* 340: 153–157. [12]

Bean, B. P. 2007. The action potential in mammalian central neurons. *Nat. Rev. Neurosci.* 8: 451–465. [7]

Beart, P. M., McDonald, D., and Gundlach, A. L. 1979. Mesolimbic dopaminergic neurones and somatodendritic mechanisms. *Neurosci. Lett.* 15:165–170. [18]

Beattie, R., and Hippenmeyer, S. 2017. Mechanisms of radial glia progenitor cell lineage progression. *FEBS Letters* 591: 3993–4008. [27]

Beckers, J. M., and Stevens, C. F. 1990. Presynaptic mechanism for long-term potentiation in the hippocampus. *Nature* 346: 724–729. [16]

Beg, A. A., and Jorgensen, E. M. 2003. EXP-1 is an excitatory GABA-gated cation channel. *Nat. Neurosci.* 6: 1145–1152. [5]

Behrens, M., Briand, L., de March, C. A., et al. 2018. Structure-function relationships of olfactory and taste receptors. *Chem Senses.* 43: 81–87. [21]

Bei, F., Lee, H., Liu, X., et al. 2016. Restoration of Visual Function by Enhancing Conduction in Regenerated Axons. *Cell* 164: 219–232. [29]

Beirowski, B., Babetto, E., Golden, J. P., et al. 2014. Metabolic regulator LKB1 is crucial for Schwann cell–mediated axon maintenance. *Nat. Neurosci.* 17: 1351–1361. [10]

Belin, S., Nawabi, H., Wang, C., et al. 2015. Injury-induced decline of intrinsic regenerative ability revealed by quantitative proteomics. *Neuron* 86: 1000–1014. [29]

Belenky, M. A., Sollars, P. J., Mount, D. B., et al. 2010. Cell-type specific distribution of chloride transporters in the rat suprachiasmatic nucleus. *Neuroscience* 165: 1519–1537. [19]

Bell, J., Bolanowski, S., and Holmes, M. H. 1994. The structure and function of Pacinian corpuscles: A review. *Prog. Neurobiol.* 42: 79–128. [21]

Bellochio, E. E., Reimer, R. J., Fremeau, R. T., and Edwards, R. H. 2000. Uptake of glutamate into synaptic vesicles by an organic phosphate transporter. *Science* 289: 957–960. [9]

Bellot-Saez, A. Kékesi, O., Morley, J. W., and Buskila. Y. 2017. Astrocytic modulation of neuronal excitability through K+ spatial buffering *Neuroscience and Biobehavioral Reviews* 77: 87–97. [10]

Belmar, J., and Eyzaguirre, C. 1966. Pacemaker site of fibrillation potentials in denervated mammalian muscle. *J. Neurophysiol.* 29: 425–441. [29]

Benagiano, V., Rizzi, A., Lorusso, L., et al. 2018. The functional anatomy of the cerebrocerebellar circuit: A review and new concepts. *J. Comp. Neurol.* 526: 769–789. [26]

Ben-Ari, Y., Gaiarsa, J. L., Tyzio, R., and Khazipov, R. 2007. GABA: A pioneer transmitter that excites immature neurons and generates primitive oscillations. *Physiol. Rev.* 87: 1215–1284. [11]

Ben-Chaim, Y., Chanda, B., Dascal, N., et al. 2006. Movement of 'gating charge' is coupled to ligand binding in a G-protein-coupled receptor. *Nature* 444: 106–109. [13]

Benardo, L. S. 1993. Characterization of cholinergic and noradrenergic slow excitatory postsynaptic potentials from rat cerebral cortical neurons. *Neuroscience* 53: 11–22. [14]

Benedetti, F., Amanzio, M., Vighetti, S., and Asteggiano, G. 2006. The biochemical and neuroendocrine bases of the hyperalgesic nocebo effect. *J. Neurosci.* 26: 12014–12022. [23]

Benians, A., Nobles, M., Hosny, S., and Tinker, A. 2005. Regulators of G-protein signaling form a quaternary complex with the agonist, receptor, and G-protein. A novel explanation for the acceleration of signaling activation kinetics. *J. Biol. Chem.* 280: 13383–13394. [12]

Bennett, M. V. 1997. Gap junctions as electrical synapses. *J. Neuro-cytol.* 26: 349–366. [11]

Bennett, M. V., and Zukin, R. S. 2004. Electrical coupling and neuronal synchronization in the mammalian brain. *Neuron* 41: 495–511. [11]

Bensmaia, S. J., and Hollins, M. 2003. The vibrations of texture. *Somatosens. Mot. Res.* 20: 33–43. [23]

Bentley, D., and Caudy, M. 1983. Navigational substrates for peripheral pioneer growth cones: Limb-axis polarity cues, limb-segment boundaries, and guidepost neurons. *Cold Spring Harb. Symp. Quant. Biol.* 48 Pt 2: 573–585. [27]

Berardi, N., and Maffei, L. 1999. From visual experience to visual function: Roles of neurotrophins. *J. Neurobiol.* 41: 119–126. [28]

Berardi, N., Cellerino, A., Domenici, L., et al. 1994. Monoclonal antibodies to nerve growth factor affect the postnatal development of the visual system. *Proc. Natl. Acad. Sci. USA* 91: 684–688. [28]

Berg, D. K., and Hall, Z. W. 1975. Increased extrajunctional acetylcholine sensitivity produced by chronic postsynaptic neuromuscular blockade. *J. Physiol.* 244: 659–676. [29]

Bergan, J. F., Ro, P., Ro, D., and Knudsen, E. I. 2005. Hunting increases adaptive auditory map plasticity in adult barn owls. *J. Neurosci.* 25: 9816–9820. [28]

Bergmann, O., Spalding, K. L., and Frisén, J. 2015. Adult neurogenesis in humans *Cold Spring Harb Perspect Biol.* 7: A018994. doi: 10.1101/cshperspect.a018994. [27]

Berlucchi, G., and Rizzolatti, G. 1968. Binocularly driven neurons in visual cortex of split-chiasm cats. *Science* 159: 308–310. [3]

Berman, D. M., and Gilman, A. G. 1998. Mammalian RGS proteins: Barbarians at the gate. *J. Biol. Chem.* 273: 1269–1272. [12]

Berne, R. M., and Levy, M. N. (Eds.). 1988. *Physiology*, 2nd ed. Mosby, St. Louis, MO. [24]

Berninger, B., Costa, M. R., Koch, U., et al. 2007. Functional properties of neurons derived from in vitro reprogrammed postnatal astroglia. *J. Neurosci.* 27: 8654–8224. [29]

Bernstein, J. 1902. Untersuchungen zur Thermodynamik der bioelektrischen Strome. *Pflügers Arch.* 92: 521–562. [6]

Bernstein, M., and Lichtman, J. W. 1999. Axonal atrophy: The retraction reaction. *Curr. Opin. Neurobiol.* 9: 364–370. [28]

Berretta, N., and Cherubini, E. 1998. A novel form of long-term depression in the CA1 area of the adult rat hippocampus independent of glutamate receptor activation. *Eur. J. Neurosci.* 10: 2957–2963. [16]

Berridge, C. W., and Waterhouse, B. D. 2003. The locus coeruleus-noradrenergic system: Modulation of behavioral state and state-dependent cognitive processes. *Brain Res. Brain Res. Rev.* 42: 33–84. [14]

Berridge, M. J. 1998. Neuronal calcium signaling. *Neuron* 21: 13–26. [17]

Berridge, M. J., Lipp, P., and Bootman, M. D. 2000. The versatility and universality of calcium signalling. *Nat. Rev. Mol. Cell Biol.* 1: 11–21. [12]

Berry, K. P., and Nedivi, E. 2017. Spine dynamics: Are they all the same? *Neuron* 96: 43–55. [17]

Berry, M. J., 2nd, Brivanlou, I. H., Jordan, T. A., and Meister, M. 1999. Anticipation of moving stimuli by the retina. *Nature* 398: 334–338. [22]

Berson, D. M. 2003. Strange vision: Ganglion cells as circadian photoreceptors. *Trends Neurosci.* 26: 314–320. [22]

Berson, D. M. 2007. Phototransduction in ganglion-cell photoreceptors. *Pflügers Arch.* 454: 849–855. [22]

Berson, D. M., Dunn, F. A., and Takao, M. 2002. Phototransduction by retinal ganglion cells that set the circadian clock. *Science* 295: 1070–1073. [19, 22]

Bertacchi, M. 2013. The positional identity of mouse ES cell-generated neurons is affected by BMP signaling. *Cell Mol. Life Sci.* 70: 1095–1111. [27]

Bertrand, N., Castro, D. S., and Guillemot, F. 2002. Proneural genes and the specification of neural cell types. *Nat. Rev. Neurosci.* 3: 517–530. [27]

Bestmann, S., Ruff, C. C., Blankenburg, F., et al. 2008. Mapping causal interregional influences with concurrent TMS-fMRI. *Exp. Brain. Res.* 191: 383–402. [1]

Bettler, B., Kaupmann, K., Mosbacher, J., and Gassmann, M. 2004. Molecular structure and physiological functions of GABA$_B$ receptors. *Physiol. Rev.* 84: 835–867. [14]

Betz, H., and Laube, B. 2006. Glycine receptors: Recent insights into their structural organization and functional diversity. *J. Neurochem.* 97: 1600–1610. [14]

Betz, W. J. 1970. Depression of transmitter release at the neuromuscular junction of the frog. *J. Physiol.* 206: 629–644. [16]

Betz, W. J., and Sakmann, B. 1973. Effects of proteolytic enzymes on function and structure of frog neuromuscular junctions. *J. Physiol.* 230: 673–688. [11]

Betz, W. J., Caldwell, J. H., and Ribchester, R. R. 1980. The effects of partial denervation at birth on the development of muscle fibres and motor units in rat lumbrical muscle. *J. Physiol.* 303: 265–279. [27]

Beurg, M., Fettiplace, R., Nam, J. H., and Ricci, A. J. 2009. Localization of inner hair cell mechanotransducer channels using high-speed calcium imaging. *Nat. Neurosci.* 12: 553–558. [21]

Bevan, S., and Yeats, J. 1991. Protons activate a cation conductance in a sub-population of rat dorsal root ganglion neurones. *J. Physiol.* 433: 145–161. [21]

Bewick, G. S. 2015. Synaptic-like vesicles and candidate transduction channels in mechanosensory terminals. *J. Anat.* 227: 194–213. [21]

Bezanilla, F. 2005. Voltage-gated ion channels. *IEEE Trans. Nanobiosci.* 4: 34–48. [7]

Bezanilla, F. 2008. How membrane proteins sense voltage. *Nat. Rev. Mol. Cell Biol.* 9: 323–332. [5, 7]

Bhadra, U., Thakkar, M., Das, P., and Bhadra, M.P. 2017. Evolution of circadian rhythms: From bacteria to human *Sleep Medicine,* 35: 49–61. [19]

Bhardwaj, R. D., Curtis, M. A., Spalding, K. L., et al. 2006. Neocortical neurogenesis in humans is restricted to development. *Proc. Natl. Acad. Sci. USA* 103: 12564–12568. [27]

Bhattacharya, S., Khatri, A., Swanger, S. A., et al. 2018. Triheteromeric GluN1/GluN2A/GluN2C NMDARs with unique single-channel properties are the dominant receptor population in cerebellar granule cells. *Neuron.* 99: 315–328. [11]

Bhattarai, J. P., Park, S. A., Park, J. B., et al. 2011. Tonic extrasynaptic GABA(A) receptor currents control gonadotropin-releasing hormone neuron excitability in the mouse. *Endocrinology* 152: 1551–1561. [19]

Bi, G. Q. et al. 1997. Kinesin- and myosin-driven steps of vesicle recruitment for Ca^{2+}-regulated exocytosis. *J. Cell Biol.* 138: 999–1008. [18]

Bi, G. Q. and Poo, M. M. 1998. Synaptic modifications in cultured hippocampal neurons: Dependence on spike timing, synaptic strength, and postsynaptic cell type. *J. Neurosci.* 18: 10464–10472. [17]

Bialek, W. 1987. Physical limits to sensation and perception. *Annu. Rev. Biophys. Biophys. Chem.* 16: 455–478. [21]

Bianchi, M. T., Botzolakis, E. J., Lagrange, A. H., and Macdonald, R. L. 2009. Benzodiazepine modulation of GABA$_A$ receptor opening frequency depends on activation context: A patch clamp and simulation study. *Epilepsy Res.* 85: 212–220. [14]

Bichet, D., Haase F. A., and Jan, L. Y. 2003. Merging functional studies with structures of inward-rectifier K(+) channels. *Nat. Rev. Neurosci.* 4: 957–967. [12]

Biel, M., Wahl-Schott, C., Michalakas, S., and Zong, X. 2009. Hyperpolarization-activated cation channels: From genes to function. *Physiol. Rev.* 89: 847–885. [6]

Biesecker, K. R. et al. 2016. Glial Cell Calcium Signaling Mediates Capillary Regulation of Blood Flow in the Retina. *J. Neurosci.* 36: 9435–9445. [18]

Biever, A., et al. 2020. Monosomes actively translate synaptic mRNAs in neuronal processes. Science 367: eaay4991. [17]

Bignami, A., and Dahl, D. 1974. Astrocyte-specific protein and neuroglial differentiation: An immunofluorescence study with antibodies to the glial fibrillary acidic protein. *J. Comp. Neurol.* 153: 27–38. [10]

Billups, B., and Attwell, D. 1996. Modulation of non-vesicular glutamate release by pH. *Nature* 379: 171–174. [10]

Bilz, F., et al. 2020. Visualization of a distributed synaptic memory code in the drosophila brain. *Neuron* 106: 1–14. [17]

Bingol, B., and Schuman, F. M. 2005. The immediate early gene *Arc/Arg3.1*: Regulation, mechanisms, and function. *Curr. Opin. Neurobiol.* 15: 536–541. [17]

Bingol, B., and Schuman, F. M. 2006. Activity-dependent dynamics and sequestration of proteasomes in dendritic spines. *Nature* 441: 1144–1148. [17]

Binotti, B., Jahn, R., and Chua, J. 2016. Functions of Rab proteins at presynaptic sites. *Cells.* doi: 10.3390/cells5010007. [13]

Bird, M. K., and Lawrence, A. J. 2009. The promiscuous mGlu5 receptor—a range of partners for therapeutic possibilities? *Trends Pharmacol. Sci.* 30: 617–623. [14]

Birder, L. A., and Perl, E. R. 1994. Cutaneous sensory receptors. *J. Clin. Neurophysiol.* 11: 534–552. [23]

Birkmayer, W., and Hornykiewicz, O. 1962. Der L-Dioxyphenylalanin (=L-DOPA)-Effekt beim Parkinson-Syndrom des Menschen: Zur Pathogenese und Behandlung def Parkinson-Akinese. *Arch. Psychiatr. Nervenkr.* 203: 560–574. [14]

Birks, R. I., and MacIntosh, F. C. 1961. Acetylcholine metabolism of a sympathetic ganglion. *Can. J. Biochem. Physiol.* 39: 787–827. [15]

Birks, R., Huxley, H. E., and Katz, B. 1960. The fine structure of the neuromuscular junction of the frog. *J. Physiol.* 150: 134–144. [13]

Birks, R., Katz, B., and Miledi, R. 1960. Physiological and structural changes at the amphibian myoneural junction in the course of nerve degeneration. *J. Physiol.* 150: 145–168. [13]

Bishop, K. M., Goudreau, G., and O'Leary, D. D. 2000. Regulation of area identity in mammalian neocortex by Emx2 and Pax 6 *Science* 288: 344–349. [27]

Bixby, J. L., and Van Essen, D. C. 1979. Competition between foreign and original nerves in adult mammalian skeletal muscle. *Nature* 282: 726–728. [29]

Björklund, A. 1991. Neural transplantation—An experimental tool with clinical possibilities. *Trends Neurosci.* 14: 319–322. [29]

Björklund, A. 2000. Cell replacement strategies for neurodegenerative disorders. *Novartis Found. Symp.* 231: 7–15. [29]

Björklund, A., and Lindvall, O. 1975. Intrastriatal implants of mesencephalic cell suspensions in weaver mutant mice: ultrastructural relationships of dopaminergic dendrites and axons issued from the graft. *Brain Res.* 83: 531–537. [18]

Björklund, A. and Lindvall, O. 2017. Replacing dopamine neurons in Parkinson's disease: How did it happen? *J. Parkinsons Dis.* 7: S21–S31. [29]

Black, J. A., and Waxman, S. G. 1988. The perinodal astrocyte. *Glia* 1: 169–183. [10]

Black, J. W., and Prichard, B. N. 1973. Activation and blockade of β adrenoceptors in common cardiac disorders. *Br. Med. Bull.* 29: 163–167. [19]

Blackman, J. G., and Purves, R. D. 1969. Intracellular recordings from the ganglia of the thoracic sympathetic chain of the guinea-pig. *J. Physiol.* 203: 173–198. [13]

Blackmer, T., Larsen, E. C., Bartleson, C., et al. 2005. G protein βδ directly regulates SNARE protein fusion machinery for secretory granule exocytosis. *Nat. Neurosci.* 8: 421–425. [14]

Blackshaw, S. E. 1981. Morphology and distribution of touch cell terminals in the skin of the leech. *J. Physiol.* 320: 219–228. [20]

Blackshaw, S. E., and Nicholls, J. G. 1995. Neurobiology and development of the leech. *J. Neurobiol.* 27: 267–276. [20]

Blackshaw, S. E., and Thompson, S. W. 1988. Hyperpolarizing responses to stretch in sensory neurones innervating leech body wall muscle. *J. Physiol.* 396: 121–137. [20, 21]

Blackshaw, S. E., Nicholls, J. G., and Parnas, I. 1982. Expanded receptive fields of cutaneous mechanoreceptor cells after single neurone deletion in leech central nervous system. *J. Physiol.* 326: 261–268. [20, 29]

Blake, D. J., Weir, A., Newey, S. E., and Davies, K. E. 2002. Function and genetics of dystrophin and dystrophin-related proteins in muscle. *Physiol. Rev.* 82: 291–329. [11]

Blake, D. T., Byl, N. N., and Merzenich, M. M. 2002. Representation of the hand in the cerebral cortex. *Behav. Brain Res.* 135: 179–184. [26]

Blakemore, C. 1977. *Mechanics of the Mind.* Cambridge University Press, Cambridge. [23]

Blakemore, C., and Van Sluyters, R. C. 1974. Reversal of the physiological effects of monocular deprivation in kittens: Further evidence for a sensitive period. *J. Physiol.* 237: 195–216. [28]

Blakemore, S. J. 2010. The developing social brain: Implications for education. *Neuron* 65: 744–747. [28]

Blanchet, C., Erostegui, C., Sugasawa, M., and Dulon, D. 1996. Acetylcholine-induced potassium current of guinea pig outer hair cells: Its dependence on a calcium influx through nicotinic-like receptors. *J. Neurosci.* 16: 2574–2584. [24]

Blankenburg, F., Ruben, J., Meyer, R., et al. 2003. Evidence for a rostral-to-caudal somatotopic organization in human primary somatosensory cortex with mirror-reversal in areas 3b and 1. *Cereb. Cortex* 13: 987–993. [23]

Blau, J., Blanchard, F., Collins, B., et al. 2007. What is there left to learn about the *Drosophila* clock? *Cold Spring Harb. Symp. Quant. Biol.* 72: 243–250. [19]

Blauert, J. 1982. Binaural localization. *Scand. Audiol. Suppl.* 15: 7–26. [24]

Blaustein, M. P., and Lederer, W. J. 1999. Sodium/calcium exchange: Its physiological implications. *Physiol. Rev.* 79: 763–854. [9]

Blaustein, M. P., Juhaszova, M., Golovina, V. A., et al. 2002. Na/Ca exchanger and PMCA localization in neurons and astrocytes: Functional implications. *Ann. N Y Acad. Sci.* 976: 356–366. [10]

Blazquez, P. M., Hirata, Y., and Highstein, S. M. 2004. The vestibulo-ocular reflex as a model system for motor learning: What is the role of the cerebellum? *Cerebellum* 3: 188–192. [24]

Bliss, T. V. P., and Lømo, T. 1973. Long-lasting potentiation of synaptic transmission in the dentate of the anesthetized rabbit following stimulation of the perforant path. *J. Physiol.* 232: 331–356. [16]

Bloomfield, S. A., and Völgyi, B. 2009. The diverse functional roles and regulation of neuronal gap junctions in the retina. *Nat. Rev. Neurosci.* 10: 495–506. [11, 18, 22]

Boadle-Biber, M. C. 1993. Regulation of serotonin synthesis. *Prog. Biophys. Mol. Biol.* 60: 1–15. [15]

Bockaert, J., Perroy, J., Bécamel, C., et al. 2010. GPCR interacting proteins (GIPs) in the nervous system: Roles in physiology and pathologies. *Annu. Rev. Pharmacol. Toxicol.* 50: 89–109. [12]

Bocquet, N., Nury, H., Baaden, M., et al. 2009. X-ray structure of a pentameric ligand-gated ion channel in the apparently open conformation. *Nature* 457: 111–114. [5]

Bodian D. 1965. A suggestive relationship of nerve cell RNA with specific synaptic sites. *Proc. Natl. Acad. Sci. USA* 53: 418–425. [17]

Bode, S., He, A. H., Soon, C. S., et al. 2011. Tracking the unconscious generation of free decisions using ultra-high field fMRI. *PLOS ONE* 6: e21612. doi: 10.1321/journal.pone.0021621. [26, 30]

Boekhoff, I., Tareilus, E., Strotmann, J., and Breer, H. 1990. Rapid activation of alternative second messenger pathways in olfactory cilia from rats by different odorants. *EMBO J.* 9: 2453–2458. [21]

Bohlhalter, S., Fretz, C., and Weder, B. 2002. Hierarchical versus parallel processing in tactile object recognition: A behavioural-neuroanatomical study of aperceptive tactile agnosia. *Brain* 125: 2537–2548. [23]

Boistel, J., and Fatt, P. 1958. Membrane permeability change during inhibitory transmitter action in crustacean muscle. *J. Physiol.* 144: 176–191. [14]

Bolanowski, S. J., Jr., Gescheider, G. A., Verrillo, R. T., and Checkosky, C. M. 1988. Four channels mediate the mechanical aspects of touch. *J. Acoust. Soc. Am.* 84: 1680–1694. [23]

Boldrini, M., Fulmore, C. A., Tartt, A. N., et al., 2018. Human hippocampal neurogenesis persists throughout aging. *Cell Stem Cell* 22: 589. [27]

Bollman, J. H., and Sakmann, B. 2005. Control of synaptic strength and timing by the release-site Ca^{2+} signal. *Nat. Neurosci.* 8: 426–434. [13]

Bonanomi, D., and Pfaff, S. L. 2010. Motor axon pathfinding. *Cold Spring Harb. Perspect. Biol.* 2: A001735. [27]

Boncinelli, E., Mallamaci, A., and Broccoli, V. 1998. Body plan genes and human malformation. *Adv. Genet.* 38: 1–29. [27]

Bond, A. M., Ming, G. L., and Song, H. 2015. Adult mammalian neural stem cells and neurogenesis: Five decades later. *Cell Stem Cell* 17: 385. [27]

Bonhoeffer, T., and Grinvald, A. 1991. Iso-orientation domains in cat visual cortex are arranged in pin-wheel-like patterns. *Nature* 353: 429–431. [3]

Bonnavion, P., and de Lecea, L. 2010. Hypocretins in the control of sleep and wakefulness. *Curr. Neurol. Neurosci. Rep.* 10: 174–179. [14]

Booth M. C., and Rolls, E. T. 1998. View-invariant representations of familiar objects by neurons in the inferior temporal visual cortex. *Cereb. Cortex* 8: 510–523. [25]

Borgdorff , A. J., and Choquet, D. Regulation of AMPA receptor lateral movements. 2002. *Nature* 417: 649–653. [16]

Borghuis, B. G., Ratliff, C. P., Smith, R. G., et al. 2008. Design of a neuronal array. *J. Neurosci.* 28: 3178–3189. [2]

Boring, E. G. 1942. *Sensation and Perception in the History of Experimental Psychology.* Appleton-Century, New York. [21]

Borodinsky, L. N. and Spitzer 2007. Activity-dependent neurotransmitter-receptor matching at the neuromuscular junction. *Proc. Natl. Acad. Sci USA* 104: 335–340. [27]

Borodinsky, L. N., Root, C. M., Cronin, J. A., et al. 2004. Activity-dependent homeostatic specification of transmitter expression in embryonic neurons. *Nature* 429: 523–530. [27]

Borroto-Escuela, D. O. et al. 2015. The role of transmitter diffusion and flow versus extracellular vesicles in volume transmission in the brain neural–glial networks. *Phil. Trans. R. Soc. B* 370: 20140183. [18]

Borst, J. G. G., and Sakmann, B. 1996. Calcium influx and transmitter release in a fast CNS synapse. *Nature* 383: 431–434. [13]

Borst, J. G. G., and Sakmann, B. 1998. Facilitation of presynaptic calcium currents in the rat brainstem. *J. Physiol.* 513: 149–155. [16]

Borst, J. G. G., Helmchen, F., and Sakmann, B. 1995. Pre- and postsynaptic whole-cell recording in the medial nucleus of the trapezoid body of the rat. *J. Physiol.* 489: 825–840. [13]

Bortolanza, M., Bariotto-Dos-Santos, K. D., Dos-Santos-Pereira, M., et al. 2016. Antidyskinetic effect of 7-nitroindazole and sodium nitroprusside associated with amantadine in a rat model of Parkinson's Disease. *Neurotox Res.* 30: 88–100. [26]

Boschat, C., Pelofi, C., Randin, O., et al. 2002. Pheromone detection mediated by a V1r vomeronasal receptor. *Nat. Neurosci.* 5: 1261–1262. [21]

Bostan, A. C., and Strick, P. L. 2018. The basal ganglia and the cerebellum: Nodes in an integrated nework. *Nature Rev. Neurosci.* doi: 10.1038/s41583-018-0002-7. [26]

Bostock, H., and Sears, T. A., and Sherratt, R. M. 1981. The effects of 4-aminopyradine and tetraethylammonium on normal and demyelinated nerve fibers. *J. Physiol.* 313: 301–315. [8]

Bouslama-Oueghlani, L., Wehrlé, R., Sotelo, C., and Dusart, I. 2003. The developmental loss of the ability of Purkinje cells to regenerate their axons occurs in the absence of myelin: An in vitro model to prevent myelination. *J. Neurosci.* 23: 8318–8329. [29]

Bowe, M. A., and Fallon, J. R. 1995. The role of agrin in synapse formation. *Annu. Rev. Neurosci.* 18: 443–462. [29]

Bowerman, R. F., and Larimer, J. L. 1976. Command neurons in crustaceans. *Comp. Biochem. Physiol. A Comp. Physiol.* 54: 1–5. [20]

Bowery, N. G., Hill, D. R., Hudson, A. L., et al. 1980. Baclofen decreases neurotransmitter release in the mammalian CNS by an action at a novel GABA receptor. *Nature* 283: 92–94. [14]

Bowling, D. B., and Michael, C. R. 1980. Projection patterns of single physiologically characterized optic tract fibers in the cat. *Nature* 286: 899–902. [3]

Bowling, D., Nicholls, J., and Parnas, I. 1978. Destruction of a single cell in the central nervous system of the leech as a means of analysing its connexions and functional role. *J. Physiol.* 282: 169–80. [20]

Bowser, D. N., and Khakh, B. S. 2004. ATP excites interneurons and astrocytes to increase synaptic inhibition in neuronal networks. *J. Neurosci.* 24: 8606–8620. [14]

Boycott, B. B., and Dowling, J. E. 1969. Organization of primate retina: Light microscopy. *Philos. Trans. R. Soc. Lond., B, Biol. Sci.* 255: 109–184. [22]

Boyd, C. A. R. 2010. Cerebellar agenesis revisited. *Brain* 133: 941–944. [26]

Boyd, I. A., and Martin, A. R. 1956. The end-plate potential in mammalian muscle. *J. Physiol.* 132: 74–91. [11, 13]

Boyden, E. S., Zhang, F., Bamberg, E., et al. 2005. Millisecond-timescale, genetically targeted optical control of neural activity *Nat. Neurosci.* 8: 1263–1268. [1]

Bozza, T., Feinstein, P., Zheng, C., and Mombaerts, P. 2002. Odorant receptor expression defines functional units in the mouse olfactory system. *J. Neurosci.* 22: 3033–3043. [21]

Bradbury, E. J., Moon, L. D., Popat, R. J., et al. 2002. Chondroitinase ABC promotes functional recovery after spinal cord injury. *Nature* 416: 636–640. [29]

Bradley, J., Resisert, J., and Frings, S. 2005. Regulation of cyclic nucleotide-gated channels. *Curr. Opin. Neurobiol.* 15: 343–349. [5]

Bradshaw, K. D., et al. 2003. A role for dendritic protein synthesis in hippocampal late LTP. *Eur. J. Neurosci.* 18: 3150–3152. [17]

Brady, S. T., Lasek, R. J., and Allen, R. D. 1982. Fast axonal transport in extruded axoplasm from squid giant axon. *Science* 218: 1129–1131. [15]

Brainard, M. S., and Knudsen, E. I. 1998. Sensitive periods for visual calibration of the auditory space map in the barn owl optic tectum. *J. Neurosci.* 18: 3929–3942. [28]

Bramham, C., and Messaoudi, E. 2005. BDNF function in adult synaptic plasticity: the synaptic consolidation hypothesis. *Prog. Neurobiol.* 76: 99–125. [17]

Brancaccio, M., Patton, A. P., Chesham, J. E., et al. 2017. Astrocytes Control Circadian Timekeeping in the Suprachiasmatic Nucleus via Glutamatergic Signaling. *Neuron* 93:1420–1435. doi: 10.1016/j.neuron.2017.02.030. [10]

Brannstrom, T. 1993. Quantitative synaptology of functionally different types of cat medial gastrocnemius α-motoneurons. *J. Comp. Neurol.* 330: 439–454. [26]

Brasch, F. E. 1922. History of Science. *Science* 55: 405–408. [30]

Bray, G. M., Villegas-Perez, M. P., Vidal-Sanz, M., et al. 1991. Neuronal and nonneuronal influences on retinal ganglion cell survival, axonal regrowth, and connectivity after axotomy. *Ann. N Y Acad. Sci.* 633: 214–228. [29]

Brecht, M., Preilowski, B., and Merzenich, M. M. 1997. Functional architecture of the mystacial vibrissae. *Behav. Brain Res.* 84: 81–97. [23]

Bredt, D. S., and Snyder, S. H. 1989. Nitric oxide mediates glutamate-linked enhancement of cGMP levels in the cerebellum. *Proc. Natl. Acad. Sci. USA* 86: 9030–9033. [12]

Breer, H., Boekhoff, I., and Tareilus, E. 1990. Rapid kinetics of second messenger formation in olfactory transduction. *Nature* 345: 65–68. [21]

Brefczynski, J. A., and DeYoe, E. A. 1999. A physiological correlate of the 'spotlight' of visual attention. *Nat. Neurosci.* 2: 370–374. [25]

Bregman, B. S., and Reier, P. J. 1986. Neural tissue transplants rescue axotomized rubrospinal cells from retrograde death. *J. Comp. Neurol.* 244: 86–95. [29]

Bregy, P., Sommer, S., and Wehner, R. 2008. Nest-mark orientation versus vector navigation in desert ants. *J. Exp. Biol.* 211: 1868–1873. [20]

Breitwieser, G. E., and Szabo, G. 1985. Uncoupling of cardiac muscarinic and β-adrenergic receptors from ion channels by a guanine nucleotide analogue. *Nature* 317: 538–540. [12]

Brejc, K., Van Dijk, W. J., Klaassen, R. V., et al. 2001. Crystal structure of an ACh-binding protein reveals the ligand-binding domain of nicotinic receptors. *Nature* 411: 269–276. [5]

Brennan, P. A., and Kendrick, K. M. 2006. *Philos. Trans. R. Soc. Lond., B, Biol. Sci.* 361: 2061–2078. [21]

Brenner, S. 1974. The genetics of *Caenorhabditis elegans*. *Genetics* 77: 71–94. [27]

Brenner, H. R., and Martin, A. R. 1976. Reduction in acetylcholine sensitivity of axotomized ciliary ganglion cells. *J. Physiol.* 260: 159–175. [29]

Brew, H., Gray, P. T., Mobbs, P., and Attwell, D. 1986. Endfeet of retinal glial cells have higher densities of ion channels that mediate K^+ buffering. *Nature* 324: 466–468. [10]

Bribián, A., Figueres-Oñate, M., Martín-López, E., and López-Mascaraque, L. 2016. Decoding astrocyte heterogeneity: New tools for clonal analysis. *Neuroscience* 323: 10–19. doi: 10.1016/j.neuroscience.2015.04.036. [1]

Brichta, A. M., Aubert, A., Eatock, R. A., and Goldberg, J. M. 2002. Regional analysis of whole cell currents from hair cells of the turtle posterior crista. *J. Neurophysiol.* 88: 3259–3278. [24]

Briggman, K. L., and Kristan, W. B. 2008. Multifunctional pattern-generating circuits. *Annu. Rev. Neurosci.* 31: 271–294. [26]

Briggman, K. L., Abarbanel, H. D., and Kristan, W. B., Jr. 2005. Optical imaging of neuronal populations during decision-making. *Science* 307: 896–901. [20]

Briggman, K. L., Kristan, W. B., González, J. E., et al. 2015. Monitoring integrated activity of individual neurons using fret-based voltage-sensitive dyes. *Adv. Exp. Med. Biol.* 859: 149–169. doi: 10.1007/978-3-319-17641-3_6. [20]

Brightman, M. W., and Reese, T. S. 1969. Junctions between intimately apposed cell membranes in the vertebrate brain. *J. Cell Biol.* 40: 668–677. [10]

Brightman, M. W., Reese, T. S., and Feder, N. 1970. Assessment with the electron microscope of the permeability to peroxidase of cerebral endothelium in mice and sharks. In E. H. Thaysen (Ed.), *Capillary Permeability* (Alfred Benzon Symposium II). Munskgaard, Copenhagen, Denmark. [10]

Brigidi, G. S., et al. 2019. Genomic decoding of neuronal depolarization by stimulus-specific NPAS4 heterodimers. *Cell* 179: 373–391. [17]

Brincat, S. L., and Connor, C. E. 2004. Underlying principles of visual shape selectivity in posterior inferotemporal cortex. *Nat. Neurosci.* 7: 880–886. [25]

Briscoe, J. 2000. A homeodomain protein code specifies progenitor cell identity and neuronal fate in the ventral neural tube. *Cell* 101: 435–445. [27]

Briscoe, J. 2009. Making a grade: Sonic Hedgehog signalling and the control of neural cell fate. *EMBO J.* 28: 457–465. [27]

Briscoe, J., and Small, S. 2015. Morphogen rules: Design principles of gradient-mediated embryo patterns. *Development* 142: 3996–4009 doi: 10.1242/dev.129452. [27]

Brittis, P. A., Lu, Q., and Flanagan, J. G. 2002. Axonal protein synthesis provides a mechanism for localized regulation at an intermediate target. Cell 110: 223–235. [27]

Brivanlou, I. H., Warland, D. K., and Meister, M. 1998. Mechanisms of concerted firing among retinal ganglion cells. *Neuron* 20: 527–539. [22, 28]

Brock, L. G., Coombs, J. S., and Eccles, J. C. 1952. The recording of potentials from motoneurones with an intracellular electrode. *J. Physiol.* 117: 431–460. [11]

Brodfuehrer, P. D., Debski, E. A., O'Gara, B. A., and Friesen, W. O. 1995. Neuronal control of leech swimming. *J. Neurobiol.* 27: 403–418. [20]

Bronner, M. 2015. Confetti clarifies controversy: Neural crest stem cells are multipotent. *Cell Stem Cell* 16: 217–218. [27]

Bronner-Fraser, M. 1985. Alterations in neural crest migration by a monoclonal antibody that affects cell adhesion. *J. Cell Biol.* 101: 610–617. [27]

Brooks, V. B. 1956. An intracellular study of the action of repetitive nerve volleys and of botulinum toxin on miniature end-plate potentials. *J. Physiol.* 134: 264–277. [13]

Brose, K., Bland, K. S., Wang, K. H., et al. 1999. Slit proteins bind Robo receptors and have an evolutionarily conserved role in repulsive axon guidance. *Cell* 96: 795–806. [27]

Brown, A. G., and Fyffe, R. E. W. 1981. Direct observations on the contacts made between Ia afferent fibers and α-motoneurones in the cat's lumbosacral spinal cord. *J. Physiol.* 313: 121–140. [26]

Brown, A. M., and Ransom, B. R. 2007. Astrocyte glycogen and brain energy metabolism. *Glia* 55: 1263–1271. [10]

Brown, D. A. 2000. Neurobiology: The acid test for resting potassium channels. *Curr. Biol.* 10: R456–459. [6]

Brown, D. A. 2010. Muscarinic acetylcholine receptors (mAChRs) in the nervous system: Some functions and mechanisms. *J. Mol. Neurosci.* 41: 340–346. [14]

Brown, D. A., and Adams, P. R. 1980. Muscarinic suppression of a novel voltage-sensitive K^+-current in a vertebrate neurone. *Nature* 283: 673–676. [12, 19]

Brown, D. A., and Passmore, G. M. 2009. Neural KCNQ (Kv7) channels. *Brit. J. Pharmacol.* 156: 1185–1195. [12, 19]

Brown, D. A., and Selyanko, A. A. 1985. Membrane currents underlying the cholinergic slow excitatory post-synaptic potential in the rat sympathetic ganglion. *J. Physiol.* 365: 365–387. [11, 15, 19]

Brown, D. A., Constanti, A., and Adams, P. R. 1983. Ca-activated potassium current in vertebrate sympathetic neurons. *Cell Calcium* 4: 407–420. [12]

Brown, D. A., Docherty, R. J., and Halliwell, J., V. 1983. Chemical transmission in the rat interpeduncular nucleus in vitro. *J. Physiol.* 341: 655–670. [14]

Brown, D. A., Hughes, S. A., Marsh, S. J., and Tinker, A. 2007. Regulation of M(Kv7.2/7.3) channels in neurons by PIP_2 and products of PIP_2 hydrolysis: Significance for receptor-mediated inhibition. *J. Physiol.* 582: 917–925. [19]

Brown, G. L. 1937. The actions of acetylcholine on denervated mammalian and frog's muscle. *J. Physiol.* 89: 438–461. [29]

Brown, H. F., DiFrancesco, D., and Noble, D. 1979. How does adrenaline accelerate the heart? *Nature* 280: 235–236. [12]

Brown, H. M., Ottoson, D., and Rydqvist, B. 1978. Crayfish stretch receptor: An investigation with voltage-clamp and ion-sensitive electrodes. *J. Physiol.* 284: 155–179. [21]

Brown, M. C. 1987. Morphology of labeled afferent fibers in the guinea pig cochlea. *J. Comp. Neurol.* 260: 591–604. [24]

Brown, M. C., Holland, R. L., and Hopkins, W. G. 1981. Motor nerve sprouting. *Annu. Rev. Neurosci.* 4: 17–42. [29]

Brown, M. C., Hopkins, W. G., and Keynes, R. J. 1982. Short- and long-term effects of paralysis on the motor innervation of two different neonatal mouse muscles. *J. Physiol.* 329: 439–450. [27]

Brown, M. C., Jansen, J. K., and Van Essen, D. 1976. Polyneuronal innervation of skeletal muscle in new-born rats and its elimination during maturation. *J. Physiol.* 261: 387–422. [27]

Brown, N., Kerby, J., Bonnert, T. P., et al. 2002. Pharmacological characterization of a novel cell line expressing human α4β3δ $GABA_A$ receptors. *Brit. J. Pharmacol.* 136: 965–974. [14]

Brown, P. K., and Wald, G. 1963. Visual pigments in human and monkey retinas. *Nature* 200: 37–43. [22]

Brown, S. P., Brenowitz, S. D., and Regehr, W. D. 2003. Brief presynaptic bursts evoke synapse-specific retrograde inhibition mediated by endogenous cannabinoids. *Nat. Neurosci.* 6: 1047–1058. [12]

Brown, T. G. 1911. The intrinsic factor in the act of progression in the mammal. *Proc. R. Soc. Lond., B, Biol. Sci.* 84: 308–319. [26]

Brownell, W. E., Bader, C. R., Bertrand, D., and de Ribaupierre, Y. 1985. Evoked mechanical responses of isolated cochlear outer hair cells. *Science* 227: 194–196. [24]

Bruening-Wright, A., Schumacher, M. A., Adelman, J. P., and Maylie, J. 2002. Localization of the activation gate for small conductance Ca^{2+}-activated K^+ channels. *J. Neurosci.* 22: 6499–6506. [5]

Brunet, L. J., Gold, G. H., and Ngai, J. 1996. General anosmia caused by a targeted disruption of the mouse olfactory cyclic nucleotide-gated cation channel. *Neuron* 17: 681–693. [21]

Brungart, D. S., Durlach, N. I., and Rabinowitz, W. M. 1999. Auditory localization of nearby sources. II. Localization of a broadband source. *J. Acoust. Soc. Am.* 106: 1956–1968. [24]

Bruni, J. E. 1998. Ependymal development, proliferation, and functions: A review. *Microsc. Res. Tech.* 41: 2–13. [18]

Bruns, D., and Jahn, R. 1995. Real-time measurement of transmitter release from single synaptic vesicles. *Nature* 377: 62–65. [18]

Bruns, D. et al. 2000. Quantal release of serotonin. *Neuron* 28: 205–220. [18]

Brusa, R., Zimmermann, F., Koh, D. S., et al. 1995. Early-onset epilepsy and postnatal lethality associated with an editing-deficient GluR-B allele in mice. *Science* 270: 1677–1680. [27]

Buckley, C. E., Marguerie, A., Alderton, W. K., and Franklin, R. J. 2010. Temporal dynamics of myelination in the zebrafish spinal cord. *Glia* 58: 802–812. [10]

Budnik, V., Ruiz-Cañada, C., and Wendler, F. 2016. Extracellular vesicles round off communication in the nervous system. *Nat. Rev. Neurosci.* 17: 160–172. [18]

Buell, T. N., and Hafter, E. R. 1988. Discrimination of interaural differences of time in the envelopes of high-frequency signals: Integration times. *J. Acoust. Soc. Am.* 84: 2063–2066. [24]

Buell, T. N., Trahiotis, C., and Bernstein, L. R. 1991. Lateralization of low-frequency tones: Relative potency of gating and ongoing interaural delays. *J. Acoust. Soc. Am.* 90: 3077–3085. [24]

Buller, A. J., Eccles, J. C., and Eccles, R. M. 1960. Interactions between motoneurones and muscles in respect of the characteristic speeds of their responses. *J. Physiol.* 150: 417–439. [29]

Bullock, T. H., and Hagiwara, S. 1957. Intracellular recording from the giant synapse of the squid. *J. Gen. Physiol.* 40: 565–577. [13]

Bult, H., Boeckxstaens, G. E., Pelckmans, P. A., et al. 1990. Nitric oxide as an inhibitory non-adrenergic non-cholinergic neurotransmitter. *Nature* 345: 346–347. [12]

Buma, P., and Nieuwenhuys, R. 1987. Ultrastructural demonstration of oxytoxin and vasopressin release sites in the neural lobe and median eminence of the rat by tannic acid and immunogold methods. *Neurosci. Lett.* 74: 151–157. [18]

Bunge, M. B. 2008. Novel combination strategies to repair the injured mammalian spinal cord. *J. Spinal Cord Med.* 31: 262–269. [29]

Bunge, M. B. 2016. Efficacy of Schwann cell transplantation for spinal cord repair is improved with combinatorial strategies. *J. Physiol.* 594: 3533–3538. [29]

Bunge, R. P. 1968. Glial cells and the central myelin sheath. *Physiol. Rev.* 48: 197–251. [10]

Burbach, J. P., Luckman, S. M., Murphy, D., and Gainer, H. 2001. Gene regulation in the magnocellular hypothalamo-neurohypophysial system. *Physiol. Rev.* 81: 1197–1267. [19]

Burdakov, D., Gerasimenko, O., and Verkhratsky, A. 2005. Physiological changes in glucose differentially modulate the excitability of hypothalamic melanin-concentrating hormone and orexin neurons in situ. *J. Neurosci.* 25: 2429–2433. [14]

Burdakov, D., Jensen, L. T., Alexopoulos, H., et al. 2006. Tandem-pore K^+ channels mediate inhibition of orexin neurons by glucose. *Neuron* 50: 711–722. [14]

Burden, S. J., Sargent, P. B., and McMahan, U. J. 1979. Acetylcholine receptors in regenerating muscle accumulate at original synaptic sites in the absence of the nerve. *J. Cell Biol.* 82: 412–425. [11, 29]

Burgen, A. S. V., and Terroux, K. G. 1953. On the negative inotropic effect in the cat's auricle. *J. Physiol.* 120: 449–464. [12]

Burgess, R. W., Nguyen, Q. T., Son, Y. J., et al. 1999. Alternatively spliced isoforms of nerve- and muscle-derived agrin: Their roles at the neuromuscular junction. *Neuron* 23: 33–44. [29]

Burgin, K. E., et al. 1990. In situ hybridization histochemistry of Ca^{2+}/calmodulin-dependent protein kinase in developing rat brain. *J. Neurosci.* 10: 1788–1798. [17]

Burke, R. E., and Glenn, L. L. 1996. Horseradish peroxidase study of the spatial and electrotonic distribution of group Ia synapses on type-identified ankle extensor motoneurons in the cat. *J. Comp. Neurol.* 372: 465–485. [26]

Burnashev, N. 1996 Calcium permeability of glutamate-gated channels in the central nervous system. *Curr. Opin. Neurobiol.* 6: 311–317. [11]

Burnashev, N., Zhou, Z., Neher, E., and Sakmann, B. 1995. Fractional calcium currents through recombinant GluR channels of the NMDA, AMPA and kainate receptor subtypes. *J. Physiol.* 485: 403–418. [12]

Burnstock, G. 1972. Purinergic nerves. *Pharmacol. Rev.* 24: 509–581. [14]

Burnstock, G. 1976. Do some nerve cells release more than one transmitter? *Neuroscience* 1: 239–248. [15]

Burnstock, G. 1995. Noradrenaline and ATP: Cotransmitters and neuromodulators. *J. Physiol. Pharmacol.* 46: 365–384. [19]

Burnstock, G., ed. 1990–99. *The Autonomic Nervous System.* 8 Vols. Harwood Academic, New Jersey. [19]

Burnstock, G. 2006. Historical review: ATP as a neurotransmitter. *Trends Pharmacol. Sci.* 27: 166–176. [19]

Burnstock, G., and Holman, M. E. 1961. The transmission of excitation from autonomic nerve to smooth muscle. *J. Physiol.* 155: 115–133. [19]

Burrell, B. D., Sahley, C. L., and Muller, K. J. 2003. Progressive recovery of learning during regeneration of a single synapse in the medicinal leech. *J. Comp. Neurol.* 457: 67–74. [20]

Burton, H., and Sinclair, R. J. 1991. Second somatosensory cortical area in macaque monkeys: 2. Neuronal responses to punctate vibrotactile stimulation of glabrous skin on the hand. *Brain Res.* 538: 127–135. [23]

Buss, R. R., Sun, W., and Oppenheim, R. W. 2006. Adaptive roles of programmed cell death during nervous system development. *Annu. Rev. Neurosci.* 29: 1–35. [27]

Buszaki, G. 1984. Feed-forward inhibition in the hippocampal formation. *Prog. Neurobiol.* 22: 131–153. [14]

Butt, A. M., and Ransom, B. R. 1993. Morphology of astrocytes and oligodendrocytes during development in the intact rat optic nerve. *J. Comp. Neurol.* 338: 141–158. [10]

Butt, A. M., Hamilton, N., Hubbard, P., et al. 2005. Synantocytes: The fifth element. *J. Anat.* 207: 695–706. [10]

Buttner, N., Siegelbaum, S. A., and Volterra, A. 1989. Direct modulation of *Aplysia* S-K$^+$ channels by a 12-lipoxygenase metabolite of arachidonic acid. *Nature* 342: 553–555. [12]

Cabelli, R. J., Shelton, D. L., Segal, R. A., and Shatz, C. J. 1997. Blockade of endogenous ligands of trkB inhibits formation of ocular dominance columns. *Neuron* 19: 63–76. [28]

Cacciatore, T. W., Rozenshteyn, R., and Kristan Jr., W. B. 2000. Kinematics and modeling of leech crawling: Evidence for an oscillatory behavior produced by propagating waves of excitation. *J. Neurosci.* 20: 1643–1655. [20]

Cadwell, C. R., et al. 2019. Development and arealization of the cerebral cortex. *Neuron* 103: 980–1004. [27]

Cain, D. P. 1998. Testing the NMDA, long-term potentiation, and cholinergic hypothesis of spatial learning. *Neurosci. Biobehav. Rev.* 22: 181–193. [16]

Cajigas, et al. 2012. The local transcriptome in the synaptic neuropil revealed by deep sequencing and high-resolution imaging. *Neuron* 74: 453–466. [17]

Calabrese, R. L., Norris, B. J., and Wenning, A. 2016. The neural control of heartbeat in invertebrates. *Curr. Opin. Neurobiol.* 41: 68–77. doi: 10.1016/j.conb.2016.08.004. [20]

Caldwell, P. C., Hodgkin, A. L., Keynes, R. D., and Shaw, T. L. 1960. The effects of injecting "energy-rich" phosphate compounds on the active transport of ions in the giant axons of *Loligo*. *J. Physiol.* 152: 561–590. [9]

Callaway, E. M. 2005. Structure and function of parallel pathways in the primate early visual system. *J. Physiol.* 566: 13–19. [3]

Calvino, M. A., and Szczupak, L. 2008. Spatial-specific action of serotonin within the leech midbody ganglion. *J. Comp. Physiol. A* 194: 523–531. [20]

Camand, E., Morel, M. P., Faissner, A., et al. 2004. Long-term changes in the molecular composition of the glial scar and progressive increase of serotoninergic fibre sprouting after hemisection of the mouse spinal cord. *Eur. J. Neurosci.* 20: 1161–1176. [29]

Cameron, J. L., Eagleson, K. L., Fox, N. A., et al. 2017. Social origins of developmental risk for mental and physical illness. *J. Neurosci.* 37: 10783–10791. [28]

Cameron, O. G. 2009 Visceral brain–body information transfer. *Neuroimage* 47: 787–794. [19]

Cammack, J. N., and Schwartz, E. A. 1993. Ions required for the electrogenic transport of GABA by horizontal cells of the catfish retina. *J. Physiol.* 472: 81–102. [9, 13]

Cammack, J. N., Rakhilin, S. V., and Schwartz, E. A. 1994. A GABA transporter operates asymmetrically and with variable stoichiometry. *Neuron* 13: 949–960. [13]

Campbell, D. S., and Holt, C. E. 2001. Chemotropic responses of retinal growth cones mediated by rapid local protein synthesis and degradation. *Neuron.* 32:1013–1026. [27]

Campbell, K., and Gotz, M. 2002. Radial glia: Multi-purpose cells for vertebrate brain development. *Trends Neurosci.* 25: 235–238. [27]

Campbell, R. R. and Wood, M. A. 2019. How the epigenome integrates information and reshapes the synapse. *Nat. Rev. Neurosci.* doi: 10.1038/s41583-019-0121-9. [17]

Campenot, R. B. 1977. Local control of neurite development by nerve growth factor. *Proc. Natl. Acad. Sci. USA* 74: 4516–4519. [27]

Campenot, R. B. 1982. Development of sympathetic neurons in compartmentalized cultures. II. Local control of neurite survival by nerve growth factor. *Dev. Biol.* 93: 13–21. [27]

Campenot, R. B. 2009. NGF uptake and retrograde signaling mechanisms in sympathetic neurons in compartmented cultures. *Results Probl. Cell Differ.* 48: 141–158. [27, 29]

Canessa, C. M., Schild, L., Buell, G., et al. 1994. Amiloride-sensitive epithelial Na+ channel is made of three homologous subunits. *Nature* 367: 463–467. [21]

Cannon, S. C. 1996. Ion channel defects and aberrant excitability in myotonia and periodic paralysis. *Trends Neurosci.* 19: 3–10. [6]

Cant, N. B., and Casseday, J. H. 1986. Projections from the anteroventral cochlear nucleus to the lateral and medial superior olivary nuclei. *J. Comp. Neurol.* 247: 457–476. [24]

Cantino, D., and Mugnani, E. 1975. The structural basis for electrotonic coupling in the avian ciliary ganglion: A study with thin sectioning and freeze-fracturing. *J. Neurocytol.* 4: 505–536. [8]

Canul-Sánchez, J. A. Hernández-Araiza, I., Hernández-García, E., et al. 2018. Different agonists induce distinct single-channel conductance states in TRPV1 channels. *J. Gen. Physiol.* 150: 1735–1746. doi: 10.1085/jgp.201812141. [5]

Cao, D., Pokorny, J., Smith, V. C., and Zele, A. J. 2008. Rod contributions to color perception: Linear with rod contrast. *Vision Res.* 48: 2586–2592. [22]

Cao, Y. Q., Mantyh, P. W., Carlson, E. J., et al. 1998. Primary afferent tachykinins are required to experience moderate to intense pain. *Nature* 392: 390–394. [14]

Capecchi, M. R. 1997. *Hox* genes and mammalian development. *Cold Spring Harb. Symp. Quant. Biol.* 62: 273–281. [27]

Capogrosso, M., Milekovic, T., Borton, D., et al. 2016. A brain-spine interface alleviating gait deficits after spinal cord injury in primates. *Nature* 539: 284–288. [29]

Capsoni, S., and Cattaneo, A. 2006. On the molecular basis linking nerve growth factor (NGF) to Alzheimer's disease. *Cell Mol. Neurobiol.* 26: 619–633. [27]

Capsoni, S., Tiveron, C., Vignone, D., et al. 2010. Dissecting the involvement of tropomyosin-related kinase A and p75 neurotrophin receptor signaling in NGF deficit-induced neurodegeneration. *Proc. Natl. Acad. Sci USA* 107: 12299–12304. [27]

Capsoni, S., Tongiorgi, E., Cattaneo, A., and Domenici, L. 1999. Dark rearing blocks the developmental down-regulation of brain-derived neurotrophic factor messenger RNA expression in layers IV and V of the rat visual cortex. *Neuroscience* 88: 393–403. [28]

Capsoni, S., Ugolini, G., Comparini, A., et al. 2000. Alzheimer-like neurodegeneration in aged antinerve growth factor transgenic mice. *Proc. Natl. Acad. Sci USA* 97: 68266831. doi: 10.1073/pnas.97.12.6826. [27]

Carafoli, E., and Brini, M. 2000. Calcium pumps: Structural basis for and mechanisms of calcium transmembrane transport. *Curr. Opin. Chem. Biol.* 4: 152–161. [9]

Caraty, A., and Skinner, D. C. 2008. Gonadotropin-releasing hormone in third ventricular cerebrospinal fluid: Endogenous distribution and exogenous uptake. *Endocrinology* 149: 5227–5234. [18]

Cariboni, A., Maggi, R., and Parnevalas, J. G. 2007. From nose to fertility: The long migratory journey of gonadotropin-releasing hormone neurons. *Trends Neurosci.* 30: 638–644. [19]

Carrillo-Reid, L., Yang, W., Bando, Y., et al. 2017. Imprinting and recalling cortical ensembles. *Science.* 353: 691–694. doi:10.1126/science.aaf7560. [2]

Carlson, M., Hubel, D. H., and Wiesel, T. N. 1986. Effects of monocular exposure to oriented lines on monkey striate cortex. *Brain Res.* 390: 71–81. [28]

Carlsson, A., Lindqvist, M., Magnusson, T., and Waldeck, B. 1958. On the presence of 3-hydroxytyramine in brain. *Science* 127: 471. [14]

Caroni, P., and Schwab, M. E. 1988. Two membrane protein fractions from rat central myelin with inhibitory properties for neurite growth and fibroblast spreading. *J. Cell Biol.* 106: 1281–1288. [10]

Caroni, P., Rotsler, S., Britt, J. C., and Brenner, H. R. 1993. Calcium influx and protein phosphorylation mediate the metabolic stabilization of synaptic acetylcholine receptors in muscle. *J. Neurosci.* 13: 1315–1325. [29]

Carrol, R. C., Lissin, D. V., von Zastrow, M., et al. 1999. Rapid redistribution of glutamate receptors contributes to long-term depression in hippocampal cultures. *Nat. Neurosci.* 2: 454–460. [16]

Castillo, P. E. 2012. Presynaptic LTP and LTD of excitatory and inhibitory synapses. *Cold Spring Harb. Perspect. Biol.* 4: a005728. [17]

Carulli, D., Buffo, A., and Strata, P. 2004. Reparative mechanisms in the cerebellar cortex. *Prog. Neurobiol.* 72: 373–398. [29]

Carvell, G. E., and Simons, D. J. 1990. Biometric analyses of vibrissal tactile discrimination in the rat. *J. Neurosci.* 10: 2638–2648. [23]

Casagrande, V. A., Yazar, F., Jones, K. D., and Ding, Y. 2007. The morphology of the koniocellular axon pathway in the macaque monkey. *Cereb. Cortex* 17: 2334–2345. [3]

Cascio, C. J., and Sathian, K. 2001. Temporal cues contribute to tactile perception of roughness. *J. Neurosci.* 21: 5289–5296. [23]

Cassell, J. F., and McLachlan, E. M. 1987. Muscarinic agonists block five different potassium conductances in guinea-pig sympathetic neurones. *Brit. J. Pharmacol.* 91: 259–261. [12]

Castellucci, V., and Kandel, E. R. 1974. A quantal analysis of the synaptic depression underlying habituation of the gill-withdrawal reflex in *Aplysia. Proc. Natl. Acad. Sci. USA* 71: 5004–5008. [16]

Castellucci, V., Pinsker, H., Kupfermann, I., and Kandel, E. R. 1970. Neuronal mechanisms of habituation and dishabituation of the gill-withdrawal reflex in *Aplysia. Science* 167: 1745–1748. [16]

Castillo, J. P., Rui, H., Basilio, D., et al. 2015. Mechanism of potassium ion uptake by the Na+/K+-ATPase. *Nature Comm.* 6: 7622 doi: 10.1038/ncomms8622. [9]

Castrén, E., Zafra, F., Thoenen, H., and Lindholm, D. 1992. Light regulates expression of brain-derived neurotrophic factor mRNA in rat visual cortex. *Proc. Natl. Acad. Sci. USA* 89: 9444–9448. [28]

Castro, J. B., Ramanathan, A., and Chennubhotla, C. S. 2013. Categorical dimensions of human odor descriptor space revealed by non-negative matrix factorization. *PLOS ONE* 8: e73289. doi: 10.1371/journal.pone.0073289. [21]

Catania, K. C. 1999. A nose that looks like a hand and acts like an eye: The unusual mechanosensory system of the star-nosed mole. *J. Comp. Physiol. A* 185: 367–372. [23]

Catania, K. C., and Kaas, J. H. 1997. Somatosensory fovea in the star-nosed mole: Behavioral use of the star in relation to innervation patterns and cortical representation. *J. Comp. Neurol.* 387: 215–233. [23]

Cattaneo, A. 2013. Immunosympathectomy as the first phenotypic knockout with antibodies. *Proc. Natl. Acad. Sci. USA* 110: 4877. [27]

Cattaneo, A., and Capsoni, S. 2018. Painless Nerve Growth Factor: A TrkA biased agonist mediating a broad neuroprotection via its actions on microglia cells. *Pharmacol Res.* 139: 17–25. 10.1016/j.phrs.2018.10.028. [27]

Cattaneo, L., and Rizzolatti, G. 2009. The mirror neuron system. *Arch. Neurol.* 66: 557–560. [26]

Catterall, W. A. 2014. Structure and function of voltage-gated sodium channels at atomic resolution. *Exp. Physiol.* 99: 35--51. [5]

Catterall, W. A., and Few, A. P. 2008. Calcium channel regulation and presynaptic plasticity. *Neuron* 59: 882–901. [16]

Caulfield, M. P., and Brown, D. A. 1992. Cannabinoid receptor agonists inhibit Ca current in NG108-15 neuroblastoma cells via a pertussis toxin-sensitive mechanism. *Brit. J. Pharmacol.* 106: 231–232. [12]

Caviness, V. S., Jr. 1982. Neocortical histogenesis in normal and reeler mice: A developmental study based upon [3H]thymidine autoradiography. *Dev. Brain Res.* 4: 293–302. [27]

Cazalis, M., Dayanithi, G., and Nordmann, J. J. 1985. The role of patterned burst and interburst interval on the excitation-coupling mechanism in the isolated rat neural lobe. *J. Physiol.* 369: 45–60. [18]

Ceccarelli, B., and Hurlbut, W. P. 1980. Vesicle hypothesis of the release of quanta of acetylcholine. *Physiol. Rev.* 60: 396–441. [13]

Celikel, T., Szostak, V. A., and Feldman, D. E. 2004. Modulation of spike timing by sensory deprivation during induction of cortical map plasticity. *Nat. Neurosci.* 7: 534–541. [23]

Cepko, C., and Pear, W. 1996. Transduction of genes using retrovirus vectors. *Curr. Protoc. Mol. Biol.* Sec. III, Unit 9.9. [27]

Cepko, C. L., Austin, C. P., Yang, X., et al. 1996. Cell fate determination in the vertebrate retina. *Proc. Natl. Acad. Sci. USA* 93: 589–595. [27]

Cesare, P., and McNaughton, P. A. 1996. A novel heat-activated current in nociceptive neurons and its sensitization by bradykinin. *Proc. Natl. Acad. Sci. USA* 93: 15435–15439. [12, 21]

Cha, A., Snyder, G. E., Selvin, P. R., and Bezanilla, F. 1999. Atomic scale movement of the voltage-sensing region in a potassium channel measured via spectroscopy. *Nature* 402: 809–813. [7]

Chakrabarti, R., Michanski, S., and Wichmann, C. 2018. Vesicle subpool organization at inner hair cell ribbon synapses. *EMBO Reports:* e44937. [24]

Chalfie, M. 2009. Neurosensory mechanotransduction. *Nat. Rev. Mol. Cell Biol.* 10: 44–52. [21]

Chalfie, M., Tu, Y., Euskirchen, G., et al. 1994. Green fluorescent protein as a marker for gene expression. *Science* 263: 802–805. [27]

Chambers, S. M., Fasano, C. A., Papapetrou, E. P., et al. 2009. Highly efficient neural conversion of human ES and iPS cells by dual inhibition of SMAD signaling. *Nat Biotech.* 27: 275–280. [27]

Chameau, P., and van Hooft, J. A. 2006. Serotonin 5-HT$_3$ receptors in the central nervous system. *Cell Tissue Res.* 326: 573–581. [14]

Champagnat, J., Morin-Surun, M. P., Fortin, G., and Thoby-Brisson, M. 2009. Developmental basis of the rostro-caudal organization of the brainstem respiratory rhythm generator. *Philos. Trans. R. Soc. Lond., B, Biol. Sci.* 364: 2469–2476. [26]

Chan, J. R., Watkins, T. A., Cosgaya, J. M., et al.2004. NGF controls axonal receptivity to myelination by Schwann cells or oligodendrocytes. *Neuron* 43: 183–191. [10]

Chanaday, N. L., and Kavalali, E. T. 2017. How do you recognize and reconstitute a synaptic vesicle after fusion? *F1000Research* 6: 1734. doi: 10.12688/f100research.12072. [13]

Chanda, B., Asamoah, O. K., Blunck, R., et al. 2005. Gating charge displacement in voltage-gated ion channels involves limited transmembrane movement. *Nature* 436: 852–856. [7]

Chandran, V., Coppola, G., Nawabi, H., et al. 2016. A Systems-Level Analysis of the Peripheral Nerve Intrinsic Axonal Growth Program. *Neuron* 89: 956–970. [29]

Chandrashekar, J., Kuhn, C., Oka, Y., et al. 2010. The cells and peripheral representation of sodium taste in mice. *Nature* 464: 297–301. [21]

Changeux, J. P. 2017. Climbing brain levels of organisation from genes to consciousness. *Trends Cog. Sci.* doi: 10.1016/j.tics.2017.01.004. [27]

Chao, M. V. 2003. Neurotrophins and their receptors: A convergence point for many signaling pathways. *Nat. Rev. Neurosci.* 4: 299–309. doi: 10.1038/nrn1078. [27]

Chao, M. V. 2019. Stoichiometry counts. *Proc. Natl. Acad. Sci. USA* www.pnas.org/cgi/doi/10.1073/pnas.1914583116. [27]

Chao, M. V., Bothwell, M. A., Ross, A. H., et al. 1986.Gene transfer and molecular cloning of the human NGF receptor. *Science* 232: 518–521. doi: 10.1126/science.3008331. [27]

Chapman, B., Stryker, M. P., and Bonhoeffer, T. 1996. Development of orientation preference maps in ferret primary visual cortex. *J. Neurosci.* 16: 6443–6453. [28]

Chapman, C. E., and Beauchamp, E. 2006. Differential controls over tactile detection in humans by motor commands and peripheral reafference. *J. Neurophysiol.* 96: 1664–1675. [23]

Charnet, P., Labarca, C., Leonard, R. J., et al. 1990. An open-channel blocker interacts with adjacent turns of α-helices in the nicotinic acetylcholine receptor. *Neuron* 4: 87–85. [5]

Chattopadhyaya, B., Di Cristo, G., Higashiyama, H., et al. 2004. Experience and activity-dependent maturation of perisomatic GABAergic innervation in primary visual cortex during a postnatal critical period. *J. Neurosci.* 24: 9598–9611. [28]

Chazal, G., and Ralston, H. J., 3rd. 1987. *J. Comp. Neurol.* 259: 317–329. doi: 10.1002/cne.902590302. [18]

Chemelli, R. M., Willie, J. T., Sinton, C. M., et al. 1999. Narcolepsy in orexin knockout mice: Molecular genetics of sleep regulation. *Cell* 98: 437–451. [14]

Chen, A., Kumar, S. M., Sahley, C. L., and Muller, K. J. 2000. Nitric oxide influences injury-induced microglial migration and accumulation in the leech CNS. *J. Neurosci.* 20: 1036–1043. [10]

Chen, C. K. 2005. The vertebrate phototransduction cascade: Amplification and termination mechanisms. *Rev. Physiol. Biochem. Pharmacol.* 154: 101–121. [22]

Chen, J., Makino, C. L., Peachey, N. S., et al. 1995. Mechanisms of rhodopsin inactivation in vivo as revealed by a COOH-terminal truncation mutant. *Science* 267: 374–377. [22]

Chen, N-H., Reith, M. E. A., and Quick, M. W. 2004. Synaptic uptake and beyond: The sodium- and chloride-dependent neurotransmitter transporter family SLC6. *Pflügers Arch.* 447: 519–531. [9]

Chen, R., Tilley, M. R., Wei, H., et al. 2006. Abolished cocaine reward in mice with a cocaine-insensitive dopamine transporter. *Proc. Natl. Acad. Sci. USA* 103: 9333–9338. [14]

Chen, X., Tomochick, D. R., Kovrigin, E., et al. 2002. Three-dimensional structure of the complexin/SNARE complex. *Neuron* 33: 397–409. [13]

Chen, Z., Gore, B. B., Long, H., et al. 2008. Alternative splicing of the Robo3 axon guidance receptor governs the midline switch from attraction to repulsion. *Neuron* 58: 325–532. [27]

Cheney, D. P., and Fetz, E. E. 1980. Functional classes of primate corticomotoneuronal cells and their relation to active force. *J. Neurophysiol.* 44: 773–791. [26]

Cheng, D., Hoogenraad, C. C., Rush, J., et al. 2006. Relative and absolute quantification of postsynaptic density proteome isolated from rat forebrain and cerebellum. *Mol. Cell. Proteomics* 5: 1158–1170. [11]

Cheng, H., and Lederer, W. J. 2008. Calcium sparks. *Physiol. Rev.* 88: 1491–1545. [12]

Cheng, K., Narendra, A., Sommer, S., and Wehner, R. 2009. Traveling in clutter: Navigation in the Central Australian desert ant *Melophorus bagoti. Behav. Processes* 80: 261–268. [20]

Cherubini, E., Gaiarsa, J. L., and Ben-Ari, Y. 1991. GABA: An excitatory transmitter in early postnatal life. *Trends Neurosci.* 14: 515–519. [19, 27]

Cherubini, E., Griguoli, M., Safiulina, V., and Lagostena, L. 2011. The depolarizing action of GABA controls early network activity in the developing hippocampus. *Mol. Neurobiol.* 43: 97–106. [27]

Chesler, A. T., Zou, D. J., Le Pichon, C. E., et al. 2007. A G protein/cAMP signal cascade is required for axonal convergence into olfactory glomeruli. *Proc. Natl. Acad. Sci. USA* 104: 1039–1044. [28]

Cheung, G. Chever, O., and Rouach, N. 2014. Connexons and pannexons: Newcomers in neurophysiology. *Frontiers in Cell Neuroscience* 8: 348. doi: 10.3389/fncel.2014.00348. [10]

Chever, O., Lee, C. Y., and Rouach, N. 2014. Astroglial connexin43 hemichannels tune basal excitatory synaptic transmission. *J. Neurosci.* 34:11228-32. doi: 10.1523/jneurosci.0015-14.2014. [10]

Chiu, S. Y., and Ritchie, J. M. 1981. Evidence for the presence of potassium channels in the paranodal region of acutely demyelinated mammalian nerve fibres. *J. Physiol.* 313: 415–437. [8]

Choi, H. J., Lee, C. J., Schroeder, A., et al. 2008. Excitatory actions of GABA in the suprachiasmatic nucleus. *J. Neurosci.* 28: 5450–5459. [19]

Choi, J. H. et al 2018. Interregional synaptic maps among engram cells underlie memory formation. *Science* 360: 430–435. [17]

Choi, K. L., Aldrich, R. W., and Yellen, G. 1991. Tetraethylammo-nium blockade distinguishes two inactivation states in voltage-gated K+ channels. *Proc. Natl. Acad. Sci. USA* 88: 5092–5095. [7]

Choquet, D., and Trille, A. 2003. The role of receptor diffusion in the organization of the postsynaptic membrane. *Nat. Rev. Neurosci.* 4: 251–265. [14]

Choquet, D. and Trille, A. 2013. The dynamic synapse. *Neuron* 80: 691. [17]

Christie, B. R., and Abraham, W. C. 1994. L-type voltage-sensitive calcium channel antagonists block heterosynaptic long-term facilitation depression in the dentate gyrus of anesthetized rats. *Neurosci. Lett.* 167: 41–45. [16]

Christmann, C., Koeppe, C., Braus, D. F., et al. 2007. A simultaneous EEG–fMRI study of painful electric stimulation. *Neuroimage* 34: 1428–1437. [23]

Cifra, A., Nani, F., Sharifullina, E., and Nistri, A. 2009. A repertoire of rhythmic bursting produced by hypoglossal motoneurons in physiological and pathological conditions. *Philos. Trans. R. Soc. Lond., B, Biol. Sci.* 364: 2493–2500. [26]

Cipelletti, B., Avanzini, G., Vitellaro-Zuccarello, L., et al. 2002. Morphological organization of somatosensory cortex in Otx1-/- mice. *Neuroscience* 115: 657–667. [27]

Civelli, O., Saito, Y., Wang, Z., et al. 2006. Orphan GPCRs and their ligands. *Pharmacol. Ther.* 110: 525–532. [14]

Clapham, D. E. 2007. Calcium signaling. *Cell* 131: 1047–1058. [12]

Clapham, D. E. 2007. Snapshot: Mammalian TRP channels. *Cell:* 129: Doi: 10.1016/j.cell.2007.03.034. [5]

Clapham, D. E., and Neer, E. J. 1997. G protein beta gamma subunits. *Annu. Rev. Pharmacol. Toxicol.* 37: 167–203. [12]

Clarey, J. C., Barone, P., and Imig, T. J. 1994. Functional organization of sound direction and sound pressure level in primary auditory cortex of the cat. *J. Neurophysiol.* 72: 2383–2405. [24]

Close, R. I. 1972. Dynamic properties of mammalian skeletal muscles. *Physiol. Rev.* 52: 129–197. [29]

Clowry, G., Molnár, Z., and Rakic, P. 2010. Renewed focus on the developing human neocortex. *J. Anat.* 217: 276–288. [27]

Cobb, S. R., Buhl, E. H., Halasy, K., et al. 1995. Synchronization of neuronal activity in hippocampus by individual GABAergic interneurons. *Nature* 378: 75–78. [14]

Cochilla, A. J., Angleson, J. K., and Betz, W. 1999. Monitoring secretory membrane with FM1-43 fluorescence. *Annu. Rev. Neurosci.* 22: 1–10. [13]

Coddington, L. T., Nietz, A. K., and Wadiche, J. I. 2014. The contribution of extrasynaptic signaling to cerebellar information processing. *Cerebellum* 13: 513–520. [18]

Coggeshall, R. E. 1972. Autoradiographic and chemical localization of 5-hydroxytryptamine in identified neurons in the leech. *Anat. Rec.* 172: 489–498. doi: 10.1002/ar.1091720303. [18]

Coggeshall, R. E., and Fawcett, D. W. 1964. The fine structure of the central nervous system of the leech, *Hirudo Medicinalis. J. Neurophysiol.* 27: 229–289. [20]

Cohen, B., Maruta, J., and Raphan, T. 2001. Orientation of the eyes to gravitoinertial acceleration. *Ann. N Y Acad. Sci.* 942: 241–258. [24]

Cohen, I., Rimer, M., Lømo, T., and McMahan, U. J. 1997. Agrin-induced postsynaptic-like apparatus in skeletal muscle fibers in vivo. *Mol. Cell. Neurosci.* 9: 237–253. [29]

Cohen, M. R., and Newsome, W. T. 2004. What electrical microstimulation has revealed about the neural basis of cognition. *Curr. Opin. Neurobiol.* 14: 169–177. [3, 25]

Cohen, M. R., and Newsome, W. T. 2009. Estimates of the contribution of single neurons to perception depend on timescale and noise correlation. *J. Neurosci.* 29: 6635–6648. [3]

Cohen, M. W. 1972. The development of neuromuscular connexions in the presence of D-tubocurarine. *Brain Res.* 41: 457–463. [29]

Cohen, M. W., Jones, O. T., and Angelides, K. J. 1991. Distribution of Ca2+ channels on frog motor nerve terminals revealed by fluorescent omega-conotoxin. *J. Neurosci.* 11: 1032–1039. [13]

Cohen, S., and Levi-Montalcini, R. 1956. A nerve growth-stimulating factor isolated from snake venom. *Proc. Natl. Acad. Sci. USA* 42: 571–574. [27]

Cohen, S., Levi-Montalcini, R., and Hamburger, V. 1954. A nerve growth-stimulating factor isolated from sarcomas 37 and 180. *Proc. Natl. Acad. Sci. USA* 40: 1014–1018. [27]

Colak, D., Ji, S. J., Porse, B. T., and Jaffrey, S. R. 2013. Regulation of axon guidance by compartmentalized nonsense-mediated mRNA decay. *Cell* 153: 1252–1265. [27]

Cole, A. E., and Nicoll, R. A. 1984. Characterization of a slow cholinergic post-synaptic potential recorded in vitro from rat hippocampal pyramidal cells. *J. Physiol.* 352: 173–188. [14]

Coleman, G. T., Bahramali, H., Zhang, H. Q., and Rowe, M. J. 2001. Characterization of tactile afferent fibers in the hand of the marmoset monkey. *J. Neurophysiol.* 85: 1793–1804. [23]

Coleman, M. P., and Freeman, M. R. 2010. Wallerian degeneration, Wld^s, and Nmnat. *Annu. Rev. Neurosci.* 33: 245–267. [29]

Colgan, L. A., Cavolo, S. L., Commons, K. G., and Levitan, E. S. 2012. Action potential-independent and pharmacologically unique vesicular serotonin release from dentrites. *J. Neurosci.* 32: 15737–15746. doi: 10.1523/jneurosci.0020–12.2012. [18]

Collett, M., Collett, T. S., and Wehner, R. 1999. Calibration of vector navigation in desert ants. *Curr. Biol.* 9: 1031–1034. [20]

Collett, M., Collett, T. S., Bisch, S., and Wehner, R. 1998. Local and global vectors in desert ant navigation. *Nature* 394: 269–272. [20]

Collett, T. S., and Baron, J. 1994. Biological compasses and the coordinate frame of landmark memories in honeybees. *Nature* 368: 137–140. [20]

Collett, T. S., and Graham, P. 2004. Animal navigation: Path integration, visual landmarks and cognitive maps. *Curr. Biol.* 14: R475–477. [20]

Collin, E., Mauborgne, A., Bourgoin, S., et al. 1991. *In vivo* tonic inhibition of spinal substance P (-like material) release by endogenous opioid(s) acting at δ receptors. *Neuroscience* 44: 725–731. [14]

Collingridge, G. L., Kehl, S. J., and McClennan, H. 1983. Excitatory amino acids in synaptic transmission in the Schaffer collateral-commissural pathway of the rat hippocampus. *J. Physiol.* 334: 33–46. [16]

Collingridge, G. L., Olsen, R. W. Peters, J., and Spedding, M. 2009. A nomenclature for ligand-gated ion channels. *Neuropharmacology* 56: 2–5. [5]

Collingridge, G. L., Peineau, S., Howland, J. C., and Wang, Y. T. 2010 Long-term depression in the CNS. *Nature Rev. Neurosci.* 11: 459–473. [16]

Collins, M. O., Husi, H., Yu, L., et al. 2006. Molecular characterization and comparison of the components and multiprotein complexes in the postsynaptic proteome. *J. Neurochem.* 97(Suppl. 1): 16–23. [11]

Colombo, M.., Raposo, G., and Théry, C. 2014. Biogenesis, secretion, and intercellular interactions of exosomes and other extracellular vesicles. *Annu. Rev. Cell. Dev. Biol.* 30: 255–289. [18]

Colquhoun, D. 2007. What have we learned from single ion channels? *J. Physiol.* 581: 425–427. [11]

Colquhoun, D. and Hawkes, A. G. 1981. On the stochastic properties of single ion channels. *Proc. R. Soc. Lond. B* 211: 205–235. [11]

Colquhoun, D., and Sakmann, B. 1981. Fluctuations in the microsecond time range of the current through single acetylcholine receptor ion channels. *Nature* 294: 464–466. [11]

Colquhoun, D., and Sakmann, B. 1985. Fast events in single-channel currents activated by acetylcholine and its analogues at the frog muscle end-plate. *J. Physiol.* 369: 501–557. [11]

Colquhoun, D., Dreyer, F., and Sheridan, R. E. 1979. The actions of tubocurarine at the frog neuromuscular junction. *J. Physiol.* 293: 247–284. [11]

Colwell, C. S. 2011. Linking neural activity and molecular oscillations in the SCN. *Nat. Rev. Neurosci.* 12: 553–569. [19]

Comb, M., Hyman, S. E., and Goodman, H. M. 1987. Mechanisms of trans-synaptic regulation of gene expression. *Trends Neurosci.* 10: 473–478. [15]

Conductier, G., Brau, F., Viola, A., et al. 2013. Melanin-concentrating hormone regulates beat frequency of ependymal cilia and ventricular volume. *Nat. Neurosci.* 16: 845–847. [18]

Congar, P., Leinekugel, X., Ben-Ari, Y., and Crépel, V. 1997. A long-lasting calcium-activated nonselective cationic current is generated by synaptic stimulation or exogenous activation of group I metabotropic glutamate receptors in CA1 pyramidal neurons. *J. Neurosci.* 17: 5366–5379. [12]

Conley, M., Penny, G. R., and Diamond, I. T. 1987. Terminations of individual optic tract fibers in the lateral geniculate nuclei of *Galago crassicaudatus* and *Tupaia belangeri*. *J. Comp. Neurol.* 256: 71–87. [2]

Connor, C. E., and Johnson, K. O. 1992. Neural coding of tactile texture: Comparison of spatial and temporal mechanisms for roughness perception. *J. Neurosci.* 12: 3414–3426. [23]

Connor, C. E., Hsiao, S. S., Phillips, J. R., and Johnson, K. O. 1990. Tactile roughness: Neural codes that account for psychophysical magnitude estimates. *J. Neurosci.* 10: 3823–3836. [23]

Connors, B. W., and Long, M. A. 2004. Electrical synapses in the mammalian brain. *Annu. Rev. Neurosci.* 27: 393–418. [11]

Consiglio, J. F., Andalib, P., and Korn, S. J. 2003. Influence of pore residues on permeation properties in the Kv2.1 potassium channel. Evidence for a selective functional interaction of K$^+$ with the outer vestibule. *J. Gen. Physiol.* 121: 111–124. [5]

Constantinidis, C., Franowicz, M. N., and Goldman-Rakic, P. S. 2001. The sensory nature of mnemonic representation in the primate prefrontal cortex. *Nat. Neurosci.* 4: 311–316. [25]

Contant, C. et al. 1996. Role of tonically-active neurons in the control of striatal function: Cellular mechanisms and behavioral correlates. *Neuroscience* 71: 937–947. [18]

Contini, M., Lin, B., Kobayashi, K., et al. 2010. Synaptic input of ON-bipolar cells onto the dopaminergic neurons of the mouse retina. *J. Comp. Neurol.* 518: 2035–2050. [18]

Contractor, A., Mulle, C., and Swanson, G. T. 2011. Kainate receptors coming of age: Milestones of two decades of research. *Trends Neurosci.* 34: 154–163. [14]

Coombs, J. S., Curtis, D. R., and Eccles, J. C. 1957. The generation of impulses in motoneurones. *J. Physiol.* 139: 232–249. [11]

Coombs, J. S., Eccles, J. C., and Fatt, P. 1955. The electrical properties of the motoneuron membrane. *J. Physiol.* 130: 291–325. [8]

Coombs, J. S., Eccles, J. C., and Fatt, P. 1955. The specific ionic conductances and the ionic movements across the motoneuronal membrane that produce the inhibitory post-synaptic potential. *J. Physiol.* 130: 326–373. [11]

Cooper, J. R., Bloom, F. E., and Roth, R. H. 2002. *The Biochemical Basis of Pharmacology*. Oxford University Press, New York. [19]

Cooper, J. R., Bloom, F. E., and Roth, R. H. 2003. *The Biochemical Basis of Neuropharmacology*, 8th ed. Oxford University Press. [14]

Corbin J. G., Nery, S., and Fishell, G. 2001 Telencephalic cells take a tangent: Non radial migration in the mammalian forebrain *Nat Neurosci* 4: 1177–1182. [27]

Corey, D. P., and Hudspeth, A. J. 1979. Ionic basis of the receptor potential in a vertebrate hair cell. *Nature* 281: 675–677. [21]

Corey, D. P., and Hudspeth, A. J. 1983. Kinetics of the receptor current in bullfrog saccular hair cells. *J. Neurosci.* 3: 962–976. [21]

Cosens, D. 1971. Blindness in a *Drosophila* mutant. *J. Insect Physiol* 17: 285–302. [5]

Cosens, D. J. and Manning, A. 1969. Abnormal electroretinogram from a *Drosophila* mutant, *Nature* 224: 285–287. [5]

Costa-Mattioli, M., et al. 2009. Translational control of long-lasting synaptic plasticity and memory. *Neuron* 61: 10–26. [17]

Coste, B., Mathur, J., Schmidt, M., et al. 2010. Piezo1 and Piezo2 are essential components of distinct mechanically activated cation channels. *Science* 330: 55–60. [5]

Courtine, G., Song, B., Roy, R. R., et al. 2008. Recovery of supraspinal control of stepping via indirect propriospinal relay connections after spinal cord injury. *Nat. Med.* 14: 69–74. [29]

Couve, A., Moss, S. J., and Pangalos, M. N. 2000. GABAB receptors: A new paradigm in G protein signaling. *Mol. Cell. Neuroscience* 16: 296–312. [14]

Cowen, P. J. 2008. Serotonin and depression: Pathophysiological mechanism or marketing myth? *Trends Pharmacol. Sci.* 29: 433–436. [14]

Cox, E. C., Muller, B., and Bonhoeffer, F. 1990. Axonal guidance in the chick visual system: Posterior tectal membranes induce collapse of growth cones from the temporal retina. *Neuron* 4: 31–37. [27]

Cox, J. J., Reimann, F., Nicholas, A. K., et al. 2006. An SCN9A channelopathy causes congenital inability to experience pain. *Nature* 2006 444: 894–898. [5]

Cox, L. J., Hengst, U., Gurskaya, N. G., et al. 2008. Intraaxonal translation and retrograde trafficking of CREB promotes neuronal survival. *Nat Cell Biol* 10: 149–159. doi: 10.1038/ncb1677. [27]

Crago, P. E., Houk, J. C., and Rymer, W. Z. 1982. Sampling of total muscle force by tendon organs. *J. Neurophysiol.* 47: 1069–1083. [26]

Craig, A. M., and Kang, Y. 2007. Neurexin–neuroligin signaling in synapse development. *Curr. Opin. Neurobiol.* 17: 43–52. [27]

Crair, M. C., Gillespie, D. C., and Stryker, M. P. 1998. The role of visual experience in the development of columns in cat visual cortex. *Science* 279: 566–570. [28]

Crawford, A. C., and Fettiplace, R. 1981. An electrical tuning mechanism in turtle cochlear hair cells. *J. Physiol.* 312: 377–412. [24]

Crawford, A. C., and Fettiplace, R. 1985. The mechanical properties of ciliary bundles of turtle cochlear hair cells. *J. Physiol.* 364: 359–379. [21]

Crawford, A. C., Evans, M. G., and Fettiplace, R. 1989. Activation and adaptation of transducer currents in turtle hair cells. *J. Physiol.* 419: 405–434. [21]

Crawford, A. C., Evans, M. G., and Fettiplace, R. 1991. The actions of calcium on the mechano-electrical transducer current of turtle hair cells. *J. Physiol.* 434: 369–398. [21]

Cregg, J. M., DePaul, M. A., Filous, A. R., et al. 2014. Functional regeneration beyond the glial scar. *Exp. Neurol.* 253: 197–207. [29]

Crepel, F., and Jaillard, D. 1991. Pairing of pre- and postsynaptic activities in cerebellar Purkinje cells induces long-term changes in synaptic efficacy in vitro. *J. Physiol.* 432: 123–141. [16]

Crick, F. H. 1979. Thinking about the brain. *Sci. Am.* 241: 219–232. [1]

Crispino, M., Chun, J. T., Cefaliello, C., et al. 2013. Local gene expression in nerve endings. *Dev. Neurobiol.* 74: 279–291. doi: 10.1002/dneu.22109. [17, 27]

Critchlow, V., and von Euler, C. 1963. Intercostal muscle spindle activity and its γ-motor control. *J. Physiol.* 168: 820–847. [26]

Crivellato, E., Nico, B., and Ribatti, D. 2008. The chromaffin vesicle: Advances in understanding the composition of a versatile, multifunctional secretory organelle. *Anat. Rec. (Hoboken)* 291: 1587–1602. [19]

Croner, L. J., and Kaplan, E. 1995. Receptive fields of P and M ganglion cells across the primate retina. *Vision Res.* 35: 7–24. [22]

Crowley, C., Spencer, S. D., Nishimura, M. C., et al.1994. Mice lacking nerve growth factor display perinatal loss of sensory and sympathetic neurons yet develop basal forebrain cholinergic neurons. *Cell* 76: 1001–1011. [27]

Crowley, J. C., and Katz, L. C. 1999. Development of ocular dominance columns in the absence of retinal input. *Nat. Neurosci.* 2: 1125–1130. [28]

Crowley, J. C., and Katz, L. C. 2000. Early development of ocular dominance columns. *Science* 290: 1321–1324. [28]

Crowley, J. C., and Katz, L. C. 2002. Ocular dominance development revisited. *Curr. Opin. Neurobiol.* 12:104–109. [28]

Cull-Candy, S., Kelly, L., and Farrant, M. 2007. Regulation of Ca^{2+}-permeable AMPA receptors: Synaptic plasticity and beyond. *Curr. Opin. Neurobiol.* 17: 277–280. [14]

Cull-Candy, S. G., Miledi, R., and Parker, I. 1980. Single glutamate-activated channels recorded from locust muscle fibres with perfused patch-clamp electrodes. *J. Physiol.* 321: 195–210. [4]

Cullen, K. E., Minor, L. B., Beraneck, M., and Sadeghi, S. G. 2009. Neural substrates underlying vestibular compensation: Contribution of peripheral versus central processing. *J. Vestib. Res.* 19: 171–182. [24]

Cully, D. S., Vassilatis, D. K., Liu, K. K., et al. 1994. Cloning of an avermectin-sensitive glutamate-gated chloride channel from *Caenorhabditis elegans*. *Nature* 371: 707–711. [5]

Cunnane, T. C., and Stjarne. L. 1984.Transmitter secretion from individual varicosities of guinea-pig and mouse vas deferens: Highly intermittent and monoquantal. *Neuroscience* 13: 1–20. [18]

Curcio, C. A., Allen, K. A., Sloan, K. R., et al. 1991. Distribution and morphology of human cone photoreceptors stained with anti-blue opsin. *J. Comp. Neurol.* 312: 610–624. [22]

Curtis, B. M., and Catterall, W. A. 1986. Reconstitution of the voltage-sensitive calcium channel purified from skeletal muscle transverse tubules. *Biochemistry* 25: 3077–3083. [12]

Curtis, D. R., and Phillis, J. W. 1958. Gamma-amino-*n*-butyric acid and spinal synaptic transmission. *Nature* 182: 323. [14]

Curtis, D. R., Phillis, J. W., and Watkins, J. C. 1959. The depression of spinal neurones by γ-amino-*n*-butyric acid and β-alanine. *J. Physiol* 146: 185–203. [14]

Curtis, D. R., Phillis, J. W., and Watkins, J. C. 1960. The chemical excitation of spinal neurones by certain acidic amino acids. *J. Physiol.* 150: 656–682. [14]

Custo Greig, L. F., Woodworth, M. B., Galazo, M. J., et al. 2013. Molecular logic of neocortical projection neuron specification, development and diversity. *Nat. Rev. Neurosci.* 14: 755–769. [27]

Cuttle, M. F., Tsujimoto, T., Forsythe, I. D., and Takahashi, T. 1998. Facilitation of the presynaptic calcium current at an auditory synapse in rat brainstem. *J. Physiol.* 512: 723–729. [16]

Cynader, M., and Mitchell, D. E. 1980. Prolonged sensitivity to monocular deprivation in dark-reared cats. *J. Neurophysiol.* 43: 1026–1040. [28]

D'Antoni, S., Berretta, A., Bonaccorso, C. M., et al. 2008. Metabotropic glutamate receptors in glial cells. *Neurochem. Res.* 33: 2436–2443. [10]

D'Arcangelo, G., Nakajima, K., Miyata, T., et al. 1997. Reelin is a secreted glycoprotein recognized by the CR-50 monoclonal antibody. *J. Neurosci.* 17: 23–31. [27]

d'Incamps, B. L., and Ascher, P. 2008. Four excitatory postsynaptic ionotropic receptors coactivated at the motoneuron-Renshaw cell synapse. *J. Neurosci.* 28: 14121–14131. [14]

Da Silva, K. M. C., Sayers, B. M., Sears, T. A., and Stagg, D. T. 1977. The changes in configuration of the rib cage and abdomen during breathing in the anaesthetized cat. *J. Physiol.* 266: 499–521. [26]

Dacke, M., and Srinivasan, M. V. 2007. Honeybee navigation: Distance estimation in the third dimension. *J. Exp. Biol.* 210: 845–853. [20]

Dacey, D. M., Crook, J. D., and Packer, O. S. 2014. Distinct synaptic mechanisms create parallel S-ON and S-OFF color opponent pathways in the primate retina. *Vis. Neurosci.* 31: 139–151. doi:10.1017/S0952523813000230. [22]

Dahlström, A., and Fuxe, K. 1964. A method for the demonstration of monoamine-containing nerve fibres in the central nervous system. *Acta Physiol. Scand.* 60: 293–294. [14]

Dahlström, A., and Fuxe, K. 1964. Evidence for the existence of monoamine-containing neurons in the central nervous system. I. Demonstration of monoamines in the cell bodies of brain stem neurons. *Acta Physiol. Scand. Suppl.* 232: 1–55. [14]

Dahlström, A. B. 2010. Fast intra-axonal transport: Beginning, development and post-genome advances. *Prog. Neurobiol.* 90: 119–145. [15]

Dale, H. H. 1914. The action of certain esters and ethers of choline, and their relation to muscarine. *J. Pharmacol. Exp. Ther.* 6: 147–190. [12]

Dale, H. H. 1933. Nomenclature of fibres in the autonomic nervous system and their effects. *J. Physiol.* 80: 10–11. [15]

Dale, H. H. 1953. *Adventures in Physiology*. Pergamon, London. [11]

Dale, H. H., Feldberg, W., and Vogt, M. 1936. Release of acetylcholine at voluntary motor nerve endings. *J. Physiol.* 86: 353–380. [11]

Dallos, P. 2008. Cochlear amplification, outer hair cells and prestin. *Curr. Opin. Neurobiol.* 18: 370–376. [24]

Dallos, P., Wu, X., Cheatham, M. A., et al. 2008. Prestin-based outer hair cell motility is necessary for mammalian cochlear amplification. *Neuron* 58: 333–339. [24]

Dan, Y., Lo, Y., and Poo, M. M. 1995. Plasticity of developing neuromuscular synapses. *Prog. Brain Res.* 105: 211–215. [29]

Dani, J. A., and Bertrand, D. 2007. Nicotinic acetylcholine receptors and nicotinic cholinergic mechanisms of the central nervous system. *Annu. Rev. Pharmacol. Toxicol.* 47: 699–729. [14]

Dani, J. W., Chernjavsky, A., Smith, S. J. 1992. Neuronal activity triggers calcium waves in hippocampal astrocyte networks. *Neuron* 8: 429–440. [18]

Daniel, P. 1946. Spinal nerve endings in the extrinsic eye muscles of man. *J. Anat.* 80: 189–193. [26]

Daniel, P. M., and Whitteridge, D. 1961. The representation of the visual field on the cerebral cortex in monkeys. *J. Physiol.* 159: 203–221. [3]

Danilova, V., Damak, S., Margolskee, R. F., and Hellekant, G. 2006. Taste responses to sweet stimuli in alpha-gustducin knockout and wild-type mice. *Chem Senses* 31: 573–580. [21]

Danjo, T., Eiraku, M., Muguruma, K., et al. 2011. Subregional specification of embryonic stem cell-derived ventral telencephalic tissues by timed and combinatory treatment with extrinsic signals. *J. Neurosci.* 31: 1919–1933. [27]

Darbon, P., Tscherter, A., Yvon, C., and Streit, J. 2003. Role of the electrogenic Na/K pump in disinhibition-induced bursting in cultured spinal networks. *J. Neurophysiol.* 90: 3119–3129. [7]

Darland, T., Heinricher, M. M., and Grandy, D. K. 1998. Orphanin FQ/nociceptin: A role in pain and analgesia, but so much more. *Trends Neurosci.* 21: 215–221. [14]

Dartnall, H. J., Bowmaker, J. K., and Mollon, J. D. 1983. Human visual pigments: Microspectrophotometric results from the eyes of seven persons. *Proc. R. Soc. Lond., B, Biol. Sci.* 220: 115–130. [22]

Darnell, J. C., and Klann, E. 2013. The translation of translational control by FMRP: Therapeutic targets for FXS. *Nat. Neurosci.* 16: 1530–1536. [17]

Dascal, N. 2001. Ion-channel regulation by G proteins. *Trends Endocrinol. Metab.* 12: 391–398. [12]

Dasen, J. S., and Jessell, T. M. 2009. Hox networks and the origins of motor neuron diversity. *Curr. Top. Dev. Biol.* 88: 169–200. [26]

DaSilva, A. F., Becerra, L., Makris, N., et al. 2002. Somatotopic activation in the human trigeminal pain pathway. *J. Neurosci.* 22: 8183–8192. [23]

Davalos, D., Grutzendler, J., Yang, G., et al. 2005. ATP mediates rapid microglial response to local brain injury in vivo. *Nat. Neurosci.* 8:752–758. [10]

David, S., and Aguayo, A. J. 1981. Axonal elongation into peripheral nervous system "bridges" after central nervous system injury in adult rats. *Science* 214: 931–933. [29]

David, S. V., Mesgarani, N., Fritz, J. B., and Shamma, S. A. 2009. Rapid synaptic depression explains nonlinear modulation of spectrotemporal tuning in primary auditory cortex by natural stimuli. *J. Neurosci.* 29: 3374–3386. [24]

Davidson, A. J., Yamazaki, S., and Menaker, M. 2003. SCN: Ringmaster of the circadian circus or conductor of the circadian orchestra? *Novartis Found. Symp.* 253: 110–121. [19]

Davidson, S. and Giesler, G. J. 2010. The multiple pathways for itch and their interactions with pain. *Trends Neurosci.* 33: 550–558. doi: 10.1016/j.tins.2010.09.002. [21]

Davies, A. M., and Lumsden, A. 1990. Ontogeny of the somatosensory system: Origins and early development of primary sensory neurons. *Annu. Rev. Neurosci.* 13: 61–73. [27]

Davies, C. H., and Collingridge, G. L. 1993. The physiological regulation of synaptic inhibition by GABAB autoreceptors in rat hippocampus. *J. Physiol.* 472: 245–265. [11]

Davies, J. G., Kirkwood, P. A., and Sears, T. A. 1985. The distribution of monosynaptic connexions from inspiratory bulbospinal neurones to inspiratory motoneurones in the cat. *J. Physiol.* 368: 63–87. [26]

Davies, K. E., and Nowak, K. J. 2006. Molecular mechanisms of muscular dystrophies: Old and new players. *Nat. Rev. Mol. Cell Biol.* 7: 762–773. [11]

Davies, P. A., Wang, W., Hales, T. G., and Kirkness, E. F. 2003. A novel class of ligand-gated ion channel is activated by Zn^{2+} *J. Biol. Chem.* 278: 712–717. [5]

Davies, S. J. A., Fitch, M. T., Memberg, S. P., et al. 1997. Regeneration of adult axons in white matter tracts of the central nervous system. *Nature* 390: 680–683. [29]

Davis, K. D. 2000. The neural circuitry of pain as explored with functional MRI. *Neurol. Res.* 22: 313–317. [23]

Davis, R., and Koelle, G. B. 1978. Electron microscope localization of acetylcholinesterase and butyrylcholinesterase in the superior cervical ganglion of the cat. I. Normal ganglion. *J. Cell Biol.* 78: 785–809. [15]

Davis, R. L., Weintraub, H., and Lassar, A. B. 1987. Expression of a single transfected cDNA converts fibroblasts to myoblasts. *Cell* 51: 987–1000. [27]

Daw, N. W. 1998. Critical periods and amblyopia. *Arch. Ophthalmol.* 116: 502–505. [28]

Daw, N. W., Jensen, R. J., and Brunken, W. J. 1990. Rod pathways in mammalian retinae. *Trends Neurosci.* 13: 110–115. [2, 18, 22]

Daw, N. W., Reid, S. N., Wang, X. F., and Flavin, H. J. 1995. Factors that are critical for plasticity in the visual cortex. *Ciba Found. Symp.* 193: 258–276; discussion 322–254. [28]

Day, J. J., and Sweatt, J. D. 2011. Epigenetic mechanisms in cognition. *Neuron* 70: 813–829. [17]

De Biase, L. M., Nishiyama, A., and Bergles, D. E. 2010. Excitability and synaptic communication within the oligodendrocyte lineage. *J. Neurosci.* 30: 3600–3611. doi: 10.1523/jneurosci.6000-09.2010. [10]

D'Este, E., Kamin, D., Balzarotti, F., and Hell, S. W. 2017. Ultrastructural anatomy of nodes of Ranvier in the peripheral nervous system as revealed by STED microscopy. *Proc. Natl. Acad. Sci. USA* 114: e191–e199. [10]

De Boysson-Bardies, B., Halle, P., Sagart, L., and Durand, C. 1989. A crosslinguistic investigation of vowel formants in babbling. *J. Child Lang.* 16: 1–17. [24]

De Felipe, C., Herrero, J. F., O'Brien, J. A., et al. 1998. Altered nociception, analgesia and aggression in mice lacking the receptor for substance P. *Nature* 392: 394–397. [14]

de Kock, C. P. et al. 2004. NMDA receptors induce somatodendritic secretion in hypothalamic neurones of lactating female rats. *J. Physiol.* 2004; 561: 53–64. [18]

de Kock, C. P. J., Cornelisse, L. N., Burnashev, N., et al. 2006. NMDA receptors trigger neurosecretion of 5-HT within dorsal raphe nucleus of the rat in the absence of action potential firing. *J. Physiol.* 577: 891–905. doi: 10.1113/jphysiol.2006.115311. [18]

de Lecea, L., Kilduff, T. S., Peyron, C., et al. 1998. The hypocretins: Hypothalamus-specific peptides with neuroexcitatory activity. *Proc. Natl. Acad. Sci. USA* 95: 322–327. [14]

De-Miguel, F. F., and Aréchiga, H. 1992. Sensory inputs mediating two opposite behavioural responses to light in the crayfish *procambarus clarkii*. *J. Exp. Biol.* 164: 153–169. [20]

De-Miguel, F. F., and Nicholls, J. G. 2015. Release of chemical transmitters from cell bodies and dendrites of nerve cells. *Philos. Trans. R Soc. Lond. B Biol. Sci.* 370: 20140181. [18]

De-Miguel, F. F., and Trueta, C. 2005. Synaptic and extrasynaptic secretion of serotonin. *Cell Mol. Neurobiol.* 25: 297–312. [15]

De-Miguel, F. F., Leon-Pinzon, C., Noguez, P., and Mendez, B. 2015. Serotonin release from the neuronal cell body and its long-lasting effects on the nervous system. Philos. Trans. *R. Soc. Lond. B Biol. Sci.* 370: 20140196. [18]

De-Miguel, F. F., Santamaría-Holek, I., Noguez, P., et al. 2012. Biophysics of active vesicle transport, an intermediate step that couples excitation and exocytosis of serotonin in the neuronal soma. *PLOS ONE* 7: e45454. (Correction: doi: 10.1371/annotation/b72afb21–407c-46e9-9870-7c59ab9e582c.) [18]

De-Miguel, F. F., Vargas-Caballero, M., García-Pérez, E. 2001. Spread of synaptic potentials through electrical synapses in Retzius neurones of the leech. *J. Exp Biol.* 204: 3241–3250. [18]

De Nadai, T., Marchetti, L., Di Rienzo, C., et al. 2015. Precursor and mature NGF live tracking: One *versus* many at a time in the axons *Scientif. Rep.* 6: 20272. doi: 10.1038/srep20272. [27]

De Potter, W. P., Smith, A. D., and De Schaepdryver, A. F. 1970. Subcellular fractionation of splenic nerve: ATP, chromogranin A, and dopamine β-hydroxylase in noradrenergic vesicles. *Tissue Cell* 2: 529–546. [15]

de Villers-Sidani, E., Chang, E. F., Bao, S., and Merzenich, M. M. 2007. Critical period window for spectral tuning defined in the primary auditory cortex (A1) in the rat. *J. Neurosci.* 27: 180–189. [28]

De Waard, M., Hering, J., Weiss, N., and Feltz, A. 2005. How do G proteins directly control neuronal Ca^{2+} channel function? *Trends Pharmacol. Sci.* 26: 427–436. [12]

Des Rosiers, M. H., Sakurada, O., Jehle, J., et al. Functional plasticity in the immature striate cortex of the monkey shown by the [14C] deoxyglucose method. 1978. . *Science* 200: 447–449. [28]

DeAngelis, G. C., Cumming, B. G., and Newsome, W. T. 1998. Cortical area MT and the perception of stereoscopic depth. *Nature* 394: 677–680. [2]

Debanne, D., and Thompson, S. M. 1996. Associative long-term depression in the hippocampus in vitro. *Hippocampus* 6: 9–16. [16]

Debby-Brafman, A., Burstyn-Cohen, T., Klar, A., and Kalcheim, C. 1999. F-Spondin, expressed in somite regions avoided by neural crest cells, mediates inhibition of distinct somite domains to neural crest migration. *Neuron* 22: 475–488. [27]

DeChiara, T. M., Vejsada, R., Poueymirou, W. T., et al. 1995. Mice lacking the CNTF receptor, unlike mice lacking CNTF, exhibit profound motor neuron deficits at birth. *Cell* 83: 313–322. [29]

Dedek, K., Kunath, B., Kananura, C., et al. 2001. Myokymia and neonatal epilepsy caused by a mutation in the voltage sensor of KCNQ2 K$^+$ channel. *Proc. Natl. Acad. Sci. USA.* 98: 12272–12277. [5]

Deeb, S. S. 2006. Genetics of variation in human color vision and the retinal cone mosaic. *Curr. Opin. Genet. Dev.* 16: 301–307. [22]

Deeb, S. S., and Kohl, S. 2003. Genetics of color vision deficiencies. *Dev. Ophthalmol.* 37: 170–187. [22]

DeFazio, R. A., Dvoryanchikov, G., Maruyama, Y., et al. 2006. Separate populations of receptor cells and presynaptic cells in mouse taste buds. *J. Neurosci.* 26: 3971–3980. [21]

Deiters, O.1859. Beiträge zur Kenntniss der Lamina spiralis membranacea der Schnecke. *Z. Wissenschaft Zool.* 1–12. [1]

Del-Bel, E., Padovan-Neto, F. E., Raisman-Vozari, R., and Lazzarini, M. 2011. Role of nitric acid in motor control: Implications for Parkinson's disease pathophysiology and treatment. *Curr. Pharm. Des.* 17: 471–488. [26]

del Castillo, J., and Katz, B. 1954. Quantal components of the end-plate potential. *J. Physiol.* 124: 560–573. [13]

del Castillo, J., and Katz, B. 1954. Statistical factors involved in neuromuscular facilitation and depression. *J. Physiol.* 124: 574–585. [16]

del Castillo, J., and Katz, B. 1954. Changes in end-plate activity produced by presynaptic polarization. *J. Physiol.* 124: 586–604. [13]

del Castillo, J., and Katz, B. 1955. On the localization of end-plate receptors. *J. Physiol.* 128: 157–181. [11]

del Castillo, J., and Katz, B. 1956. Biophysical aspects of neuromuscular transmission. *Prog. Biophys. Biophys. Chem.* 6: 121–170. [13]

del Castillo, J., and Stark, L. 1952. The effect of calcium ions on the motor end-plate potentials. *J. Physiol.* 116: 507–515. [13]

del Río-Hortega, P. 1920. La microglia y su transformacion celulas en basoncito y cuerpos granulo-adiposos. *Trab. Lab. Invest. Biol. Madrid* 18: 37–82. [10]

Dell'Anno, M. T., Wang, X., Onorati, M., et al. 2018. Human neuroepithelial stem cell regional specificity enables spinal cord repair through a relay circuit. *Nat. Comm.* 9: 3419. doi:10.1038/s41467-018-05844-8. [29]

Deller, T., Haas, C. A., Freiman, T. M., et al. 2006. Lesion-induced axonal sprouting in the central nervous system. *Adv. Exp. Med. Biol.* 557: 101–121. [29]

Delmas, P., and Brown, D. A. 2005. Pathways modulating neural KCNQ/M (Kv7) potassium channels. *Nat. Rev. Neurosci.* 6: 850–862. [19]

Delmas, P., Brown, D. A., Dayrell, M., et al. 1998. On the role of endogenous G-protein beta gamma subunits in N-type Ca^{2+} current inhibition by neurotransmitters in rat sympathetic neurones. *J. Physiol.* 506: 319–329. [12]

Delmas, P., Crest, M., and Brown, D. A. 2004. Functional organization of PLC signaling microdomains in neurons. *Trends Neurosci.* 27: 41–47. [12]

Delmas, P., Wanaverbecq, N., Abogadie, F. C., et al. 2002. Signaling microdomains define the specificity of receptor-mediated InsP(3) pathways in neurons. *Neuron* 34: 209–220. [12]

DeLong, M., and Wichmann, T. 2009. Update on models of basal ganglia function and dysfunction. *Parkinsonism Relat Disord.* 15(Suppl. 3): S247–240. [26]

Denda, S., and Reichardt, L. F. 2007. Studies on integrins in the nervous system. *Methods Enzymol.* 426: 203–221. [27]

Deniz, S., Wersinger, E., Schwab, Y., et al. 2011. Mammalian retinal horizontal cells are unconventional GABAergic neurons. *J. Neurochem.* 116: 350–362. [22]

Denk, W., Holt, J. R., Shepherd, G. M., and Corey, D. P. 1995. Calcium imaging of single stereocilia in hair cells: Localization of transduction channels at both ends of tip links. *Neuron* 15: 1311–1321. [21]

Denk, W., Sugimori, M., and Llinas, R. 1995. Two types of calcium response limited to single spines in cerebellar Purkinje cells. *Proc. Natl. Acad. Sci. USA* 92: 8279–8282. [12]

Dennis, M. J., and Miledi, R. 1974. Characteristics of transmitter release at regenerating frog neuromuscular junctions. *J. Physiol.* 239: 571–594. [13]

Dennis, M. J., and Sargent, P. B. 1979. Loss of extrasynaptic acetylcholine sensitivity upon reinnervation of parasympathetic ganglion cells. *J. Physiol.* 289: 263–275. [29]

Dennis, M. J., and Yip, J. W. 1978. Formation and elimination of foreign synapses on adult salamander muscle. *J. Physiol.* 274: 299–310. [29]

Dennis, M. J., Harris, A. J., and Kuffler, S. W. 1971. Synaptic transmission and its duplication by focally applied acetylcholine in parasympathetic neurons in the heart of the frog. *Proc. Roy. Soc. Lond., B, Biol. Sci.* 177: 509–539. [11]

Denton, R. M., Mckormack, J. G., and Edgell, N. J. 1990. The hormonal regulation of pyruvate dehydrogenase complex. *Physiol. Rev.* 70: 391–425. [18]

Denzer, A. J., Schulthess, T., Fauser, C., et al. 1998. Electron microscopic structure of agrin and mapping of its binding site in laminin-1. *EMBO J.* 17: 335–343. [29]

Derijck, A. A., Van Erp, S., and Pasterkamp, R. J. 2010. Semaphorin signaling: Molecular switches at the midline. *Trends Cell Biol.* 20: 568–576. [27]

Desai, A. R., and McConnell, S. K. 2000. Progressive restriction in fate potential by neural progenitors during cerebral cortical development. *Development* 127: 2863–2872. [27]

Descarries, L. et al. 1996. The structural bases of the regulation of neuron sensitivity. *J. Comp. Neurol.* 375: 167–186. [18]

Descarries, L., Gisiger, V., and Steriade, M. 1997. Diffuse transmission by acetylcholine in the CNS. *Prog. Neurobiol.* 53: 603–625. [14]

Desimone, R., Albright, T. D., Gross, C. G., and Bruce, C. 1984. Stimulus-selective properties of inferior temporal neurons in the macaque. J. Neurosci. 4: 2051–2062. [25]

Des Rosiers, M. H., Sakurada, O., Jehle, J., et al. Functional plasticity in the immature striate cortex of the monkey shown by the [14C] deoxyglucose method. 1978. *Science* 200: 447–449. [28]

Devaux, J. J., Kleopas, K. A., Cooper, E. C., and Scherer, S. S. 2004. KCNQ2 is a nodal K$^+$ channel. *J. Neurosci.* 24: 1236–1244. [8]

DeVries, S. H. 2000. Bipolar cells use kainate and AMPA receptors to filter visual information into separate channels. *Neuron* 28: 847–856. [22]

DeVries, S. H., and Baylor, D. A. 1995. An alternative pathway for signal flow from rod photoreceptors to ganglion cells in mammalian retina. *Proc. Natl. Acad. Sci. USA* 92: 10658–10662. [22]

DeVries, S. H., and Schwartz, E. A. 1989. Modulation of an electrical synapse between solitary pairs of catfish horizontal cells by dopamine and second messengers. *J. Physiol.* 414: 351–375. [18]

Deyoe, E. A., Hockfield, S., Garren, H., Van Essen, D. C. 1990. Antibody labeling of functional subdivisions in visual cortex: Cat-301 immunoreactivity in striate and extrastriate cortex of the macaque monkey. *Vis. Neurosci.* 5: 67–81. [3]

Diamond, M. E., Armstrong-James, M., and Ebner, F. F. 1993. Experience-dependent plasticity in adult rat barrel cortex. *Proc. Natl. Acad. Sci. USA* 90: 2082–2086. [23]

Diamond, M. E., Huang, W., and Ebner, F. F. 1994. Laminar comparison of somatosensory cortical plasticity. *Science* 265: 1885–1888. [23]

Diamond, M. E., von Heimendahl, M., Knutsen, P. M., et al. 2008. 'Where' and 'what' in the whisker sensorimotor system. *Nat. Rev. Neurosci.* 9: 601–612. [23]

Diana, M., and Tepper, J. M. 2002. Electrophysiological pharmacology of mesencephalic dopaminergic neurons. In *Handbook of Experimental Pharmacology*, Vol. 154, part 1. Springer-Verlag, Berlin, pp. 1–62. [14]

Díaz-García, C. M., Mongeon, R., Lahmann, C., et al. 2017. Neuronal stimulation triggers neuronal glycolysis and not lactate uptake. *Cell Metab.* 26: 361–374. doi: 10.1016/j.cmet.2017.06.021. [10]

Díaz-Hernández, E. 2018. The thalamostriatal projections contribute to the initiation and execution of a sequence of movements. *Neuron* 100: 739–752. [26]

Dibaj, P., Nadrigny, F., Steffens, H., et al. 2010. NO mediates microglial response to acute spinal cord injury under ATP control in vivo. *Glia* 58: 1133–1144. [10]

Dib-Hajj, S. D., Yang, Y., Black, J. A., and Waxman, S. G. 2013. The NaV1.7 sodium channel: *Nature Rev Neurosci* 14: 49–62. [5]

DiCarlo, J. J., and Cox, D. D. 2007. Untangling invariant object recognition. *Trends Cogn. Sci.* 11: 333–341. [25]

DiCarlo, J. J., and Johnson, K. O. 2000. Spatial and temporal structure of receptive fields in primate somatosensory area 3b: Effects of stimulus scanning direction and orientation. *J. Neurosci.* 20: 495–510. [23]

DiCarlo, J. J., and Johnson, K. O. 2002. Receptive field structure in cortical area 3b of the alert monkey. *Behav. Brain Res.* 135: 167–178. [23]

DiCarlo, J. J., Johnson, K. O., and Hsiao, S. S. 1998. Structure of receptive fields in area 3b of primary somatosensory cortex in the alert monkey. *J. Neurosci.* 18: 2626–2645. [23]

DiCarlo, J. J., Zoccolan D., and Rust, N. C. 2012. How does the brain solve visual object recognition? *Neuron* 73: 415–434. doi: 10.1016/j.neuron.2012.01.010. [25]

Dickinson-Nelson, A., and Reese, T. S. 1983. Structural changes during transmitter release at synapses in the frog sympathetic ganglion. *J. Neurosci.* 3: 42–52. [13]

Dickson, B. J., and Gilestro, G. F. 2006. Regulation of commissural axon pathfinding by slit and its Robo receptors. *Annu. Rev. Cell. Dev. Biol.* 22: 651–675. [27]

Diesseroth, K. 2011. Optogenetics. *Nat. Methods* 8: 26–29. [14]

Dietrichs, E. 2008. Clinical manifestation of focal cerebellar disease as related to the organization of neural pathways. *Acta Neurol Scand. Suppl.* 188: 6–11. [26]

Dietzel, I., Heinemann, U., and Lux, H.D. 1989. Relations between slow extracellular potential changes, glial potassium buffering, and electrolyte and cellular volume changes during neuronal hyperactivity in cat brain. *Glia* 2: 25–44. [10]

DiFrancesco, D., and Tortura, D. P. 1991. Direct activation of cardiac pacemaker channels by intracellular cyclic AMP. *Nature* 351: 145–147. [12]

Dimou, L. and Goetz, M. 2014. Glial cells as progenitors and stem cells: New roles in the healthy and diseased brain. *Physiol. Rev.* 94: 709–737. [29]

Dimou, L., and Gallo, V. 2015. NG2-glia and their functions in the central nervous system. *Glia* 63: 1429–1451. [29]

Dimou, L., and Goetz, M. 2014. Glial cells as progenitors and stem cells: New roles in the healthy and diseased brain. *Physiol. Rev.* 94: 709–737. [27]

Dingledine, R., Borges, K., Bowie, D., and Traynelis, S. F. 1999. The glutamate receptor ion channels. *Pharmacol. Rev.* 51: 7–61. [5]

Dionne, V. E., and Leibowitz, M. D. 1982. Acetylcholine receptor kinetics. A description from single-channel currents at the snake neuromuscular junction. *Biophys. J.* 39: 253–261. [11]

DiPaola, M., Czajkowski, C., and Karlin, A. 1989. The sidedness of the COOH terminus of the acetylcholine receptor δ subunit. *J. Biol. Chem.* 264: 15457–15463. [5]

Diss, J. K. J., Fraser, S. P., and Djamgoz, M. B. A. 2004. Voltage-gated Na+ channels: Multiplicity of expression, plasticity, functional implications and pathophysiological aspects. *Eur. Biophys. J.* 33: 180–193. [5]

Do, M. T. H. 2019. Melanopsin and the intrinsically photosensitive retinal ganglion cells: Biophysics to behavior. *Neuron* 104: 205–226. [22]

Do, M. T., Kang, S. H., Xue, T., et al. 2009. Photon capture and signalling by melanopsin retinal ganglion cells. *Nature* 457: 281–287. [19]

Dodd, J., and Horn, J. P. 1983. A reclassification of B and C neurones in the ninth and tenth paravertebral sympathetic ganglia of the bullfrog. *J. Physiol.* 334: 255–269. [12]

Dodd, J., and Horn, J. P. 1983. Muscarinic inhibition of sympathetic C cells in the bullfrog. *J Physiol.* 334: 271–291. [12]

Dodge, F. A., Jr., and Rahamimoff, R. 1967. Co-operative action of calcium ions in transmitter release at the neuromuscular junction. *J. Physiol.* 193: 419–432. [13]

Doe, C. Q., Kuwada, J. Y., and Goodman, C. S. 1985. From epithelium to neuroblasts to neurons: The role of cell interactions and cell lineage during insect neurogenesis. *Philos. Trans. R. Soc. Lond., B, Biol. Sci.* 312: 67–81. [27]

Doerrbaum, A. R., et al. 2018. Local and global influences on protein turnover in neurons and glia. *eLife* 7: e34202. [17]

Domenici, L., Berardi, N., Carmignoto, G., et al. 1991. Nerve growth factor prevents the amblyopic effects of monocular deprivation. *Proc. Natl. Acad. Sci. USA* 88: 8811–8815. [28]

Domenici, L., Cellerino, A., Berardi, N., et al. 1994. Antibodies to nerve growth factor (NGF) prolong the sensitive period for monocular deprivation in the rat. *Neuroreport* 5: 2041–2044. [28]

Domenici, M. R., Berretta, N., and Cherubini, E. 1998. Two distinct forms of long-term depression co-exist at the mossy fiber-CA3 synapse in the hippocampus during development. *Proc. Natl. Acad. Sci. USA* 95: 8310–8315. [16]

Doron, K. W., and Gazzaniga, M. S. 2008. Neuroimaging techniques offer new perspectives on callosal transfer and interhemispheric communication. *Cortex* 44: 1023–1029. [3]

Dougherty, K. J., and Kiehn, O. 2010. Functional organization of V2a-related locomotor circuits in the rodent spinal cord. *Ann. NY Acad. Sci.* 1198: 85–93. [26]

Doupnik, C. A., Davidson, N., Lester, H. A., and Kofuji, P. 1997. RGS proteins reconstitute the rapid gating kinetics of gbetagamma-activated inwardly rectifying K+ channels. *Proc. Natl. Acad. Sci. USA* 94: 10461–10466. [12]

Dowdall, M. J., Boyne, A. F., and Whittaker, V. P. 1974. Adenosine triphosphate: A constituent of cholinergic synaptic vesicles. *Biochem. J.* 140: 1–12. [15]

Dowling, J. E. 1987. *The Retina: An Approachable Part of the Brain.* Harvard University Press, Cambridge, MA. [22]

Dowling, J. E., and Boycott, B. B. 1966. Organization of the primate retina: Electron microscopy. *Proc. R. Soc. Lond., B, Biol. Sci.* 166: 80–111. [2, 18, 22]

Downing, P. E., Chan, A. W., Peelen, M. V., et al. 2006. Domain specificity in visual cortex. *Cereb. Cortex* 16: 1453–1461. [25]

Doyle, M., and Kleber, M. A. 2011. Mechanisms of dendritic mRNA transport and its role in synaptic tagging. *EMBO J.* 30: 3540–3552. [17]

Doyle, D. A., Cabral, J. M., Pfeutzner, A. K., et al. 1998. The structure of the potassium channel: Molecular basis of K+ conductance and selectivity. *Science* 280: 69–77. [5]

Drachman, D. B. 1994. Myasthenia gravis. *New England J. Med.* 330: 1797–1810. [13]

Dreifuss, J. J. et al. 1971. Action potentials and release of neurohypophysial hormones *in vitro. J. Physiol.* 215: 805–817. [18]

Drescher, U., Kremoser, C., Handwerker, C., et al. 1995. In vitro guidance of retinal ganglion cell axons by RAGS, a 25 kDa tectal protein related to ligands for Eph receptor tyrosine kinases. *Cell* 82: 359–370. [27]

Driver, J., and Halligan, P. W. 1991. Can visual neglect operate in object-centred co-ordinates? An affirmative single case study. *Cogn. Neuropsychol.* 8: 475–496. [30]

Droz, B., and Leblond, C. P. 1963. Axonal migration of proteins in the central nervous system and peripheral nerves as shown by radioautography. *J. Comp. Neurol.* 121: 325–346. [15]

Du Bois-Reymond, E. 1848. *Untersuchungen über thierische Electricität.* Reimer, Berlin. [11]

Du Vigneaud, V. 1955. Hormones of the posterior pituitary gland: Oxytocin and vasopressin. *Harvey Lect.* 50: 1–26. [14]

Duan, Y., Panoff, J., Burrell, B. D., et al. 2005. Repair and regeneration of functional synaptic connections: Cellular and molecular interactions in the leech. *Cell Mol. Neurobiol.* 25: 441–450. [20]

Duan, Y., Sahley, C. L., and Muller, K. J. 2009. ATP and NO dually control migration of microglia to nerve lesions. *Dev. Neurobiol.* 69: 60–72. [10]

Dubois, J. M. 1983. Potassium currents in the frog node of Ranvier. *Prog. Biophys. Mol. Biol.* 42: 1–20. [8]

Dubouic, D. 2007. The rise and fall of *Hox* gene clusters. *Development* 134: 2549–2560. [27]

Dubreuil, V., Barhanin, J., Goridis, C., and Brunet, J. F. 2009 Breathing with *phox2b. Philos. Trans. R. Soc. Lond., B Biol. Sci.* 364: 2477–2483. [26]

Dudar, J. D., and Szerb, J. C. 1969. The effect of topically applied atropine on resting and evoked cortical acetylcholine release. *J. Physiol.* 203: 741–762. [14]

Dudek, S. M., and Bear, M. F. 1992. Homosynaptic long-term depression in area CA1 of hippocampus and the effects of *N*-methyl-D-aspartate receptor blockade. *Proc. Natl. Acad. Sci. USA* 89: 4363–4367. [16]

Dudek, S. M. and Fields, R. D. 2002. Somatic action potentials are sufficient for late-phase LTP-related cell signaling. *Proc. Natl. Acad. Sci. USA* 99: 3962–3967. [17]

Dudel, J., and Kuffler, S. W. 1961. Presynaptic inhibition at the crayfish neuromuscular junction. *J. Physiol.* 155: 543–562. [11]

Dugué, G. P., Brunel, N., Hakim, V., et al. 2009. Electrical coupling mediates tunable low-frequency oscillations and resonance in the cerebellar Golgi cell network. *Neuron* 61: 126–139. [11]

Dulac, C., and Axel, R. 1995. A novel family of genes encoding putative pheromone receptors in mammals. *Cell* 83: 195–206. [21]

Dulcis, D., Jamshidi, P., Leutgeb, S., and Spitzer, N. C. 2013. Neurotransmitter switching in the adult brain regulates behavior. *Science* 340: 449–453. [27]

Dun, N. J., and Minota, S. 1982. Post-tetanic depolarization in sympathetic neurones of the guinea-pig. *J. Physiol.* 323: 325–337. [18]

Dunnett, S. B., Björklund, A., and Stenevi, U. 1983. Dopamine-rich transplants in experimental parkinsonism. *Trends Neurosci.* 6: 266–270. [29]

Dunwiddie, T. V., and Masino, S. A. 2001. The role and regulation of adenosine in the central nervous system. *Annu. Rev. Neurosci.* 24: 31–55. [14, 15]

Dupin, E., Ziller, C., and Le Douarin, N. M. 1998. The avian embryo as a model in developmental studies: Chimeras and *in vitro* clonal analysis. *Curr. Top. Dev. Biol.* 36: 1–35. [27]

Durbaba, R., Taylor, A., Ellaway, P. H., and Rawlinson, S. 2003. The influence of bag$_2$ and chain intrafusal muscle fibers on secondary spindle afferents in the cat. *J. Physiol.* 550: 263–278. [26]

Durbeej, M. 2010. Laminins. *Cell Tissue Res.* 339: 259–268. [27]

Durkee, C. A., and Araque, A. 2019. Diversity and specificity of astrocyte–neuron communication. *Neuroscience* 396: 73–78. [18]

Dursteler, R. M., Wurtz, R. H., and Newsome, W. T. 1987. Directional pursuit deficits following lesions of the foveal representation within the superior temporal sulcus of the macaque monkey. *J. Neurophysiol.* 57: 1262–1287. [25]

Dusart, I., Ghoumari, A., Wehrle, R., et al. 2005. Cell death and axon regeneration of Purkinje cells after axotomy: Challenges of classical hypotheses of axon regeneration. *Brain Res. Brain Res. Rev.* 49: 300–316. [29]

Dutton, A., and Dyball, R. E. 1979. Phasic firing enhances vasopressin release from the rat neurohypophysis. *J. Physiol.* 290: 433–440. [18]

Dwyer, T. M., Adams, D. J., and Hille, B. 1980. The permeability of the endplate channel to organic ions in frog muscle. *J. Gen. Physiol.* 75: 469–492. [5]

Dykes, I. M., Freeman, F. M., Bacon, J. P., and Davies, J. A. 2004. Molecular basis of gap junctional communication in the CNS of the leech *Hirudo medicinalis*. *J. Neurosci.* 24: 886–894. [11]

Eatock, R. A., Rusch, A., Lysakowski, A., Saeki, M. 1998. Hair cells in mammalian utricles. *Otolaryngol. Head Neck Surg.* 119: 172–181. [24]

Eatock, R. A., Xue, J., and Kalluri, R. 2008. Ion channels in mammalian vestibular afferents may set regularity of firing. *J. Exp. Biol.* 211: 1764–1774. [24]

Ebert, D. H. and Greenberg M. E. 2013. Activity-dependent neuronal signalling and autism spectrum disorder. *Nature* 493: 327–337. [17]

Ebert, R., et al. 2009. Induced pluripotent stem cells from a spinal muscular atrophy patient. *Nature* 457: 277. [27]

Eccles, J. 1976. From electrical to chemical transmission in the central nervous system. *Notes Rec. R Soc. Lond.* 30: 219–230. [18]

Eccles, J. C. 1981. Physiology of motor control in man. *Appl. Neurophysiol.* 44: 5–15. [26]

Eccles, J. C., and O'Connor, W. J. 1939. Responses which nerve impulses evoke in mammalian striated muscles. *J. Physiol.* 97: 44–102. [11]

Eccles, J. C., and Sherrington, C. S. 1930. Numbers and contraction-values of individual motor-units examined in some muscles of the limb. *Proc. R. Soc. Lond., B, Biol. Sci.* 106: 326–357. [26]

Eccles, J. C., Eccles, R. M., and Magni, F. 1961. Central inhibitory action attributable to presynaptic depolarization produced by muscle afferent volleys. *J. Physiol.* 159: 147–166. [11]

Eccles, J. C., Fatt, P., and Koketsu, K. 1954. Cholinergic and inhibitory synapses in a pathway from motor-axon collaterals to motoneurones. *J. Physiol.* 126: 524–562. [14, 15]

Eccles, J. C., Katz, B., and Kuffler, S. W. 1941. Nature of the "endplate potential" in curarized muscle. *J. Neurophysiol.* 4: 362–387. [11]

Eccles, J. C., Katz, B., and Kuffler, S. W. 1942. Effects of eserine on neuromuscular transmission. *J. Neurophysiol.* 5: 211–230. [11]

Eccles, J. C. et al. (Eds.). 1986. In *Progress in Brain Research*, Vol. 680 Elsevier Science Publishers B.V. (Biomedical Division). [18]

Edin, B. B., and Vallbo, A. B. 1990. Muscle afferent responses to isometric contractions and relaxations in humans. *J. Neurophysiol.* 63: 1307–1313. [26]

Edmonds, B., Gibb, A. J., and Colquhoun, D. 1995. Mechanisms of activation of glutamate receptors and the time course of excitatory synaptic currents. *Annu. Rev. Physiol.* 57: 495–519. [11]

Edwards, C., Ottoson, D., Rydqvist, B., and Swerup, C. 1981. The permeability of the transducer membrane of the crayfish stretch receptor to calcium and other divalent cations. *Neuroscience* 6: 1455–1460. [21]

Edwards, D. H., Jr. 1984. Crayfish extraretinal photoreception. I. Behavioral and motorneuronal responses to abdominal illumination. *J. Exp. Biol.* 109: 291–306. [20]

Edwards, D. H., Heitler, W. J., and Krasne, F. B. 1999. Fifty years of a command neuron: The neurobiology of escape behavior in the crayfish. *Trends Neurosci.* 22: 153–161. [18, 20]

Edwards, F. A., Gibb, A. J., and Colquhoun, D. 1992. ATP receptor-mediated synaptic currents in the central nervous system. *Nature* 359: 144–147. [14]

Edwards, F. A., Konnerth, A., and Sakmann, B. 1990. Quantal analysis of inhibitory synaptic transmission in the dentate gyrus of rat hippocampal slices: A patch-clamp study. *J. Physiol.* 430: 213–249. [13]

Edwards, R. H. 2007. The neurotransmitter cycle and quantal size. *Neuron* 55: 835–858. [9, 15]

Egan, T. M., Henderson, G., North, R. A., and, Williams, J. T. 1983. Noradrenaline-mediated synaptic inhibition in rat locus coeruleus neurones. *J. Physiol.* 345: 477–88. [14]

Eggan, K., Baldwin, K., Tackett, M., et al. 2004. Mice cloned from olfactory sensory neurons. *Nature* 428: 44–49. [27]

Eggermann, E., and Feldmeyer, D. 2009. Cholinergic filtering in the recurrent excitatory microcircuit of cortical layer 4. *Proc. Natl. Acad. Sci. USA* 106: 11753–11758. [14]

Ehringer, H., and Hornykiewicz, O. 1960. Verteilung von Noradrenalin und Dopamin (3 -Hydroxytyramin) im Gehirn des Menschen und ihr Verhalten bei Erkrankungen des extrapyramidalen Systems. *Klin. Wochenschr.* 38: 1236–1239. [14]

Eiden, L. E. 1998. The cholinergic gene locus. *J. Neurochem.* 70: 2227–2240. [15]

Eiden, L. E., Schäfer, M. K.-H., Weihe, E., and Schütz, B. 2004. The vesicular amine transporter family (SLC18): Amine/proton antiporters required for vesicular accumulation and regulated exocytotic secretion of monoamines and acetylcholine. *Pflügers Arch.* 447: 636–640. [9]

Eikeles, N., and Esler, M. 2005. The neurobiology of human obesity. *Exp. Physiol.* 90: 673–682. [19]

Eilers, J., Plant, T., and Konnerth, A. 1996. Localized calcium signaling and neural integration in cerebellar Purkinje neurons. *Cell Calcium* 20: 215–226. [12]

Eiraku, M., et al. 2008. Self-organized formation of polarized cortical tissues from ESCs and its active manipulation by extrinsic signals. *Cell Stem Cell* 3, 519–532. [27]

Eiraku, M., Takata, N., Ishibashi, H., et al. 2011. Self-organizing optic-cup morphogenesis in three-dimensional culture. *Nature* 472: 51–56. [1]

Elbert, T., Pantev, C., Wienbruch, C., et al. 1995. Increased cortical representation of the fingers of the left hand in string players. *Science* 270: 305–307. [23]

Elden, L. E., Schäfer, M. K.-H., Weihe, E., and Schütz, B. 2004. The vesicular amine transporter family (SLC18): Amine/proton antiporters required for vesicular accumulation and regulated exocytotic secretion of monoamines and acetylcholine. *Pflügers Arch.* 447: 636–640. [9]

Elgersma, Y., and Silva, A. J. 1999. Molecular mechanisms of synaptic plasticity. *Curr. Opin. Neurobiol.* 9: 209–213. [16]

Elgoyhen, A. B., Johnson, D. S., Boulter, J., et al. 1994. α9: An acetylcholine receptor with novel pharmacological properties expressed in rat cochlear hair cells. *Cell* 79: 705–715. [24]

Elgoyhen, A. B., Vetter, D. E., Katz, E., et al. 2001. α10: A determinant of nicotinic cholinergic receptor function in mammalian vestibular and cochlear mechanosensory hair cells. *Proc. Natl. Acad. Sci. USA* 98: 3501–3506. [24]

Elhamdani, A., Azizi, F., and Artalejo, C. R. 2006. Double patch clamp reveals that transient fusion (kiss-and-run) is a major mechanism of secretion in calf adrenal chromaffin cells: High calcium shifts the mechanism from kiss-and-run to complete fusion. *J. Neurosci.* 26: 3030–3036. [13]

Elliott, T. R. 1904. On the action of adrenalin. *J. Physiol.* 31: (Proc.) xx–xxi. [11]

Elliott, T. R. 1904. On the innervation of the ileo-colic sphincter. *J. Physiol.* 31: 157–168. doi: 10.1113/jphysiol.1904.sp001028. [18]

Elliott, E. J., and Muller, K. J. 1983. Sprouting and regeneration of sensory axons after destruction of ensheathing glial cells in the leech central nervous system. *J. Neurosci.* 3: 1994–2006. [20]

Ellis-Davies, G. C. R. 2008. Neurobiology with caged calcium. *Chem. Rev.* 108: 1603–1613. [13]

Engel, J., Braig, C., Ruttiger, L., et al. 2006. Two classes of outer hair cells along the tonotopic axis of the cochlea. *Neuroscience* 143: 837–849. [24]

Engert, F., and Bonhoeffer, T. 1999. Dendritic spine changes associated with hippocampal long-term synaptic plasticity. *Nature* 399: 66–70. [16. 17]

England, J. D., Levinson, S. R., and Shrager, P. 1996. Immunocytochemical investigations of sodium channels along nodal and internodal portions of demyelinating axons. *Microsc. Res. Tech.* 34: 445–451. [8]

Ercan-Sencicek, A. G., Stillman, A. A., Ghosh, A. K., et al. 2010. L-histidine decarboxylase and Tourette's syndrome. *New England J. Med.* 362: 1901–1908. [14]

Erickson, J. D., De Gois, S., Varoqui, H., et al. 2006. Activity-dependent regulation of vesicular glutamate and GABA transporters: A means to scale quantal size. *Neurochem. Int.* 48: 643–649. [15]

Erickson, J. D., Varoqui, H., Schäfer, M. K., et al. 1994. Functional identification of a vesicular acetylcholine transporter and its expression from a "cholinergic" gene locus. *J. Biol. Chem.* 269: 21929–21932. [15]

Ericson, J., Muhr, J., Placzek, M., et al. 1995. Sonic hedgehog induces the differentiation of ventral forebrain neurons: A common signal for ventral patterning within the neural tube. *Cell* 81: 747–756. [27]

Eriksson, P., et al., 1998. Neurogenesis in the adult human hippocampus. *Nature Med.* 4: 1313–1317. [27]

Erlander, M. G., Tillakaratne, N. J. K., Feldblum, S., et al. 1991. Two genes encode distinct glutamate decarboxylases. *Neuron* 7: 91–100. [15]

Ernsberger, U. 2009. Role of neurotrophin signalling in the differentiation of neurons from dorsal root ganglia and sympathetic ganglia. *Cell Tissue Res.* 336: 349–384. [27]

Ernst, A., Alkass, K., Bernard, S., et al., 2014. Neurogenesis in the striatum of the adult human brain. *Cell* 156: 1072–1083. [27]

Ertel, E. A., Campbell, K. P., Harpold, M. M., et al. 2000. Nomenclature of voltage-gated calcium channels. *Neuron* 25: 533–525. [5]

Erxleben, C. F. 1993. Calcium influx through stretch-activated cation channels mediates adaptation by potassium current activation. *Neuroreport* 4: 616–618. [21]

Erxleben, C., and Kriebel, M. E. 1988. Subunit composition of the spontaneous miniature end-plate currents at the mouse neuromuscular junction. *J. Physiol.* 400: 659–676Erzurumlu, R. S. 2010. Critical period for the whisker-barrel system. *Exp. Neurol.* 222: 10–12. [28]

Erzurumlu R. S. 2010. Critical period for the whisker-barrel system. *Exp. Neurol.* 222: 10-12. [28]

Erzurumlu, R. S., and Gaspar, P. 2012. Development and critical period plasticity of the barrel cortex. *Eur. J. Neurosci.* 35: 1540–1553. [28]

Escher, P., Lacazette, E., Courtet, M., et al.2005. Synapses form in skeletal muscles lacking neuregulin receptors. *Science* 308: 1920–1923. [29]

Eshed-Eisenbach, Y. and Peles, E. 2013. The making of a node: A co-production of neurons and glia. *Curr. Opin. Neurobiol.* 23:1049–1056. doi: 10.1016/j.conb.2013.06.003. [10]

Esmaeili, V., and Diamond, M. E. 2019. Neuronal correlates of tactile working memory in prefrontal and vibrissal somatosensory cortex. *Cell Reports* 27: 3167–3181.e5. [25]

Espinosa-Medina, I., Saha, O., Boismoreau, F., et al. 2016.The sacral autonomic outflow is sympathetic. *Science.* 354: 893–897. [19]

Espuny-Camacho, I., Michelsen, K. A., Gall, D., et al., 2013. Pyramidal neurons derived from human pluripotent stem cells integrate efficiently into mouse brain circuits in vivo. *Neuron* 77: 440–456. [27]

Eugenin, J., and Nicholls, J. G. 1997. Chemosensory and cholinergic stimulation of fictive respiration in isolated CNS of neonatal opossum. *J. Physiol.* 501: 425–437. [26]

Eugenin, J., Nicholls, J. G., Cohen, L. B., and Muller, K. J. 2006. Optical recording from respiratory pattern generator of fetal mouse brainstem reveals a distributed network. *Neuroscience* 137: 1221–1227. [26]

Evans, M. G. 1996. Acetylcholine activates two currents in guinea-pig outer hair cells. *J. Physiol.* 491: 563–578. [24]

Evans, W. H., and Martin, P. E. M. 2002: Gap junctions: Structure and function. *Mol. Membr. Biol.* 19: 121–136. [8]

Evarts, E. V. 1965. Relation of discharge frequency to conduction velocity in pyramidal neurons. *J. Neurophysiol.* 28: 216–228. [26]

Evarts, E. V. 1966. Pyramidal tract activity associated with a conditioned hand movement in the monkey. *J. Neurophysiol.* 29: 1011–1027. [26]

Evers, J., Laser, M., Sun, Y. A., et al. 1989. Studies of nerve–muscle interactions in *Xenopus* cell culture: Analysis of early synaptic currents. *J. Neurosci.* 9: 1523–1539. [27, 29]

Eyzaguirre, C., and Kuffler, S. W. 1955. Processes of excitation in the dendrites and in the soma of single isolated sensory nerve cells of the lobster and crayfish. *J. Gen. Physiol.* 39: 87–119. [21]

Fagg, A. H., Hatsopoulos, N. G., de Lafuente, V., et al. 2007. Biomimetic brain machine interfaces for the control of movement. *J. Neurosci.* 27: 11842–11846. [25]

Fagiolini, M., and Hensch, T. K. 2000. Inhibitory threshold for critical-period activation in primary visual cortex. *Nature* 404: 183–186. [28]

Fain, G. L., Matthews, H. R., and Cornwall, M. C. 1996. Dark adaptation in vertebrate photoreceptors. *Trends Neurosci.* 19: 502–507. [22]

Faissner, A., and Steindler, D. 1995. Boundaries and inhibitory molecules in developing neural tissues. *Glia* 13: 233–254. [10]

Falck, B., Hillarp, N. A., Thieme, G., and Torp, A. 1962. Fluorescence of catecholamines and related compounds condensed with formaldehyde. *J. Histochem. Cytochem.* 10: 348–354. [14]

Falkenburger, B. H., Jensen, J. B., and Hille, B. 2010. Kinetics of M1 muscarinic receptor and G protein signaling to phospholipase C in living cells. *J. Gen. Physiol.* 135: 81–97. [12]

Falkenburger, B. H., Jensen, J. B., and Hille, B. 2010. Kinetics of PIP_2 metabolism and KCNQ2/3 channel regulation studied with a voltage-sensitive phosphatase in living cells. *J. Gen. Physiol.* 135: 99–114. [12]

Falker, B., and Adelman, J. P. 2008. Control of K_{Ca} channels by calcium nano-microdomains. *Neuron* 59: 873–881. [5]

Fallon, J. B., Irvine, D. R., and Shepherd, R. K. 2008. Cochlear implants and brain plasticity. *Hear Res.* 238: 110–117. [28]

Fambrough, D. M. 1979. Control of acetylcholine receptors in skeletal muscle. *Physiol. Rev.* 59: 165–227. [29]

Famiglietti, E. V., Jr., and Kolb, H. 1975. A bi-stratified amacrine cell and synaptic circuitry in the inner plexiform layer of the retina. *Brain Res.* 84: 293–300. [22]

Fania, C., et al. 2017. Polymerase-free measurement of microRNA-122 with single base specificity using single molecule arrays: Detection of drug-induced liver injury. *PLOS ONE* 12: e0179280. [18]

Fanselow, M. S., and Kim, J. J. 1994. Acquisition of contextual Pavlovian fear conditioning is blocked by application of an NMDA receptor antagonist D,L-2-amino-5-Phosphonovaleric acid to the basolateral amygdala. *Behav. Neurosci.* 108: 210–212. [16]

Färber, K., and Kettenmann, H. 2005. Physiology of microglial cells. *Brain Res. Brain Res. Rev.* 48: 133–143. [10]

Farbman, A. I. 1994. Developmental biology of olfactory sensory neurons. *Semin. Cell Biol.* 5: 3–10. [21]

Farinas, I., Yoshida, C. K., Backus, C., and Reichardt, L. F. 1996. Lack of neurotrophin-3 results in death of spinal sensory neurons and premature differentiation of their precursors. *Neuron* 17: 1065–1078. [27]

Farrant, M., and Nusser, Z. 2005. Variations on an inhibitory theme: Phasic and tonic activation of GABA_A receptors. *Nat. Rev. Neurosci.* 6: 215–229. [14]

Farris, S., et al. 2014. Memory and executive function in aging and AD. *J. Neurosci.* 34: 448–443. [17]

Fassihi, A., Akrami A., Esmaeili, V., and Diamond, M. E. 2014. Tactile perception and working memory in rats and humans. *Proc. Natl. Acad. Sci. USA* 111: 2331–2336. [25]

Fatt, P., and Ginsborg, B. L. 1958. The ionic requirements for the production of action potentials in crustacean muscle fibres. *J. Physiol.* 142: 516–543. [7]

Fatt, P., and Katz, B. 1951. An analysis of the end-plate potential recorded with an intra-cellular electrode. *J. Physiol.* 115: 320–370. [6, 11, 15]

Fatt, P., and Katz, B. 1952. Spontaneous subthreshold potentials at motor nerve endings. *J. Physiol.* 117: 109–128. [13]

Fatt, P., and Katz, B. 1953. The effect of inhibitory nerve impulses on a crustacean muscle fibre. *J. Physiol.* 121: 374–389. [11]

Fawcett, J. 2009. Molecular control of brain plasticity and repair. *Prog. Brain Res.* 175: 501–509. [28]

Fawcett, J. W. 2015. The extracellular matrix in plasticity and regeneration after CNS injury and neurodegenerative disease. *Progr. Brain Res.* 218: 213–226. [29]

Fawcett, J. W., and Keynes, R. J. 1990. Peripheral nerve regeneration. *Annu. Rev. Neurosci.* 13: 43–60. [29]

Fawcett, J. W., and Verhaagen, J. 2018. Intrinsic determinants of axon regeneration. *Dev. Neurobiol.* 78: 890–897. DOI 10.1002/dneu22637. [29]

Feinberg, K., Eshed-Eisenbach, Y., Frechter, S., et al. 2010. A glial signal consisting of gliomedin and NrCAM clusters axonal Na+ channels during the formation of nodes of Ranvier. *Neuron* 65: 490–502. [10]

Fekete, D. M., Rouiller, E. M., Liberman, M. C., and Ryugo, D. K. 1984. The central projections of intracellularly labeled auditory nerve fibers in cats. *J. Comp. Neurol.* 229: 432–450. [24]

Feldberg, W. 1945. Present views of the mode of action of acetylcholine in the central nervous system. *Physiol. Rev.* 25: 596–642. [11]

Feldberg, W. 1950. The role of acetylcholine in the central nervous system. *Br. Med. Bull.* 6: 312–321. [14]

Feldheim, D. A., and O'Leary, D. D. 2010. Visual map development: Bidirectional signaling, bifunctional guidance molecules, and competition. *Cold Spring Harb. Perspect. Biol.* 2: A001768. [27]

Feldman, D. E., and Knudsen, E. I. 1997. An anatomical basis for visual calibration of the auditory space map in the barn owl's midbrain. *J. Neurosci.* 17: 6820–6837. [28]

Feldman, J. L., Mitchell, G. S., and Nattie, E. E. 2003. Breathing: Rhythmicity, plasticity, chemosensitivity. *Annu. Rev. Neurosci.* 26: 249–266. [26]

Feller, M. B. 2009. Retinal waves are likely to instruct the formation of eye-specific retinogeniculate projections. *Neural Dev.* 4: 24. [28]

Fellman, D. J., and Van Essen, D. C. 1991. Distributed hierarchical processing in the primate cerebral cortex. *Cereb. Cortex* 1: 1–47. [25]

Felmy, F., Neher, E., and Schneggenberger, R. 2003. The timing of phasic transmitter release is Ca2+-dependent and lacks direct influence of presynaptic terminal membrane potential. *Proc. Natl. Acad. Sci. USA* 100: 15200–15205. [13]

Feng, D., Kim, T., Ozkan, E., et al. 2010. Molecular and structural insight into proNGF engagement of p75NTR and sortilin. *J. Mol. Biol.* 396: 967–984. [27]

Ferguson, I. A. et al. 1991. Receptor-mediated retrogade transport in CNS neurons after intraventricular administration of NGF and growth factors. *J. Comp Neurol.* 313: 680–692. [18]

Fernandez-Fernandez, J. M., Abogadie, F. C., Milligan, G., et al. 2001. Multiple pertussis toxin-sensitive G-proteins can couple receptors to GIRK channels in rat sympathetic neurons when expressed heterologously, but only native G(i)-proteins do so in situ. *Eur. J. Neurosci.* 14: 283–292. [12]

Fernandez-Fernandez, J. M., Wanaverbecq, N., Halley, P., et al. 1999. Selective activation of heterologously expressed G protein-gated K+ channels by M2 muscarinic receptors in rat sympathetic neurones. *J. Physiol.* 515: 631–637. [12]

Fernandez-Liero, R. and Scheres, S. H. W. 2016. Unravelling biological macromolecules with cryo-electron microscopy. *Nature* 537: 339–346. [5]

Fernández, M. de L., Chan, Y. B., Yew, J. Y., et al. 2010. Pheromonal and behavioral cues trigger male-to-female aggression in *Drosophila*. *PLOS Biol.* 8: e1000541. [30]

Ferrington, D. G., and Rowe, M. 1980. Differential contributions to coding of cutaneous vibratory information by cortical somatosensory areas I and II. *J. Neurophysiol.* 43: 310–331. [23]

Ferster, D., Chung, S., and Wheat, H. 1996. Orientation selectivity of thalamic input to simple cells of cat visual cortex. *Nature* 380: 249–252. [2]

Fertuck, H. C., and Salpeter, M. M. 1974. Localization of acetylcholine receptor by 125I-labeled α-bungarotoxin binding at mouse motor endplates. *Proc. Natl. Acad. Sci. USA* 71: 1376–1378. [11]

Fesenko, E. E., Kolesnikov, S. S., and Lyubarsky, A. L. 1985. Induction by cyclic GMP of cationic conductance in plasma membrane of retinal rod outer segment. *Nature* 313: 310–313. [22]

Fettiplace, R. 1987. Electrical tuning of hair cells in the inner ear. *Trends Neurosci.* 10: 421–425. [24]

Fettiplace, R. 2016. Is TMC1 the Hair Cell Mechanotransducer channel? *Biophys. J.* 111: 3–9. [5]

Fiacco, A., and McCarthy, K. D. 2004. Intracellular astrocyte calcium waves in situ increase the frequency of spontaneous AMPA receptor currents in CA1 pyramidal neurons. *J. Neurosci.* 24: 722–732. [10]

Fiacco, T. A., Agulhon, C., and McCarthy, K. D. 2009. Sorting out astrocyte physiology from pharmacology. *Annu. Rev. Pharmacol. Toxicol.* 49: 151–174. [10]

Fiddes, I. T., et al. 2018. Human-specific NOTCH2NL genes affect notch signaling and cortical neurogenesis. *Cell* 173: 1356–1369. [27]

Fields, R. D., and Burnstock, G. 2006. Purinergic signaling in neuron glial interactions. *Nat. Rev. Neurosci.* 7: 423–436. [14]

Fierro, L., and Llano, I. 1996. High endogenous calcium buffering in Purkinje cells from rat cerebellar slices. *J. Physiol.* 496: 617–625. [12]

Figueres-Oñate, M., García-Marqués, J., and López-Mascaraque, L. 2016. UbC-StarTrack, a clonal method to target the entire progeny of individual progenitors. *Sci Rep.* 6: 33896. doi: 10.1038/srep33896. [10]

Filip, M., and Bader, M. 2009. Overview on 5-HT receptors and their role in physiology and pathology of the central nervous system. *Pharmacol Rep.* 61: 761–777. [14]

Filippov, A. K., Choi, R. C., Simon, J., et al. 2006. Activation of P2Y_1 nucleotide receptors induces inhibition of the M-type K+ current in rat hippocampal pyramidal neurons. *J. Neurosci.* 26: 9340–9348. [14]

Filippov, A. K., Couve, A., Pangalos, M. N., et al. 2000. Heteromeric assembly of GABA_BR1 and GABA_BR2 receptor subunits inhibits Ca2+ current in sympathetic neurons. *J. Neurosci.* 20: 2867–2874. [14]

Fillenz, M. 2005. In vivo neurochemical monitoring and the study of behaviour. *Neurosci. Biobehav. Rev.* 29: 949–962. [1]

Fillenz, M. 2005. The role of lactate in brain metabolism. *Neurochem. Int.* 47: 413–417. [10]

Finelli, M. J., Wong, J. K., and Zou, H. Epigenetic regulation of sensory axon regeneration after spinal cord injury. *J. Neurosci.* 33: 19664–19676. [29]

Finger, T. E., Danilova, V., Barrows, J., et al. 2005. ATP signaling is crucial for communication from taste buds to gustatory nerves. *Science* 310: 1495–1499. [21]

Fink, K. L., López-Giráldez, F., Kim, I. J., et al. 2017. Identification of Intrinsic Axon Growth Modulators for Intact CNS Neurons after Injury. *Cell Rep.* 18: 2687–2701. [29]

Finn, I. M., and Ferster, D. 2007. Neural connections and receptive field properties in the primary visual cortex. *J. Neurosci.* 27: 9638–9648. [2]

Finn, I. M., Priebe, N. J., and Ferster, D. 2007. The emergence of contrast-invariant orientation tuning in simple cells of cat visual cortex. *Neuron* 54: 137–152. [2]

Firestein, S., Shepherd, G. M., and Werblin, F. S. 1990. Time course of the membrane current underlying sensory transduction in salamander olfactory receptor neurones. *J. Physiol.* 430: 135–158. [21]

Fischbach, G. D., and Rosen, K. M. 1997. ARIA: A neuromuscular junction neuregulin. *Annu. Rev. Neurosci.* 20: 429–458. [29]

Fischer, W., Bjorklund, A., Chen, K., and Gage, F. H. 1991. NGF improves spatial memory in aged rodents as a function of age. *J. Neurosci.* 11: 1889–1906. [27]

Fischmeister, R., and Hartzell, H. C. 1986. Mechanism of action of acetylcholine on calcium current in single cells from frog ventricle. *J. Physiol.* 376: 183–202. [12]

Fischmeister, R., Castro, L. R., Abi-Gerges, A., et al. 2006. Compartmentation of cyclic nucleotide signaling in the heart: The role of cyclic nucleotide phosphodiesterases. *Circ. Res.* 99: 816–828. [12]

Fishell, G. and Heintz, N. 2013. The neuron identity problem: Form meets function. *Neuron* 80: 602–612. [27]

Fisher, S. K., and Boycott, B. B. 1974. Synaptic connections made by horizontal cells within the outer plexiform layer of the retina of the cat and the rabbit. *Proc. R. Soc. Lond., B, Biol. Sci.* 186: 317–331. [1]

Fitch, M. T., and Silver, J. 1999. Beyond the glial scar: Cellular and molecular mechanisms by which glial cells contribute to CNS regenerative failure. In M. H. Tuszynski and J. H. Kordower (Eds.), *CNS Regeneration: Basic Science and Clinical Advances.* Academic Press, San Diego, pp. 55–88. [29]

Fitzpatrick, J. S., Haggenston, A. S., Hertle, D. N., et al. 2009. Inositol-1,4,5-trisphosphate receptor-mediated Ca^{2+} waves in pyramidal neuron dendrites propagate through hot spots and cold spots. *J. Physiol.* 587: 1439–1459. [12]

Flavell, S. W., and Greenberg, M. E. 2008. Signaling mechanisms linking neuronal activity to gene expression and plasticity of the nervous system. *Annu. Rev. Neurosci.* 31: 563–590. [12, 17]

Fleischmann, P. N., Grob, R., Wehner, R., and Rössler, W. 2017. Species-specific differences in the fine structure of learning walk elements in *Cataglyphis* ants. *J. Exp. Biol.* 220: 2426–2435. doi: 10.1242/jeb.158147. [20]

Fleishman, S. J., Ungar, V. M., Yeager, M., and Ben-Tal, N. 2004. A C$^{\alpha}$ model for the transmembrane α helices of gap junction intercellular channels. *Mol. Cell* 15: 879–888. [8]

Flock, A. 1965. Transducing mechanisms in the lateral line canal organ receptors. *Cold Spring Harb. Symp. Quant. Biol.* 30: 133–145. [21]

Flock, A., and Russell, I. 1976. Inhibition by efferent nerve fibres: Action on hair cells and afferent synaptic transmission in the lateral line canal organ of the burbot *Lota lota. J. Physiol.* 257: 45–62. [24]

Flock, A., Flock, B., and Murray, E. 1977. Studies on the sensory hairs of receptor cells in the inner ear. *Acta Otolaryngol.* 83: 85–91. [21]

Flockerzi, V., Oeken, H-J., Hofmann, F., et al. 1986. Purified dihydropyridine-binding site from skeletal muscle t-tubules is a functional calcium channel. *Nature* 323: 66–68. [12]

Florey, E. 1954. An inhibitory and an excitatory factor of mammalian central nervous system, and their action on a single sensory neuron. *Arch. Int. Physiol.* 62: 33–53. [14]

Florio, M., Albert, M., Taverna, E., et al. 2015. Human-specific gene ARHGAP11B promotes basal progenitor amplification and neocortex expansion, *Science* 347: 1465–1470. doi: 10.1126/science.aaa1975. [27]

Flynn, G. E., Johnson, J. P., Jr., and Zagotta, W. N. 2001. Cyclic nucleotide-gated channels: Shedding light on the openings of a channel pore. *Nat. Rev. Neurosci.* 2: 643–652. [5]

Fogassi, L., and Luppino, G. 2005. Motor functions of the parietal lobe. *Curr. Opin. Neurobiol.* 15: 626–631. [26]

Fonseca, R. et al. 2004. Competing for memory: hippocampal LTP under regimes of reduced protein synthesis. *Neuron* 44: 1011. [17]

Fonseca, R., Vabulas, R., Hartl, F. U., et al. 2006. A balance of protein synthesis and proteasome-dependent degradation determines the maintenance of LTP. *Neuron* 52: 239–245. [17]

Fonseca, R., et al., 2006. Neuronal activity determines the protein synthesis dependence of long-term potentiation. *Nat. Neurosci.* 9: 478–480. [17]

Fontaine, B., and Changeux, J-P. 1989. Localization of nicotinic acetylcholine receptor α-subunit transcripts during myogenesis and motor endplate development in the chick. *J. Cell Biol.* 108: 1025–1037. [29]

Foote, S. L., Bloom, F. E., and Aston-Jones, G. 1983. Nucleus locus ceruleus: New evidence of anatomical and physiological specificity. *Physiol. Rev.* 63: 844–914. [14]

Forman, D. S., Padjen, A. L., and Siggins, G. R. 1977. Axonal transport of organelles visualized by light microscopy: Cinemicrographic and computer analysis. *Brain Res.* 136: 197–213. [15]

Forscher, P., and Smith, S. J. 1988. Actions of cytochalasins on the organization of actin filaments and microtubules in a neuronal growth cone. *J. Cell Biol.* 4: 1505–1516. [27]

Förster, E., Bock, H. H., Herz, J., et al. 2010. Emerging topics in Reelin function. *Eur. J. Neurosci.* 31: 1511–1518. [27]

Forsythe, I. D. 1994. Direct patch recording from identified presynaptic terminals mediating glutaminergic EPSCs in the rat CNS *in vitro. J. Physiol.* 479: 381–387. [13]

Forsythe, I. D., Tsujimoto, T., Barnes-Davies, M., et al. 1998. Inactivation of presynaptic calcium current contributes to synaptic depression at a fast central synapse. *Neuron* 20: 797–807. [16]

Foster, R. G., Provencio, I., Hudson, D., et al. 1991. Circadian photoreception in the retinally degenerate mouse (rd/rd). *J. Comp. Physiol. A* 169: 39–50. [22]

Fournier, A. E., GrandPre, T., and Strittmatter, S. M. 2001. Identification of a receptor mediating Nogo-66 inhibition of axonal regeneration. *Nature* 409: 341–346. [29]

Foust, A., Popovic, M., Zecevic, D., and McCormick, D. A. 2009. Action potentials initiate in the axon initial segment and propagate through axon collaterals reliably in cerebellar Purkinje neurons. *Neuroscience* 162: 836–851. [26]

Fowler, C. E., Aryal, P., Suen, K. F., and Slesinger, P. A. 2007. Evidence for association of GABA$_B$ receptors with Kir3 channels and regulators of G protein signalling (RGS4) proteins. *J. Physiol.* 580: 51–65. [12]

Fowler, C. J., Griffiths, D., de Groat, W. C. 2008. The neural control of micturition. *Nat. Rev. Neurosci.* 9: 453–466. [19]

Frade, J. M., Rodriguez-Tebar, A., Barde, Y. A. 1996. Induction of cell death by endogenous nerve growth factor through its p75 receptor. *Nature* 383: 166–168. [27]

Franchini, L. F., and Elgoyhen, A. B. 2006. Adaptive evolution in mammalian proteins involved in cochlear outer hair cell electromotility. *Mol. Phylogenet. Evol.* 41: 622–635. [24]

Francis, N. J., and Landis, S. C. 1999. Cellular and molecular determinants of sympathetic neuron development. *Annu. Rev. Neurosci.* 22: 541–566. [27]

Francois, J. 1979. Late results of congenital cataract surgery. *Ophthalmology* 86: 1586–1598. [28]

Frank, K., and Fuortes, M. G. F. 1957. Presynaptic and postsynaptic inhibition of monosynaptic reflexes. *Fed. Proc.* 16: 39–40. [11]

Frank, T., Khimich, D., Neef, A., and Moser, T. 2009. Mechanisms contributing to synaptic Ca^{2+} signals and their heterogeneity in hair cells. *Proc. Natl. Acad. Sci. USA* 106: 4483–4488. [24]

Frankenhaeuser, B., and Hodgkin, A. L. 1957. The actions of calcium on the electrical properties of squid axons. *J. Physiol.* 137: 218–244. [7]

Franks, N. P. 2008. General anaesthesia: From molecular targets to neuronal pathways of sleep and arousal. *Nat. Rev. Neurosci.* 9: 370–386. [14]

Fraser, J. A., and Huang, C. L. H. 2004. A quantitative analysis of cell volume and resting potential determination and regulation of excitable cells. *J. Physiol.* 559: 459–478. [6]

Freedman, M. S., Lucas, R. J., Soni, B., et al. 1999. Regulation of mammalian circadian behavior by non-rod, non-cone, ocular photoreceptors. *Science* 284: 502–504. [22]

Freeman, A. W., and Johnson, K. O. 1982. Cutaneous mechanoreceptors in macaque monkey: Temporal discharge patterns evoked by vibration, and a receptor model. *J. Physiol.* 323: 21–41. [23]

Freiwald, W. A., Tsao, D. Y., and Livingstone, M. S. 2009. A face feature space in the macaque temporal lobe. *Nat. Neurosci.* 12: 1187–1196. [25]

Fremeau, Jr., R. T., Burman, J., Qureshi, T., et al. 2002. The identification of vesicular glutamate transporter 3 suggests novel modes of signaling by glutamate. *Proc. Natl. Acad. Sci. USA* 99: 14488–14493. [9]

Fremeau, Jr., R. T., Kam, K., Qureshi, T., et al. 2004. Vesicular glutamate transporters 1 and 2 target to functionally distinct synaptic release sites. *Science* 304: 1815–1819. [9]

French, C. R., Sah, P., Buckett, K. J., and Gage, P. W. 1990. A voltage-dependent persistent sodium current in mammalian hippocampal neurons. *J. Gen. Physiol.* 95: 1139–1157. [7]

French, K. A., and Muller, K. J. 1986. Regeneration of a distinctive set of axosomatic contacts in the leech central nervous system. *J. Neurosci.* 6: 318–324. [20]

French, R. J., and Zamponi, G. W. 2005. Voltage-gated sodium and calcium channels in nerve, muscle, and heart. *IEEE Trans. Nanobioscience* 4: 58–69. [5]

Frenkel, M. Y., Sawtell, N. B., Diogo, A. C., et al. 2006. Instructive effect of visual experience in mouse visual cortex. *Neuron* 51: 339–349. [28]

Frey, U., et al. 1996. Influence of actinomycin D, a RNA synthesis inhibitor, on long-term potentiation in rat hippocampal neurons in vivo and in vitro. *J. Physiol* 490: 703. [17]

Frey, U. and Morris R. G. M. 1997.Synaptic tagging and long-term potentiation. *Nature* 385: 533–536. [17]

Frey, U. and Morris, R. G.M. 1998. Synaptic tagging: Implications for late maintenance of hippocampal long-term potentiation. *TINS* 21: 181. [17]

Fried, S. I., Munch, T. A., and Werblin, F. S. 2002. Mechanisms and circuitry underlying directional selectivity in the retina. *Nature* 420: 411–414. [22]

Friesen, W. O., and Kristan, W. B. 2007. Leech locomotion: Swimming, crawling, and decisions. *Curr. Opin. Neurobiol.* 17: 704–711. [18, 20]

Fritsch, G., and Hitzig, E. 1870. Ueber die electrische Erregbarkeit des Grosshirns. *Arch. Anat. Physiol. Wiss. Med.* 37: 300–332. [26]

Fritschy, J. M., Harvey, R. J., and Schwarz, G. 2008. Gephyrin: Where do we stand, where do we go? *Trends Neurosci.* 31: 257–264. [11]

Fu, Y., and Yau, K. W. 2007. Phototransduction in mouse rods and cones. *Pflügers Arch.* 454: 805–819. [22]

Fu, Y., Liao, H. W., Do, M. T., and Yau, K. W. 2005. Non-image forming ocular photoreception in vertebrates. 2005. *Curr. Opin. Neurobiol.* 15: 415–422. [2]

Fuchs, P. A., and Getting, P. A. 1980. Ionic basis of presynaptic inhibitory potentials at crayfish claw opener. *J. Neurophysiol.* 43: 1547–1557. [11]

Fuchs, P. A., and Murrow, B. W. 1992. Cholinergic inhibition of short (outer) hair cells of the chick's cochlea. *J. Neurosci.* 12: 800–809. [12, 24]

Fuchs, P. A., Nicholls, J. G., and Ready, D. F. 1981. Membrane properties and selective connecions of identified leech neurones in culture. *J. Physiol.* 316: 203–233. [18]

Fucile, S. 2004. Ca^{2+} permeability of nicotinic acetylcholine receptors. *Cell Calcium* 35: 1–8. [12]

Fuentealba, L. C., Obernier, K., and Alvarez-Buylla, A. 2012. Adult neural stem cells bridge their niche *Cell Stem Cell* 10: 698–708. [27]

Fujisawa, H. 2004. Discovery of semaphorin receptors, neuropilin and plexin, and their functions in neural development. *J. Neurobiol.* 59: 24–33. [27]

Fukami, Y., and Hunt, C. C. 1977. Structures in sensory region of snake spindles and their displacement during stretch. *J. Neurophysiol.* 40: 1121–1131. [21]

Fuller, J. L. 1967. Experimental deprivation and later behavior. *Science* 158: 1645–1652. [28]

Fullerton, S. M., Strittmatter, W. J., and Matthew, W. D. 1998. Peripheral sensory nerve defects in apolipoprotein E knockout mice. *Exp. Neurol.* 153: 156–163. [29]

Fulop, T., Radabaugh, S., and Smith, C. 2005. Activity-dependent differential transmitter release in mouse adrenal chromaffin cells. *J. Neurosci.* 25: 7324–7332. [19]

Fuortes, M. G., and Poggio, G. F. 1963. Transient responses to sudden illumination in cells of the eye of *Limulus*. *J. Gen. Physiol.* 46: 435–452. [22]

Furchgott, R. F., and Zawadzki, J. V. 1980. The obligatory role of the endothelial cells in the relaxation of arterial smooth muscle by acetylcholine. *Nature* 288: 373–376. [12]

Furness, D. N., Dehnes, Y., Akhtar, A. Q., et al. 2008. A quantitative assessment of glutamate uptake into hippocampal synaptic terminals and astrocytes: New insights into a neuronal role for excitatory amino acid transporter 2 (EAAT2). *Neuroscience* 157: 80–94. [10]

Furness, J. B., Bornstein, J. C., Murphy, R., and Pompolo, S. 1992. Roles of peptides in transmission in the enteric nervous system. *Trends Neurosci.* 15: 66–71. [14]

Furshpan, E. J., and Potter, D. D. 1959. Transmission at the giant motor synapses of the crayfish. *J. Physiol.* 145: 289–325. [11]

Furshpan, E. J., MacLeish, P. R., O'Lague, P. H., and Potter, D. D. 1976. Chemical transmission between rat sympathetic neurons and cardiac myocytes developing in microcultures: Evidence for cholinergic, adrenergic, and dual-function neurons: *Proc. Natl. Acad. Sci. USA* 73: 4225–4229. [27]

Fuxe, K., Dahlström, A., Höistad, M., et al. 2007. From the Golgi-Cajal mapping to the transmitter-based characterization of the neuronal networks leading to two modes of brain communication: Wiring and volume transmission. *Brain Res Rev.* 55: 17–54. [14, 18]

Fuxe, K., Dahlström, A. B., Jonsson, G., et al. 2010. The discovery of central monoamine neurons gave volume transmission to the wired brain. *Prog. Neurobiol.* 90: 82–100. [14]

Gaddum, J. H. 1943. Symposium on chemical constitution and pharmacological action. *Trans. Faraday Soc.* 39: 323–332. [11]

Gage, F. H., Armstrong, D. M., Williams, L. R., and Varon, S. 1988. Morphological response of axotomized septal neurons to nerve growth factor. *J. Comp. Neurol.* 269: 147–155. [27]

Gähwiler, B. H., and Brown, D. A. 1985. Functional innervation of cultured hippocampal neurones by cholinergic afferents from co-cultured septal explants. *Nature* 313: 577–579. [14]

Gähwiler, B. H., and Brown, D. A. 1985. GABA$_B$-receptor-activated K+ current in voltage-clamped CA3 pyramidal cells in hippocampal cultures. *Proc. Natl. Acad. Sci. USA* 82: 1558–1562. [14]

Galambos, R. 1956. Suppression of auditory nerve activity by stimulation of efferent fibers to the cochlea. *J. Neurophysiol.* 19: 424–437. [24]

Gallagher, J. P., Higashi, H., and Nishi, S. 1978. Characterization and ionic basis of GABA-induced depolarizations recorded in vitro from cat primary afferent neurones. *J. Physiol.* 275: 263–282. [11]

Galli, L., and Maffei, L. 1988. Spontaneous impulse activity of rat retinal ganglion cells in prenatal life. *Science* 242: 90–91. [28]

Gallo, G., and Letourneau, P. C. 2004. Regulation of growth cone actin filaments by guidance cues. *J. Neurobiol.* 58: 92–102. [27]

Galzi, J. L., Devillers-Thiery, A., Hussey, N., et al. 1992. Mutations in the channel domain of a neuronal nicotinic receptor convert ion selectivity from cationic to anionic. *Nature* 359: 500–505. [5]

Gamal El-Din, T. M., Heldstab, H., Lehmann, C., and Greef, N. G. 2010. Double gaps along *Shaker* S4 demonstrate omega currents at three different closed states. *Channels* 4: 1–8. [7]

Gamper, N., and Ooi, L. 2015. Redox and nitric oxide-mediated regulation of sensory neuron ion channel function. *Antioxid Redox Signal.* 22: 486–504. [12]

Gamper, N. S., and Shapiro, M. S. 2007. Regulation of ion transport proteins by membrane phosphoinositides. *Nat. Rev. Neurosci.* 8: 1–14. [12]

Gamzu, E., and Ahissar, E. 2001. Importance of temporal cues for tactile spatial-frequency discrimination. *J. Neurosci.* 21: 7416–7427. [23]

Gandhi, S. P., and Stevens, C. F. 2003. Three modes of synaptic vesicular recycling revealed by single-vesicle imaging. *Nature* 423: 607–613. [13]

Gao, P., et al. 2014. Deterministic progenitor behavior and unitary production of neurons in the neocortex. *Cell* 159: 775–788. [27]

Gao, T., Yatani, A., Dell'Acqua, M. L., Sako, H., et al. 1997. cAMP-dependent regulation of cardiac L-type Ca^{2+} channels requires membrane targeting of PKA and phosphorylation of channel subunits. *Neuron* 19: 185–196. [12]

García-Anoveros, J., and Corey, D. P. 1997. The molecules of mechanosensation. *Annu. Rev. Neurosci.* 20: 567–594. [21]

García-Pérez, E., Vargas-Caballero, M., Velazquez-Ulloa, et al. 2004. Synaptic integration in electrically coupled neurons. *Biophys. J.* 86: 646–655. doi: 10.1016/S0006-3495(04)74142-9. [18]

Gardner, E. P., Palmer, C. I., Hamalainen, H. A., and Warren, S. 1992. Simulation of motion on the skin. V. Effect of stimulus temporal frequency on the representation of moving bar patterns in primary somatosensory cortex of monkeys. *J. Neurophysiol.* 67: 37–63. [23]

Garfield, A. S., and Heisler, L. K. 2009. Pharmacological targeting of the serotonergic system for the treatment of obesity. *J. Physiol.* 587: 49–60. [14]

Garner, A. R. et al. 2012. Generation of a synthetic memory trace. *Science* 335: 1513. [17]

Garner, C. C., et al. 1988. Selective localization of messenger RNA for cytoskeletal protein MAP2 in dendrites. *Nature* 336: 674–677. [17]

Garthwaite, J. 2008. Concepts of neural nitric oxide-mediated transmission. *Eur. J. Neurosci.* 27: 2783–2802. [12]

Garthwaite, J., Charles, S. L., and Chess-Williams, R. 1988. Endothelium-derived relaxing factor release on activation of NMDA receptors suggests role as intercellular messenger in the brain. *Nature* 336: 385–388. [12]

Gasnier, B. 2004. The SLC32 transporter, a key protein for the synaptic release of inhibitory amino acids. *Pflügers Arch.* 447: 756–759. [9]

Gaspard, N., Bouschet, T., Dimidschstein, J., et al. 2008. An intrinsic mechanism of corticogenesis from embryonic stem cells. *Nature* 455: 351–357. [27]

Gautam, M., Noakes, P. G., Moscoso, L., et al. 1996. Defective neuromuscular synaptogenesis in agrin-deficient mutant mice. *Cell* 85: 525–535. [29]

Gautvik, K. M., de Lecea, L., Gautvik, V. T., et al. 1998. Overview of the most prevalent hypothalamus-specific mRNAs, as identified by directional tag PCR subtraction. *Proc. Natl. Acad. Sci. USA* 93: 8733–8738. [14]

Gazzaniga, M. S. 2005. Forty-five years of split-brain research and still going strong. *Nat. Rev. Neurosci.* 6: 653–659. [3]

Gehring, W. J., Kloter, U., and Suga, H. 2009. Evolution of the *Hox* gene complex from an evolutionary ground state. *Curr. Top. Dev. Biol.* 88: 35–61. [27]

Geiger, J. R., Lübke, J., Roth, A., Frotscher, M., and Jonas, P. 1997. Submillisecond AMPA receptor-mediated signaling at a principal neuron-interneuron synapse. *Neuron* 18: 1009–1023. [14]

Georgopoulos, A. P., Merchant, H., Naselaris, T., and Amirikian, B. 2007. Mapping of the preferred direction in the motor cortex. *Proc. Natl. Acad. Sci. USA* 104: 11068–1072. [26]

Georgopoulos, A. P., Schwartz, A. B., and Kettner, R. E. 1986. Neuronal population coding of movement direction. *Science* 243: 1416–1419. [26]

Geppetti, P., Veldhuis, N. A., Lieu, T. M., and Bunnett, N. G. 2015. G protein-coupled receptors: Dynamic machines for signaling pain and itch. *Neuron.* 88; 635–639. [21]

Gerencser, G. A., and Zhang, J. 2003. Existence and nature of the chloride pump. *Biochim. Biophys. Acta* 1618: 133–139. [9]

Gether, U., Andersen, P. H., Larsson, O. M., and Schousboe, A. 2006. Neurotransmitter transporters: Molecular function of important drug targets. *Trends Pharmacol. Sci.* 27: 375–383. [9, 15]

Ghosh, A., and Greenberg, M. E. 1995. Calcium signaling in neurons: Molecular mechanisms and cellular consequences. *Science* 268: 239–247. [12]

Gibbins, I. L., and Morris, J. L. 2006. Structure of peripheral synapses: Autonomic ganglia. *Cell Tissue Res.* 326: 205–220. [19]

Giepmans, B. N., Adams, S. R., Ellisman, M. H., and Tsien, R. Y. 2006. The fluorescent toolbox for assessing protein location and function. *Science* 312: 217–224. [27]

Gil, J. M., and Rego, A. C. 2008. Mechanisms of neurodegeneration in Huntington's disease. *Eur. J. Neurosci.* 27: 2803–2820. [26]

Gilbert, C. D., and Wiesel, T. N. 1979. Morphology and intracortical projections of functionally characterised neurones in the cat visual cortex. *Nature* 280: 120–125. [2, 3]

Gilbert, C. D., and Wiesel, T. N. 1981. Laminar specialization and intracortical connections in cat primary visual cortex. In F. O. Schmitt, F. G. Worden, and F. Dennis (Eds.), *The organization of the cerebral cortex.* MIT Press, Cambridge, pp. 163–198. [3]

Gilbert, C. D., and Wiesel, T. N. 1983. Cluster intrinsic connections in cat visual cortex. *J. Neurosci.* 3: 1116–1133. [3]

Gilbert, C. D., and Wiesel, T. N. 1989. Columnar specificity of intrinsic horizontal and corticocortical connections in cat visual cortex. *J. Neurosci.* 9: 2432–2442. [3]

Gilbert, S. F. and Barresi M. J. F. 2016. *Developmental Biology*, 11th ed. Oxford University Press/Sinauer, Sunderland, MA. [27]

Gilbertson, T. A., Roper, S. D., and Kinnamon, S. C. 1993. Proton currents through amiloride-sensitive Na$^+$ channels in isolated hamster taste cells: Enhancement by vasopressin and cAMP. *Neuron* 10: 931–942. [21]

Gillespie, J. S., Liu, X. R., and Martin, W. 1989. The effects of L-arginine and NG-monomethyl L-arginine on the response of the rat anococcygeus muscle to NANC nerve stimulation. *Brit. J. Pharmacol.* 98: 1080–1082. [12]

Gillespie, P. G., and Muller, U. 2009. Mechanotransduction by hair cells: Models, molecules, and mechanisms. *Cell* 139: 33–44. [21]

Gillespie, P. G., Wagner, M. C., and Hudspeth, A. J. 1993. Identification of a 120 kd hair-bundle myosin located near stereociliary tips. *Neuron* 11: 581–594. [21]

Gilman, A. G. 1987. G proteins: Transducers of receptor-generated signals. *Annu. Rev. Biochem.* 56: 615–649. [12]

Giniatullin, R., Nistri, A., and Fabbretti, E. 2008. Molecular mechanisms of sensitization of pain-transducing P2X3 receptors by the migraine mediators CGRP and NGF. *Mol. Neurobiol.* 37: 83–90. [19]

Giorgi, C., Yeo, G. W., Stone, M. E., et al. 2007. The EJC Factor eIF4AIII modulates synaptic strength and neuronal protein expression. *Cell* 130: 179–191. [17, 27]

Giraudat, J., Dennis, M., Heidmann, T., et al. 1986. Structure of the high-affinity binding site for noncompetitive blockers of the acetylcholine receptor: Serine 262 of the delta subunit is labeled by [3H] chlorpromazine. *Proc. Natl. Acad. Sci. USA* 83: 2719–2723. [5]

Giraudat, J., Dennis, M., Heidmann, T., et al. 1987. Structure of the high-affinity binding site for noncompetitive blockers of the acetylcholine receptor: [3H] chlorpromazine labels homologous residues in the beta and delta chains. *Biochemistry* 26: 2410–2418. [5]

Girouard, H., Bonev, A. D., Hannah, R. M., et al. 2010. Astrocytic endfoot Ca^{2+} and BK channels determine both arteriolar dilation and constriction. *Proc. Natl. Acad. Sci. USA.* 107: 3811–3816. [10]

Gitik, M., Reichert, F., and Rotshenker, S. 2010. Cytoskeleton plays a dual role of activation and inhibition in myelin and zymosan phagocytosis by microglia. *FASEB J.* 24: 2211–2221. [29]

Giuditta, A., et al. 1986. Rapid important paper: Messenger RNA in squid axoplasm. *Proc. Natl. Acad. Sci. USA* 59: 1284–1287. [17, 27]

Giuditta, A., et al. 2002.Axonal and presynaptic protein synthesis: new insights into the biology of the neuron. *Trends Neurosci.* 25: 400–404. [17]

Giuditta, A., Chun, J. T., Eyman, M., et al. 2008. Local gene expression in axons and nerve endings: The glia-neuron unit. *Physiol. Rev.* 88: 515–555. [15]

Giuditta, A., Dettbarn, W. D., and Brzin, M. 1968. Protein synthesis in the isolated giant axon of the squid. *Proc. Natl. Acad. Sci. USA* 59: 1284–1287. [17, 27]

Glanzman, D. L. 2009. Habituation in *Aplysia*: The cheshire cat of neurobiology. *Neurobiol. Learn. Mem.* 92: 147–154. [16, 20]

Glavic, A., Gómez-Skarmeta, and Mayor, R. 2002. The homeoprotein *Xiro1* is required for midbrain-hindbrain boundary formation. *Development* 129: 1609–21. [27]

Glickstein, M., and Berlucchi, G. 2008. Classical disconnection studies of the corpus callosum. *Cortex* 44: 914–927. [3]

Glickstein, M., Sultan, F., and Voogd, J. 2011. Functional localization in the cerebellum. *Cortex* 47: 59–80. [26]

Glock, C., et al. 2017. mRNA transport and local translation in neurons. *Curr. Op. Neurobiol.* 45: 169–177. [17]

Glover, J. C., and Kramer, A. P. 1982. Serotonin analog selectively ablates identified neurons in the leech embryo. *Science* 216: 317–319. [20]

Glowatzki, E., and Fuchs, P. A. 2002. Transmitter release at the hair cell ribbon synapse. *Nat. Neurosci.* 5: 147–154. [24]

Glowatzki, E., Cheng, N., Hiel, H., et al. 2006. The glutamate-aspartate transporter GLAST mediates glutamate uptake at inner hair cell afferent synapses in the mammalian cochlea. *J. Neurosci.* 26: 7659–7664. [9]

Glusman, S., and Kravitz, E. A. 1982. The action of serotonin on excitatory nerve terminals in lobster nerve-muscle preparations. *J. Physiol.* 325: 223–241. [18]

Goard, M., and Dan, Y. 2009. Basal forebrain activation enhances cortical coding of natural scenes. *Nat. Neurosci.* 12: 1444–1449. [14]

Gobbo, F., et al. 2017. Activity-dependent expression of Channelrhodopsin at neuronal synapses. *Nat. Comm.* 8: 1629. [17]

Godde, B., Diamond, M., and Braun, C. 2010. Feeling for space or for time: Task-dependent modulation of the cortical representation of identical vibrotactile stimuli. *Neurosci. Lett.* 480: 143–147. [25]

Godecke, I., and Bonhoeffer, T. 1996. Development of identical orientation maps for two eyes without common visual experience. *Nature* 379: 251–254. [28]

Gogolla, N., Caroni, P., Lüthi, A., and Herry, C. 2009. Perineuronal nets protect fear memories from erasure. *Science* 325: 1258–1261. [28]

Gold, J. I., and Knudsen, E. I. 1999. Hearing impairment induces frequency-specific adjustments in auditory spatial tuning in the optic tectum of young owls. *J. Neurophysiol.* 82: 2197–2209. [28]

Gold, M. R., and Martin, A. R. 1983. Characteristics of inhibitory post-synaptic currents in brain-stem neurones of the lamprey. *J. Physiol.* 342: 85–98. [13]

Gold, M. R., and Martin, A. R. 1983. Analysis of glycine-activated inhibitory post-synaptic channels in brain-stem neurones of the lamprey. *J. Physiol.* 342: 99–117. [6, 11]

Gold, M. R., and Martin, A. R. 1984. γ-Aminobutyric acid and glycine activate Cl⁻ channels having different characteristics in CNS neurones. *Nature* 308: 639–641. [14]

Gold T. Hearing. II. 1948. The physical basis of the action of the cochlea. *Proc. R. Soc. Lond. B Biol. Sci.* 135: 492–498. [24]

Goldberg, J. M. 2000. Afferent diversity and the organization of central vestibular pathways. *Exp. Brain Res.* 130: 277–297. [24]

Goldin, A. L., Barchi, R. L., Caldwell, J. H., et al. 2000. Nomenclature of sodium channels. *Neuron* 28: 365–368. [5]

Goldman, D. E. 1943. Potential, impedance and rectification in membranes. *J. Gen. Physiol.* 27: 37–60. [6]

Goldman, S. A. 2016. Stem and Progenitor Cell-Based Therapy of the Central Nervous System: Hopes, Hype, and Wishful Thinking. *Cell Stem Cell* 18: 174–188. [29]

Goldsmith, T. H., and Wehner, R. 1977. Restrictions on rotational and translational diffusion of pigment in the membranes of a rhabdomeric photoreceptor. *J. Gen. Physiol.* 70: 453–490. [20]

Goldstein, S. A. N., Bockenhauer, D., O'Kelly, I., and Zilberberg, N. 2001. Potassium leak channels and the KCNK family of two-P-domain subunits. *Nat. Rev. Neurosci.* 2: 175–184. [5, 6]

Golgi, C. 1903. *Opera Omnia*, Vols. 1 and 2. U. Hoepli, Milan, Italy. [10]

Gollisch, T., and Meister, M. 2008. Rapid neural coding in the retina with relative spike latencies. *Science* 319: 1108–1111. [2]

Golomb, D., Yue, C., and Yaari, Y. 2006. Contribution of persistent Na⁺ current and M-type K⁺ current to somatic bursting in CA1 pyramidal cells: Combined experimental and modeling study. *J. Neurophysiol.* 96: 1912–1926. [7]

Gomeza, J., Hälsmann, S., Ohno, K., et al. 2003. Inactivation of the glycine transporter 1 gene discloses vital role of glial glycine uptake in glycinergic inhibition. *Neuron* 40: 785–796. [10]

Goncalves, J. T., Schafer, S. T., and Gage, F. H. 2016. Adult neurogenesis in the hippocampus: From stem cells to behavior *Cell* 167: 897–914. [27]

Goodman, C. S., Raper, J. A., Chang, S., and Ho, R. 1983 Grasshopper growth cones: Divergent choices and labelled pathways *Prog. Brain Res.* 58: 283–304. [27]

Gorin, P. D., and Johnson, E. M. 1979. Experimental autoimmune model of nerve growth factor deprivation: Effects on developing peripheral sympathetic and sensory neurons. *Proc. Natl. Acad. Sci. USA* 76: 5382–5386. [27]

Götz, M., and Barde, Y. A. 2005. Radial glial cells defined and major intermediates between embryonic stem cells and CNS neurons. *Neuron* 46: 369–372. [10]

Götz, M., Nakafuku, M., and Petrik, D. 2016. Neurogenesis in the developing and adult brain-similarities and key differences. *Cold Spring Harb. Perspect. Biol.* doi: 10.1101/cshperspect.a018853. [27]

Gourine, A. V., Kasymov, V., Marina, N., et al. 2010. Astrocytes control breathing through pH-dependent release of ATP. *Science* 329: 571–575. [10, 14]

Govek, E. E., Hatten, M. E., and Van Aelst, L. 2011. The role of Rho GTPase proteins in CNS neuronal migration. *Dev. Neurobiol.* 71: 528–553. [27]

Grade, S. and Goetz, M. 2017. Neuronal replacement therapy: Previous achievements and challenges ahead. *NPJ Regen. Med.* 2: 29. doi:10.1038/s41536-017-0033-0. [29]

Gradinaru, V., Mogri, M., Thompson, K. R., et al. 2009. Optical deconstruction of parkinsonian neural circuitry. *Science* 324: 354–359. [30]

Gradinaru, V., Zhang, F., Ramakrishnan, C., et al. 2010. Molecular and cellular approaches for diversifying and extending optogenetics. *Cell* 141: 154–165. [14]

Grafstein, B., and Forman, D. S. 1980. Intracellular transport in neurons. *Physiol. Rev.* 60: 1167–1283. [15]

Granseth, B., Odermaatt, B., Royle, S. J., and Lagnado, L. 2006. Clathrin-mediated endocytosis is the dominant mechanism of vesicle retrieval at hippocampal synapses. *Neuron* 51: 773–786. [13]

Grant, L., Yi, E., and Glowatzki, E. 2010. Two modes of release shape the postsynaptic response at the inner hair cell ribbon synapse. *J. Neurosci.* 30: 4210–4220. [24]

Grassi, F., and Lux, H. D. 1989. Voltage-dependent GABA-induced modulation of calcium currents in chick sensory neurons. *Neurosci. Lett.* 105: 113–119. [12]

Graybiel, A. M. 2008. Habits, rituals, and the evaluative brain. *Annu. Rev. Neurosci.* 31: 359–387. [26]

Greene, L. A., and Shooter, E. M. 1980. The nerve growth factor: Biochemistry, synthesis, and mechanism of action. *Annu. Rev. Neurosci.* 3: 353–402. [27]

Greer, P. L., et al. 2010. The Angelman Syndrome protein Ube3A regulates synapse development by ubiquitinating arc. *Cell* 140: 704–716. [17]

Greitz, D. 1993. Cerebrospinal fluid circulation and associated intracranial dynamics. A radiologic investigation using MR imaging and radionuclide cisternography. *Acta Radiol. Suppl.* 386: 1–23. [18]

Grichtchenko, I. I., Choi, I., Zhong, X., et al. 2001. Cloning, characterization, and chromosomal mapping of a human electroneutral Na⁺-driven Cl-HCO₃ exchanger. *J. Biol. Chem.* 276: 8358–8363. [9]

Griesinger, C. B., Richards, C. D., and Ashmore, J. F. 2005. Fast vesicle replenishment allows indefatigable signalling at the first auditory synapse. *Nature* 435: 212–215. [24]

Griffin, J. W., and Thompson, W. J. 2008. Biology and pathology of nonmyelinating Schwann cells. *Glia* 56: 1518–1531. [29]

Griffiths, T. D., Buchel, C., Frackowiak, R. S., and Patterson, R. D. 1998. Analysis of temporal structure in sound by the human brain. *Nat. Neurosci.* 1: 422–427. [24]

Grill-Spector, K., and Malach, R. 2004. The human visual cortex. *Annu. Rev. Neurosci.* 27: 649–677. [25]

Grill-Spector, K., Knouf, N., and Kanwisher, N. 2004. The fusiform face area subserves face perception, not generic within-category identification. *Nat. Neurosci.* 7: 555–562. [25]

Grill-Spector, K., Kushnir, T., Edelman, S., et al. 1999. Differential processing of objects under various viewing conditions in the human lateral occipital complex. *Neuron* 24: 187–203. [25]

Grill-Spector, K., Kushnir, T., Hendler, T., et al.1998. A sequence of object-processing stages revealed by fMRI in the human occipital lobe. *Hum. Brain Mapp.* 6: 316–328. [25]

Grimes, W. N., Zhang, J., Graydon, C. W., et al. Retinal parallel processors: More than 100 independent microcircuits operate within a single interneuron. *Neuron* 65: 873–885. [22]

Grinnell, A. D., and Rheuben, M. B. 1979. The physiology, pharmacology and trophic effectiveness of synapses formed by autonomic preganglionic nerves on frog skeletal muscles. *J. Physiol.* 289: 219–240. [29]

Grinvald, A., Lieke, E., Frostig, R. D., et al. 1986. Functional architecture of cortex revealed by optical imaging of intrinsic signals. *Nature* 324: 361–364. [3]

Groh, J. M., Born, R. T., and Newsome, W. T. 1997. How is a sensory map read out? Effects of microstimulation in visual area MT on saccades and smooth pursuit eye movements. *J. Neurosci.* 17: 4312–4330. [25]

Gross, C. G., Rocha-Miranda, C. E., and Bender, D. B. 1972. Visual properties of neurons in inferotemporal cortex of the Macaque. *J. Neurophysiol.* 35: 96–111. [25]

Grumbacher-Reinert, S., and Nicholls, J. 1992. Influence of substrate on retraction of neurites following electrical activity of leech Retzius cells in culture. *J. Exp. Biol.* 167: 1–14. [27]

Grutzendler, J., et al. 2002. Long-term dendritic spine stability in the adult cortex. *Nature* 420: 812. [17]

Grynkiewicz, G., Poenie, M., and Tsien, R. Y. 1985. A new generation of Ca^{2+} indicators with greatly improved fluorescence properties. *J. Biol. Chem.* 260: 3440–3450. [12]

Gu, X. N., Macagno, E. R., and Muller, K. J. 1989. Laser microbeam axotomy and conduction block show that electrical transmission at a central synapse is distributed at multiple contacts. *J. Neurobiol.* 20: 422–434. [8]

Gu, Y. et al. 2010. Neuronal soma-satellite glial cell interactions in sensory ganglia and the participation of purinergic receptors. *Neuron Glia Biol.* 6: 53–62. [18]

Guedes-Dias, P., and Holzbauer, E. L. F. 2019. Axonal transport: Driving synaptic function. *Science* 366: 199. doi: 10.1126/science.aaw9997. [15]

Guertin, P. A. 2009. The mammalian central pattern generator for locomotion. *Brain Res. Rev.* 62: 45–56. [26]

Guertin, P. A., and Hounsgaard, J. 1998. Chemical and electrical stimulation induce rhythmic motor activity in an in vitro preparation of the spinal cord from adult turtles. *Neurosci. Lett.* 245: 5–8. [26]

Guic-Robles, E., Jenkins, W. M., and Bravo, H. 1992. Vibrissal roughness discrimination is barrelcortex-dependent. *Behav. Brain Res.* 48: 145–152. [23]

Guidry, G., Willison, B. D., Blakely, R. D., et al. 2005. Developmental expression of the high affinity choline transporter in cholinergic sympathetic neurons. *Auton. Neurosci.* 123: 54–61. [19]

Guillery, R. W. 1970. The laminar distribution of retinal fibers in the dorsal lateral geniculate nucleus of the rat: A new interpretation. *J. Comp. Neurol.* 138: 339–368. [3]

Guillery, R. W. 2005. Anatomical pathways that link perception and action. *Prog. Brain Res.* 149: 235–256. [2]

Guillery, R. W., and Stelzner, D. J. 1970. The differential effects of unilateral lid closure upon the monocular and binocular segments of the dorsal lateral geniculate nucleus in the cat. *J. Comp. Neurol.* 139: 413–421. [28]

Güler, A. D., Ecker, J. L., Lall, G. S., et al. 2008. Melanopsin cells are the principal conduits for rod-cone input to non-image-forming vision. *Nature* 453: 102–105. [19]

Gulledge, A. T., and Stuart, G. J. 2005. Cholinergic inhibition of neonatal pyramidal neurons. *J. Neurosci.* 28: 10305–10320. [12]

Gulledge, A. T., Bucci, D. J., Zhang, S. S., et al. 2009. M1 receptors mediate cholinergic modulation of excitability in neocortical pyramidal neurons. *J. Neurosci.* 29: 9888–9902. [14]

Gundersen, R. W. and Barret, J. N. 1979 Neuronal chemotaxis: Chick dorsal root axons turn toward high concentrations of nerve growth factor. *Science* 206: 1079–1080. [27]

Gunthorpe, M. J., and Lummis, S. C. R. 2001. Conversion of the ion selectivity of the 5-HT$_{3A}$ receptor from cationic to anionic reveals a conserved feature of the ligand-gated ion channel superfamily. *J. Biol. Chem.* 276: 10977–10983. [5]

Guo, Z., Zhang, L., Wu, Z., et al. 2014. In vivo direct reprogramming of reactive glial cells into functional neurons after brain injury and in an Alzheimer's disease model. *Cell Stem Cell* 14: 188–202. [29]

Gurdon, J. 1962. The developmental capacity of nuclei taken from intestinal epithelium cells of feeding tadpoles. *J. Embryol. Exp. Morphol* 10: 622. [27]

Gurdon, J. 2012. The egg and the nucleus: A battle for supremacy (Nobel Lecture). *Development* 140: 2449–2456. [27]

Gurdon, J. B., and Melton, D. A. 2008. Nuclear reprogramming in cells. *Science* 322: 1811–1815. [27]

Gustincich, S., Feigenspan, A., Wu, D. K., et al. 1997. Control of dopamine release in the retina: A transgenic approach to neural networks. *Neuron* 18: 723–736. [18]

Guth, L. 1968. "Trophic" influences of nerve. *Physiol. Rev.* 48: 645–687. [29]

Gutierrez, R. 2015. The plastic neurotransmitter phenotype of the hippocampal granule cells and of the moss in their messy fibers. *J. Chem. Neuroanat.* 13: 9–20. [15]

Guzowski, J. F., et al. 1999. Environment-specific expression of the immediate-early gene *Arc* in hippocampal neuronal ensembles. *Nat. Neurosci.* 2: 1120–1124. [17]

Haas, H., and Panula, P. 2003. The role of histamine and the tuberomamillary nucleus in the nervous system. *Nat. Rev. Neurosci.* 4: 121–130. [14]

Haas, H. L., and Konnerth, A. 1983. Histamine and noradrenaline decrease calcium-activated potassium conductance in hippocampal pyramidal cells. *Nature* 302: 432–434. [14]

Haas, H. L., and Selbach, O. 2000. Functions of neuronal adenosine receptors. *Naunyn Schmiedebergs Arch. Pharmacol.* 362: 375–381. [14]

Haas, H. L., Sergeeva, O. A., and Selbach, O. 2008. Histamine in the nervous system. *Physiol. Rev.* 88: 1183–1241. [14]

Habas, C. 2010. Functional imaging of the deep cerebellar nuclei: A review. *Cerebellum* 9: 22–28. [26]

Habets, R. L., and Borst, J. G. 2005. Post-tetanic potentiation in the rat calyx of Held synapse. *J. Physiol.* 564: 173–187. [16]

Habets, R. L., and Borst, J. G. 2006. An increase in calcium influx contributes to post-tetanic potentiation at the rat calyx of Held synapse. *J. Neurophysiol.* 96: 2868–2876. [16]

Habets, R. L., and Borst, J. G. 2007. Dynamics of the readily releasable pool during post-tetanic potentiation in the rat calyx of Held synapse. *J. Physiol.* 581: 467–478. [16]

Hackett, T. A., Preuss, T. M., and Kaas, J. H. 2001. Architectonic identification of the core region in auditory cortex of macaques, chimpanzees, and humans. *J. Comp. Neurol.* 441: 197–222. [24]

Hadaczek, P. et al. 2006. The "perivascular pump" driven by arterial pulsation is a powerful mechanism for the distribution of therapeutic molecules within the brain. *Mol. Ther.* 14: 69–78. [18]

Hafner, A. S., Donlin-Asp, P. G., Leitch, B., et al. 2019. Local protein synthesis is a ubiquitous feature of neuronal pre- and postsynaptic compartments. *Science* 364: eaau3644. [1, 17]

Hagenston, A. M., and Bading, H. 2011. Calcium signaling in synapse-to-nucleus communication. *Cold Spring Harb. Perspect. Biol.* 3: a004564. [17]

Hagiwara, S., and Byerly, L. 1981. Calcium channel. *Annu. Rev. Neurosci.* 4: 69–125. [7]

Halassa, M. M., and Haydon, P. G. 2010. Integrated brain circuits: Astrocytic networks modulate neuronal activity and behavior. *Annu. Rev. Physiol.* 72: 335–55. [10]

Halder, G., Callaerts, P., and Gehring, W. J. 1995. Induction of ectopic eyes by targeted expression of the eyeless gene in *Drosophila*. *Science* 267: 1788–1792. [1]

Hall, Z. W., Bownds, M. D., and Kravitz, E. A. 1970. The metabolism of γ-aminobutyric acid in the lobster nervous system. *J. Cell Biol.* 46: 290–299. [15]

Halliwell, J. V., and Adams, P. R. 1982. Voltage-clamp analysis of muscarinic excitation in hippocampal neurons. *Brain Res.* 250: 71–92. [14]

Halliwell, J. V., and Horne, A. L. 1998. Evidence for enhancement of gap junctional coupling between rat island of Calleja granule cells *in vitro* by the activation of dopamine D$_3$ receptors. *J. Physiol.* 506: 175–194. [11]

Hallock, P. T., Xu, C. F., Park, T. J., et al. 2010. Dok-7 regulates neuromuscular synapse formation by recruiting Crk and Crk-L. *Genes Dev.* 24: 2451–2461. [29]

Hamburger, V. 1934. The effects of wing bud extirpation on the development of the central nervous system in chick embryos. *J. Exp. Zool.* 68: 449–494. [27]

Hamburger, V., and Levi-Montalcini, R. 1949. Proliferation, differentiation and degeneration in the spinal ganglia of the chick embryo under normal and experimental conditions. *J. Exp. Zool.* 111:457–501. [27]

Hamill, M. B., and Koch, D. D. 1999. Pediatric cataracts. *Curr. Opin. Ophthalmol.* 10: 4–9. [28]

Hamill, O. P., and Sakmann, B. 1981. Multiple conductance of single acetylcholine receptor channels in embryonic muscle cells. *Nature* 294: 462–464. [4]

Hamill, O. P., Marty, A., Neher, E., et al. 1981. Improved patch-clamp techniques for high-resolution current recording from cells and cell-free membrane patches. *Pflügers Arch.* 391: 85–100. [4]

Hamilton, N. B., and Attwell, D. 2010. Do astrocytes really exocytose neurotransmitters? *Nat. Rev. Neurosci.* 11: 227–238. [10]

Hamon, M., Bourgoin, S., Artaud, F., and El Mestikawy, S. 1981. The respective roles of tryptophan uptake and tryptophan hydroxylase in the regulation of serotonin synthesis in the central nervous system. *J. Physiol. (Paris)* 77: 269–279. [15]

Han, G. A., Malintan, N. T., Collins, B. M., et al. 2010. Munc18-1 as a key regulator of neurosecretion. *J. Neurochem.* 115: 1–10. [13]

Han, J-H., et al. 2009. Selective erasure of a fear memory. *Science* 323: 1492. [17]

Han, T. W., et al. 2012. Cell-free formation of RNA granules: Bound RNAs identify features and components of cellular assemblies. *Cell* 149: 768–779. [17]

Han, Y. K., Kover, H., Insanally, M. N., et al. 2007. Early experience impairs perceptual discrimination. *Nat. Neurosci.* 10: 1191–1197. [28]

Hanlon, M. R., and Wallace, B. A. 2002. Structure and function of voltage-dependent ion channel regulatory β subunits. *Biochemistry* 41: 2886–2894. [5]

Hanover, J. L., Huang, Z. J., Tonegawa, S., and Stryker, M. P. 1999. Brain-derived neurotrophic factor overexpression induces precocious critical period in mouse visual cortex. *J. Neurosci.* 19: RC40. [28]

Hansen, D. V., Lui, J. H., Parker, P. R., and Kriegstein, A. R. 2010. Neurogenic radial glia in the outer subventricular zone of human neocortex. *Nature* 464: 554–561. [10, 27]

Hansen, H. H., Waroux, O., Seutin, V., et al. 2008. Kv7 channels: Interaction with dopaminergic and serotonergic neurotransmission in the CNS. *J. Physiol.* 586: 1823–1832. [19]

Hansen, K. B., Yi, F., Perszyk, R. E., et al. 2018. Structure, function, and allosteric modulation of NMDA receptors. *J. Gen. Physiol.* 150: 1081–1105. [11]

Hansen, S. M., Berezin, V., and Bock, E. 2008. Signaling mechanisms of neurite outgrowth induced by the cell adhesion molecules NCAM and N-cadherin. *Cell Mol. Life Sci.* 65: 3809–3821. [27]

Hanus, C., and Schuman, E. M. 2013. Proteostasis in complex dendrites. *Nat. Rev. Neurosci.* 14: 638–648. [17]

Harauzov, A., Spolidoro, M., DiCristo, G., et al. 2010. Reducing intracortical inhibition in the adult visual cortex promotes ocular dominance plasticity. *J. Neurosci.* 30: 361–371. [28]

Hardie, R. C. and Minke, B. 1992. The *trp* gene is essential for a light-activated Ca^{2+} channel in *Drosophila* photoreceptors, *Neuron* 8: 643–651. [5]

Hardingham, G. E., et al. 2002. Extrasynaptic NMDARs oppose synaptic NMDARs by triggering CREB shut-off and cell death pathways. *Nat. Neurosci.* 5: 405. [17]

Hardingham, A. M., and Bading, H. 2010. Synaptic versus extrasynaptic NMDA receptor signalling: Implications for neurodegenerative disorders. *Nat. Rev. Neurosci.* 11: 682–696. [17]

Harik, S. I. 1984. Locus ceruleus lesion by local 6-hydroxydopamine infusion causes marked and specific destruction of noradrenergic neurons, long-term depletion of norepinephrine and the enzymes that synthesize it, and enhanced dopaminergic mechanisms in the ipsilateral cerebral cortex. *J. Neurosci.* 4: 699–707. [14]

Harlow, H. F., and Woolsey, C. N. 1958. *Biological and Biochemical Bases of Behavior.* University of Wisconsin Press, Madison. [23]

Harlow, J. M. 1868. Recovery from passage of an iron bar through the head. *Publ. Mass. Med. Soc.* 2: 328–334. [28]

Harlow, M. L., Ress, D., Stoschek, A., et al. 2001. The architecture of active zone material at the frog's neuromuscular junction. *Nature* 409: 479–484. [13]

Harris, A. J., Kuffler, S. W., and Dennis, M. L. 1971. Differential chemosensitivity of synaptic and extrasynaptic areas on the neuronal surface membrane in parasympathetic neurones of the frog, tested by microapplication of acetylcholine. *Proc. R. Soc. Lond., B, Biol. Sci.* 177: 541–553. [29]

Harris, G. W., and Ruf, K. B. 1970. Luteinizing hormone releasing factor in rat hypophysial portal blood collected during electrical stimulation of the hypothalamus. *J. Physiol.* 208: 243–250. [19]

Harris, J. A., Harris, I. M., and Diamond, M. E. 2001. The topography of tactile learning in humans. *J. Neurosci.* 21: 1056–1061. [23]

Harris, J. A., Petersen, R. S., and Diamond, M. E. 1999. Distribution of tactile learning and its neural basis. *Proc. Natl. Acad. Sci. USA* 96: 7587–7591. [1, 23]

Harris, K. M., and Landis, D. M. M. 1986. Membrane structure at synaptic junctions in area CA1 of the rat hippocampus. *Neuroscience* 19: 857–872. [13]

Harris, W. A., Holt, C. E., and Bonhoeffer, F. 1987. Retinal axons with and without their somata, growing to and arborizing in the tectum of *Xenopus* embryos: A time-lapse video study of single fibres in vivo. *Development* 101: 123–133. [27]

Hartline, H. K. 1940. The receptive fields of optic nerve fibers. *Am. J. Physiol.* 130: 690–699. [2, 20]

Hartshorn, R. P., and Catterall, W. A. 1984. The sodium channel from rat brain: Purification and subunit composition. *J. Biol. Chem.* 259: 1667–1675. [5]

Harward, S. C., Hedrick, N. G., Hall, C. E., et al., 2016. Autocrine BDNF-TrkB signalling within a single dendritic spine. *Nature* 538: 99–103. [17]

Harwell, C. C., et al. 2015. Wide dispersion and diversity of clonally related inhibitory interneurons. *Neuron* 87: 999–1007. [27]

Hashimoto, H., Robin, F. B., Sherrard, K. M., et al. 2015. Sequential Contraction and exchange of apical junctions drives zippering and neural tube closure in a simple chordate. *Develop. Cell* 32: 241–255. [27]

Hashimotodani, Y., Ohno-Shosaku, T., and Kano, M. 2007. Endocannabinoids and synaptic function in the CNS. *Neuroscientist* 13: 127–137. [12]

Hashimotodani, Y., Ohno-Shosaku, T., Tsubokawa, H., et al. 2005. Phospholipase Cbeta serves as a coincidence detector through its Ca^{2+} dependency for triggering retrograde endocannabinoid signal. *Neuron* 45: 257–268. [12]

Hasselmo, M. E. 2006. The role of acetylcholine in learning and memory. *Curr. Opin. Neurobiol.* 16: 710–715. [14]

Hasson, U., Hendler, T., Ben Bashat, D., and Malach, R. 2001. Vase or face? A neural correlate of shape-selective grouping processes in the human brain. *J. Cogn. Neurosci.* 13: 744–753. [25]

Hata, Y., Tsumoto, T., and Stryker, M. P. 1999. Selective pruning of more active afferents when cat visual cortex is pharmacologically inhibited. *Neuron* 22: 375–381. [28]

Hattar, S., Liao, H. W., Takao, M., et al. 2002. Melanopsin-containing retinal ganglion cells: Architecture, projections, and intrinsic photosensitivity. *Science* 295: 1065–1070. [18, 19]

Hatten, M. E. 1990. Riding the glial monorail: A common mechanism for glial-guided neuronal migration in different regions of the developing mammalian brain. *Trends Neurosci.* 13: 179–184. [10, 23]

Hatten, M. E. 1999. Central nervous system neuronal migration. *Annu. Rev. Neurosci.* 22: 511–539. [10]

Hatten, M. E., Liem, R. K., and Mason, C. A. 1986. Weaver mouse cerebellar granule neurons fail to migrate on wild-type astroglial processes *in vitro. J. Neurosci.* 6: 2676–2683. [27]

Hawkins, J., and Blakeslee, S. 2004. *On Intelligence.* Times Books, New York. [1]

Hayashi-Takagi, A., et al. 2015. Labelling and optical erasure of synaptic memory traces in the motor cortex. *Nature* 525: 333–338. [17]

Hayworth, C. R., Moody, S. E., Chodosh, L. A., et al. 2006. Induction of neuregulin signaling in mouse Schwann cells in vivo mimics responses to denervation. *J. Neurosci.* 26: 6873–6884. [29]

He, L., and Wu, L-G. 2007. The debate on the kiss-and-run fusion at synapses. *Trends Neurosci.* 30: 447–455. [13]

He, L., Wu, X-S., Mohan, R., and Wu, L-G. 2006. Two modes of fusion pore opening revealed by cell-attached recordings at a synapse. *Nature* 444: 102–105. [13]

Hebb, D. O. 1949. *The Organization of Behavior: A Neuropsychological Theory.* Wiley, New York. [16]

Hedgecock, E. M., Culotti, J. G., and Hall, D. H. 1990. The *unc-5, unc-6,* and *unc-40* genes guide circumferential migrations of pioneer axons and mesodermal cells on the epidermis in *C. elegans. Neuron* 4: 61–85. [27]

Hediger, M. A., Romero, M. F., Peng, J. B., et al. 2004. The ABCs of solute carriers: Physiological, pathological and therapeutic implications of human membrane transport proteins. *Pflügers Arch.* 447: 465–468. [15]

Hefti, F. 1986. Nerve growth factor promotes survival of septal cholinergic neurons after fimbrial transections. *J. Neurosci.* 6: 2155–2162. [27]

Heidelberger, R., and Matthews, G. 1992. Calcium influx and calcium current in single synaptic terminals of goldfish retinal bipolar neurons. *J. Physiol.* 447: 235–256. [13]

Heidelberger, R., Thoreson, W. B., and Witkovsky, P. 2005. Synaptic transmission at retinal ribbon synapses. Prog. Retin. Eye Res. 24: 682–720. [22]

Heil, P., Rajan, R., and Irvine, D. R. 1994. Topographic representation of tone intensity along the isofrequency axis of cat primary auditory cortex. *Hear. Res.* 76: 188–202. [24]

Heiligenberg, W. 1989. Coding and processing of electrosensory information in gymnotiform fish. *J. Exp. Biol.* 146: 255–275. [21]

Hein, P., Frank, M., Hoffmann, C., Lohse, M. J., and Bünemann, M. 2005. Dynamics of receptor/G protein coupling in living cells. *EMBO J.* 24: 4106–4114. [12]

Heinemann, S. H., Terlau, H., Stühmer, W., et al. 1992. Calcium channel characteristics conferred on the sodium channel by single mutations. *Nature* 356: 441–443. [5]

Heinrich, C., et al. 2014. Sox2-mediated conversion of NG2 glia into induced neurons in the injured adult cerebral cortex. *Stem Cell Rep.* 3: 1000–1014. [29]

Heins, N., Malatesta, P., Cecconi, F., et al. 2002. Glial cells generate neurons: The role of the transcription factor Pax6. *Nat. Neurosci.* 5: 308–315. [29]

Helmholtz, H. von. 1889. *Popular Scientific Lectures.* Longmans, London. [1]

Helmholtz, H. von. 1962/1924. *Helmholtz's Treatise on Physiological Optics.* Dover, New York. [22]

Hemmati-Brivanlou, A., and Melton, D. A. 1997. Vertebrate embryonic cells will become nerve cells unless told otherwise. *Cell* 88: 13–17. [27]

Hemmati-Brivanlou, A., and Melton, D. 1997. Vertebrate neural induction. *Annu. Rev. Neurosci.* 20: 43–60. [27]

Henderson, L. P. 1983. The role of 5-hydroxytyptamine as a transmitter between identified leech neurones in culture. *J. Physiol. (Lond.)* 339: 309–324. [18]

Henderson, R. 2013 Ion channel seen by electron microscopy. *Nature* 504: 93–94. [5]

Henderson, T. A., Woolsey, T. A., and Jacquin, M. F. 1992. Infraorbital nerve blockade from birth does not disrupt central trigeminal pattern formation in the rat. *Brain Res. Dev. Brain Res.* 66: 146–152. [28]

Hendry, I. A., Ktöckel, K., Thoenen, H., and Iversen, L. L. 1974. The retrograde axonal transport of nerve growth factor. *Brain Res.* 68: 103–121. [27]

Hendry, S. H. C., and Calkins, D. J. 1998. Neuronal chemistry and functional organization in the primate visual system. *Trends Neurosci.* 21: 344–349. [2, 3]

Henneberger, C., Papouin, T., Oliet, S. H., and Rusakov, D. A. 2010. Long-term potentiation depends on release of D-serine from astrocytes. *Nature* 463: 232–236. [10]

Henneman, E., Somjen, G., and Carpenter, D. O. 1965. Functional significance of cell size in spinal motoneurons. *J. Neurophysiol.* 28: 560–580. [26]

Hensch, T. K. 2004. Critical period regulation. *Annu. Rev. Neurosci.* 27: 549–579. [28]

Hensch, T. K., and Quinlan, E. M. 2018. Critical periods in amblyopia. *Visual Neurosci.* 35: e014. [28]

Hensch, T. K., and Stryker, M. P. 2004. Columnar architecture sculpted by GABA circuits in developing cat visual cortex. *Science* 303: 1678–1681. [28]

Hensch, T. K., Fagiolini, M., Mataga, N., et al. 1998. Local GABA circuit control of experience-dependent plasticity in developing visual cortex. *Science* 282: 1504–1508. [28]

Herbert, A. L. and Monk, K. R. 2017. Advances in myelinating glial cell development. *Curr. Opin. Neurobiol.* 42: 53–60. doi: 10.1016/j.conb.2016.11.003. [10]

Herbert, S. C., Mount, D. B., and Gamba, G. 2004. Molecular physiology of cation-coupled Cl⁻ cotransport. *Pflügers Arch.* 447: 580–593. [9]

Herbst, W. A. and Martin, K. C. 2017. Regulated transport of signaling proteins from synapse to nucleus. *Curr. Op. Neurobiol.* 45: 78–84. [17]

Herlitze, S., Garcia, D. E., Mackie, K., et al. 1996. Modulation of Ca^{2+} channels by G-protein beta gamma subunits. *Nature* 380: 258–262. [12]

Herlitze, S., Villarroel, A., Witzemann, V., et al. 1996. Structural determinants of channel conductance in fetal and adult rat muscle acetylcholine receptors. *J. Physiol.* 492: 775–787. [11]

Hernandez, A., Salinas, E., Garcia, R., and Romo, R. 1997. Discrimination in the sense of flutter: New psychophysical measurements in monkeys. *J. Neurosci.* 17: 6391–6400. [25]

Hernandez, A., Zainos, A., and Romo, R. 2000. Neuronal correlates of sensory discrimination in the somatosensory cortex. *Proc. Natl. Acad. Sci. USA* 97: 6191–6196. [25]

Hernandez, A., Zainos, A., and Romo, R. 2002. Temporal evolution of a decision-making process in medial premotor cortex. *Neuron* 33: 959–972. [25]

Hernandez, C. C., Zaika, O., Tolstykh, G. P., and Shapiro, M. S. 2008. Regulation of neural KCNQ channels: Signalling pathways, structural motifs and functional implications. *J. Physiol.* 586: 1811–1821. [19]

Hernandez, R. E., Rikhof, H. A., Bachmann, R., and Moens, C. B. 2004. vhnf1 integrates global RA patterning and local FGF signals to direct posterior hindbrain development in zebrafish. *Development* 131: 4511–4520. [27]

Hernández-Falcón, J. et al. 2005. Changes in heart rate associated with contest outcome in agonistic encounters in lobsters. *Cell Mol. Neurobiol.* 25: 329–343. [18]

Herrada, G., and Dulac, C. 1997. A novel family of putative pheromone receptors in mammals with a topographically organized and sexually dimorphic distribution. *Cell* 90: 763–773. [21]

Herrero, J. L., Roberts, M. J., Delicato, L. S., et al. 2008. Acetylcholine contributes through muscarinic receptors to attentional modulation in V1. *Nature* 454: 1110–1114. [14]

Hertting, G., and Axelrod, J. 1961. Fate of tritiated noradrenaline at the sympathetic nerve endings. *Nature* 192: 172–173. [15]

Hertting, G., Axelrod, J., Kopin, I. J., and Whitby, L. J. 1961. Lack of uptake of catecholamines after chronic denervation of sympathetic nerves. *Nature* 189: 66. [15]

Hertz L. 2004. Intercellular metabolic compartmentation in the brain: Past, present and future. *Neurochem. Int.* 45: 285–296. [15]

Hestrin, S., and Galarreta, M. 2005. Electrical synapses define networks of neocortical GABAergic neurons. *Trends Neurosci.* 28: 304–309. [11]

Heuser, J. E. 1989. Review of electron microscopic evidence favouring vesicle exocytosis as the structural basis for quantal release during synaptic transmission. *Quart. J. Exp. Physiol.* 74: 1051–1069. [13]

Heuser, J. E., and Reese, T. S. 1973. Evidence for recycling of synaptic vesicle membrane during transmitter release at the frog neuromuscular junction. *J. Cell Biol.* 57: 315–344. [13]

Heuser, J. E., and Reese, T. S. 1981. Structural changes after transmitter release at the frog neuromuscular junction. *J. Cell Biol.* 88: 564–580. [13]

Heuser, J. E., Reese, T. S., and Landis, D. M. D. 1974. Functional changes in frog neuromuscular junction studied with freeze-fracture. *J. Neurocytol.* 3: 109–131. [13]

Heuser, J. E., Reese, T. S., Dennis, M. J., et al. 1979. Synaptic vesicle exocytosis captured by quick freezing and correlated with quantal transmitter release. *J. Cell Biol.* 81: 275–300. [13]

Hevner, R. F. 2006. From radial glia to pyramidal-projection neuron: Transcription factor cascades in cerebral cortex development. *Mol. Neurobiol.* 33: 33–50. [10]

Higashida, H., Lopatina, O., Yoshihara, T., et al. 2010. Oxytocin signal and social behaviour: Comparison among adult and infant oxytocin, oxytocin receptor and CD38 gene knockout mice. *J. Neuroendocrin.* 22: 373–379. [14]

Highstein, S. M. 1991. The central nervous system efferent control of the organs of balance and equilibrium. *Neurosci. Res.* 12: 13–30. [24]

Highstein, S. M., Rabbitt, R. D., Holstein, G. R., and Boyle, R. D. 2005. Determinants of spatial and temporal coding by semicircular canal afferents. *J. Neurophysiol.* 93: 2359–2370. [24]

Higuchi, M., Maas, S., Single, F. N., et al. 2000. Point mutation in an AMPA receptor gene rescues lethality in mice deficient in the RNA-editing enzyme ADAR2. *Nature* 406: 78–81. [27]

Hilaire, G. G., Nicholls, J. G., and Sears, T. A. 1983. Central and proprioceptive influences on the activity of levator costae motoneurones in the cat. *J. Physiol.* 342: 527–548. [26]

Hilf, R. J., and Dutzler, R. 2008. X-ray structure of a prokaryotic pentameric ligand-gated ion channel. *Nature* 452: 375–379. [5]

Hilf, R. J., and Dutzler, R. 2009 Structure of a potentially open state of a proton-activated pentameric ligand-gated ion channel. *Nature* 457: 115–118. [Hill, R. 2000. NK1 (substance P) receptor antagonists— why are they not analgesic in humans? *Trends Pharmacol. Sci.* 21: 244–246. [14]

Hille, B. 1970. Ionic channels in nerve membranes. *Prog. Biophys. Mol. Biol.* 21: 1–32. [7]

Hille, B. 1994. Modulation of ion-channel function by G-protein-coupled receptors. *Trends Neurosci.* 17: 531–536. [12]

Hille, B. 2001. *Ion Channels in Excitable Membranes*, 3rd ed. Sinauer Associates, Sunderland MA. [4, 7, 11]

Hirano, T. 1990. Depression and potentiation of the synaptic transmission between a granule cell and a Purkinje cell in rat cerebellar culture. *Neurosci. Lett.* 119: 141–144. [16]

Hirano, T. 1990. Effects of postsynaptic depolarization in the induction of synaptic depression between a granule cell and a Purkinje cell in rat cerebellar culture. *Neurosci. Lett.* 119: 145–147. [16]

Hirasawa, H., Contini, M., and Raviola, E. 2015. Extrasynaptic release of GABA and dopamine by retinal dopaminergic neurons. *Philos. Trans. R. Soc. Lond. B Biol. Sci.* 370: 20140186. [18]

Hirasawa, H., Puopolo, M., and Raviola, E. 2009. Extrasynaptic release of GABA by retinal dopaminergic neurons. *J. Neurophysiol.* 102: 146–158. doi: 10.1152/jn.00130.2009. [18]

Hirokawa, N. 1998. Kinesin and dynein superfamily proteins and the mechanism of organelle transport. *Science* 279: 519–552. [15]

Hirokawa, N., Niwa, S., and Tanaka, Y. 2010. Molecular motors in neurons: Transport mechanisms and roles in brain function, development, and disease. *Neuron* 68: 610–638. [15]

Hirokawa, N., Terada, S., Funakoshi, T., and Takeda, S. 1997. Slow axonal transport: The subunit transport model. *Trends Cell Biol.* 7: 382–388. [15]

Hirsch, J. A., and Martinez, L. M. 2006. Circuits that build visual cortical receptive fields. *Trends Neurosci.* 29: 30–39. [2]

Hirsch, J. A., Gallagher, C. A., Alonso, J. M., and Martinez, L. M. 1998. Ascending projections of simple and complex cells in layer 6 of the cat striate cortex. *J. Neurosci.* 18: 8086–8094. [3]

Ho, R. K. 1992. Cell movements and cell fate during zebrafish gastrulation. *Dev. Suppl.* 65–73. [27]

Hobert, O. 2010. Neurogenesis in the nematode *Caenorhabditis elegans*. *WormBook.* 4: 1–24. [27]

Hochedlinger, K., and Jaenisch, R. 2015. Induced pluripotency and epigenetic reprogramming *Cold Spring Harbour Perspect. Biol.* 7: A019448. [29]

Hodgkin, A. L. 1964. *The Conduction of the Nervous Impulse.* Liverpool University Press, Liverpool, England. [1]

Hodgkin, A. L. 1973. Presidential address. *Proc. R. Soc. Lond., B, Biol. Sci.* 183: 1–19. [6]

Hodgkin, A. L. and Horowicz, P. 1959. The influence of potassium and chloride ions on the membrane potential of single muscle fibres. *J. Physiol.* 145: 405–432. [6]

Hodgkin, A. L. and Huxley, A. F. 1952. Propagation of electrical signals along giant nerve fibres. *Proc. Roy. Soc. Lond. B* 140: 177–183. [7]

Hodgkin, A. L., and Huxley, A. F. 1952. Currents carried by sodium and potassium ion through the membrane of the giant axon of *Loligo*. *J. Physiol.* 116: 449–472. [7]

Hodgkin, A. L., and Huxley, A. F. 1952. The components of the membrane conductance in the giant axon of *Loligo*. *J. Physiol.* 116: 473–496. [7]

Hodgkin, A. L., and Huxley, A. F. 1952. The dual effect of membrane potential on sodium conductance in the giant axon of *Loligo*. *J. Physiol.* 116: 497–506. [7]

Hodgkin, A. L., and Huxley, A. F. 1952e. A quantitative description of membrane current and its application to conduction and excitation in nerve. *J. Physiol.* 117: 500–544. [7]

Hodgkin, A. L., and Katz, B. 1949. The effect of sodium ions on the electrical activity of the giant axon of the squid. *J. Physiol.* 108: 37–77. [6]

Hodgkin, A. L., and Keynes, R. D. 1955. Active transport of cations in giant axons from *Sepia* and *Loligo*. *J. Physiol.* 128: 28–60. [9]

Hodgkin, A. L., and Keynes, R. D. 1956. Experiments on the injection of substances into squid giant axons by means of a microsyringe. *J. Physiol.* 131: 592–617. [6]

Hodgkin, A. L., and Keynes, R. D. 1957. Movements of labelled calcium in squid giant axons. *J Physiol.* 138: 253–281. [6, 12]

Hodgkin, A. L., and Rushton, W. A. H. 1946. The electrical constants of a crustacean nerve fiber. *Proc. R. Soc. Lond., B, Biol. Sci.* 133: 444–479. [8]

Hodgkin, A. L., Huxley, A. F., and Katz, B. 1952. Measurement of current-voltage relations in the membrane of the giant axon of *Loligo*. *J. Physiol.* 116: 424–448. [7]

Hofer, H., Singer, B., and Williams, D. R. 2005. Different sensations from cones with the same photopigment. *J. Vision* 5: 5. [22]

Hofer, S. B., Mrsic-Flogel, T. D., Bonhoeffer, T., and Hübener, M. 2009. Experience leaves a lasting structural trace in cortical circuits. *Nature* 457: 313–317. [17, 28]

Hofmann, F., Biel, M., and Flockerzi, V. 1994. Molecular basis for Ca^{2+} channel diversity. *Annu. Rev. Neurosci.* 17: 399–418. [5]

Hofmann, L., and Palczewski, K. 2015. Advances in understanding the molecular basis of the first steps in color vision. *Prog. Retin. Eye Res.* 49: 46–66. [22]

Hökfelt, T. 1968. In vitro studies on central and peripheral monoamine neurons at the ultrastructural level. *Z. Zellforsch Mikrosk Anat.* 91: 1–74. [18]

Hökfelt, T. et al. 2018. Neuropeptide and small transmitter coexistence: Fundamental studies and relevance to mental illness. *Front. Neural Circuit.* 12: 106. [18]

Hökfelt, T., Broberger, C., Xu, Z. Q., et al. 2000. Neuropeptides— an overview. *Neuropharmacology* 39: 1337–1356. [14]

Hökfelt, T., Johansson, O., Llungdahl, A., et al. 1980. Peptidergic neurons. *Nature* 284: 515–521. [14]

Hökfelt, T., Kellerth, J. O., Nilsson, G., and Pernow, B. 1975. Substance P: Localization in the central nervous system and in some primary sensory neurons. *Science* 190: 889–890. [14]

Hökfelt, T., Ljungdahl, A., Terenius, L., et al.1977. Immunohistochemical analysis of peptide pathways possibly related to pain and analgesia: Enkephalin and substance P. *Proc. Natl. Acad. Sci. USA* 74: 3081–3085. [14]

Hollins, M., and Bensmaia, S. J. 2007. The coding of roughness. *Can. J. Exp. Psychol.* 61: 184–195. [23]

Hollins, M., Fox, A., and Bishop, C. 2000. Imposed vibration influences perceived tactile smoothness. *Perception* 29: 1455–1465. [23]

Hollis, E. R., 2nd, Ishiko, N., Yu, T., et al. 2016. Ryk controls remapping of motor cortex during functional recovery after spinal cord injury. *Nat. Neurosci* 19: 697–705. [29]

Hollman, M., and Heinemann, S. 1994. Cloned glutamate receptors. *Annu. Rev. Neurosci.* 17: 31–108. [14]

Hollmann, M., Hartley, M., and Heinemann, S. 1991. Ca^{2+} permeability of KA–AMPA-gated glutamate receptor channels depends on subunit composition. *Science* 252: 851–853. [27]

Hollmann, M., Maron, C., and Heinemann, S. 1994. N-Glycosylation sit tagging suggests a three transmembrane domain topology for the glutamate receptor GluR1. *Neuron* 13: 1331–1343. [5]

Hollyday, M., and Hamburger, V. 1976. Reduction of the naturally occurring motor neuron loss by enlargement of the periphery. *J. Comp. Neurol.* 170: 311–320. [27]

Hölscher, C. 1999. Synaptic plasticity and learning and memory: LTP and beyond. *J. Neurosci. Res.* 58: 62–75. [16]

Holt, J. C., Chatlani, S., Lysakowski, A., and Goldberg, J. M. 2007. Quantal and nonquantal transmission in calyx-bearing fibers of the turtle posterior crista. *J. Neurophysiol.* 98: 1083–1101. [24]

Holtmaat, A. and Svoboda K. 2009. Experience-dependent structural synaptic plasticity in the mammalian brain. *Nat. Rev. Neurosci.* 10: 647–658. [17]

Holton, P. 1959. The liberation of adenosine triphosphate on antidromic stimulation of sensory nerves. *J. Physiol.* 145: 494–504. [14]

Homma, Y., Baker, B. J., Jin, L., et al. 2009. Wide-field and two-photon imaging of brain activity with voltage- and calcium-sensitive dyes. *Philos. Trans. R. Soc. Lond., B, Biol. Sci.* 364: 2453–2467. [1]

Hong, E. J., et al. 2008. A biological function for the neuronal activity-dependent component of *Bdnf* transcription in the development of cortical inhibition. *Neuron* 60: 610–624. [17]

Hooks, B. M., and Chen, C. 2007. Critical periods in the visual system: Changing views for a model of experience-dependent plasticity. *Neuron* 56: 312–326. [28]

Horisberger, J. D. 2004. Recent insights into the structure and mechanism of the sodium pump. *Physiology* 19: 377–387. [9]

Horn, R., and Marty, A. 1988. Muscarinic activation of ionic currents measured by a new whole-cell recording method. *J. Gen. Physiol.* 92: 145–149. [4]

Hörner, M., Weiger, W. A., Edwards, D. H., and Kravitz, E. A. 1997. Excitation of identified serotonergic neurons by escape command neurons in lobsters. *J. Exp Biol.* 200: 2017–2033. [18]

Horton, J. C., and Hocking, D. R. 1996. Pattern of ocular dominance columns in human striate cortex in strabismic amblyopia. *Vis. Neurosci.* 13: 787–795. [28]

Horton, J. C., and Hocking, D. R. 1997. Timing of the critical period for plasticity of ocular dominance columns in macaque striate cortex. *J. Neurosci.* 17: 3684–3709. [28]

Horton, J. C., and Hocking, D. R. 1998. Effect of early monocular enucleation upon ocular dominance columns and cytochrome oxidase activity in monkey and human visual cortex. *Vis. Neurosci.* 15: 289–303. [28]

Hoshi, T., Zagotta, W. N., and Aldrich, R. W. 1990. Biophysical and molecular mechanisms of *Shaker* potassium channel inactivation. *Science* 250: 533–550. [7]

Hoshi, T., Zagotta, W. N., and Aldrich, R. W. 1991. Two types of inactivation in *Shaker* K^+ channels: Effects of alterations in the carboxyl terminal region. *Neuron* 7: 547–566. [7]

Hosie, A. M., Wilkins, M. E., da Silva, H. M., and Smart, T. G., 2006. Endogenous neurosteroids regulate GABAA receptors through two discrete transmembrane sites. *Nature* 444: 486–489. [14]

Hosoya, T., Baccus, S. A., and Meister, M. 2005. Dynamic predictive coding by the retina. *Nature* 436: 71–77. [22]

Housley, G. D., and Ashmore, J. F. 1991. Direct measurement of the action of acetylcholine on isolated outer hair cells of the guinea pig cochlea. *Proc. R. Soc. Lond., B, Biol. Sci.* 244: 161–167. [24]

Howard, J., and Hudspeth, A. J. 1988. Compliance of the hair bundle associated with gating of mechanoelectrical transduction channels in the bullfrog's saccular hair cell. *Neuron* 1: 189–199. [21]

Howard, J., Hudspeth, A. J., and Vale, R. D. 1989. Movement of microtubules by single kinesin molecules. *Nature* 342: 154–158. [15]

Howe, C. L., and Mobley, W. C. 2005. Long-distance retrograde neurotrophic signaling. *Curr. Opin. Neurobiol.* 15: 40–48. [27]

Howe, W. M., and Kenny, P. J. 2018. Burst firing sets the stage for depression. *Nature* 554: 304–305. [14]

Howes, O. D., and Kapur, S. 2009. The dopamine hypothesis of schizophrenia: Version III—the final common pathway. *Schizophr. Bull.* 35: 549–562. [14]

Hrvatin, S., et al. 2018. Single-cell analysis of experience-dependent transcriptomic states in the mouse visual cortex. *Nat. Neurosci.* 21: 120–129. [17]

Hu, F., and Strittmatter, S. M. 2004. Regulating axon growth within the postnatal central nervous system. *Semin. Perinatol.* 28: 371–378. [29]

Huang, C.-L., Slesinger, P. A., Casey, P. J., et al. 1995. Evidence that direct binding of Gβγ to the GIRK1 G protein-gated inwardly rectifying K^+ channel is important for channel activation. *Neuron* 15: 1133–1143. [12]

Huang, E. J., and Reichardt, L. F. 2001. Neurotrophins: Roles in neuronal development and function. *Annu. Rev. Neurosci.* 246: 77–136. [27]

Huang, H. P. et al. 2007. Number of neurotransmitter molecules in vesicle. *Proc. Natl. Acad. Sci. USA* 104: 1401–1406. [18]

Huang, H. P. et al. 2012. Physiology of quantal norepinephrine release from somatodendritic sites of neurons in locus coeruleus. *Front. Mol. Neurosci.* 5: 29. [18]

Huang, L. Y., and Neher, E. 1996. Ca(2+)-dependent exocytosis in the somata of dorsal root ganglion neurons. *Neuron* 17: 135–145. [18]

Huang, Y., Jellies, J., Johansen, K. M., and Johansen, J. 1998. Development and pathway formation of peripheral neurons during leech embryogenesis. *J. Comp. Neurol.* 397: 394–402. [20]

Huang, Y. J., Maruyama, Y., Lu, K. S., et al. 2005. Mouse taste buds use serotonin as a neurotransmitter. *J. Neurosci.* 25: 843–847. [21]

Huang, Z. J., Kirkwood, A., Pizzorusso, T., et al. 1999. BDNF regulates the maturation of inhibition and the critical period of plasticity in mouse visual cortex. *Cell* 98: 739–755. [28]

Huang, Z. L., Qu, W. M., Li, W. D., et al. 2001. Arousal effect of orexin A depends on activation of the histaminergic system. *Proc. Natl. Acad. Sci. USA* 98: 9965–9970. [14]

Hubel, D. H. 1981. Evolution of ideas on the primary visual cortex, 1955–1978: A biased historical account. Nobel Lecture. www.nobelprize.org/prizes/medicine/1981/hubel/lecture/ [2]

Hubel, D. H. 1982. Exploration of the primary visual cortex. *Nature* 299: 515–524. [2]

Hubel, D. H. 1988. *Eye, Brain and Vision.* Scientific American Library, New York. [2, 3, 28]

Hubel, D. H., and Wiesel, T. N. 1959. Receptive fields of single neurons in the cat's striate cortex. *J. Physiol.* 148: 574–591. [1, 2, 3]

Hubel, D. H., and Wiesel, T. N. 1961. Integrative action in the cat's lateral geniculate body. *J. Physiol.* 155: 385–398. [2]

Hubel, D. H., and Wiesel, T. N. 1962. Receptive fields, binocular interaction and functional architecture in the cat's visual cortex. *J. Physiol.* 160: 106–154. [2, 3]

Hubel, D. H., and Wiesel, T. N. 1963. Receptive fields of cells in striate cortex of very young, visually inexperienced kittens. *J. Neurophysiol.* 26: 994–1002. [28]

Hubel, D. H., and Wiesel, T. N. 1965. Binocular interaction in striate cortex of kittens reared with artificial squint. *J. Neurophysiol.* 28: 1041–1059. [28]

Hubel, D. H., and Wiesel, T. N. 1965. Receptive fields and functional architecture in two non-striate visual areas (18 and 19) of the cat. *J. Neurophysiol.* 28: 229–289. [2, 3]

Hubel, D. H., and Wiesel, T. N. 1967. Cortical and callosal connections concerned with the vertical meridian of visual field in the cat. *J. Neurophysiol.* 30: 1561–1573. [3]

Hubel, D. H., and Wiesel, T. N. 1968. Receptive fields and functional architecture of monkey striate cortex. *J. Physiol.* 195: 215–243. [2, 3]

Hubel, D. H., and Wiesel, T. N. 1970. The period of susceptibility to the physiological effects of unilateral eye closure in kittens. *J. Physiol.* 206: 419–436. [28]

Hubel, D. H., and Wiesel, T. N. 1972. Laminar and columnar distribution of geniculo-cortical fibers in the macaque monkey. *J. Comp. Neurol.* 146: 421–450. [2, 3]

Hubel, D. H., and Wiesel, T. N. 1974. Sequence regularity and geometry of orientation columns in the monkey striate cortex. *J. Comp. Neurol.* 158: 267–294. [3]

Hubel, D. H., and Wiesel, T. N. 1977. Functional architecture of macaque monkey visual cortex (Ferrier Lecture). *Proc. R. Soc. Lond., B, Biol. Sci.* 198: 1–59. [1, 3, 28]

Hubel, D. H., and Wiesel, T. N. 2005. *Brain and Visual Perception.* Oxford University Press, New York, USA. [2]

Hubel, D. H., Wiesel, T. N., and LeVay, S. 1977. Plasticity of ocular dominance columns in monkey striate cortex. *Philos. Trans. R. Soc. Lond., B, Biol. Sci.* 278: 377–409. [28]

Hubener, M., Shoham, D., Grinvald, A., and Bonhoeffer, T. 1997. Spatial relationships among three columnar systems in cat area 17. *J. Neurosci.* 17: 9270–9284. [3]

Huber, K. M., et al. 2000. Role for rapid dendritic protein synthesis in hippocampal mGluR-dependent long-term depression. *Science* 288: 1254–1257. [17]

Huber, R. et al. 1997. Biogenic amines and aggression: experimental approaches in crustaceans. *Brain Behav. Evol.* 50: 60–68. [18]

Huber, R., and Knaden, M. 2018. Desert ants possess distinct memories for food and nest odors. *Proc. Natl. Acad. Sci. USA.* 115: 10470–10474. doi: 10.1073/pnas.1809433115. [20]

Hübner, C. A., Stein, V., Hermans-Borgmeyer, I., et al. 2001. Disruption of KCC2 reveals an essential role of K-Cl cotransport already in early synaptic inhibition. *Neuron* 30: 515–524. [11]

Huckstepp, R. T., id Bihi, R., Eason, R., et al. 2010. Connexin hemichannel-mediated CO_2-dependent release of ATP in the medulla oblongata contributes to central respiratory chemosensitivity. *J. Physiol.* 588: 3901–3920. [26]

Hudspeth, A. J. 1982. Extracellular current flow and the site of transduction by vertebrate hair cells. *J. Neurosci.* 2: 1–10. [21]

Hudspeth, A. J., and Corey, D. P. 1977. Sensitivity, polarity, and conductance change in the response of vertebrate hair cells to controlled mechanical stimuli. *Proc. Natl. Acad. Sci. USA* 74: 2407–2411. [21]

Hudspeth, A. J., and Gillespie, P. G. 1994. Pulling springs to tune transduction: Adaptation by hair cells. *Neuron* 12: 1–9. [21]

Hudspeth, A. J., and Jacobs, R. 1979. Stereocilia mediate transduction in vertebrate hair cells (auditory system/cilium/vestibular system). *Proc. Natl. Acad. Sci. USA* 76: 1506–1509. [21]

Hudspeth, A. J., and Lewis, R. S. 1988. Kinetic analysis of voltage- and ion-dependent conductances in saccular hair cells of the bull-frog, *Rana catesbeiana. J. Physiol.* 400: 237–274. [24]

Hudspeth, A. J., Poo, M. M., and Stuart, A. E. 1977. Passive signal propagation and membrane properties in median photoreceptors of the giant barnacle. *J. Physiol.* 272: 25–43. [21]

Huebner, E. A., and Strittmatter, S. M. 2009. Axon regeneration in the peripheral and central nervous systems. *Results Probl. Cell Differ.* 48: 339–351. [29]

Hughes, J. 1975. Isolation of an endogenous compound from the brain with pharmacological properties similar to morphine. *Brain Res.* 88: 295–308. [14]

Hughes, J., Smith, T. W., Kosterlitz, H. W., et al. 1975. Identification of two related pentapeptides from the brain with potent opiate agonist activity. *Nature* 258: 577–580. [14]

Hughes, S., Marsh, S. J., Tinker, A., and Brown, D. A. 2007. PIP_2-dependent inhibition of M-type (Kv7.2/7.3) potassium channels: Direct on-line assessment of PIP_2 depletion by Gq-coupled receptors in single living neurons. *Pflügers Arch.* 455: 115–124. [12]

Hultborn, H. 2006. Spinal reflexes, mechanisms and concepts: From Eccles to Lundberg and beyond. *Prog. Neurobiol.* 78: 215–242. [26]

Humphrey, A. L., Sur, M., Uhlrich, D. J., and Sherman, S. M. 1985. Projection patterns of individual X- and Y-cell axons from the lateral geniculate nucleus to cortical area 17 in the cat. *J. Comp. Neurol.* 233: 159–189. [28]

Hunt, C. C., Wilkinson, R. S., and Fukami, Y. 1978. Ionic basis of the receptor potential in primary endings of mammalian muscle spindles. *J. Gen. Physiol.* 71: 683–698. [21]

Hurlemann, R., Patin, A., Onur, O. A., et al. 2010. Oxytocin enhances amygdala-dependent, socially reinforced learning and emotional empathy in humans. *J. Neurosci.* 30: 4999–5007. [14]

Hutchins, B. I., and Kalil, K. 2008. Differential outgrowth of axons and their branches is regulated by localized calcium transients. *J. Neurosci.* 28: 143–153. [27]

Hutter, O. F., and Trautwein, W. 1956. Vagal and sympathetic effects on the pacemaker fibers in the sinus venosus of the heart. *J. Gen. Physiol.* 39: 715–733. [12]

Huxley, A. 1928. *Point Counter Point.* Harper Collins, New York. [24]

Hyvarinen, J., Poranen, A., and Jokinen, Y. 1980. Influence of attentive behavior on neuronal responses to vibration in primary somatosensory cortex of the monkey. *J. Neurophysiol.* 43: 870–882. [23]

Hyvarinen, J., Sakata, H., Talbot, W. H., and Mountcastle, V. B. 1968. Neuronal coding by cortical cells of the frequency of oscillating peripheral stimuli. *Science* 162: 1130–1132. [23]

Ichida, J. M., and Casagrande, V. A. 2002. Organization of the feedback pathway from striate cortex (V1) to the LGN (LGN) in the owl monkey (*Aotus trivirgatus*). *J. Comp. Neurol.* 454: 272–283. [2]

Igelhorst, B. A., Niederkinkhaus, V., Karus, et al. 2015. Regulation of neuronal excitability by release of proteins from glial cells. *Philos Trans R Soc Lond B Biol Sci.*370: 20140194. doi: 10.1098/rstb.2014.0194. [10]

Iggo, A., and Muir, A. R. 1969. The structure and function of a slowly adapting touch corpuscle in hairy skin. *J. Physiol.* 200: 763–796. [23]

Iglesias, R., Dahl, G., Qiu, F., et al. 2009. Pannexin 1: The molecular substrate of astrocyte "hemichannels." *J. Neurosci.* 29: 7092–7097. [10]

Ignarro, J. 1990. Biosynthesis and metabolism of endothelium-derived nitric oxide. *Annu. Rev. Physiol.* 30: 535–560. [12]

Ikeda, S. R. 1996. Voltage-dependent modulation of N-type calcium channels by G-protein beta gamma subunits. *Nature* 380: 255–258. [12]

Ikoma, A., Rukwied, R., Stander, S., Steinhoff, M., Miyachi Y., and Schmelz, M. 2003. Neurophysiology of pruritus: Interaction of itch and pain. *Arch. Dermatol.* 139: 1475–1478. [23]

Imamoto, Y., and Shichida, Y. 2014. Cone visual pigments. *Biochim Biophys Acta.* 1837: 664–673. doi:10.1016/j.bbabio.2013.08.009. [22]

Imoto, K., Busch, C., Sakmann, B., et al. 1998. Rings of negatively charged amino acids determine the acetylcholine receptor conductance. *Nature* 335: 645–648. [5]

Imoto, K., Konno, T., Nakai, J., et al. 1991. A ring of uncharged polar amino acids as a component of channel constriction in the nicotinic acetylcholine receptor. *FEBS Lett.* 289: 193–200. [5]

Ingber, D. E. 2006. Cellular mechanotransduction: Putting all the pieces together again. *FASEB J.* 20: 811–827. [21]

Inoue, S. 1981. Video image processing greatly enhances contrast, quality and speed in polarization-based microscopy. *J. Cell Biol.* 89: 346–356. [15]

Insanally, M. N., Kover, H., Kim, H., and Bao, S. 2009. Feature-dependent sensitive periods in the development of complex sound representation. *J. Neurosci.* 29: 5456–5462. [28]

Isaac, J. T., Nicoll, R. A., and Malenka, R. C. 1995. Evidence for silent synapses: Implications for the expression of LTP. *Neuron* 15: 427–434. [16]

Isaac, R. E., Bland, N. D., and Shirras, A. D. 2009. Neuropeptidases and the metabolic inactivation of insect neuropeptides. *Gen. Comp. Endocrinol.* 162: 8–17. [15]

Isaacson, J. S., Solís, J. M., and Nicoll, R. A. 1993. Local and diffuse synaptic actions of GABA in the hippocampus. *Neuron* 10: 165–175. [18]

Isbister, C. M., and O'Connor, T. P. 1999. Filopodial adhesion does not predict growth cone steering events *in vivo. J. Neurosci.* 19: 2589–2600. [27]

Ishikawa, T., Sahara, Y., and Takahashi, T. 2002. A single packet of transmitter does not saturate postsynaptic glutamate receptors. *Neuron* 34: 613–621. [15]

Ito, M. 1972. Neural design of the cerebellar motor control system. *Brain Res.* 40: 81–84. [24]

Ito, M. 1984. *The Cerebellum and Neural Control.* Raven, New York. [26]

Ito, M., and Simpson, J. I. 1971. Discharges in Purkinje cell axons during climbing fiber activation. *Brain Res.* 31: 215–219. [26]

Ito, M., Sakurai, M., and Tongroach, P. 1982. Climbing fibre induced depression of both mossy fibre responsiveness and glutamate sensitivity of cerebellar Purkinje cells. *J. Physiol.* 324: 113–134. [16]

Ito, M., Tamura, H., Fujita, I., and Tanaka, K. 1995. Size and position invariance of neuronal responses in monkey inferotemporal cortex. *J. Neurophysiol.* 73: 218–226. [25]

Iulita, M. F., and Cuello, A. C. 2014. Nerve growth factor metabolic dysfunction in Alzheimer's disease and Down syndrome. *Trends in Pharmacol. Sci.* 35: 338–348. [27]

Ivanov, A. and Purves, D. 1989. Ongoing electrical activity of superior cervical ganglion cells in mammals of different size. *J. Comp. Neurol.* 284: 398–404. [19]

Iversen, L. 2003. Cannabis and the brain. *Brain* 126: 1252–1270. [12]

Iversen, L. 2006. Neurotransmitter transporters and their impact on the development of psychopharmacology. *Brit. J. Pharmacol.* 147(Suppl. 1): S82–88. [15]

Iversen, L. L. 1971. Role of transmitter uptake mechanisms in synaptic neurotransmission. *Brit. J. Pharmacol.* 41: 571–591. [14]

Iversen, L. L., Iverson, S. D., Bloom, F. E., and Roth, R. H. 2009. *Introduction to Neuropsychopharmacology.* Oxford University Press, New York. [9]

Iwafuchi-Doi, M., and Zaret, K. S. 2014. Pioneer transcription factors in cell reprogramming. *Genes Dev.* 28:2679–2692. [27]

Iwase, S., et al. 2017. Epigenetic etiology of intellectual disability. *J. Neurosci.* 37: 10773–10782. [17]

Izquierdo, I., and Medina, J. H. 1995. Correlation between the pharmacology of long-term potentiation and the pharmacology of memory. *Neurobiol. Learn. Mem.* 63: 19–32. [16]

Jackson, C. R. et al. 2009. Essential roles of dopamine D_4 receptors and the type 1 adenylyl cyclase in photic control of cyclic AMP in photoreceptor cells. *J. Neurochem.* 109: 148e157. [18]

Jacobs, B. L., and Azmitia, E. C. 1992. Structure and function of the brain serotonin system. *Physiol. Rev.* 72: 165–229. [14]

Jacobs, G. H. 2008. Primate color vision: A comparative perspective. *Vis. Neurosci.* 25: 619–633. [22]

Jadzinsky, P. D., and Baccus, S. A. 2015. Synchronized amplification of local information transmission by peripheral retinal input. *eLife* 4: e09266. doi: 10.7554/eLife.09266. [22]

Jaffe, E. H. et al. 1998. Extrasynaptic vesicular transmitter release from the somata of substantia nigra neurons in rat midbrain slices. *J. Neurosci.* 18: 3548–3553. [18]

Jan, Y. N., Jan, L. Y., and Kuffler, S. W. 1979. A peptide as a possible transmitter in sympathetic ganglia of the frog. *Proc. Natl. Acad. Sci. USA* 76: 1501–1505. [19]

Jan, Y. N., Jan, L. Y., and Kuffler, S. W. 1980. Further evidence for peptidergic transmission in sympathetic ganglia. *Proc. Natl. Acad. Sci. USA* 77: 5008–5012. [19]

Jänig, W., and McLachlan, E. M. 1992. Characteristics of function-specific pathways in the sympathetic nervous system. *Trends Neurosci.* 15: 475–481. [19]

Jänig, W., Keast, J. R., McLachlan, E. M., et al. 2017. Renaming all spinal autonomic outflows as sympathetic is a mistake. *Auton. Neurosci.* 206: 60–62. [19]

Jansen, J. K. S., and Matthews, P. B. C. 1962. The central control of the dynamic response of muscle spindle receptors. *J. Physiol.* 161: 357–378. [21]

Jansen, J. K. S., and Nicholls, J. G. 1973. Conductance changes, an electrogenic pump and the hyperpolarization of leech neurones following impulses. *J. Physiol.* 229: 635–655. [7]

Jansen, J. K. S., Lømo, T., Nicholaysen, K., and Westgaard, R. H. 1973. Hyperinnervation of skeletal muscle fibers: Dependence on muscle activity. *Science* 181: 559–561. [29]

Jaramillo, F., and Hudspeth, A. J. 1991. Localization of the hair cell's transduction channels at the hair bundle's top by iontophoretic application of a channel blocker. *Neuron* 7: 409–420. [21]

Jarvilehto, T., Hamalainen, H., and Laurinen, P. 1976. Characteristics of single mechanoreceptive fibres innervating hairy skin of the human hand. *Exp. Brain Res.* 25: 45–61. [23]

Jarvis, M. F., and Khakh, B. S. 2009. ATP-gated P2X channels. *Neuropharmacology* 56: 208–215. [5]

Jasper, H., and Penfield, W. 1954. *Epilepsy and the Functional Anatomy of the Human Brain*, 2nd ed. Boston: Little, Brown and Co. [23]

Jasser, A., and Guth, P. S. 1973. The synthesis of acetylcholine by the olivo-cochlear bundle. *J. Neurochem.* 20: 45–53. [24]

Jeanmonod, D., Rice, F. L., and van Der Loos, H. 1977. Mouse somatosensory cortex: Development of the alterations in the barrel field which are caused by injury to the vibrissal follicles. *Neurosci. Lett.* 6: 151–156. [23]

Jenkinson, D. H. 1960. The antagonism between tubocurarine and substances which depolarize the motor end-plate. *J. Physiol.* 152: 309–324. [11]

Jenkinson, D. H. 2006. Potassium channels—multiplicity and challenges. *Brit. J. Pharmacol.* 147: S63–S71. [7]

Jenkinson, D. H. 2011. Classical approaches to the study of drug-receptor interactions. In J. C. Foreman, T. Johansen, and A. J. Gibb (Ed.), *Textbook of Receptor Pharmacology*, 3rd ed. CRC Press, London, U. K, pp. 3–76. [11]

Jenkinson, D. H., and Nicholls, J. G. 1961. Contractures and permeability changes produced by acetylcholine in depolarized denervated muscle. *J. Physiol.* 159: 111–127. [11]

Jennings, E. A., Ryan, R. M., and Christie, M. J. 2004. Effects of sumatriptan on rat medullary dorsal horn neurons. *Pain* 111: 30–37. [14]

Jentsch, T. J. 2000. Neuronal KCNQ potassium channels: Physiology and role in disease. *Nat. Rev. Neurosci.* 1: 21–30. [30]

Jessel, T. M. 2000. Neuronal specification in the spinal cord: Inductive signal and transcriptional codes. *Nat. Rev. Genet.* 1: 20–29. [27]

Ji, G., Feldman, M. E., Deng, K. Y., et al. 2004. Ca^{2+}-sensing transgenic mice: Postsynaptic signaling in smooth muscle. *J. Biol. Chem.* 279: 21461–21468. [1]

Ji, T. H., Grossmann, M., and Ji, I. 1998. G protein–coupled receptors. I. Diversity of receptor-ligand interactions. *J. Biol. Chem.* 273: 17299–17302. [12]

Jiang, G. J., Zidanic, M., Michaels, R. L., et al. 1997. CSlo encodes calcium-activated potassium channels in the chick's cochlea. *Proc. R. Soc. Lond., B, Biol. Sci.* 264: 731–737. [24]

Jiang, Y., Ruta, V., Chen, J., et al. 2003. The principle of gating charge movement in a voltage-dependent K^+ channel. *Nature* 423: 42–48. [7]

Jin, N. G., and Ribelayga, C. P. 2016. Direct evidence for daily plasticity of electrical coupling between rod photoreceptors in the mammalian retina. *J. Neurosci.* 36: 178–184. [18]

Jin, J., Wang, Y., Swadlow, H. A., and Alonso, J. M. 2011. Population receptive fields of ON and OFF thalamic inputs to an orientation column in visual cortex. *Nat. Neurosci.* 14:232–238. doi: 10.1038/nn.2729. [2]

Jo, Y. H., and Role, L. W. 2002. Coordinate release of ATP and GABA at *in vitro* synapses of lateral hypothalamic neurons. *J. Neurosci.* 22: 4794–4804. [14]

Joh, T. H., Park, D. H., and Reis, D. J. 1978. Direct phosphorylation of brain tyrosine hydroxylase by cyclic AMP-dependent protein kinase: Mechanism of enzyme activation. *Proc. Natl. Acad. Sci. USA* 75: 4744–4748. [15]

Johansson, C. B. et al. 1999. Identification of a neural stem cell in the adult mammalian central nervous system. *Cell* 96: 25–34. [18]

Johansen, J. P., et al. 2010. Optical activation of lateral amygdala pyramidal cells instructs associative fear learning. *Proc. Natl. Acad. Sci. USA* 107: 12692–12697. [17]

Johansson, P. A., Dziegielewska, K. M., Liddelow, S. A., and Saunders, N. R. 2008. The blood-CSF barrier explained: When development is not immaturity. *Bioessays* 30: 237–248. [10]

Johansson, R. S., and Vallbo, A. B. 1979. Detection of tactile stimuli. Thresholds of afferent units related to psychophysical thresholds in the human hand. *J. Physiol.* 297: 405–422. [23]

Johansson, R. S., and Vallbo, A. B. 1983. Tactile sensory coding in the glabrous skin of the human hand. *Trends Neurosci.* 6: 27–32. [23]

Johnson, E. W., and Wernig, A. 1971. The binomial nature of transmitter release at the crayfish neuromuscular junction. *J. Physiol.* 218: 757–767. [13]

Johnson, F. H., Eyring, H., and Polissar, M. J. 1954. *The Kinetic Basis of Molecular Biology.* Wiley, New York. [4]

Johnson, J. W., and Ascher, P. 1987. Glycine potentiates the NMDA response in cultured mouse brain neurons. *Nature* 325: 529–531. [11]

Johnson, M. H. 2005. Subcortical face processing. *Nat. Rev. Neurosci.* 6: 766–774. [25]

Jomphe, C., Bourque, M. J., Fortin, G. D., et al. 2005. Use of TH-EGFP transgenic mice as a source of identified dopaminergic neurons for physiological studies in postnatal cell culture. *J. Neurosci. Methods* 146: 1–12. [14]

Jonas, P., Bischofberger, J., and Sandkühler, J. 1998. Corelease of two fast neurotransmitters at a central synapse. *Science* 281: 419–424. [14, 15]

Jonas, P., Major, G., and Sakmann, B. 1993. Quantal components of unitary EPSCs at the mossy fibre synapse on CA3 pyramidal cells of rat hippocampus. *J. Physiol.* 472: 615–663. [13]

Jones, E. M., Gray-Keller, M., and Fettiplace, R. 1999. The role of Ca²⁺-activated K⁺ channel spliced variants in the tonotopic organization of the turtle cochlea. *J. Physiol.* 518: 653–665. [24]

Jones, E. M., Laus, C., and Fettiplace, R. 1998. Identification of Ca²⁺-activated K⁺ channel splice variants and their distribution in the turtle cochlea. *Proc. R. Soc. Lond., B, Biol. Sci.* 265: 685–692. [24]

Jones, S. W., and Adams, P. R. 1987. In *Neuromodulation: The Biochemical Control of Neuronal Excitability*. Oxford University Press, New York, pp. 159–186. [19]

Jones, T. A., Leake, P. A., Snyder, R. L., et al. 2007. Spontaneous discharge patterns in cochlear spiral ganglion cells before the onset of hearing in cats. *J. Neurophysiol.* 98: 1898–1908. [28]

Jope, R. 1979. High-affinity choline uptake and acetylcholine production in the brain. Role in regulation of ACh synthesis. *Brain Res. Rev.* 1: 313–344. [15]

Jorgensen, P. L., Hakansson, K. O., and Karlish, S. J. D. 2003. Structure and mechanism of the Na,K-ATPases: Functional sites and their interactions. *Annu. Rev. Physiol.* 65: 817–849. [9]

Josselyn, S. A., et al. 2015. Finding the engram. *Nat. Rev. Neurosci.* 16: 521. [17]

Josselyn, S. A., and Frankland, P. W. 2018. Memory allocation: Mechanisms and function. *Annu. Rev. Neurosci.* 41: 389–413 2018. [17]

Joyner, A. L., Liu, A., and Millet, S. 2000. Otx2, Gbx2 and Fgf8 interact to position and maintain a mid-hindbrain organizer. *Curr. Opin. Cell Biol.* 12: 736–741. [27]

Juge, N., Gray, J. A., Omote, H., et al. 2010. Metabolic control of vesicular glutamate transport and release. *Neuron* 68: 99–112. [15]

Jung, H., Yoon, B. C., and Holt, C. E. 2012 Axonal mRNA localization and local protein synthesis in nervous system assembly, maintenance and repair. *Nat Rev. Neurosci* 13: 308. [27]

Jung, S., Aliberti, J., Graemmel, P., et al. 2000. Analysis of fractalkine receptor CX(3)CR1 function by targeted deletion and green fluorescent protein reporter gene insertion. *Mol. Cell Biol.* 20: 4106–4114. [10]

Jung, H., et al. 2014. Remote control of gene function by local translation. *Cell* 157: 26–40. [17]

Kaas, J. H. 1983. What, if anything, is, S. I.? Organization of first somatosensory area of cortex. *Physiol. Rev.* 63: 206–231. [23]

Kadoya, K., Lu, P., Nguyen, K., et al. 2016. Spinal cord reconstitution with homologous neural grafts enables robust corticospinal regeneration. *Nat. Med.* 22: 479–487. [29]

Kalb, R. 2005. The protean actions of neurotrophins and their receptors on the life and death of neurons. *Trends Neurosci.* 28: 5–11. [27]

Kalivas, P. W., and Duffy, P. 1990. Effect of acute and daily cocaine treatment on extracellular dopamine in the nucleus accumbens. *Synapse* 5: 48–58. [14]

Kallen, R. G., Sheng, Z-H., Yang, J., Chen, L., et al. 1990. Primary structure and expression of a sodium channel characteristic of denervated and immature rat skeletal muscle. *Neuron* 4: 233–342. [29]

Kalmijn, A. J. 1982. Electric and magnetic field detection in elasmobranch fishes. *Science* 218: 916–918. [21]

Kanai, Y., and Hediger, M. A. 2004. The glutamate/neutral amino acid transporter family SLC1: Molecular, physiological, and pharmacological aspects. *Pflügers Arch.* 447: 469–479. [9]

Kanai, R., Ogawa, H., Vilsen, B., et al. 2013. Crystal structure of a Na⁺-bound Na⁺-, K⁺-ATP-ase preceding the e1P state. *Nature* 502: 201–206. [9]

Kandel, E. R. 2001. The molecular biology of memory storage: A dialogue between genes and synapses. *Science* 294: 1030–1038. [20]

Kaneko, A. 1970. Physiological and morphological identification of horizontal, bipolar and amacrine cells in goldfish retina. *J. Physiol.* 207: 623–633. [22]

Kaneko, A. 1971. Electrical connexions between horizontal cells in the dogfish retina. *J. Physiol.* 213: 95–105. [22]

Kaneko, A., and Hashimoto, H. 1969. Electrophysiological study of single neurons in the inner nuclear layer of the carp retina. *Vision Res.* 9: 37–55. [1, 22]

Kaneko, A., and Tachibana, M. 1986. Effects of gamma-aminobutyric acid on isolated cone photoreceptors of the turtle retina. *J. Physiol.* 373: 443–461. [22]

Kang, H., and Schuman E. 1996. A requirement for local protein synthesis in neurotrophin-induced hippocampal synaptic plasticity. *Science* 273: 1402–1406. [17]

Kang Miller, J., Ayzenshtat, I., Carrillo-Reid, L., and Yuste, R. 2014. Visual stimuli recruit intrinsically generated cortical ensembles. *Proc. Natl. Acad. Sci. USA.* 111: e4053–e4061. doi: 10.1073/pnas.1406077111. [2]

Kanning, K. C., Kaplan, A., and Henderson, C. E. 2010. Motor neuron diversity in development and disease. *Annu. Rev. Neurosci.* 33: 409–440. [26]

Kano, M., Ohno-Shosaku, T., Hashimotodani, Y., et al. 2009. Endocannabinoid-mediated control of synaptic transmission. *Physiol. Rev.* 89: 309–380. [12]

Kanold, P. O., and Shatz, C. J. 2006. Subplate neurons regulate maturation of cortical inhibition and outcome of ocular dominance plasticity. *Neuron* 51: 627–638. [27]

Kanwal, J. S., and Rauschecker, J. P. 2007. Auditory cortex of bats and primates: Managing species-specific calls for social communication. *Front. Biosci.* 12: 4621–4640. [24]

Kanwisher, N., and Yovel, G. 2006. The fusiform face area: A cortical region specialized for the perception of faces. *Philos. Trans. R. Soc. Lond., B, Biol. Sci.* 361: 2109–2128. [25]

Kaplan, D. R., Hempstead, B. L., Martin-Zanca, D., et al. 1991. The trk proto-oncogene product: A signal transducing receptor for nerve growth factor. *Science* 252: 554–558. doi: 10.1126/science.1850549. [27]

Kaplan, E., and Shapley, R. M. 1986. The primate retina contains two types of ganglion cells, with high and low contrast sensitivity. *Proc. Natl. Acad. Sci. USA* 83: 2755–2757. [22]

Kapur, M., et al. 2017. Regulation of mRNA translation in neurons-a matter of life and death. *Neuron* 96: 616–637. [17]

Káradóttir, R., Cavelier, P., Bergersen, L. H., and Attwell, D. 2005. NMDA receptors are expressed in oligodendrocytes and activated in ischaemia. *Nature* 438: 1162–1166. [10]

Káradóttir, R., Hamilton, N. B., Bakiri, Y. and Attwell, D. 2008. Spiking and non-spiking classes of oligodendrocyte precursor glia in CNS white matter. *Na.t Neurosci.* 11: 450–456. doi: 10.1038/nn2060. [10]

Karlin, A. 2002. Emerging structure of nicotinic acetylcholine receptors. *Nat. Rev. Neurosci.* 3: 102–114. [5]

Karplus, M., and Petsko, G. A. 1990. Molecular dynamics simulations in biology. *Nature* 347: 631–639. [4]

Kasai, H. 1999. Comparative biology of Ca²⁺-dependent exocytosis: Implications of kinetic diversity for secretory function. *Trends Neurosci.* 22: 88–93. [13]

Kasakov, L., Ellis, J., Kirkpatrick, K., et al. 1988. Direct evidence for concomitant release of noradrenaline, adenosine 5′-triphosphate and neuropeptide Y from sympathetic nerve supplying the guinea-pig vas deferens. *J. Auton. Nerv. Syst.* 22: 75–82. [19]

Kask, K., Zamanillo, D., Rozov, A., et al. 1998. The AMPA receptor subunit GluR-B in its Q/R site-unedited form is not essential for brain development and function. *Proc. Natl. Acad. Sci. USA* 95: 13777–13782. [27]

Kaspar, J., Schor, R. H., and Wilson, V. J. 1988. Response of vestibular neurons to head rotations in vertical planes. II. Response to neck stimulation and vestibular–neck interactions. *J. Neurophysiol.* 60: 1765–1768. [26]

Kastner, D. B., and Baccus, S. A. 2013. Spatial segregation of adaptation and predictive sensitization in retinal ganglion cells. *Neuron* 79: 541–554. [22]

Kastner, S., Pinsk, M. A., De Weerd, P., et al. 1999. Increased activity in human visual cortex during directed attention in the absence of visual stimulation. *Neuron* 22: 751–761. [25]

Kastner, S., Schneider, K. A., and Wunderlich, K. 2006. Beyond a relay nucleus: Neuroimaging views on the human LGN. *Prog. Brain Res.* 155: 125–143. [2]

Katona, I., Sperlágh, B., Maglóczky, Z., et al. 2000. GABAergic interneurons are the targets of cannabinoid actions in the human hippocampus. *Neuroscience* 100: 797–804. [12]

Katsuki, Y. 1961. Neural mechanisms of auditory sensation in cats. In W. A. Rosenblith (Ed.), *Sensory Communication*. MIT Press, Cambridge, MA, pp. 561–583. [24]

Katz, B. 1950. Depolarization of sensory terminals and the initiation of impulses in the muscle spindle. *J. Physiol.* 111: 261–282. [21]

Katz, B. 1971. Quantal mechanism of neural transmitter release. *Science* 173: 123–126. [1]

Katz, B., and Miledi, R. 1964. The development of acetylcholine sensitivity in nerve-free segments of skeletal muscle. *J. Physiol.* 170: 389–396. [29]

Katz, B., and Miledi, R. 1965. The effect of temperature on the synaptic delay at the neuromuscular junction. *J. Physiol.* 181: 656–670. [13]

Katz, B., and Miledi, R. 1967. The timing of calcium action during neuromuscular transmission. *J. Physiol.* 189: 535–544. [13]

Katz, B., and Miledi, R. 1967. A study of synaptic transmission in the absence of nerve impulses. *J. Physiol.* 192: 407–436. [13]

Katz, B., and Miledi, R. 1968. The role of calcium in neuromuscular facilitation. *J. Physiol.* 195: 481–492. [16]

Katz, B., and Miledi, R. 1972. The statistical nature of the acetylcholine potential and its molecular components. *J. Physiol.* 224: 665–699. [4, 13]

Katz, B., and Miledi, R. 1973. The binding of acetylcholine to receptors and its removal from the synaptic cleft. *J. Physiol.* 231: 549–574. [11, 15]

Katz, B., and Miledi, R. 1975. The nature of the prolonged endplate depolarization in anti-esterase treated muscle. *Proc. R. Soc. Lond. B.* 192: 27–38. [15]

Katz, L. C., and Crowley, J. C. 2002. Development of cortical circuits: Lessons from ocular dominance columns. *Nat. Rev. Neurosci.* 3: 34–42. doi: 10.1038/nrn703. [28]

Kaufman, C. M., and Menaker, M. J. 1993. Effect of transplanting suprachiasmatic nuclei from donors of different ages into completely SCN lesioned hamsters. *J. Neural Transplant. Plast.* 4: 257–265. [19]

Kaupp, U. B., and Seifert, R. 2002. Cyclic nucleotide-gated ion channels. *Physiol. Rev.* 82: 769–824. [22]

Kaur, G., Han, S. J., Yang, I., and Crane, C. 2010. Microglia and central nervous system immunity. *Neurosurg. Clin. N. Am.* 21: 43–51. [10]

Kaushalya, S. K., Desai, R., Arumugam, S., et al. 2008. Three-photon microscopy shows that somatic release can be a quantitatively significant component of serotonergic neurotransmission in the mammalian brain. *J. Neurosci. Res.* 86: 3469–3480. doi: 10.1002/jnr.21794. [18]

Kawashima, T., et al. 2013. Functional labeling of neurons and their projections using the synthetic activity-dependent promoter E-SARE. *Nat. Methods* 10: 889–895. [17]

Kazmierczak, P., Sakaguchi, H., Tokita, J., et al. 2007. Cadherin 23 and protocadherin 15 interact to form tip-link filaments in sensory hair cells. *Nature* 449: 87–91. [21]

Keirstead, H. S., and Miller, R. F. 1997. Metabotropic glutamate receptor agonists evoke calcium waves in isolated Müller cells. *Glia* 21: 194–203. [10]

Keirstead, H. S., Dyer, J. K., Sholomenko, G. N., et al. 1995. Axonal regeneration and physiological activity following transection and immunological disruption of myelin within the hatchling chick spinal cord. *J. Neurosci.* 15: 6963–6974. [29]

Kelleher, R. J., Govindarajan, A., and Tonegawa, S. 2004. Translational regulatory mechanisms in persistent forms of synaptic plasticity. *Neuron* 44: 59–73. [17]

Kellenberger, S. West, J. W., Catterall W. A., and Scheuer, T. 1997. Molecular analysis of potential hinge residues in the inactivation gate of brain type IIA Na$^+$ channels. *J. Gen. Physiol.* 109: 607–617. [7]

Kellenberger, S., West, J. W., Scheuer, T., and Catterall, W. A. 1997. Molecular analysis of a putative inactivation particle in the inactivation gate of brain type IIA sodium channels *J. Gen Physiol.* 109: 589–605. [7]

Kelley, S. P., Dunlop, J. I., Kirkness, E. F., et al. 2003. A cytoplasmic region determines single channel conductance in 5HT$_3$ receptors. *Nature* 424: 321–324. [5]

Kelly, R. M., and Strick, P. L.; Strick. 2000. Rabies as a transneuronal tracer of circuits in the central nervous system. *J. Neurosci. Methods* 103: 63–71. [1]

Kelsch, W., Sim, S., and Lois, C. 2010. Watching synaptogenesis in the adult brain. *Annu. Rev. Neurosci.* 33: 131–149. [27]

Kemp, D. T. 1978. Stimulated acoustic emissions from within the human auditory system. *J. Acoust. Soc. Am.* 64: 1386–1391. [21]

Kempermann, G., Song,H., and Gage, F.H. 2015. Neurogenesis in the adult hippocampus. *Cold Spring Harb. Perspect. Biol.* 7: A018812. [27]Kennedy, P. R. 1990. Corticospinal, rubrospinal and rubro-olivary projections: A unifying hypothesis. *Trends Neurosci.* 13: 474–479. [26]

Kennedy, T. E., Serafini, T., de la Torre, J. R., and Tessier-Lavigne, M. 1994. Netrins are diffusible chemotropic factors for commissural axons in the embryonic spinal cord. *Cell* 78: 425–435. [27]

Kenshalo, D. R., Iwata, K., Sholas, M., and Thomas, D. A. 2000. Response properties and organization of nociceptive neurons in area 1 of monkey primary somatosensory cortex. *J. Neurophysiol.* 84: 719–729. [23]

Keramidas, A., Moorhouse, A. J., French, C. R., et al. 2000. M2 pore mutations convert the glycine receptor channel from being anion- to cation-selective. *J. Biophys.* 78: 247–259. [5]

Keramidas, A., Moorhouse, A. J., Schofield, P. R., and Barry, P. H. 2004. Ligand-gated ion channels: Mechanisms underlying ion selectivity. *Prog. Biophys. Mol. Biol.* 86: 161–204. [5]

Kerchner, G. A., and Nicoll, R. A. 2008. Silent synapses and the emergence of a postsynaptic mechanism for LTP. *Nat. Neurosci.* 9: 813–825. [16, 18]

Kerem, B., Rommens, J. M., Buchanan, J. A., et al. 1989. Identification of the cystic fibrosis gene: Genetic analysis. *Science* 245: 1073–1080. [30]

Kessels, H. W., and Malinow, R. 2009. Synaptic AMPA receptor plasticity and behavior. *Neuron* 61: 340–350. [16]

Kettenmann, H., and Ransom, B. R. (Eds.). 2005. *Neuroglia*, 2nd ed. Oxford University Press, New York. [10]

Keuroghlian, A. S., and Knudsen, E. I. 2007. Adaptive auditory plasticity in developing and adult animals. *Prog. Neurobiol.* 82: 109–121. [28]

Keynes, R. D., and Lumsden, A. 1990. Segmentation and the origin of regional diversity in the vertebrate central nervous system. *Neuron* 2: 1–9. [27]

Keynes, R. D., and Rojas, E. 1974. Kinetics and steady-state properties of the charged system controlling sodium conductance in the squid giant axon. *J. Physiol.* 239: 393–434. [7]

Kheirbek, M. A. and Hen, R. 2013. (Radioactive) neurogenesis in the human hippocampus. *Cell* 153: 1183. [27]

Khirug, S., Yamada, J., Afzalov, R., et al. 2008. GABAergic depolarization of the axon initial segment in cortical principal neurons is caused by the Na-K-2Cl cotransporter NKCC1. *J. Neurosci.* 28: 4635–4639. [11]

Kiang, N. Y., Rho, J. M., Northrop, C. C., et al. 1982. Hair-cell innervation by spiral ganglion cells in adult cats. *Science* 217: 175–177. [24]

Kiani, R., Esteky, H., and Tanaka, K. 2004. Differences in onset latency of macaque inferotemporal neural responses to primate and non-primate faces. *J. Neurophysiol.* 94: 1587–1596. [25]

Kiecker, C., and Lumsden, A. 2005. Compartments and their boundaries in vertebrate brain development. *Nat. Rev. Neurosci.* 6: 553–564. [27]

Kieffer, B. L., and Gavériaux-Ruff, C. 2002. Exploring the opioid system by gene knockout. *Prog. Neurobiol.* 66: 285–306. [14]

Kier, C. K., Buchsbaum, G., and Sterling, P. 1995. How retinal microcircuits scale for ganglion cells of different size. *J. Neurosci.* 15: 7673–7683. [22]

Kikkawa, S., Nakagawa, M., Iwasa, T., et al. 1993. GTP-binding protein couples with metabotropic glutamate receptor in bovine retinal on-bipolar cell. *Biochem. Biophys. Res. Commun.* 195: 374–379. [22]

Kim, D. S., and Bonhoeffer, T. 1994. Reverse occlusion leads to a precise restoration of orientation preference maps in visual cortex. *Nature* 370: 370–372. [28]

Kim, E., and Sheng, M. 2004. PDZ domain proteins of synapses. *Nat. Rev. Neurosci.* 5: 771–781. [11]

Kim, J. H., and Richter, J. D. 2006. Opposing polymerase-deadenylase activities regulate cytoplasmic polyadenylation. *Mol. Cell* 24: 173–183. [17]

Kim, J. M., Beyer, R., Morales, M., et al. 2010. Expression of BK-type calcium-activated potassium channel splice variants during chick cochlear development. *J. Comp. Neurol.* 518: 2554–2569. [24]

Kim, N., Stiegler, A. L., Cameron, T. O., et al. 2008. Lrp4 is a receptor for Agrin and forms a complex with MuSK. *Cell* 135: 334–342. [29]

Kinnamon, S. C., Dionne, V. E., and Beam, K. G. 1988. Apical localiza-tion of K+ channels in taste cells provides the basis for sour taste transduction. *Proc. Natl. Acad. Sci. USA* 85: 7023–7027. [21]

Kirkeby, A., and Barker, R. A. 2018. Parkinson disease and growth factors: Is GDNF good enough? *Nat. Rev Neurol.* 15: 312–314. doi: 10.1038/s41582-019-0180-6. [27]

Kirkwood, P. A., and Sears, T. A. 1982. Excitatory postsynaptic poten-tials from single muscle spindle afferents in external intercostal motoneurones of the cat. *J. Physiol.* 322: 287–314. [26]

Kirsch, J., Wolters, I., Triller, A., and Betz, H. 1993. Gephyrin antisense oligonucleotides prevent glycine receptor clustering in spinal neu-rons. *Nature* 366: 745–748. [11]

Kirshner, N. 1969. Storage and secretion of adrenal catecholamines. *Adv. Biochem. Psychopharmacol.* 1: 71–89. [13]

Klaus, J., et al. 2019. Altered neuronal migratory trajectories in human cerebral organoids derived from individuals with neuronal heteroto-pia. *Nat. Med.* 25: 561–568. [27]

Klausberger, T., and Somogyi, P. 2008. Neuronal diversity and temporal dynamics: The unity of hippocampal circuit operations. *Science* 321: 53–57. [14]

Kleene, S. J. 2008. The electrochemical basis of odor transduction in vertebrate olfactory cilia. *Chem. Senses.* 33: 839–859. [21]

Kleene, S. J., and Gesteland, R. C. 1991. Calcium-activated chloride con-ductance in frog olfactory cilia. *J. Neurosci.* 11: 3624–3629. [21]

Klein, R., et al. 1991. The trk proto-oncogene encodes a receptor for nerve growth factor. *Cell* 65: 189–197. [27]

Klyachko, V. A., and Jackson, M. B. 2002. Capacitance steps and fusion pores of small and large-dense-core vesicles in nerve terminals. *Nature* 418: 89–92. [13]

Knapp, A. G., and Dowling, J. E. 1987. Dopamine enhances excitatory amino acid-gated conductances in cultured retinal horizontal cells. *Nature* 325: 437–439. [18]

Kneussel, M., and Loebrich, S. 2007. Trafficking and synaptic anchoring of ionotropic inhibitory neurotransmitter receptors. *Biol. Cell* 99: 297–309. [11]

Knöpfel, T., Lin, M. Z., Levskaya, A., et al. 2010. Toward the second gen-eration of optogenetic tools. *J. Neurosci.* 30: 14998–15004. [28]

Knudsen, E. I. 1998. Capacity for plasticity in the adult owl auditory sys-tem expanded by juvenile experience. *Science* 279: 1531–1533. [28]

Knudsen, E. I. 1999. Mechanisms of experience-dependent plasticity in the auditory localization pathway of the barn owl. *J. Comp. Physiol. A* 185: 305–321. [28]

Knudsen, E. I., and Knudsen, P. F. 1990. Sensitive and critical periods for visual calibration of sound localization by barn owls. *J. Neurosci.* 10: 222–232. [28]

Kodera, N., Yamamoto, D., Ishikawa, R., and Ando, T. 2010. Video imaging of walking myosin V by high-speed atomic force micros-copy. *Nature* 468: 72–76. [15]

Koehler, R. C., Roman, R. J., and Harder, D. R. 2009. Astrocytes and the regulation of cerebral blood flow. *Trends Neurosci.* 32: 160–169. [10]

Koehnle, T. J., and Brown, A. 1999. Slow axonal transport of neurofila-ment protein in cultured neurons. *J. Cell Biol.* 144: 447–458. [15]

Koelle, G. B. 1962. A new general concept of the neurohumoral func-tions of acetylcholine and acetylcholinesterase *J. Pharm. Pharmacol.* 14: 65–90. [19]

Koelle, G. B., and Friedenwald, J. S. 1949. A histochemical method for localizing cholinesterase activity. *Proc. Soc. Exp. Biol. Med.* 70: 617–622. [14]

Koenig, D., and Hofer, H. 2011. The absolute threshold of cone vision. *J. Vision* 11: 21. doi:10.1167/11.1.21. [22]

Kofuji, P., and Newman, E. A. 2004. Potassium buffering in the central nervous system. *Neuroscience* 129: 1045–1056. [10]

Kofuji, P., Ceelen, P., Zahs, K. R., et al. 2000. Genetic inactivation of an inwardly rectifying potassium channel (Kir4.1 subunit) in mice: Phenotypic impact in retina. *J. Neurosci.* 20: 5733–5740. [10]

Köhler, M., Burnashev, N., Sakmann, B., and Seeburg, P. H. 1993. Determinants of Ca^{2+} permeability in both TM1 and TM2 of high-affinity kainate receptor channels: Diversity by RNA editing. *Neuron* 10: 491–500. [5]

Koike, C., Numata, T., Ueda, H., Mori, Y., and Furukawa, T. 2010. TRPM1: A vertebrate TRP channel responsible for retinal ON bipolar function. *Cell Calcium* 48: 95–101. [22]

Kolb, H. 1997. Amacrine cells of the mammalian retina: Neurocircuitry and functional roles. *Eye (Lond.)* 11 (Pt 6): 904–923. [22]

Koles, K., Nunnari, J., Korkut, C., et al. 2012. Mechanism of evenness interrupted (evi)-exosome release at synaptic boutons *J. Biol. Chem.* 287: 16820–16834. [18]

Kolodkin, A. L. 1996 Growth cones and the cues that repel them. *Trends Neurosci.* 19: 507–513. [27]

Kolodkin, A. L., and Tessier-Lavigne, M. 2011. Mechanisms and mol-ecules of neuronal wiring: A primer. *Cold Spring Harb. Perspect. Biol.* 3: A001727. [27]

Kong, J-H., Adelman, J. P., and Fuchs, P. A. 2008. Expression of the SK2 calcium-activated potassium channel is required for cholinergic function in mouse cochlear hair cells *J. Physiol.* 586: 5471–5485. [12]

Kononenko, N. I., Kuehl-Kovarik, M. C., Partin, K. M., and Dudek, F. E. 2008. Circadian difference in firing rate of isolated rat suprachiasmatic nucleus neurons *Neurosci. Lett.* 436: 314–316. [19]

Konopka, R. J. and Benzer, S. 1971. Clock mutants of Drosophila mela-nogaster. *Proc. Natl. Acad. Sci., USA* 68: 2112–2116. [19]

Kopin, I. J. 1968. False adrenergic transmitters. *Annu. Rev. Pharmacol.* 8: 377–394. [15]

Kopin, I. J., Breese, G. R., Krauss, K. R., and Weise, V. K. 1968. Selective release of newly synthesized norepinephrine from the cat spleen during sympathetic nerve stimulation. *J. Pharmacol. Exp. Ther.* 161: 271–278. [13]

Koppl, C. 1997. Phase locking to high frequencies in the auditory nerve and cochlear nucleus magnocellularis of the barn owl, *Tyto alba. J. Neurosci.* 17: 3312–3321. [24]

Korkut, C. et al. 2009. Trans-synaptic transmission of vesicular Wnt signals through Evi/Wntless. *Cell* 139: 393–404. [18]

Korn, S. J., and Trapani, J. G. 2005. Potassium channels. *IEEE Trans. Nanobiosci.* 4: 21–33. [5]

Kornack, D. R., and Rakic, P. 1999. Continuation of neurogenesis in the hippocampus of the adult macaque monkey. *Proc. Natl. Acad. Sci. USA* 96: 5768–5773. [27]

Korogod, N., Lou, X., and Schneggenburger, R. 2005. Presynaptic Ca^{2+} requirements and developmental regulation of posttetanic potentia-tion in the calyx of Held. *J. Neurosci.* 25: 5127–5137. [16]

Kosik, K. 2016. Life at low copy number: How dendrites manage with so few mRNAs. *Neuron* 92: 1168–1180. [17]

Kosslyn, S. M., Pascual-Leone, A., Felician, O., et al. 1999. The role of area 17 in visual imagery: Convergent evidence from PET and rTMS. *Science* 284: 167–170. [25]

Kosterin, P., Kim, G. H., Muschol, M., et al. 2005. Changes in FAD and NADH fluorescence in neurosecretory terminals are triggered by calcium entry and by ADP production. *J. Membr. Biol.* 208: 113–124. [19]

Koutalos, Y., and Yau, K. W. 1996. Regulation of sensitivity in vertebrate rod photoreceptors by calcium. *Trends Neurosci.* 19: 73–81. [22]

Kovalchuk, Y., Holthoff, K., and Konnerth, A. 2004. Neurotrophin action on a rapid timescale. *Curr. Opin. Neurobiol.* 14: 558–563. [27]

Kozlov, A., Huss, M., Lansner, A., et al. 2009. Simple cellular and net-work control principles govern complex patterns of motor behavior. *Proc. Natl. Acad. Sci. USA* 106: 20027–20032. [26]

Kral A. 2013. Auditory critical periods: A review from system's perspective. *Neuroscience* 247: 117–133. [28]

Kramer, A. P., and Weisblat, D. A. 1985. Developmental neural kinship groups in the leech. *J. Neurosci.* 5: 388–407. [27]

Krauthammer, C. 2000. Restoration, reality and Christopher Reeve. *Time* February 14: 76. [30]

Kravitz, A. V., Freeze, B. S., Parker, P. R. L., et al. 2010. Regulation of parkinsonian motor behaviours by optogenetic control of basal ganglia circuitry. *Nature* 466: 622–626. [14]

Kravitz, E. A. 1988. Hormonal control of behavior: Amines and the biasing of behavioral output in lobsters. *Science* 241: 1775–1781. [18]

Kravitz, E. A. 2000. Serotonin and aggression: Insights gained from a lobster model system and speculations on the role of amine neurons in a complex behavior. *J. Comp. Physiol. A* 186: 221–238. [14]

Kreitzer, A. C. 2009. Physiology and pharmacology of striatal neurons. *Annu. Rev. Neurosci.* 32: 127–147. [26]

Kreitzer, A. C., and Malenka, R. C. 2008. Striatal plasticity and basal ganglia circuit function. *Neuron* 60: 543–554. [26]

Kreitzer, A. C., and Regehr, W. G. 2001. Retrograde inhibition of presynaptic calcium influx by endogenous cannabinoids at excitatory synapses onto Purkinje cells. *Neuron* 29: 717–727. [12]

Kremkow, J., and Alonso, J. M. 2018. Thalamocortical circuits and functional architecture. *Ann. Rev. Vis. Sci.* 4: 5.1–5.23. [2]

Kretschmar, K., and Watt, F. M. 2012. Lineage tracing. *Cell* 148: 33. [27]

Kriebel, M. E., and Gross, C. E. 1974. Multimodal distribution of frog miniature endplate potentials in adult denervated and tadpole leg muscles. *J. Gen. Physiol.* 64: 85–103. [13]

Kriegstein, A., and Alvarez-Buylla, A. 2009. The glial nature of embryonic and adult neural stem cells. *Annu. Rev. Neurosci.* 32: 149–184. [27]

Kristan, W. B., Jr., Calabrese, R. L., and Friesen, W. O. 2005. Neuronal control of leech behavior. *Prog. Neurobiol.* 76: 279–327. [20]

Krizhevsky, A., Sutskever, I., and Hinton, G. E. 2012. ImageNet classification with deep convolutional neural networks. In *Advances in Neural Information Processing Systems 25.* Pereira, F., et al. (Eds.). Curran Associates, Inc., pp. 1097–1105. [25]

Krnjevic, K., and Phillis, J. W. 1963. Iontophoretic studies of neurones in the mammalian cerebral cortex. *J. Physiol.* 165: 274–304. [14]

Krnjevic, K., and Schwartz, S. 1967. The action of γ-aminobutyric acid on cortical neurons. *Exp. Brain Res.* 3: 320–336. [14]

Kros, C. J. 2007. How to build an inner hair cell: Challenges for regeneration. *Hear. Res.* 227: 3–10. [24]

Krug, M., Muller-Welde, P., Wagner, M., et al. 1985. Functional plasticity in two afferent systems of the granule cells in the rat dentate area: Frequency-related changes, long-term potentiation and heterosynaptic depression. *Brain. Res.* 360: 264–272. [16]

Krüger, J., Caruana, F., Volta, R. D., and Rizzolatti, G. 2010. Seven years of recording from monkey cortex with a chronically implanted multiple microelectrode. *Front. Neuroeng.* 3: 6. [26]

Kubisch, C., Schroeder, B. C. Friedrich, T., et al. 1999 KCNQ4, a novel potassium channel expressed in sensory outer hair cells, is mutated in dominant deafness. *Cell.* 96: 437–446. [5]

Kubo, Y., Adelman, J. P., Clapham, D. E., et al. 2005. International Union of Pharmacology. LIV. Nomenclature and molecular relationships of inwardly rectifying potassium channels. *Pharmacol. Rev.* 57: 509–526. [5]

Kubota, Y., Ito, C., Sakurai, E., et al. 2002. Increased methamphetamine-induced locomotor activity and behavioral sensitization in histamine-deficient mice. *J. Neurochem.* 83: 837–845. [14]

Kubota, T., Durek, T., Dang, B., et al. 2017. Mapping of voltage sensor positions in resting and inactivated mammalian sodium channels by LRET. *Proc. Natl. Acad. Sci. USA* 114: e1857–e1865. [5]

Kuffler, D. P., Nicholls, J., and Drapeau, P. 1987. *J. Comp. Neurol.* 256: 516–526. doi: 10.1002/cne.902560404. [18]

Kuffler, S. W. 1953. Discharge patterns and functional organization of the mammalian retina. *J. Neurophysiol.* 16: 37–68. [1, 2, 20]

Kuffler, S. W. 1980. Slow synaptic responses in autonomic ganglia and the pursuit of a peptidergic transmitter. *J. Exp. Biol.* 89: 257–286. [14, 19]

Kuffler, S. W., and Edwards, C. 1958. Mechanism of gamma aminobutyric acid (GABA) action and its relation to synaptic inhibition. *J. Neurophysiol.* 21: 589–610. [14]

Kuffler, S. W., and Eyzaguirre, C. 1955. Processes of excitation in the dendrites and in the soma of single isolated sensory nerve cells of the lobster and crayfish. *J. Gen. Physiol.* 39: 87–119. [8]

Kuffler, S. W., and Eyzaguirre, C. 1955. Synaptic inhibition in an isolated nerve cell. *J. Gen. Physiol.* 39: 155–184. [11]

Kuffler, S. W., and Nicholls, J. G. 1966. The physiology of neuroglial cells. *Ergeb. Physiol.* 57: 1–90. [10]

Kuffler, S. W., and Potter, D. D. 1964. Glia in the leech central nervous system: Physiological properties and neuron-glia relationship. *J. Neurophysiol.* 27: 290–320. [10, 20]

Kuffler, S. W., and Yoshikami, D. 1975. The distribution of acetylcholine sensitivity at the post-synaptic membrane of vertebrate skeletal twitch muscles: Iontophoretic mapping in the micron range. *J. Physiol.* 244: 703–730. [11]

Kuffler, S. W., and Yoshikami, D. 1975. The number of transmitter molecules in a quantum: An estimate from iontophoretic application of acetylcholine at the neuromuscular synapse. *J. Physiol.* 251: 465–482. [13]

Kuffler, S. W., Dennis, M. J., and Harris, A. J. 1971. The development of chemosensitivity in extrasynaptic areas of the neuronal surface after denervation of parasympathetic ganglion cells in the heart of the frog. *Proc. R. Soc. Lond., B, Biol. Sci.* 177: 555–563. [29]

Kuffler, S. W., Hunt, C. C., and Quilliam, J. P. 1951. Function of medullated small-nerve fibers in mammalian ventral roots: Efferent muscle spindle innervation. *J. Neurophysiol.* 14: 29–51. [26]

Kuffler, D. P., Nicholls, J., and Drapeau, P. 1987. Transmitter localization and vesicle turnover at a serotoninergic synapse between identified leech neurons in culture. J. Comp. Neurol. 256: 516–526. [18]

Kuffler, S. W., Nicholls, J. G., and Orkand, R. K. 1966. Physiological properties of glial cells in the central nervous system of amphibia. *J. Neurophysiol.* 29: 768–787. [10]

Kukley, M., Capetillo-Zarate, E., and Dietrich, D. 2007. Vesicular glutamate release from axons in white matter. *Nat. Neurosci.* 10: 311–320. Epub 2007 Feb 11. [10]

Kuljis, R. O., and Rakic, P. 1990. Hypercolumns in primate visual cortex can develop in the absence of cues from photoreceptors. *Proc. Natl. Acad. Sci. USA* 87: 5303–5306. [28]

Kullmann, P. H. and, Horn, J. P. 2006. Excitatory muscarinic modulation strengthens virtual nicotinic synapses on sympathetic neurons and thereby enhances synaptic gain. *J. Neurophysiol.* 96.3104–3113. [19]

Kumamaru, H., Kadoya, K., Adler, A. F., et al. 2018. Generation and post-injury integration of human spinal cord neural stem cells. *Nat. Methods* 15: 723–731. doi.org/10.1038/s41592-018-0074-3. [29]

Kumar, S., Porcu, P., Werner, D. F., et al. 2009. The role of GABA$_A$ receptors in the acute and chronic effects of ethanol: A decade of progress. *Psychopharmacology (Berl.)* 205: 529–564. [14]

Kummer, T. T., Misgeld, T., and Sanes, J. R. 2006. Assembly of the post-synaptic membrane at the neuromuscular junction: Paradigm lost. *Curr. Opin. Neurobiol.* 16: 74–82. [29]

Kunisch, M., Haenlin, M., and Campos-Ortega, J. A. 1994. Lateral inhibition mediated by the Drosophila neurogenic gene delta is enhanced by proneural proteins. *Proc. Natl. Acad. Sci. USA* 91: 10139–10143. [27]

Kuno, M. 1964. Quantal components of excitatory synaptic potentials in spinal motoneurones. *J. Physiol.* 175: 81–99. [13]

Kuno, M. 1964. Mechanism of facilitation and depression of the excitatory synaptic potential in spinal motoneurones. *J. Physiol.* 175: 100–112. [11, 16]

Kuno, M. 1971. Quantum aspects of central and ganglionic synaptic transmission in vertebrates. *Physiol. Rev.* 51: 647–678. [26]

Kupchik, Y. M., Rashkovan, G., Ohana, L., et al. 2008. Molecular mechanisms that control initiation and termination of physiological depolarization-evoked transmitter release. *Proc. Natl. Acad. Sci. USA* 105: 4435–4440. [12, 13]

Kupfermann, I. 1991. Functional studies of cotransmission. *Physiol. Rev.* 71: 683–732. [15]

Kurahashi, T., and Yau, K. W. 1993. Co-existence of cationic and chloride components in odorant-induced current of vertebrate olfactory receptor cells. *Nature* 363: 71–74. [21]

Kuriyama, S., and Mayor, R. 2008. Molecular analysis of neural crest migration. *Philos. Trans. R Soc. Lond. Ser B Biol. Sci.* 363: 1349–1362. [27]

Kurth-Nelson, Z. L., Mishra, A., Newman, E. A. 2009. Spontaneous glial calcium waves in the retina develop over early adulthood. *J. Neurosci.* 29: 11339–11346. [10]

Kushmerick, C., Price, G. D., Taschenberger, H., et al. 2004. Retroinhibition of presynaptic Ca^{2+} currents by endocannabinoids released via postsynaptic mGluR activation at a calyx synapse. *J. Neurosci.* 24: 5955–5965. [12]

Kuwada, S., Fitzpatrick, D. C., Batra, R., and Ostapoff, E. M. 2006. Sensitivity to interaural time differences in the dorsal nucleus of the lateral lemniscus of the unanesthetized rabbit: Comparison with other structures. *J. Neurophysiol.* 95: 1309–1322. [24]

Kuypers, H. G. J. M., and Ugolini, G. 1990. Viruses as trans-neuronal tracers. *Trends Neurosci.* 13: 71–75. [15]

Kuzhandaivel, A., Margaryan, G., Nistri, A., and Mladinic, M. 2010. Extensive glial apoptosis develops early after hypoxic-dysmetabolic insult to the neonatal rat spinal cord in vitro. *Neuroscience* 169: 325–338. [29]

Kwak, S., and Kawahara, Y. 2005. Deficient RNA editing of GluR2 and neuronal death in amyotropic lateral sclerosis. *J. Mol. Med.* 83: 110–120. [27]

Kwan, K. Y., and Corey, D. P. 2009. Burning cold: Involvement of TRPA1 in noxious cold sensation. *J. Gen. Physiol.* 133: 251–256. [21]

Kwan, K. Y., Allchorne, A. J., Vollrath, M. A., et al. 2006. TRPA1 contributes to cold, mechanical, and chemical nociception but is not essential for hair-cell transduction. *Neuron* 50: 277–289. [21]

Kyrousi, C., Lygerou, Z., and Taraviras, S. 2017. How a radial glial cell decides to become a multiciliated ependymal cell. *Glia.* 65: 1032–1042. doi: 10.1002/glia.23118. Epub 2017 Feb 7. [10]

Kyte, J., and Doolittle, R. F. 1982. A simple method for displaying the hydrophobic character of a protein. *J. Mol. Biol.* 157: 105–132. [5]

Labay, V., Weichert, R. M., Makishima, T., and Griffith, A. J. 2010. Topology of transmembrane channel-like gene 1 protein. *Biochemistry* 409: 8592–8598. [5]

Labhart, T. 1988. Polarization-opponent interneurons in the insect visual system. *Nature* 331: 435–437. [20]

Labhart, T. 2000. Polarization-sensitive interneurons in the optic lobe of the desert ant *Cataglyphis bicolor*. *Naturwissenschaften* 87: 133–136. [20]

Labhart, T., Petzold, J., and Helbling, H. 2001. Spatial integration in polarization-sensitive interneurones of crickets: A survey of evidence, mechanisms and benefits. *J. Exp. Biol.* 204: 2423–2430. [20]

Lagostena, L., Rosato-Siri, M., D'Onofrio, M., et al. 2010. In the adult hippocampus, chronic nerve growth factor deprivation shifts GABAergic signaling from the hyperpolarizing to the depolarizing direction. *J. Neurosci.* 30: 885–893. [12]

Lak, A., Arabzadeh, E., and Diamond, M. E. 2008. Enhanced response of neurons in rat somatosensory cortex to stimuli containing temporal noise. *Cereb. Cortex* 18: 1085–1093. [25]

Lak, A., Arabzadeh, E., Harris, J., and Diamond, M. 2010. Correlated physiological and perceptual effects of noise in a tactile stimulus. *Proc. Natl. Acad. Sci. USA* 17: 7981–7986. [25]

Lamas, J. A., Reboreda, A., and Codesido, V. 2002. Ionic basis of the membrane potential in cultured rat sympathetic neurons. *Neuroreport* 13: 585–591. [6]

Lamb, T. D. 2009. Evolution of vertebrate retinal photoreception. *Philos. Trans. R. Soc. Lond., B, Biol. Sci.* 364: 2911–2924. [22]

Lamotte d'Incamps, B., and Ascher, P. 2008. Four excitatory postsynaptic ionotropic receptors coactivated at the motoneuron-Renshaw cell synapse. *J. Neurosci.* 28: 14121–14131. [15]

LaMotte, R. H., and Mountcastle, V. B. 1975. Capacities of humans and monkeys to discriminate vibratory stimuli of different frequency and amplitude: A correlation between neural events and psychological measurements. *J. Neurophysiol.* 38: 539–559. [23, 25]

Lampl, I., Anderson, J. S., Gillespie, D. C., and Ferster, D. 2001. Prediction of orientation selectivity from receptive field architecture in simple cells of cat visual cortex. *Neuron* 30: 263–274. [2]

Lancaster, M., et al. 2013. Cerebral organoids model human brain development and microcephaly. *Nature* 501: 373. [27]

Lancaster, M. A. 2019. An electric take on neural fate and cortical development. *Developmental Cell* 48: 1–2. [27]

Land, M. F. 2009. Vision, eye movements, and natural behavior. *Vis. Neurosci.* 26: 51–62. [24]

Lane, M. A., Truettner, J. S., Brunschwig, J. P., et al. 2007. Age-related differences in the local cellular and molecular responses to injury in developing spinal cord of the opossum, *Monodelphis domestica. Eur. J. Neurosci.* 25: 1725–1742. [29]

Lang, T., Wacker, I., Steyer, J., Kaether, C., et al. 1997. Ca^{2+}-triggered peptide secretion in single cells imaged with green fluorescent protein and evanescent-wave microscopy. *Neuron* 18: 857–863. [13]

Langer, P., Grunder, S., and Rusch, A. 2003. Expression of Ca^{2+}-activated BK channel mRNA and its splice variants in the rat cochlea. *J. Comp. Neurol.* 455: 198–209. [24]

Langley, J. N. 1907. On the contraction of muscle, chiefly in relation to the presence of "receptive" substances. *J. Physiol.* 36: 347–384. [11]

Langley, J. N., and Anderson, H. K. 1904. The union of different kinds of nerve fibres. *J. Physiol.* 31: 365–391. [29]

Lapato, A. S. and Tiwari-Woodruff, S. K. 2018. Connexins and pannexins: At the junction of neuro-glial homeostasis and disease. *J. Neurosci. Res.* 96: 31–44. doi: 10.1002/jnr.24088. [10]

Larkum, M. E., Zhu, J. J., and Sakmann, B. 1999. A new cellular mechanism for coupling inputs arriving at different cortical layers. *Nature* 398: 338–341. [8]

Larrson, H. P., Baker, O. S., Dhillon, D. S., and Isacoff, E. Y. 1996. Transmembrane movement of the *Shaker* K^+ channel S4. *Neuron* 16: 387–397. [5]

Laverty, D., Thomas, P., Field, M., et al. 2017. Crystal structures of a $GABA_A$-receptor chimera reveal new endogenous neurosteroid-binding sites. *Nat Struct Mol Biol.* 24: 977–985. doi: 10.1038/nsmb.3477. PMID: 28967882. [14]

Lawrence, D. G., and Kuypers, H. G. J. M. 1968. The functional organization of the motor system in the monkey. I. The effects of bilateral pyramidal lesions. *Brain* 91: 1–14. [26]

Lawrence, J. J. 2008. Cholinergic control of GABA release: Emerging parallels between neocortex and hippocampus. *Trends Neurosci.* 31: 317–327. [14]

Lazarini, F., and Lledo, P. M. 2011. Is adult neurogenesis necessary for olfaction? *Trends Neurosci.* 34: 20–30. [27]

Le Douarin, N. M., et al. 1975. Cholinergic differentiation of presumptive adrenergic neuroblasts in interspecific chimeras after heterotopic transplantation. *Proc. Natl. Acad. Sci USA* 72: 728–732. [27]

Le Douarin, N. M. 1986. Cell line segregation during peripheral nervous system ontogeny. *Science* 231: 1515–1522. [27]

Le Douarin, N. M. 2008. Developmental patterning deciphered in avian chimeras. *Dev. Growth Differ.* 50(Suppl. 1): S11–28. [27]

Le Douarin, N. M., Calloni, G. W., and Dupin, E. 2008. The stem cells of the neural crest. *Cell Cycle* 7: 1013–1019. [27]

Lebedev, M. A., and Nelson, R. J. 1996. High-frequency vibratory sensitive neurons in monkey primary somatosensory cortex: Entrained and nonentrained responses to vibration during the performance of vibratory-cued hand movements. *Exp. Brain Res.* 111: 313–325. [23]

Lebedev, M. A., Mirabella, G., Erchova, I., and Diamond, M. E. 2000. Experience-dependent plasticity of rat barrel cortex: Redistribution of activity across barrel-columns. *Cereb. Cortex.* 10: 23–31. [28]

LeBlanc, J. J., and Fagiolini, M. 2011. Autism: A "critical period" disorder? *Neural Plast.* Epub 2011: 921680. doi: 10.1155/2011/921680 [28]

Leblanc, P. et al. 1988. *Neuroendocrinology* 48: 482–488. [18]

Ledent, C., Vaugeois, J. M., Schiffmann, S. N., et al. 1997. Aggressiveness, hypoalgesia and high blood pressure in mice lacking the adenosine A_{2a} receptor. *Nature* 388: 674–678. [14]

Lee, B. B., Martin, P. R., and Grunert, U. Retinal connectivity and primate vision. *Prog. Retin. Eye Res.* 29: 622–639. [22]

Lee, C. C., and Winer, J. A. 2005. Principles governing auditory cortex connections. *Cereb. Cortex* 15: 1804–1814. [24]

Lee, H-K., Kameyama, K., Huganir, R. L., and Bear, M. F. 1998. NMDA induces long-term synaptic depression and dephosphorylation of the GluR1 subunit of AMPA receptors in hippocampus. *Neuron* 21: 1151–1162. [16]

Lee, H. S., Ghetti, A., Pinto-Duarte, A., et al. 2014. Astrocytes contribute to gamma oscillations and recognition memory. *Proc. Natl. Acad. Sci. USA* 111: e3343–e3352. doi: 10.1073/pnas.1410893111. [10]

Lee, J. K., Geoffroy, C. G., Chan, A. F., et al. 2010. Assessing spinal axon regeneration and sprouting in Nogo-, MAG-, and OMgp-deficient mice. *Neuron* 66: 663–670. [29]

Lee, L. J., Chen, W. J., Chuang, Y. W., and Wang, Y. C. 2009. Neonatal whisker trimming causes long-lasting changes in structure and function of the somatosensory system. *Exp. Neurol.* 219: 524–532. [28]

Lee, R., et al. 2001. Regulation of cell survival by secreted proneurotrophins. *Science* 294: 1945–1948. [27]

Lee, S. J., Escobedo-Lozoya, Y., Szatmari, E. M., and Yasuda, R. 2009. Activation of CaMKII in single dendritic spines during long-term potentiation. *Nature* 458: 299–304. [12]

Lee, V. H., Lee, L. T., and Chow, B. K. 2008. Gonadotropin-releasing hormone: Regulation of the GnRH gene. *FEBS J.* 275: 5458–5478. [19]

Lee, Y., Morrison, B. M., Li, Y., et al. 2012. Oligodendroglia metabolically support axons and contribute to neurodegeneration. *Nature.* 487: 443–448. [10]

Lehrer, M., and Collett, T. S. 1994. Approaching and departing bees learn different cues to the distance of a landmark. *J. Comp. Physiol. A* 175: 171–177. [20]

Leksell, L. 1945. The action potential and excitatory effects of the small ventral root fibres to skeletal muscle. *Acta Physiol. Scand.* 10(Suppl. 31): 1–84. [26]

Lemon, R. N. 2008. Descending pathways in motor control. *Annu. Rev. Neurosci.* 31: 195–218. [26]

Lendvai, B., and Vizi, E. S. 2008. Nonsynaptic chemical transmission through nicotinic acetylcholine receptors. *Physiol. Rev.* 88: 333–349. [14]

Leon-Pinzon, C., Cercós, M. G., Noguez, P., et al. 2014. Exocytosis of serotonin from the neuronal soma is sustained by a serotonin and calcium-dependent feedback loop. *Front. Cell Neurosci.* 8: 169. doi: 10.3389/fncel.2014.00169. [18]

Leonard, R. J., Labarca, C. G., Charnet, P., et al. 1988. Evidence that the M2 membrane-spanning region lines the ion channel pore of a nicotinic receptor. *Science* 242: 1578–1581. [5]

Lerner, Y., Hendler, T., Ben-Bashat, D., et al. 2001. A hierarchical axis of object processing stages in the human visual cortex. *Cereb. Cortex* 11: 287–297. [25]

Lester, H. A., Dibas, M. I., Dahan, D. S., et al. 2004. Cys-loop receptors: New twists and turns. *Trends Neurosci.* 27: 329–336. [5]

Leung, K. M., van Horck, F. P., Lin, A. C., et al. 2006. Asymmetrical beta-actin mRNA translation in growth cones mediates attractive turning to netrin-1. *Nat. Neurosci.* 9: 1247–1256. [27]

LeVay, S., Connolly, M., Houde, J., and Van Essen, D. C. 1985. The complete pattern of ocular dominance stripes in the striate cortex and visual field of the macaque monkey. *J. Neurosci.* 5: 486–501. [3]

LeVay, S., Hubel, D. H., and Wiesel, T. N. 1975. The pattern of ocular dominance columns in macaque visual cortex revealed by a reduced silver stain. *J. Comp. Neurol.* 159: 559–576. [3]

LeVay, S., Stryker, M. P., and Shatz, C. J. 1978. Ocular dominance columns and their development in layer IV of the cat's visual cortex: A quantitative study. *J. Comp. Neurol.* 179: 223–244. [28]

LeVay, S., Wiesel, T. N., and Hubel, D. H. 1980. The development of ocular dominance columns in normal and visually deprived monkeys. *J. Comp. Neurol.* 191: 1–51. [28]

Levenes, C., Daniel, H., and Crepel, F. 1998. Long-term depression of synaptic transmission in the cerebellum: Cellular and molecular mechanisms revisited. *Prog. Neurobiol.* 55: 79–91. [16]

Levi-Montalcini, R. 1952. Effects of mouse tumor transplantation on the nervous system. *Ann. NY Acad. Sci.* 55: 330–344. [27]

Levi-Montalcini, R. 1982. Developmental neurobiology and the natural history of nerve growth factor. *Annu. Rev. Neurosci.* 5: 341–362. [27]

Levi-Montalcini, R. 1987 The Nerve Growth Factor thirty-five years later. *Science* 237: 1154–1162. [27]

Levi-Montalcini, R. 1989. *In praise of Imperfection*. Sloan Foundation Science Series.

Levi-Montalcini, R., and Booker, B. 1960. Destruction of the sympathetic ganglia in mammals by an antiserum to a nerve-growth protein. *Proc. Natl. Acad. Sci. USA* 46: 384–391. [27]

Levi-Montalcini, R., and Cohen, S. 1956. In vitro and in vivo effects of a nerve growth-stimulating agent isolated from snake venom. *Proc. Natl. Acad. Sci. USA* 42: 695–699. [27]

Levi-Montalcini., R., and Hamburger, V. 1953. A diffusible agent of mouse sarcoma, producing hyperplasia of sympathetic ganglia and hyperneurotization of viscera in the chick embryo. *J. Exp. Zool.* 123: 233–287. [27]

Levi-Montalcini, R., and Levi, G. 1942. Les conséquences de la destruction d'un territoire d'innervation périphérique sur le développement des centres nerveux correspondants dans l'embryon de poulet. *Arch. Biol. (Liege)* 53: 537–545. [27]

Levi-Montalcini, R., and Levi, G. 1943. Recherches quantitatives sur la marche du processus de différenciation des neurones dans les ganglions spinaux de l'embryon de poulet. *Arch. Biol. (Liege)* 54: 189–206. [27]

Levi-Montalcini, R., Meyer, H., and Hamburger, V. 1954. In vitro experiments on the effects of mouse sarcomas 180 and 37 on the spinal and sympathetic ganglia of the chick embryo. *Cancer Res.* 14: 49–57. [27]

Levitan, I. B. 1994. Modulation of ion channels by protein phosphorylation and dephosphorylation. *Annu. Rev. Physiol.* 56: 193–212. [12]

Levitan, I. B. 2006. Signaling protein complexes associated with neuronal ion channels. *Nat. Neurosci.* 9: 305–310. [12]

Levy, W.B. and Steward, O. 1983. Temporal contiguity requirements for long-term associative potentiation/depression in the hippocampus. *Neuroscience* 8: 791–793. [16]

Lewcock, J. W., and Reed, R. R. 2004. A feedback mechanism regulates monoallelic odorant receptor expression. *Proc. Natl. Acad. Sci. USA* 101: 1069–1074. [21]

Lewis, E. B.1978. A gene complex controlling segmentation in *Drosophila. Nature* 76: 565–570. [27]

Lewis, J. E., and Kristan, W. B., Jr. 1998. A neuronal network for computing population vectors in the leech. *Nature* 391: 76–79. [20]

Lewis, K. E., and Eisen, J. S. 2003. From cells to circuits: Development of the zebrafish spinal cord. *Prog. Neurobiol.* 69: 419–449. [10]

Lewis, P. R., and Shute, C. C. 1967. The cholinergic limbic system: Projections to hippocampal formation, medial cortex, nuclei of the ascending cholinergic reticular system, and the subfornical organ and supra-optic crest. *Brain* 90: 521–540. [14]

Lewis, R. S., and Hudspeth, A. J. 1983. Voltage- and ion-dependent conductances in solitary vertebrate hair cells. *Nature* 304: 538–541. [24]

Lewis, T. L., and Maurer, D. 2005. Multiple sensitive periods in human visual development: Evidence from visually deprived children. *Dev. Psychobiol.* 46: 163–183. [28]

LeWitt, P. A. 2008. Levodopa for the treatment of Parkinson's disease. *New England J. Med.* 359: 2468–2476. [14]

Li, C.-L., and Jasper, H. H. 1953. Microelectrode studies of the electrical activity in the cerebral cortex of the cat. *J. Physiol.* 121: 117–140. [8]

Li, N., and DiCarlo, J. J. 2008. Unsupervised natural experience rapidly alters invariant object representation in visual cortex. *Science* 321: 1502–1507. [25]

Li, Q., and Burrell, B. D. 2009. Two forms of long-term depression in a polysynaptic pathway in the leech CNS: One NMDA receptor-dependent and the other cannabinoid-dependent. *J. Comp. Physiol. A* 195: 831–841. [20]

Li, W., et al. 2017. REM sleep selectively prunes and maintains new synapses in development and learning. *Nat. Neurosci.* 20: 427–437. [17]

Li, X. J., Blackshaw, S., and Snyder, S. H. 1994. Expression and localization of amiloride-sensitive sodium channel indicate a role for non-taste cells in taste perception. *Proc. Natl. Acad. Sci. USA* 91: 1814–1818. [21]

Li, Y., Atkin, G. M., Morales, M. M., et al. 2009. Developmental expression of BK channels in chick cochlear hair cells. *BMC Dev. Biol.* 9: 67. [24]

Li, Y., Du, X. F., Liu, C. S., et al. 2012. Reciprocal regulation between resting microglial dynamics and neuronal activity in vivo. *Dev. Cell* 23: 1189–202. doi: 10.1016/j.devcel.2012.10.027. [10]

Li, Y., Field, P. M., and Raisman, G. 1998. Regeneration of adult corticospinal axons induced by transplanted olfactory ensheathing cells. *J. Neurosci.* 18: 10514–10524. [29]

Li, Y., Gamper, N., Hilgemann, D. W., and Shapiro, M. S. 2005. Regulation of Kv7 (KCNQ) K⁺ channel open probability by phosphatidylinositol 4,5-bisphosphate. *J. Neurosci.* 25: 9825–9835. [12]

Li, Y., Muffat, J., Omer, A., et al. 2017. Induction of expansion and folding in human cerebral organoids. *Cell Stem Cell* 20: 385. [27]

Liang, J., Williams, D. R., and Miller, D T. 1997. Supernormal vision and high-resolution retinal imaging through adaptive optics. *J. Opt. Soc. Am. A* 14: 2884–2892. [22]

Liao, D., Hessler, N. A., and Malinow, R. 1995. Activation of postsynaptically silent synapses during pairing-induced LTP in the CA1 region of hippocampal slice. *Nature* 375: 400–404. [16]

Libby, R. T., and Steel, K. P. 2000. The roles of unconventional myosins in hearing and deafness. *Essays Biochem.* 35: 159–174. [21]

Liberles, S. D., and Buck, L. B. 2006. A second class of chemosensory receptors in the olfactory epithelium. *Nature* 442: 645–650. [21]

Liberman, M. C. 1982. Single-neuron labeling in the cat auditory nerve. *Science* 216: 1239–1241. [24]

Liberman, M. C. 1988. Response properties of cochlear efferent neurons: Monaural vs. binaural stimulation and the effects of noise. *J. Neurophysiol.* 60: 1779–1798. [24]

Libet, B., Gleason, C. A., Wright, E.W., and Pearl, D. K. 1983. Time of conscious intention to act in relation to onset of cerebral activity (readiness potential). The unconscious initiation of a freely voluntary act. *Brain* 106: 623–642. [26, 30]

Liley, A. W. 1956. The quantal components of the mammalian end-plate potential. *J. Physiol.* 133: 571–587. [16]

Lim, M. M., Wang, Z., Olazábal, D. E., Ren, X., Terwilliger, E. F., and Young, L. J. 2004. Enhanced partner preference in a promiscuous species by manipulating the expression of a single gene. *Nature* 429: 754–757. [14]

Lima, S. Q., and Miesenboeck, G. 2005. Remote control of behavior through genetically targeted photostimulation of neurons. *Cell* 121: 141–152. [1]

Lin, A. C., and Holt, C. E. 2007. Local translation and directional steering in axons. *EMBO J.* 26: 3729–3736. [27]

Lin, D. M., Wang, F., Lowe, G., Gold, G. H., Axel, R., Ngai, J., and Brunet, L. 2000. Formation of precise connections in the olfactory bulb occurs in the absence of odorant-evoked neuronal activity. *Neuron* 26: 69–80. [28]

Lin, J. H., and Rydqvist, B. 1999. The mechanotransduction of the crayfish stretch receptor neurone can be differentially activated or inactivated by local anaesthetics. *Acta Physiol. Scand.* 166: 65–74. [21]

Lin, J. S. 2000. Brain structures and mechanisms involved in the control of cortical activation and wakefulness, with emphasis on the posterior hypothalamus and histaminergic neurons. *Sleep Med. Rev.* 4: 471–503. [14]

Lin, L., Faraco, J., Li, R., et al. 1999. The sleep disorder canine narcolepsy is caused by a mutation in the hypocretin (orexin) receptor 2 gene. *Cell* 98: 365–376. [14]

Lin, S., Landmann, L., Ruegg, M. A., and Brenner, H. R. 2008. The role of nerve- versus muscle-derived factors in mammalian neuromuscular junction formation. *J. Neurosci.* 28: 3333–3340. [29]

Linden, D. J. 1994. Long-term synaptic depression in the mammalian brain. *Neuron.* 12: 457–472. [16]

Linden, D. J., and Connor, J. A. 1995. Long-term synaptic depression. *Annu. Rev. Neurosci.* 18: 319–357. [16]

Ling, G., and Gerard, R. W. 1949. The normal membrane potential of frog sartorius fibers. *J. Cell Comp. Physiol.* 34: 383–396. [4, 11]

Link, W., et al., 1995. Somatodendritic expression of an immediate early gene is regulated by synaptic activity. *Proc. Natl. Acad. Sci. USA* 92: 5734–5738. [17]

Lippe, W. R. 1994. Rhythmic spontaneous activity in the developing avian auditory system. *J. Neurosci.* 14: 1486–1495. [28]

Lipscombe, D., Kongsamut, S., and Tsien, R. W. 1989. α-Adrenergic inhibition of sympathetic neurotransmitter release mediated by modulation of N-type calcium-channel gating. *Nature* 340: 639–642. [12]

Lisberger, S. G. 2009. Internal models of eye movement in the floccular complex of the monkey cerebellum. *Neuroscience* 162: 763–776. [24]

Lisman, J. E. 2009. The pre/post LTP debate. *Neuron* 63: 281–284. [16]

Lisman, J. E., Pi, H. J., Zhang, Y., and Otmakhova, N. A. 2010. A thalamo-hippocampal-ventral tegmental area loop may produce the positive feedback that underlies the psychotic break in schizophrenia. *Biol. Psychiatry* 68: 17–24. [30]

Lisman, J., et al. 2018. Memory formation depends on both synapse-specific modifications of synaptic strength and cell-specific increases in excitability. *Nat. Neurosci.* 21: 309–314. [17]

Listerud, M., Brussaard, A. B., Devay, P., Colman, D. R., and Role., L. W. 1992. Functional contribution of neuronal AChR subunits revealed by antisense oligonucleotides. *Science.* 254: 1518–1521. [19]

Little, S. C., and Mullins, M. C. 2006. Extracellular modulation of BMP activity in patterning the dorsoventral axis. *Birth Defects Res. C Embryo Today* 78: 224–242. [27]

Liu, B. P., Cafferty, W. B., Budel, S. O., and Strittmatter, S. M. 2006. Extracellular regulators of axonal growth in the adult central nervous system. *Philos. Trans. R. Soc. Lond., B, Biol. Sci.* 361: 1593–1610. [27]

Liu, C. R., Xu, L., Zhong, Y. M., et al. 2009. Expression of connexin 35/36 in retinal horizontal and bipolar cells of carp. *Neuroscience* 164: 1161–1169. [22]

Liu, K., Lu, Y., Lee, J. K., et al. 2010. PTEN deletion enhances the regenerative ability of adult corticospinal neurons. *Nat Neurosci.* 13: 1075–1081. [29]

Liu, N., Varma, S., Shooter, E. M., and Tolwani, R. J. 2005. Enhancement of Schwann cell myelin formation by K252a in the Trembler-J mouse dorsal root ganglion explant culture. *J. Neurosci. Res.* 79: 310–317. [10]

Liu, Q., Tang, Z., Surdenikova, L., et al. 2009. Sensory neuron-specific GPCR Mrgprs are itch receptors mediating chloroquine-induced pruritus. *Cell* 139: 1353–1365. [21]

Liu, X., et al. 2012. Optogenetic stimulation of a hippocampal engram activates fear memory recall. *Nature* 484: 381–385. [17]

Liu, Y., and Joho, R. H. 1998. A side chain in S6 influences both open-state stability and ion permeation in a voltage-gated K⁺ channel. *Pflügers Arch.* 435: 654–661. [5]

Liu, Y., Jurman, M. E., and Yellen, G. 1997. Gated access to the pore of a voltage-dependent K⁺ channel. *Neuron* 19: 175–184. [5]

Liu, Y., Miao, Q., Yuan, J., et al. 2015. Ascl1 Converts Dorsal Midbrain Astrocytes into Functional Neurons In Vivo. *J. Neurosci.* 35: 9336–9355. [29]

Livesey, F. J., and Cepko, C. L. 2001. Vertebrate neural cell-fate determination: Lessons from the retina. *Nature Rev Neurosci* 2: 109. [27]

Livet, J., Weissman, T. A., Kang, H., et al. 2007. Transgenic strategies for combinatorial expression of fluorescent proteins in the nervous system. *Nature* 450: 56–62. [30]

Livingstone, M. S., Harris-Warrick, R. M., and Kravitz, E. A. 1980. *Science* 208: 76–79. [18]

Livingstone, M. S., and Hubel, D. H. 1984. Anatomy and physiology of a color system in the primate visual cortex. *J. Neurosci.* 4: 309–356. [3]

Livingstone, M. S., and Hubel, D. H. 1987. Connections between layer 4B of area 17 and the thick cytochrome oxidase stripes of area 18 in the squirrel monkey. *J. Neurosci.* 7: 3371–3377. [3]

Livingstone, M. S., and Hubel, D. H. 1988. Segregation of form, color, movement, and depth: Anatomy, physiology, and perception. *Science* 240: 740–749. [3]

Livingstone, P. D., and Wonnacott, S. 2009. Nicotinic acetylcholine receptors and the ascending dopamine pathways. *Biochem. Pharmacol.* 78: 744–755. [14]

Llano, I., Leresche, N., and Marty, A. 1991. Calcium entry increases the sensitivity of cerebellar Purkinje cells to applied GABA and decreases inhibitory synaptic currents. *Neuron* 6: 564–674. [12]

Lledo, P. M., Alonso, M., and Grubb, M. S. 2006. Adult neurogenesis and functional plasticity in neuronal circuits. *Nat. Rev. Neurosci.* 7: 179–193. [27]

Llewellyn, L. E. 2009. Sodium channel inhibiting marine toxins. *Prog. Mol. Subcell. Biol.* 46: 67–87. [7]

Llinás, R. 1982. Calcium in synaptic transmission. *Sci. Am.* 247: 56–65. [13]

Llinás, R., and Sugimori, M. 1980. Electrophysiological properties of *in vitro* Purkinje cell dendrites in mammalian cerebellar slices. *J. Physiol.* 305: 197–213. [7, 8]

Llinás, M., Sugimori, M., and Silver, R. B. 1992. Microdomains of high calcium concentration in a presynaptic nerve terminal. *Science* 256: 677–679. [13]

Llinás, R., Leznik, E., and Makarenko, V. I. 2002. On the amazing olivo-cerebellar system. *Ann. N Y Acad. Sci.* 978: 258–272. [26]

Llinás, R., Sugimori, M., and Silver, R. B. 1992. Microdomains of high calcium concentration in a presynaptic terminal. *Science* 256: 677–679. [12, 13]

Llobet, A., Beaumont, V., and Lagnado, L. 2003. Real-time measurements of exocytosis at synapses and neuroendocrine cells using interference reflection microscopy. *Neuron* 40: 1075–1086. [13]

Lloyd, I. C., Ashworth, J., Biswas, S., and Abadi, R. V. 2007. Advances in the management of congenital and infantile cataract. *Eye (Lond).* 21: 1301–1309. [28]

Lockery, S. R., and Kristan, W. B., Jr. 1990. Distributed processing of sensory information in the leech. II. Identification of interneurons contributing to the local bending reflex. *J. Neurosci.* 10: 1816–1829. [20]

Lodato, S., et al. 2011. Excitatory projection neuron subtypes control the distribution of local inhibitory interneurons in the cerebral cortex. *Neuron* 69: 763–779. [27]

Lodato, S., and Arlotta, P. 2015. Generating neuronal diversity in the mammalian cerebral cortex. *Annu. Rev. Cell Dev. Biol.* 31: 11.1–11.22. [27]

Lodge, D. 2009. The history of the pharmacology and cloning of ionotropic glutamate receptors and the development of idiosyncratic nomenclature. *Neuropharmacology* 56: 6–21. [5, 14]

Loewenstein, O., and Wersall, J. 1959. A functional interpretation of the electron-microscopic structure of the sensory hairs in the cristæ of the elasmobranch Raja clavata in terms of directional sensitivity. *Nature* 184: 1807–1808. [21]

Loewenstein, W. 1981. Junctional intercellular communication: The cell-to-cell membrane channel. *Physiol. Rev.* 61: 829–913. [11]

Loewenstein, W. R. 1999. *The Touchstone of Life*. Oxford University Press, New York. [10]

Loewenstein, W. R., and Mendelson, M. 1965. Components of receptor adaptation in a Pacinian corpuscle. *J. Physiol.* 177: 377–397. [21]

Loewi, O. 1921. Über humorale Übertragbarkeit der Herznervenwirkung. *Pflügers Arch.* 189: 239–242. [11]

Logothetis, N. K., Pauls, J., and Poggio, T. 1995. Shape representation in the inferior temporal cortex of monkeys. *Curr. Biol.* 5: 552–563. [25]

Logothetis, N. K., Pauls, J., Bulthoff, H. H., and Poggio, T. 1994. View-dependent object recognition by monkeys. *Curr. Biol.* 4: 401–414. [25]

Lomeli, J., Quevedo, J., Linares, P., and Rudomin, P. 1998. Local control of information flow in segmental and ascending collaterals of single afferents. *Nature* 395: 600–604. [11]

Lømo T. 2003. The discovery of long-term potentiation. *Philos. Trans. R. Soc. Lond., B, Biol. Sci.* 358: 617–620. [16]

Lømo, T., and Rosenthal, J. 1972. Control of ACh sensitivity by muscle activity in the rat. *J. Physiol.* 221: 493–513. [29]

Long, S. B., Campbell, E. B., and MacKinnon, R. 2005. Crystal structure of a mammalian voltage-dependent *Shaker* family K+ channel. *Science* 309: 897–903. [5]

Long, S. B., Campbell, E. B., and MacKinnon, R. 2005. Voltage sensor of Kv1.2: Structural basis of electromechanical coupling. *Science* 309: 903–908. [5]

Lonsbury-Martin, B. L., and Martin, G. K. 2003. Otoacoustic emissions. *Curr. Opin. Otolaryngol. Head Neck Surg.* 11: 361–366. [21]

Lorente de No, R. 1933. Vestibular ocular reflex arc. *Arch. Neurol. Psychiatry.* 30: 245–291. [24]

Lorenz, K. 1970. *Studies in Animal and Human Behavior*. Harvard Press, Cambridge, MA. [28]

Loring, R. H., and Salpeter, M. M. 1980. Denervation increases turnover rate of junctional acetylcholine receptors. *Proc. Natl. Acad. Sci. USA* 77: 2293–2297. [11]

Lottem, E., and Azouz, R. 2009. Mechanisms of tactile information transmission through whisker vibrations. *J. Neurosci.* 29: 11686–11697. [23]

LoTurco, J. J., et al. 1995. GABA and glutamate depolarize cortical progenitor cells and inhibit DNA synthesis. *Neuron* 15: 1287–1298. [27]

Love, F. M., Son, Y. J., and Thompson, W. J. 2003. Activity alters muscle reinnervation and terminal sprouting by reducing the number of Schwann cell pathways that grow to link synaptic sites. *J. Neurobiol.* 54: 566–576. [10, 29]

Lowel, S., and Singer, W. 1992. Selection of intrinsic horizontal connections in the visual cortex by correlated neuronal activity. *Science* 255: 209–212. [28]

Lowenstein, O., Osborne, M. P., and Thornhill, R. A. 1968. The anatomy and ultrastructure of the labyrinth of the lamprey (*Lampetra fluviatilis* L.). *Proc. R. Soc. Lond., B, Biol. Sci.* 170: 113–134. [24]

Lowery, L. A., and Van Vactor, D. 2009. The trip of the tip: Understanding the growth cone machinery. *Nat. Rev. Mol. Cell Biol.* 10: 332–343. [27]

Lowrey, P. L., and Takahashi, J. S. 2004. Mammalian circadian biology: Elucidating genome-wide levels of temporal organization. *Annu. Rev. Genomics Hum. Genet.* 5: 407–441. [19]

Lu, B., Su, Y., Das, S., Liu, J., Xia, J., and Ren, D. 2007. The neuronal channel NALCN contributes resting sodium permeability and is required for normal respiratory rhythm. *Cell* 129: 371–383. [6]

Lu, H. D., and Roe, A. W. 2008. Functional organization of color domains in V1 and V2 of macaque monkey revealed by optical imaging. *Cereb. Cortex* 18: 516–533. [3]

Lu, J., Karadsheh, M., and Delpire, E. 1999. Developmental regulation of the neuronal-specific isoform of K-Cl cotransporter KCC2 in postnatal rat brains. *J. Neurobiol.* 39: 558–568. [9]

Lu, P., Wang, Y., Graham, L.et al. 2012. Long-distance growth and connectivity of neural stem cells after severe spinal cord injury. *Cell* 150: 1264–1273. [29]

Lu, P., Woodruff, G., Wang, Y., et al. 2014. Long-distance axonal growth from human induced pluripotent stem cells after spinal cord injury. *Neuron* 83: 789–796. [29]

Lu, P., Yang, H., Culbertson, M., et al. 2006. Olfactory ensheathing cells do not exhibit unique migratory or axonal growth-promoting properties after spinal cord injury. *J. Neurosci.* 26: 11120–11130. [29]

Lu, T., Nguyen, B., Zhang, X., and Yang, J. 1999. Architecture of a K+ channel inner pore revealed by stoichiometric covalent modification. *Neuron* 22: 571–580. [5]

Lu, T., Ting, A. Y., Mainland, J., et al. 2001. Probing ion permeation and gating in a K+ channel with backbone mutations in the selectivity filter. *Nat. Neurosci.* 4: 239–246. [5]

Lu, Y., et al. 2011. TrkB as a potential synaptic and behavioral tag. *J. Neurosci.* 31: 11762–11771. [17]

Lu, Z. 2004. Mechanism of rectification in inward-rectifier K+ channels. *Annu. Rev. Physiol.* 66: 103–129. [5]

Lucas, S. M., and Binder, M. D. 1984. Topographic factors in distribution of homonymous group Ia-afferent input to cat medial gastrocnemius motoneurons. *J. Neurophysiol.* 51: 50–63. [26]

Ludwig, M., and Leng, G. 2006. Dendritic peptide release and peptide-dependent behaviours. *Nat. Rev. Neurosci.* 7: 126–136. [18]

Ludwig, M., Sabatier, N., Bull, P. M., et al. 2002. Intracellular calcium stores regulate activity-dependent neuropeptide release from dendrites. *Nature* 418: 85–89. [18]

Ludwig, M., and Stern, J. 2015. Multiple signalling modalities mediated by dendritic exocytosis of oxytocin and vasopressin. *Philos. Trans. R. Soc. Lond. B Biol. Sci.* 370: 20140182. [18]

Luebke, A. E., and Robinson, D. A. 1994. Gain changes of the cat's vestibulo-ocular reflex after flocculus deactivation. *Exp. Brain Res.* 98: 379–390. [24]

Luff, S. E. 1996. Ultrastructure of sympathetic axons and their structural relationship with vascular smooth muscle. *Anat. Embryol. (Berl).* 193: 515–531. [18]

Lui, J. H., et al. 2011. Development and evolution of the human neocortex. *Cell* 146: 18. [27]

Lumpkin, E. A., and Hudspeth, A. J. 1995. Detection of Ca^{2+} entry through mechanosensitive channels localizes the site of mechanoelectrical transduction in hair cells. *Proc. Natl. Acad. Sci. USA* 92: 10297–10301. [21]

Lumsden, A., and Krumlauf, R. 1996. Patterning the vertebrate neuroaxis. *Science* 274: 1109–1115. [27]

Lumsden, A. G., and Davies, A. M. 1986. Chemotropic effect of specific target epithelium in the developing mammalian nervous system. *Nature* 323: 538–539. [27]

Lundberg, A., and Quilisch, H. 1953. On the effect of calcium on presynaptic potentiation and depression at the neuromuscular junction. *Acta Physiol. Scand.* 30(Suppl. III): 121–129. [16]

Lundstrom, R. J. 1986. Responses of mechanoreceptive afferent units in the glabrous skin of the human hand to vibration. *Scand. J. Work Environ. Health.* 12: 413–416. [23]

Luo, D. G., Xue, T., and Yau, K. W. 2008. How vision begins: An odyssey. *Proc. Natl. Acad. Sci. USA* 105: 9855–9862. [22]

Luo, L., and O'Leary, D. D. 2005. Axon retraction and degeneration in development and disease. *Annu. Rev. Neurosci.* 28: 127–156. [27]

Luskin, M. B. 1993. Restricted proliferation and migration of postnatally generated neurons derived from the forebrain subventricular zone. *Neuron* 11: 173–189. [27]

Luskin, M. B. 1998. Neuroblasts of the postnatal mammalian forebrain: Their phenotype and fate. *J. Neurobiol.* 36: 221–233. [10]

Luskin, M. B., and Shatz, C. J. 1985. Neurogenesis of the cat's primary visual cortex. *J. Comp. Neurol.* 242: 611–631. [27]

Luskin, M. B., and Shatz, C. J. 1985. Studies of the earliest generated cells of the cat's visual cortex: Cogeneration of subplate and marginal zones. *J. Neurosci.* 5: 1062–1075. [27]

Lustig, L. R. 2006. Nicotinic acetylcholine receptor structure and function in the efferent auditory system *Anat. Rec.* 288A: 424–234. [12]

Lustig, L. R. 2010. In *The Oxford Handbook of Auditory Science: The Ear.* Oxford University Press: New York. pp. 15–47. [28]

Lustig, L. R., Leake, P. A., Snyder, R. L., and Rebscher, S. J. 1994. Changes in the cat cochlear nucleus following neonatal deafening and chronic intracochlear electrical stimulation. *Hear. Res.* 74: 29–37. [28]

Lyckman, A. W., Horng, S., Leamey, C. A., et al. 2008. Gene expression patterns in visual cortex during the critical period: Synaptic stabilization and reversal by visual deprivation. *Proc. Natl. Acad. Sci. USA* 105: 9409–9414. [28]

Lyford, G. L., et al., 1995. Arc, a growth factor and activity-regulated gene, encodes a novel cytoskeleton-associated protein that is enriched in neuronal dendrites. *Neuron* 14: 433–445. [17]

Lynch, G. S., Dunwiddie, T., and Gribkoff, V. 1977. Heterosynaptic depression: A postsynaptic correlate of long-term potentiation. *Nature* 266: 737–739. [16]

Lynch, J. W. 2009. Native glycine receptor subtypes and their physiological roles. *Neuropharmacol.* 56: 303–309. [5]

Lynch, M. A. 2004. Long-term potentiation and memory. *Physiol. Rev.* 84: 87–136. [16]

Lyons, M. R., and West, A. E. 2011. Mechanisms of specificity in neuronal activity-regulated gene transcription. *Prog. Neurobiol.* 94: 259–295. [17]

Ma, J., et al. 2018. Neural lineage tracing in the mammalian brain. *Curr. Opin. Neurobiol.* 50: 7–16. [27]

Ma, K. H., Hung, H. A., and Svaren, J. 2016. Epigenomic Regulation of Schwann Cell Reprogramming in Peripheral Nerve Injury. *J. Neuroscience.* 36: 9135–9147. [29]

Ma, M., and Dahl, G. 2006. Cosegregation of permeability and single channel conductance in chimeric connexins. *Biophys. J.* 90: 151–163. [8]

Ma, P. M., Beltz, B. S., and Kravitz, E. A. 1992. Serotonin-containing neurons in lobsters: Their role as gain-setters in postural control mechanisms. *J. Neurophysiol.* 1992 68:1, 36–54. [18]

Ma, W., Ribeiro-da-Silva, A., De Koninck, Y., et al. 1997. Substance P and enkephalin immunoreactivities in axonal boutons presynaptic to physiologically identified dorsal horn neurons. An ultrastructural multiple-labeling study in the cat. *Neuroscience* 77: 793–811. [14]

Mabb, A. M., and Ehlers, M. D. 2010. Ubiquitination in postsynaptic function and plasticity. *Annu. Rev. Cell Dev. Biol.* 26: 179–210. [27]

Mabb, A. M. and Ehlers, A. D. 2017. Arc ubiquitination in synaptic plasticity. *Sem. in Cell Develop. Biol.* 77: 10–16. [17]

Macagno, E. R. 1980. Number and distribution of neurons in leech segmental ganglia. *J. Comp. Neurol.* 190: 283–302. [20]

Macagno, E. R., Muller, K. J., and Pitman, R. M. 1987. Conduction block silences parts of a chemical synapse in the leech central nervous system. *J. Physiol.* 387: 649–664. doi: 10.1113/jphysiol.1987.sp016593. [20]

Macaluso, E., Frith, C. D., and Driver, J. 2000. Modulation of human visual cortex by crossmodal spatial attention. *Science* 289: 1206–1208. [25]

MacDermott, A. B., Connor, E. A., Dionne, V. E., and Parsons, R. L. 1980. Voltage clamp study of fast excitatory synaptic currents in bullfrog sympathetic ganglion cells. *J. Gen. Physiol.* 75: 39–60. [15]

MacInnis, B. L., and Campenot, R. B. 2002. Retrograde support of neuronal survival without retrograde transport of nerve growth factor. *Science* 295: 1536–1539. [27]

MacKie, K., and Hille, B. 1992. Cannabinoids inhibit N-type calcium channels in neuroblastoma–glioma cells. *Proc. Natl. Acad. Sci. USA* 89: 3825–3829. [12]

MacLennan, D. H., Abu-Abed, M., and Kang, C. H. 2002. Structure-function relationships in Ca^{2+} cycling proteins. *J. Mol. Cell. Cardiol.* 34: 897–918. [9]

MacMillan, S. J., Mark, M. A., and Duggan, A. W. 1998. The release of beta-endorphin and the neuropeptide-receptor mismatch in the brain. *Brain Res.* 794: 127–136. [18]

MacNeil, M. A., Heussy, J. K., Dacheux, R. F., et al. 1999. The shapes and numbers of amacrine cells: Matching of photofilled with Golgi-stained cells in the rabbit retina and comparison with other mammalian species. *J. Comp. Neurol.* 413: 305–326. [22]

Macpherson, P. C., Cieslak, D., and Goldman, D. 2006. Myogenin-dependent nAChR clustering in aneural myotubes. *Mol. Cell. Neurosci.* 31: 649–660. [29]

Madduri, S., and Gander, B. 2010. Schwann cell delivery of neurotrophic factors for peripheral nerve regeneration. *J. Peripher. Nerv. Syst.* 15: 93–103. [29]

Madison, D. V., and Nicoll, R. A. 1986. Actions of noradrenaline recorded intracellularly in rat hippocampal CA1 pyramidal neurones, in vitro. *J. Physiol.* 372: 221–244. [14]

Madison, D. V., and Nicoll, R. A. 1986. Cyclic adenosine 3′,5′-monophosphate mediates beta-receptor actions of noradrenaline in rat hippocampal pyramidal cells. *J. Physiol.* 372: 245–259. [14]

Madison, D. V., Lancaster, B., and Nicoll, R. A. 1987. Voltage clamp analysis of cholinergic action in the hippocampus. *J. Neurosci.* 7: 733–741. [14]

Maeda, S., Nakagawa, S., Suga, M., Yamashita, E., Oshima, A., Fujiyoshi, Y., and Tsukihara, T. 2009. Structure of the connexin 26 gap junction channel at 3.5 Å resolution. *Nature* 458: 597–604. [8]

Maeno, T., Edwards, C., and Anraku, M. 1977. Permeability of the end-plate membrane activated by acetylcholine to some organic cations. *J. Neurobiol.* 8: 173–184. [5]

Maffei, L., Berardi, N., Domenici, L., Parisi, V., and Pizzorusso, T. 1992. Nerve growth factor (NGF) prevents the shift in ocular dominance distribution of visual cortical neurons in monocularly deprived rats. *J. Neurosci.* 12: 4651–4662. [28]

Maffei, L., and Galli-Resta, L. 1990. Correlation in the discharges of neighboring rat retinal ganglion cells during prenatal life. *Proc. Natl. Acad. Sci. USA* 87: 2861–2864. [22, 28]

Magee, J. C., and Johnston, D. 1997. A synaptically controlled, associative signal for Hebbian plasticity in hippocampal neurons. *Science* 275: 209. [17]

Magistretti, P. J. 2009. Role of glutamate in neuron-glia metabolic coupling. *Am. J. Clin. Nutr.* 90: 875–880. [10]

Magleby, K. L., and Stevens, C. F. 1972. The effect of voltage on the time course of end-plate currents. *J. Physiol.* 223: 151–171. [11]

Magleby, K. L. and Stevens, C. F. 1972. A quantitative description of end-plate currents. *J. Physiol.* 223: 173–197. [11]

Magleby, K. L., and Terrar, D. A. 1975. Factors affecting the time course of decay of end-plate currents: A possible cooperative action of acetylcholine on receptors at the frog neuromuscular junction. *J. Physiol.* 244: 467–495. [11]

Magleby, K. L., and Weinstock, M. M. 1980. Nickel and calcium ions modify the characteristics of the acetylcholine receptor-channel complex at the frog neuromuscular junction. *J. Physiol.* 299: 203–218. [13]

Magleby, K. L., and Zengel, J. E. 1976. Augmentation: A process that acts to increase transmitter release at the frog neuromuscular junction. *J. Physiol.* 257: 449–470. [16]

Maguire, G., and Werblin, F. 1994. Dopamine enhances a glutamate-gated ionic current in OFF bipolar cells of the tiger salamander retina. *J. Neurosci.* 14: 6094–16101. [18]

Mahaut-Smith, M. P., Martinez-Pinna, J., and Gurung, I. S. 2008. A role for membrane potential in regulating GPCRs? *Trends Pharmacol. Sci.* 29: 421–429. [12]

Mahns, D. A., Perkins, N. M., Sahai, V., et al. 2006. Vibrotactile frequency discrimination in human hairy skin. *J. Neurophysiol.* 95: 1442–1450. [23]

Maienschein, J. 1978. Cell lineage, ancestral reminiscence, and the biogenetic law. *J. Hist. Biol.* 11: 129–158. [20]

Mains, R. E., and Eipper, B. A. 1999. In *Basic Neurochemistry: Molecular, Cellular, and Medical Aspects*, 6th ed. Lippincott-Raven, Philadelphia, pp. 363–382. [15]

Mains, R. E., and Patterson, P. H. 1973. Primary cultures of dissociated sympathetic neurons. I. Establishment of long-term growth in culture and studies of differentiated properties. *J. Cell Biol.* 59: 329–345. [27]

Maiti, S., Shear, J. B., Williams, R. M., et al. 1997. Measuring serotonin distribution in live cells with three-photon excitation. *Science* 275: 530–532. [1]

Majdan, M., and Shatz, C. J. 2006. Effects of visual experience on activity-dependent gene regulation in cortex. *Nat. Neurosci.* 9: 650–659. [28]

Majewski, H., and Iannazzo, L. 1998. Protein kinase C: A physiological mediator of enhanced transmitter output. *Prog. Neurobiol.* 55: 463–476. [12]

Makino, H., and Malinow, R. 2009. AMPA receptor incorporation into synapses during LTP: The role of lateral movement and exocytosis. *Neuron* 64: 381–390. [16]

Malach, R., Ebert, R., and Van Sluyters, R. C. 1984. Recovery from effects of brief monocular deprivation in the kitten. *J. Neurophysiol.* 51: 538–551. [28]

Malatesta, P. 2000. Isolation of radial glial cells by fluorescent-activated cell sorting reveals a neuronal lineage. *Development* 157: 5253–5263. [27]

Malaviya, R., Morrison, A. R., and Pentland, A. P. 1996. Histamine in human epidermal cells is induced by ultraviolet light injury. *J. Invest. Dermatol.* 106: 785–789. [21]

Malenka, R. C., and Nicoll, R. A. 1999. Long-term potentiation—A decade of progress? *Science* 285: 1870–1874. [16]

Malenka, R. C., Kauer, J. A., Perkel, D. J., et al. 1989. An essential role for postsynaptic calmodulin and protein kinase activity in long-term potentiation. *Nature* 340: 554–557. [16]

Malinow, R., and Malenka, R. C. 2002. AMPA receptor trafficking and synaptic plasticity. *Annu. Rev. Neurosci.* 25: 103–126. [16]

Malinow, R., and Tsien, R. W. 1990. Presynaptic enhancement shown by whole-cell recordings of long-term potentiation in hippocampal slices. *Nature* 346: 177–180. [16]

Malinow, R., Schulman, H., and Tsien, R. W. 1989. Inhibition of postsynaptic PKC or CaMKII blocks induction but not expression of LTP. *Science* 245: 862–866. [16]

Mallamaci, A., et al. 2000. . Area identity shifts in the early cerebral cortex of Emx2$^{-/-}$ mutant mice. *Nat. Neurosci.* 3: 679–686. [27]

Mallamaci, A. 2011. Molecular bases of cortico-cerebral regionalization. *Prog. Brain Res.* 189: 37–64. [27]

Mallart, A., and Martin, A. R. 1967. Analysis of facilitation of transmitter release at the neuromuscular junction of the frog. *J. Physiol.* 193: 679–697. [16]

Mallart, A., and Martin, A. R. 1968. The relation between quantum content and facilitation at the neuromuscular junction of the frog. *J. Physiol.* 196: 593–604. [16]

Mallo, M. and Alonso, C. R. 2013. The regulation of Hox gene expression during animal development. *Development* 140: 3951–3963. [27]

Malmierca, M. S. 2003. The structure and physiology of the rat auditory system: An overview. *Int. Rev. Neurobiol.* 56: 147–211. [24]

Malonek, D., Tootell, R. B. H., and Grinvald, A. 1994. Optical imaging reveals the functional architecture of neurons processing shape and motion in owl monkey area MT. *Proc. R. Soc. Lond., B, Biol. Sci.* 258: 109–119. [25]

Malpeli, J. G., Lee, D., and Baker, F. H. 1996. Laminar and retinotopic organization of the macaque LGN: Magnocellular and parvocellular magnification functions. *J. Comp. Neurol.* 375: 363–377. [2]

Mandelkow, E., and Hoenger, A. 1999. Structures of kinesin and kinesin-microtubule interactions. *Curr. Opin. Cell Biol.* 11: 34–44. [15]

Mandolesi, G., Menna, E., Harauzov, A., et al. 2005. A role for retinal brain-derived neurotrophic factor in ocular dominance plasticity. *Curr. Biol.* 15: 2119–2124. [28]

Mangel, S. C., and Dowling, J. E. 1987. The interplexiform-horizontal cell system of the fish retina: Effects of dopamine, light stimulation and time in the dark. *Proc. R. Soc. Lond. B Biol. Sci.* 231: 91–121. [18]

Manita, S., and Ross, W. N. 2009. Synaptic activation and membrane potential changes modulate the frequency of spontaneous elementary Ca^{2+} release events in the dendrites of pyramidal neurons. *J. Neurosci.* 29: 7833–7845. [12]

Manley, G. A. 2000. Cochlear mechanisms from a phylogenetic viewpoint. *Proc. Natl. Acad. Sci. USA* 97: 11736–11743. [24]

Mano, T., Iwase, S., and Toma, S. 2006. Microneurography as a tool in clinical neurophysiology to investigate peripheral neural traffic in humans. *Clin. Neurophysiol.* 117: 2357–2384. [23]

Mansour, A., Khachaturian, H., Lewis, M. E., et al. 1988. Anatomy of CNS opioid receptors. *Trends Neurosci.* 11: 308–314. [14]

Mansvelder, H. D., Keath, J. R., and McGehee, D. S. 2002. Synaptic mechanisms underlie nicotine-induced excitability of brain reward areas. *Neuron* 33: 905–919. [14]

Marban, E., Yamagishi, T., and Tomaselli, G. F. 1998. Structure and function of voltage-gated sodium channels. *J. Physiol.* 508: 647–657. [5]

Marcaggi, P., and Attwell, D. 2004. Role of glial amino acid transporters in synaptic transmission and brain energetics. *Glia* 47: 217–25. [10]

Marchand-Pauvert, V., Nicolas, G., Marque, P., et al. 2005. Increase in group II excitation from ankle muscles to thigh motoneurones during human standing. *J. Physiol.* 566: 257–271. [26]

Marchetti, L., et al. 2019. Fast-diffusing p75^{NTR} monomers support apoptosis and growth cone collapse by neurotrophin ligands. *Proc. Natl. Acad. Sci. USA.* doi: 10.1073/ pnas.1902790116. [27]

Marcus, D. C., Wu, T., Wangemann, P., and Kofuji, P. 2002. KCNJ10 (Kir4.1) potassium channel knockout abolishes endocochlear potential. *Am. J. Physiol. Cell Physiol.* 282: C403–407. [24]

Marder, E., and Bucher, D. 2007. Understanding circuit dynamics using the stomatogastric nervous system of lobsters and crabs. *Annu. Rev. Physiol.* 69: 291–316. [20]

Marder, E., Manor, Y., Nadim, F., et al. 1998. Frequency control of a slow oscillatory network by a fast rhythmic input: Pyloric to gastric mill interactions in the crab stomatogastric nervous system. *Ann. NY Acad. Sci.* 860: 226–238. [20]

Mariani, J. and Vaccarino, F. M. 2019. Breakthrough moments: Yoshiki Sasai's discoveries in the 3rd dimension. *Cell Stem Cell* 24: 837. [27]

Marin-Burgin, A., Kristan, W. B., Jr., and French, K. A. 2008. From synapses to behavior: Development of a sensory-motor circuit in the leech. *Dev. Neurobiol.* 68: 779–787. [20]

Marín O. 2012. Interneuron dysfunction in psychiatric disorders. *Nat. Rev. Neurosci.* 13: 107–120. https://doi.org/10.1038/nrn3155 [28]

Marín O. 2016. Developmental timing and critical windows for the treatment of psychiatric disorders. *Nat. Med.* 22: 1229–1238. https://doi.org/10.1038/nm.4225 [28]

Marín, O., and Rubenstein, J. L. 2003. Cell migration in the forebrain. *Annu. Rev. Neurosci.* 26: 441–483. [27]

Marín, O., Valiente, M., Ge, X., and Tsai, L. H. 2010. Guiding neuronal cell migrations. *Cold Spring Harb. Perspect. Biol.* 2: A001834. [27]

Marker, C. L., Luján, R., Colón, J., and Wickman, K. 2006. Distinct populations of spinal cord lamina II interneurons expressing G-protein-gated potassium channels. *J. Neurosci.* 26: 12251–12259. [14]

Markram, H., Lubke, J., Frotscher, M., and Sakmann, B. 1997. Regulation of synaptic efficacy by coincidence of postsynaptic APs and EPSPs. *Science* 275: 213–215. [8, 17]

Marks, W. B., Dobelle, W. H., and Macnichol, E. F., Jr. 1964. Visual pigments of single primate cones. *Science* 143: 1181–1183. [22]

Marmont, G. 1949. Studies on the axon membrane; a new method. *J. Cell. Comp. Physiol.* 34: 351–382. [7]

Martin, A. R., and Fuchs, P. A. 1992. The dependence of calcium-activated potassium currents on membrane potential. *Proc. R. Soc. Lond., B, Biol. Sci.* 250: 71–76. [24]

Martin, A. R., and Levinson, S. R. 1985. Contribution of the Na^+-K^+ pump to membrane potential in familial periodic paralysis. *Muscle Nerve* 8: 354–362. [6]

Martin, A. R., and Pilar, G. 1963. Dual mode of synaptic transmission in the avian ciliary ganglion. *J. Physiol.* 168: 443–463. [11, 13]

Martin, A. R., and Pilar, G. 1964. Quantal components of the synaptic potential in the ciliary ganglion of the chick. *J. Physiol.* 175: 1–16. [13]

Martin, A. R., and Pilar, G. 1964. Presynaptic and postsynaptic events during post-tetanic potentiation and facilitation in the avian ciliary ganglion. *J. Physiol.* 175: 16–30. [16]

Martin, D. L. 1987. Regulatory properties of brain glutamate decarboxylase. *Cell. Mol. Neurobiol.* 7: 237–253. [15]

Martin, D. P., Schmidt, R. E., DiStefano, P. S., et al. 1988. Inhibitors of protein synthesis and RNA synthesis prevent neuronal death caused by nerve growth factor deprivation. *J. Cell Biol.* 106: 829–844. [27]

Martin, D. W. 2005. Structure-function relationships in the Na^+, K^+-pump. *Semin. Nephrol.* 25: 282–281. [9]

Martin, K. C., and Kosik, K. S. 2002. Synaptic tagging—who's it? *Nat. Rev. Neurosci.* 3: 813. [17]

Martin, P., Mehta, A. D., and Hudspeth, A. J. 2000. Negative hair-bundle stiffness betrays a mechanism for mechanical amplification by the hair cell. *Proc. Natl. Acad. Sci. USA* 97: 12026–12031. [21]

Martin, S. J., et al. 2000. Synaptic plasticity and memory: an evaluation of the hypothesis. *Annu. Rev. Neurosci.* 23: 649–711. [17]

Martinello, K., Huang, Z., Lujan, R., et al. 2015. Cholinergic afferent stimulation induces axonal plasticity in adult hippocampal granule cells. *Neuron* 85: 346–363. [14]

Martinez, J. L., Jr., and Derrick, B. E. 1996. Long-term potentiation and learning. *Annu. Rev. Psychol.* 47: 173–203. [16]

Martinez, L. M., and Alonso, J. M. 2001. Construction of complex receptive fields in cat primary visual cortex. *Neuron* 32: 515–525. [2]

Marvizón, J. C., Chen, W., and Murphy, N. 2009. Enkephalins, dynorphins, and β-endorphin in the rat dorsal horn: An immunofluorescence colocalization study. *J. Comp. Neurol.* 517: 51–68. [14]

Masland, R. H. 1988. Amacrine cells. *Trends Neurosci.* 11: 405–410. [22]

Masland, R. H. 2001. Neuronal diversity in the retina. *Curr. Opin. Neurobiol.* 11: 431–436. [22]

Masland, R. H. 2001. The fundamental plan of the retina. *Nat. Neurosci.* 4: 877–886. [22]

Mason, A., and Muller, K. J. 1996. Accurate synapse regeneration despite ablation of the distal axon segment. *Eur. J. Neurosci.* 8: 11–20. [20]

Masserdotti, G., Gascón, S., and Götz, M. 2016. Direct neuronal reprogramming: Learning from and for development *Development* 143: 2494–2510. [29]

Masu, M., Iwakabe, H., Tagawa, Y., et al. 1995. Specific deficit of the ON response in visual transmission by targeted disruption of the mGluR6 gene. *Cell* 80: 757–765. [22]

Mathie, A. A., Cull-Candy, S. G., and Colquhoun, D. 1991. Conductance and kinetic properties of single nicotinic acetylcholine receptor channels in rat sympathetic neurons. *J. Physiol.* 439: 717–750. [19]

Matsuda, L., Lolait, S. J., Brownstein, M. J., Young, A. C., and Bonner, T. I. 1990. Structure of a cannabinoid receptor and functional expression of the cloned cDNA. *Nature* 346: 561–564. [12]

Matsunami, H., and Buck, L. B. 1997. A multigene family encoding a diverse array of putative pheromone receptors in mammals. *Cell* 90: 775–784. [21]

Matsunami, H., Montmayeur, J. P., and Buck, L. B. 2000. A family of candidate taste receptors in human and mouse. *Nature* 404: 601–604. [21]

Matsuzaki, M., Honkura, N., Ellis-Davies, G. C., and Kasai, H. 2004. Structural basis of long-term potentiation in single dendritic spines. *Nature* 429: 761–766. [16, 17]

Matthews, G., and Fuchs, P. 2010. The diverse roles of ribbon synapses in sensory neurotransmission. *Nat. Rev. Neurosci.* 11: 812–822. [13, 24]

Matthews, G., and Wickelgren, W. O. 1979. Glycine, GABA and synaptic inhibition of reticulospinal neurones of the lamprey. *J. Physiol.* 293: 393–414. [6]

Matthews, M. R., and Nelson, V. H. 1975. Detachment of structurally intact nerve endings from chromatolytic neurones of rat superior cervical ganglion during the depression of synaptic transmission induced by postganglionic axotomy. *J. Physiol.* 245: 91–135. [29]

Matthews, P. B. 1981. Evolving views on the internal operation and functional role of the muscle spindle. *J. Physiol.* 320: 1–30. [21]

Matthews, P. B. C. 1964. Muscle spindles and their motor control. *Physiol. Rev.* 44: 219–288. [21]

Matthews, P. B. C. 1972. *Mammalian Muscle Receptors and Their Central Action.* Edward Arnold, London. [26]

Matthey, R. 1925. Récupération de la vue après résection des nerfs optiques chez le triton. *C. R. Soc. Biol.* 93: 904–906. [29]

Matulef, K., and Zagotta, W. N. 2003. Cyclic nucleotide-gated channels. *Annu. Rev. Cell. Dev. Biol.* 19: 23–44. [5]

Maturana, H. R., Lettvin, J. Y., McCulloch, W. S., and Pitts, W. H. 1960. Anatomy and physiology of vision in the frog (*Rana pipiens*). *J. Gen. Physiol.* 43: 129–175. [2]

Maue, R. A., and Dionne, V. E. 1987. Patch-clamp studies of isolated mouse olfactory receptor neurons. *J. Gen. Physiol.* 90: 95–125. [21]

Maunsell, J. H., and Newsome, W. T. 1987. Visual processing in monkey extrastriate cortex. *Annu. Rev. Neurosci.* 10: 363–401. [3, 25]

Maunsell, J. H. R., and Van Essen, D. C. 1983. Functional properties of neurons in the middle temporal visual area (MT) of the macaque monkey. I. Selectivity for stimulus direction, speed and orientation. *J. Neurophysiol.* 49: 1127–1147. [25]

May, B. J., and Huang, A. Y. 1996. Sound orientation behavior in cats. I. Localization of broadband noise. *J. Acoust. Soc. Am.* 100: 1059–1069. [24]

Mayer, C., et al. 2015. Clonally related forebrain interneurons disperse broadly across both functional areas and structural boundaries. *Neuron* 87: 989–998. [27]

Mayer, M. L., Westbrook, G. L., and Guthrie, P. B. 1984. Voltage-dependent block by Mg^{2+} of NMDA responses in spinal cord neurones. *Nature* 309: 261–263. [11, 16]

Mayford, M., et al. 1996. The 3′-untranslated region of CaMKIIα is a cis-acting signal for the localization and translation of mRNA in dendrites. *Proc. Natl. Acad. Sci. USA* 93: 13250–13255. [17]

Maylie, J., Bond, C. T., Herson, P. S., Lee, W. S., and Adelman, J. P. 2004. Small conductance Ca^{2+}-activated K^+ channels and calmodulin. *J. Physiol.* 554: 255–261. [12]

Mayser, W. Schloss, P., and Betz, H. 1992. Primary structure and functional expression of a choline transporter expressed in the rat nervous system. *FEBS Lett.* 305: 31–36. [9]

Mazzoni, E. O., et al. 2013. Saltatory remodeling of Hox chromatin in response to rostrocaudal patterning signals. *Nat. Neurosci.* 16: 1191–1198. [27]

McConnell, S. K. 1995. Constructing the cerebral cortex: Neurogenesis and fate determination. *Neuron* 15: 761–768. [27]

McCormack, E. J., Egnor, M. R., and Wagshul, M. E. 2007. Improved cerebrospinal fluid flow measurements using phase contrast balanced steady-state free precession. *Magn. Reson. Imaging* 25: 172–182. [18]

McCormick, D. A., and Williamson, A. 1989. Convergence and divergence of neurotransmitter action in human cerebral cortex. *Proc. Natl. Acad. Sci. USA* 86: 8098–8102. [14]

McCrea, P. D., Popot, J. L., and Engleman, D. M. 1987. Transmembrane topography of the nicotinic acetylcholine receptor subunit. *EMBO J.* 6: 3619–3626. [5]

McDonald, T. F., Pelzer, S., Trautwein, W., and Pelzer, D. J. 1994. Regulation and modulation of calcium channels in cardiac, skeletal, and smooth muscle cells. *Physiol. Rev.* 74: 365–507. [12]

McGehee, D. S., Heath, M. J., Gelber, S., et al. 1995. Nicotine enhancement of fast excitatory synaptic transmission in CNS by presynaptic receptors. *Science* 269: 1692–1696. [14]

McGinnis, W. et al 1984. A conserved DNA sequence in homoeotic genes of the *Drosophila* Antennapedia and bithorax complexes. *Nature* 308: 428–433. [27]

McGinty, D. J., and Harper, R. M. 1976. Dorsal raphe neurons: depression of firing during sleep in cats. *Brain Res.* 101: 569–575. [18]

McGlade-McCulloh, E., Morrissey, A. M., Norona, F., and Muller, K. J. 1989. Individual microglia move rapidly and directly to nerve lesions in the leech central nervous system. *Proc. Natl. Acad. Sci. USA.* 86: 1093–1097. [10]

McGlone, F., Vallbo, A. B., Olausson, H., et al. 2007. Discriminative touch and emotional touch. *Can. J. Exp. Psychol.* 61: 173–183. [23]

McGraw, L. A., and Young, L. J. 2010. The prairie vole: An emerging model organism for understanding the social brain. *Trends Neurosci.* 33: 103–109. [14]

McIntire, S. L., Reimer, R. J., Schuske, K., Edwards, R. H., and Jorgensen, E. M. 1997. Identification and characterization of the vesicular GABA transporter. *Nature* 389: 870–876. [9]

McIntyre, A. 1980. Biological seismography. *Trends Neurosci.* 3: 202–205. [21]

McKenna, M. P., and Raper, J. A. 1988. Growth cone behavior on gradients of substratum bound laminin. *Dev. Biol.* 130: 232–236. [27]

McKernan, D. P., and Cotter, T. G. 2007. A critical role for Bim in retinal ganglion cell death. *J. Neurochem.* 102: 922–930. [29]

McKernan, M. G., and Shinnick-Gallagher, P. 1997. Fear conditioning induces a lasting potentiation of synaptic currents in vitro. *Nature* 390: 607–611. [16]

McLachlan, E. M., ed. 1995. *Autonomic Ganglia.* Gordon and Breach, London. [19]

McLaughlin, S. K., McKinnon, P. J., and Margolskee, R. F. 1992. Gustducin is a taste-cell-specific G protein closely related to the transducins. *Nature* 357: 563–569. [21]

McMahan, U. J. 1990. The agrin hypothesis. *Cold Spring Harb. Symp. Quant. Biol.* 55: 407–418. [11, 29]

McMahan, U. J., and Slater, C. R. 1984. The influence of basal lamina on the accumulation of acetylcholine receptors at synaptic sites in regenerating muscle. *J. Cell Biol.* 98: 1453–1473. [29]

McMahan, U. J., and Wallace, B. G. 1989. Molecules in basal lamina that direct the formation of synaptic specializations at neuromuscular junctions. *Dev. Neurosci.* 11: 227–247. [29]

McMahan, U. J., Edgington, D. R., and Kuffler, D. P. 1980. Factors that influence regeneration of the neuromuscular junction. *J. Exp. Biol.* 89: 31–42. [29]

McMahan, U. J., Sanes, J. R., and Marshall, L. M. 1978. Cholinesterase is associated with the basal lamina at the neuromuscular junction. *Nature* 271: 172–174. [15]

McMahan, U. J., Spitzer, N. C., and Peper, K. 1972. Visual identification of nerve terminals in living isolated skeletal muscle. *Proc. Roy. Soc. Lond., B, Biol. Sci.* 181: 421–430. [11]

McRae, P. A., Rocco, M. M., Kelly, G., Brumberg, J. C., and Matthews, R. T. 2007. Sensory deprivation alters aggrecan and perineuronal net expression in the mouse barrel cortex. *J. Neurosci.* 27: 5405–5413. [28]

McShane et al. 2015. Cellular basis of neuroepithelial bending during mouse spinal neural tube closure. *Dev. Biol.* 404: 113–124. [27]

Mehta, A. D. et al. 1999. Myosin-V is a processive actin-based motor. *Nature* 400: 590–593. [18]

Meier, J. C., Henneberger, C., Melnik, I., et al. 2005. RNA editing produces glycine receptor alpha3 (P185L), resulting in high agonist potency. *Nature Neurosci.* 8: 736–744. [5]

Meier, J. D., Aflalo, T. N., Kastner, S., and Graziano, M. S. A. 2008. Complex organization of human primary motor cortex: A high-resolution fMRI study. *J. Neurophysiol.* 100: 1800–1812. [26]

Meis, S. 2003. Nociceptin/orphanin FQ: Actions within the brain. *Neuroscientist* 9: 158–168. [14]

Meissirel, C., Wikler, K. C., Chalupa, L. M., and Rakic, P. 1997. Early divergence of magnocellular and parvocellular functional subsystems in the embryonic primate visual system. *Proc. Natl. Acad. Sci. USA* 94: 5900–5905. [28]

Meister, M., and Berry, M. J., 2nd. 1999. The neural code of the retina. *Neuron* 22: 435–450. [22]

Meister, M., Lagnado, L., and Baylor, D. A. 1995. Concerted signaling by retinal ganglion cells. *Science* 270: 1207–1210. [2, 22]

Meister, M., Wong, R. O., Baylor, D. A., and Shatz, C. J. 1991. Synchronous bursts of action potentials in ganglion cells of the developing mammalian retina. *Science* 252: 939–943. [28]

Meladinic, M., Bechetti, A., Didelon, F., et al. 1999. Low expression of the CLC-2 chloride channel during postnatal development: A mechanism for the paradoxical depolarizing action of GABA and glycine in the hippocampus. *Proc. Roy. Soc. Lond., B, Biol. Sci.* 266: 1207–1213. [6]

Meldolesi, J. 2018. Exosomes and ectosomes in intercellular communication. *Curr. Biol.* 28: R435–R444. doi: 10.1016/j.cub.2018.01.059. [18]

Mellios, N., Sugihara, H., Castro, J., et al. 2011. miR-132, an experience-dependent microRNA, is essential for visual cortex plasticity. *Nat. Neurosci.* 14: 1240–1242. [28]

Melzack, R. 1973. *The Puzzle of Pain.* Harmondsworth: Penguin Books. [23]

Mendell, L. M., and Henneman, E. 1971. Terminals of single Ia fibers: Location, density, and distribution within a pool of 300 homonymous motoneurons. *J. Neurophysiol.* 34: 171–187. [26]

Mendez, J. A. et al. 2011. Somatodendritic dopamine release requires synaptotagmin 4 and 7 and the participation of voltage-gated calcium channels. *J. Biol. Chem.* 286: 23928–23937. [18]

Menei, P., Montero-Menei, C., Whittemore, S. R., et al. 1998. Schwann cells genetically modified to secrete human BDNF promote enhanced axonal regrowth across transected adult rat spinal cord. *Eur. J. Neurosci.* 10: 607–621. [29]

Menesini-Chen, M. L., Chen, J. S., Levi-Montalcini, R. 1978. Sympathetic nerve fibers ingrowth in the central nervous system of neonatal rodent upon intracerebral NGF injections. *Arch. Ital. Biol.* 116: 53–84. [27]

Menini, A., Picco, C., and Firestein, S. 1995. Quantal-like current fluctuations induced by odorants in olfactory receptor cells. *Nature* 373: 435–437. [21]

Mercado, A., Mount, D. B., and Gamba, G. 2004. Electroneutral cation-chloride cotransporters in the central nervous system. *Neurochem. Res.* 29: 17–25. [9]

Merchant, H., Naselaris, T., and Georgopoulos, A. P. 2008. Dynamic sculpting of directional tuning in the primate motor cortex during three-dimensional reaching. *J. Neurosci.* 28: 9164–9172. [26]

Merigan, W. H., and Maunsell, J. H. R. 1993. How parallel are the primate visual pathways? *Annu. Rev. Neurosci.* 16: 369–402. [3, 25]

Merkle, T., and Wehner, R. 2008. Landmark guidance and vector navigation in outbound desert ants. *J. Exp. Biol.* 211: 3370–3377. [20]

Merzenich, M. M., Kaas, J. H., Sur, M., and Lin, C. S. 1978. Double representation of the body surface within cytoarchitectonic areas 3b and 1 in "SI" in the owl monkey (*Aotus trivirgatus*). *J. Comp. Neurol.* 181: 41–73. [23]

Merzenich, M. M., Knight, P. L., and Roth, G. L. 1975. Representation of cochlea within primary auditory cortex in the cat. *J. Neurophysiol.* 38: 231–249. [24]

Mesce, K. A., Esch, T., and Kristan, W. B., Jr. 2008. Cellular substrates of action selection: A cluster of higher-order descending neurons shapes body posture and locomotion. *J. Comp. Physiol. A.* 194: 469–481. [20]

Mesgarani, N., David, S. V., Fritz, J. B., and Shamma, S. A. 2008. Phoneme representation and classification in primary auditory cortex. *J. Acoust. Soc. Am.* 123: 899–909. [24]

Mesulam, M. 2004. The cholinergic lesion of Alzheimer's disease: Pivotal factor or side show? *Learn. Mem.* 11: 43–49. [14]

Metea, M. R., and Newman, E. A. 2006. Calcium signaling in specialized glial cells. *Glia* 54: 650–655. [10]

Metea, M. R., and Newman, E. A. 2006. Glial cells dilate and constrict blood vessels: A mechanism of neurovascular coupling. *J. Neurosci.* 26: 2862–2870. [10, 18]

Metea, M. R., Kofuji, P., and Newman, E. A. 2007. Neurovascular coupling is not mediated by potassium siphoning from glial cells. *J. Neurosci.* 27: 2468–2471. [10]

Meunier, J. C., Mollereau, C., Toll, L., et al. 1995. Isolation and structure of the endogenous agonist of opioid receptor-like ORL₁ receptor. *Nature* 377: 532–535. [14]

Meves, H. 2008. Arachidonic acid and ion channels: An update. *Brit. J. Pharmacol.* 155: 4–16. [12]

Meyer, A. C., Frank, T., Khimich, D., et al. 2009. Tuning of synapse number, structure and function in the cochlea. *Nat. Neurosci.* 12: 444–453. [24]

Meyer, G. 2010. Building a human cortex: The evolutionary differentiation of Cajal-Retzius cells and the cortical hem. *J. Anat.* 217: 334–343. [27]

Meyer, M., Matsuoka, I., Wetmore, C., et al. 1992. Enhanced synthesis of brain-derived neurotrophic factor in the lesioned peripheral nerve: Different mechanisms are responsible for the regulation of BDNF and NGF mRNA. *J. Cell Biol.* 119: 45–54. [29]

Middlebrooks, J. C., Dykes, R. W., and Merzenich, M. M. 1980. Binaural response-specific bands in primary auditory cortex (AI) of the cat: Topographical organization orthogonal to isofrequency contours. *Brain. Res.* 181: 31–48. [24]

Mikoshiba, K. 2007. IP3 receptor/Ca^{2+} channel: From discovery to new signaling concepts. *J. Neurochem.* 102: 1426–1446. [12]

Miledi, R. 1960. The acetylcholine sensitivity of frog muscle fibers after complete or partial denervation. *J. Physiol.* 151: 1–23. [29]

Miledi, R. 1960. Junctional and extra-junctional acetylcholine receptors in skeletal muscle fibres. *J. Physiol.* 151: 24–30. [11]

Miledi, R., Parker, I., and Sumikawa, K. 1983. Recording single γ-aminobutyrate- and acetylcholine-activated receptor channels translated by exogenous mRNA in Xenopus oocytes. *Proc. R. Soc. Lond., B, Biol. Sci.* 218: 481–484. [5]

Miledi, R., Stefani, E., and Steinbach, A. B. 1971. Induction of the action potential mechanism in slow muscle fibres of the frog. *J. Physiol.* 217: 737–754. [29]

Milhorat, T. H. 1975. The third circulation revisited. *J. Neurosurg.* 42: 628–645. [18]

Millar, N. S., and Gotti, C. 2009. Diversity of vertebrate nicotinic acetylcholine receptors. *Neuropharmacology* 56: 237–246. [5, 14]

Miller, C., and White, M. M. 1984. Dimeric structure of single chloride channels from Torpedo electroplax. Proc. Nat. Acad. Sci. USA 81: 2772–2775. [5]

Miller, J., Agnew, W. S., and Levinson S. R. 1985. Principal glycopeptide of the tetrodotoxin/saxitoxin binding protein from *Electrophorus electricus*: Isolation and partial chemical and physical purification. *Biochemistry* 22: 462–470. [5]

Miller, S., et al. 2002. Disruption of dendritic translation of CaMKIIalpha impairs stabilization of synaptic plasticity and memory consolidation. *Neuron* 36: 507–519. [17]

Milner, A. D., Perrett, D. I., Johnston, R. S., et al. 1991. Perception and action in "visual form agnosia." *Brain* 114: 405–428. [25]

Mineo, M., Jolley, T., and Rodriguez, G. 2004. Leech therapy in penile replantation: A case of recurrent penile self-amputation. *Urology* 63: 981–983. [20]

Mink, J. W., and Thach, W. T. 1991. Basal ganglia motor control. III. Pallidal ablation: Normal reaction time, muscle co-contraction, and slow movement. *J. Neurophysiol.* 65: 330–351. [26]

Mink, J. W., and Thach, W. T. 1993. Basal ganglia intrinsic circuits and their role in behavior. *Curr. Opin. Neurobiol.* 3: 950–957. [26]

Minor, L. B. 2005. Clinical manifestations of superior semicircular canal dehiscence. *Laryngoscope* 115: 1717–1727. [24]

Miserendino, M. J., Sananes, C. B., Melia, K. R., and Davis, M. 1990. Blocking acquisition but not expression of conditioned fear-potentiated startle by NMDA antagonists in the amygdala. *Nature* 345: 716–718. [16]

Mishina, M., Takai, T., Imoto, K., et al. 1986. Molecular distinction between fetal and adult forms of muscle acetylcholine receptor. *Nature* 321: 406–411. [11, 29]

Mitchell, E. A., Herd, M. B., Gunn, B. G., et al. 2008. Neurosteroid modulation of GABA$_A$ receptors: Molecular determinants and significance in health and disease. *Neurochem. Int.* 52: 588–595. [14]

Miyakawa, H., Lev-Ram, V., Lasser-Ross, N., and Ross, W. N. 1992. Calcium transients evoked by climbing fiber and parallel fiber synaptic inputs in guinea pig cerebellar Purkinje neurons. *J. Neurophysiol.* 68: 1178–1189. [26]

Miyata, T. and Ogawa, M. 2007. Cell migration: Catapulting neurons from the ventricular zone? *Curr. Biol.* 17: 146. [27]

Miyata, T., et al. 2001. Asymmetric inheritance of radial glial fibers by cortical neurons. *Neuron* 31: 727–741. [27]

Miyata, T., et al. 2015. Interkinetic nuclear migration generates and opposes ventricular-zone crowding: insight into tissue mechanics. *Front. Cell Neurosci.* 8: 473. [27]

Miyawaki, A., Llopis, J., Heim, R., et al. 1997. Fluorescent indicators for Ca^{2+} based on green fluorescent proteins and calmodulin. *Nature* 388: 882–887. [12]

Mladinic, M., Lefèvre, C., Del Bel, E., et al. 2010. Developmental changes of gene expression after spinal cord injury in neonatal opossums. *Brain Res.* 1363: 20–39. [29]

Mladinic, M., Muller, K. J., and Nicholls. J. G. 2009. Central nervous system regeneration: From leech to opossum. *J. Physiol.* 587: 2775–2782. [29]

Mladinic, M., Wintzer, M., Casseler, C., et al. 2005. Differential expression of genes at stages when regeneration can and cannot occur after injury to immature mammalian spinal cord. *Cell. Mol. Neurobiol.* 25: 405–424. [29]

Mochida, S., Few, A. P., Scheuer, T., and Catterall, W. A. 2008. Regulation of presynaptic Ca$_V$2.1 channels by Ca^{2+} sensor proteins mediates short-term synaptic plasticity. *Neuron* 57: 210–216. [16]

Modney, B. K., Sahley, C. L., and Muller, K. J. 1997. Regeneration of a central synapse restores nonassociative learning. *J. Neurosci.* 17: 6478–6482. [20]

Moeller, F. G., Dougherty, D. M., Swann, A. C., et al. 1996. Tryptophan depletion and aggressive responding in healthy males. *Psychopharmacology (Berl)* 126: 96–103. [15]

Moens, C. B., and Prince, V. E. 2002. Constructing the hindbrain: Insights from the zebrafish. *Dev. Dyn.* 224: 1–17. [27]

Möhler, H. 2006. GABA(A) receptor diversity and pharmacology. *Cell Tissue Res.* 326: 505–516. [14]

Moiseff, A. 1989. Bi-coordinate sound localization by the barn owl. *J. Comp. Physiol. A* 164: 637–644. [28]

Moller, A. R. 2006. History of cochlear implants and auditory brainstem implants. *Adv. Otorhinolaryngol.* 64: 1–10. [28]

Mombaerts, P., Wang, F., Dulac, C., et al. 1996. Visualizing an olfactory sensory map. *Cell* 87: 675–686. [21]

Mongillo, G., et al. 2017. Intrinsic volatility of synaptic connections - a challenge to the synaptic trace theory of memory. *Curr. Op. Neurobiol.* 46: 7–13. [17]

Montal, M. O., Iwamoto, T., Tomich, J. M., and Montal, M. 1993. Design, synthesis, and functional characterization of a pentameric channel protein that mimics the presumed pore structure of the nicotinic cholinergic receptor. *FEBS Lett.* 320: 261–266. [5]

Montell, C. and Rubin, G. M. 1989 Molecular characterization of the *Drosophila trp* locus: A putative integral membrane protein required for phototransduction, *Neuron* 2:1313–1323. [5]

Montero, M., Brini, M., Marsault, R., et al. 1995. Monitoring dynamic changes in free Ca^{2+} concentration in the endoplasmic reticulum of intact cells. *EMBO J.* 14: 5467–5475. [12]

Monyer, H., Burnashev, N., Laurie, D. J., et al. 1994. Developmental and regional expression in the rat brain and functional properties of four NMDA receptors. *Neuron* 12: 529–540. [11]

Mooney, R. 2009. Neurobiology of song learning. *Curr. Opin. Neurobiol.* 19: 654–660. [28]

Moore, D. L., Blackmore, M. G., Hu, Y., et al. 2009. KLF family members regulate intrinsic axon regeneration ability. *Science* 326: 298–301. [29]

Moore, M. J., and Caspary, D. M. 1983. Strychnine blocks binaural inhibition in lateral superior olivary neurons. *J. Neurosci.* 3: 237–242. [24]

Moos, F. et al. 1989. Release of oxytocin within the supraoptic nucleus during the milk ejection reflex in rats. *Exp. Brain Res.* 76: 593–602. [18]

Moransard, M., Borges, L. S., Willmann, R., et al. 2003. Agrin regulates rapsyn interaction with surface acetylcholine receptors, and this underlies cytoskeletal anchoring and clustering. *J. Biol. Chem.* 278: 7350–7359. [29]

Moreno-Jimenez, E. P., et al. 2019. Adult hippocampal neurogenesis is abundant in neurologically healthy subjects and drops sharply in patients with Alzheimer's disease. *Nat. Med.* 25: 55. [27]

Moreno-Manzano, V. 2019. Ependymal cells in the spinal cord as neuronal progenitors. *Curr. Opin. Pharmacol.* 50: 82–87. [18]

Morgans, C. W., El Far, O., Berntson, A., et al. 1998. Calcium extrusion from mammalian photoreceptor terminals. *J. Neurosci.* 18: 2467–2474. [22]

Morishita, H., Miwa, J. M., Heintz, N., and Hensch, T. K. 2010. Lynx1, a cholinergic brake, limits plasticity in adult visual cortex. *Science* 330: 1238–1240. [28]

Morita, K., and Barrett, E. F. 1990. Evidence for two calcium-dependent potassium conductances in lizard motor nerve terminals. *J. Neurosci.* 10: 2614–2625. [13]

Morris, J. F., and Ludwig, M. 2004. Magnocellular dendrites: Prototypic Receiver/Transmitters. *J. Neuroendocrinol.* 16: 403–408. doi: 10.1111/j.0953-8194.2004.01182.x. [18]

Morrison, A. D. 1998. 1 + 1 = r4 and much much more. *Bioessays* 20: 794–797. [27]

Mörschel, M., and Dutschmann, M. 2009. Pontine respiratory activity involved in inspiratory/expiratory phase transition. *Philos. Trans. R. Soc. Lond., B, Biol. Sci.* 364: 2517–2526. [26]

Morton, N. E. 1991. Genetic epidemiology of hearing impairment. *Ann. N Y Acad. Sci.* 630: 16–31. [28]

Moser, E. I., Krobert, K. A., Moser, M.-B., and Morris, R. G. M. 1998. Impaired spatial learning after saturation of long-term potentiation. *Science* 281: 2038–2042. [16]

Moser, E., Moser, M., and Andersen, P. 1993. Spatial learning impairment parallels the magnitude of dorsal hippocampal lesions, but is hardly present following ventral lesions. *J. Neurosci.* 13: 3916–3925. [16]

Mosko, S. S., and Jacobs, B. L. 1974. Midbrain raphe neurons: Spontaneous activity and response to light. *Physiol. Behav.* 13: 589–593. [18]

Moss, S. J., and Smart, T. G. 2001. Constructing inhibitory synapses. *Nat. Rev. Neurosci.* 2: 240–250. [11]

Moulton, E. A., Pendse, G., Morris, S., et al. 2009. Segmentally arranged somatotopy within the face representation of human primary somatosensory cortex. *Hum. Brain Mapp.* 30: 757–765. [23]

Mountcastle, V. B. 1957. Modality and topographic properties of single neurons of cat's somatic sensory cortex. *J. Neurophysiol.* 20: 408–434. [3]

Mudge, A. W., Leeman, S. E., and Fischbach, G. D. 1979. Enkephalin inhibits release of substance P from sensory neurons in culture and decreases action potential duration. *Proc. Natl. Acad. Sci. USA* 76: 526–530. [14]

Mufson, E. J., Ginsberg, S. D., Ikonomovic, M. D., and DeKosky, S. T. 2003. Human cholinergic basal forebrain: Chemoanatomy and neurologic dysfunction. *J. Chem. Neuroanat.* 26: 233–242. [27]

Mulkey, R. M., and Malenka, R. C. 1992. Mechanisms underlying induction of homosynaptic long-term depression in area CA1 of the hippocampus. *Neuron* 9: 967–975. [16]

Muller, D., Joly, M., and Lynch, G. 1988. Contributions of quisqualate and NMDA receptors to the induction and expression of LTP. *Science* 242: 1694–1697. [16]

Muller, K. J. 1973. Photoreceptors in the crayfish compound eye: Electrical interactions between cells as related to polarized-light sensitivity. *J. Physiol.* 232: 573–595. [20]

Muller, K. J. 1981. Synapses and synaptic transmission. In K. J. Muller, J. G. Nicholls, and G. S. Stent (Eds.), *Neurobiology of the Leech*. Cold Spring Harbor Laboratory, Cold Spring Harbor, NY, pp. 79–111. [20]

Muller, K. J., and Carbonetto, S. 1979. The morphological and physiological properties of a regenerating synapse in the C. N. S. of the leech. *J. Comp. Neurol.* 185: 485–516. [20]

Muller, K. J., and McMahan, U. J. 1976. The shapes of sensory and motor neurones and the distribution of their synapses in ganglia of the leech: A study using intracellular injection of horseradish peroxidase. *Proc. R. Soc. Lond., B, Biol. Sci.* 194: 481–499. [20]

Muller, K. J., and Nicholls, J. G. 1974. Different properties of synapses between a single sensory neurone and two different motor cells in the leech CNS. *J. Physiol.* 238: 357–369. [20]

Muller, K. J., Nicholls, J. G., and Stent, G. S. (Eds.). 1981. *Neurobiology of the Leech.* Cold Spring Harbor Laboratory, Cold Spring Harbor, NY. [20]

Muller, K. J., Tsechpenakis, G., Homma, R., Nicholls, J. G., Cohen, L. B., and Eugenin, J. 2009. Optical analysis of circuitry for respiratory rhythm in isolated brainstem of foetal mice. *Philos. Trans. R. Soc. Lond., B, Biol. Sci.* 364: 2485–2491. [20]

Müller, M., and Schlue, W. R. 1998. Macroscopic and single-channel chloride currents in neuropile glial cells of the leech central nervous system. *Brain Res.* 781: 307–19. [10]

Müller, M., and Wehner, R. 1994. The hidden spiral: Systematic search and path integration in desert ants, *Cataglyphis fortis. J. Comp. Physiol. A* 175: 525–530. [20]

Müller, M., and Wehner, R. 2007. Wind and sky as compass cues in desert ant navigation. *Naturwissenschaften* 94: 589–594. [20]

Müller, M., and Wehner, R. 2010. Path integration provides a scaffold for landmark learning in desert ants. *Curr. Biol.* 20: 1368–1371. [20]

Mullins, L. J. 1975. Ion selectivity of carriers and channels. *J. Biophys.* 15: 921–931. [5]

Mullins, L. J., and Noda, K. 1963. The influence of sodium-free solutions on membrane potential of frog muscle fibers. *J. Gen. Physiol.* 47: 117–132. [6]

Mullins, O. J., and Friesen, W. O. 2012. The brain matters: Effects of descending signals on motor control. *J. Neurophysiol.* 107: 2730–2741. [20]

Munch, T. A., and Werblin, F. S. 2006. Symmetric interactions within a homogeneous starburst cell network can lead to robust asymmetries in dendrites of starburst amacrine cells. *J. Neurophysiol.* 96: 471–477. [22]

Munk, H. 1881. *Ueber die Functionen der Grosshirnrinde; gesammelte Mittheilungen aus den Jahren 1877–80.* Hirschwald, Berlin. [25]

Murashima, M., and Hirano, T. 1999. Entire course and distinct phases of day-lasting depression of miniature EPSC amplitudes in cultured Purkinje neurons. *J. Neurosci.* 19: 7326–7333. [16]

Murphy, P. C., and Sillitoe, A. M. 1991. Cholinergic enhancement of direction sensitivity in the visual cortex of the cat. *Neuroscience* 40: 13–20. [14]

Nabavi et al. 2014. Engineering a memory with LTD and LTP. *Nature* 511: 348. [17]

Nadella, K. M., Roš, H., Baragli, C., et al. 2016. Random-access scanning microscopy for 3D imaging in awake behaving animals. *Nat. Meth.* 13: 1001–1004. [30]

Nader, K. 2015. Reconsolidation and the dynamic nature of memory. *Cold Spring Harb. Perspect. Biol.* 7: a021782. [17]

Nader, K., et al. 2000. Fear memories require protein synthesis in the amygdala for reconsolidation after retrieval. *Nature* 406: 722–726. [17]

Nagatsu, T. 1995. Tyrosine hydroxylase: Human isoforms, structure and regulation in physiology and pathology. *Essays Biochem.* 30: 15–35. [15]

Nagatsu, T., and Ichinose, H. 1999. Regulation of pteridine-requiring enzymes by the cofactor tetrahydrobiopterin. *Mol. Neurobiol.* 19: 79–96. [15]

Nagel, G., Ollig, D., Fuhrmann, M., et al. 2002. Channelrhodopsin-1: A light-gated proton channel in green algae *Science* 296: 2395–2398. [1]

Nagelhus, E. A., and Ottersen, O. P. 2013. Physiological roles of aquaporin-4 in brain. *Physiol. Rev.* 93:1543–1562. doi:10.1152/physrev.00011.2013. [10]

Nagerl, U. V., et al. 2004. Bidirectional activity-dependent morphological plasticity in hippocampal neurons. *Neuron* 44: 759–767. [17]

Nakajima, S., and Onodera, K. 1969. Adaptation of the generator potential in the crayfish stretch receptors under constant length and constant tension. *J. Physiol.* 200: 187–204. [21]

Nakajima, S., and Onodera, K. 1969. Membrane properties of the stretch receptor neurones of crayfish with particular reference to mechanisms of sensory adaptation. *J. Physiol.* 200: 161–185. [21]

Nakajima, S., and Takahashi, K. 1966. Post-tetanic hyperpolarization and electrogenic Na pump in stretch receptor neurone of crayfish. *J. Physiol.* 187: 105–127. [21]

Nakajima, Y., Tisdale, A. D., and Henkart, M. P. 1973. Presynaptic inhibition at inhibitory nerve terminals: A new synapse in the crayfish stretch receptor. *Proc. Natl. Acad. Sci. USA* 70: 2462–2466. [11]

Nakamura, T., and Gold, G. H. 1987. A cyclic nucleotide-gated conductance in olfactory receptor cilia. *Nature* 325: 442–444. [21]

Nakamura, T., et al. 1999. Synaptically activated Ca^{2+} release from internal stores in CNS neurons. *Neuron* 24: 727–737. [17]

Nakanishi, S., Nakajima, Y., Masu, M., et al. 1998. Glutamate receptors: Brain function and signal transduction. *Brain Res. Brain Res. Rev.* 26: 230–235. [22]

Nakano, T., Ando, S., Takata, N., et al. 2012. Self-formation of optic cups and storable stratified neural retina from human ESCs. *Cell Stem Cell* 10: 771–785. [1, 27]

Namer, B., and Handwerker, H. O. 2009. Translational nociceptor research as guide to human pain perceptions and pathophysiology. *Exp. Brain Res.* 196: 163–172. [23]

Nargeot, J., Nerbonne, J. M., Engels, J., and Lester, H. A. 1983. Time course of the increase in the myocardial slow inward current after a photochemically generated concentration jump of intracellular cAMP. *Proc. Natl. Acad. Sci. USA* 80: 2385–2399. [12]

Nastuk, W. L. 1953. Membrane potential changes at a single muscle endplate produced by transitory application of acetylcholine with an electrically controlled microjet. *Fed. Proc.* 12: 102. [11]

Nathans, J. 1987. Molecular biology of visual pigments. *Annu. Rev. Neurosci.* 10: 163–194. [22]

Nathans, J. 1989. The genes for color vision. *Sci. Am.* 260: 42–49. [22]

Nathans, J. 1999. The evolution and physiology of human color vision: Insights from molecular genetic studies of visual pigments. *Neuron* 24: 299–312. [22]

Nathans, J., and Hogness, D. S. 1984. Isolation and nucleotide sequence of the gene encoding human rhodopsin. *Proc. Natl. Acad. Sci. USA* 81: 4851–4855. [22]

Nathans, J., Piantanida, T. P., Eddy, R. L., et al. 1986. Molecular genetics of inherited variation in human color vision. *Science* 232: 203–210. doi:10.1126/science.3485310. [22]

Navaratnam, D. S., Bell, T. J., Tu, T. D., et al. 1997. Differential distribution of Ca^{2+}-activated K^+ channel splice variants among hair cells along the tonotopic axis of the chick cochlea. *Neuron* 19: 1077–1085. [24]

Navarrete, M., and Araque, A. 2010. Endocannabinoids potentiate synaptic transmission through stimulation of astrocytes. *Neuron* 68: 113–126. [12]

Nave, K. A., and Trapp, B. D. 2008. Axon-glial signaling and the glial support of axon function. *Annu. Rev. Neurosci.* 31: 535–561. [10]

Naya, Y., Sakai, K., and Miyashita, Y. 1996. Activity of primate inferotemporal neurons related to a sought target in pair-association task. *Proc. Natl. Acad. Sci. USA* 93: 2664–2669. [25]

Naya, Y., Yoshida, M., and Miyashita, Y. 2001. Backward spreading of memory-retrieval signal in the primate temporal cortex. *Science* 291: 661–664. [25]

Neher, E., and Augustine, G. J. 1992. Calcium gradients and buffers in bovine chromaffin cells. *J. Physiol.* 450: 273–301. [12]

Neher, E., and Sakaba, T. 2008. Multiple roles of calcium ions in the regulation of neurotransmitter release. *Neuron* 59: 861–872. [16]

Neher, E., and Sakmann, B. 1976. Single channel currents recorded from membrane of denervated frog muscle fibres. *Nature* 260: 799–802. [11]

Neher, E., Sakmann, B., and Steinbach, J. H. 1978. The extracellular patch clamp: A method for resolving currents through individual open channels in biological membranes. *Pflügers Arch.* 375: 219–228. [4]

Neil, E. 1954. Reflexogenic areas of the circulation. *Arch. Middlesex Hosp.* 4: 16. (Modified from Berne, M., and Levy, M. N. 1990. *Principles of Physiology.* Wolfe, London.) [19]

Nelken, I. 2004. Processing of complex stimuli and natural scenes in the auditory cortex. *Curr. Opin. Neurobiol.* 14: 474–480. [24]

Nelken, I., and Bar-Yosef, O. 2008. Neurons and objects: The case of auditory cortex. *Front. Neurosci.* 2: 107–113. [24]

Nelken, I., Rotman, Y., and Bar Yosef, O. 1999. Responses of auditory-cortex neurons to structural features of natural sounds. *Nature* 397: 154–157. [24]

Nelson, C. A., 3rd, Zeanah, C. H., Fox, N. A., et al. 2007. Cognitive recovery in socially deprived young children: The Bucharest Early Intervention Project. *Science.* 318: 1937–1940. [28]

Nelson, N., and Lill, H. 1994. Porters and neurotransmitter transporters. *J. Exp. Biol.* 196: 213–228. [9]

Nestler, E. J., et al. 2016. Epigenetic basis of mental illness. *Neuroscientist* 22: 447–463. [17]

Neves, G., et al. 2008. Synaptic plasticity, memory and the hippocampus: a neural network approach to causality. *Nat. Rev. Neurosci.* 9: 65–75. [17]

Newman, E. A. 1986. High potassium conductance in astrocyte endfeet. *Science* 275: 844–847. [10]

Newman, E. A. 1987. Distribution of potassium conductance in mammalian Müller (glial) cells: A comparative study. *J. Neurosci.* 7: 2423–2432. [10]

Newman, E. A. 2003. Glial cell inhibition of neurons by release of ATP. *J. Neurosci.* 23: 1659–1666. [10]

Newman, E. A. 2004. A dialogue between glia and neurons in the retina: Modulation of neuronal excitability. *Neuron Glia Biol.* 1: 245–252. [10]

Newman, E. A. 2013. Functional hyperemia and mechanisms of neurovascular coupling in the retinal vasculature. *J. Cereb. Blood Flow Metab.* 33:1685–1695. [18]

Newman, E. A. 2015. Glial cell regulation of neuronal activity and blood flow in the retina by release of gliotransmitters. *Philos. Trans. R. Soc. Lond. B Biol. Sci.* 370: 20140195. [18]

Newsome, W. T., and Pare, E. B. 1988. A selective impairment of motion perception following lesions of the middle temporal visual area (MT). *J. Neurosci.* 8: 2201–2211. [25]

Newsome, W. T., and Wurtz, R. H. 1988. Probing visual cortical function with discrete chemical lesions. *Trends Neurosci.* 11: 394–400. [25]

Nguyen, M. D., Mushynski, W. E., and Julien, J. P. 2002. Cycling at the interface between neurodevelopment and neurodegeneration. *Cell Death Differ.* 9: 1294–1306. [27]

Nguyen, P. V., et al. 1994. Requirement of a critical period of transcription for induction of a late phase of LTP. *Science* 264: 1104–1107. [17]

Nguyen, T. et al. 2001. Intracellular pathways regulating ciliary beating of rat brain ependymal cells. *J. Physiol.* 531: 131–140. [18]

Nicholls, C. G., and Lopatin, A. N. 1997. Inward rectifier potassium channels. *Annu. Rev. Physiol.* 59: 171–191. [5]

Nicholls, J. G. 2007. How acetylcholine gives rise to current at the motor end-plate. *J. Physiol.* 578: 621–622. [11]

Nicholls, J. G., and Baylor, D. A. 1968. Specific modalities and receptive fields of sensory neurons in the CNS of the leech. *J. Neurophysiol.* 31: 740–756. [6, 20]

Nicholls, J. G., and Purves, D. 1972. A comparison of chemical and electrical synaptic transmission between single sensory cells and a motoneurone in the central nervous system of the leech. *J. Physiol.* 225: 637–656. [11, 20]

Nicholls, J. G., and Saunders, N. 1996. Regeneration of immature mammalian spinal cord after injury. *Trends Neurosci.* 19: 229–234. [29]

Nicholls, J. G., and Van Essen, D. 1974. The nervous system of the leech. *Sci Am.* 230: 38–48. [20]

Nicholls, J. G., and Wallace, B. G. 1978. Modulation of transmission at an inhibitory synapse in the central nervous system of the leech. *J. Physiol.* 281: 157–170. [11]

Nicholls, J. G., Stewart, R. R., Erulkar, S. D., and Saunders, N. R. 1990. Reflexes, fictive respiration, and cell division in the brain and spinal cord of the newborn opossum, *Monodelphis domestica*, isolated and maintained *in vitro. J. Exp. Biol.* 152: 1–15. [26]

Nicola, S. M., Surmeier, D. J., and Malenka, R. C. 2000. Dopaminergic modulation of neuronal excitability in the striatum and nucleus accumbens. *Annu. Rev. Neurosci.* 23: 185–215. [14]

Nikolaienko, O., et al. 2017. Arc protein: a flexible hub for synaptic plasticity and cognition. *Semin. Cell Dev. Biol.* doi: 10.1016/j.semcdb.2017.09.006. [17]

Nicoll, R. A. 1985. The septo-hippocampal projection: A model cholinergic pathway. *Trends Neurosci.* 8: 533–536. [14]

Nicoll, R. A. 2004. My close encounters with GABA$_B$ receptors. *Biochem. Pharmacol.* 68: 1667–1674. [14]

Nicoll, R. A., and Schmitz, D. 2005. Synaptic plasticity at hippocampal mossy fibre synapses. *Nat. Rev. Neurosci.* 6: 863–876. [16]

Nicoll, R. A., Eccles, J. C., Oshima, T., and Rubia, F. 1975. Prolongation of hippocampal inhibitory postsynaptic potentials by barbiturates. *Nature* 258: 625–627. [14]

Nicoll, R. A., Tomita, S., and Bredt, D. S. 2006. Auxiliary subunits assist AMPA-type glutamate receptors. *Science* 311: 1253–1256. [14]

NIDCD. 2016. NIDCD Fact Sheet: *Cochlear Implants.* National Institute on Deafness and Other Communication Disorders. Publication No. 00–4798. (www.nidcd.nih.gov/sites/default/files/Documents/health/hearing/CochlearImplants.pdf) [28]

Niell, C. M. 2015. Cell types, circuits, and receptive fields in the mouse visual cortex. *Annu. Rev. Neurosci.* 38: 413–431. doi: 10.1146/annurev-neuro-071714-033807. [3]

Nielsen, J. B., and Sinkjaer, T. 2002. Afferent feedback in the control of human gait. *J. Electromyogr. Kinesiol.* 12: 213–217. [26]

Nielsen, S., Nagelhus, E. A., Amiry-Moghaddam, M., et al. 1997. Specialized membrane domains for water transport in glial cells: High-resolution immunogold cytochemistry of aquaporin-4 in rat brain. *J. Neurosci.* 17: 171–180. doi:10.1523/JNEUROSCI.17-01-00171.1997. [10]

Niesler, B., Frank, B., Kapeller, J., and Rappold, G. A. 2003. Cloning, physical mapping and expression analysis of the human 5-HT$_3$ serotonin receptor-like genes *HTR3C*, *HTR3D* and *HTR3E*. *Gene* 310: 101–111. [5]

Nikbakht, N., Tafreshiha, A., Zoccolan, D., and Diamond, M. E. 2018 Supralinear and supramodal integration of visual and tactile signals in rats: Psychophysics and neuronal mechanisms. *Neuron* 97: 626–639. e8. [25]

Nikolaienko, O., et al. 2017. Arc protein: A flexible hub for synaptic plasticity and cognition. *Semin. Cell Dev. Biol.* doi: 10.1016/j.semcdb.2017.09.006. [17]

Nikolopoulou, E., et al. 2017. Neural tube closure: Cellular, molecular and biomechanical mechanisms. *Development* 144: 552–566. [27]

Nilius, B., and Voets, T. 2005. TRP Channels: A TR(I)P through the world of multifunctional cation channels. *Pflügers Arch.* 451: 1–10. [5]

Nimigean, C. M., Chappie, J. S., and Miller, C. 2003. Electrostatic tuning of ion conductance in potassium channels. *Biochemistry* 42: 9263–9268. [5]

Nimmerjahn, A., Kirchhoff, F., and Helmchen.F. 2005. Resting microglial cells are highly dynamic surveillants of brain parenchyma in vivo. *Science* 308: 1314–1318. doi: 10.1126/science.1110647. [10]

Niparko, J. K., and Marlowe, A. 2010. Hearing aids and cochlear implants. In P. A. Fuchs (Ed.), *The Oxford University Handbook of Auditory Science: The Ear.* Oxford University Press, New York, pp. 409–436. [28]

Niparko, J. K., Tobey, E. A., Thal, D. J., et al. 2010. Spoken language development in children following cochlear implantation. *JAMA* 303: 1498–1506. [24]

Nirenberg et al., 1996. The dopamine transporter is localized to dendritic and axonal plasma membranes of nigrostriatal dopaminergic neurons. *J. Neurosci.* 16: 436–447. [18]

Nirenberg, M. J. et al. 1996. Ultrastructural localization of the vesicular monoamine transporter-2 in midbrain dopaminergic neurons: Potential sites for somatodendritic storage and release of dopamine. *J. Neurosci.* 16: 4135–4145. [18]

Nishiyama, A., Boshans, L., Goncalves, C. M., et al. 2016. Lineage, fate, and fate potential of NG2-glia. *Brain Res.* 1638: 116–128. doi: 10.1016/j.brainres.2015.08.013. Epub 2015 Aug 21. [10]

Niswender, C., and Conn, P. J. 2010. Metabotropic glutamate receptors: Physiology, pharmacology, and disease. *Annu. Rev. Pharmacol. Toxicol.* 50: 295–322. [14]

Nja, A., and Purves, D. 1978. The effects of nerve growth factor and its antiserum on synapses in the superior cervical ganglion of the guinea-pig. *J. Physiol.* 277: 55–75. [29]

Noakes, P. G., Gautam, M., Mudd, J., et al. 1995. Aberrant differentiation of neuromuscular junctions in mice lacking s-laminin/laminin β2. *Nature* 374: 258–262. [29]

Noctor, S. C., Flint, A. C., Weissman, T. A., et al. 2001. Neurons derived from radial glial cells establish radial units in neocortex. *Nature* 409: 714–720. [27]

Noda, M., Shimizu, S., Tanabe, T., et al. 1984. Primary structure of *Electrophorus electricus* sodium channel deduced from cDNA sequence. *Nature* 312: 121–127. [5]

Noda, M., Suzuki, H., Numa, S. and Stühmer, W. 1989. A single point mutation confers tetrodotoxin and saxitoxin insensitivity on sodium channel II. *FEBS Lett.* 259: 213–216. [5]

Noda, M., Takahashi, H., Tanabe, T., et al. 1982. Primary structure of α-subunit precursor of *Torpedo californica* acetylcholine receptor deduced from cDNA sequence. *Nature* 299: 793–797. [5]

Noda, M., Takahashi, H., Tanabe, T., et al. 1983. Primary structure of β- and δ-subunit precursors of *Torpedo californica* acetylcholine receptor deduced from cDNA sequences. *Nature* 301: 251–255. [5]

Noda, M., Takahashi, H., Tanabe, T., et al. 1983. Structural homology of *Torpedo californica* acetylcholine receptor subunits. *Nature* 302: 528–532. [5]

Noguez, P., Rubí, J. M., and De-Miguel, F. F. 2019. Thermodynamic efficiency of somatic exocytosis of serotonin. *Front Physiol.* 10: 473. [18]

Nolte, J. 1988. *The Human Brain*, 2nd ed. Mosby, St. Louis, Mo. [27]

Nomura, A., Shigemoto, R., Nakamura, Y., et al. 1994. Developmentally regulated postsynaptic localization of a metabotropic glutamate receptor in rat rod bipolar cells. *Cell* 77: 361–369. [22]

North, R. A. 2002. Molecular physiology of P2X receptors. *Physiol. Rev.* 82: 1013–1067. [14]

North, R. A., Williams, J. T., Surprenant, A., and Christie, M. J. 1987. μ and δ receptors belong to a family of receptors that are coupled to potassium channels. *Proc. Natl. Acad. Sci. USA* 84: 5487–5491. [12]

Nottebohm, F. 1989. From bird song to neurogenesis. *Sci. Am.* 260: 74–79. [27]

Notterpek, L., Shooter, E. M., and Snipes, G. J. 1997. Up-regulation of the endosomal-lysosomal pathway in the trembler. *J. Neurosci.* 17: 4190–4200. [10]

Nowak, L., Bregestovski, P., Ascher, P., et al. 1984. Magnesium gates glutamate-activated channels in mouse central neurones. *Nature* 307: 462–465. [11, 16]

Numa, S., Noda, M., Takahashi, H., et al. 1983. Molecular structure of the nicotinic acetylcholine receptor. *Cold Spring Harb. Symp. Quant. Biol.* 48: 57–69. [5]

Numano, R., Yamazaki, S., Umeda, N., et al. 2006. Constitutive expression of the *Period1* gene impairs behavioral and molecular circadian rhythms. *Proc. Natl. Acad. Sci. USA* 103: 3716–3721. [19]

Nusbaum, M. P., Blitz, D. M., and Marder, E. 2017. Functional consequences of neuropeptide and small-molecule co-transmission. *Nat. Rev. Neurosci.* 18: 389–403. [18]

Nusslein-Volhard, C. 2012. The zebrafish issue of Development. *Development* 139: 4099–4103. [27]

Nykjaer, A., et al. 2004. Sortilin is essential for proNGF-induced neuronal cell death. *Nature* 427: 843–848. [27]

O'Connor, R., and Tessier-Lavigne, M. 1999. Identification of maxillary factor, a maxillary process-derived chemoattractant for developing trigeminal sensory axons. *Neuron* 24, 165–178. [27]

O'Craven, K. M., Downing, P. E., and Kanwisher, N. 1999. fMRI evidence for objects as the units of attentional selection. *Nature* 401: 584–587. [25]

O'Donnell, P., and Grace, A. A. 1993. Dopaminergic modulation of dye coupling between neurons in the core and shell regions of the nucleus accumbens. *J. Neurosci.* 13: 3456–3471. [11]

O'Malley, J., Moore, C. T., and Salpeter, M. M. 1997. Stabilization of acetylcholine receptors by exogenous ATP and its reversal by cAMP and calcium. *J. Cell Biol.* 138: 159–165. [29]

O'Rourke, N. A., Sullivan, D. P., Kaznowski, C. E.,et al. 1995. Tangential migration of neurons in the developing cerebral cortex. *Development* 121: 2165–2176. [27]

O'Sullivan, B. P., and Freedman, S. D. 2009. Cystic fibrosis. *Lancet* 373: 1891–1904. [30]

Obaid, A. L., Nelson, M. E., Lindstrom, J., and Salzberg, B. M. 2005. Optical studies of nicotinic acetylcholine receptor subtypes in the guinea-pig enteric nervous system. *J. Exp. Biol.* 208: 2891–3001. [19]

Obata, K., Ito, M., Ochi, R., and Sato, N. 1967. Pharmacological properties of the postsynaptic inhibition by Purkinje cell axons and the action of gamma-aminobutyric acid on Deiters NEURONES. *Exp. Brain Res.* 4: 43–57. [14]

Ochoa, J., and Torebjork, E. 1983. Sensations evoked by intraneural microstimulation of single mechanoreceptor units innervating the human hand. *J. Physiol.* 342: 633–654. [23]

Ochoa, J., and Torebjork, E. 1989. Sensations evoked by intraneural microstimulation of C nociceptor fibres in human skin nerves. *J. Physiol.* 415: 583–599. [23]

Odette, L. L., and Newman, E. A. 1988. Model of potassium dynamics in the central nervous system. *Glia* 1: 198–210. [10]

Ohata, S., and Alvarez-Buylla, A. 2016. Planar organization of multiciliated ependymal (E1) cells in the brain ventricular epithelium. *Trends Neurosci.* 39: 543–551. [18]

Oheim, M., and Stühmer, W. 2000. Tracking chromaffin granules on their way through the actin cortex. *Eur. Biophys. J.* 29: 67–89. doi: 10.1007/s002490050253. [18]

Oheim, M., Kirchhoff, F., and Stühmer, W. 2006 Calcium microdomains in regulated exocytosis. *Cell Calcium* 40: 423–439. [10, 12]

Ohki, K., Chung, S., Ch'ng, Y. H., et al. 2005. Functional imaging with cellular resolution reveals precise micro-architecture in visual cortex. *Nature* 433: 597–603. [3]

Ohki, K., Chung, S., Kara, P., et al. 2006. Highly ordered arrangement of single neurons in orientation pinwheels. *Nature* 442: 925–928. [3]

Ohmori, H. 1985. Mechano-electrical transduction currents in isolated vestibular hair cells of the chick. *J. Physiol.* 359: 189–217. [21]

Ohno-Shosaku, T., Maejima, T., and Kano, A. 2001 Endogenous cannabinoids mediate retrograde signals from depolarized postsynaptic neurons to presynaptic terminals. *Neuron* 29: 729–738. [12]

Okada, K., Inoue, A., Okada, M., et al. 2006. The muscle protein Dok-7 is essential for neuromuscular synaptogenesis. *Science* 312: 1802–1805. [29]

Okada, Y., Miyamoto, T., and Sato, T. 1994. Activation of a cation conductance by acetic acid in taste cells isolated from the bullfrog. *J. Exp. Biol.* 187: 19–32. [21]

Okano, H., and Yamanaka, S. 2014. iPS cell technologies: Significance and applications to CNS regeneration and disease. *Mol. Brain.* 7: 22. [29]

Okano, T., Kojima, D., Fukada, Y., et al. 1992. Primary structures of chicken cone visual pigments: Vertebrate rhodopsins have evolved out of cone visual pigments. *Proc. Natl. Acad. Sci. USA* 89: 5932–5936. [22]

Okita, K., Ichisaka, T., and Yamanaka, S. 2007. Generation of germline-competent induced pluripotent stem cells. *Nature* 448: 313–317. [27]

Okuno, H., et al. 2012. Inverse synaptic tagging of inactive synapses via dynamic interaction of Arc/Arg3.1 with CaMKIIβ *Cell* 149: 886–898. [17]

Okuno, H., Minatohara, K., and Bito, H. 2018. Inverse synaptic tagging: An inactive synapse-specific mechanism to capture activity-induced Arc/arg3.1 and to locally regulate spatial distribution of synaptic weights. *Sem. Cell Dev. Biol.* 77: 43–50. [17]

Oldham, W. H., and Hamm, H. E. 2008. Heterotrimeric G protein activation by G-protein-coupled receptors. *Nat. Rev. Mol. Cell. Biol.* 459: 356–363. [12]

Oliet, S., Malenka, R. C., and Nicoll, R. A. 1996. Bidirectional control of quantal size by synaptic activity in the hippocampus. *Science* 271: 1294–1297. [16]

Oliver, D., Klöcker, N., Schuck, J., et al. 2000. Gating of Ca^{2+}-activated K$^+$ channels controls fast inhibitory synaptic transmission at auditory outer hair cells. *Neuron* 26: 595–601. [12]

Olivera, B. M., Miljanich, G. P., Ramachandran, J., and Adams, M. E. 1994. Calcium channel diversity and neurotransmitter release: The omega-conotoxins and omega-agatoxins. *Annu. Rev. Biochem.* 63: 823–867. [12]

Olsen, R. W., and Sieghart, W. 2008. International Union of Pharmacology. LXX. Subtypes of γ-aminobutyric acid$_A$ receptors: Classification on the basis of subunit composition, pharmacology, and function. Update. *Pharmacol. Rev.* 60: 243–260. [14]

Olsen, R. W., and Sieghart, W. 2009. GABAA receptors: Subtypes provide diversity of function and pharmacology. *Neuropharmacology* 56: 141–148. [5]

Olveczky, B. P., Baccus, S. A., and Meister, M. 2007. Retinal adaptation to object motion. *Neuron* 56: 689–700. [22]

Oray, S., Majewska, A., and Sur, M. 2004. Dendritic spine dynamics are regulated by monocular deprivation and extracellular matrix degradation. *Neuron* 44: 1021–1030. [28]

Orban, G. A., Van Essen, D., and Vanduffel, W. 2004. Comparative mapping of higher visual areas in monkeys and humans. *Trends. Cogn. Sci.* 8: 315–324. [3]

Orkand, R. K., Nicholls, J. G., and Kuffler, S. W. 1966. Effect of nerve impulses on the membrane potential of glial cells in the central nervous system of amphibia. *J. Neurophysiol.* 29: 788–806. [10]

O'Shea, T. M., Burda, J. E., and Sofroniew, M. V. 2017. Cell Biology of spinal cord injury and repair. *J. Clin. Investig.* 127: 3259–3270. [29]

Oshima, A., Matsuzawa., T., Murata, K., et al. 2016. Hexadecameric structure of an invertebrate gap junction channel . *J. Mol. Biol.* 428: 1227–1236. [11]

Osterberg, G. 1935. Topography of the layer of rods and cones in the human retina. *Acta Ophthalmologica Supplement* 6: 1–103. [22]

Ostroff, L. E., et al. 2002. Polyribosomes redistribute from dendritic shafts into spines with enlarged synapses during LTP in developing rat hippocampal slices. *Neuron.* 35: 535–545. [17]

Otsuka, M., and Yoshioka, K. 1993. Neurotransmitter functions of mammalian tachykinins. *Physiol. Rev.* 73: 229–308. [14]

Otsuka, M., Iversen, L. L., Hall, Z. W., and Kravitz, E. A. 1966. Release of γ-aminobutyric acid from inhibitory nerves of lobster. *Proc. Natl. Acad. Sci. USA* 56: 1110–1115. [14]

Ottoson, D. 1956. Analysis of the electrical activity of the olfactory epithelium. *Acta Physiol. Scand.* 35: 1–83. [21]

Ouyang, K., Zheng, H., Qin, X., et al. Ca^{2+} sparks and secretion in dorsal root ganglion neurons. *Proc. Natl. Acad. Sci. USA* 102: 12259–12264. [12]

Oyster, C. W., and Barlow, H. B. 1967. Direction-selective units in rabbit retina: Distribution of preferred directions. *Science* 155: 841–842. [2]

Ozair, M. Z. et al 2013. Neural induction and early patterning in vertebrates. *Wiley Interdiscip. Rev. Dev. Biol.* 2: 479–498. [27]

Pack, C. C., Livingstone, M. S., Duffy, K. R., and Born, R. T. 2003. End-stopping and the aperture problem: Two-dimensional motion signals in macaque V1. *Neuron* 39: 671–680. [2]

Packard, M. et al. 2002. The *Drosophila* Wnt, wingless, provides an essential signal for pre- and postsynaptic differentiation. *Cell* 111: 319–330. [18]

Palacin, M., Estévez, R., Bertran, J., and Zorzano, A. 1998. Molecular biology of mammalian plasma membrane amino acid transporters. *Physiol. Rev.* 78: 969–1054. [9]

Palczewski, K., Kumasaka, T., Hori, T., et al. 2000. Crystal structure of rhodopsin: A G protein-coupled receptor. *Science.* 289:739–745. [22]

Palmada, M., and Centelles, J. J. 1998. Excitatory amino acid neurotransmission. Pathways for metabolism, storage and reuptake of glutamate in brain. *Front. Biosci.* 3: 701–718. [15]

Palmer, A. M. 2010. The role of the blood-CNS barrier in CNS disorders and their treatment. *Neurobiol. Dis.* 37: 3–12. [10]

Palmer, A. R., and Russell, I. J. 1986. Phase-locking in the cochlear nerve of the guinea-pig and its relation to the receptor potential of inner hair-cells. *Hear. Res.* 24: 1–15. [24]

Palmer, R. M. J., Ferrige, J., and Moncada, S. 1987. Nitric oxide release accounts for the biological activity of endothelium-derived relaxing factor. *Nature* 324: 524–526. [12]

Pandi-Perumal, S. R., Srinivasan, V., Maestroni, G. J., et al. 2006. Melatonin: Nature's most versatile biological signal? *FEBS J.* 273: 2813–2838. [19]

Pangrsic, T., Potokar, M., Stenovec, M., et al. 2007. Exocytotic release of ATP from cultured astrocytes. *J. Biol. Chem.* 282: 28749–28758. [10]

Panayotis, N., et al. 2015. Macromolecular transport in synapse to nucleus communication. *Trends Neurosci.* 38: 108–116. [17]

Pankratov, Y., Lalo, U., Verkhratsky, A., and North, R. A. 2006. Vesicular release of ATP at central synapses. *Pflügers Arch.* 452: 589–597. [14]

Pannasch, U., Vargová, L., Reingruber, J., et al. 2011. Astroglial networks scale synaptic activity and plasticity. *Proc. Natl. Acad. Sci. USA* 108: 8467–8472. doi: 10.1073/pnas.1016650108. [10]

Paolicelli, R. C., et al. 2011. Synaptic pruning by microglia is necessary for normal brain development. *Science* 333: 1456–1458. [17]

Papardia, S., and Hardingham, G. E. 2007. The dichotomy of NMDA receptor signalling. *Neuroscientist* 13: 572–579. [14]

Papazian, D. M., Timpe, L. C., Yan, Y. N., and Yan, L. Y. 1987. Cloning and complementary DNA from *Shaker,* a putative potassium channel gene from *Drosophila. Science* 237: 749–753. [5]

Papouin, T., Ladepeche, L., Ruel, J., et al. 2012. Synaptic and extrasynaptic NMDA receptors are gated by different endogenous coagonists. *Cell.* 150: 633–646. [11]

Pare, M., Smith, A. M., and Rice, F. L. 2002. Distribution and terminal arborizations of cutaneous mechanoreceptors in the glabrous finger pads of the monkey. *J. Comp. Neurol.* 445: 347–359. [23]

Pareek, S., Notterpek, L., Snipes, G. J., et al. 1997. Neurons promote the translocation of peripheral myelin protein 22 into myelin. *J. Neurosci.* 17: 7754–7762. [10]

Parekh, A. B. 2008. Ca^{2+} microdomains near plasma membrane Ca^{2+} channels: Impact on cell function. *J. Physiol.* 586: 3043–3054. [12]

Park, H. and Poo M. 2013. Neurotrophin regulation of neural circuit development and function. *Nat. Rev. Neurosci.* 14: 7–23. [17]

Park, K. K., Liu, K., Hu, Y., et al. 2008. Promoting axon regeneration in the adult CNS by modulation of the PTEN/mTOR pathway. *Science* 322: 963–966. [29]

Parkhurst et al. 2013. Microglia promote learning-dependent synapse formation through brain-derived neurotrophic factor. *Cell* 155: 1596. [17]

Parker, A. J., and Newsome, W. T. 1998. Sense and the single neuron: Probing the physiology of perception. *Annu. Rev. Neurosci.* 21: 227–277. [25]

Parnas, H., and Parnas, I. 2007. The chemical synapse goes electric: Ca^{2+}- and voltage-sensitive GPCRs control neurotransmitter release. *Trends Neurosci.* 30: 54–61. [12]

Parnas, I., and Parnas, H. 2010 Control of neurotransmitter release: From Ca^{2+} to voltage dependent G-protein coupled receptors. *Pflügers Arch.* 460: 975–990. [13]

Parsons, S. M., Prior, C., and Marshall, I. G. 1993. Acetylcholine transport, storage, and release. *Int. Rev. Neurobiol.* 35: 279–390. [15]

Paschal, B. M., and Vallee, R. B. 1987. Retrograde transport by the microtubule associated protein MAP 1C. *Nature* 330: 181–183. [15]

Pastor, J., Soria, B., and Belmonte, C. 1996. Properties of the nociceptive neurons of the leech segmental ganglion. *J. Neurophysiol.* 75: 2268–2279. [20]

Pastrana, E. 2011. Optogenetics: Controlling cell function with light. *Nat. Methods* 8: 24–25. [14]

Patapoutian, A., Peier, A. M., Story, G. M., and Viswanath, V. 2003. ThermoTRP channels and beyond: Mechanisms of temperature sensation. *Nat. Rev. Neurosci.* 4: 529–539. [21]

Paton, W.D., Vizi, E. S. 1969. The inhibitory action of noradrenaline and adrenaline on acetylcholine output by guinea-pig ileum longitudinal muscle strip. *Brit. J. Pharmacol.* 35: 10–28. [18]

Paulson, O. B., and Newman, E. A. 1987. Does the release of potassium from astrocyte endfeet regulate cerebral blood flow? *Science* 237: 896–898. [10]

Payne, J. A., Rivera, C., Voipio, J., and Kaila, K. 2003. Cation-chloride co-transporters in neuronal communication, development and trauma. Trends Neurosci. 26: 199–206. [11]

Payton, W. B. 1981. History of medicinal leeching and early medical references. In Muller, K. J., Nicholls, J. G., and Stent, G. S. (Eds.) *Neurobiology of the Leech.* Cold Spring Harbor Laboratory, Cold Spring Harbor, NY, pp. 27–34. [20]

Pearson, K. 1976. The control of walking. *Sci. Am.* 235: 72–86. [26]

Pearson, K. G. 2008. Role of sensory feedback in the control of stance duration in walking cats. *Brain Res. Rev.* 57: 222–227. [26]

Peinado, A., Juste, R., and Kayz, L. C. 1993. Extensive dye coupling between rat neocortical neurons during the period of circuit formation. *Neuron* 10: 103–114. [11]

Peirson, S. N., Halford, S., and Foster, R. G. 2009. The evolution of irradiance detection: Melanopsin and the non-visual opsins. *Philos. Trans. R. Soc. Lond., B, Biol. Sci.* 364: 2849–2865. [22]

Penfield, W. 1924. Oligodendroglia and its relation to classical neuroglia. *Brain* 47: 430–452. [10]

Penfield, W. 1932. *Cytology and Cellular Pathology of the Nervous System,* Vol. 2. Hafner, New York. [10]

Penfield, W., and Rasmussen, T. 1950. *The Cerebral Cortex of Man. A Clinical Study of Localization of Function.* Macmillan, New York. [26]

Penington, N. J., Kelly, J. S., and Fox, A. P. 1993. Whole-cell recordings of inwardly rectifying K^+ currents activated by $5\text{-}HT_{1A}$ receptors on dorsal raphe neurones of the adult rat. *J. Physiol.* 469: 387–405. [14]

Penn, A. A., Riquelme, P. A., Feller, M. B., and Shatz, C. J. 1998. Competition in retinogeniculate patterning driven by spontaneous activity. *Science* 279: 2108–2112. [28]

Penner, R., and Neher, E. 1988. The role of calcium in stimulus-secretion coupling in excitable and non-excitable cells. *J. Exp. Biol.* 139: 329–345. [13]

Penner, R., and Neher, E. 1989. The patch-clamp technique in the study of secretion. *Trends Neurosci.* 12: 159–163. [13]

Peper, K., and McMahan, U. J. 1972. Distribution of acetylcholine receptors in the vicinity of nerve terminals on skeletal muscle of the frog. *Proc. R. Soc. Lond., B, Biol. Sci.* 181: 431–440. [11]

Peper, K., Dreyer, F., Sandri, C., et al. 1974. Structure and ultrastructure of the frog motor end-plate: A freeze-etching study. *Cell Tissue Res.* 149: 437–455. [13]

Pepperberg, D. R., Okajima, T. L., Wiggert, B., et al. 1993. Interphotoreceptor retinoid-binding protein (IRBP). Molecular biology and physiological role in the visual cycle of rhodopsin. *Mol, Neurobiol.* 7: 61–85. [22]

Perea, G., and Araque, A. 2010. Glia modulates synaptic transmission. *Brain Res. Rev.* 63: 93–102. [10]

Perea, G., Navarrete, M., and Araque, A. 2009. Tripartite synapses: Astrocytes process and control synaptic information. *Trends Neurosci.* 32: 421–431. [10]

Peretz, I. 2006. The nature of music from a biological perspective. *Cognition* 100: 1–32. [25]

Perez, C. A., Engineer, C. T., Jakkamsetti, V., et al. 2012. Different timescales for the neural coding of consonant and vowel sounds. *Cereb. Cortex* 23: 670–683. [24]

Pernía-Andrade, A. J., Kato, A., Witschi, R., et al. 2009. Spinal endocannabinoids and CB1 receptors mediate C-fiber-induced heterosynaptic pain sensitization. *Science* 325: 760–764. [12]

Perrett, D. I., Rolls, E. T., and Caan, W. 1982. Visual neurones responsive to faces in the monkey temporal cortex. *Exp. Brain Res.* 47: 329–342. [25]

Perrett, D. I., Smith, P. A., Potter, D. D., et al. 1984. Neurones responsive to faces in the temporal cortex: Studies of functional organization, sensitivity to identity and relation to perception. *Hum. Neurobiol.* 3: 197–208. [25]

Perry, V. H., Nicoll, J. A., and Holmes, C. 2010. Microglia in neurodegenerative disease. *Nat. Rev. Neurol.* 6: 193–201. [10]

Pert, C. B., and Snyder, S. H. 1973. Opiate receptor: Demonstration in nervous tissue. *Science* 179: 1011–1014. [23]

Peters, A., Palay, S. L., and Webster, H. de F. 1991. *The Fine Structure of the Nervous System: Neurons and Their Supporting Cells,* 3rd ed. Oxford University Press, New York. [10]

Peters, J. A., Hales, T. G., and Lambert, J. J. 2006. Molecular determinants of single-channel conductance and ion selectivity in the Cys-loop family: Insights from the $5\text{-}HT_3$ receptor. *Trends Pharmacol. Sci.* 26: 587–594. [5]

Petersen, R. S., and Diamond, M. E. 2000. Spatial–temporal distribution of whisker-evoked activity in rat somatosensory cortex and the coding of stimulus location. *J. Neurosci.* 20: 6135–6143. [23]

Petrovic, P., Dietrich, T., Fransson, P., et al. 2005. Placebo in emotional processing—induced expectations of anxiety relief activate a generalized modulatory network. *Neuron* 46: 957–969. [23]

Pette, D. 2001. Historical perspectives: Plasticity of mammalian skeletal muscle. *J. Appl. Physiol.* 90: 1119–1124. [29]

Pevsner, J., Reed, R. R., Feinstein, P. G., and Snyder, S. H. 1988. Molecular cloning of odorant-binding protein: Member of a ligand carrier family. *Science* 241: 336–339. [21]

Pfaffinger, P. J., Martin, J. M., Hunter, D. D., et al. 1985. GTP-binding proteins couple cardiac muscarinic receptors to a K channel. *Nature* 317: 536–538. [12]

Pfeffer, S. E., and Wittlinger, M. 2016. Optic flow odometry operates independently of stride integration in carried ants. *Science* 353: 1155–1157. [20]

Pfrieger, F. W., and Barres, B. A. 1996. New views on synapse-glia interactions. *Curr. Opin. Neurobiol.* 6: 615–621. [10]

Phelan, K. A., and Hollyday, M. 1990. Axon guidance in muscleless chick wings: The role of muscle cells in motoneuronal pathway selection and muscle nerve formation. *J. Neurosci.* 10: 2699–2716. [27]

Phelan, P., Bacon, J. P., Davies, J. A., et al. 1998. Innexins: A family of invertebrate gap-junction proteins. *Trends Genet.* 14: 348–349. [11]

Phelan, P., Goulding, L. A., Tam, J. L., et al. 2008. Molecular mechanism of rectification at identified electrical synapses in the *Drosophila* giant fiber system. *Curr. Biol.* 18: 1955–1960. [11]

Philippidou, P., and Dasen, J. S. 2013. Hox genes: Vhoreographers in neural development, architects of circuit organization. *Neuron* 80: 12. [27]

Philipson, K. D., and Nicoll, D. A. 2000. Sodium–calcium exchange: A molecular perspective. *Annu. Rev. Physiol.* 62: 111–133. [9]

Piccolino, M., Neyton, J., and Gerschenfeld, H. M. 1984. Decrease of gap junction permeability induced by dopamine and cyclic adenosine 3':5'-monophosphate in horizontal cells of turtle retina. *J. Neurosci.* 4: 2477–2488. doi: 10.1523/JNEUROSCI.04-10-02477.1984. [18]

Pickles, J. O., Comis, S. D., and Osborne, M. P. 1984. Cross-links between stereocilia in the guinea pig organ of Corti, and their possible relation to sensory transduction. *Hear. Res.* 15: 103–112. [21]

Pierrot-Deseilligny, C. 2009. Effect of gravity on vertical eye position. *Ann. NY Acad. Sci.* 1164: 155–165. [26]

Pietrobon, D. 2010. CaV2.1 channelopathies. *Pflügers Arch.* 460: 375–393. [30]

Pifferi, S., Boccaccio, A., and Menini, A. 2006. Cyclic nucleotide-gated ion channels in sensory transduction. *FEBS Lett.* 580: 2853–2859. [21]

Pifferi, S., Dibattista, M., Sagheddu, C., et al. 2009. Calcium-activated chloride currents in olfactory sensory neurons from mice lacking bestrophin-2. *J. Physiol.* 587: 4265–4279. [21]

Piggins, H. D., and London, A. 2005. Circadian Biology: Clocks within Clocks. *Curr. Biol.* 15: 455–457. [19]

Piñeyro, G., and Blier, P. 1999. Autoregulation of serotonin neurons: Role in antidepressant actions. *Pharmacol. Rev.* 51: 533–591. [14]

Pinheiro, P. S., and Mulle, C. 2008. Presynaptic glutamate receptors: Physiological functions and mechanisms of action. *Nat. Rev. Neurosci.* 9: 423–436. [11]

Piomelli, D. 2001. The ligand that came from within. *Trends Neurosci.* 22: 17–19. [12]

Piomelli, D., Volterra, A., Dale, N., et al. 1987. Lipoxygenase metabolites of arachidonic acid as second messengers for presynaptic inhibition of Aplysia sensory cells. *Nature* 328: 38–43. [12]

Piper, M., et al. 2006. Signaling mechanisms underlying Slit2-induced collapse of *Xenopus* retinal growth cones. *Neuron* 49: 215–228. [27]

Pitler, T. A., and Alger, B. E. 1992. Postsynaptic spike firing reduces synaptic GABA$_A$ responses in hippocampal pyramidal cells. *J. Neurosci.* 12: 4122–4132. [12]

Pittman, A., and Chien, C. B. 2002 *Neuron* 35: 409–411. [27]

Pizzorusso, T., Fagiolini, M., Fabris, M., et al. 1994. Schwann cells transplanted in the lateral ventricles prevent the functional and anatomical effects of monocular deprivation in the rat. *Proc. Natl. Acad. Sci. USA* 91: 2572–2576. [28]

Pizzorusso, T., Medini, P., Berardi, N., et al. 2002. Reactivation of ocular dominance plasticity in the adult visual cortex. *Science* 298: 1248–1251. [28]

Placzek, M., Yamada, T., Tessier-Lavigne, M., et al. 1991. Control of dorsoventral pattern in vertebrate neural development: Induction and polarizing properties of the floor plate. *Development* 113(Suppl. 2): 105–122. [27]

Plotkin, M. D., Kaplan, M. R., Peterson, L. N., et al. 1997. Expression of the Na^+-K^+-2Cl^- cotransporter BSC2 in the nervous system. *Am. J. Physiol. Cell Physiol.* 272: C173–C183. [9]

Polley, D. B., Steinberg, E. E., and Merzenich, M. M. 2006. Perceptual learning directs auditory cortical map reorganization through top-down influences. *J. Neurosci.* 26: 4970–4982. [28]

Pollo, A., Amanzio, M., Arslanian, A., et al. 2001. Response expectancies in placebo analgesia and their clinical relevance. *Pain* 93: 77–84. [23]

Poo, M. M. 2015. What is memory? The present state of the engram. *BMC Biology* doi: 10.1186/s12915-016-0261-6. [17]

Pooya, S., Liu, X., Kumar, V. B., et al. 2015. The tumour suppressor LKB1 regulates myelination through mitochondrial metabolism. *Nat. Commun.* 5: 1–15. [10]

Poritsky, R. 1969. Two- and three-dimensional ultrastructure of boutons and glial cells on the motoneural surface in the cat spinal cord. *J. Comp. Neurol.* 135: 423–452. [1]

Porro, C. A., Francescato, M. P., Cettolo, V., et al. 1996. Primary motor and sensory cortex activation during motor performance and motor imagery: A functional magnetic resonance imaging study. *J. Neurosci.* 16: 7688–7698. [26]

Port, F., and Basler, K. 2010. Wnt trafficking: New insights into Wnt maturation, secretion and spreading. *Traffic* 11: 1265–1271. [27]

Porter, C. W., and Barnard, E. A. 1975. The density of cholinergic receptors at the postsynaptic membrane: Ultrastructural studies in two mammalian species. *J. Membr. Biol.* 20: 31–49. [13]

Potter, L. T. 1970. Synthesis, storage, and release of [^{14}C]acetylcholine in isolated rat diaphragm muscles. *J. Physiol.* 206: 145–166. [13, 15]

Pouille, F., and Scanziani, M. 2001. Enforcement of temporal fidelity in pyramidal cells by somatic feed-forward inhibition. *Science* 293: 1159–1163. [14]

Pow, D. V., and Morris, J. F. 1989. Dendrites of hypothalamic magnocellular neurons release neurohypophysial peptides by exocytosis. *Neuroscience* 32: 435–439. [18]

Powell, T. P., and Mountcastle, V. B. 1959 Some aspects of the functional organization of the cortex of the postcentral gyrus of the monkey: A correlation of findings obtained in a single unit analysis with cytoarchitecture. *Bull. Johns Hopkins Hosp.* 105: 133–162. [23, 25]

Prado, M. A., Reis, R. A., Prado, V. F., et al. 2002. Regulation of acetylcholine synthesis and storage. *Neurochem. Int.* 41: 291–299. [15]

Prather, J. F., Peters, S., Nowicki, S., and Mooney, R. 2010. Persistent representation of juvenile experience in the adult songbird brain. *J. Neurosci.* 30: 10586–10598. [28]

Preuss, T. M., and Coleman, G. Q. 2002. Human-specific organization of primary visual cortex: Alternating compartments of dense Cat-301 and calbindin immunoreactivity in layer 4A. *Cereb. Cortex* 12: 671–691. [3]

Preuss, T. M., Stepniewska, I., and Kaas, J. H. 1996. Movement representation in the dorsal and ventral premotor areas of owl monkeys: A microstimulation study. *J. Comp. Neurol.* 371: 649–676. [26]

Price, D. J., Jarman, A. P., Mason, J. O., and Kind, P. C. 2011. *Building Brains: An Introduction to Neural Development,* Wiley Blackwell, Oxford, UK. [27]

Price, G. D., and Trussell, L. O. 2006. Estimate of the chloride concentration in a central glutamatergic terminal: A gramicidin perforated-patch study on the calyx of Held. *J. Neurosci.* 26: 11432–11436. [11]

Priebe, N. J., and Ferster, D. 2008. Inhibition, spike threshold, and stimulus selectivity in primary visual cortex. *Neuron* 57: 482–497. [2]

Priebe, N. J., and Ferster, D. 2012. Mechanisms of neuronal computation in mammalian visual cortex. *Neuron* 75: 194–208. [2]

Provencio, I., Jiang, G., De Grip, W. J., et al. 1998. Melanopsin: An opsin in melanophores, brain, and eye. *Proc. Natl. Acad. Sci. USA* 95: 340–345. [22]

Prud'homme, M. J., Houdeau, E., Serghini, R., et al. 1999. Small intensely fluorescent cells of the rat paracervical ganglion synthesize adrenaline, receive afferent innervation from postganglionic cholinergic neurones, and contain muscarinic receptors. *Brain Res.* 821: 141–149. [19]

Puhl, J. G., Masino, M. A., and Mesce, K. A. 2012. Necessary, sufficient and permissive: A single locomotor command neuron important for intersegmental coordination. *J. Neurosci.* 32:17646–17657. [20]

Pun, R. Y. K., and Lecar, H. 2001. Patch clamp techniques and analysis. In: N. Sperelakis (Ed.), *Cell Physiology Source Book*, 3rd ed. Academic Press, San Diego, pp. 441–453. [4]

Puopolo, M., Hochstetler, S. E., Gustincich, S., et al. 2001. Extrasynaptic release of dopamine in a retinal neuron: Activity dependence and transmitter modulation. *Neuron* 30: 211–225. [18]

Purali, N. 2005. Structure and function relationship in the abdominal stretch receptor organs of the crayfish. *J. Comp. Neurol.* 488: 369–383. [21]

Purkinje, J. 1825. Beobachtungen und Versuche zur Physiologie der Sinne. Zweites Bändchem (Observations and Experimentations Investigating the Physiology of Senses). In *Neue Beträge zur Kenntnis des Sehens in Subjektiver Hinsicht*. Reimer: Berlin. [22]

Purves, D. 1975. Functional and structural changes in mammalian sympathetic neurones following interruption of their axons. *J. Physiol.* 252: 429–463. [29]

Purves, D., and Sakmann, B. 1974. Membrane properties underlying spontaneous activity of denervated muscle fibers. *J. Physiol.* 239: 125–153. [29]

Purves, D., Augustine, G. J., Fitzpatrick, D., et al. 1997. *Neuroscience.* Oxford University Press/Sinauer, Sunderland MA. [8]

Pusch, M., and Jentsch, T. J. 2005. Unique structure and function of chloride transporting CLC proteins. *IEEE Trans. Nanobiosci.* 4: 49–57. [5]

Pusch, M., Noda, M., Stühmer, W., et al. 1991. Single point mutations of the sodium channel drastically reduce the pore permeability without preventing its gating. *Eur. Biophys. J.* 20: 127–133. [5]

Putignano, E., Lonetti, G., Cancedda, L., et al. 2007. Developmental downregulation of histone posttranslational modifications regulates visual cortical plasticity. *Neuron* 53: 747–759. [28]

Puzzolo, E., and Mallamaci, A. 2010. Cortico-cerebral histogenesis in the opossum *Monodelphis domestica*: Generation of a hexalaminar neocortex in the absence of a basal proliferative compartment. *Neural Development.* 5: 8. [1, 27]

Qian, H., Malchow, R. P., Chappell, R. L., and Ripps, H. 1996. Zinc enhances ionic currents induced in skate Müller (glial) cells by the inhibitory neurotransmitter GABA. *Proc. R. Soc. Lond., B, Biol. Sci.* 263: 791–796. [10]

Qian, X., Shen, Q., Goderie, S. K., et al. 2000. Timing of CNS cell generation: A programmed sequence of neuron and glial cell production from isolated murine cortical stem cells. *Neuron* 28: 69–80. [27]

Quian Quiroga, R. 2013. Gnostic cells in the 21st century. *Acta Neurobiol. Exp.* 73: 463–471. [30]

Quian Quiroga, R., Mukamel, R., Isham, E. A., and Fried, I. 2008. Human single-neuron responses at the threshold of conscious recognition. *Proc. Natl. Acad. Sci. USA* 105: 3599–3604. [30]

Quian Quiroga, R., Reddy, L., Kreiman, G., et al. 2005. Invariant visual representation by single neurons in the human brain. *Nature* 435: 1102–1107. [30]

Quilliam, T. A., and Armstrong, J. 1963. Mechanoreceptors. *Endeavour* 22: 55–60. [21]

Quiroga, R. Q., Reddy, L., Kreiman, G., et al. 2005. Invariant visual representation by single neurons in the human brain. *Nature* 435: 1102–1107. [25]

Raff, M. 1996. Neural development: Mysterious no more? *Science* 274: 1063. [30]

Raftery, M. A., Hunkapiller, M. W., Strader, C. D., and Hood, L. E. 1980. Acetylcholine receptor: Complex of homologous subunits. *Science* 208: 1454–1457. [5]

Raggenbass, M. 2001. Vasopressin- and oxytocin-induced activity in the central nervous system: Electrophysiological studies using in-vitro systems. *Prog. Neurobiol.* 64: 307–326. [14]

Rahmouni, K., Haynes, W. G., and Mark, A. L. 2004. In D. Robertson (Ed.), *Primer on the Autonomic Nervous System*. Academic Press, London pp. 86–89. [19]

Raisman, G. 2007. Repair of spinal cord injury by transplantation of olfactory ensheathing cells. *C. R. Biol.* 330: 557–560. [29]

Rajan, R. 1995. Frequency and loss dependence of the protective effects of the olivocochlear pathways in cats. *J. Neurophysiol.* 74: 598–615. [24]

Rakic P. 2003. Elusive radial glial cells: Historical and evolutionary perspective. *Glia* 43: 19–32. [10]

Rakic, P. 1974. Neurons in rhesus monkey visual cortex: Systematic relation between time of origin and eventual disposition. *Science* 183: 425–427. [27]

Rakic, P. 1977. Prenatal development of the visual system in rhesus monkey. *Philos. Trans. R. Soc. Lond., B, Biol. Sci.* 278: 245–260. [28]

Rakic P. 1976. Prenatal genesis of connections subserving ocular dominance in the rhesus monkey. *Nature* 261: 467–471. [28]

Rakic, P. 1981. Neuronal-glial interaction during brain development. *Trends Neurosci.* 4: 184–187. [10, 27]

Rakic, P. 2002. Adult neurogenesis in mammals: An identity crisis. *J. Neurosci.* 22: 614–618. [27]

Rakic, P. 2003. Developmental and evolutionary adaptations of cortical radial glia. *Cereb. Cortex.* 13: 541–549. [10]

Rakic, P. 2006. A century of progress in corticoneurogenesis: From silver impregnation to genetic engineering. *Cereb. Cortex.* 16(Suppl. 1): I3–i17. [28]

Rakic, P. 2006. Neuroscience. No more cortical neurons for you. *Science* 313: 928–929. [27]

Ralph, M. R., Foster, R., Davis, F. C., and Menaker, M. 1990. Transplanted suprachiasmatic nucleus determines circadian period. *Science* 247: 975–978. [19]

Ramachandran, R., Davis, K. A., and May, B. J. 1999. Single-unit responses in the inferior colliculus of decerebrate cats. I. Classification based on frequency response maps. *J. Neurophysiol.* 82: 152–163. [24]

Raman, I. M., Sprunger, L. K., Meisler, M. H., and Bean, B. P. 1997. Altered subthreshold sodium currents and disrupted firing patterns in Purkinje neurons of *Scn8a* mutant mice. *Neuron* 19: 881–891. [7]

Ramanathan, K., Michael, T. H., Jiang, G. J., et al. 1999. A molecular mechanism for electrical tuning of cochlear hair cells. *Science* 283: 215–217. [24]

Ramirez, S., et al. 2013. Creating a false memory in the hippocampus. *Science* 341: 387–391. [17]

Ramón y Cajal, S. [1909–1911] 1995. *Histology of the Nervous System*, 2 Vols. Translated by Neely Swanson and Larry Swanson. Oxford University Press, New York. [10, 26]

Ramón y Cajal, S. 1911. *Histologie du Système Nerveux*, Vol. 2. Maloine, Paris. [1]

Ramón y Cajal, S. 1955. *Histologie du Système Nerveux*, Vol. 2. C.S.I.C., Madrid. [3]

Ranade, S. S., Syeda, R., and Patapoutian, A. 2015. Mechanically activated ion channels. *Neuron* 87: 1162–1179. [5]

Randall, A., and Tsien, R. W. 1995. Pharmacological dissection of multiple types of calcium channel currents in rat cerebellar granule neurons. *J. Neurosci.* 15: 2995–3012. [5]

Randlett, O., Norden, C., and Harris, W. A. 2011. The vertebrate retina: A model for neuronal polarization *in vivo. Dev. Neurobiol.* 71: 567–583. [27]

Randolph, M., and Semmes, J. 1974. Behavioral consequences of selective subtotal ablations in the postcentral gyrus of *Macaca mulatta. Brain Res.* 70: 55–70. [23]

Rang, H. P. 1981. The characteristics of synaptic currents and responses to acetylcholine of rat submandibular ganglion cells. *J. Physiol.* 311: 23–55. [15, 19]

Ranganathan, R., Cannon, S. C., and Horvitz, H. R. 2000. MOD-1 is a serotonin-gated chloride channel that modulates locomotory behaviour in *C. elegans. Nature* 408: 470–475. [5]

Rangaraju, V., et al. 2019. Spatially stable mitochondrial compartments fuel local translation during plasticity. *Cell* 176: 73–84. [17]

Ransohoff, R. M., and Perry, V. H. 2009. Microglial physiology: Unique stimuli, specialized responses. *Annu. Rev. Immunol.* 27: 119–145. [10]

Ransom, B. R., and Goldring, S. 1973. Slow depolarization in cells presumed to be glia in cerebral cortex of cat. *J. Neurophysiol.* 36: 869–878. [10]

Ransom, B. R., and Sontheimer, H. 1992. The neurophysiology of glial cells. *J. Clin. Neurophysiol.* 9: 224–251. [10]

Rasband, M. N., Trimmer, J. S., Schwartz, T. L., et al. 1998. Potassium channel distribution, clustering, and function in remyelinating rat axons. *J. Neurosci.* 18: 36–47. [8]

Rasmussen, G. 1946. The olivary peduncle and other fiber projections of the superior olivary complex. *J. Comp. Neurol.* 84: 141–219. [24]

Rav-Acha, M., Sagiv, N., Segev, I., et al. 2005. Dynamic and spatial features of the inhibitory pallidal GABAergic synapses. *Neuroscience* 135: 791–802. [26]

Raveh, A., Riven, I., and Reuvenny, E. 2009. Elucidation of the gating of the GIRK channel using a spectroscopic approach. *J. Physiol.* 587: 5331–5335. [12]

Raymond, C. R. 2007. LTP forms 1, 2, and 3: Different mechanisms for the "long" in long-term potentiation. *Trends Neurosci.* 30: 167–175. [16]

Raymond, C. R., and Redman S. J. 2006. Spatial segregation of neuronal calcium signals encodes different forms of LTP in rat hippocampus. *J. Physiol.* 570: 97–111. [16]

Razak, K. A., Richardson, M. D., and Fuzessery, Z. M. 2008. Experience is required for the maintenance and refinement of FM sweep selectivity in the developing auditory cortex. *Proc. Natl. Acad. Sci. USA* 105: 4465–4470. [28]

Ready, D. F., Hanson, T. E., and Benzer, S. 1976. Development of the *Drosophila* retina, a neurocrystalline lattice. *Dev. Biol.* 53: 217–240. [27]

Reale, R. A., and Imig, T. J. 1980. Tonotopic organization in auditory cortex of the cat. *J. Comp. Neurol.* 192: 265–291. [24]

Rebsam, A., Seif, I., and Gaspar, P. 2005. Dissociating barrel development and lesion-induced plasticity in the mouse somatosensory cortex. *J. Neurosci.* 25: 706–710. [28]

Recanzone, G. H., Merzenich, M. M., and Schreiner, C. E. 1992. Changes in the distributed temporal response properties of S. I. cortical neurons reflect improvements in performance on a temporally based tactile discrimination task. *J. Neurophysiol.* 67: 1071–1091. [23]

Recanzone, G. H., Merzenich, M. M., Jenkins, W. M., et al. 1992. Topographic reorganization of the hand representation in cortical area 3b owl monkeys trained in a frequency-discrimination task. *J. Neurophysiol.* 67: 1031–1056. [23]

Reddy, V. B., Azimi, E., Chu, L., and Lerner, E. A. 2018. Mas-related G-protein coupled receptors and cowhage-induced itch. *J. Invest. Dermatol.* 138: 461–464. doi: 10.1016/j.jid.2017.05.042. [21]

Redfern, P. A. 1970. Neuromuscular transmission in new-born rats. *J. Physiol.* 209: 701–709. [27]

Redman, S. 1990. Quantal analysis of synaptic potentials in neurons of the central nervous system. *Physiol. Rev.* 70: 165–198. [13]

Redmond, S. A., Mei, F., Eshed-Eisenbach, Y., et al. 2016. Somatodendritic expression of JAM2 inhibits oligodendrocyte myelination. *Neuron.* 91: 824–836. doi: 10.1016/j.neuron.2016.07.021. [10]

Redondo, R. L. and Morris R. 2011. Making memories last: the synaptic tagging and capture hypothesis. *Nat. Rev. Neurosci.* 12: 17. [17]

Redondo, R. L., et al. 2010. Synaptic tagging and capture: Differential role of distinct calcium/calmodulin kinases in protein synthesis-dependent long-term potentiation. *J. Neurosci.* 30: 4981–4989. [17]

Reed, R. R. 2004. After the Holy Grail: Establishing a molecular basis for mammalian olfaction. *Cell* 116: 329–336. [21]

Reese, T. S., and Karnovsky, M. J. 1967. Fine structural localization of a blood-brain barrier to exogenous peroxidase. J. Cell Biol. 34: 207–217. [10]

Reger, J. F. 1958. The fine structure of neuromuscular synapses of gastrocnemii from mouse and frog. *Anat. Rec.* 130: 7–23. [13]

Reichardt, L. F. 2006. Neurotrophin-regulated signalling pathways. *Philos. Trans. R. Soc. Lond., B, Biol. Sci.* 361: 1545–1564. [27]

Reid, G. 2005. ThermoTRP channels and cold sensing: What are they really up to? *Pflügers Arch.* 451: 250–263. [21]

Reier, P. J., Stokes, B. T., Thompson, F. J., and Anderson, D. K. 1992. Fetal cell grafts into resection and contusion/compression injuries of the rat and cat spinal cord. *Exp. Neurol.* 115: 177–188. [29]

Reijmers et al. 2007. Localization of a stable neural correlate of associative memory. *Science* 317: 1230. [17]

Reinscheid, R. K., Nothacker, H. P., Bourson, A., et al. 1995. Orphanin FQ: A neuropeptide that activates an opioidlike G protein-coupled receptor. *Science* 270: 792–794. [14]

Reiser, G., and Miledi, R. 1988. Characteristics of Schwann-cell miniature end-plate currents in denervated frog muscle. *Pflügers Arch.* 412: 22–28. [10]

Reiser, G., and Miledi, R. 1989. Changes in the properties of synaptic channels opened by acetylcholine in denervated frog muscle. *Brain Res.* 479: 83–97. [13]

Reist, N. E., Werle, M. J., and McMahan, U. J. 1992. Agrin released by motor neurons induces the aggregation of acetylcholine receptors at neuromuscular junctions. *Neuron* 8: 865–868. [27]

Reist, N. E., and Smith, S. J. 1992. Neurally evoked calcium transients in terminal Schwan cells at the neuromuscular junction. *Proc. Natl. Acad. Sci. USA* 89:7625–7629. [18]

Reiter, H. O., Waitzman, D. M., and Stryker, M. P. 1986. Cortical activity blockade prevents ocular dominance plasticity in the kitten visual cortex. *Exp. Brain Res.* 65: 182–188. [28]

Rennels, M. L. et al. 1985. Evidence for a "paravascular" fluid circulation in the mammalian central nervous system, provided by the rapid distribution of tracer protein throughout the brain from the subarachnoid space. *Brain Res.* 326: 47–63. [18]

Ress, D., Backus, B. T., and Heeger, D. J. 2000. Activity in primary visual cortex predicts performance in a visual detection task. *Nat. Neurosci.* 3: 940–945. [25]

Ressler, K. J., Sullivan, S. L., and Buck, L. B. 1993. A zonal organization of odorant receptor gene expression in the olfactory epithelium. *Cell* 73: 597–609. [21]

Restrepo, D., Miyamoto, T., Bryant, B. P., and Teeter, J. H. 1990. Odor stimuli trigger influx of calcium into olfactory neurons of the channel catfish. *Science* 249: 1166–1168. [21]

Reuter, H. 1974. Localization of β adrenergic receptors, and effects of noradrenaline and cyclic nucleotides on action potentials, ionic currents and tension in mammalian cardiac muscle. *J. Physiol.* 242: 429–451. [12]

Reuter, H., Cachelin, A. B., DePeyer, J. E., and Kokubun, S. 1983. Modulation of calcium channels in cultured cardiac cells by isoproternenol and 8-bromo-cAMP. *Cold Spring Harb. Symp. Quant. Biol.* 48: 193–200. [12]

Reuveny, E., Slesinger, P. A., Inglese, J., et al. 1994. Activation of the cloned muscarinic potassium channel by G protein βγ subunits. *Nature* 370: 143–146. [12]

Reynolds, B. A., and Weiss, S. 1996. Clonal and population analyses demonstrate that an EGF-responsive mammalian embryonic CNS precursor is a stem cell. *Dev. Biol.* 175: 1–13. [27]

Rheaume, B.A., Jereen, A., Bolisetty, M., et al. 2018. Single cell transcriptome profiling of retinal ganglion cells identifies cellular subtypes. *Nat. Comm.* 9: 2759. doi: 10.1038/s41467-018-05134-3. [1]

Rhinn, M., Lun, K., Luz, M., et al. 2005. Positioning of the midbrain-hindbrain boundary organizer through global posteriorization of the neuroectoderm mediated by Wnt8 signaling. *Development* 132: 1261–1272. [27]

Ribchester, R. R., and Taxt, T. 1983. Motor unit size and synaptic competition in rat lumbrical muscles reinnervated by active and inactive motor axons. *J. Physiol.* 344: 89–111. [27]

Ribelayga, C., Cao, Y., and Mangel, S. C. 2008. The circadian clock in the retina controls rod-cone coupling. *Neuron* 59: 790–801. [18]

Ricci, A. J., and Fettiplace, R. 1997. The effects of calcium buffering and cyclic AMP on mechano-electrical transduction in turtle auditory hair cells. *J. Physiol.* 501(Pt 1): 111–124. [21]

Rice, F. L., Mance, A., and Munger, B. L. 1986. A comparative light microscopic analysis of the sensory innervation of the mystacial pad. I. Innervation of vibrissal follicle-sinus complexes. *J. Comp. Neurol.* 252: 154–174. [24]

Rice, J. J., May, B. J., Spirou, G. A., Young, E. D. 1992. Pinna-based spectral cues for sound localization in cat. *Hear. Res.* 58: 132–152. [24]

Richards, D. A. 2009. Vesicular release mode shapes the postsynaptic response at hippocampal synapses. *J. Physiol.* 587: 5073–5080. [13]

Richards, D. A., Gautimosime, D., Rizzoli, S., and Betz, W. J. 2003. Synaptic vesicle pools at the frog neuromuscular junction. *Neuron* 39: 529–541. [13]

Richardson, P. M., McGuinness, U. M., and Aguayo, A. J. 1980. Axons from CNS neurones regenerate into PNS grafts. *Nature* 284: 264–265. [29]

Richardson, W. D., Young, K. M., Tripathi, R. B. and McKenzie, I. 2011. NG2-glia as multipotent neural stem cells: Fact or fantasy? *Neuron* 70: 661–673. [10]

Richter, J. D. 2007. CPEB: A life in translation. *Trends Biochem. Sci.* 32: 279–285. [17]

Rieke, F., and Baylor, D. A. 1998. Origin of reproducibility in the responses of retinal rods to single photons. *Biophys. J.* 75: 1836–1857. [22]

Riesen, A. H., and Aarons, L. 1959. Visual movement and intensity discrimination in cats after early deprivation of pattern vision. *J. Comp. Physiol. Psychol.* 52: 142–149. [28]

Righi, M., et al. 2000. Brain-derived neurotrophic factor (BDNF) induces dendritic targeting of BDNF and tyrosine kinase B mRNAs in hippocampal neurons through a phosphatidylinositol-3 kinase-dependent pathway. *J. Neurosci.* 20: 3165. [17]

Rijntjes, M., Dettmers, C., Buchel, C., et al. 1999. A blueprint for movement: Functional and anatomical representations in the human motor system. *J. Neurosci.* 19: 8043–8048. [26]

Rimer, M. 2010. Modulation of agrin-induced acetylcholine receptor clustering by extracellular signal-regulated kinases 1 and 2 in cultured myotubes. *J. Biol. Chem.* 285: 32370–32377. [29]

Riozzoli, S. O. and Betz, W. J. 2005. Synaptic vesicle pools. *Nature Rev. Neurosci.* 6: 57–69. [13]

Ritchie, J. M. 1987. Voltage-gated cation and anion channels in mammalian Schwann cells and astrocytes. *J. Physiol. (Paris)* 82: 248–257. [10]

Ritchie, J. M., Black, J. A., Waxman, S. G., and Angelides, K. J. 1990. Sodium channels in the cytoplasm of Schwann cells. *Proc. Natl. Acad. Sci. USA.* 87: 9290–9294. [10]

Rivera, C., Voipio, J., Payne, J. A., et al. 1999. The K^+/Cl^- co-transporter KCC2 renders GABA hyperpolarizing during neuronal maturation. *Nature.* 397: 251–255. [9]

Riviere, S., Challet, L., Fluegge, D., et al. 2009. Formyl peptide receptor-like proteins are a novel family of vomeronasal chemosensors. *Nature* 459: 574–577. [21]

Rizo, J. 2018. Mechanism of transmitter release coming into focus. *Protein Sci.* 27: 1364–1391. doi: 10.1002/pro.3445. PMID 29893445. [13]

Rizzi, C., et al. 2018. NGF steers microglia toward a neuroprotective phenotype. *Glia* doi: 10.1002/glia.23312. [27]

Rizzolatti, G., and Wolpert, D. M. 2005. Motor systems. *Curr. Opin. Neurobiol.* 15: 624–625. [26]

Rizzuto, R., and Pozzan, T. 2006. Microdomains of intracellular Ca^{2+}: Molecular determinants and functional consequences. *Physiol. Rev.* 86: 369–408. [9]

Robbins, J., Passmore, G. M., Abogadie, F. C., et al. 2013 Effects of KCNQ2 gene truncation on M-type Kv7 potassium currents. *PLOS ONE.* 8:e71809. doi: 10.1371/journal.pone.0071809. [5]

Roberts, A., and Bush, B. M. 1971. Coxal muscle receptors in the crab: The receptor current and some properties of the receptor nerve fibres. *J. Exp. Biol.* 54: 515–524. [21]

Roberts, E., and Frankel, S. 1950. γ-Aminobutyric acid in brain: Its formation from glutamic acid. *J. Biol. Chem.* 187: 55–63. [14]

Robertson, D., ed. 2004. *Primer on the Autonomic Nervous system.* Academic Press, London. [19]

Robertson, S. J., and Edwards, F. A. 1998. ATP and glutamate are released from separate neurones in the rat medial habenula nucleus: Frequency dependence and adenosine-mediated inhibition of release. *J. Physiol.* 508: 691–701. [14]

Robinson, D. A., and Fuchs, A. F. 1969. Eye movement evoked by stimulation of frontal eye fields. *J. Neurophysiol.* 32: 637–648. [25]

Robitaille, R., Adler, E. M., and Charlton, M. P. 1990. Strategic location of calcium channels at release sites of frog neuromuscular synapses. *Neuron* 5: 773–779. [13]

Rodieck, R. W. 1989. Starburst amacrine cells of the primate retina. *J. Comp. Neurol.* 285: 18–37. [22]

Rodieck, R. W., and Marshak, D. W. 1992. Spatial density and distribution of choline acetyltransferase immunoreactive cells in human, macaque, and baboon retinas. *J. Comp. Neurol.* 321: 46–64. [22]

Rodríguez, E. M. et al. 2005. Hypothalamic tanycytes: A key component of brain-endocrine interaction. *Int. Rev. Cytol.* 247: 89–164. [18]

Rodriguez, M. J., Perez-Etchegoyen, C. B., and Szczupak, L. 2009. Premotor nonspiking neurons regulate coupling among motoneurons that innervate overlapping muscle fiber population. *J. Comp. Physiol. A* 195: 491–500. [20]

Roehm, P. C., Xu, N., Woodson, E. A., et al. 2008. Membrane depolarization inhibits spiral ganglion neurite growth via activation of multiple types of voltage sensitive calcium channels and calpain. *Mol. Cell Neurosci.* 37: 376–387. [27]

Roelink, H., Porter, J. A., Chiang, C., et al. 1995. Floor plate and motor neuron induction by different concentrations of the amino-terminal cleavage product of Sonic hedgehog autoproteolysis. *Cell* 81: 445–455. [27]

Rogan, M. T., Staubil, U. V., and LeDoux, J. E. 1997. Fear conditioning induces associative long-term potentiation in the amygdala. *Nature* 390: 604–607. [16]

Rogers, M., and Sargent, P. B. 2003. Rapid activation of presynaptic nicotinic acetylcholine receptors by nerve-released transmitter. *Eur. J. Neurosci.* 18: 2946–2956. [19]

Rojas, L., and Orkand, R. K. 1999. K^+ channel density increases selectively in the endfoot of retinal glial cells during development of Rana catesbiana. *Glia* 25: 199–203. [10]

Rokni, D., Llinas, R., and Yarom, Y. 2008. The morpho/functional discrepancy in the cerebellar cortex: Looks alone are deceptive. *Front. Syst. Neurosci.* 2: 192–198. [26]

Role, L. W., and Berg, D. K. 1996. Nicotinic receptors in the development and modulation of CNS synapses. *Neuron* 16: 1077–1085. [14]

Rollema, H., Coe, J. W., Chambers, L. K., et al. 2007. Rationale, pharmacology and clinical efficacy of partial agonists of $\alpha_4\beta_2$ nACh receptors for smoking cessation. *Trends Pharmacol. Sci.* 28: 316–325. [14]

Rolls, A., Shechter, R., and Schwartz, M. 2009. The bright side of the glial scar in CNS repair. *Nat. Rev. Neurosci.* 10: 235–241. [29]

Rolls, E. T. 1984. Neurons in the cortex of the temporal lobe and in the amygdala of the monkey with responses selective for faces. *Hum. Neurobiol.* 3: 209–222. [25]

Romanski, L. M., and Averbeck, B. B. 2009. The primate cortical auditory system and neural representation of conspecific vocalizations. *Annu. Rev. Neurosci.* 32: 315–346. [24]

Romero, M. F., Fulton, C. M., and Boron, W. F. 2004. The SLC4 family of HCO_3^- transporters. *Pflügers Arch.* 447: 495–509. [9]

Romo, R., and Salinas, E. 2003. Flutter discrimination: Neural codes, perception, memory and decision making. *Nat. Rev. Neurosci.* 4: 203–218. [25]

Romo, R., Hernández, A., and Zainos, A. 2004. Neuronal correlates of a perceptual decision in ventral premotor cortex. *Neuron* 41: 165–173. [25]

Romo, R., Hernández, A., Zainos, A., et al. 2000. Sensing without touching: Psychophysical performance based on cortical microstimulation. *Neuron* 26: 273–278. [25]

Romo, R., Hernández, A., Zainos, A., et al. 2002. Exploring the cortical evidence of a sensory-discrimination process. *Philos. Trans. R. Soc. Lond. B Biol. Sci.* 357: 1039–1051. [25]

Romo, R., Merchant, H., Zainos, A., and Hernández, A. 1997. Categorical perception of somesthetic stimuli: Psychophysical measurements correlated with neuronal events in primate medial premotor cortex. *Cereb. Cortex* 7: 317–326. [25]

Roorda A., and Williams D. R. 1999. The arrangement of the three cone classes in the living human eye. *Nature* 397: 520–522. doi:10.1038/17383. [22]

Roorda, A., Romero-Borja, F., Donnelly, W. J., III, et al. 2002. Adaptive optics scanning laser ophthalmoscopy. *Opt. Express* 10: 405–412. [22]

Roper, J., and Schwarz, J. R. 1989. Heterogeneous distribution fast and slow potassium channels in myelinated rat nerve. *J. Physiol.* 416: 93–110. [8]

Roper, S. D. 2015. The taste of table salt. *Pflügres Arch.* 467: 457–463. [21]

Rose, C. R., Ransom, B. R., and Waxman, S. G. 1997. Pharmacological characterization of Na^+ influx via voltage-gated Na^+ channels in spinal cord astrocytes. *J. Neurophysiol.* 78: 3249–3258. [10]

Rosenbaum, D. M., Rasmussen, S. G., and Kobilka, B. K. 2009. The structure and function of G-protein-coupled receptors. *Nature* 459: 356–363. [12]

Rosenblatt, K. P., Sun, Z. P., Heller, S., and Hudspeth, A. J. 1997. Distribution of Ca^{2+}-activated K^+ channel isoforms along the tonotopic gradient of the chicken's cochlea. *Neuron* 19: 1061–1075. [24]

Rosenthal, J. L. 1969. Post-tetanic potentiation at the neuromuscular junction of the frog. *J. Physiol.* 203: 121–133. [16]

Rosenzweig, E. S., Brock, J. H., Lu, P., et al. 2018. *Nat. Med.* 24: 484–490. doi:10.1038/nm.4502. [29]

Rosenzweig, E. S., Salegio, E. A., Liang, J. J., et al. 2019. Chondroitinase improves anatomical and functional outcomes after primate spinal cord injury. *Nat. Neurosci.* 22: 1269–1275. [29]

Rosenzweig, M. R., and Bennett, E. L. 1996. Psychobiology of plasticity: Effects of training and experience on brain and behavior. *Behav. Brain Res.* 78: 57–65. [28]

Roska, B., and Werblin, F. 2003. Rapid global shifts in natural scenes block spiking in specific ganglion cell types. *Nat. Neurosci.* 6: 600–608. [22]

Ross, C. A., and Tabrizi, S. J. 2011. Huntington's disease: From molecular pathogenesis to clinical treatment. *Lancet Neurol.* 10: 83–98. [30]

Ross, W. N. 2012. Understanding calcium waves and sparks in central neurons. *Nat. Rev. Neurosci.* 13: 157–168. [17]

Ross, W. N., and Werman, R. 1987. Mapping calcium transients in the dendrites of Purkinje cells form the guinea pig cerebellum in vitro. *J. Physiol.* 389: 319–336. [16]

Ross, W. N., Arechiga, H., and Nicholls, J. G. 1988. Influence of substrate on the distribution of calcium channels in identified leech neurons in culture. *Proc. Natl. Acad. Sci. USA* 85: 4075–4078. [12]

Ross, W. N., Lasser-Ross, N., and Werman, R. 1990. Spatial and temporal analysis of calcium-dependent electrical activity in guinea pig Purkinje cell dendrites. *Proc. R. Soc. Lond., B, Biol. Sci.* 240: 173–185. [7]

Ross, W. N., Salzberg, B. M., Cohen, L. B., and Davila, H. V. 1974 A large change in dye absorption during the action potential. *Biophys. J.* 14: 983–986. [1]

Rossant, J. 1985. Interspecific cell markers and lineage in mammals. *Philos. Trans. R. Soc. Lond., B, Biol. Sci.* 312: 91–100. [27]

Rossi, D. J., Oshima, T., and Attwell, D. 2000. Glutamate release in severe brain ischemia is mainly by reversed uptake. *Nature.* 403: 316–321. [9]

Rossi, S. L., and Keirstead, H. S. 2009. Stem cells and spinal cord regeneration. *Curr. Opin. Biotechnol.* 20: 552–562. [29]

Rothwell, J. C., Traub, M. M., Day, B. L., et al. 1982. Manual motor performance in a deafferented man. *Brain* 105: 515–542. [26]

Rotshenker, S. 1988. Multiple modes and sites for the induction of axonal growth. *Trends Neurosci.* 11: 363–366. [29]

Rotshenker, S. 2009 The role of Galectin-3/MAC-2 in the activation of the innate-immune function of phagocytosis in microglia in injury and disease. *J. Mol. Neurosci.* 39: 99–103. [10, 29]

Rouiller, E. M., Moret, V., Tanne, J., and Boussaoud, D. 1996. Evidence for direct connections between the hand region of the supplementary motor area and motoneurons in the macaque monkey. *Eur. J. Neurosci.* 8: 1055–1059. [26]

Roux, I., Safieddine, S., Nouvian, R., et al. 2006. Otoferlin, defective in a human deafness form, is essential for exocytosis at the auditory ribbon synapse. *Cell* 127: 277–289. [24]

Rovainen, C. M. 1967. Physiological and anatomical studies on large neurons of the central nervous system of the sea lamprey (*Petromyzon marinus*). II. Dorsal cells and giant interneurons. *J. Neurophysiol.* 30: 1024–1042. [11]

Roy, C. S., and Sherrington, C. S. 1890. On the regulation of the blood-supply of the brain. *J. Physiol.* 11: 85–108, 158-7-158-17. [18]

Rozanski, G. M., Li, Q., Kim, H., and Stanley, E. F. 2012. *Eur. J. Neurosci.* 37: 359–365. doi: 10.1111/ejn.12082. [18]

Roy, S., and Field, G. D. 2019. Dopaminergic modulation of retinal processing from starlight to sunlight. *J. Pharmacol. Sci.* 140: 86–93. [18]

Roy, S., Jayakumar, J., Martin, P. R., Dreher, B., et al. 2009. Segregation of short-wavelength-sensitive (S) cone signals in the macaque dorsal lateral geniculate nucleus. *Eur. J. Neurosci.* 30: 1517–1526. [3, 22]

Rubin, E. 1915. *Synsoplevede figurer, studier i psykologisk analyse.* København og Kristiania, Gyldendal, Nordisk forlag. [25]

Rude, S., Coggeshall, E., Van, Orden, L. S. III 1969. Chemical and ultrastructural identification of 5-hydroxytryptamine in an identified neuron. *J. Cell Biol.* 41: 832–854. [18]

Rudolf, R., Mongillo, M., Rizutto, R., and Pozzan, T. 2003. Looking forward to seeing calcium. *Nat. Rev. Mol. Cell Biol.* 4: 579–586. [13]

Rudomin, P. 2009. In search of lost presynaptic inhibition. *Exp. Brain Res.* 196: 139–151. [11]

Rudy, J. W. 2020. *The Neurobiology of Learning and Memory,* 3rd ed. Oxford University Press/Sinauer, Sunderland, MA. [17]

Rueter, S. M., Burns, C. M., Coode, S. A., et al. 1995. Glutamate receptor RNA editing in vitro by enzymatic conversion of adenosine to inosine. *Science* 267: 1491–1494. [27]

Ruiz, M. L., and Karpen, J. W. 1997. Single cyclic nucleotide-gated channels locked in different ligand-bound states. *Nature* 389: 389–392. [22]

Russell, I. J., and Murugasu, E. 1997. Medial efferent inhibition suppresses basilar membrane responses to near characteristic frequency tones of moderate to high intensities. *J. Acoust. Soc. Am.* 102: 1734–1738. [24]

Russell, J. M. 2000. Sodium–potassium–chloride cotransport. *Physiol. Rev.* 80: 211–276. [9]

Russell, J. M., and Boron, W. F. 1976. Role of chloride transport in regulation of intracellular pH. *Nature* 264: 73–74. [9]

Rust, G., Burgunder, J. M., Lauterburg, T. E., and Cachelin, A. B.1994. Expression of neuronal nicotinic acetylcholine receptor subunit genes in the rat autonomic nervous system. *Eur. J. Neurosci.* 6: 478–485. [19]

Rutherford, M. A., and Roberts, W. M. 2006. Frequency selectivity of synaptic exocytosis in frog saccular hair cells. *Proc. Natl. Acad. Sci. USA* 103: 2898–2903. [24]

Ryan, C. A., and Salvesen, G. S. 2003. Caspases and neuronal development. *Biol. Chem.* 384: 855–861. [27]

Ryan, T. J. et al 2015. Engram cells retain memory under retrograde amnesia. *Science* 348: 1007–1013. [17]

Ryba, N. J., and Tirindelli, R. 1997. A new multigene family of putative pheromone receptors. *Neuron* 19: 371–379. [21]

Rydqvist, B., and Purali, N. 1993. Transducer properties of the rapidly adapting stretch receptor neurone in the crayfish (*Pacifastacus leniusculus*). *J. Physiol.* 469: 193–211. [21]

Ryugo, D. K., Kretzmer, E. A., and Niparko, J. K. 2005. Restoration of auditory nerve synapses in cats by cochlear implants. *Science* 310: 1490–1492. [28]

Saab, A., Tzvetavona, I. D., Trevisiol, A., et al. 2016. Oligodendroglial NMDA receptors regulate glucose import and axonal energy metabolism. *Neuron.* 91: 119–132. [10]

Sabesan, R., Schmidt, B. P., Tuten, W. S., and Roorda, A. 2016. The elementary representation of spatial and color vision in the human retina. *Sci. Adv.* 2: e1600797. doi: 10.1126/sciadv.1600797. [22]

Sachdev, R. N., and Catania, K. C. 2002. Receptive fields and response properties of neurons in the star-nosed mole's somatosensory fovea. *J. Neurophysiol.* 87: 2602–2611. [23]

Sachs, M. B. 1984. Neural coding of complex sounds: Speech. *Annu. Rev. Physiol.* 46: 261–273. [24]

Sacktor, T. C. and Hell, J. W. 2017. The genetics of PKMζ and memory maintenance. *Science Signal* 10, eaao2327. [17]

Sadagopan, S., and Wang, X. 2008. Level invariant representation of sounds by populations of neurons in primary auditory cortex. *J. Neurosci.* 28: 3415–3426. [24]

Saez, J. C., Berthoud, V. M., Branes, M. C., et al. 2003. Plasma membrane channels formed by connexins: Their regulation and functions. *Physiol. Rev.* 83: 1359–1400. [11]

Saez, L., Meyer, P., and Young, M. W. 2007. A PER/TIM/DBT interval timer for *Drosophila*'s circadian clock. *Cold Spring Harb. Symp. Quant. Biol.* 72: 69–74. [19]

Safieddine, S., and Wenthold, R. J. 1999. SNARE complex at the ribbon synapses of cochlear hair cells: Analysis of synaptic vesicle- and synaptic membrane-associated proteins. *Eur. J. Neurosci.* 11: 803–812. [24]

Safiulina V. F., Fattorini, G., Conti, F., and Cherubini, E. 2006. GABAergic signaling at mossy fiber synapses in neonatal rat hippocampus. *J. Neurosci* 26: 597–608. [27]

Sagne, C., El Mestikaway, S., Isambert, M. F., et al. 1997. Cloning of a functional vesicular GABA and glycine transporter by screening genome databases. *FEBS Lett.* 417: 177–183. [9]

Sah, P., Hestrin, S., and Nicoll, R. A. 1990. Properties of excitatory postsynaptic currents recorded in vitro from rat hippocampal interneurones. *J. Physiol.* 430: 605–616. [11]

Sahley, C. L., Modney, B. K., Boulis, N. M., and Muller, K. J. 1994. The S cell: An interneuron essential for sensitization and full dishabituation of leech shortening. *J. Neurosci.* 14: 6715–6721. [20]

Sahni, V., and Kessler, J. A. 2010. Stem cell therapies for spinal cord injury. *Nat. Rev. Neurol.* 6: 363–372. [29]

Sajikumar, S. et al. 2014. Competition between recently potentiated synaptic inputs reveals a winner-take-all phase of synaptic tagging and capture. *Proc. Natl. Acad. Sci USA* 111: 12217–12221. [17]

Sakmann, B. 1992. Elementary steps in synaptic transmission revealed by currents through single ion channels. *Neuron* 8: 613–629. [11]

Sakmann, B., Noma, A., and Trautwein, W. 1983. Acetylcholine activation of single muscarinic K^+ channels in isolated pacemaker cells of the mammalian heart. *Nature* 303: 250–253. [12]

Sakuma, K., and Yamaguchi, A. 2010. The functional role of calcineurin in hypertrophy, regeneration, and disorders of skeletal muscle. *J. Biomed. Biotechnol.* 2010: 721219. [29]

Sakurai, M. 1987. Synaptic modification of parallel fibre-Purkinje cell transmission in *in vitro* guinea-pig cerebellar slices. *J. Physiol.* 394: 463–480. [16]

Sakurai, M. 1990. Calcium is an intracellular mediator of the climbing fiber induction of cerebellar long-term depression. *Proc. Natl. Acad. Sci. USA* 87: 3383–3385. [16]

Sakurai, T., Amemiya, A., Ishii, M., et al. 1998. Orexins and orexin receptors: A family of hypothalamic neuropeptides and G protein-coupled receptors that regulate feeding behavior. *Cell* 92: 573–585. [14]

Sale, A., Berardi, N., and Maffei, L. 2014. Environment and brain plasticity: Towards an endogenous pharmacotherapy. *Physiol. Rev.* 94: 189–234. [28]

Sale, A., Berardi, N., Spolidoro, M., et al. 2010. GABAergic inhibition in visual cortical plasticity. Front .Cell Neurosci. 4: 10. doi: 10.3389/fncel.2010.00010. [28]

Sala, C., O'Malley, J., Xu, R., et al. 1997. ε subunit-containing acetylcholine receptors in myotubes belong to the slowly degrading population. *J. Neurosci.* 17: 8937–8944. [29]

Salinas, E., Hernández, A., Zainos, A., and Romo, R. 2000. Periodicity and firing rate as candidate neural codes for the frequency of vibrotactile stimuli. *J. Neurosci.* 20: 5503–5515. [25]

Salio, C., Lossi, L., Ferrini, F., and Merighi, A. 2006. Neuropeptides as synaptic transmitters. *Cell Tissue Res.* 326: 583–598. [14, 15]

Salkoff, L., Baker, K., Butler, A., et al. 1992. An essential "set" of K^+ channels conserved in flies, mice and humans. *Trends Neurosci.* 15: 161–166. [5]

Salmons, S., and Sreter, F. A. 1975. The role of impulse activity in the transformation of skeletal muscle by cross innervation. *J. Anat.* 120: 412–415. [29]

Salpeter, M. M. 1987. Vertebrate neuromuscular junctions: General morphology, molecular organization, and functional consequences. In M. M. Salpeter (Ed.), *The Vertebrate Neuromuscular Junction.* Alan R. Liss, New York, pp. 1–54. [11, 15]

Salpeter, M. M., and Loring, R. H. 1985. Nicotinic acetylcholine receptors in vertebrate muscle: Properties, distribution and neural control. *Prog. Neurobiol.* 25: 297–325. [29]

Salpeter, M. M., and Marchaterre, M. 1992. Acetylcholine receptors in extrajunctional regions of innervated muscle have a slow degradation rate. *J. Neurosci.* 12: 35–38. [29]

Salter, M. W. and Beggs, S. 2014. Sublime microglia: Expanding roles for the guardians of the CNS. *Cell.* 158: 15–24. doi: 10.1016/j.cell.2014.06.008. [10]

Sámano, C., Zetina, M. E., Marín, M. A., et al. 2006. Choline acetyltransferase and neuropeptide immunoreactivities are colocalized in somata, but preferentially localized in distinct axon fibers and boutons of cat sympathetic preganglionic neurons. *Synapse* 60: 295–306. [19]

Sambandan, S., et al. 2017. Activity-dependent spatially localized miRNA maturation in neuronal dendrites. *Science* 355: 634–637. [17]

Samuels, S. E., Lipitz, J. B., Dahl, G., and Muller, K. J. 2010. Neuroglial ATP release through innexin channels controls microglial cell movement to a nerve injury. *J. Gen. Physiol.* 136: 425–442. [10, 14, 29]

Sandler, V. M., and Ross, W. N. 1999. Serotonin modulates spike back-propagation and associated $[Ca^{2+}]_i$ changes in the apical dendrites of hippocampal CA1 pyramidal neurons. *J. Neurophysiol.* 81: 216–224. [8]

Sandyk, R. 1992. L-Tryptophan in neuropsychiatric disorders: A review. *Int. J. Neurosci.* 67: 127–144. [15]

Sanes, D. H., and Bao, S. 2009. Tuning up the developing auditory CNS. *Curr. Opin. Neurobiol.* 19: 188–199. [28]

Sanes, D. H., Reh, T. A., and Harris, W. A. 2011. *Development of the Nervous System,* 3rd ed. Academic Press. Burlington, VT. [27]

Sanes, J. R., and Lichtman, J. W. 1999. Development of the vertebrate neuromuscular junction. *Annu. Rev. Neurosci.* 22: 389–442. [29]

Sanes, J. R., and Lichtman, J. W. 2001. Induction, assembly, maturation and maintenance of a postsynaptic apparatus. *Nat. Rev. Neurosci.* 2: 791–805. [11]

Sanes, J. R. and Masland, R. H. 2015 The types of retinal ganglion cells: Current status and implications for neuronal classification. *Annual Review of Neuroscience* 38: 221–246. [22]

Sanes, J. R., and Zipursky, S. L. 2010. Design principles of insect and vertebrate visual systems. *Neuron* 66: 15–36. [27]

Sanes, J. R., Marshall, L. M., and McMahan, U. J. 1978. Reinnervation of muscle fiber basal lamina after removal of muscle fibers. *J. Cell Biol.* 78: 176–198. [29]

Sanhueza, M., and Lisman J. 2013. The CaMKII/NMDAR complex as a molecular memory. *Mol. Brain* 6:10. [17]

Sankaranarayanan, S., and Ryan, T. A. 2000. Real time measurements of vesicle SNARE recycling in synapses of the central nervous system. *Nat. Cell Biol.* 2: 197–204. [13]

Santello, M., et al. 2019. Astrocyte function from information processing to cognition and cognitive impairment. *Nat. Neurosci.* 22: 154–166. [17]

Saper, C. B. 2002. The central autonomic nervous system: Conscious visceral perception and autonomic pattern generation. *Annu. Rev. Neurosci.* 25: 433–469. [19]

Saper, C. B., and Fuller, P. M. 2007. Inducible clocks: Living in an unpredictable world. *Cold Spring Harb. Symp. Quant. Biol.* 72: 543–550. [19]

Sara, S. J. 2008. The locus coeruleus and noradrenergic modulation of cognition. *Nat. Rev. Neurosci.* 10: 211–223. [14]

Sarfati, J., Dodé, C., and Young, J. 2010. Kallmann syndrome caused by mutations in the PROK2 and PROKR2 genes: Pathophysiology and genotype-phenotype correlations. *Front. Horm. Res.* 39: 121–32. [27]

Sargent, P. B. 1993. The diversity of neuronal nicotinic acetylcholine receptors. *Annu. Rev. Neurosci.* 16: 403–443. [14]

Sargent, P. B., and Pang, D. Z. 1989. Acetylcholine receptor-like molecules are found in both synaptic and extrasynaptic clusters on the surface of neurons in the frog cardiac ganglion. *J. Neurosci.* 9: 1062–1072. [29]

Sargent, P. B., Bryan, G. K., Streichert, L. C., and Garrett, E. N. 1991. Denervation does not alter the number of neuronal bungarotoxin binding sites on autonomic neurons in the frog cardiac ganglion. *J. Neurosci.* 11: 3610–3623. [29]

Sarkar, B., Das, A. K., Arumugam, S., et al. 2012. The dynamics of somatic exocytosis in monoaminergic neurons. *Front. Physiol.* 3: 414. doi: 10.3389/fphys.2012.00414. [18]

Sarter, M., Hasselmo, M. E., Bruno, J. P., and Givens, B. 2005. Unraveling the attentional functions of cortical cholinergic inputs: Interactions between signal-driven and cognitive modulation of signal detection. *Brain Res. Brain Res. Rev.* 48: 98–111. [14]

Sasai, Y. 1998. Identifying the missing links: Genes that connect neural induction and primary neurogenesis in vertebrate embryos. *Neuron* 21: 455–458. [27]

Saunders, N. R., Ek, C. J., Habgood, M. D., and Dziegielewska, K. M. 2008. Barriers in the brain: A renaissance? *Trends Neurosci.* 31: 279–286. [10]

Saunders, N. R., Kitchener, P., Knott, G. W., et al. 1998. Development of walking, swimming and neuronal connections after complete spinal cord transection in the neonatal opossum, *Monodelphis domestica*. *J. Neurosci.* 18: 339–355. [29]

Savchenko, A., Barnes, S., and Kramer, R. H. 1997. Cyclic-nucleotide-gated channels mediate synaptic feedback by nitric oxide. *Nature* 390: 694–698. [12]

Sawada, K., Echigo, N., Juge, N., et al. 2008. Identification of a vesicular nucleotide transporter. *Proc. Natl. Acad. Sci. USA* 105: 5683–5686. [15]

Scanziani, M. 2000. GABA spillover activates postsynaptic $GABA_B$ receptors to control rhythmic hippocampal activity. *Neuron* 25: 673–681. [14]

Scemes, E., Suadicani, S. O., Dahl, G., and Spray, D. C. 2007. Connexin and pannexin mediated cell-cell communication. *Neuron Glia Biol.* 3: 199–208. [10]

Scarpa, E., and Mayor, R. 2016. Collective cell migration in development. *J. Cell Biol.* 212: 143–155. [27]

Schafer, D. P., et al. 2012. Microglia sculpt postnatal neural circuits in an activity and complement-dependent manner. *Neuron* 74: 691–705. [17]

Schafer D. P., Lehrman E. K., and Stevens B. 2013. The "quad-partite" synapse: Microglia-synapse interactions in the developing and mature CNS. *Glia.* 61: 24–36. [10]

Schaller, K. L., Krzemien, D. M., Yarowsky, P. J., et al. 1995. A novel, abundant sodium channel expressed in neurons and glia. *J. Neurosci.* 15: 3231–3242. [7]

Schalling, M., Stieg, P. E., Lindquist, C., et al. 1989. Rapid increase in enzyme and peptide mRNA in sympathetic ganglia after electrical stimulation in humans. *Proc. Natl. Acad. Sci. USA* 86: 4302–4305. [15]

Schecterson, L. C., and Bothwell, M. 2010. Neurotrophin receptors: Old friends with new partners. *Dev. Neurobiol.* 70: 332–338. [27]

Scheutze, S. M., and Role, L. M. 1987. Developmental regulation of nicotinic acetylcholine receptors. *Annu. Rev. Neurosci.* 10: 403–457. [29]

Schikorski, T., and Stevens, C. F. 1997. Quantitative ultrastructural analysis of hippocampal excitatory synapses. *J. Neurosci.* 17: 5858–5867. [13]

Schiller, P. H. Parallel information processing channels created in the retina. *Proc. Natl. Acad. Sci. USA* 107: 17087–17094. [22]

Schliebs, R., and Arendt, T. 2006. The significance of the cholinergic system in the brain during aging and in Alzheimer's disease. *J. Neural Transm.* 113: 1625–1644. [14]

Schmelz, M., Schmidt, R., Weidner, C., et al. 2003. Chemical response pattern of different classes of C-nociceptors to pruritogens and algogens. *J. Neurophysiol.* 89: 2441–2448. [23]

Schmidt, B. P., Sabesan, R., Tuten, et al. 2018. Sensations from a single M-cone depend on the activity of surrounding S-cones. *Sci Rep 8*: 8561. doi: 10.1038/s41598-018-26754-1. [22]

Schmidt, R. F. 1971. Presynaptic inhibition in the vertebrate central nervous system. *Ergeb. Physiol.* 63: 20–101. [11]

Schmitt, S. 2003. Homeosis and atavistic regeneration: The "biogenetic law" in Entwicklungsmechanik. *Hist. Philos. Life Sci.* 25: 193–210. [27]

Schmolesky, M. T., Wang, Y., Hanes, D. P., et al. 1998. Signal timing across the macaque visual system. *J. Neurophysiol.* 79: 3272–3278. [25]

Schnapf, J. L., and Baylor, D. A. 1987. How photoreceptor cells respond to light. *Sci. Am.* 256: 40–47. [22]

Schnapf, J. L., Kraft, T. W., Nunn, B. J., and Baylor, D. A. 1988. Spectral sensitivity of primate photoreceptors. *Vis. Neurosci.* 1: 255–261. [22]

Schnapp, B. J., Vale, R. D., Sheetz, M. P., and Reese, T. S. 1985. Single microtubules from squid axoplasm support bidirectional movement of organelles. *Cell* 40: 455–462. [15]

Schnell, L., and Schwab, M. E. 1990. Axonal regeneration in the rat spinal cord produced by an antibody against myelin-associated neurite growth inhibitors. *Nature* 343: 269–272. [29]

Schnetkamp, P. P. 2004. The *SLC24* Na^+/Ca^{2+}- K^+ exchanger family: Vision and beyond. *Pflügers Arch.* 447: 683–688. [9]

Schnitzer, M. J., and Block, S. M. 1997. Kinesin hydrolyses one ATP per 8-nm step. *Nature* 388: 386–390. [18]

Schnitzer, M. J., and Meister, M. 2003. Multineuronal firing patterns in the signal from eye to brain. *Neuron* 37: 499–511. [22]

Schnupp, J. W., Hall, T. M., Kokelaar, R. F., and Ahmed, B. 2006. Plasticity of temporal pattern codes for vocalization stimuli in primary auditory cortex. *J. Neurosci.* 26: 4785–4795. [24]

Scholfield, C. N. 1978. A barbiturate induced intensification of the inhibitory potential in slices of guinea-pig olfactory cortex. *J. Physiol.* 275: 559–566. [14]

Scholfield, C. N. 1980. Potentiation of inhibition by general anaesthetics in neurones of the olfactory cortex in vitro. *Pflügers Arch.* 383: 249–255. [14]

Schonweiler, R., Ptok, M., and Radu, H. J. 1998. A cross-sectional study of speech- and language-abilities of children with normal hearing, mild fluctuating conductive hearing loss, or moderate to profound sensoneurinal hearing loss. *Int. J. Pediatr. Otorhinolaryngol.* 44: 251–258. [28]

Schramm, M., and Selinger, Z. 1984. Message transmission: Receptor controlled adenylate cyclase system. *Science* 225: 1350–1356. [12]

Schratt, G., et al. 2006. A brain-specific microRNA regulates dendritic spine development. *Nature* 439: 283–289. [17]

Schratt, G. 2009. microRNAs at the synapse. *Nat. Rev. Neurosci.* 10: 842–849. doi: 10.1038/nrn2763. [17]

Schreiner, C. E., and Winer, J. A. 2007. Auditory cortex mapmaking: Principles, projections, and plasticity. *Neuron* 56: 356–365. [24, 27]

Schuldiner, S., Schirvan, A., and Linial, M. 1995. Vesicular neurotransmitter transporters: From bacteria to humans. *Physiol. Rev.* 75: 369–392. [9]

Schulman, H. 1995. Protein phosphorylation in neuronal plasticity and gene expression. *Curr. Opin. Neurobiol.* 5: 375–381. [16]

Schultz, W., Dayan, P., and Montague, R. R. 1997. A neural substrate of prediction and reward. *Science* 275: 1593–1599. [14]

Schummers, J., Yu, H., and Sur, M. 2008. Tuned responses of astrocytes and their influence on hemodynamic signals in the visual cortex. *Science* 320: 1638–1643. [10]

Schwab, M. E. 2004. Nogo and axon regeneration. *Curr. Opin. Neurobiol.* 14: 118–1124. [10]

Schwab, M. E., and Caroni, P. 1988. Oligodendrocytes and CNS myelin are nonpermissive substrates for neurite growth and fibroblast spreading in vitro. *J. Neurosci.* 8: 2381–2393. [29]

Schwab, M. E., and Strittmatter, S. M. 2014. Nogo limits neural plasticity and recovery from injury. *Curr. Op. Neurobiol.* 27: 53–60. [29]

Schwartz, E. A. 1987. Depolarization without calcium can release gamma-aminobutyric acid from a retinal neuron. *Science* 238: 350–355. [13, 22]

Schwartzman, R. J., and Semmes, J. 1971. The sensory cortex and tactile sensitivity. *Exp. Neurol.* 33: 147–158. [23]

Schwarz, J. R., Glassmeier, G., Cooper, E. C., et al. 2006. KCNQ channels mediate I_{Ks}, a slow K^+ current regulating excitability in the rat node of Ranvier. *J. Physiol.* 573: 17–34. [8]

Scott, S. H. 2008. Inconvenient truths about neural processing in primary motor cortex. *J. Physiol.* 586: 1217–1224. [26]

Seabrook, T. A., Burbridge, T. J., Crair, M. C., and Huberman, A. D. 2017. Architecture, Function, and Assembly of the Mouse Visual System. *Annu. Rev. Neurosci.* 40: 499–538. [28]

Seal, R. P., and Edwards, R. H. 2006. Functional implications of neurotransmitter co-release: Glutamate and GABA share the load. *Curr. Opin. Pharmacol.* 6: 114–119. [15]

Seal, R. P., Akil, O., Yi, E., et al. 2008. Sensineuronal deafness and seizures in mice lacking vesicular glutamate transporter 3. *Neuron* 24: 173–174. [9]

Seamans, J. K., and Yang, C. R. 2004. The principal features and mechanisms of dopamine modulation in the prefrontal cortex. *Prog. Neurobiol.* 74: 1–58. [14]

Sears, T. A. 1964. Efferent discharges in alpha and fusimotor fibers of intercostal nerves of the cat. *J. Physiol.* 174: 295–315. [26]

Seeburg, P. H., and Hartner, J. 2003. Regulation of ion channel/neurotransmitter receptor function by RNA editing. *Curr. Opin. Neurobiol.* 13: 279–283. [14]

Seeburg, P. H., Single, F., Kuner, T., et al. 2001. Genetic manipulation of key determinants of ion flow in glutamate receptor channels in the mouse. *Brain Res.* 907: 233–243. [27]

Seeger, M., Tear, G., Ferres-Marco, D., and Goodman, C. S. 1993. Mutations affecting growth cone guidance in *Drosophila*: Genes necessary for guidance toward or away from the midline. *Neuron* 10: 409–426. [27]

Seidah, N. G., and Chretien, M. 1997. Eukaryotic protein processing: Endoproteolysis of precursor proteins. *Curr. Opin. Biotechnol.* 8: 602–607. [15]

Sekine, Y., Lin-Moore, A., Chenette, D. M., et al. 2018. Functional Genome-wide Screen Identifies Pathways Restricting Central Nervous System Axonal Regeneration. *Cell Rep.* 23: 415–428. [29]

Selverston, A. I., and Ayers, J. 2006. Oscillations and oscillatory behavior in small neural circuits. *Biol. Cybern.* 95: 537–554. [19]

Selyanko, A. A., Derkach, V., and Skok, V. I. 1979. Fast excitatory postsynaptic currents in voltage-clamped mammalian sympathetic ganglion neurons. *J. Auton. Ner. Syst.* 1: 127–137. [19]

Semmes, J., Porter, L., and Randolph, M. C. 1974. Further studies of anterior postcentral lesions in monkeys. *Cortex* 10: 55–68. [23]

Semon, R. 1904. *Die Mneme als erhaltendes Prinzip im Wechsel des organischen Geschehens.* Wilhelm Engelmann, Leipzig, 1904. [17]

Sengpiel, F., Stawinski, P., and Bonhoeffer, T. 1999. Influence of experience on orientation maps in cat visual cortex. *Nat Neurosci.* 2: 727–732. [28]

Serizawa, S., Miyamichi, K., Nakatani, H., et al. 2003. Negative feedback regulation ensures the one receptor-one olfactory neuron rule in mouse. *Science* 302: 2088–2094. [21]

Severini, C., Improta, G., Falconieri-Erspamer, G., et al. 2002. The tachykinin peptide family. *Pharmacol. Rev.* 54: 285–322. [14]

Shackleton, T. M., Skottun, B. C., Arnott, R. H., and Palmer, A. R. 2003. Interaural time difference discrimination thresholds for single neurons in the inferior colliculus of Guinea pigs. *J. Neurosci.* 23: 716–724. [24]

Shah, M. M., Migliore, M., Valencia, I., et al. 2008. Functional significance of K_v7 channels in hippocampal pyramidal neurons. *Proc. Natl. Acad. Sci. USA.* 22: 7869–7874. [8, 14]

Shain, D. H., ed. 2009. *Annelids in Modern Biology.* Wiley-Blackwell, Hoboken, NJ. [20]

Shain, D. H., Stuart, D. K., Huang, F. Z., and Weisblat, D. A. 2000. Segmentation of the central nervous system in leech. *Development* 127: 735–744. [27]

Shapiro, L., Love, J., and Colman, D. R. 2007. Adhesion molecules in the nervous system: Structural insights into function and diversity. *Annu. Rev. Neurosci.* 30: 451–474. [27]

Shapovalov, A. I., and Shiriaev, B. I. 1980. Dual mode of junctional transmission at synapses between single primary afferent fibres and motoneurones in the amphibian. *J. Physiol.* 306: 1–15. [11]

Sharpee, T. O. 2016. How invariant feature selectivity is achieved in cortex. *Front. Synaptic Neurosci.* 8: 26. doi: 10.3389/fnsyn.2016.00026) [25]

Sharuna, N., Harlow, M. L., Jung, J. H., et al. 2009. Macromolecular connections of active zone material to docked synaptic vesicles and presynaptic membrane at neuromuscular junctions of the mouse. *J. Comp. Neurol.* 513: 457–468. [13]

Shatz, C. J. 1977. Anatomy of interhemispheric connections in the visual system. *J. Comp. Neurol.* 173: 497–518. [3]

Shatz, C. J. 1996. Emergence of order in visual system development. *Proc. Natl. Acad. Sci. USA* 93: 602–608. [28]

Shatz, C. J., and Luskin, M. B. 1986. The relationship between the geniculocortical afferents and their cortical target cells during development of the cat's primary visual cortex. *J. Neurosci.* 6: 3655–3668. [27]

Shatz, C. J., and Stryker, M. P. 1978. Ocular dominance in layer IV of the cat's visual cortex and the effects of monocular deprivation. *J. Physiol.* 281: 267–283. [28]

Sheetz, M. P. 1999. Motor and cargo interactions. *Eur. J. Biochem.* 262: 19–25. [15]

Shekhar, K., Lapan, S. W., Whitney, I. E., et al. 2016. Comprehensive classification of retinal bipolar neurons by single-cell transcriptomics. *Cell* 166: 1308–1323.e30. doi: 10.1016/j.cell.2016.07.054. [22]

Shen, H., Jhou, Q., Pan, X., et al. 2017. Structure of a eukaryotic voltage-gated sodium channel at near-atomic resolution. *Science* 355,eaal4326. doi: 10.1126/science,aal4326. [5]

Shen, K., Fetter, R. D., and Bargmann, C. I. 2004. Synaptic specificity is generated by the synaptic guidepost protein SYG-2 and its receptor, SYG-1. *Cell* 116: 869–881. [27]

Shen, Q., et al. 2006. The timing of cortical neurogenesis is encoded within lineages of individual progenitor cells. *Nat. Neurosci.* 9: 743. [27]

Shen, W., Hamilton, S. E., Nathanson, N. M., and Surmeier, D. J. 2005. Cholinergic suppression of KCNQ channel currents enhances excitability of striatal medium spiny neurons. *J. Neurosci.* 25: 7449–7458. [12, 14]

Sheng, M., and Lee, S. H. 2000. Growth of the NMDA receptor industrial complex. *Nat. Neurosci.* 3: 633–635. [11]

Shepard, R. N. 1990. *Mind Sights: Original Visual Illusions, Ambiguities, and other Anomalies.* W. H. Freeman, New York. [3]

Sherman, S. M. 2007. The thalamus is more than just a relay. *Curr. Opin. Neurobiol.* 17: 417–422. [2]

Sherrington, C. S. 1906. *The Integrative Action of the Nervous System.* Reprint, Yale University Press, New Haven, CT, 1966. [1]

Sherrington, C. S. 1906. *The Integrative Action of the Nervous System,* 1961 ed. Yale University Press, New Haven, CT. [26]

Sherrington, C. S. 1910. Flexor-reflex of the limb, crossed extension reflex, and reflex stepping and standing (cat and dog). *J. Physiol.* 40: 28–121. [26]

Sherrington, C. S. 1933. *The brain and Its Mechanism.* Cambridge University Press, London. [26]

Sherrington, C. S. 1951. *Man on His Nature.* Cambridge University Press, Cambridge. [2, 22]

Shi, S.-H., Hayashi, Y., Esteban, J. A., and Malinowm R. 2001. Subunit-specific rules governing AMPA receptor trafficking to synapses in hippocampal pyramidal neurons. *Cell* 105: 331–343. [16]

Shi, S-H., Hayashi, Y., Petralia, R. S., et al. 1999. Rapid spine delivery and redistribution of AMPA receptors after synaptic NMDA receptor activation. *Science* 284: 1811–1816. [16]

Shibuya, I. et al. 1998. PACAP increases the cytosolic $Ca2'$ concentration and stimulatcs somatodendritic vasopressin release in rat supraoptic neurones. *J. Neuroendocrinol.* 10: 31–42. [18]

Shichida, Y., Imai, H., Imamoto, Y., et al. 1994. Is chicken green-sensitive cone visual pigment a rhodopsin-like pigment? A comparative study of the molecular properties between chicken green and rhodopsin. *Biochemistry,* 33: 9040–9044. [22]

Shigeoka, T., Jung, H., Jung, J., et al. 2016. Dynamic axonal translation in developing and mature visual circuits. *Cell* 166: 181–192. [1, 17]

Shigeoka, T., et al. 2019. On-site ribosome remodeling by locally synthesized ribosomal proteins in axons. *Cell Rep.* 29: 3605. [17]

Shik, M. L., and Orlovsky, G. N. 1976. Neurophysiology of locomotor automatism. *Physiol. Rev.* 56: 465–501. [26]

Shimomura, O., and Johnson, F. H. 1970. Calcium binding, quantum yield, and emitting molecule in aequorin bioluminescence. *Nature* 227: 1356–1357. [12]

Shiogemua, N. and Ninomiya, Y. 2016. Recent advances in molecular mechanisms of taste signaling and modifying. *Int. Rev. Cell. Mol. Biol.* 23: 71–106. [21]

Shlens, J., Rieke, F., and Chichilnisky, E. 2008. Synchronized firing in the retina. *Curr. Opin. Neurobiol.* 18: 396–402. [22]

Shmuel, A., Korman, M., Sterkin, A., et al. 2005. Retinotopic axis specificity and selective clustering of feedback projections from V2 to V1 in the owl monkey. *J. Neurosci.* 25: 2117–2131. [3]

Shooter, E. M. 2001. Early days of the nerve growth factor proteins. *Annu. Rev. Neurosci.* 24: 601–629. [27]

Shotwell, S. L., Jacobs, R., and Hudspeth, A. J. 1981. Directional sensitivity of individual vertebrate hair cells to controlled deflection of their hair bundles. *Ann. NY Acad. Sci.* 374: 1–10. [21]

Shoykhet, M., Doherty, D., and Simons, D. J. 2000. Coding of deflection velocity and amplitude by whisker primary afferent neurons: Implications for higher level processing. *Somatosens. Mot. Res.* 17: 171–180. [23]

Shrager, P., Chiu, S. Y., and Ritchie, J. M. 1985. Voltage-dependent sodium and potassium channels in mammalian cultured Schwann cells. *Proc. Natl. Acad. Sci. USA.* 82: 948–952. [10]

Shyng, S.-L., Xu, R., and Salpeter, M. M. 1991. Cyclic AMP stabilizes the degradation of original junctional acetylcholine receptors in denervated muscle. *Neuron* 6: 469–475. [29]

Si, K., Lindquist, S., and Kandel, E. 2004. A possible epigenetic mechanism for the persistence of memory. *Cold Spring Harb. Symp. Quant. Biol.* 69: 497–498. [20]

Sidorov, M. S., Auerbach, B. D., and Bear, M. F. 2013. Fragile X mental retardation protein and synaptic plasticity. *Mol.Brain* 6: 15. [17]

Siegel, G. J., Agranoff, B. W., Albers, R. W., and Molinoff, P. B. 1994. Basic *Neurochemistry: Molecular, Cellular and Medical Aspects* 5th edition. Lippincott-Raven: Philadelphia, PA. [15]

Siepka, S. M., Yoo, S. H., Park, J., et al. 2007. Genetics and neurobiology of circadian clocks in mammals. *Cold Spring Harb. Symp. Quant. Biol.* 72: 251–259. [19]

Sierra, A., de Castro, F., del Río-Hortega, J., et al. 2016. The "Big-Bang" for modern glial biology: Translation and comments on Pío del Río-Hortega 1919 series of papers on microglia. *Glia.* 64: 1801–1840. doi: 10.1002/glia.23046. [10]

Sigworth, F. J. 1994. Voltage gating of ion channels. *Q. Rev. Biophys.* 27: 1–40. [5]

Sigworth, F. J., and Neher, E. 1980. Single Na⁺ channel currents observed in cultured rat muscle cells. *Nature* 287: 447–449. [7]

Silinsky, E. M., and Redman, R. S. 1996. Synchronous release of ATP and neurotransmitter within milliseconds of a motor-nerve impulse in the frog. *J. Physiol.* 492: 815–822. [13]

Silva, A. J., et al. 1998. CREB and memory. *Ann. Rev. Neurosci.* 21: 127–148. [17]

Silver, J. 2010. Much Ado about Nogo. *Neuron* 66: 619–621. [29]

Silver, J. 2016. The glial scar is more than just astrocytes. *Exp. Neurol.* 286: 147–149. doi/10.1016/j.expneurol.2016.06.018. [29]

Silver, R. A. et al. 1996. Deactivation and desensitization of non-NMDA receptors in patches and the time course of EPSCs in rat cerebellar granule cells. *J. Physiol.* 493: 167–173. [18]

Simakov, O., Marletaz, F., Cho, S. J., et al. 2013. Insights into bilaterian evolution from three spiralian genomes. *Nature* 493: 526–531. doi: 10.1038/nature11696. [20]

Simmons, M. L. et al. 1995. L-type calcium channels mediate dynorphin neuropeptide release from dendrites but not axons of hippocampal granule cells. *Neuron* 14: 1265–1272. [18]

Simões, G. F., and Oliveira, A. L. 2010. Alpha motoneurone input changes in dystrophic MDX mice after sciatic nerve transection. *Neuropathol. Appl. Neurobiol.* 36: 55–70. [29]

Simon, E. J., Hiller, J. M., and Edelman, I. 1973. Stereospecific binding of the potent narcotic analgesic [³H]Etorphine to rat-brain homogenate. *Proc. Natl. Acad. Sci. USA* 70: 1947–1949. [23]

Simon, H., Hornbruch, A., and Lumsden, A. 1995. Independent assignment of antero-posterior and dorso-ventral positional values in the developing chick hindbrain. *Curr. Biol.* 5: 205–214. [27]

Simons, D. J. 1978. Response properties of vibrissa units in rat S. I. somatosensory neocortex. *J. Neurophysiol.* 41: 798–820. [23]

Sims, T. J., Waxman, S. G., Black, J. A., and Gilmore, S. A. 1985. Perinodal astrocytic processes at notes of Ranvier in developing normal and glial cell deficient rat spinal cord. *Brain Res.* 337: 321–331. [10]

Sincich, L. C., and Horton, J. C. 2005. The circuitry of V₁ AND V₂: Integration of color, form, and motion. *Ann. Rev. Neurosci.* 28: 303–326. [3]

Sincich, L. C., Jocson, C. M., and Horton, J. C. 2007. Neurons in V1 patch columns project to V2 thin stripes. *Cereb. Cortex* 17: 935–941. [3]

Sincich, L. C., Park, K. F., Wohlgemuth, M. J., and Horton, J. C. 2004. Bypassing V1: A direct geniculate input to area MT. *Nat. Neurosci.* 7: 1123–1128. [3]

Sinclair, R. J., and Burton, H. 1993. Neuronal activity in the second somatosensory cortex of monkeys (*Macaca mulatta*) during active touch of gratings. *J. Neurophysiol.* 70: 331–350. [23]

Singer, W. 1995. Development and plasticity of cortical processing architectures. *Science* 270: 758–764. [28]

Sive, H. L., Grainger, R. M., and Harland, R. M. 2010. Microinjection of *Xenopus* embryos. *Cold Spring Harb. Protoc.* 2010: Pdb ip81. [27]

Sivilotti, L. 2010. What single-channel analysis tells us of the activation mechanism of ligand-gated channels: The case of the glycine receptor. *J. Physiol.* 588: 45–58. [14]

Sivilotti, L., and Colquhoun, D. 1995. Acetylcholine receptors: Too many channels, too few functions. *Science* 269: 1681–1682. [14]

Sivilotti, L., and Colquhoun, D. 2016. In praise of single channel kinetics. *J. Gen. Physiol.* 148: 79–88. [11]

Sjöqvist, M. and Andersson, E. R. 2019. Do as I say, Not(ch) as I do: Lateral control of cell fate. *Dev. Biology* 447: 58–70. [27]

Skene, J. H. P., and Shooter, E. M. 1983. Denervated sheath cells secrete a new protein after nerve injury. *Proc. Natl. Acad. Sci. USA* 80: 4169–4173. [29]

Skinner, D. C. et al. 1997. Simultaneous measurement of gonadotropin-releasing hormone in the third ventricular cerebrospinal fluid and hypophyseal portal blood of the ewe. *Endocrinology* 138: 4699–4704. [18]

Skipor, J., and Thiery, J. C. 2008. The choroid plexus--cerebrospinal fluid system: Undervaluated pathway of neuroendocrine signaling into the brain. *Acta Neurobiol. Exp. (Wars)* 68: 414–428. [18]

Skou, J. C. 1957. The influence of some cations on an adenosine triphosphatase from peripheral nerves. *Biochim. Biophys. Acta* 23: 394–401. [9]

Skou, J. C. 1988. Overview: The Na,K pump. *Methods Enzymol.* 156: 1–25. [9]

Slobodov, U., Reichert, F., Mirski, R., and Rotshenker, S. 2009. The role of Galectin-3/MAC-2 in the activation of the innate-immune function of phagocytosis in microglia in injury and disease. *J. Mol. Neurosci.* 39: 99–103. [10]

Smart, T. G., Hosie, A. M., and Miller, P. 2004. Zn²⁺ ions: Modulators of excitatory and inhibitory synaptic activity. *Neuroscientist* 10: 432–442. [14]

Smeyne, R. J., Klein, R., Schnapp, A., et al. 1994. Severe sensory and sympathetic neuropathies in mice carrying a disrupted Trk/NGF receptor gene. *Nature* 368: 246–249. [27]

Smith, A. D., de Potter, W. P., Moerman, E. J., and Schaepdryver, A. F. 1970. Release of dopamine β-hydroxylase and chromogranin A upon stimulation of the splenic nerve. *Tissue Cell* 2: 547–568. [13]

Smith, R. J., Bale, J. F., Jr., and White, K. R. 2005. Sensorineural hearing loss in children. *Lancet* 365: 879–890. [28]

Snyder, S. H., Jaffrey, S. R., and Zakhary, R. 1998. Nitric oxide and carbon monoxide: Parallel roles as neural messengers. *Brain Res. Brain Res. Rev.* 26: 167–175. [12]

So, I., Ashmole, I., Davies, N. W., et al. The K⁺ channel signature sequence of murine Kir 2.1: Mutations that affect microscopic gating but not ion selectivity. *J. Physiol.* 531.1: 37–50. [5]

Sobkowicz, H. M., Rose, J. E., Scott, G. L., and Slapnick, S. M. 1982. Ribbon synapses in the developing intact and cultured organ of Corti in the mouse. *J. Neurosci.* 2: 942–957. [24]

Soderling, T. 2000. CaM-kinases: Modulators of synaptic plasticity. *Curr Opin. Neurobiol.* 10: 375–380. [12]

Soejima, M., and Noma, A. 1984. Mode of regulation of the ACh-sensitive K-channel by the muscarinic receptor in rabbit atrial cells. *Pflügers Arch.* 400: 424–431. [12]

Soghomonian, J. J., and Martin, D. L. 1998. Two isoforms of glutamate decarboxylase: Why? *Trends Pharmacol. Sci.* 19: 500–505. [15]

Söhl, G., Maxeiner, S., and Willecke, K. 2005. Expression and functions of neuronal gap junctions. *Nat. Rev. Neurosci.* 6: 191–200. [11]

Sokoloff, L. 1977. Relation between physiological function and energy metabolism in the central nervous system. *J. Neurochem.* 29: 13–26. [3]

Sokolov, S., Scheuer, T., and Catterall, W. A. 2005. Ion permeation through a voltage-sensitive gating pore in brain sodium channels having voltage sensor mutations. *Neuron* 47: 183–189. [7]

Sokolov, S., Scheuer, T., and Catterall, W. A. 2007. Gating pore currents in an inherited ion channelopathy. *Nature* 446: 76–78. [6]

Sokolove, P. G., and Cooke, I. M. 1971. Inhibition of impulse activity in a sensory neuron by an electrogenic pump. *J. Gen. Physiol.* 57: 125–163. [21]

Sokolowski, B., Duncan, R. K., Chen, S., et al. 2009. The large-conductance Ca²⁺-activated K⁺ channel interacts with the apolipoprotein ApoA1. *Biochem. Biophys. Res. Commun.* 387: 671–675. [24]

Soldner, F., et al. 2011. Generation of isogenic pluripotent stem cells differing exclusively at two early onset Parkinson point mutations. *Cell* 146: 318. [27]

Soldovieri, M. S., Miceli, F. and Taglialatela, M. 2011 Driving with no brakes: Molecular pathophysiology of Kv7 potassium channels. *Physiology* 26: 365–376. [5]

Solecki, D. J., Model, L., Gaetz, J., et al. 2004. Par6alpha signaling controls glial-guided neuronal migration. *Nat. Neurosci.* 7: 1169–1170. [10]

Sommer, B., Kohler, M., Sprengle, R., and Seeburg, P. H. 1991. RNA editing in brain controls a determinant of ion flow in glutamate-gated channels. *Cell* 67: 11–19. [5]

Son, Y. J., and Thompson, W. J. 1995. Schwann cell processes guide regeneration of peripheral axons. *Neuron* 14: 125–132. [10, 29]

Son, Y. J., and Thompson, W. J. 1995. Nerve sprouting in muscle is induced and guided by processes extended by Schwann cells. *Neuron* 14: 133–141. [10, 29]

Son, Y. J., Trachtenberg, J. T., and Thompson, W. J. 1996. Schwann cells induce and guide sprouting and reinnervation of neuromuscular junctions. *Trends Neurosci.* 19: 280–285. [10]

Sorg, B. A., Berretta, S., Blacktop, J. M., et al. 2016. Casting a Wide Net: Role of Perineuronal Nets in Neural Plasticity. *J. Neurosci.* 36: 11459–11468. [28]

Soshnikova, N., and Duboule, D. 2009. Epigenetic regulation of vertebrate *Hox* genes: A dynamic equilibrium. *Epigenetics* 4: 537–540. [27]

Sosinsky, G. E., and Nicholson, B. J. 2005. Structural organization of gap junction channels. *Biochim. Biophys. Acta* 1711: 99–125. [8]

Sossin, W. S. and Costa-Mattioli, M. 2018. Translational control in the brain in health and disease. *Cold Spring Harb. Perspect. Biol.* doi: 10.1101/cshperspect. a032912. [17]

Sossin, W. S., Fisher, J. M., and Scheller, R. H. 1989. Cellular and molecular biology of neuropeptide processing and packaging. *Neuron* 2: 1407–1417. [15]

Sotelo, C., and Alvarado-Mallart, R. M. 1991. The reconstruction of cerebellar circuits. *Trends Neurosci.* 14: 350–355. [29]

Sotelo, C., Alvarado-Mallart, R. M., Frain, M., and Vernet, M. 1994. Molecular plasticity of adult Bergmann fibers is associated with radial migration of grafted Purkinje cells. *J. Neurosci.* 14: 124–133. [29]

Sotelo, C., Llinás, R., and Baker, R. 1974. Structural study of inferior olivary nucleus of the cat: Morphological correlates of electrotonic coupling. *J. Neurophysiol.* 37: 541–559. [8]

Soto, F., Garcia-Guzman, M., and Stühmer, W. 1997. Cloned ligand-gated channels activated by extracellular ATP (P2X receptors). *J. Membr. Biol.* 160: 91–100. [19]

Sousa, A. M. M., et al. 2017. Evolution of the human nervous system function, structure, and development. *Cell* 170: 226–247. [27]

Southwell, D. G., Froemke, R. C., Alvarez-Buylla, A., et al. 2010. Cortical plasticity induced by inhibitory neuron transplantation. *Science* 327: 1145–1148. [28]

Spacek, J., and Harris, K. M. 1998. Three-dimensional organization of cell adhesion junctions at synapses and dendritic spines in area CA1 of the rat hippocampus. *J. Comp. Neurol.* 393: 58–68. [11]

Spalding, K. L., et al., 2013. Dynamics of hippocampal neurogenesis in adult humans. *Cell* 153: 1219–1227. [27]

Specht, S., and Grafstein, B. 1973. Accumulation of radioactive protein in mouse cerebral cortex after injection of [3H]-fucose into the eye. *Exp. Neurol.* 41: 705–722. [3]

Spemann, H., and Mangold, H. 1924. Induction of embryonic primordia by implantation of organizers from a different species. *Arch. Mikr. Anat. EntwMech* 100: 599–638. [27]

Sperry, R. W. 1963. Chemoaffinity in the orderly growth of nerve fiber patterns and connections. *Proc. Natl. Acad. Sci. USA* 50: 703–710. [27, 29]

Sperry, R. W. 1970. Perception in the absence of neocortical commissures. *Proc. Res. Assoc. Nerv. Ment. Dis.* 48: 123–138. [3]

Spiegel, I., et al. 2014. Npas4 regulates excitatory-inhibitory balance within neural circuits through cell-type-specific gene programs. *Cell* 157: 1216–1229. [17]

Spillane, J., Kullmamm, D. M., and Hanna, M. G. 2016. Genetic neurological channelopathies: Molecular genetics and clinical phenotypes. *J.Neurol. Neurosurg. Psychiatry* 87: 37–48. [5]

Spitzer, N. 2017. Neurotransmitter switching in the developing and adult brain. *Annu. Rev. Neurosci.* 40: 1–19. [27]

Spoendlin, H. 1969. Innervation patterns in the organ of corti of the cat. *Acta Otolaryngol.* 67: 239–254. [24]

Spruston, N. 2008. Pyramidal neurons: Dendritic structure and synaptic integration. *Nat. Rev. Neurosci.* 9: 206–221. [11]

Spyer, K. M., and Gourine, A. V. 2009. Chemosensory pathways in the brainstem controlling cardiorespiratory activity. *Philos. Trans. R. Soc. Lond., B, Biol. Sci.* 364: 2603–2610. [19, 26]

Sretavan, D. W., and Shatz, C. J. 1986. Prenatal development of retinal ganglion cell axons: Segregation into eye-specific layers within the cat's lateral geniculate nucleus. *J. Neurosci.* 6: 234–251. [28]

Sretavan, D. W., Shatz, C. J., and Stryker, M. P. 1988. Modification of retinal ganglion cell axon morphology by prenatal infusion of tetrodotoxin. *Nature* 336: 468–471. [28]

Srinivasan, M., Zhang, S., Lehrer, M., and Collett, T. 1996. Honeybee navigation en route to the goal: Visual flight control and odometry. *J. Exp. Biol.* 199: 237–244. [20]

Srivastava, D. and DeWitt, N. 2016. In vivo cellular reprogramming: The next generation. *Cell* 166: 1386–1396. [29]

Staley, K., Smith, R., Schaak, J., et al. 1996. Alteration of GABA_A receptor function following gene transfer of the CLC-2 chloride channel. *Neuron* 17: 543–551. [6]

Stanke, M., Duong, C. V., Pape, M., et al. 2006. Target-dependent specification of the neurotransmitter phenotype: Cholinergic differentiation of sympathetic neurons is mediated in vivo by gp 130 signaling. *Development* 133: 141–150. [27]

Starling, E. H. 1941. *Starling's Principles of Human Physiology*. Churchill, London. [19]

Steinbach, J. H., and Akk, G. 2001. Modulation of GABA_A receptor channel gating by pentobarbital. *J. Physiol.* 537: 715–733. [14]

Steindler, D. A., Cooper, N. G., Faissner, A., and Schachner, M. 1989. Boundaries defined by adhesion molecules during development of the cerebral cortex: The J1/tenascin glycoprotein in the mouse somatosensory cortical barrel field. *Dev. Biol.* 131: 243–260. [10]

Steiner, D. F., 1998. The proprotein convertases. *Curr. Opin. Chem. Biol.* 2: 31–39. [15]

Steinert, J. R., Kopp-Scheinpflug, C., Baker, C., et al. 2008. Nitric oxide is a volume transmitter regulating postsynaptic excitability at a glutamatergic synapse. *Neuron* 60: 642–656. [12]

Stelzner, D. J. 2008. Short-circuit recovery from spinal injury. *Nat. Med.* 14: 19. [29]

Stent, G. S., and Weisblat, D. A. 1985. Cell lineage in the development of invertebrate nervous systems. *Annu. Rev. Neurosci.* 8: 45–70. [10]

Stent, G. S., Kristan, W. B., Jr., Friesen, W. O., et al. 1978. Neuronal generation of the leech swimming movement. *Science* 200: 1348–1357. [20]

Stephan, A. B., Shum, E. Y., Hirsh, S., et al. 2009. ANO2 is the cilial calcium-activated chloride channel that may mediate olfactory amplification. *Proc. Natl. Acad. Sci. USA* 106: 11776–11781. [12]

Sterling, P., and Demb, J. B. 2003. In G. M. Shepherd, *Synaptic Organization of the Brain*. Oxford University Press, New York. [22]

Stern, C. D. 2007. Neural induction: old problem, new findings, yet more questions. *Development* 132: 2007. [27]

Stern, K., and McClintock, M. K. 1998. Regulation of ovulation by human pheromones. *Nature* 392: 177–179. [21]

Stettler, D. D., Das A., Bennett, J., and Gilbert, C. D. 2002. Lateral connectivity and contextual interactions in macaque primary visual cortex. *Neuron* 36: 739–750. [2, 3]

Stevens, C. F., and Wang, Y. 1993. Reversal of long-term potentiation by inhibitors of haem oxygenase. *Nature* 364: 147–149. [12]

Stevens, C. F., and Wesseling, J. F. 1999. Augmentation is a potentiation of the exocytotic process. *Neuron* 22: 139–146. [16]

Steward, O. and Lewy 1982. Preferential localization of polyribosomes under the base of dendritic spines in granule cells of the dentate gyrus. *J. Neurosci.* 2: 284–291. [17]

Steward, O., and Worley, P. 2001. A cellular mechanism for targeting newly synthesized mRNAs to synaptic sites on dendrites. *Proc. Natl. Acad. Sci USA* 98: 7062–7068. [17]

Steward, O., and Worley, P. F. 2001. Selective targeting of newly synthesized Arc mRNA to active synapses requires NMDA receptor activation. *Neuron* 30: 227–40. doi: 10.1016/s0896-6273(01)00275-6. [17]

Steward, O. Sharp, K. G., and Matsudaira Yee, K. 2014. Long distance migration and colonization of transplanted neural stem cells. *Cell* 156: 385. [29]

Steward, O. Sharp, K., Selvan, G., et al. 2006. A re-assessment of the consequences of delayed transplantation of olfactory lamina propria following complete spinal cord transection in rats. *Exp. Neurol.* 198: 483–499. [29]

Steward, O., Wallace, C. S., Lyford, G. L., and Worley, P. F. 1998. Synaptic activation causes the mRNA for the IEG Arc to localize selectively near activated postsynaptic sites on dendrites. *Neuron* 21: 741–751. [17]

Steward, O., et al. 2015. Localization and local translation of *Arc/Arg3.1* mRNA at synapses: some observations and paradoxes. *Front. Mol. Neurosci.* 7: 1–15. [17]

Steyer, J. A., Horstmann, H., and Almers, W. 1997. Transport, docking and exocytosis of single secretory granules in live chromaffin cells. *Nature* 388: 474–478. [13]

Stoney, S. D., Jr., Thompson, W. D., and Asanuma, H. 1968. Excitation of pyramidal tract cells by intracortical microstimulation: Effective extent of stimulating current. *J. Neurophysiol.* 31: 659–669. [25]

Streb, H., Irvine, R. F., Berridge, M. J., and Schulz, I. 1983. Release of Ca^{2+} from a nonmitochondrial intracellular store in pancreatic acinar cells by inositol-1,4,5-trisphosphate. *Nature* 306: 67–69. [12]

Streisinger, G., Walker, C., Dower, N., et al. 1981. Production of clones of homozygous diploid zebra fish (*Brachydanio rerio*). *Nature* 291: 293–296. [27]

Strick, P. L., Dum, R. P., and Fiez, J. A. 2009. Cerebellum and nonmotor function. *Annu. Rev. Neurosci.* 32: 413–434. [26]

Stryer, L. 1987. The molecules of visual excitation. *Sci. Am.* 257: 42–50. [22]

Stryer, L., and Bourne, H. R. 1986. G proteins: A family of signal transducers. *Annu. Rev. Cell Biol.* 2: 391–419. [22]

Stryker, M. P., and Harris, W. A. 1986. Binocular impulse blockade prevents the formation of ocular dominance columns in cat visual cortex. *J. Neurosci.* 6: 2117–2133. [28]

Stuart, A. E. 1970. Physiological and morphological properties of motoneurones in the central nervous system of the leech. *J. Physiol.* 209: 627–646. [20]

Stuart, A. E., Borycz, J., and Meinertzhagen, I. A. 2007. The dynamics of signaling at the histaminergic photoreceptor synapse of arthropods. *Prog. Neurobiol.* 82: 202–227. [14]

Stuart, G. J. and Sakmann, B. 1994. Active propagation of somatic action potentials into neocortical pyramidal cell dendrites. *Nature* 367: 69–72. [17]

Stuart, G., Schiller, J., and Sakmann, B. 1997. Action potential initiation and propagation in rat neocortical pyramidal neurons. *J. Physiol.* 505: 617–632. [8]

Stuart, G., Spruston, N., Sakmann, B., and Hausser, M. 1997. Action potential initiation and backpropagation in neurons of the mammalian CNS. *Trends Neurosci.* 20: 125–131. [8]

Stuber, G. D., Hnasko, T. S., Britt, J. P., et al. 2010. Dopaminergic terminals in the nucleus accumbens but not the dorsal striatum corelease glutamate. *J. Neurosci.* 30: 8229–8233. [14]

Stühmer, W., Conti, F., Suzuki, H., et al. 1989. Structural parts involved in activation and inactivation of the sodium channel. *Nature* 239: 597–603. [5]

Su, M., Li, L., Wang, J., et al. 2019. Kv7.4 channel contribute to projection-specific auto-inhibition of dopamine neurons in the ventral tegmental area. *Front. Cell Neurosci.* 13: 557. [18]

Su, Z., Niu, W., Liu, M. L., et al. 2014. In vivo conversion of astrocytes to neurons in the injured adult spinal cord. *Nat. Comm.* 5: 3338. [29]

Subramanian, M., et al. 2011. G-quadruplex RNA structure as a signal for neurite mRNA targeting. *EMBO Rep.* 12: 697–704. [17]

Sudhof, T. C. 2008. Neuroligins and neurexins link synaptic function to cognitive disease. *Nature* 455: 903–911. [27]

Sudhof, T. C. 2013. Neurotransmitter release: The last millisecond in the lie of a synaptic vesicle. *Neuron* 80: 675–690. [13]

Sudhof, T. 2017. Synaptic neurexin complexes: A molecular code for the logic of neural circuits. *Cell* 171: 745. [27]

Suga, M., Maeda, S., Nakagawa, S., et al. 2009. A description of the structural determination procedures of a gap junction channel at 3.5 A resolution. *Acta Crystallogr. D Biol. Crystallogr.* 65: 758–766. [11]

Sugiura, Y., Woppmann, A., Miljanich, G. P., and Ko, C-P. 1995. A novel omega-conopeptide for the presynaptic localization of calcium channels at the mammalian neuromuscular junction. *J. Neurocytol.* 24: 15–27. [13]

Sugiyama, S., Di Nardo, A. A., Aizawa, S., et al. 2008. Experience-dependent transfer of Otx2 homeoprotein into the visual cortex activates postnatal plasticity. *Cell.* 134: 508–520. [28]

Suh, B. C., and Hille, B. 2008. PIP_2 is a necessary cofactor for ion channel function: How and why? *Annu. Rev. Biophys.* 37: 175–195. [19]

Suh, B. C., Horowitz, L. F., Hirdes, W., et al. 2004. Regulation of KCNQ2/KCNQ3 current by G protein cycling: The kinetics of receptor-mediated signaling by Gq. *J. Gen. Physiol.* 123: 663–683. [12]

Suh, B. C., Inoue, T., Meyer, T., and Hille, B. 2006. Rapid chemically induced changes of PtdIns(4,5)P2 gate KCNQ ion channels. *Science* 314: 1454–1457. [12]

Sullivan, J. M. 2007. A simple depletion model of the readily releasable pool of synaptic vesicles cannot account for paired-pulse depression. *J. Neurophysiol.* 97: 948–950. [16]

Sulzer, D., Joyce, M. P., Lin, L., et al. 1998. Dopamine neurons make glutamatergic synapses in vitro. *J. Neurosci.* 18: 4588–4602. [15]

Sun, F., Park, K. K., Belin, S., et al. 2011. Sustained axon regeneration induced by co-deletion of PTEN and SOCS3. *Nature* 480: 372–375. [29]

Sun, Y. A., and Poo, M.-M. 1987. Evoked release of acetylcholine from the growing embryonic neuron. *Proc. Natl. Acad. Sci. USA* 84: 2540–2544. [18]

Surmeier, D. J., Ding, J., Day, M., et al. 2007. D1 and D2 dopamine-receptor modulation of striatal glutamatergic signaling in striatal medium spiny neurons. *Trends Neurosci.* 30: 228–245. [26]

Surprenant, A., and North, R. A. 2009. Signaling at purinergic P2X receptors. *Annu. Rev. Physiol.* 71: 333–359. [14]

Susuki, K., and Rasband, M. N. 2008. Molecular mechanisms of node of Ranvier formation. *Curr. Opin. Cell Biol.* 20: 616–623. [8, 10]

Suter, D. M., Errante, L. D., Belotserkovsky, V., and Forscher, P. 1998. The Ig superfamily cell adhesion molecule, apCAM, mediates growth cone steering by substrate-cytoskeletal coupling. *J. Cell Biol.* 141: 227–240. [27]

Sutherland, E. W. 1972. Studies on the mechanism of hormone action. *Science* 177: 401–408. [12]

Sutter, M. L., and Schreiner, C. E. 1995. Topography of intensity tuning in cat primary auditory cortex: Single-neuron versus multiple-neuron recordings. *J. Neurophysiol.* 73: 190–204. [24]

Suzuki, I. K., and Vanderhaeghen, P. 2015. Is this a brain which I see before me? Modeling human neural development with pluripotent stem cells. *Development* 142: 3138–3150. [27]

Suzuki, I. K., et al. 2018. Human-Specific NOTCH2NL Genes Expand Cortical Neurogenesis through Delta/Notch Regulation. *Cell* 173: 1370. [27]

Suzuki, R., Hunt, S. P., and Dickenson, A. H. 2003. The coding of noxious mechanical and thermal stimuli of deep dorsal horn neurones is attenuated in NK1 knockout mice. *Neuropharmacology* 45: 1093–1100. [14]

Svoboda, K. and Yasuda, R. 2006. Principles of two-photon excitation microscopy and its applications to neuroscience. *Neuron* 50: 823–839. [17]

Svoboda, K., Helmchen, F., Denk, W., and Tank, D. W. 1999. Spread of dendritic excitation in layer 2/3 pyramidal neurons in rat barrel cortex in vivo. *Nat. Neurosci.* 2: 65–73. [8]

Svoboda, K., Schmidt, C. F., Schnapp, B. J., and Block, S. M. 1993. Direct observation of kinesin stepping by optical trapping interferometry. *Nature* 365: 721–727. [15]

Sweatt, J. D. 2013. The emerging field of neuroepigenetics. *Neuron* 80: 624–632. [17]

Swindale, N. V., Matsubara, J. A., and Cynader, M. S. 1987. Surface organization of orientation and direction selectivity in cat area 18. *J. Neurosci.* 7: 1414–1427. [3]

Szabo, A., and Mayor, R. 2018. Mechanisms of neural crest migration. *Annu. Rev. Genet.* 52: 43–63. [27]

Szallasi, A., and Blumberg, P. M. 1996. Vanilloid receptors: New insights enhance potential as a therapeutic target. *Pain* 68: 195–208. [21]

Szczot, M., Pogorzala, L. A., Solinski, H. J., et al. 2017. Cell-type-specific splicing of Piezo2 regulates mechanotransduction. *Cell Reports* 21: 2760–2771. [21]

Szentágothai J. 1973. Neuronal and Synaptic Architecture of the Lateral Geniculate Nucleus. In Jung R. (Eds.) *Visual Centers in the Brain. Handbook of Sensory Physiology (Central Processing of Visual Information Part B)*, Vol. 7/3/3B. Springer, Berlin, Heidelberg. [2]

Szmajda, B. A., Buzás, P., Fitzgibbon, T., and Martin, P. R. 2006. Geniculocortical relay of blue-off signals in the primate visual system. *Proc. Nat. Acad. Sci. USA.* 103: 19512–19517. [22]

Szule, J. A. Harlow, M. L., Jung, J. H., et al. 2012. Regulation of synaptic vesicle docking by different classes of macromolecules in active zone material. *PLOS ONE* 7: 333333. doi: 10.1371/journal pone 0033333. [13]

Szule, J. A., Jung, J. H., and McMahan, U. J. 2015. The structure and function of "active zone material" at synapses. *Phil. Trans. R. Soc. B* 370: 2014.0189. [13]

Taccola, G., and Nistri, A. 2006. Oscillatory circuits underlying locomotor networks in the rat spinal cord. *Crit. Rev. Neurobiol.* 18: 25–36. [26]

Tachibana, S., Takeuchi, M., and Fujiwara, T. 1985. Visualization of autonomic varicose terminal axons by scanning electron microscopy. *J. Electron Microsc. (Tokyo)* 34: 136–138. [18]

Tadenev, A. L., Kulaga, H. M., May-Simera, H. L., et al. 2011. Loss of Bardet-Biedl syndrome protein-8 (BBS8) perturbs olfactory function, protein localization, and axon targeting. *Proc. Natl. Acad. Sci. USA* 108(25): 10320–10325. [21]

Takahashi, K., and Yamanaka, S. 2006. Induction of pluripotent stem cells from mouse embryonic and adult fibroblast cultures by defined factors. *Cell* 126: 663–676. [27]

Takahashi, K., Lin, J. S., and Sakai, K. 2006. Neuronal activity of histaminergic tuberomammillary neurons during wake-sleep states in the mouse. *J. Neurosci.* 26: 10292–10298. [14]

Takahashi, T., Kajikawa, Y., and Tsujimoto, T. 1998. G-protein-coupled modulation of presynaptic calcium currents and transmitter release by a GABA$_B$ receptor. *J. Neurosci.* 18: 3138–3146. [12, 14]

Takai, T., Noda, M., Mishina, M., et al. 1985. Cloning, sequencing, and expression of cDNA for a novel subunit of acetylcholine receptor from calf muscle. *Nature* 315: 761–764. [5]

Takamori, S. 2006. VGLUTs: "Exciting" times for glutamate research? *Neurosci. Res.* 55: 343–351. [9]

Takeda, H., Inazu, M., and Matsumiya, T. 2002. Astroglial dopamine transport is mediated by norepinephrine transporter. *Naunyn Schmiedebergs Arch Pharmacol.* 366: 620–623. [10]

Takeoka, A., Vollenweider, I., Courtine, G., and Arber, S. 2014. Muscle spindle feedback directs locomotor recovery and circuit reorganization after spinal cord injury. *Cell* 159: 1626–1639. [29]

Takeuchi, A., and Takeuchi, N. 1959. Active phase of frog's end-plate potential. *J. Neurophysiol.* 22: 395–411. [11]

Takeuchi, A., and Takeuchi, N. 1960. On the permeability of the end-plate membrane during the action of transmitter. *J. Physiol.* 154: 52–67. [11]

Takeuchi, A., and Takeuchi, N. 1964. The effect on crayfish muscle of iontophoretically applied glutamate. *J. Physiol.* 170: 296–317. [14]

Takeuchi, A., and Takeuchi, N. 1966. On the permeability of the presynaptic terminal of the crayfish neuromuscular junction during synaptic inhibition and the action of γ-aminobutyric acid. *J. Physiol.* 183: 433–449. [11]

Takeuchi, A., and Takeuchi, N. 1967. Anion permeability of the inhibitory post-synaptic membrane of the crayfish neuromuscular junction. *J. Physiol.* 191: 575–590. [11]

Takeuchi, N. 1963. Some properties of conductance changes at the end-plate membrane during the action of acetylcholine. *J. Physiol.* 167: 128–140. [11]

Takeuchi, T., et al. 2013. The synaptic plasticity and memory hypothesis: encoding, storage and persistence. *Phil Transact. Roy, Soc. B.* 369: 20130288. [17]

Takumi, Y., Matsubara, A., Rinvik, E., and Otterson, O. P. 1999. The arrangement of glutamate receptors in excitatory synapses. *Ann. NY Acad. Sci.* 868: 474–481. [16]

Takumi, Y., Ramirez-Leon, V., Laake, P., et al. 1999. Different modes of expression of AMPA and NMDA receptors in hippocampal synapses. *Nat. Neurosci.* 2: 618–624. [16]

Talbot, S. A., and Marshall, W. H. 1941. Physiological studies on neural mechanisms of visual localization and discrimination. *Am. J. Ophthalmol.* 24: 1255–1264. [3]

Tan, J., Epema, A. H., and Voogd, J. 1995. Zonal organization of the flocculovestibular nucleus projection in the rabbit: A combined axonal tracing and acetylcholinesterase study. *J. Comp. Neurol.* 356: 51–71. [26]

Tanabe, T. Takashima, H., Mikami, A., et al. 1987. Primary structure of receptors for calcium channel blockers from skeletal muscle. *Nature* 328: 313–318. [5]

Tanaka, J-I., et al. 2008. Protein synthesis and neurotrophin-dependent structural plasticity of single dendritic spines. *Science* 319: 1683. [17]

Tang, Y-G., and Zucker, R. S. 1997. Mitochondrial involvement in posttetanic potentiation of synaptic transmission. *Neuron* 18: 483–491. [16]

Tank, D. W., Huganir, R. L., Greengard, P., and Webb, W. W. 1983. Patch-recorded single-channel currents of the purified and reconstituted *Torpedo* acetylcholine receptor. *Proc. Natl. Acad. Sci. USA.* 80: 5129–5133. [5]

Tao-Cheng, J. H., Nagy, Z., and Brightman, M. W. 1987. Tight junctions of brain endothelium in vitro are enhanced by astroglia. *J. Neurosci.* 7: 3293–3299. [10]

Taranda, J., Maison, S. F., Ballestero, J. A., et al. 2009. A point mutation in the hair cell nicotinic cholinergic receptor prolongs cochlear inhibition and enhances noise protection. *PLOS Biol.* 7: e18. [24]

Tardin, C., Cognet, L., Bats, C., et al. 2003. Direct imaging of lateral movements of AMPA receptors inside synapses. *EMBO J.* 22: 4656–4665. [14]

Tarozzo, G., De Andrea, M., Feuilloley, M., et al. 1998. Molecular and cellular guidance of neuronal migration in the developing olfactory system of rodents. *Ann. NY Acad. Sci.* 839: 196–200. [19]

Tarozzo, G., Peretto, P., Biffo, S., et al. 1995. Development and migration of olfactory neurones in the nervous system of the neonatal opossum. *Proc. R. Soc. Lond., B, Biol. Sci.* 262: 95–101. [19]

Tasic, B. 2018. Single cell transcriptomics in neuroscience: Cell classification and beyond. *Curr. Op Neurobiol.* 50: 242–249. [27]

Tasic, B., Yao, Z., Graybuck, L. T., et al. 2018. Shared and distinct transcriptomic cell types across neocortical areas. *Nature* 563: 72–78. [3]

Taylor, A. R., Gifondorwa, D. J., Newbern, J. M., et al. 2007. Astrocyte and muscle-derived secreted factors differentially regulate motoneuron survival. *J. Neurosci.* 27: 634–644. [29]

Taylor, W. R., and Baylor, D. A. 1995. Conductance and kinetics of single cGMP-activated channels in salamander rod outer segments. *J. Physiol.* 483 (Pt 3): 567–582. [22]

Teillet, M. A., Ziller, C., and Le Douarin, N. M. 2008. Quail–chick chimeras. *Methods Mol. Biol.* 461: 337–350. [27]

Terenius, L. 1973. Stereospecific interaction between narcotic analgesics and a synaptic plasm a membrane fraction of rat cerebral cortex. *Acta Pharmacol. Toxicol. (Copenh.)* 32: 317–320. [23]

Terlau, H., and Olivera, B. M. 2004. *Conus* Venoms: A rich source of novel ion channel-targeted peptides. *Physiol. Rev.* 84: 41–68. [7]

Tessier-Lavigne, M., Placzek, M., Lumsden, A. G., et al. 1988. Chemotropic guidance of developing axons in the mammalian central nervous system. *Nature* 336: 775–778. [27]

Tettamanti, G., Cattaneo, A. G., Gornati, R., et al. 2010. Phylogenesis of brain-derived neurotrophic factor (BDNF) in vertebrates. *Gene* 450: 85–93. [27]

Teune, T. M., van der Burg, J., de Zeeuw, C. I., et al. 1998. Single Purkinje cell can innervate multiple classes of projection neurons in the cerebellar nuclei of the rat: A light microscopic and ultrastructural triple-tracer study in the rat. *J. Comp. Neurol.* 392: 164–178. [15]

Thach, W. T. 2007. On the mechanism of cerebellar contributions to cognition *Cerebellum* 6: 163–167. [26]

Thach, W. T., Goodkin, H. G., and Keating, J. G. 1992. The cerebellum and the adaptive coordination of movement. *Annu. Rev. Neurosci.* 15: 403–442. [26]

Thevenau, E., et al. 2013. Chase-and-run between adjacent cell populations promotes directional collective migration. *Nat. Cell Biol.* 15: 763–772. [27]

Thiele, A. 2013. Muscarinic signaling in the brain. *Annu. Rev. Neurosci.* 36: 271–294. [14]

Thion, M.S., et al. 2018. Microglia and early brain development: An intimate journey. *Science* 362: 185–189. [27]

Thoenen, H. 1991. The changing scene of neurotrophic factors. *Trends Neurosci.* 14: 165–170. [17]

Thoenen, H., Mueller, R. A., and Axelrod, J. 1969. Increased tyrosine hydroxylase activity after drug-induced alteration of sympathetic transmission. *Nature* 221: 1264. [15]

Thoenen, H., et al. 1970. Phase difference in the induction of tyrosine hydroxylase in cell body and nerve terminals of sympathetic neurones. *Proc. Natl. Acad. Sci USA* 65: 58–62. [27]

Thoenen, H., Otten, U., and Schwab, M. 1979. Orthograde and retrograde signals for the regulation of neuronal gene expression: The peripheral sympathetic nervous system as a model. In *The Neurosciences: Fourth Study Program*. MIT Press, Cambridge, MA, pp. 911–928. [15]

Thomas, R. C. 1969. Membrane currents and intracellular sodium changes in a snail neurone during extrusion of injected sodium. *J. Physiol.* 201: 495–514. [9]

Thomas, R. C. 1972. Intracellular sodium activity and the sodium pump in snail neurones. *J. Physiol.* 220: 55–71. [9]

Thomas, R. C. 1977. The role of bicarbonate, chloride and sodium ions in the regulation of intracellular pH in snail neurones. *J. Physiol.* 273: 317–338. [9]

Thomas, R. C. 2009. The plasma membrane calcium ATPase (PMCA) of neurones is electroneutral and exchanges 2 H+ for each Ca^{2+} or Ba^{2+} ion extruded. *J. Physiol.* 87: 315–327. [9]

Thompson, L. H., and Björklund, A. 2009. Transgenic reporter mice as tools for studies of transplantability and connectivity of dopamine neuron precursors in fetal tissue grafts. *Prog. Brain Res.* 175: 53–79. [29]

Thompson, W. 1983. Synapse elimination in neonatal rat muscle is sensitive to pattern of muscle use. *Nature* 302: 614–616. [27]

Thoreson, W. B. 2007. Kinetics of synaptic transmission at ribbon synapses of rods and cones. *Mol. Neurobiol.* 36: 205–223. [22]

Thorn, P., et al. 2016. Exocytosis in non-neuronal cells. *J. Neurochem.* 137: 849–859. [18]

Thorpe, S. J., Fize, D., and Marlot, C. 1996. Speed of processing in the human visual system. *Nature* 381: 520–522. [25]

Thyssen, A., Hirnet, D., Wolburg, H., et al. 2010. Ectopic vesicular neurotransmitter release along sensory axons mediates neurovascular coupling via glial calcium signaling. *Proc. Natl. Acad. Sci. USA* 107: 15258–15263. [14]

Tian, N., and Copenhagen, D. R. 2003. Visual stimulation is required for refinement of ON and OFF pathways in postnatal retina. *Neuron* 39: 85–96. [28]

Timpe, L. C., Schwartz, T. L., Tempel, B. L., et al. 1988. Expression of functional potassium channels from *Shaker* cDNA in *Xenopus* oocytes. *Nature* 331: 143–145. [5]

Tirindelli, R., Dibattista, M., Pifferi, S., and Menini, A. 2009. From pheromones to behavior. *Physiol. Rev.* 89: 921–956. [21]

Tobin, V. A., and Ludwig, M. 2007. The role of the actin cytoskeleton in oxytocin and vasopressin release from rat supraoptic nucleus neurons. *J. Physiol.* 582: 1337–1348. [18]

Tobin, V., Leng, G., and Ludwig, M. 2012. The involvement of actin, calcium channels and exocytosis proteins in somato-dendritic oxytocin and vasopressin release. *Front. Physiol.* 3: 261. [18]

Tobin, V. A., Douglas, A. J., Leng, G., and Ludwig, M. 2011. The involvement of voltage-operated calcium channels in somato-dendritic oxytocin release. *PLOS ONE* 6: e25366. doi: 10.1371/journal.pone.0025366. [18]

Toda, M., and Okamura, T. 2003. The pharmacology of nitric oxide in the peripheral nervous system of blood vessels. *Pharmacol. Rev.* 55: 271–324. [19]

Tonegawa, S., et al. 2015. Memory engram cells have come of age. *Neuron* 87: 918. [17]

Togashi, H., Sakisaka, T., and Takai, Y. 2009. Cell adhesion molecules in the central nervous system. *Cell Adh. Migr.* 3: 29–35. [27]

Tognini, P., Napoli, D., Tola, J., et al. 2015. *Nat. Neurosci.* 18: 956–958. [28]

Tognini, P., Putignano, E., Coatti, A., and Pizzorusso, T. 2011. Experience-dependent expression of miR-132 regulates ocular dominance plasticity. *Nat. Neurosci.* 14: 1237–1239. [28]

tom Dieck, S., and Brandstatter, J. H. 2006. Ribbon synapses of the retina. *Cell Tissue Res.* 326: 339–346. [22]

Tombola, F., Pathak, M. M., and Isacoff, E. E. 2005. Voltage-sensing arginines in a potassium channel permeate and occlude cation-selective pores. *Neuron* 45: 379–388. [7]

Tomita, H., Ohbayashi, M., Nakahara, K., et al. 1999. Top-down signal from prefrontal cortex in executive control of memory retrieval. *Nature* 401: 699–703. [25]

Tongiorgi, E. 2008. Activity-dependent expression of brain-derived neurotrophic factor in dendrites: Facts and open questions. *Neurosci. Res.* 61: 335–346. [27]

Tongiorgi, E., et al. 1997. Activity-dependent dendritic targeting of BDNF and TrkB mRNAs in hippocampal neurons. *J. Neurosci.* 17: 9492–9505. [17]

Tongiorgi, E., Armellin, M., Giulianini, P. G., et al., 2004. Brain-derived neurotrophic factor mRNA and protein are targeted to discrete dendritic laminas by events that trigger epileptogenesis. *J. Neurosci.* 24: 6842–6852. [17]

Tootell, R. B., and Hadjikhani, N. 2000. Attention—brains at work! *Nat. Neurosci.* 3: 206–208. [25]

Torebjork, E. 1985. Nociceptor activation and pain. *Philos. Trans. R. Soc. Lond., B, Biol. Sci.* 308: 227–234. [23]

Tornqvist, K., Yang, X. L., and Dowling, J. E. 1988. Modulation of cone horizontal cell activity in the teleost fish retina. III. Effects of prolonged darkness and dopamine on electrical coupling between horizontal cells. *J. Neurosci.* 8: 2279–2288. [22]

Torper, O., Ottosson, D. R., Pereira, M., et al. 2015. In vivo reprogramming of striatal NG2 glia into functional neurons that integrate into local host circuitry. *Cell Rep* 12: 474–481. [29]

Torre, V., Ashmore, J. F., Lamb, T. D., and Menini, A. 1995. Transduction and adaptation in sensory receptor cells. *J. Neurosci.* 15: 7757–7768. [22]

Torres, G. E., and Amara, S. G. 2007. Glutamate and monamine transporters: New visions of form and function. *Curr. Opin. Neurobiol.* 17: 304–312. [9, 15]

Torre, E. R. and Steward O. 1992. Demonstration of local protein synthesis within dendrites using a new cell culture system that permits the isolation of living axons and dendrites from their cell bodies. *J. Neurosci.* 12: 762–772. [17]

Torregrosa-Hetland, C. J., et al. 2011. The F-actin cortical network is a major factor influencing the organization of the secretory machinery in chromaffin cells. *J. Cell Sci.* 124: 727–734. [18]

Tovar, A. de la Rosa, Mishra, P. K. and De-Miguel, F. F. 2016. On the basis of synaptic integration constancy during growth of a neuronal circuit. *Front. Cell. Neurosci.* doi: 10.3389/fncel.2016.00198. [11]

Tovote, P., et al. 2015. Neuronal circuits for fear and anxiety. *Nat. Rev. Neurosci.* 16: 317. [17]

Town, S. M., Wood, K. C., and Bizley, J. K. 2018. Sound identity is represented robustly in auditory cortex during perceptual constancy. *Nat. Comm.* 9: 4786. [24]

Townes-Anderson, E., MacLeish, P. R., and Raviola E. 1985. Rod cells dissociated from mature salamander retina: Ultrastructure and uptake of horseradish peroxidase. *J. Cell Bio.* 100: 175–188. [22]

Toyoshima, C., and Unwin, N. 1988. Ion channel of acetylcholine receptor reconstituted from images of postsynaptic membranes. *Nature* 336: 247–250. [5]

Toyoshima, C., Nakasako, M., Nomura, H., and Ogawa, H. 2000. Crystal structure of the calcium pump of the sarcoplasmic reticulum at 2.6 A resolution. *Nature* 405: 647–655. [9]

Trachtenberg, J., et al. 2002. Long-term in vivo imaging of experience-dependent synaptic plasticity in adult cortex. *Nature* 420: 788. [17]

Tricoire, H. et al. 2003. Origin of cerebrospinal fluid melatonin and possible function in the integration of photoperiod. *Reprod. Suppl.* 61: 311–321. [18]

Trautwein, W., Osterrieder, W., and Noma, A. 1981. Potassium channels and the muscarinic receptor in the sino-atrial node of the heart. In N. J. M. Birdsall (Ed.), in *Drug Receptors and their Effectors*. London: MacMillan, pp. 5–22. [12]

Trautwein, W., Taniguchi, J., and Noma, A. 1982. The effect of intracellular cyclic nucleotides and calcium on the action potential and acetylcholine response of isolated cardiac cells. *Pflügers Arch.* 392: 307–314. [12]

Travaglia, A., Bisaz, R., Sweet, E. S., et al. 2016. Infantile amnesia reflects a developmental critical period for hippocampal learning. *Nat. Neurosci.*19: 1225–1233. [28]

Trigo, F. F., Marty, A., and Stell, B. M. 2008. Axonal GABA$_A$ receptors. *Eur. J. Neurosci.* 28: 841–848. [11]

Tritsch, N. X., and Bergles, D. E. 2010. Developmental regulation of spontaneous activity in the mammalian cochlea. *J. Neurosci.* 30: 1539–1550. [28]

Tritsch, N. X., Yi, E., Gale, J. E., et al. 2007. The origin of spontaneous activity in the developing auditory system. *Nature* 450: 50–55. [28]

Tropea, D., Van Wart, A., and Sur, M. 2009. Molecular mechanisms of experience-dependent plasticity in visual cortex. *Philos. Trans. R. Soc. Lond., B, Biol. Sci.* 364: 341–355. [28]

Trouslard, J., Marsh, S. J., and Brown, D. A. 1993. Calcium entry through nicotinic receptor channels and calcium channels in cultured rat superior cervical ganglion cells. *J. Physiol.* 481: 251–271. [12]

Trueta, C., and De-Miguel, F. F. 2012. Extrasynaptic exocytosis and its mechanisms: A source of molecules mediating volume transmission in the nervous system. *Front. Physiol.* 3: 319. [18]

Trueta, C., Kuffler, D. P., and De-Miguel, F. F. 2012. Cycling of dense core vesicles involved in somatic exocytosis of serotonin by leech neurons. *Front. Physiol.* 3: 175. doi: 10.3389/fphys.2012.00175. [18]

Trueta, C., Méndez, B., and De-Miguel, F. F. 2003. Somatic exocytosis of serotonin mediated by L-type calcium channels in cultured leech neurones. *J. Physiol.* 547: 405–416. [20]

Truman, J. W., Thorn, R. S., and Robinow, S. 1992. Programmed neuronal death in insect development. *J. Neurobiol.* 23: 1295–1311. [27]

Ts'o, D. Y., and Gilbert, C. D. 1988. The organization of chromatic and spatial interactions in the primate striate cortex. *J. Neurosci.* 8: 1712–1727. [3]

Ts'o, D. Y., Frostig, R. D., Lieke, E. E., and Grinvald, A. 1990. Functional organization of primate visual cortex revealed by high resolution optical imaging. *Science* 249: 417–420. [3]

Ts'o, D. Y., Gilbert, C. D., and Wiesel, T. N. 1986. Relationships between horizontal interactions and functional architecture in cat striate cortex as revealed by cross-correlation analysis. *J. Neurosci.* 6: 1160–1170. [3]

Ts'o, D. Y., Roe, A. W., and Gilbert, C. D. 2001. A hierarchy of the functional organization for color, form and disparity in primate visual area V2. *Vision Res.* 41: 1333–1349. [3]

Ts'o, D. Y., Zarella, M., and Burkitt, G. 2009. Whither the hypercolumn? *J. Physiol.* 587: 2791–2805. [3]

Tsai, L., and Barnea, G. 2014. A critical period defined by axon-targeting mechanisms in the murine olfactory bulb. *Science.* 344: 197–200. [28]

Tsao, D. Y., and Livingstone, M. S. 2008. Mechanisms of face perception. *Annu. Rev. Neurosci.* 31: 411–437. [3]

Tsao, D. Y., Freiwald, W. A., Tootell, R. B., and Livingstone, M. S. 2006. A cortical region consisting entirely of face-selective cells. *Science* 311: 670–674. [3, 25]

Tschopp, P., and Duboule, D. 2011. A regulatory 'landscape effect' over the *HoxD* cluster. *Dev. Biol.* 351: 288–296. [27]

Tsetlin, V., and Hucho, F. 2009. Nicotinic acetylcholine receptors at atomic resolution. *Curr. Opin. Pharmacol.* 9: 306–310. [5]

Tsien, R. W. 1987. Calcium currents in heart cells and neurons. In *Neuromodulation: The Biochemical Control of Neuronal Excitability*. Oxford University Press, New York, pp. 206–242. [12]

Tsien, R. Y. 1989. Fluorescent probes of cell signaling. *Annu. Rev. Neurosci.* 12: 227–253. [13]

Tsubokawa, H., and Ross, W. N. 1996. IPSPs modulate spike backpropagation and associated [Ca^{2+}]$_i$ changes in the dendrites of hippocampal CA1 pyramidal neurons. *J. Neurophysiol.* 76: 2896–2906. [8]

Tsuda, M., Tozaki-Saitoh, H., and Inoue, K. 2010. Pain and purinergic signaling. *Brain Res. Rev.* 63: 222–232. [14]

Tsujino, N., and Sakurai, T. 2009. Orexin/hypocretin: A neuropeptide at the interface of sleep, energy homeostasis, and reward system. *Pharmacol. Rev.* 61: 162–176. [14]

Tsunoo, A., Yoshii, M., and Narahashi, T. 1986: Block of calcium channels by enkephalin and somatostatin in neuroblastoma-glioma hybrid NG108-15 cells. *Proc. Nat. Acad. Sci. USA* 83: 9832–9836. [12]

Tsuzuki, K., and Suga, N. 1988. Combination-sensitive neurons in the ventroanterior area of the auditory cortex of the mustached bat. *J. Neurophysiol.* 60: 1908–1923. [24]

Tu, Y.-H., Cooper, A. J., Teng, B., et al. 2018. An evolutionarily conserved gene family encodes protein-selective ion channels. *Science* 359:1047–1050. [21]

Tucker, K. L., Meyer, M., and Barde, Y. A. 2001. Neurotrophins are required for nerve growth during development. *Nat. Neurosci.* 4: 29–37. [27]

Turner, D. L., and Cepko, C. L. 1987. A common progenitor for neurons and glia persists in rat retina late in development. *Nature* 328: 131–136. [27]

Turrini, P., Casu, M. A., Wong, T. P., et al. 2001. Cholinergic nerve terminals establish classical synapses in the rat cerebral cortex: Synaptic pattern and age-related atrophy. *Neuroscience* 105: 277–285. [14]

Tyrrell, L., Renganathan, M., Dib-Hajj, S. D., and Waxman, S. G. 2001. Glycosylation alters steady-state inactivation of sodium channel Na$_v$1.9/NaN in dorsal root ganglion neurons and is developmentally regulated. *J. Neurosci.* 21: 9629–9637. [5]

Tyssowsky, K. M., et al. 2018. Different neuronal activity patterns induce different gene expression programs. *Neuron* 98: 530–546. [17]

Tyzio, R., Allene, C., Nardou, R., et al. 2011. Depolarizing actions of GABA in immature neurons depend neither on ketone bodies nor on pyruvate. *J. Neurosci.* 31: 34–45. [27]

Udenfriend, S. 1950. Identification of γ-aminobutyric acid in brain by the isotope derivative method. *J. Biol. Chem.* 187: 65–69. [14]

Uğurbil, K., Hu, X., Chen, W., et al. 1999. Functional mapping in the human brain using high magnetic fields. *Philos. Trans. R. Soc. Lond., B, Biol. Sci.* 354: 1195–1213. [1]

Ullian, E. M., McIntosh, J. M., and Sargent, P. B. 1997. Rapid synaptic transmission in the avian ciliary ganglion is mediated by two distinct classes of nicotinic receptors. *J. Neurosci.* 17: 7210–7219. [19]

Umbriaco, D., Watkins, K. C., Descarries, L., et al. 1994. Ultrastructural and morphometric features of the acetylcholine innervation in adult rat parietal cortex: An electron microscopic study in serial sections. *J. Comp. Neurol.* 348: 351–373. [14]

Umbriaco, D. et al. 1995. Relational features of acetylcholine, noradrenaline, serotonin and GABA axon terminals in the stratum radiatum of adult rat hippocampus (CA1). *Hippocampus* 5: 605–620. [18]

Ungerstedt, U. 1971. Stereotaxic mapping monoamine pathways in the rat brain. *Acta Physiol. Scand. Suppl.* 367: 1–49. [14]

Unwin, N. 1995. Acetylcholine receptor imaged in the open state. *Nature* 373: 37–43. [5]

Unwin, N. 2005. Refined structure of the nicotinic acetylcholine receptor at 4Å resolution. *J. Mol. Biol.* 346: 967–989. [5]

Unwin, N. and Fujiyoshi, Y. 2012. Gating movement of acetylcholine receptor caught by plunge-freezing. *J. Mol. Biol.* 422: 617–634. [5]

Unwin, N., Miyazawa, A., Li, J., and Fujiyoshi, Y. 2002. Activation of the nicotinic acetylcholine receptor involves a switch in conformation of the alpha subunits. *J. Mol. Biol.* 319: 1165–1176. [5]

Unwin, N., Toyoshima, C., and Kubalek, E. 1988. Arrangement of acetylcholine receptor subunits in the resting and desensitized states, determined by cryoelectron microscopy of crystallized *Torpedo* postsynaptic membranes. *J. Cell Biol.* 107: 1123–1138. [5]

Vabnick, I., and Shrager, P. 1998. Ion channel redistribution and function during development of the myelinated axon. *J. Neurobiol.* 37: 80–96. [8]

Vale, R. D., and Fletterick, R. J. 1997. The design plan of kinesin motors. *Annu. Rev. Cell Dev. Biol.* 13: 745–777. [15]

Vallbo, A. B., and Hagbarth, K. E. 1968. Mechnoreceptor activity recorded from human peripheral nerves. *Electroencephalogr. Clin. Neurophysiol.* 25: 407. [23]

Vallee, R. B., and Bloom, G. S. 1991. Mechanisms of fast and slow axonal transport. *Annu. Rev. Neurosci.* 14: 59–92. [15]

Vallee, R. B., and Gee, M. A. 1998. Make room for dynein. *Trends Cell Biol.* 8: 490–494. [15]

Vallee, R. B., Shpetner, H. S., and Paschal, B. M. 1989. The role of dynein in retrograde axonal transport. *Trends Neurosci.* 12: 66–70. [15]

Van Boven, R. W., Hamilton, R. H., Kauffman, T., et al. 2000. Tactile spatial resolution in blind Braille readers. *Neurology* 54: 2230–2236. [23]

Van den Ameele, J., et al. 2014. Thinking out of the dish: what to learn about cortical development using pluripotent stem cells. *Trends Neurosci.* 37: 334–342. [27]

van den Brand, R., Heutschi, J., Barraud, Q., et al. 2012. Restoring voluntary control of locomotion after paralyzing spinal cord injury. *Science* 336: 1182–1185. [29]

van den Pol, A. N. 2010. Excitatory neuromodulator reduces dopamine release, enhancing prolactin secretion. *Neuron* 65: 147–149. [14]

van der Loos, H., and Dorfl, J. 1978. Does the skin tell the somatosensory cortex how to construct a map of the periphery? *Neurosci. Lett.* 7: 23–30. [23]

van der Loos, H., and Woolsey, T. A. 1973. Somatosensory cortex: Structural alterations following early injury to sense organs. *Science* 179: 395–398. [28]

van der Loos, H., Dorfl, J., and Welker, E. 1984. Variation in pattern of mystacial vibrissae in mice. A quantitative study of ICR stock and several inbred strains. *J. Hered.* 75: 326–336. [23]

Van Driesche, S. J. and Martin, K. C. 2018. New frontiers in RNA transport and local translation in neurons. *Dev. Neurobiol.* 78: 331–339. [17]

Van Essen, D. C. 1997. A tension based theory of morphogenesis and compact wiring in the central nervous system. *Nature* 385: 313–318. [3]

Van Essen, D. C., and Drury, H. A. 1997. Structural and functional analyses of human cerebral cortex using a surface-based atlas. *J. Neurosci.* 17: 7079–7102. [3]

Van Essen, D., and Jansen, J. K. 1974. Reinnervation of rat diaphragm during perfusion with α-bungarotoxin. *Acta Physiol. Scand.* 91: 571–573. [29]

Van Essen, D., and Kelly, J. 1973. Correlation of cell shape and function in the visual cortex of the cat. *Nature* 241: 403–405. [10]

van Hooft, J. A., Spier, A. D., Yakel, J. L., et al. 1998. Promiscuous coassembly of serotonin 5-HT$_3$ and nicotinic α4 receptor subunits into Ca^{2+}-permeable ion channels. *Proc. Natl. Acad. Sci. USA* 95: 11456–11461. [14]

van Middendorp, J. J., Sanchez, G. M., and Burridge, A. L. 2010. The Edwin Smith papyrus: A clinical reappraisal of the oldest known document on spinal injuries. *Eur. Spine J.* 19: 1815–1823. [29]

van Westen, D., Fransson, P., Olsrud, J., et al. 2004. Fingersomatotopy in area 3b: An fMRI-study. *BMC Neurosci.* 5: 28. [23]

Vandermaelen, C. P., and Aghajanian, G. K. 1983. Electrophysiological and pharmacological characterization of serotonergic dorsal raphe neurons recorded extracellularly and intracellularly in rat brain slices. *Brain Res.* 289: 109–119. [14]

Vandermeeren Y, Bastings, E., Good, D., et al. 2003. Plasticity of motor maps in primates: Recent advances and therapeutical perspectives. *Rev. Neurol. Paris* 159: 259–275. [26]

Varga, Z. M., Bandtlow, C. E., Erulkar, S. D., et al. 1995. The critical period for repair of CNS of neonatal opossum (*Monodelphis domestica*) in culture: Correlation with development of glial cells, myelin and growth-inhibitory molecules. *Eur. J. Neurosci.* 7: 2119–2129. [29]

Varma, N., Carlson, G. C., Ledent, C., and Alger, B. E. 2001. Metabotropic glutamate receptors drive the endocannabinoid system in hippocampus. *J. Neurosci.* 21: RC188 (1–5). [12]

Vassar, R., Ngai, J., and Axel, R. 1993. Spatial segregation of odorant receptor expression in the mammalian olfactory epithelium. *Cell* 74: 309–318. [21]

Vautrin, J., and Kriebel, M. E. 1991. Characteristics of slow-miniature end plate currents show a subunit composition. *Neuroscience* 41: 71–88. [13]

Veening, J. G., and Barendregt, H. P. 2010. The regulation of brain states by neuroactive substances distributed via the cerebrospinal fluid; a review. *Cerebrospinal Fluid Res.* 7: 1. [18]

Velázquez-Ulloa, N., Blackshaw, S. E., Szczupak, L., et al. 2003. Convergence of mechanosensory inputs onto neuromodulatory serotonergic neurons in the leech. *J. Neurobiol.* 54: 604–617. doi: 10.1002/neu.10184. [18]

Ventre-Dominey, J. 2014. Vestibular function in the temporal and parietal cortex: Distinct velocity and inertial processing pathways. *Front. Integ. Neurosci.* 8: 53–53. [24]

Venugopalan, P., Wang, Y., Nguyen, T., et al. 2016. Transplanted neurons integrate into adult retinas and respond to light. *Nat. Commun.* 7: 10472. doi: 10.138/ncomms10472. [29]

Vergara, C., Latorre, R. Marrion, N. V., and Adelman, J. P. 1998. Calcium-activated potassium channels. *Curr. Opin. Neurobiol.* 8: 321–329. [5]

Verkhratsky, A., Krishtal, O. A., and Burnstock, G. 2009. Purinoceptors on neuroglia. *Mol. Neurobiol.* 39: 190–208. [10]

Veronin, L. L., and Cherubini, E. 2004. "Deaf, mute and whispering" silent synapses: Their role in synaptic plasticity. *J. Physiol.* 557: 3–12. [16]

Veruki, M. L., and Wässle, H. 1996. Immunohistochemical Localization of Dopamine D Receptors in Rat Retina. *Eur. J. Neurosci.* 8: 2286–2297. [18]

Vessal, M., and Darian-Smith, C. 2010. Adult neurogenesis occurs in primate sensorimotor cortex following cervical dorsal rhizotomy. *J. Neurosci.* 30: 8613–8623. [27]

Vetere, G., et al. 2019. Memory formation in the absence of experience. *Nat. Neurosci.* 22: 933. [17]

Vetter, R. J., Williams, J. C., Hetke, J. F., et al. 2004. Chronic neural recording using silicon-substrate microelectrode arrays implanted in cerebral cortex. *IEEE Trans. Biomed. Eng.* 51:896–904. [1]

Vickers, C. A., et al. 2005. Induction and maintenance of late-phase long-term potentiation in isolated dendrites of rat hippocampal CA1 pyramidal neurons. *J. Physiol.* 568.3: 803–813. [17]

Vidal-Sanz, M., Bray, G. M., and Aguayo, A. J. 1991. Regenerated synapses in the superior colliculus after the regrowth of retinal ganglion cell axons. *J. Neurocytol.* 20: 940–952. [29]

Viganò, F., and Dimou, L. 2016. The heterogeneous nature of NG2-glia. Brain Research 1638: 129–137. [10]

Vignoli, B., et al. 2016. Peri-synaptic glia recycles brain-derived neurotrophic factor for LTP Stabilization and memory retention. *Neuron* 92: 873. [17]

Viktorin, G., Chiuchitu, C., Rissler, M., et al. 2009. Emx3 is required for the differentiation of dorsal telencephalic neurons. *Dev. Dyn.* 238: 1984–1998. [27]

Villanueva, S., Fiedler, J., and Orrego, F. 1990. A study in rat brain cortex synaptic vesicles of endogenous ligands for *N*-methyl-D-aspartate receptors. *Neuroscience* 37: 23–30. [13]

Villarroel, A., Herlitze, S., Koenen, M., and Sakmann, B. 1991. Location of threonine residue in the α-subunit M2 transmembrane segment that determines the ion flow through the acetylcholine receptor channel. *Proc. R. Soc. Lond., B, Biol. Sci.* 243: 69–74. [5]

Vincent, S. B. 1912. The function of the vibrissae in the behavior of the white rat. *Behav. Monogr:* 1–82. [23]

Virchow, R. 1959. *Cellularpathologie.* (F. Chance, trans.) Hirschwald, Berlin. (Excerpts are from pp. 310, 315, and 317.) [10]

Virkki, L. V., Choi, I., Davis, B. A., and Boron, W. F. 2003. Cloning of a Na$^+$-driven Cl-HCO$_3$ exchanger from squid giant fiber lobe. *Am. J. Physiol.* 285: C771–C780. [9]

Vitale, M. L., Seward, E. P., and Trifaró, J. M. 1995. Chromaffin cell cortical actin network dynamics control the size of the release-ready vesicle pool and the initial rate of exocytosis. *Neuron* 14: 353–363. [18]

Vizi, E. S., Kiss, J. P., and Lendvai, B. 2004. Nonsynaptic communication in the central nervous system. *Neurochem. Int.* 45: 443–451. [18]

Voderholzer, U., Hornyak, M., Thiel, B., et al. 1998. Impact of experimentally induced serotonin deficiency by tryptophan depletion on sleep EEG in healthy subjects. *Neuropsychopharmacology* 18: 112–124. [15]

Voigt, T., and Wässle, H. 1987. Dopaminergic innervation of A II amacrine cells in mammalian retina. *J. Neurosci.* 7: 4115–4128. [18]

Vollrath, M. A., Kwan, K. Y., and Corey, D. P. 2007. The micromachinery of mechanotransduction in hair cells. *Annu. Rev. Neurosci.* 30: 339–365. [21]

von Bekesy, G. 1960. *Experiments in Hearing.* McGraw-Hill, New York. [24]

von Euler, U. S. 1956. *Noradrenaline.* Charles Thomas, Springfield, IL. [19]

Von Euler, U. S., and Gaddum, J. H. 1931. An unidentified depressor substance in certain tissue extracts. *J. Physiol.* 72: 74–87. [14]

von Heimendahl, M., Itskov, P. M., Arabzadeh, E., and Diamond, M. E. 2007. Neuronal activity in rat barrel cortex underlying texture discrimination. *PLOS Biol* 5: e305. [23]

Vugler, A. A. 2010. Progress toward the maintenance and repair of degenerating retinal circuitry. *Retina* 30: 983–1001. [30]

Vyskocil, F., Malomouzh, A. I., and Nikolsky, E. E. 2009. Non-quantal acetylcholine release at the neuromuscular junction. *Physiol. Res.* 58: 763–784. [13]

Wada, Y., and Yamamoto, T. 2001. Selective impairment of facial recognition due to a haematoma restricted to the right fusiform and lateral occipital region. *J. Neurol. Neurosurg. Psychiatry* 71: 254–257. [25]

Wagenaar, D. A. 2015. A classic model animal in the 21st century: Recent lessons from the leech nervous system. *J. Exp. Biol.* 218: 3353–3359. doi: 10.1242/jeb.113860. [20]

Wager, T. D., Rilling, J. K., Smith, E. E., et al. 2004. Placebo-induced changes in fMRI in the anticipation and experience of pain. *Science* 303: 1162–1167. [23]

Wagner, F. B., Mignardot, J. B., Le Goff-Mignardot, C. G., et al. 2018. Targeted neurotechnology restores walking in humans with spinal cord injury. *Nature* 563: 65–71. [29]

Wagner, J. A., Carlson, S. S., and Kelly, R. B. 1978. Chemical and physical characterization of cholinergic synaptic vesicles. *Biochemistry* 17: 1199–1206. [13]

Wagner, S., Castel, M., Gainer, H., and Yarom, Y. 1997. GABA in the mammalian suprachiasmatic nucleus and its role in diurnal rhythmicity. *Nature* 387: 598–603. [19]

Wagner, S., Sagiv, N., and Yarom, Y. 2001. GABA-induced current and circadian regulation of chloride in neurones of the rat suprachiasmatic nucleus. *J. Physiol.* 537: 853–869. [19]

Wagshul, M. E. et al. 2006. Amplitude and phase of cerebrospinal fluid pulsations: experimental studies and review of the literature. *J. Neurosurg.* 104: 810–819. [18]

Wahl-Schott, C., and Biel, M. 2009. HCN channels: Structure, cellular regulation and physiological function. *Cell. Mol. Life Sci.* 66: 470–494. [12]

Wainer, B. H., Levey, A. I., Mufson, E. J., and Mesulam, M. M. 1984. Cholinergic systems in mammalian brain identified with antibodies against choline acetyltransferase. *Neurochem. Int.* 6: 163–182. [14]

Waite, A., Tinsley, C. L., Locke, M., and Blake, D. J. 2009. The neurobiology of the dystrophin-associated glycoprotein complex. *Ann. Med.* 41: 344–359. [11]

Waldmann, R., Champigny, G., Bassilana, F., et al. 1997. A proton-gated cation channel involved in acid-sensing. *Nature* 386: 173–177. [21]

Walker, D., and De Waard, M. 1998. Subunit interaction sites in voltage-dependent Ca^{2+} channels: Role in channel function. *Trends Neurosci.* 21: 148–154. [5]

Wallace, C. S., Lyford, G. L., Worley. P. F., and Steward, O. 1998. Differential Intracellular Sorting of Immediate Early Gene mRNAs Depends on Signals in the mRNA Sequence. *J. Neurosci.* 18: 26–35. [17]

Wallner, M., Hanchar, H. J., and Olsen, R. W. 2003. Ethanol enhances $\alpha_4\beta_3\delta$ and $\alpha_6\beta_3\delta$ γ-aminobutyric acid type A receptors at low concentrations known to affect humans. *Proc. Natl. Acad. Sci. USA* 100: 15218–1522. [14]

Walsh, E. J., and McGee, J. 1987. Postnatal development of auditory nerve and cochlear nucleus neuronal responses in kittens. *Hear Res.* 28: 97–116. [28]

Walter, J., Henke-Fahle, S., and Bonhoeffer, F. 1987. Avoidance of posterior tectal membranes by temporal retinal axons. *Development* 101: 909–913. [27]

Walter, J., Kern-Veits, B., Huf, J., et al. 1987. Recognition of position-specific properties of tectal cell membranes by retinal axons *in vitro.* *Development* 101: 685–696. [27]

Walters, E. T., and Cohen, L. B. 1997. Functions of the LE sensory neurons in *Aplysia.* *Invert. Neurosci.* 3: 15–25. [20]

Walum, H., Westberg, L., Henningsson, S., et al. 2008. Genetic variation in the vasopressin receptor 1a gene (*AVPR1A*) associates with pair-bonding behavior in humans. *Proc. Natl. Acad. Sci. USA* 105: 14153–14156. [14]

Wandell, B. 1995. *Foundations of Vision.* Oxford University Press/Sinauer, Sunderland, MA. [22]

Wang, C., et al. 2020. Microglia mediate forgetting via complement-dependent synaptic elimination. *Science* 367: 688–694. [17]

Wang, D. O., Kim, S. M., Zhao, Y., et al. 2009. Synapse- and stimulus-specific local translation during long-term neuronal plasticity. *Science* 324: 1536–1540. [12]

Wang, F., Nemes, A., Mendelsohn, M., and Axel, R. 1998. Odorant receptors govern the formation of a precise topographic map. *Cell* 93: 47–60. [28]

Wang, H.-S., and McKinnon, D. 1995. Potassium currents in rat prevertebral and paravertebral sympathetic neurones: Control of firing properties. *J. Physiol.* 485: 319–325. [19]

Wang, H.-S., Pan, Z., Shi, W., et al. 1998. KCNQ2 and KCNQ3 potassium channel subunits: Molecular correlates of the M-channel. *Science* 282: 1890–1893. [12]

Wang, H., and Macagno, E. R. 1997. The establishment of peripheral sensory arbors in the leech: *In vivo* time-lapse studies reveal a highly dynamic process. *J. Neurosci.* 17: 2408–2419. [20]

Wang, H., and Macagno, E. R. 1998. A detached branch stops being recognized as self by other branches of a neuron. *J. Neurobiol.* 35: 53–64. [20]

Wang, H., Kunkel, D. D., Martin, T. M., et al. 1993. Heteromultimeric K$^+$ channels in terminal and juxtaparanodal regions of neurons. *Nature* 365: 75–79. [8]

Wang, H. S. Pan, Z., Shi, W., et al. 1998 KCNQ2 and KCNQ3 potassium channel subunits: Molecular correlates of the M-channel. *Science* 282: 1890–1893. [5]

Wang, Q., Curran, M. E. Splawski, I., et al. 1996. Positional cloning of a novel potassium channel gene: KVLQT1 mutations cause cardiac arrhythmias. *Nat. Genet.* 12: 17–23. [5]

Wang, R. Y., and Aghajanian, G. K. 1977. Antidromically identified serotonergic neurons in the rat midbrain raphe: Evidence for collateral inhibition. *Brain Res.* 132: 186–193. [14]

Wang, T., and Montell, C. 2007. Phototransduction and retinal degeneration in *Drosophila.* *Pflügers Arch.* 454: 821–847. [22]

Wang, X., and Kadia, S. C. 2001. Differential representation of species-specific primate vocalizations in the auditory cortices of marmoset and cat. *J. Neurophysiol.* 86: 2616–2620. [24]

Wang, Y. F., and Hatton, G. I. 2006. Mechanisms underlying oxytocin-induced excitation of supraoptic neurons: Prostaglandin mediation of actin polymerization. *J. Neurophysiol.* 3933–3947. [18]

Wang, Z., Gerstein, M., and Snyder, M. 2009. RNA-Seq: A revolutionary tool for transcriptomics. *Nat. Rev. Genet.* 10: 57–63. doi: 10.1038/nrg2484. [1]

Wangemann, P. 2006. Supporting sensory transduction: Cochlear fluid homeostasis and the endocochlear potential. *J. Physiol.* 576: 11–21. [24]

Ward, N. S., and Frackowiak, R. S. 2004. Towards a new mapping of brain cortex function. *Cerebrovasc. Dis.* 17(Suppl 3): 35–38. [1, 26]

Warr, W. B. 1975. Olivocochlear and vestibular efferent neurons of the feline brain stem: Their location, morphology and number determined by retrograde axonal transport and acetylcholinesterase histochemistry. *J. Comp. Neurol.* 161: 159–181. [24]

Warr, W. B., Guinan J. J., and White J. S. 1986. Organization of the efferent fibers: The later and medial olivocochlear systems. In Altschuler, R. A., Hoffman, D. W., and Bobbin, R. P. (Eds.), *Neurobiology of Hearing: The Cochlea.* Raven Press, New York, pp. 333–348. [24]

Waselus, M., Van Bockstaele, E. J. 2007. Co-localization of corticotropin-releasing factor and vesicular glutamate transporters within axon terminals of the rat dorsal raphe nucleus. *Brain Res.* 1174: 53–65. [14]

Wässle, H. 2004. Parallel processing in the mammalian retina. *Nat. Rev. Neurosci.* 5: 747–757. [22]

Watanabe, H., Nagata, E., Kosakai, A., et al. 2000. Disruption of the epilepsy KCNQ2 gene results in neural hyperexcitability. *J. Neurochem.* 75: 28–33. [5]

Waters, J., Schaefer, A., and Sakmann, B. 2005. Backpropagating action potentials in neurones: Measurement, mechanisms, and potential functions. *Prog. Biophys. Mol. Biol.* 87: 145–170. [8]

Watkins, J. C., and Evans, R. H. 1981. Excitatory amino acid transmitters. *Annu. Rev. Pharmacol. Toxicol.* 21: 165–204. [11]

Watters, M. R. 2005 Tropical marine neurotoxins: Venoms to drugs. *Semin. Neurol.* 25: 278–289. [7]

Weatherbee, S. D., Anderson, K. V., and Niswander, L. A. 2006. LDL-receptor-related protein 4 is crucial for formation of the neuromuscular junction. *Development* 133: 4993–5000. [29]

Weber, E., Evans, C. J., and Barchas, J. D. 1983. Multiple endogenous ligands for opioid receptors. *Trends Neurosci.* 6: 333–336. [14]

Webster, H., and Aström, K. E. 2009. Gliogenesis: Historical perspectives, 1839–1985. *Adv. Anat. Embryol. Cell Biol.* 202: 1–109. [10]

Wehner, R. 1989. Neurobiology of polarization vision. *Trends Neurosci.* 12: 353–359. [20]

Wehner, R. 1994. Himmelsbild und kompassauge—neurobiologie eines Navigationssystems, *Verhand. Deutsch. Zool. Ges.* 87: 9–37. [20]

Wehner, R. 1994. The polarization-vision project: Championing organismic biology. *Fortschr. Zool.* 31: 11–53. [20]

Wehner, R. 1996. Polarisationsmuster analyse bei Insekten. *Nova Acta Leoplodina NF* 72: 159–183. [20]

Wehner, R. 1997. The ant's celestial compass: Spectral and polarization channels. In Lehrer, M. (Ed.) *Orientation and Communication in Arthropods.* Birkhauser, Basel, Switzerland, pp. 145–185. [20]

Wehner, R., and Bernard, G. D. 1993. Photoreceptor twist: A solution to the false-color problem. *Proc. Natl. Acad. Sci. USA* 90: 4132–4135. [20]

Wehner, R., and Muller, M. 2006. The significance of direct sunlight and polarized skylight in the ant's celestial system of navigation. *Proc. Natl. Acad. Sci. USA* 103: 12575–12579. [20]

Wei, A. D., Gutman, G. A., Aldrich, R., et al. 2005. International Union of Pharmacology. LII. Nomenclature and molecular relationships of calcium-activated potassium channels. *Pharmacol. Rev.* 57: 463–472. [5]

Weidner, N., Ner, A., Salimi, N., and Tuszynski, M. H. 2001. Spontaneous corticospinal axonal plasticity and functional recovery after adult central nervous system injury. *Proc. Natl. Acad. Sci. USA* 98: 3513–3518. [29]

Weiner, N., and Rabadjija, M. 1968. The effect of nerve stimulation on the synthesis and metabolism of norepinephrine from cat spleen during sympathetic nerve stimulation. *J. Pharmacol. Exp. Ther.* 160: 61–71. [15]

Weinfeld, A. B., Yuksel, E., Boutros, S., et al. 2000. Clinical and scientific considerations in leech therapy for the management of acute venous congestion: An updated review. *Ann. Plast. Surg.* 45: 207–212. [20]

Weinhard, L., et al. 2018. Microglia remodel synapses by presynaptic trogocytosis and spine head filopodia induction. *Nat. Comm.* 9: 1228. [17]

Weinreich, D. 1970. Ionic mechanisms of post-tetanic potentiation at the neuromuscular junction of the frog. *J. Physiol.* 212: 431–446. [16]

Weinstein, S., Semmes, J., Ghent, L., and Teuber, H. L. 1958. Roughness discrimination after penetrating brain injury in man: Analysis according to locus of lesion. *J. Comp. Physiol. Psychol.* 51: 269–275. [23]

Weisblat, D. A., and Kuo, D.-H. 2009. *Helobdella* (Leech), a model for developmental studies. In *Emerging Model Organisms, a Laboratory Manual.* Cold Spring Harbor Laboratory, Cold Spring Harbor, NY, pp. 245–274. [20]

Weisblat, D. A., and Shankland, M. 1985. Cell lineage and segmentation in the leech. *Philos. Trans. R. Soc. Lond., B, Biol. Sci.* 312: 39–56. [27]

Weisblat, D. A., Zackson, S. L., Blair, S. S., and Young, J. D. 1980. Cell lineage analysis by intracellular injection of fluorescent tracers. *Science* 209: 1538–1541. [27]

Weiss, P., and Hiscoe, H. B. 1948. Experiments of the mechanism of nerve growth. *J. Exp. Zool.* 107: 315–395. [15]

Weissman, T. A., Riquelme, P. A., Ivic, L., et al. 2004. Calcium waves propagate through radial glial cells and modulate proliferation in the developing neocortex. *Neuron* 43: 647–661. [10]

Weissmann, C. 2009. Thoughts on mammalian prion strains. *Folia Neuropathol.* 47: 104–113. [30]

Weitsen, H. A., and Weight, F. F. 1977. Synaptic innervation of sympathetic ganglion cells in the bullfrog. *Brain Res.* 128: 197–211. [15]

Welker, C. 1976. Receptive fields of barrels in the somatosensory neocortex of the rat. *J. Comp. Neurol.* 166: 173–189. [23]

Welker, E., and van der Loos, H. 1986. Quantitative correlation between barrel-field size and the sensory innervation of the whiskerpad: A comparative study in six strains of mice bred for different patterns of mystacial vibrissae. *J. Neurosci.* 6: 3355–3373. [23]

Werker, J. F., and Tees, R. C. 2005. Speech perception as a window for understanding plasticity and commitment in language systems of the brain. *Dev. Psychobiol.* 46: 233–251. [28]

Werman, R., Davidoff, R. A., and Aprison, M. H. 1968. Inhibitory action of glycine on spinal neurons in the cat. *J. Neurophysiol.* 31: 81–95. [14]

Werner, R., Levine, E., Rabadan-Diehl, C., and Dahl, G. 1989. Formation of hybrid cell-cell channels. *Proc. Natl. Acad. Sci. USA* 86: 5380–5384. [11]

Wersinger, E., McLean, W. J., Fuchs, P. A., and Pyott, S. J. 2010. BK channels mediate cholinergic inhibition of high frequency cochlear hair cells. *PLOS ONE* 5: e13836. [24]

Wes, P. D. Chevesich, J., Jeromin, A., et al. 1995. TRPC1, a human homolog of a *Drosophila* store-operated channel. *Proc.Natl. Acad. Sci. USA* 92: 9652–9656. [5]

Wessberg, J., Olausson, H., Fernström, K. W., and Vallbo, A. B. 2003. Receptive field properties of unmyelinated tactile afferents in the human skin. *J. Neurophysiol.* 89: 1567–1575. [23]

West, A. E., and Greenberg, M. E. 2011. *Cold Spring Harb. Perspect. Biol.* 3: a005744. [17]

Westheimer, G. 2009. The third dimension in the primary visual cortex. *J. Physiol.* 587: 2807–2816. [3]

Weston, J. A. 1970. The migration and differentiation of neural crest cells. *Adv. Morphog.* 8: 41–114. [27]

Weyand, T. 2015. The multifunctional lateral geniculate nucleus. *Rev. Neurosci.* 27: 135–157. [3]

Whim, M. D., Church, P. J., and Lloyd, P. E. 1993. Functional roles of peptide cotransmitters at neuromuscular synapses in *Aplysia. Mol. Neurobiol.* 7: 335–347. [15]

Whitfield, I. C. 1979. The object of the sensory cortex. *Brain Behav. EVol.* 16: 129–154. [25]

Whittington, M. A., and Traub, R. D. 2003. Interneuron diversity series: Inhibitory interneurons and network oscillations *in vitro. Trends Neurosci.* 26: 676–682. [11, 14]

Wickelgren, W. O., Leonard, J. P., Grimes, M. J., and Clark, R. D. 1985. Ultrastructural correlates of transmitter release in presynaptic areas of lamprey reticulospinal axons. *J. Neurosci.* 5: 1188–1201. [13]

Wickman, K. D., Iñiguez-Lluhi, J. A., Davenport, P. A., et al. 1994. Recombinant G-protein βγ subunits activate the muscarinic-gated atrial potassium channel. *Nature* 368: 255–257. [12]

Wictorin, K., and Bjorklund,O . 1992. Axon outgrowth from grafts of human embryonic spinal cord in the lesioned adult rat spinal cord. *Neuroreoport* 3: 1045–1048. [29]

Wiech, K., Preissl, H., and Birbaumer, N. 2001. Neural networks and pain processing. New insights from imaging techniques. *Anaesthesist* 50: 2–12. [23]

Wiederhold, M. L., and Kiang, N. Y. 1970. Effects of electric stimulation of the crossed olivocochlear bundle on single auditory-nerve fibers in the cat. *J. Acoust. Soc. Am.* 48: 950–965. [24]

Wiersma, C. A., and Yamaguchi, T. 1966. The neuronal components of the optic nerve of the crayfish as studied by single unit analysis. *J. Comp. Neurol.* 128: 333–358. [20]

Wiese, K., ed. 2002. *The Crustacean Nervous System*. Berlin, Germany. [20]

Wiesel, T. N. 1982. Postnatal development of the visual cortex and the influence of environment. *Nature* 299: 583–591. [27, 28]

Wiesel, T. N., and Hubel, D. H. 1963. Effects of visual deprivation on morphology and physiology of cells in the cats lateral geniculate body. *J. Neurophysiol.* 26: 978–993. [28]

Wiesel, T. N., and Hubel, D. H. 1963. Single-cell responses in striate cortex of kittens deprived of vision in one eye. *J. Neurophysiol.* 26: 1003–1017. [28]

Wiesel, T. N., and Hubel, D. H. 1965. Comparison of the effects of uni-lateral and bilateral eye closure on cortical unit responses in kittens. *J. Neurophysiol.* 28: 1029–1040. [28]

Wiesel, T. N., and Hubel, D. H. 1974. Ordered arrangement of orienta-tion columns in monkeys lacking visual experience. *J. Comp. Neurol.* 158: 307–318. [3, 28]

Willard, A. L. 1981. Effects of serotonin on the generation of the motor program for swimming by the medicinal leech. *J. Neurosci.* 1: 936–944. [20]

Williams, J. T., North, R. A., Shefner, S. A., et al. 1984. Membrane prop-erties of rat locus coeruleus neurones. *Neurosience* 13: 137–156. [14]

Williams, K. W., Scott, M. M., and Elmquist, J. K. 2009. From observa-tion to experimentation: Leptin action in the mediobasal hypothala-mus. *Am. J. Clin. Nutr.* 89: 9855–9905. [19]

Williams, P. R., Suzuki, S. C., Yoshimatsu, T., et al. 2010. In vivo devel-opment of outer retinal synapses in the absence of glial contact. *J. Neurosci.* 30: 11951–11961. [10]

Williamson, R., and Chrachri, A. 2007. A model biological neural net-work: The cephalopod vestibular system. *Philos. Trans. R. Soc. Lond., B, Biol. Sci.* 362: 473–481. [24]

Wilmut, I., et al. 1997. Viable offspring derived from fetal and adult mammalian cells. *Nature* 385: 810–813. [27]

Wilson Horch, H. L., and Sargent, P. B. 1995. Perisynaptic surface dis-tribution of multiple classes of nicotinic acetylcholine receptors on neurons in the chicken ciliary ganglion. *J. Neurosci.* 15: 7778–7795. [29]

Wilson Horch, H. L., and Sargent, P. B. 1996. Effects of denervation on acetylcholine receptor clusters on frog cardiac ganglion neurons as revealed by quantitative laser scanning confocal microscopy. *J. Neurosci.* 16: 1720–1729. [29]

Wilson, L., and Maden, M. 2005. The mechanisms of dorsoventral pat-terning in the vertebrate neural tube. *Dev. Biol.* 282: 1–13. [27]

Wilson, P. M., Fryer, R. H., Fang, Y., and Hatten, M. E. 2010. Astn2, a novel member of the astrotactin gene family, regulates the trafficking of ASTN1 during glial-guided neuronal migration. *J. Neurosci.* 30: 8529–8540. [27]

Wilson, R. I., and Nicoll, R. A. 2001. Endogenous cannabinoids mediate retrograde signalling at hippocampal synapses. *Nature* 410: 588–592. [12]

Wilson, R. I., and Nicoll, R. A. 2002. Endocannabinoid signaling in the brain. *Science* 296: 678–682. [12]

Wilson, S. I. and Edlund, T. 2001. Neural induction: Toward a unifying mechanism. *Nat. Neurosci. Suppl.* 4: 1161–1168. [27]

Windhorst, U. 2007. Muscle proprioceptive feedback and spinal net-works. *Brain. Res. Bull.* 73: 155–202. [26]

Winer, J. A., and Lee, C. C. 2007. The distributed auditory cortex. *Hear. Res.* 229: 3–13. [24]

Winks, J. S., Hughes, S., Filippov, A. K., et al. 2005. Relationship between membrane phosphatidylinositol-4,5-bisphosphate and receptor-mediated inhibition of native neuronal M channels. *J. Neurosci.* 25: 3400–3413. [12]

Winslow, J. T., Hastings, N., Carter, C. S., et al. 1993. A role for central vasopressin in pair bonding in monogamous prairie voles. *Nature* 365: 545–548. [14]

Winslow, R. L., and Sachs, M. B. 1987. Effect of electrical stimulation of the crossed olivocochlear bundle on auditory nerve response to tones in noise. *J. Neurophysiol.* 57: 1002–1021. [24]

Wise, A., Jupe, S. C., and Rees, S. 2004. The identification of ligands at orphan G-protein coupled receptors. *Annu. Rev. Pharmacol. Toxicol.* 44: 43–66. [14]

Wise, D. S., Schoenborn, B. P., and Karlin, A. 1981. Structure of acetyl-choline receptor dimer determined by neutron scattering and elec-tron microscopy. *J. Biol. Chem.* 256: 4124–4126. [5]

Witkovsky, P. et al. 2009. Immunocytochemical identification of proteins involved in dopamine release from the somatodendritic compartment of nigral dopaminergic neurons. *Neuroscience* 164: 488–496. [18]

Wittlinger, M., Wehner, R., and Wolf, H. 2006. The ant odometer: Stepping on stilts and stumps. *Science* 312: 1965–1967. [20]

Wittlinger, M., Wehner, R., and Wolf, H. 2007. The desert ant odom-eter: A stride integrator that accounts for stride length and walking speed. *J. Exp. Biol.* 210: 198–207. [20]

Witzemann, V., Brenner, H-R., and Sakmann, B. 1991. Neural factors regulate AChR subunit mRNAs at rat neuromuscular synapses. *J. Cell Biol.* 114: 125–141. [11, 29]

Wojciulik, E., Kanwisher, N., and Driver, J. 1998. Covert visual attention modulates face-specific activity in the human fusiform gyrus: FMRI study. *J. Neurophysiol.* 79: 1574–1578. [25]

Wolburg, H., and Paulus, W. 2010. Choroid plexus: Biology and pathol-ogy. *Acta. Neuropathol.* 119: 75–88. [10]

Wolburg, H., Noell, S., Mack, A., et al. 2009. Brain endothelial cells and the glio-vascular complex. *Cell Tissue Res.* 335: 75–96. [10]

Wolfe, J., Hill, D. N., Pahlavan, S., et al. 2008. Texture coding in the rat whisker system: Slip-stick versus differential resonance. *PLOS Biol* 6: e215. [23]

Wollmuth, L. P., and Sobolevsky, A. I. 2004. Structure and gating of the glutamate receptor ion channel. *Trends Neurosci.* 27: 321–328. [5, 11]

Womac, A. D., Burkeen, J. F., Neuendorff, N., et al. 2009. Circadian rhythms of extracellular ATP accumulation in suprachiasmatic nucleus cells and cultured astrocytes. *Eur. J. Neurosci.* 30: 869–876. [10]

Wong-Riley, M. 1989. Cytochrome oxidase: An endogenous metabolic marker for neuronal activity. *Trends Neurosci.* 12: 94–101. [3]

Wong, R. O. 1999. Retinal waves and visual system development. *Annu. Rev. Neurosci.* 22: 29–47. [28]

Woolf, N. J. 1991. Cholinergic systems in mammalian brain and spinal cord. *Prog. Neurobiol.* 37: 475–524. [14]

Woolsey, T. A., and van der Loos, H. 1970. The structural organization of layer IV in the somatosensory region (SI) of mouse cerebral cor-tex. The description of a cortical field composed of discrete cytoar-chitectonic units. *Brain Res.* 17: 205–242. [23]

Wotring, V. E., Miller, T. S., and Weiss, D. S. 2003. Mutations in the GABA receptor selectivity filter: A possible role for effective charges. *J. Physiol.* 548: 527–540. [5]

Wray, S. 2010. From nose to brain: Development of gonadotrophin-releasing hormone-1 neurones. *J. Neuroendocrinol.* 22: 743–753. [27]

Wray, S., Grant, P., and Gainer, H. 1989. Evidence that cells express-ing luteinizing hormone-releasing hormone mRNA in mouse are derived from progenitor cells in the olfactory placode. *Proc. Natl. Acad. Sci. USA* 86: 8132–8136. [19, 27]

Wright, B. D., Sen, K., Bialek, W. and Doupe, A. J. 2002. Spike tim-ing and the coding of naturalistic sounds in a central auditory area of songbirds. In *Advances in Neural Information Processing 14*, T. G. Dietterich, S. Becker, and Z. Ghahramani (Eds.). MIT Press, Cambridge, MA, pp. 309–316. [1]

Wu, J., Lewis, A. H., and Grandi, J. 2017. Touch, tension and transduction: The function and regulation of Piezo ion channels. *Trends in Biochem. Sci.* 42: 57–71. [5]

Wu, J., Yan, Z., Li, Z., et al. 2016. Structure of the voltage-gated calcium channel Ca(v)1.1 at 3.6 Å resolution. *Nature* 537: 191–196. [5]

Wu, L.-G., and Saggau, P. 1997. Presynaptic inhibition of elicited neurotransmitter release. *Trends Neurosci.* 20: 204–212. [14]

Wu, L.-G., Ryan, T. A., and Lagnado, L. 2007. Modes of synaptic vesicle retrieval at ribbon synapses, calyx-type synapses, and small central synapses. *J. Neuosci.* 27: 11793–11802. [13]

Wu, L.-J. Sweet, T.-B., and Clapham, D. E. 2010. International Union of Basic and Clinical Pharmacology. LXXVI. Current Progress in the Mammalian TRP Ion Channel Family. *Pharmacol. Rev.* 62: 381–404. [5]

Wu, W., and Wu, L. G. 2007. Rapid bulk endocytosis and its kinetics of fission pore closure at a central synapse. *Proc. Natl. Acad. Sci. USA* 104: 10234–10239. [13]

Wu, W., Li, L., Yick, L. W., et al. 2003. GDNF and BDNF alter the expression of neuronal NOS, c-Jun, and p75 and prevent motoneuron death following spinal root avulsion in adult rats. *J. Neurotrauma* 20: 603–612. [27]

Wurmser, A. E., Nakashima, K., Summers, R. G., et al. 2004. Cell fusion-independent differentiation of neural stem cells to the endothelial lineage. *Nature* 430: 350–356. [27]

Xerri, C., Coq, J. O., Merzenich, M. M., and Jenkins, W.M 1996. Experience-induced plasticity of cutaneous maps in the primary somatosensory cortex of adult monkeys and rats. *J. Physiol. Paris* 90: 277–280. [26]

Xerri, C., Stern, J. M., and Merzenich, M. M. 1994. Alterations of the cortical representation of the rat ventrum induced by nursing behavior. *J. Neurosci.* 14: 1710–1721. [23]

Xiao, C., Nashmi, R., McKinney, S., et al. 2009. Chronic nicotine selectively enhances $\alpha_4\beta_2^*$ nicotinic acetylcholine receptors in the nigrostriatal dopamine pathway. *J Neurosci.* 29: 12428–12439. [14]

Xiao, J., Kilpatrick, T. J., and Murray, S. S. 2009. The role of neurotrophins in the regulation of myelin development. *Neurosignals* 17: 265–276. [10]

Xin, D., Bloomfield, S. A. 1999. Dark- and light-induced changes in coupling between horizontal cells in mammalian retina. *J. Comp. Neurol.* 405: 75–87. [18]

Xu, J., Du, Y., and Deng, H. 2015. Direct lineage reprogramming: Strategies, mechanisms and applications. *Cell Stem Cell* 16: 119–134. [29]

Xu, J., and Wu, L-G. 2005. The decrease in the presynaptic calcium current is a major cause of short-term depression at a calyx-type synapse. *Neuron* 46: 633–645. [16]

Xu, J., He, L., and Wu, L-G. 2007. Role of calcium channels in short-term synaptic plasticity. *Curr. Opin. Neurobiol.* 17: 352–359. [16]

Xu, K., and Terakawa, S. 1999. Fenestration nodes and the wide submyelinic space form the basis for unusually fast impulse conduction of shrimp myelinated axons. *J. Exp. Biol.* 202: 1979–1989. [8]

Xu, R., and Salpeter, M. M. 1995. Protein kinase A regulates the degradation rate of Rs acetylcholine receptors. *J. Cell. Physiol.* 165: 30–39. [29]

Xu, T., et al. 2009. Rapid formation and selective stabilization of synapses for enduring motor memories. *Nature* 462: 915–919. [17]

Yamada, T., Placzek, M., Tanaka, H., et al. 1991. Control of cell pattern in the developing nervous system: Polarizing activity of the floor plate and notochord. *Cell* 64: 635–647. [27]

Yamamori, T., Fukada, K., Aebersold, R., et al. 1989. The cholinergic neuronal differentiation factor from heart cells is identical to leukemia inhibitory factor. *Science* 246: 1412–1416. [27]

Yamane, Y., Carlson, E. T., Bowman, K. C., et al. 2008. A neural code for three-dimensional object shape in macaque inferotemporal cortex. *Nat. Neurosci.* 11: 1352–1360. [25]

Yamasaki, M., Matsui, M., and Watanabe, M. 2010. Preferential localization of muscarinic M_1 receptor on dendritic shaft and spine of cortical pyramidal cells and its anatomical evidence for volume transmission. *J. Neurosci.* 30: 4408–4418. [14]

Yamashita, A., Singh, S. K., Kawate, T., et al. 2005. Crystal structure of a bacterial homologue of Na^+/Cl^--dependent neurotransmitter transporters. *Nature* 437: 215–223. [9]

Yamashita, M., and Wässle, H. 1991. Responses of rod bipolar cells isolated from the rat retina to the glutamate agonist 2-amino-4-phosphonobutyric acid (APB). *J. Neurosci.* 11: 2372–2382. [22]

Yamins, D. L., and DiCarlo, J. J. 2016. Using goal-driven deep learning models to understand sensory cortex. *Nat. Neurosci.* 19: 356–365. doi: 10.1038/nn.4244. [25]

Yan, T. C., Hunt, S. P., and Stanford, S. C. 2009. Behavioural and neurochemical abnormalities in mice lacking functional tachykinin-1 (NK1) receptors: A model of attention deficit hyperactivity disorder. *Neuropharmacology* 57: 627–635. [14]

Yang, G., et al. 2009. Stably maintained dendritic spines are associated with lifelong memories. *Nature* 462: 920–924. [17]

Yang, J., Ellinor, P. T., Sather, W. A., et al. 1993. Molecular determinants of Ca^{2+} selectivity and ion permeation in L-type calcium channels. *Nature* 366: 158–161. [5]

Yang, N., George, A. L., and Horn, R. 1996. Molecular basis of charge movement in voltage-gated sodium channels. *Neuron* 16: 113–122. [5]

Yang, X. F., Miao, Y., Ping, Y., et al. 2011. Melatonin inhibits tetraethylammonium-sensitive potassium channels of rod ON type bipolar cells via MT2 receptors in rat retina. *Neuroscience* 173: 19–29. [22]

Yang, X. L., Gao, F., and Wu, S. M. 1999. Modulation of horizontal cell function by $GABA_A$ and $GABA_C$ receptors in dark- and light-adapted tiger salamander retina. *Vis. Neurosci.* 16: 967–979. [22]

Yao, J., et al. 2006.An essential role for beta-actin mRNA localization and translation in Ca^{2+}-dependent growth cone guidance. *Nat. Neurosci.* 9: 1265–1273. [27]

Yap, E-L., and Greenberg, M. E. 2018. Activity-regulated transcription: Bridging the gap between neural activity and behavior. *Neuron* 100: 330. [17]

Yarom, Y., Sugimori, M., and Llinás, R. 1985. Ionic currents and firing patterns or mammalian vagal motoneurons *in vitro. Neuroscience* 16: 719–737. [7]

Yates, B. J., and Miller, A. D. 1994. Properties of sympathetic reflexes elicited by natural vestibular stimulation: Implications for cardiovascular control. *J. Neurophysiol.* 71: 2087–2092. [24]

Yau, K. W. 1976. Physiological properties and receptive fields of mechanosensory neurones in the head ganglion of the leech: Comparison with homologous cells in segmental ganglia. *J. Physiol.* 263: 489–512. [20]

Yau, K. W., and Nakatani, K. 1985. Light-suppressible, cyclic GMP-sensitive conductance in the plasma membrane of a truncated rod outer segment. *Nature* 317: 252–255. [22]

Ye, W., Shimamura, K., Rubenstein, J. L., et al. 1998. FGF and Shh signals control dopaminergic and serotonergic cell fate in the anterior neural plate. *Cell* 93: 755–766. [27]

Yeh, C. I., Stoelzel, C. R., Weng, C., and Alonso, J. M. 2009. Functional consequences of neuronal divergence within the retinogeniculate pathway. *J. Neurophysiol.* 101: 2166–2185. [2]

Yellen, G., Jurman, M. E., Abramson, T., and MacKinnon, R. 1991. Mutations affecting internal TEA blockade identify the probable pore-forming region of a K^+ channel. *Science* 251: 939–942. [5]

Yernool, D., Boudker, O., Jin, Y., and Gouaux, E. 2004. Structure of a glutamate transporter homologue from *Pyrococcus horikoshil. Nature* 431: 811–818. [9]

Yi, J. J., and Ehlers, M. D. 2005. Ubiquitin and protein turnover in synapse function. *Neuron* 47: 629–632. [17]

Yool, A. J., and Schwartz, T. L. 1991. Alterations in ionic selectivity of a K^+ channel by mutation of the H5 region. *Nature* 349: 700–704. [5]

Yoshimura, M., and Furue, H. 2006. Mechanisms for the anti-nociceptive actions of the descending noradrenergic and serotonergic systems in the spinal cord. *J. Pharmacol. Sci.* 101: 107–117. [14]

Young, E. D. 2008. Neural representation of spectral and temporal information in speech. *Philos. Trans. R. Soc. Lond., B, Biol. Sci.* 363: 923–945. [24]

Young, E. D., and Sachs, M. B. 1979. Representation of steady-state vowels in the temporal aspects of the discharge patterns of populations of auditory-nerve fibers. *J. Acoust. Soc. Am.* 66: 1381–1403. [24]

Young, J. Z. 1936. The giant nerve fibres and epistellar body of cephalopods. *Q. J. Microsc. Sci.* 78: 367–386. [6]

Young, L. J. 2009. Love: Neuroscience reveals all. *Nature* 457: 148. [14]

Young, L. J., Nilsen, R., Waymire, K. G., et al. 1999. Increased affiliative response to vasopressin in mice expressing the V_{1a} receptor from a monogamous vole. *Nature* 400: 766–768. [14]

Young, N. A., Vuong, J., and Teskey, G. C. 2012. Development of motor maps in rats and their modulation by experience. *J. Neurophysiol.* 108: 1309–1317. [26]

Younts, T. J., Monday, H. R., Dudok, B., et al. 2016. Presynaptic Protein Synthesis Is Required for Long-Term Plasticity of GABA Release. *Neuron* 92: 479–492. [16, 17]

Yu, F. H., and Catterall, W. A. 2003. Overview of the voltage-gated sodium channel family. *Genome Biol.* 4: 207.1–207.7. [5]

Yu, F. H., Westenbroek, R. E., Silos-Santiago, I., et al. 2003. Sodium channel β4, a new disulfide-linked auxiliary subunit with similarity to β2. *J. Neurosci.* 23: 7577–7585. [5]

Yu, W. M., Yu, H., and Chen, Z. L. 2007. Laminins in peripheral nerve development and muscular dystrophy. *Mol. Neurobiol.* 35: 288–297. [10]

Yue, W. W. S., Silverman, D. Ren, X., et al. 2019. Elementary response triggered by transducin in retinal rods. *Proc. Nat. Acad. Sci. USA* 116: 5144–5153. [22]

Yurek, D. M., and Sladek, J. R., Jr. 1990. Dopamine cell replacement: Parkinson's disease. *Annu. Rev. Neurosci.* 13: 415–440. [14]

Zagha, E., Manita, S., Ross, W. N., and Rudy, B. 2010. Dendritic Kv3.3 potassium channels in cerebellar purkinje cells regulate generation and spatial dynamics of dendritic Ca^{2+} spikes. *J. Neurophysiol.* 103: 3516–3525. [26]

Zagotta, W. N., Hoshi, T., and Aldrich, R. W. 1990. Restoration of inactivation in mutants of *Shaker* potassium channels by a peptide derived from ShB. *Science* 250: 568–571. [7]

Zagrebelsky, M., Buffo, A., Skerra, A., et al. 1998. Retrograde regulation of growth-associated gene expression in adult rat Purkinje cells by myelin-associated neurite growth inhibitory proteins. *J. Neurosci.* 18: 7912–7929. [29]

Zamparo, I., Francia, S., Franchi, S. A., et al. 2019. Axonal Odorant Receptors Mediate Axon Targeting. *Cell Rep.* 29: 4334–4348. [28]

Zanazzi, G., and Matthews, G. 2009. The molecular architecture of ribbon presynaptic terminals. *Mol. Neurobiol.* 39: 130–148. [13, 22]

Zeanah, C. H., Egger, H. L., Smyke, A. T., et al. 2009. Institutional rearing and psychiatric disorders in Romanian preschool children. *Am. J. Psych.* 166: 777–785. [28]

Zehring, W. A., Wheeler, D. A., Reddy, P., et al. 1984. P-element transformation with period locus DNA restores rhythmicity to mutant, arrhythmic *Drosophila melanogaster*. *Cell* 39: 369–376. [19]

Zeki, S. 1990. Colour visions and functional specialization in the visual cortex. *Disc. Neurosci.* 6: 1–64. [3]

Zeki S. 2005. The Ferrier Lecture 1995 Behind the Seen: The functional specialization of the brain in space and time. *Phil. Trans. R. Soc.* B3601145–1183. [2]

Zeki, S. 2007. The neurobiology of love. *FEBS Lett.* 581: 2575–2579. [14]

Zeki, S., Watson, J. D., Lueck, C. J., et al. 1991. A direct demonstration of functional specialization in human visual cortex. *J. Neurosci.* 11: 641–649. [3]

Zeki, S. M. 1974. Functional organization of a visual area in the posterior bank of the superior temporal sulcus of the rhesus monkey. *J. Physiol.* 236: 549–573. [25]

Zelenin, P. V., Beloozerova, I. N., Sirota, M. G., et al. 2010. Activity of red nucleus neurons in the cat during postural corrections. *J. Neurosci.* 30: 14533–14542. [26]

Zemelman, B. V., Lee, G. A., Ng, M., and Miesenböck, G. 2002. Selective photostimulation of genetically ChARGed neurons. *Neuron* 33: 15–22. [1]

Zenisek, D., Steyer, J. A., Feldman, M. E., and Almers, W. 2002. A membrane marker leaves synaptic vesicles in milliseconds in retinal bipolar cells. *Neuron* 35: 1085–1097. [13]

Zha, D., Chen, F., Ramamoorthy, S., et al. 2012. In vivo outer hair cell length changes expose the active process in the cochlea. *PLOS ONE* 7:e32757. [24]

Zhai, S., et al. 2013. Long-distance integration of nuclear ERK signaling triggered by activation of a few dendritic spines. *Science* 342: 1107–1111. [17]

Zhang, A. J., Jacoby, R., and Wu. S. M. 2011. Light- and dopamine-regulated receptive field plasticity in primate horizontal cells. *J. Comp. Neurol.* 519: 2125–2134. [3]

Zhang, B., Luo, S., Wang, Q., et al. 2008. LRP4 serves as a coreceptor of agrin. *Neuron* 60: 285–297. [29]

Zhang, H. Q., Murray, G. M., Coleman, et al. 2001. Functional characteristics of the parallel SI- and SII-projecting neurons of the thalamic ventral posterior nucleus in the marmoset. *J. Neurophysiol.* 85: 1805–1822. [23]

Zhang, J., Carver, C. M., Choveau, F. S. and Shapiro, M. S. 2016. Clustering and functional coupling of diverse ion channels and signaling proteins revealed by super-resolution STORM microscopy in neurons. *Neuron* 92: 461–478. [12]

Zhang, Q., Li, Y., and Tsien, R. W. 2009. The dynamic control of kiss-and-run and vesicle reuse probed with single nanoparticles. *Science* 323: 1449–1453. [13]

Zhang, W., Basile, A. S., Gomeza, J., et al. 2002. Characterization of central inhibitory muscarinic autoreceptors by the use of muscarinic acetylcholine receptor knock-out mice. *J. Neurosci.* 22: 1709–1717. [14]

Zhang, Y., Buonanno, A., Vertes, R. P., et al. 2012. NR2C in the thalamic reticular nucleus; effects of the NR2C knockout. *PLOS ONE* 7:e41908. [11]

Zhang, Y., Hoon, M. A., Chandrashekar, J., et al. 2003. Coding of sweet, bitter, and umami tastes: Different receptor cells sharing similar signaling pathways. *Cell* 112: 293–301. [21]

Zhang, Z., Zhao, Z., Margolskee, R., and Liman, E. 2007. The transduction channel TRPM5 is gated by intracellular calcium in taste cells. *J. Neurosci.* 27: 5777–5786. [21]

Zhao, S., and Frotscher, M. 2010. Go or stop? Divergent roles of Reelin in radial neuronal migration. *Neuroscientist* 16: 421–434. [27]

Zhao, X., Stafford, B. K., Godin, A. L., et al. 2014. Photoresponse diversity among the five types of intrinsically photosensitive retinal ganglion cells. *J. Physiol.* 592: 1619–1636. doi: 10.1113/jphysiol.2013.262782. [22]

Zheng, C., Heintz, N., and Hatten, M. E. 1996. CNS gene encoding astrotactin, which supports neuronal migration along glial fibers. *Science* 272: 417–419. [27]

Zheng, J., Shen, W., He, D. Z., et al. 2000. Prestin is the motor protein of cochlear outer hair cells. *Nature* 405: 149–155. [24]

Zhou, F. M., Liang, Y., Salas, R., et al. 2005. Corelease of dopamine and serotonin from striatal dopamine terminals. *Neuron* 46: 65–74. [15]

Zhou, F. M., Wilson, C. J., and Dani, J. A. 2002. Cholinergic interneuron characteristics and nicotinic properties in the striatum. *J. Neurobiol.* 53: 590–605. [14]

Zhou, J., Shapiro, M. S., and Hille, B. 1997. Speed of Ca^{2+} channel modulation by neurotransmitters in rat sympathetic neurons. *J. Neurophysiol.* 77: 2040–2048. [12]

Zhou, Q., et al. 2004. Shrinkage of dendritic spines associated with long-term depression of hippocampal synapses. Neuron 44: 749–757. [17]

Zhou, W., Raisman, G., and Zhou, C. 1998. Transplanted embryonic entorhinal neurons make functional synapses in adult host hippocampus. *Brain Res.* 788: 202–206. [29]

Zhou, Z. J. 1998. Direct participation of starburst amacrine cells in spontaneous rhythmic activities in the developing mammalian retina. *J. Neurosci.* 18: 4155–4165. [28]

Zhu, X., Bergles, D. E., and Nishiyama, A. 2008. NG2 cells generate both oligodendrocytes and gray matter astrocytes. *Development* 135:145–157. doi:10.1242/dev.004895, [10]

Zhu, X., Chu, P. B., Peyton, M., and Birnbaumer, L. 1995.Molecular cloning of a widely expressed human homo logue for the *Drosophila trp* gene. *FEBS Lett, 373*: 193–198. [5]

Zhu, X., Hill, R. A., and Nishiyama, A. 2008. NG2 cells generate oligodendrocytes and gray matter astrocytes in the spinal cord. *Neuron Glia Biol.* 4: 19–26. doi:10.1017/S1740925X09000015. [10]

Zhuo, M., Small, S. A., Kandel, E. R., and Hawkins, R. D. 1993. Nitric oxide and carbon monoxide produce activity-dependent long-term synaptic enhancement in hippocampus. *Science* 260: 1946–1950. [12]

Zigmond, R. E., Schwarzchild, M. A., and Rittenhouse, A. R. 1989. Acute regulation of tyrosine hydroxylase by nerve activity and by neurotransmitters via phosphorylation. *Annu. Rev. Neurosci.* 12: 415–461. [15]

Zihl, J., Von Cramon, D., and Mai, N. 1983. Selective disturbance of movement vision after bilateral brain damage. *Brain* 106: 313–340. [25]

Zimmermann, H. 2006. Ectonucleotidases in the nervous system. In *Novartis Foundation Symposium 276: Purinergic Signalling in Neuron-Glial Interactions.* Wiley, Chichester, UK, pp. 113–128. [15]

Zimmermann, H., and Denston, C. R. 1977. Recycling of synaptic vesicles in the cholinergic synapses of the *Torpedo* electric organ during induced transmitter release. *Neuroscience* 2: 695–714. [13]

Zimmermann, H., and Denston, C. R. 1977. Separation of synaptic vesicles of different functional states from the cholinergic synapses of the *Torpedo* electric organ. *Neuroscience* 2: 715–730. [13]

Ziskin, J. L., Nishiyama, A., Rubio, M., et al. 2007. Vesicular release of glutamate from unmyelinated axons in white matter. *Nat. Neurosci.* 10: 321–330. doi: 10.1038/nn1854. [10]

Zito, K., Knott, G., Shepherd, G. M., et al. 2004. Induction of spine growth and synapse formation by regulation of the spine actin cytoskeleton. *Neuron* 44: 321–334. [11]

Zoccolan, D., Kouh, M., Poggio, T., and DiCarlo, J. J. 2007. Trade-off between object selectivity and tolerance in monkey inferotemporal cortex. *J. Neurosci.* 27: 12292–12307. [25]

Zollikofer, C., Wehner, R., and Fukushi, T. 1995. Optical scaling in conspecific *Cataglyphis* ants. *J. Exp. Biol.* 198: 1637–1646. [20]

Zou, D. J., Feinstein, P., Rivers, A. L., et al. 2004. Postnatal refinement of peripheral olfactory projections. *Science* 304: 1976–1979. [28]

Zubieta, J. K., and Stohler, C. S. 2009. Neurobiological mechanisms of placebo responses. *Ann. NY Acad. Sci.* 1156: 198–210. [23]

Zubieta, J. K., Bueller, J. A., Jackson, L. R., et al. 2005. Placebo effects mediated by endogenous opioid activity on μ-opioid receptors. *J. Neurosci.* 25: 7754–7762. [23]

Zucker, R. S., and Regehr, W. G. 2002. Short-term synaptic plasticity. *Annu. Rev. Physiol.* 64: 355–405. [16]

Zuo, Y., Lubischer, J. L., Kang, H., et al. 2004. Fluorescent proteins expressed in mouse transgenic lines mark subsets of glia, neurons, macrophages, and dendritic cells for vital examination. *J. Neurosci.* 24: 10999–11009. [10]

Zuo, Y., Perkon, I., and Diamond, M. E. 2011. Whisking and whisker kinematics during a texture classification task. *Philos. Trans. R. Soc. Lond., B, Biol. Sci.* 366: 3058–3069. [23]

Zweifel, L. S., Kuruvilla, R., and Ginty, D. D. 2005. Functions and mechanisms of retrograde neurotrophin signaling. *Nat. Rev. Neurosci.* 6: 615–625. [27]

Index

in direct chemical transmission, 187, 189, 190, 215, 218
end plate potential in, 255–258
exocytosis process in, 160, 179, 247, 261, 262–267, 269, 276, 310
extrasynaptic, 18, 187, 250, 289, 387, 389–390
factors regulating, 16, 18, 253
by glial cells, 178–179
G protein inhibition of calcium channels in, 224–226
kiss-and-run process in, 269, 270, 273, 274, 275
in light response, 18
long-term depression of, 327, 330, 340–343, 345
long-term potentiation of, 187, 327, 330, 333–340, 345
measurement of, 16
of motoneurons, 17, 587
and nerve terminal ultrastructure, 261–262
nonquantal, 247, 260, 276
post-tetanic potentiation and augmentation of, 327, 329–330, 331–332, 345
presynaptic action potential in, 187
presynaptic autoreceptors in, 253
presynaptic inhibition of, 208, 209
quantal. *See* Quantal release of neurotransmitters
and recovery, 157, 159
and recycling, 247, 271, 272–275
releasable pool size in, 332
in retina, 16, 491
from ribbon synapses, 270–271, 545
short-term facilitation and depression of, 328–329, 330, 331, 345
somatic and synaptic release compared, 405
in spillover leak, 390, 405–407
subquantal, 269
and synaptic vesicle attachments, 267–268, 269
and transport. *See* Neurotransmitter transport
and uptake, 157, 159–160, 163, 165, 178, 271–272, 323
without full vesicle fusion, 269, 270
Neurotransmitter transport, 149, 157–160, 163, 307, 323
axonal, 307, 318–321, 324
direction of, 160
in glial cells, 170, 178
hydrogen exchange system in, 157, 163
reversal of, 160, 178
into synaptic vesicles, 157–158
transport molecules in, 157–160, 162, 316
and uptake, 157, 159–160, 163, 165, 178, 271–272, 323
Neurotrophic factor, brain-derived. *See* Brain-derived neurotrophic factor
Neurotrophins, 173, 179, 652–655, 681
Neurovascular coupling in retina, 409–411
Neurulation, 624
Neutrality, electrical, 105
Newborn animals, visual system in, 182, 667, 668–672
Newman, E. A., 176, 410
Newsome, W. T., 57, 574

NG2 cells, 19, 165, 167, 168, 170, 179, 721
direct reprogramming of, 728–729
Nicholls, John, 404, 450
Nicoll, R. A., 338, 405
Nicotine, 194, 196, 290, 297
Nicotinic acetylcholine receptors, 77, 78–79, 80, 82, 101, 194, 195
activation of, 84
in autonomic nervous system, 80, 421, 422
and α-bungarotoxin, 78, 290
in central nervous system, 80, 290, 293
chlorpromazine binding sites, 83
in closed and open states, 84, 85
curare blocking, 224
developmental changes in, 646
in hair cells, 542–543
high-resolution imaging of, 83–84
intracellular and extracellular domains of, 83–84
ion selectivity and conductance, 85–86
mapping distribution of, 197, 198
molecular structure of, 83–84
in myasthenia gravis, 97
opening in bursts, 203
and plasticity in adult visual cortex, 693
pore size, 85
presynaptic, 290
structure of pore lining, 82, 83
subunit diversity, 100
Night vision, 23, 24, 491, 494
Nigrostriatal pathway, 296, 610
Nimodipine, 396, 408
Nissl substance, 701
Nitric oxide, 217, 238–239, 610
in autonomic nervous system, 239, 417, 423
and calcium as second messenger, 240
and microglial cell migration, 180
in retina, 504
synthesis of, 308
as tertiary messenger, 217, 243, 244
Nitric oxide synthase, 211, 212, 238, 239
and calcium as second messenger, 240, 243
S-Nitrosylation, nitric oxide mediated, 239
NK receptors, 300
NMDA glutamate receptors, 94, 95, 204–205
activation of, 178, 392
calcium permeability of, 205, 241, 285, 336
in central nervous system, 204–205, 239, 285
in critical periods of development, 682, 695
and excitatory postsynaptic currents, 204
extrasynaptic, 352, 353, 392, 397
localization of, 212
and long-term synaptic depression, 341, 342
and long-term synaptic potentiation, 336, 337, 338, 339, 344, 362, 369
and nitric oxide signaling, 239
structure of, 204
synaptic, 351, 352, 353
Nocebo effect, 513, 521
Nociceptin, 302
Nociception, 97, 484, 521. *See also* Pain sensations
Nociceptors, 466, 484, 521
Nodes of Ranvier, 135, 141, 171, 172, 174
formation of, 175
and internodal region, 141, 175

potassium channels in, 141, 143, 174, 175
sodium channels in, 141, 143, 175
Noggin, 621
Nogo protein, 716
Noise analysis, ion channel, 67, 68, 259
Non-adrenergic, non-cholinergic (NANC) fibers, 239
Nonquantal neurotransmitter release, 247, 260, 276
Nonsense mediated decay, 651
NOP receptor, 302
Norepinephrine, 434, 644
and adrenergic receptors, 219, 227, 228, 420
and calcium channel activity, 225, 226, 227
in CNS, 279, 280, 281, 292–294, 305
conversion of dopamine to, 296
discovery of, 425
feedback inhibition, 225, 312
and heart rate, 227, 231
localization of, 424
in locus coeruleus, 292–294, 303
release of, 225, 235, 263, 309, 317, 417, 419
storage of, 316
in sympathetic postganglionic transmission, 424
synthesis of, 308, 310–312, 314, B3
transport of, 158, 312, 316, 323
uptake of, 157, 159, 162, 178, 323
Notch-Delta pathway, 618, 622, 623, 662
in adult neurogenesis, 638
in lateral inhibition, 618, 622, 623, 662
Notochord, 627–628, 629
Noxious stimuli, response of leech N cells to, 451–454, 456–457, 458–459
Npas4 transcription factor, 357
N-type calcium channels, 225, 226
N-type inactivation of potassium channels, 128
Nuclear bag fibers, 470
Nuclear chain fibers, 470
Nuclear migration, interkinetic, 630, 632
Nucleus accumbens, 290, 296, 297, 305
Numa, S., 79, 80

O

Object cells, 738
Object perception and recognition, 557–558, 567–573, 581, 738–740
adaptation in, 571
associations between image pairs in, 578–579
coding mechanisms in, 577–578
in complex shapes, 577
deficits in, 568–569
face recognition in. *See* Face recognition
invariance in, 570–573, 581
multiple sensory modalities in, 579–580
orientation categorization tasks in, 579–580
processing speed in, 577
top-down inputs in, 578
ventral visual pathway in, 567–568, 581
Occipital lobe, 45, 47, 558, 568, 581
Octopamine, 389
Ocular dominance columns, 43, 44, 47–50, 58, 667
age dependence of, 670
axon branching patterns in, 670
cell layers of, 48, 669
critical periods in development, 667, 671, 672, 675, 681–682, 684, 693, 696